Present Knowledge in Nutrition

Present Knowledge in Nutrition

Seventh Edition

Ekhard E. Ziegler and L. J. Filer, Jr., Editors

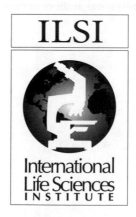

ILSI PRESS
Washington, DC
1996

ILSI PRESS
International Life Sciences Institute/ILSI North America
1126 Sixteenth Street, N.W.
Washington, D.C. 20036-4810

Library of Congress Catalog Number 96-77097

ISBN 0-944398-72-3

Printed in the United States of America

Contents

Foreword

The International Life Sciences Institute is a nonprofit, worldwide foundation established in 1978 to advance the understanding of scientific issues relating to nutrition, food safety, toxicology, risk assessment, and the environment. By bringing together scientists from academia, government, industry, and the public sector, ILSI seeks a balanced approach to solving problems of common concern for the well-being of the general public.

Since its inception ILSI has had a major interest in nutrition issues as they relate to public health and safety. The ILSI Human Nutrition Institute has programs in micronutrient malnutrition, complex carbohydrates, child nutrition and physical activity, and other areas. The ILSI Allergy and Immunology Institute supports research to advance the understanding, prevention, and treatment of food allergy. ILSI's worldwide branches and its focal point in China have sponsored activities pertaining to nutrition and food safety, including dietary fats and carbohydrates, functional foods, dietary fiber, antioxidants, macronutrient substitutes, nutritional epidemiology, aging, obesity, and improved detection and control of such foodborne pathogens as *Listeria monocytogenes* and *Escherichia coli* O157:H7.

ILSI participated in the 1992 International Conference on Nutrition and is implementing a number of the recommendations in the Plan of Action resulting from that landmark meeting, including the alleviation of micronutrient deficiencies and creation of a process that individual countries can use to create dietary guidelines appropriate for their populations. ILSI is working with the World Health Organization and the Food and Agriculture Organization of the United Nations to develop food-based strategies to improve micronutrient nutrition.

ILSI publishes the premier review journal in nutrition science and policy. *Nutrition Reviews,* edited at Tufts University and published monthly, monitors and reports on major developments for its global readership of nutrition and dietetics professionals and students.

Given ILSI's extensive involvement in nutrition issues, I am especially pleased to make available the seventh edition of *Present Knowledge in Nutrition,* with its comprehensive and up-do-date examination of nutrition science today. First published in 1953, *Present Knowledge in Nutrition* has become a standard reference work in classrooms, laboratories, clinics, and practitioners' offices around the world. With previous editions translated into Spanish, Japanese, Indonesian, Korean, and Chinese, *Present Knowledge in Nutrition* has become one of the most widely used authoritative reference works on nutrition published.

I am confident that the information contained in this latest edition will contribute to understanding the complex and rapidly evolving science of nutrition.

Alex Malaspina, President
International Life Sciences Institute

Preface

The seventh edition of *Present Knowledge in Nutrition* reflects the growth in the science base and application of nutrition science to a wide variety of related disciplines. As medicine has evolved from a focus on treatment to prevention, principles of nutrition have evolved from the identification of specific nutrients and understanding of their role in preventing deficiency states to the prevention of chronic rather than acute disease states.

The principles of nutrition have driven the development of advances in food safety, food technology, biotechnology, disease prevention, and public policy as the latter relates to assessment of the health and well-being of population groups, nutrition education programs, and public assistance programs.

This growth process has dictated, and will continue to dictate, the size and content of the seventh and future editions of *Present Knowledge in Nutrition*. Four chapters published in the sixth edition were eliminated; however, 13 new chapters were prepared for the seventh edition to accommodate the expanding information base and present the cutting edge of the nutrition sciences.

The fact that the majority of chapters were prepared by authors residing in North America reflects the primary readership of the text and its use in educational programs. There is no question that each chapter is current and comprehensive, and written to both inform and challenge the reader. The information in the book has been organized and presented to maximize its usefulness as both a text and a reference for students, researchers, and practitioners in basic nutrition sciences, clinical nutrition, dietetics, and related areas.

It would not have been possible to develop and finalize this edition of *Present Knowledge in Nutrition* without the unselfish support of the author or authors of each chapter who gave generously of their time and expertise to produce this insightful volume. The editors are deeply indebted to each of these contributors. Initial guidance provided by an editorial panel was helpful in the identification of chapter titles and potential authors.

Lastly, we acknowledge the support and efforts of Lisa Schomberg, who provided support services for the editorial work at the University of Iowa; Roberta Gutman, managing editor of ILSI Press, who managed the editorial and production activity at ILSI; and Judith Dickson, who undertook the herculean task of coordinating the copyediting effort to produce this comprehensive text and reference.

As editors, we experienced our share of highs and lows as we brought the volume into being and completion. We were both relieved and pleased with the end result. To all of the authors we extend our heartfelt thanks and appreciation for a job well done.

Ekhard E. Ziegler
L. J. Filer, Jr.
Editors

Contributors

Editors

Ekhard E. Ziegler, M.D.
Department of Pediatrics
College of Medicine
University of Iowa
Iowa City, Iowa 52242

L. J. Filer, Jr., M.D, Ph.D.
Department of Pediatrics
College of Medicine
University of Iowa
Iowa City, IA 52242

Chapter Authors

Nobuyuki Amano
National Institutes of Health
9000 Rockville Pike
Bethesda, MD 20892

G. Harvey Anderson, Ph.D.
Department of Nutritional Sciences
University of Toronto
Toronto, Ontario, Canada M5S 1A8

Michael C. Archer, Ph.D., D.Sc.
Department of Nutritional Sciences
University of Toronto
Toronto, Canada M5S 1A8

Claude D. Arnaud, M.D.
Program of Osteoporosis and Bone Biology
University of California
San Francisco, CA 94115-3004

Eldon W. Askew, Ph.D.
Division of Foods and Nutrition
University of Utah
Salt Lake City, UT 84112

John L. Beard, Ph.D.
Nutrition Department
Pennsylvania State University
University Park, PA 16802-0001

Philip R. Becket, Ph.D.
Section of Pediatric Endocrinology
Department of Pediatrics
Baylor University
Houston, TX 77030-2600

Carolyn D. Berdanier, Ph.D.
Department of Food and Nutrition
University of Georgia
Athens, GA 30602

Warren P. Bishop, M.D.
Department of Pediatrics
College of Medicine
University of Iowa
Iowa City, IA 52242

George A. Bray, M.D.
Pennington Biomedical Research Center
Baton Rouge, LA 70808-4124

Ronette Briefel, Dr.P.H.
Nutrition Monitoring and Related Research
National Health and Nutrition Examination Survey
Department of Health and Human Services
Hyattsville, MD 20782

Stephanie Brooks, M.S., R.D., C.N.S.D.
Santa Clara Valley Medical Center
San Jose, CA 95128

Raymond F. Burk, Jr., M.D.
Department of Medicine and Center in Molecular
    Toxicology
Vanderbilt University School of Medicine
Nashville, TN 37232-2279

Elsworth R. Buskirk, Ph.D.
Applied Physiology Human Performance Laboratory
Pennsylvania State University
University Park, PA 16802-6902

Robert Cousins, Ph.D.
Center for Nutritional Sciences
University of Florida
Gainesville, FL 32611

Yasmin S. Cypel, Ph.D.
Survey Systems/Food Consumption Laboratory
Agricultural Research Service
U.S. Department of Agriculture
Riverdale, MD 20737

Peter R. Dallman, M.D.
2201 Ninth Ave.
San Francisco, CA 94116

Johanna T. Dwyer, D.Sc.
Frances Stern Nutrition Center
Tufts University School of Medicine
Boston, MA 02111

John W. Finley, Ph.D.
R.M. Schaeberle Technology Center
Nabisco Inc.
East Hanover, NJ 07936-1944

Josef E. Fischer, M.D.
Department of Surgery
University of Cincinnati Medical Center
Cincinnati, OH 45267-0558

Gilbert B. Forbes, M.D.
University of Rochester Medical Center
Rochester, NY 14642

Pamela J. Fraker, Ph.D.
Department of Biochemistry
Michigan State University
East Lansing, MI 48824-1319

Daniel Gallaher, Ph.D.
College of Agriculture and Environmental Sciences
University of California
Davis, CA 95616-4789

Phillip J. Garry, Ph.D.
Clinical Nutrition Laboratory
University of New Mexico School of Medicine
Albuquerque, NM 87131-0001

Scott M. Grundy, M.D., Ph.D.
Center for Human Nutrition.
University of Texas Southwestern Medical Center
Dallas, TX 75235-9052

Barry Halliwell, Ph.D., D.Sc.
Pharmacology Group
University of London King's College, Chelsea
London SW3 6LX, United Kingdom

Charles H. Halsted, M.D.
Division of Clinical Nutrition and Metabolism
School of Medicine
University of California
Davis, CA 95616

William C. Heird, M.D.
Department of Pediatrics
USDA/ARS Children's Nutrition Research Center
Baylor University
Houston, TX 77030

Victor Herbert, M.D., J.D.
Bronx Veterans Affairs Medical Center
Bronx, NY 10468-3904

Edward S. Horton, M.D.
Joslin Diabetes Center
Boston, MA 02215

Sheila M. Innis, Ph.D.
Department of Pediatrics
University of British Columbia
Vancouver, BC, Canada V5Z 4H4

Robert A. Jacob, Ph.D.
USDA Human Nutrition Research Center
Presidio San Francisco
San Francisco, CA 94129-0602

John M. James, M.D.
Department of Pediatrics
Arkansas Children's Hospital
Little Rock, AR 72202-3591

Timothy D. Kane, M.D.
Department of Surgery
University of Cincinnati Medical Center
Cincinnati, OH 45267-0558

Patrick Kearns, M.D.
Santa Clara Valley Medical Center
San Jose, CA 95128

Carl L. Keen, Ph.D.
Department of Nutrition
University of California
Davis, CA 95616

Saulo Klahr, M.D.
Department of Medicine
Washington University School of Medicine
Jewish Hospital
St. Louis, MO 63113

Howard R. Knapp, M.D., Ph.D.
Department of Internal Medicine
College of Medicine
University of Iowa
Iowa City, Iowa 52242

Oran Kwon, Ph.D.
National Institutes of Health
9000 Rockville Pike
Bethesda, MD 20892

James E. Leklem, Ph.D.
Department of Nutrition and Food Management
Oregon State University
Corvallis, OR 97331-5103

Orville A. Levander, Ph.D.
Agricultural Research Service
U.S. Department of Agriculture
Beltsville, MD 20705

Gilbert Leveille, Ph.D.
R.M. Schaeberle Technology Center
Nabisco Inc.
East Hanover, NJ 07936-1944

Mark A. Levine, M.D.
National Institutes of Health
9000 Rockville Pike
Bethesda, MD 20892

Alice H. Lichtenstein, D.Sc.
USDA Human Nutrition Research Center on Aging
Tufts University
Boston, MA 02111

Maria C. Linder, Ph.D.
Department of Chemistry and Biochemistry
California State University
Fullerton, CA 92634

Friedrich C. Luft, M.D.
Franz Volhard Klinik
Free University of Berlin
13122 Berlin, Germany

Donald M. Mock, M.D., Ph.D.
Department of Pediatrics
Arkansas Children's Hospital
Little Rock, AR 72202-3591

Linda V. Muir, M.D.
Department of Pediatrics
College of Medicine
University of Iowa
Iowa City, IA 52242

Raffaele Napoli, M.D.
Joslin Diabetes Center
Boston, MA 02215

Forrest H. Nielsen, Ph.D.
Grand Forks Human Nutrition Research Center
Agricultural Research Service
U.S. Department of Agriculture
Grand Forks, ND 58202-9034

Anthony W. Norman, Ph.D.
Department of Biomedical Sciences and Biochemistry
University of California
Riverside, CA 92521-0129

James A. Olson, Ph.D.
Department of Biochemistry and Biophysics
Iowa State University
Ames, IA 50011-3260

Eleanor M. Pao, Ph.D. (Retired)
Nutrition Monitoring Division
Human Nutrition Information Service
U.S. Department of Agriculture
Sebring, OH 44672

Michael W. Pariza, Ph.D.
Food Research Institute
Department of Food Microbiology and Toxicology
University of Wisconsin
Madison, WI 53706-1187

Jae Park, Ph.D.
National Institutes of Health
9000 Rockville Pike
Bethesda, MD 20892

Kathy Phipps, Dr.P.H.
Oregon Pacific Area Health Education Center
Newport, OR 97365

Mary Frances Picciano, Ph.D.
Department of Nutrition
Pennsylvania State University
State College, PA 16802-0001

Nora Plesofsky-Vig, Ph.D.
Department of Plant Biology
University of Minnesota
St. Paul, MN 55108

Peter John Reeds, Ph.D.
USDA/ARS Children's Nutrition Research Center
Department of Pediatrics
Baylor University
Houston, TX 77071

William J. Rhead, M.D., Ph.D.
Department of Pediatrics
College of Medicine
University of Iowa
Iowa City, Iowa 52242

Prof. Gianguido Rindi
Istituto di Fisiologia Umana
Universita di Pavia
27100 Pavia, Italy

Richard S. Rivlin, M.D.
Memorial Sloan-Kettering Cancer Center
New York, NY 10021

Irwin H. Rosenberg, M.D.
USDA Human Nutrition Research Center
    on Aging
Tufts University
Boston, MA 02111

Steven Rumsey, Ph.D.
National Institutes of Health
9000 Rockville Pike
Bethesda, MD 20892

Sarah D. Sanchez, M.S.
Program of Osteoporosis and Bone Biology
University of California
San Francisco, CA 94115-3004

Kathleen D. Sanders, M.D.
Department of Pediatrics
University Hospitals and Clinics
University of Iowa
Iowa City, IA 52242

Barbara O. Schneeman, Ph.D.
College of Agriculture and Environmental
    Sciences
University of California
Davis, CA 95616-4789

Jacob Selhub, Ph.D.
USDA Human Nutrition Research Center
    on Aging
Tufts University
Boston, MA 02111

Maurice E. Shils, M.D., Sc.D.
Winston-Salem, NC 27106

Ronald J. Sokol, M.D.
Children's Hospital
Denver, CO 80218

MaryFran Sowers, Ph.D.
Department of Epidemiology
School of Public Health
University of Michigan
Ann Arbor, MI 48109-0001

John B. Stanbury, M.D.
International Council for the Control of Iodine
    Deficiency Disorders
Brussels, Belgium

Barbara J. Stoecker, Ph.D., R.D.
Department of Nutritional Sciences
Oklahoma State University
Stillwater, OK 74078-0337

John W. Suttie, Ph.D.
Department of Nutritional Sciences
University of Wisconsin
Madison, WI 53706-1569

Marian E. Swenseid, Ph.D.
Department of Community Health Science
School of Public Health
University of California
Los Angeles, CA 90024-3531

Béla Szepesi, Ph.D.
Bowie, MD 20715

Valerie Tarasuk, Ph.D.
Department of Nutritional Sciences
Faculty of Medicine
University of Toronto
Toronto, Ontario, Canada M5S 1A8

Bruno J. Vellas, M.D.
Centre Geriatric
Toulouse, France

Yaohui Wang, Ph.D.
National Institutes of Health
9000 Rockville Pike
Bethesda, MD 20892

Susan Welsh, Ph.D.
Cooperative State Research, Education, and Extension
    Service
U.S. Department of Agriculture
Washington, D.C. 20250

Wei Xu, Ph.D.
National Institutes of Health
9000 Rockville Pike
Bethesda, MD 20892

Ray Yip, M.D.
Division of Nutrition
Centers for Disease Control and Prevention
Atlanta, GA 30333

Sheri Zidenberg-Cherr, Ph.D.
Department of Nutrition
University of California
Davis, CA 95616-4789

Chapter 1

Energy Requirements

Raffaele Napoli and Edward S. Horton

Undernutrition remains a leading cause of mortality and morbidity in developing countries worldwide. It has been estimated that >400 million people worldwide are undernourished, and this number is expected to increase as overpopulation continues.[1] In the United States inadequate nutrition continues to be of concern for many segments of the population, such as pregnant women, young children, elderly adults, and those living below the poverty level. National and international health policies are attempting to address the critical issue of uneven distribution of food supplies among various segments of the population.

In industrialized countries such as the United States, the major nutritional problem is one of surfeit, with excess dietary energy and fat contributing to the disproportionate increase in metabolic disease prevalent in our society. The gift of modernization and technological advancements may, like the Trojan horse, carry the seeds of destruction for societies that traditionally have been free from the diseases of plenitude (obesity, non-insulin-dependent diabetes mellitus, hypertension, and hyperlipidemias). The toll for overindulgence is great in both human and financial terms.

Energy Needs

How efficiently a person can convert the potential energy available in foodstuffs into body energy stores is subject to individual variation and may explain the propensity toward or resistance to weight gain in different subjects over a long period of time. The so-called thrifty gene that may have had survival value for American Indians subject to harsh desert conditions with limited food sources may be considered maladaptive in present-day America, where food is plentiful and obesity is nearly endemic. Differences between lean and obese individuals in Na^+,K^+-ATPase pump activity, thermogenic responses to various hormonal and environmental stimuli, and possibly in substrate cycle activity may help us understand the biochemical nature of this metabolic efficiency.[2] Several studies in animals have indicated a role for the β_3-adrenoreceptor in the regulation of energy expenditure and fat accumulation.[3] There-

fore, the identification of increased frequencies of mutations in the β_3-adrenoreceptor gene in populations of obese people suggests that abnormalities in the activity of this receptor may be involved in the susceptibility to obesity in humans.[4-6] Recently, the discovery of the genetic abnormality responsible for obesity in *ob/ob* mice has indicated interesting new directions for the search for the defect or defects responsible for human obesity.[7] However, as emphasized by Sims,[8] any discussion of obesity must acknowledge the heterogeneity present in obese individuals that may help to explain some of the divergent results reported in various studies.

Energy Balance

Food is required as a fuel for the maintenance of energy-requiring processes that sustain life. Energy is required for maintaining the physicochemical environment of the intact animal, the so-called internal milieu, and for sustaining the electromechanical activities that define the organism. In the late 18th century, Lavoisier made the landmark discovery that the life-sustaining process of respiration was merely a form of chemical combustion and as such could be measured precisely. By the end of the next century, Rubner[9] was measuring the excretion rates of expired carbon dioxide and urinary nitrogen to estimate energy expenditure in human subjects. This method, known as indirect calorimetry, estimates metabolic rate from measurements of oxygen consumption and carbon dioxide production. When urinary nitrogen excretion is also measured, net rates of substrate oxidation can be calculated by using the tables of Lusk.[10]

For measurements of resting metabolic rate (RMR) in a supine, resting subject, the ventilated-hood system was shown to be accurate (2–5% error) with minimal inconvenience to the subject during relatively long-term measurements (several hours).[11] A steady state of carbon dioxide production and respiratory exchange must be reached, and subjects should have normal acid-base balance. For longer time periods, indirect calorimetry chambers are used. This technique was described by Ravussin et al.[12] The chambers are large enough to allow subjects to move freely and perform normal daily activities (i.e., sleeping, eating, and mild exercise) and to allow for precise measurement of energy expenditure over 24 hours. An advantage of the chamber is the ability to estimate physical activity with a radar-detection device.

The doubly labeled water technique, in which water is labeled with ^{2}H and ^{18}O, has been shown to measure energy expenditure in free-living subjects accurately over a period of several weeks.[13] This technique offers the potential for more studies of prolonged duration in subjects engaged in normal daily activities but is not widely available because of cost and the requirement for an isotope-ratio mass-spectrometry facility.

Direct calorimetry is probably the most accurate method for measuring energy expenditure (only 1–2% error) but is not widely used because of cost, limited chamber size, and slow response time. In addition, since the time of Atwater and Benedict,[14] many investigators have shown the close correlation between direct and indirect calorimetric measurements. Consequently, the former method is seldom used in present-day research studies. A novel version of the direct calorimeter, the space suit described by Webb et al.,[15] is intriguing but is still in the experimental stage.

Energy intake. Energy intake is a highly variable component of the energy balance equation and may be important in the causation and maintenance of the obese state. Danforth[16] emphasized the importance of the composition of food intake in addition to total energy intake in the pathogenesis of obesity.

Energy expenditure. Energy expenditure includes several components: RMR, the thermic effect of exercise (TEE), the thermic effect of food (TEF, formerly known as specific dynamic action), and facultative thermogenesis (also known as adaptive thermogenesis).

Resting metabolic rate. RMR is usually the greatest contributor (60–75%) to total daily energy expenditure. RMR is a measurement of the energy expended for maintenance of normal body functions and homeostasis plus a component for activation of the sympathetic nervous system. RMR is measured with the subject in a supine or sitting position in a comfortable environment several hours after a meal or significant physical activity. The basal metabolic rate, originally defined by Boothby and Sandiford,[17] is measured in the morning upon awakening, before any physical activity, and 12–18 hours after a meal. It may be slightly lower than RMR, but the difference is small and RMR is now the more commonly used measurement. Several factors are known to influence the RMR, including nutritional state, thyroid function, and sympathetic nervous system activity. Differences in RMR due to differences in body size, sex, or age are largely corrected if the data are related to fat-free mass (FFM).[12] Most studies do not find a difference

between lean and obese subjects when RMR is expressed per kilogram FFM. This lack of difference highlights the importance of accurate body composition measurements when different groups of subjects are compared in the ongoing search for clues to explain and correct the obese state. The decrease in RMR with age is explained largely, but not exclusively,[18] by a decrease in lean body mass. Women have lower RMRs than do men because of smaller body size and lower lean body mass, although RMR seems to vary with the menstrual cycle.[19]

It was shown that differences in FFM, age, and sex may account for 83% of the variance in RMR between different individuals.[12] Of great importance, family membership contributes an additional 11% to the variance in RMR per kilogram FFM. Similar findings of a genetic component to RMR were reported in studies of monozygotic twins and in retrospective studies of adopted children in Denmark.[20,21] Subjects with lower RMRs appear to be more susceptible to weight gain over the period of follow-up in both adult and pediatric populations.[22,23] The authors speculate that weight gain in such subjects would reach a plateau once the increase in lean body mass and energy cost of bodily movement brought subjects into energy balance. This theory suggests one mechanism for positive energy balance and weight gain over a long period of time in genetically susceptible individuals.

RMR is dependent also on thyroid hormone status and sympathetic nervous system (SNS) activity. The major clinical use of energy-expenditure measurements during the early part of this century was to diagnose over- and underactivity of the thyroid gland. Recent studies showed a relationship between RMR and rates of norepinephrine turnover by use of infusions of radioactive norepinephrine, which is a better index of SNS activity than is measurement of catecholamine concentration in plasma. Chronic administration (2 weeks) of the β-adrenergic agonist terbutaline increases RMR by 8% in humans,[24] whereas pharmacological blockade of the SNS by the acute administration of α- and β-blocking drugs appears to have little effect on RMR.[25] It was shown in animals that β_3-adrenergic stimulation, obtained by administration of specific β_3-agonists, induces an increase in RMR.[3] The identification of mutations in the β_3-adrenoreceptor gene associated with human obesity suggests that the abnormalities in RMR seen in obesity might be linked to inefficient β_3-adrenergic stimulation.[4–6]

Thermic effect of exercise. TEE is the second largest component of energy expenditure. It represents the cost of physical activity above basal levels. In a moderately active individual it comprises 15–30% of total energy requirements. Of all the components of energy expenditure, TEE is most variable and therefore most amenable to alteration. Increases in energy expenditure 10–15 times above the RMR can be achieved with intense exercise. Few, if any, factors appear to affect TEE except the amount of work done. Several studies compared TEE in lean and obese subjects, and in most cases no differences in the efficiency of exercise were found when the energy cost of moving the increased body weight of obese subjects was taken into account.[26] Previous exercise may increase metabolic rate for at least 18 hours and potentiates the thermic response to insulin-glucose infusions for >14 hours.[27,28]

The degree of spontaneous physical activity appears to be another variable that may allow for positive energy balance and weight gain in subjects prone to obesity. Earlier studies suggested that obese girls were less active during periods of recreation than were their lean schoolmates.[29] Using the indirect calorimetry chamber, Ravussin et al.[12] demonstrated a wide range in spontaneous physical activity, termed "fidgeting," among individuals. Fidgeting accounted for between 418 and 3347 kJ/d (between 100 and 800 kcal/d) in their subjects.

Thermic effect of food. TEF refers to the increase in energy expenditure above RMR that occurs for several hours after the ingestion of a meal. The earlier term "specific dynamic action" was initially applied to dietary protein, but it is now recognized that ingestion of each macronutrient (protein, fat, and carbohydrate) results in a thermogenic effect. TEF is the result of energy expended to digest, transport, metabolize, and store food. On average TEF accounts for ≈10% of daily energy expenditure and varies depending on the metabolic fate of ingested substrate. The cost of storing the fat contained in a meal in adipose tissue amounts to only 3% of the energy content of a meal. If glucose is directly oxidized, all the energy is available, whereas if it is first stored as glycogen, 7% of the available energy is lost.[30] Evidence suggests that only about one-third of liver glycogen repletion in rats starved for 24 hours occurs via the direct pathway from glucose; the remainder comes from triose phosphate intermediates and other mechanisms.[31] The cost of the indirect pathway of glycogenesis from triose phosphate intermediates is greater than the cost of direct synthesis of glycogen from glucose.

Theoretically, excess dietary carbohydrate can result in de novo lipogenesis, resulting in an increase in adipose tissue fat stores. However, this process is energy inefficient, requiring 26% of the ingested energy.[30] In addition, it was shown that carbohydrate overfeeding results in very little net lipogenesis over 24 hours.[32] Thus, fat balance remains negative at least in the short term after carbohydrate overfeeding because lipid oxidation continues. These considerations led Danforth[16] to conclude that the composition of the diet is at least as important as its energy content in determining whether a positive fat balance is maintained. Of the three macronutrients, dietary protein produces the greatest TEF.[33] This effect appears to be due to the high energy cost of protein degradation and synthesis, which require ≈24% of available energy.

The SNS appears to play an important role in TEF, especially after carbohydrate ingestion. Glucose ingestion and intravenous glucose-insulin infusions result in a 5–7% increase in energy expenditure above RMR, and up to 70% of this increase can be inhibited by administration of β-adrenergic–blocking drugs such as propranolol.[25,34] Increases in norepinephrine turnover correlate with the thermic response to a meal. TEF is also increased during treatment with β_3-agonists in rats, suggesting a possible role of β_3-adrenoreceptors in the regulation of this component of energy expenditure, in addition to their role in the regulation of RMR.[3]

Although subjects with insulin resistance demonstrate a decreased TEF, this impairment becomes normal if either insulin or glucose concentrations are increased sufficiently to result in normal rates of glucose disposal.[35] TEF after ingestion of fructose, which does not require insulin for cellular uptake, is normal in insulin-resistant subjects, again suggesting that the major determinant of TEF after carbohydrate ingestion is substrate metabolism rather than insulin secretion or action per se. Whether previous studies showed a decreased TEF in obese compared with lean subjects may have depended on the degree of insulin resistance present in the obese group.[35] Insulin is capable of stimulating Na^+,K^+-ATPase pump activity directly, and may exert thermogenic effects by direct stimulation of insulin-sensitive areas of the hypothalamus.[36]

TEF varies greatly among individuals, and even repeated measurements in the same individual under the same laboratory and nutrient intake conditions show a high degree of variability. Therefore, studies comparing TEF between different populations, such as lean and obese subjects, must be interpreted cautiously.

Facultative thermogenesis. The final component of energy expenditure, facultative thermogenesis, is readily demonstrable in animals but is less well described in humans. It appears to account for ≤10–15% of total daily energy expenditure but may have significant effects on long-term weight changes. Facultative thermogenesis is the change in energy expenditure induced by changes in ambient temperature, food intake, emotional stress, and other factors. The best-described version of facultative thermogenesis is nonshivering thermogenesis in rodents exposed to cold environments, during which heat production is increased via SNS stimulation of brown adipose tissue (BAT). BAT mitochondria have a unique proton conductance mechanism that allows them to reversibly uncouple oxidation from ADP phosphorylation.[37] Under stimulation by the SNS, the intracellular concentration of free fatty acids is increased and proton conductance is uncoupled. Both thyroid hormone and insulin are required for norepinephrine to increase BAT thermogenesis.[38] Glucagon may contribute to thermogenesis directly or indirectly by increasing catecholamine concentrations. The role of BAT in facultative thermogenesis in adult humans is questionable and is probably small in magnitude,[39] although BAT was histologically identified in adults chronically exposed to cold outdoor temperatures.[40] Use of immunocytochemical techniques revealed the presence of a mitochondrial uncoupling protein with a molecular weight of 32,000 in adult humans.[41] Intriguingly, elevated catecholamine concentrations in pheochromocytoma were shown to increase thermogenesis in the intraabdominal adipose tissue sites that are the same sites containing BAT in infants.[42]

Another form of facultative thermogenesis that is consistently shown in man occurs with altered nutritional intakes. Decreased energy intakes for prolonged periods result in a progressive decrease in RMR that is greater than can be accounted for by decreases in FFM. Associated with decreased energy intake is reduced insulin secretion and reduced activity of 5'-monodeiodinase, which converts the primary thyroid gland secretagogue 3,3',5,5'-tetraiodothyronine (T_4) to the metabolically active thyroid hormone 3,3',5-triiodothyronine (T_3).[43] Dietary carbohydrate is the primary nutrient regulating plasma concentrations of T_3. Recently, Danforth[44] showed that energy balance is more important than the absolute rate of energy intake or expenditure in altering T_3 concentrations. The decrease in T_3 is not entirely responsible for the decreased RMR during fasting, because restoring T_3 concentration to normal does not increase the RMR of starved rats.[45] Both an increase in T_3 and in nutrient ingestion are required for the increase in RMR to occur with refeeding. Underfeeding decreases the activity of the SNS, as determined by norepinephrine-turnover studies.[46] The finding that RMR may remain depressed for prolonged periods after dietary stabilization following rapid weight-reduction programs sounds a cautionary note regarding the clinical application of very-low-energy diets.[47] Furthermore, the maintenance of a reduced body weight in obese people is associated with compensatory changes in energy expenditure that oppose the maintenance of a body weight different from the usual weight.[48] These compensatory changes may account for the poor long-term efficacy of treatment of obesity.[48]

Experimental overfeeding in man has provided some valuable insights. Neumann[49] first used the term "luxus consumption" in 1902 and in the same year Rubner[9] in studies in dogs described the process whereby overfed lean animals were able to dissipate increased energy intake through heat loss. Although the convincing demonstration of this process in long-term studies has been difficult, studies yielding negative results have been criticized for inadequate duration or magnitude of overfeeding. As pointed out by Garrow[50] there appears to be a threshold of ≈84 MJ (≈20,000 kcal) of excess intake for the demonstration of luxus consumption, or diet-induced thermogenesis, in humans. In a review of earlier studies of overfeeding, Webb[51] concluded that only about one-half of the weight gain predicted from energy intake actually occurred. The Vermont study of experimental overfeeding of prisoners showed that previously lean subjects required about twice the daily energy intake of the spontaneously obese to maintain increased body weight, although there was a large degree of individual variation.[52] In addition, maintenance of an increased body weight, similar to that which occurs in maintenance of a reduced body weight, is associated with compensatory changes in energy expenditure opposing the change from the usual body weight.[48]

Increases in thyroid hormone concentrations and SNS activity appear to play important roles in the mechanisms of luxus consumption. As mentioned above, carbohydrate is the major nutrient increasing T_3 production. Current attention is being focused on the activity of substrate cycles, such as the Cori cycle (glucose to lactate to glucose) and the glucose (glucose to glucose-6-phosphate) and fructose (fructose-1-phosphate to fructose-1,6-diphosphate) cycles to explain differences in energetics with altered nutritional states. Newsholme[53] points out that such cycles, formerly called futile cycles, are far from futile and probably play important roles in finely regulating substrate fluxes in opposing directions. Recent studies demonstrated increased activity of glucose and fructose cycles in experimental hyperthyroidism and increased activity of the lipid cycle (lipolysis to reesterification) in burn patients.[54,55] The latter was shown to be partly under the influence of the SNS and was partially inhibited by administration of propranolol. As mentioned above, the Na^+,K^+-ATPase pump is under the influence of hormonal regulation; thyroid hormones, insulin, phosphatidylinositol, and possibly norepinephrine exert effects on pump activity.[56]

The extent to which defective facultative thermogenesis can contribute to or maintain the obese state was briefly mentioned in relation to TEF. Impairments in TEF during feeding or insulin-glucose infusions in obesity appear to be largely secondary to insulin resistance and decreased glucose disposal and are improved by treatments such as diet and exercise, which improve insulin sensitivity.[57] Whether differences in substrate-cycle activity in either the fasting or postprandial state can explain a tendency toward weight gain in obesity requires further studies.

Perspectives

It was recently discovered that fat deposition in an animal model of obesity is regulated by a previously unknown protein, called leptin (from the Greek leptos, meaning thin).[7] The administration of leptin to obese *ob/ob* mice, which do not produce this protein because of a genetic defect, rapidly normalizes their body weight.[58-60] This normalization occurs through an action on both components of the energy balance, i.e, reduction in food intake and increase in energy expenditure.[58,59] Interestingly, leptin production in normal mice increases after food ingestion, suggesting that a fine regulation of the appetite might be due to this protein.[60] In addition, increases in serum insulin, but not in glucose, stimulate the production of leptin.[61] One mechanism through which leptin acts in regulating food intake is inhibition of the synthesis and release by the hypothalamus of neuropeptide-Y, a substance involved in regulation of appetite.[62] Although an analogue of leptin was identified in humans, caution should be used in the extrapolation of animal data to humans for several reasons. First, human obesity is a heterogeneous disease, whereas obesity in *ob/ob* mice is due to a single gene defect. Second, resistance to the effect of leptin has been already described in *db/db* mice, and is likely due to a postulated defect in the leptin receptor present in these animals; similarly, resistance to leptin action might be present in humans. Third, human obesity seems to be associated with increased, rather than decreased, leptin plasma levels and leptin expression in fat cells, suggesting a more complicated regulatory role for this molecule.[63-65] However, the discovery of leptin has provided a new key for our understanding of the molecular mechanisms of obesity and it will be important to test the therapeutic effect of leptin in human obesity.

Summary

Although there are large interindividual differences in energy requirements, much of the variance can be accounted for by FFM, age, sex, and amount of physical activity. Genetic factors also appear to play an important role. Determining which factors help to explain the development or perpetuation of the obese state requires further investigation, but greater understanding will likely follow the improvements in technical capabilities and better-designed and controlled long-term studies in obese subjects. Because of an epidemic of obesity-associated metabolic diseases in Western societies, this improved understanding is essential for the health of the population.

References

1. Hegsted DM (1984) Energy requirements. In Olson RE, Broquist HP, Chichester CO, et al (eds), Present knowledge in nutrition, 5th ed. The Nutrition Foundation, Washington, DC, pp 1–6
2. DeLuise M, Blackburn GL, Flier JS (1980) Reduced activity of the red-cell sodium-potassium pump in human obesity. N Engl J Med 303:1017–1022
3. Himms-Hagen J, Cui J, Danforth E Jr, et al (1994) Effect of CL-316,243, a thermogenic β_3-agonist, on energy balance and brown and white adipose tissues in rats. Am J Physiol 266:R1371–R1382
4. Walston J, Silver K, Bogardus C, et al (1995) Time of onset of non-insulin-dependent diabetes mellitus and genetic variation in the β_3-adrenergic-receptor gene. N Engl J Med 333:343–347
5. Widen E, Lehto M, Kannen T, et al (1995) Association of polymorphism in the β_3-adrenergic-receptor gene with features of the insulin resistance syndrome in Finns. N Engl J Med 333:348–351
6. Clement K, Vaisse C, Manning BJK, et al (1995) Genetic variation of the β_3-adrenergic receptor and an increased capacity to gain weight in patients with morbid obesity. N Engl J Med 333:352–354
7. Zhang Y, Proenca R, Maffei M, et al (1994) Positional cloning of the mouse obese gene and its human homologue. Nature 372:425–432
8. Sims EAH (1982) Characterization of the syndromes of obesity. In Brodoff BN, Bleicher SJ (eds), Diabetes mellitus and obesity. Williams and Wilkins, Baltimore, MD, pp 219–226
9. Rubner M (1902) Die Gesetze des Energieverbrauchs bei der Ernährung. Deutiche, Leipzig
10. Lusk G (1924) Animal calorimetry: analysis of the oxidation of mixtures of carbohydrate and fat. J Biol Chem 59:41–42
11. Jequier E (1981) Long-term measurement of energy expenditure in man: direct or indirect calorimetry? In Bray GA (ed), Recent advances in obesity research III. Newman, London, pp 130–135
12. Ravussin E, Lillioja S, Anderson TE, et al (1986) Determinants of 24-hour energy expenditure in man: methods and results using a respiratory chamber. J Clin Invest 78:1568–1578
13. Schoeller DA, Webb P (1986) Five-day comparison of the doubly labeled water method with respiratory gas exchange. Am J Clin Nutr 40:153–158
14. Atwater WO, Benedict FG (1905) A respiration calorimeter with appliances for the direct determination of oxygen. Publication 42. Carnegie Institution of Washington, Washington, DC
15. Webb P, Annis JF, Troutman SJ (1980) Energy balance in man measured by direct and indirect calorimetry. Am J Clin Nutr 33:1287–1298
16. Danforth E (1985) Diet and obesity. Am J Clin Nutr 41:1132–1145
17. Boothby WM, Sandiford I (1929) Normal values for standard metabolism. Am J Physiol 90:290–291
18. Poehlman ET, Bere EM, Joseph JR, et al (1992) The influence of aerobic capacity, body composition, and thyroid hormones on the age-related decline in resting metabolic rate. Metabolism 41:915–921
19. Solomon SJ, Kurzer MS, Calloway DH (1982) Menstrual cycle and basal metabolic rate in women. Am J Clin Nutr 36:611–616
20. Bouchard C, Tremblay A, Despres JP, et al (1988) Sensitivity to overfeeding: the Quebec experiment with identical twins. Prog Food Nutr Sci 12:45–72
21. Stunkard AJ, Scrensen TIA, Hanis C, et al (1986) An adoption study of human obesity. N Engl J Med 314:193–198
22. Ravussin E, Lillioja S, Knowler WC, et al (1988) Reduced rate of energy expenditure as a risk factor for body-weight gain. N Engl J Med 318:467–472
23. Roberts SB, Savage J, Coward WA, et al (1988) Energy

expenditure and intake in infants born to lean and over-weight mothers. N Engl J Med 317:461–466

24. Scheidegger K, O'Connell M, Robbins DC, et al (1984) Effects of chronic beta-receptor stimulation on sympathetic nervous system activity, energy expenditure, and thyroid hormones. J Clin Endocrinol Metab 58:895–903

25. DeFronzo RA, Thorin D, Feiber J, et al (1984) Effect of beta and alpha adrenergic blockade on glucose-induced thermogenesis in man. J Clin Invest 73:633–639

26. Bray GA, Whipp BJ, Koyal SN (1974) The acute effects of food intake on energy expenditure during cycle ergometry. Am J Clin Nutr 27:254–259

27. Bielinski R, Schutz Y, Jequier E (1985) Energy metabolism during the postexercise recovery in man. Am J Clin Nutr 42:69–82

28. Devlin JT, Horton ES (1986) Potentiation of the thermic effect of insulin by exercise: differences between lean, obese, and non-insulin-dependent men. Am J Clin Nutr 43:884–890

29. Bullen BA, Reed RB, Mayer J (1964) Physical activity of obese and nonobese adolescent girls appraised by motion picture sampling. Am J Clin Nutr 14:211–223

30. Flatt JP (1987) Dietary fat, carbohydrate balance, and weight maintenance: effects of exercise? Am J Clin Nutr 45:296–306

31. Katz J, McGarry JD (1984) The glucose paradox: is glucose a substrate for liver metabolism. J Clin Invest 74:1901–1909

32. Acheson K, Schultz T, Bessard E, et al (1984) Nutritional influences on lipogenesis and thermogenesis after a carbohydrate meal. Am J Physiol 246:E62–E70

33. Nair KS, Halliday D, Garrow JS (1983) Thermic response to isoenergetic protein, carbohydrate or fat meals in lean and obese subjects. Clin Sci 65:307–312

34. Acheson K, Jequier E, Wahren J (1983) Influence of beta adrenergic blockade on glucose-induced thermogenesis in man. J Clin Invest 72:981–986

35. Ravussin E, Acheson KJ, Vernet O, et al (1985) Evidence that insulin resistance is responsible for the decreased thermic effect of glucose in human obesity. J Clin Invest 76:1268–1273

36. Rosic NK, Standaert ML, Pollet RJ (1985) The mechanism of insulin stimulation of (Na+,K+)-ATPase transport activity in muscle. J Biol Chem 260:6206–6212

37. Nicholls DG, Locke R (1984) Thermogenic mechanisms in brown fat. Physiol Rev 64:1–64

38. Himms-Hagen J (1984) Thermogenesis in brown adipose tissue as an energy buffer. N Engl J Med 311:1549–1558

39. Astrup AJ, Bulow J, Madsen J, et al (1985) Contribution of BAT and skeletal muscle to thermogenesis induced by ephedrine in man. Am J Physiol 248:E507–E515

40. Heaton JM (1972) The distribution of brown adipose tissue in the human. J Anat 112:35–39

41. Lean MEJ, James WPT (1983) Uncoupling proteins in human brown adipose tissue mitochrondria: isolation and detection by specific antiserum. FEBS Lett 163:235–240

42. Lean MEJ, James WPT, Jennings G, et al (1986) Brown adipose tissue in patients with phaechromo. Int J Obes 10:219–227

43. Burger A, O'Connell M, Scheidegger K, et al (1987) Monodeiodination of triiodothyronine and reverse triiodothyronine during low and high calorie diets. J Clin Endocrinol Metab 65:829–835

44. Danforth E (1989) Hormonal adaption to energy balance and imbalance and the regulation of energy expenditure. In Lardy HA, Stratman F (eds), Hormones, thermogenesis, and obesity. Elsevier, New York, pp 19–31

45. Burger AG, Berger M, Wimpfheimer K, et al (1980) Interre-

46. Bazelmans J, Nestel PJ, O'Dea K, et al (1985) Blunted norepinephrine responses to changing energy states in obese subjects. Metabolism 34:154–160

47. Greissler CA, Miller DS, Shah M (1987) The daily metabolic rate of the postobese and the lean. Am J Clin Nutr 45:914–920

48. Leibel RL, Rosenbaum M, Hirsch J (1995) Changes in energy expenditure resulting from altered body weight. N Engl J Med 332:621–628

49. Neumann RO (1902) Experimentalle Beiträge zur Lehre von dem taglichen Nährungsbedarf der Menschen unter besonder Berucksichtigung der notwendigen Eisewissmenge. Arch Hyg 45:1–2

50. JS Garrow (1978) The regulation of energy expenditure in man. In Bray GA (ed), Recent advances in obesity research II. Newman, London, pp 200–236

51. Webb P (1980) The measurement of energy exchange in man: an analysis. Am J Clin Nutr 33:1299–1310

52. Sims EAH (1976) Experimental obesity, dietary induced thermogenesis and their clinical implications. Clin Endocrinol Metab 5:377–395

53. Newsholme EA (1980) A possible metabolic basis for the control of body weight. N Engl J Med 302:400–405

54. Shulman GI, Landenson PW, Wolfe MH, et al (1985) Substrate cycling between gluconeogenesis and glycolysis in euthyroid, hypothyroid, and hyperthyroid man. J Clin Invest 76:757–764

55. Wolfe RR, Hemdon DN, Jahoor F, et al (1987) Effect of severe burn injury on substrate cycling by glucose and fatty acids. N Engl J Med 317:403–408

56. Simmons DA, Kern EFO, Winegrad AI, et al (1986) Basal phosphatidylinositol turnover controls aortic Na+/K+ ATP activity. J Clin Invest 77:503–513

57. Ravussin E, Bogardus C, Schwartz RS, et al (1983) Thermic effect of infused glucose and insulin in man: decreased response with increased insulin resistance in obesity and non-insulin dependent diabetes mellitus. J Clin Invest 72:893–902

58. Pelleymounter MA, Cullen MJ, Baker MB, et al (1995) Effects of the obese gene product on body weight regulation in ob/ob mice. Science 260:540–541

59. Halaas JL, Gajiwala KS, Maffei M, et al (1995) Weight-reducing effects of the plasma protein encoded by the obese gene. Science 269:543–546

60. Campfield LA, Smith FJ, Guisez Y, et al (1995) Recombinant mouse ob protein: evidence for a peripheral signal linking adiposity and central neural networks. Science 269:546–547

61. Saladin R, DeVos P, Guerre-Millo M, et al (1995) Transient increase in obese gene expression after food intake or insulin administration. Nature 377:527–529

62. Stephens TW, Basinski M, Bristow PK, et al (1995) The role of neuropeptide Y in the antiobesity action of the obese gene product. 377:530–532

63. Maffei M, Halass J, Ravussin E, et al (1995) Leptin levels in human and rodent: measurement of plasma leptin and ob RNA in obese and weight-reduced subjects. Nature Med 1:115–116

64. Lonnqvist F, Arner P, Nordfors L, Schalling M (1995) Overexpression of the obese (ob) gene in adipose tissue of human obese subjects. Nature Med 1:950–953

65. Hamilton BS, Paglia D, Kwan AYM, Deitel M (1995) Increased obese mRNA expression in omental fat cells from massively obese humans. Nature Med 1:953–956

Chapter 2

Body Composition

Gilbert B. Forbes

Biochemists in the late 19th century and early 20th century realized that neutral fat did not bind water or electrolytes and so suggested that tissue composition be calculated on a fat-free basis. Assuming that fat-free body mass (FFM) (or as some prefer, lean body mass) has a constant composition, the size of the FFM can be estimated by assaying the body content of one of its components, such as water, potassium, or nitrogen, whence body fat is determined by subtraction. Body density, computerized axial tomography (CAT), dual-energy x-ray absorptiometry (DEXA), and magnetic resonance imaging (MRI) provide estimates of both FFM and body fat. The last three techniques, as well as neutron activation, yield estimates of skeletal size. Skinfold thickness measurements (really a double layer of skin and subcutaneous tissue) provide an estimate of body fat content; these together with various body circumferences can provide information on body fat distribution.

As a result of the widespread application of these techniques, we now have a great deal of information on body composition throughout the life span of humans. The application of some newer techniques is now being vigorously pursued. It has been known for a long time that the metabolic-balance technique (element based; intake minus outgo) can estimate changes in body content of a number of elements.

Fat-free mass is defined as body weight minus ether-extractable fat and so excludes the small amounts of structural lipids in cell walls and nerve elements but includes the stroma and nonlipid components of adipose tissue. Body cell mass consists of the cellular components of muscle, viscera, blood, and brain and is considered to be proportional to body potassium content.

There are books that provide details of the body composition techniques now in use.[1-4] It is essential for those who use these techniques to become thoroughly familiar with them and to recognize their limitations.

Methods

Some methods are best suited to the research laboratory, whereas others are more appropriate for studies of large numbers of individuals (Table 1). The latter include skinfold thickness measurements, body circumferences, weight, and height.

Because FFM comprises 70–90% of body weight in children and adults, it is obvious that FFM and weight will be related. In subjects with widely varied fat content, one can anticipate that body fat and weight will also be related (assuming, of course, that age and sex are defined).

Indeed, the body mass index (BMI, expressed in kg/m²), defined as weight divided by height squared, has proven useful in estimating body fat percentage, providing that age and sex are taken into account. This is because most of the weight differences among individuals of a given age and sex comprise body fat. Exceptions are body builders, pregnant women, patients with anorexia nervosa, and those with massive obesity. Average BMI values are the same (BMI = 20–25) for young adult men and women even though the women have more fat and less muscle.

Cross-sectional areas of the muscle-bone component and the fat component of the arm can be calculated from arm circumference and skinfold thickness, and tables of normal values are published.[5] Normative data for the ratio of waist circumference to hip circumference are also published.[6] Supranormal ratios are considered to constitute a risk of ill health. The cross-sectional area of the second metacarpal bone cortex, as determined from standard roentgenograms, provides a rough estimate of skeletal size.

Body density. Body density is usually determined by weighing the subject in air and then underwater, with corrections for residual lung volume and an assumed value for intestinal gas. By use of a principle first described by Archimedes, density of the whole body (D) is obtained. The relative proportions of lean and fat (in adults D = 1.100 and 0.900 g/cm³, respectively) can be calculated from the observed density of the whole body. The usual formula is

$$\text{Fraction fat} = (4.95/D) - 4.50.$$

It is likely that the density of the FFM in children and in elderly adults differs from that of young and middle-aged adults.

Table 1. Body composition techniques: advantages and disadvantages[a]

	Advantages	Disadvantages
Density	Estimates FFM and fat simultaneously, nonhazardous	Subject cooperation necessary, unsuitable for young children and elderly people, error from intestinal gas
Dilution methods	Estimate body fluid volumes; great variety: determine Na, K, Cl(Br), H_2O, extracellular fluid	Radiation exposure (some materials); blood samples needed (some materials); incomplete equilibration of Na, K; overestimation by deuterium, tritium; value for extracellular fluid depends on method used; ^{18}O assay requires elaborate equipment
^{40}K counting	No hazard, minimal subject cooperation needed	Instrument expensive, proper calibration necessary, problem in interpretation in subjects with K deficiency
Metabolic balance	No hazard, suitable for many elements, can detect small changes in body content (<1%)	Measures only change in body composition, meticulous subject cooperation required, metabolic ward expensive, error from unmeasured skin losses
Creatinine excretion	No hazard, estimate of muscle mass	Meticulous subject cooperation required, Influenced by diet, collection time critical, day-to-day variation (c.v. 5–10%)
Anthropometry (skinfold thickness, circumference)	Inexpensive, direct estimate of body fat and regional muscle, fat distribution	Poor precision in obese subjects and in those with firm subcutaneous tissue, regional variation in subcutaneous fat layer, uncertainty ratio subcutaneous fat: total fat
CAT scan	Delineates organ size, fat distribution, bone size	Instrument expensive, radiation exposure
TOBEC	No hazard, estimate of FFM	Apparatus expensive
Bioelectrical conductivity	Apparatus inexpensive, no hazard, estimate of total body H_2O	Many prediction formulas
Neutron activation	Minimal subject cooperation needed; body content of Ca, P, N, Na, Cl	Apparatus very expensive, calibration very difficult, radiation exposure minimal
MRI	Delineates organ size, muscle, fat, fat distribution, total body water	Apparatus very expensive
DEXA	Estimates bone mineral content, total and regional; body fat, soft tissue lean	Expensive, radiation exposure minimal

[a]Abbreviations: FFM, fat-free mass; CAT, computerized axial tomography; TOBEC, total-body electrical conductivity; MRI, magnetic resonance imaging, also nuclear magnetic resonance; DEXA, dual-energy x-ray absorptiometry.

Dilution techniques. Plasma volume can be estimated with Evans blue dye (T-1824) or ^{131}I-labeled albumin, and total erythrocyte mass can be estimated with erythrocytes tagged with ^{51}Cr, ^{55}Fe, or ^{59}Fe. Materials for extracellular fluid volume estimation are inulin, SCN–, Br–, ^{82}Br–, $^{35}S_2O_3$–, or $^{35}SO_4^{2-}$; estimations vary somewhat with these materials. Total body water is estimated by deuterium, tritium, or oxygen-18 dilution or by dilution of alcohol, or N-acetyl-4-aminopyrine. Intracellular fluid volume is calculated by difference. Because 73% of FFM consists of water, its size can be estimated from total body water; body fat is weight minus FFM.

^{40}K counting. The body contains enough of this naturally occurring isotope ($t_{1/2}$ 1.3×10^9 y, body content 4 kBq) to permit its detection and quantitation by low-background scintillation counters. From the known abundance of ^{40}K (0.012%), one can calculate total body potassium content. Several types of detectors have been used; each instrument requires calibration. Once body potassium content has been determined, FFM is calculated under the assumption that this body component has a relatively constant potassium content; body fat is the difference between body weight and FFM.

By cadaver analysis, the potassium content of the FFM is 68 mmol/kg. Some investigators have used this value for adult males and 64.2 for adult females, whereas others use 64.5 and 58 mmol/kg, respectively. FFM composition of infants differs from that of adults: water content is higher whereas potassium content and density are lower.

Urinary creatinine excretion. The assumption that urinary creatinine is an index of muscle mass is supported by the work of Schutte et al.[7] in dogs. Studies of human subjects of widely varied body size have also shown a good relationship between creatinine excretion and FFM. On the basis of human and animal data, fat-free skeletal muscle, on average, makes up 49% of total fat-free weight. However, all of the published regressions of urinary creatinine excretion on FFM have positive intercepts on the y axis, so the creatinine-to-FFM ratio (and hence the creatinine-to-muscle mass ratio) is somewhat lower for individuals who excrete large amounts of creatinine than for those who excrete smaller amounts. The urine collections must be timed accurately, and the excretion rate can be affected by diet. For individuals consuming a meat-free diet, the relationship between muscle mass (MM) and creatinine excretion (Cr) is[3]

$$MM \text{ (kg)} = 11.8 \text{ Cr (g/d)} + 10.1.$$

Metabolic balance. Although the metabolic-balance technique cannot estimate body content per se, it can detect small changes in body content of a number of elements. For example, a change in body nitrogen content of 16 g, equivalent to 0.5 kg FFM, is easily detected, although such a change is well within the error of body composition techniques. The drawbacks are the meticulous cooperation required of the subject, the need for a fore period to allow adjustment to a given diet, the need to estimate cutaneous losses (which are most difficult to measure), and the nonrandom nature of the intake and excretion variables, the result being that positive balances tend to be overestimated and negative balances underestimated, never the reverse.

Other techniques. These include total-body electrical conductivity (TOBEC), bioelectrical impedance, DEXA, CAT, and nuclear magnetic resonance (or MRI). The last three provide certain advantages (which are gained at considerable expense) in that skeletal weight and body fat distribution, both internal and subcutaneous, can be estimated.

The TOBEC instrument generates an oscillating radio frequency current (5 MHz) in a large solenoidal coil. The degree to which the induced electrical current is perturbed by a subject placed in the coil is proportional to the water content of the subject and thus to lean body weight.

The bioelectrical impedance technique consists of passing a weak alternating current (800 µA, 50 kHz) through the body. The observed impedance is an inverse function of total body water and a direct function of height squared. Precision is improved by adding weight, age, and sex to the equation, whereupon results are highly correlated with those of other techniques. Modern instruments measure body impedance at more than one current frequency; at low frequencies impedance is said to be a function of extracellular water whereas at high frequencies it provides an estimate of total body water.[8] There are many published equations for estimating body composition from bioimpedance; most are population specific.[9] The simplicity of the technique makes it easy to use, but it has failed in some hands to adequately predict changes in body composition. There is some question as to whether it is superior to careful anthropometric measurements.

DEXA consists of scanning the body with x-rays of differing energy. The attenuation of these rays by body tissues is subjected to computer analysis to yield estimates of total bone mineral, total body fat-free soft tissue, and body fat. The instrument can also estimate vertebral bone mineral and femoral bone mineral separately if desired. The radiation dose is very small and the ability of the instruments to measure bone, as well as soft tissue lean and fat, is a distinct advantage. However, some questions remain as to its ultimate accuracy.[10,11]

CAT can delineate organ size, regional fat depots, and skeletal size. Multiple cuts are needed to assess the entire body, so the radiation exposure is appreciable.[12]

Neutron activation involves exposing the entire body to a known flux of neutrons and measuring the induced radioactivity. This can yield estimates of total-body calcium, phosphorus, nitrogen, sodium, chlorine, and carbon. The apparatus is intricate, expensive, and difficult to calibrate; there are only a few such instruments in operation worldwide. Surprisingly, the radiation dose to subjects is rather small.

The principle of MRI is beyond the scope of this article. It offers the opportunity of delineating organ size and structure, body fat distribution, total body water, and muscle size, all without radiation exposure. It is, of course, very expensive.

All of these techniques are subject to technical error, variously estimated at 2–6%. None is foolproof, and each demands practice and attention to detail to achieve worthwhile results. Each technique involves assumptions that may be different in different populations; for example, the water content of the FFM is greater in infants than adults.

Efforts are now being made to improve body composition estimates by measuring in rapid succession total body water, bone mineral, and body density (and in some instances potassium or nitrogen), to provide a multicompartmental analysis of the body.[13,14] Such complicated procedures are best suited to the research laboratory.

Variations in FFM and Body Fat

Age and sex. Table 2 lists average values for selected age groups. The onset of puberty is accompanied by a spurt in FFM, which is more intense in boys, and an increase in body fat, especially in girls. The result is that adult women have only about two-thirds as much FFM as men while having a larger percentage body fat. Indeed, in young adults the average sex difference in FFM (M-F ratio 1.4) is relatively greater than the difference in stature (ratio 1.08) or in body weight (ratio 1.25). Recent data obtained by dual-photon absorptiometry show a similar trend for total bone mineral; a definite sex difference appears at midpuberty, reaching an M-F ratio of about 1.3 in the early adult years.[15] The sex ratio for urinary creatinine excretion (an index of muscle

Table 2. Average values for weight, FFM, and percent fat as a function of age

	Newborn	10-year-old boy	10-year-old girl	15-year-old boy	15-year-old girl	Adult man	Adult woman
Weight (kg)	3.4	31	32	60	54	72	58
FFM (kg)	2.9	27	26	51	40	61	42
Percent fat	14	13	19	13	26	15	28

mass) is 1.5. During the later adult years, both sexes experience a modest decline in FFM. These are, of course, average values, and it has been established that both FFM and body fat show some variability. However, when subjects of a given age, sex, and height are analyzed, FFM exhibits much less variability than does body fat; hence, it is fat that accounts for much of the variability in body weight.

Stature. At all ages thus far examined, FFM is a function of stature. On average, the regression slope is 0.69 kg FFM/cm in adult males and a 0.48 kg/cm in adult females. Skeletal size is also a function of height, as is total-body calcium, the regression slope being 20 g calcium/cm height. On the basis of these findings, a 186-cm male would be expected to have 1370 g calcium in his body and a 154-cm woman to have only 730 g calcium.

Race. Orientals are usually shorter and lighter than Caucasians, so it is to be expected that they would have a smaller lean weight. African Americans, on the other hand, tend to have a slightly larger FFM and more total-body calcium than do Caucasians.[16]

Heredity. It is well known that weight and height are under genetic influence. Studies have shown that the same is true for FFM, total body fat, and skinfold thickness.[17,18]

Pregnancy. Of the total weight gain during pregnancy, some 12–13 kg on average, the fetus, placenta, and amniotic fluid together comprise 4.2 kg; the remaining 8 kg is maternal tissue per se. Plasma volume and extracellular and intracellular fluid volumes all increase. Because the ratio of body water to body potassium increases, the increase in extracellular fluid volume is proportionately greater than that of intracellular fluid volume, which is in keeping with the observation that many pregnant women have mild edema. A portion of the weight gain (variously estimated at 2–4 kg) consists of fat.

Some Correlates of Body Composition

Because adult females have only about two-thirds as much FFM as do males, protein and energy requirements are correspondingly less. The recommended dietary allowances of the National Research Council reflect this sex difference. Basal metabolic rate is more closely related to FFM than it is to body weight, and studies of adult women have shown that total energy needs are directly proportional to the size of the fat-free body; the significance of this relationship is enhanced by the fact that the intercepts of the regression lines are close to zero.[19] It would seem prudent to adjust the dose of certain drugs, i.e., those that do not distribute in body fat, on the basis of FFM rather than body weight.

Body fat stores are important during energy deprivation. It is well known that obese individuals can tolerate much longer fasts than can those who are thin. In individuals given low-energy diets, FFM accounts for a smaller fraction of the total weight loss in those who are obese than in those who are thin.[20] Obese individuals preferentially burn fat and so tend to conserve lean tissue when faced with an energy deficit.

Henry[21] described a good relationship between protein and energy metabolism. The ratio of urinary nitrogen loss (and hence FFM loss) to basal metabolic rate does not change during the course of fasting, and is distinctly lower in obese than in thin individuals.

Careful studies have shown that skeletal mass is proportional to FFM.[22] Hence, individuals with subnormal FFM may be at risk for fractures.

Influence of Nutrition

The availability of modern body-composition techniques has made it possible to study the long-term changes in body composition without having to deal with the technical problems inherent in the metabolic-balance method. It is the long-term change, whether it be weight loss or weight gain, that deserves consideration. Of paramount importance to the modern nutritional scene is the matter of energy balance.

Energy deficit. Generally speaking, the rate of weight loss is proportional to the energy deficit; individuals who fast lose weight more rapidly than do those given submaintenance amounts of food. Careful studies of underfed subjects have shown that weight reduction involves a loss of both FFM and fat. The relative contribution of each of these components to the total weight loss depends on two factors: the initial body fat content and the size of the energy deficit. For example, thin individuals who fast lose twice as much nitrogen per kilogram of weight loss as do obese individuals, and thin individuals consuming 5.9–7.9 MJ (1400–1900 kcal) diets have a relatively greater loss of FFM per unit weight loss than do obese individuals.

Table 3. Reference man and woman; total body content[a]

Substance	Male	Female
Water	2500 mol (45,000 g)	1700 mol (31,000 g)
Hydrogen, nonaqueous	1000 mol (2000 g)	—
Oxygen, nonaqueous	90 mol (2900 g)	—
Carbon	1333 mol (16,000 g)	—
Nitrogen	64 mol (1800 g)	46 mol (1300 g)
Calcium	27 mol (1100 g)	21 mol (830 g)
Phosphorus	16 mol (500 g)	13 mol (400 g)
Potassium	3600 mmol (140 g)	2560 mmol (100 g)
Sodium	4170 mmol (100 g)	3200 mmol (77 g)
Chlorine	2680 mmol (95 g)	2000 mmol (70 g)
Sulfur	4400 mmol (140 g)	—
Magnesium	780 mmol (19 g)	—
Silicon	640 mmol (18 g)	—
Iron	75 mmol (4.2 g)	—
Fluorine	140 mmol (2.6 g)	—
Zinc	35 mmol (2.3 g)	—
Copper	1.1 mmol (0.07 g)	—
Manganese	180 μmol (0.01 g)	—
Iodine	79 μmol (0.01 g)	—

[a]Seventeen additional elements (all < 330 mg) are listed in reference 25. For many, the body content is a function of diet.

The second factor is equally important: for all categories of initial body fat content studied to date, the ratio of change in FFM to change in weight is directly related to the size of the energy deficit. This ratio is highest in those who fast and progressively decreases with increasing energy intake, i.e., more lean is conserved as more food is consumed. One searches in vain for well-controlled studies showing that body nitrogen and FFM can be completely preserved on low-energy diets, a conclusion reached many years ago by Calloway and Spector.[23] Such losses do tend to diminish with time; however, so does the rate of weight loss.

Obese patients subjected to intestinal bypass or gastric stapling operations also lose FFM as they lose weight. In various studies FFM comprises 15–40% of the total weight loss.

Energy excess. When undernourished individuals are induced to gain weight, both FFM and fat increase. The same thing happens when normal individuals are overfed. A compilation of studies from several sources shows that the amount of weight gain experienced during deliberate overfeeding of normal adults is directly proportional to the total excess energy consumed during the overfeeding period. The average energy cost of the weight gain is 33.5 kJ/g (8 kcal/g) gain. Moreover, about one-third of the gain consists of FFM. It goes without saying that such diets must be adequate in protein and other essentials.

When observations on diet-induced weight loss and weight gain are considered in total, it is apparent that FFM and fat are, in a sense, companions. A change in one is accompanied by a change in the other, although not always in the same proportion.[24]

Body composition in obesity. Except in rare instances, human obesity can develop only in the face of a positive energy balance; so, in this sense, obesity is a nutritional disease. Obese children tend to be tall for age, and studies of obese children, adolescents, and adults show that a portion of their excess weight (10–30%) consists, for the majority, of fat-free tissue. Such data can only be interpreted to mean that obese individuals are overnourished. The exceptions are individuals with increased adrenocortical activity and those given diets that are high in energy and very low in protein; under these circumstances, body fat increases at the expense of the FFM. Patients with the Prader-Willi syndrome (obesity associated with hypogonadism, mental retardation, and tendency for diabetes mellitus caused by a partial deletion of chromosome 15) differ in having a reduced FFM.

The situation is quite different in animals that become obese after experimentally induced hypothalamic lesions and in Zucker rats. These animals tend to be stunted and to have a smaller FFM than do controls and thus cannot serve as proper models for human obesity.

Body composition in undernutrition. Patients with anorexia nervosa have a reduction in both body fat and FFM. Generally, extracellular fluid volume tends to be better preserved than intracellular fluid volume in undernourished states so that the ratio of extracellular to intracellular fluid volume is increased. In severe malnutrition, especially when complicated by trauma or infection, body cells have reduced amounts of potassium, phosphorus, and magnesium and increased amounts of sodium.

Other influences. Physical activity contributes to the stability of the FFM. FFM tends to diminish during bed rest and in the absence of gravity. Vigorous and sustained exercise results in an increase in FFM (though the changes are of modest degree) and a decrease in body fat, provided body weight is sustained. If much weight is lost, FFM will decline.[23] The larger FFM and smaller body fat content of many athletes probably represents the combined influences of heredity and prolonged physical training. The most striking effects are those produced by the administration of anabolic steroids, large doses of which result in greater increases in FFM than any recorded thus far from exercise alone.

Table 3 lists the multitude of elements to be found in the body of a male adult (the so-called reference man) as compiled by the International Commission on Radiation Protection.[25] I have added some values for certain elements for the average woman as determined by body composition assays.

References

1. Davies PSW, Cole TJ, eds (1995) Body composition techniques in health and disease. Cambridge University Press, Cambridge, UK
2. Shephard RJ (1991) Body composition in biological anthropology. Cambridge University Press, New York
3. Forbes GB (1987) Human body composition: growth, aging, nutrition and activity. Springer Verlag, New York
4. Moore FD, Olesen KH, McMurray JD, et al (1963) The body cell mass and its supporting environment: body composition in health and disease. WB Saunders, Philadelphia
5. Frisancho AR (1981) New norms of upper limb fat and muscle areas for assessment of nutritional status. Am J Clin Nutr 34:2450–2545
6. Forbes GB (1990) The abdomen: hip ratio. Normative data and observations on selected patients. Int J Obes 14:149–157
7. Schutte JE, Longhurst JC, Gaffney FA, et al (1981) Total plasma creatinine: an accurate measure of total striated muscle. J Appl Physiol 51:762–766
8. Deurenberg P (1995) Multi-frequency impedance as a measure of body water compartments. In Davies PSW, Cole TJ (eds), Body composition techniques in health and disease. Cambridge University Press, Cambridge, UK, pp 45–56
9. Kushner RF (1992) Bioelectrical impedance analysis: a review of principles and applications. J Am Coll. Nutr 11:199–209
10. Jebb SA, Goldberg GR, Jennings G, et al (1995) Dual-energy x-ray absorptiometry measurements of body composition: effects of depth and tissue thickness including comparisons with direct analysis. Clin Sci 88:319–324
11. Ellis KJ, Shypailo RJ, Pratt JA, et al (1994) Accuracy of dual-energy x-ray absorptiometry for body composition measurements in children. Am J Clin Nutr 60:660–665
12. Krist H, Chowdhury B, Sjöström L, et al (1988) Adipose tissue volume determination in males by computed tomography and ^{40}K. Int J Obes 12:249–266
13. Jebb SA, Elia M (1995) Multi-compartment models for the assessment of body composition in health and disease. In Davies PSW, Cole TJ (eds), Body composition techniques in health and disease. Cambridge University Press, Cambridge, UK, pp 240–254
14. Heymsfield SB, Waki M (1991) Body composition in humans: advances in the development of multi-compartment models. Nutr Rev 49:97–108
15. Ogle GD, Allen JR, Humphries LRJ, et al (1995) Body composition assessment by dual-energy X-ray absorptiometry in subjects aged 4-26 y. Am J Clin Nutr 61:746–753
16. Cohn SH, Abesamis C, Zanzi I, et al (1977) Body elemental composition: comparison between black and white adults. Am J Physiol 232:E419–E422
17. Bouchard C, Savard R, Després J-P, et al (1985) Body composition in adopted and biological siblings. Hum Biol 57:61–75
18. Forbes GB, Sauer EP, Weitkamp LR (1995) Lean body mass in twins. Metabolism 44:1442–1446
19. Forbes GB (1989) Maintenance energy needs for women as a function of body size and composition. Am J Clin Nutr 50:404–405
20. Forbes GB (1987) Lean body mass—body fat interrelationships in humans. Nutr Rev 45:225–231
21. Henry CJK (1995) Influence of body composition on protein and energy requirements: some new insights. In Davies PSW, Cole TJ (eds), Body composition techniques in health and disease. Cambridge University Press, Cambridge, UK, pp 85–99
22. Aloia JF, Vaswani A, Ma R, et al (1995) To what extent is bone mass determined by fat-free or fat mass? Am J Clin Nutr 61:1110–1114
23. Calloway DH, Spector H (1954) Nitrogen balance as related to caloric and protein intake in active young men. Am J Clin Nutr 2:405–412
24. Forbes GB (1993) The companionship of lean and fat. In Ellis KJ, Eastman JD (eds), Human body composition. Plenum Press, New York, pp 1–14
25. International Commission on Radiation Protection (1975) Report of the Task Force Group on Reference Man, no. 23. Pergamon Press, Oxford

Chapter 3

Hunger, Appetite, and Food Intake

G. Harvey Anderson

The determinants of food selection and food intake in humans are many and are both physiological and psychological in origin.[1] In all of these processes the brain is the organizer and integrator of the signals, balancing expenditure and storage of energy with the intake of food.[2]

A fundamental question remains to be answered, however. That is, how do the complex processes of hunger, appetite, and satiation lead to energy balance (or energy imbalance and obesity) and adequate nutrient intake?

The purpose of this review is to provide an overview of factors thought to regulate food intake.

From Initiation to Termination of Food Intake

Under strictly physiological circumstances, hunger initiates food-seeking behavior, although the specific origins of hunger and meal initiation have not been determined.[1,2] At the simplest level of description one can say that when the body needs food the characteristic sensations of hunger increase in intensity as long as the need is not satisfied. The sensations may be relatively weak if the person has eaten recently, or relatively strong and unpleasant if the person has not eaten for some time. However, the sensations may be modified by many factors, including the cephalic phase of appetite, which is the response to the thought, sight, taste, or smell of food.

Appetite, a desire for food, may be accentuated by hunger and is generally associated with pleasurable aspects of food choice and ingestion. The term appetite is frequently used to discuss signals that guide selection and consumption of specific foods and nutrients.[1] Thus, appetite can be expressed by different behaviors. It may lead to the specific intake of energy to satisfy body energy deficits, or to the selection of foods to meet the specific nutrient requirements of the organism, or to meet a hedonic desire for a specific taste (e.g., savory or sweet).

With the initiation of food ingestion a progression of psychological and physiological responses occurs, leading to satiation and the termination of food intake. If the hunger sensations are driven by an energy deficit then the sensations can be decreased and satisfied by the ingestion of food containing the macronutrients fat, carbohydrate, or protein, which provide energy. The ingestion of these nutrients as well as many micronutrients, also satisfies nutrient specific appetites. These nutrient-specific appetites are not as easily demonstrated as is the overriding demand for energy, but they are factors in determining food choice in experimental animals and perhaps in humans.[3]

The amount of food ingested depends upon sensory and cognitive responses of the consumer as well as upon the energy and nutrient content of the food.[1] In humans, cultural and social conventions are significant modifiers of the signals arising from internal metabolic and physiological conditions. Psychological factors, such as the presence of others eating, social factors, such as occasion, culture, and religious beliefs, and hedonic factors will all contribute to the relative state of satiation or the process of terminating hunger.[1,4] If hunger is weak, food intake can be enhanced by cognitive and sensory factors that are pleasant. Conversely, even when hunger signals are strong, sufficient food may not be ingested to bring about satiety. For example, food that is unfamiliar, unpleasant, or forbidden for religious beliefs can result in the failure to respond to the hunger signals.[4]

Following the satiety signals arising from sensory and cognitive factors, postingestive and postabsorptive satiation signals begin to arise from the food ingested.[2] Bulk, composition, rate of absorption, and metabolic responses all affect the time frame in which satiety ultimately occurs. The duration of satiety and the interval to the next ingestion of food depend on a complex system of neuronal responses integrated in the central nervous system.

Food Composition and Energy Intake

Meeting energy requirements appears to be the primary reason for food ingestion by animals. However, regulation of energy intake and balance of body energy are determined by both the energy content of the food and the source of the energy. The sources of dietary energy are the three macronutrients, fat, carbohydrate, and protein, and each has unique effects on food intake regulatory mechanisms. Food selection studies in experimental animals suggest that there are specific regulatory systems for the intake of these nutrients, and much recent effort has been directed toward studying the significance of macronutrient-specific appetites in the determination of energy balance.

Fat and food intake. Fat consumption gives rise to signals that contribute to the process of satiation during a meal and, as well, may satisfy fat-specific appetites.

Fat appetites have been observed in experimental animals, and their physiological origin has been supported by both food selection studies and by identification of specific brain neuropeptides (e.g., galanin) that regulate fat intake.[5,6] Similarly in humans the presence of a "fat tooth" has been proposed on the basis of preference by obese subjects for sweet-fat foods, although the origins of this preference may be primarily hedonic.[7]

Of the three macronutrients, fat has the highest energy density (37.66 kJ/g, or 9 kcal/g) and requires the least amount of energy for storage in the body. Both its metabolism and storage may provide indications of the energy balance in the system.[8,9] Fat ingestion leads to the release of cholecystokinin, which slows gastric emptying and also provides a direct satiation signal to central food intake regulatory mechanisms.[10]

While fat ingestion gives rise to satiety it is currently considered to be the dietary energy source that is most likely to lead to obesity, for four reasons. First, given the energetics of fat metabolism and storage, there is good reason to suspect that ingesting fat is more likely to lead to excess body fat than ingesting carbohydrate.[11] Second, experimental studies have confirmed these predictions by showing that overfed human subjects stored 75–85% of the excess energy from carbohydrate and 90–95% of the excess energy from fat.[12] Third, fat has a weaker effect than carbohydrate on satiety in humans and experimental animals. This relative insensitivity to fat in meal feeding studies has been suggested to be a factor in the development and maintenance of obesity in humans.[13] Fourth, epidemiologic studies suggest a positive association between high fat consumption and frequency of obesity.[14]

Additional evidence of the importance of fat to the regulatory mechanisms of food intake is provided by rat studies in which the composition of dietary fat is a factor in determining macronutrient selection. Rats increase protein and decrease carbohydrate intake after ingestion of diets containing beef tallow compared to diets containing soybean oil or corn oil.[15,16,17]

Carbohydrate and food intake. Carbohydrate ingestion gives rise to satiety. But according to the concept of carbohydrate-specific appetites, carbohydrate intake may determine some obesity.

Carbohydrate-specific appetites have been proposed for both experimental animals and humans.[3] In humans, these appetites have been suggested as the cause of obesity in individuals defined as "carbohydrate cravers," a condition attributed to low levels of the neurotransmitter serotonin in the brain.[18] Serotonin has an inhibitory effect on food intake. Thus it has been hypothesized that overeating occurs as an attempt to normalize brain content of serotonin because metabolic responses to carbohydrate ingestion lead to increased brain uptake of tryptophan, the precursor of serotonin.[3] More recently, neuropeptide Y has been identified as a regulator of carbohydrate intake in rats, offering further support for carbohydrate-specific appetites and control mechanisms.[5]

There is little doubt that carbohydrate ingestion affects intake regulatory systems and leads to satiety. In experimental animals short-term energy intake is decreased in a dose-dependent manner after starch or sugar preloads are given intragastrically.[19,20] The type of carbohydrate fed also appears to influence the time course and precision of compensation of food intake in rats. For example, after intragastric preloads of sucrose and corn starch, food intake was suppressed more by sucrose during the first one and a half hours of feeding, but after three and a half hours total food intake was identical for both treatments.[21] Fructose preloads decrease the size of the next meal more than preloads of other carbohydrates.[20] In humans, a variety of carbohydrates including glucose, fructose, sucrose, maltodextrins, and polysaccharides when given in preloads or meals have been shown to suppress later food intake, but fructose is more effective than glucose in reducing mealtime intake and the desire to eat.[22,23] Similarly, other carbohydrates that are slowly absorbed and cause a small but sustained increase of blood glucose have greater satiety value than rapidly absorbed carbohydrates.[24]

The role of sugars in appetite control has been of considerable interest, because of the hypothesis that their sweet taste in some way overrides normal satiety responses expected of carbohydrates.[25] However, experimental studies show that sugars suppress food intake to an extent similar to rapidly absorbed starch.[22,26] Epidemiologic data also show inverse associations between sugar intake and the frequency of obesity, thus suggesting that fat, not carbohydrate, is the macronutrient most associated with obesity in a population.[27]

As with fat, evidence for specific regulatory mechanisms controlling carbohydrate intake has been provided by food selection studies. In rats given diet choices, a carbohydrate preload leads to a preference for a low-carbohydrate, high-protein diet.[28,29]

Protein and food intake. Protein is a dietary source of energy but it is an unlikely candidate for causing excess energy intake even though protein-specific appetites have been demonstrated. Because protein provides not only energy but also essential amino acids, there would seem to be some logical basis for a protein appetite driven by amino acid requirements.[30] Indeed, quantitative regulation of protein intake in animals given dietary choices has been demonstrated for rats, mice, dogs, and chickens. Evidence for a protein-specific appetite in humans is suggested by the 14–16% of dietary energy consumed as protein whenever a diverse and adequate food supply is available.[30,31]

Protein-induced suppression of food intake in both experimental animals and humans is greater than can be explained by its energy content alone, suggesting that there is a direct effect of protein, or of its amino acid constituents, in regulating satiety.[31] Rats given a preload of protein by gavage or as a meal will suppress their food intake for several hours and to a greater extent than if a similar energy load is given as fat or carbohydrate and, if provided a choice, will select a low-protein diet for their next meal.[21,28,32] In humans, protein ingestion also leads to less food intake in the next meal than can be accounted for by protein energy content alone.[33,34]

Control Mechanisms of Food Intake

The events associated with processing ingested food, including diet-induced thermogensis (DIT) and the release of many preabsorptive and postabsorptive signals, are detected by the central nervous system and operate in the process of satiation.[2]

The brain and neural pathways of hunger and satiety. The brain regulates food intake. Historically, recognition of the brain's function began with lesion studies that identified the roles of the ventromedial hypothalamus (VMH) and the lateral hypothalamus (LH).[2] The VMH was identified as the satiety center when lesions to this area caused hyperphagia and an increase in body weight in rats.[35] The LH was identified as the hunger center because lesions to this area caused aphagia and a loss of body weight in rats.[36] It is now known that several anatomical sites in the brain participate in regulating food intake through complex neural networks, many neurotransmitters, and neuropeptides.[2,37] The amino acid γ-aminobutyric acid and possibly glutamate and the monoamine neurotransmitters, including serotonin, the catecholamines, and histamine, are well-established components of food intake control mechanisms. In the past 20 years the importance of neuropeptides to feeding behavior has been recognized. These peptides, which include neuropeptide Y, galanin, opioids, and growth hormone–releasing factor, affect feeding primarily through their action on the medial hypothalamus.[37,38]

It is not known how the brain integrates the wealth of internal and external signals to balance energy and possibly macronutrient intake with requirements. It seems that there is considerable redundancy in the system, which is fortunate in a system essential to the survival of the organism. Redundancy may explain why it has been so difficult to assign a primary role to any specific control system, signal, or neurotransmitter, or to identify a specific genetic factor or metabolic error that accounts for energy imbalance in either experimental animals or humans.

A brief review of the major physiological signals that are believed to be received by the brain and used in the initiation and termination of feeding is presented below.

Thermogenesis, hunger, and appetite. It is clear that a primary determinant of total food intake is the energy required by the body. Thus the role of thermogenesis in both the initiation and termination of feeding is of interest.

For ≈4–6 hours after meal initiation diet-induced thermogenesis (DIT) generates heat by obligatory and facultative responses to food ingestion and burns 6–15% of the energy consumed.[39] Up to 75% of the heat production in DIT results from the obligatory work of digestion, absorption, transport, and metabolism of ingested food. The facultative component, 25% or more, appears to result from activation of the sympathetic nervous system through insulin-mediated stimulation and other mechanisms.[40]

The original thermostatic hypothesis of feeding control was stated in 1953 by Strominger and Brobeck as follows: "There is no simple correlation between energy needs and food intake which is valid under all conditions, and it is our purpose to present the hypothesis that the important factor in regulation of food intake is not its energy value, but rather the amount of extra heat released in its assimilation."[41] Thus it was proposed that during food consumption heat released through DIT increases body core temperature and results in termination of feeding. Conversely, as thermogenesis subsides, body temperature decreases and the decrease is the cue that initiates food intake.

Recently, Rampone and Reynolds concluded that the hypothesis has not been adequately tested, perhaps because in recent years the focus on DIT has been on its role in energy expenditure as an indicator of metabolic efficiency, and not its role in food intake control. They suggest that very small increases in DIT can be sensed by temperature-sensitive neurons in the rostral hypothalamus, which are linked to the brain's food intake–regulating mechanism via the ventromedial nucleus.[42,43]

The thermostatic hypothesis linked to the glucostatic hypothesis has been invoked as an explanation for the feeding behavior of newborn infants. Himms-Hagen suggests a link among brown adipose tissue (in young humans and animals a heat-producing organ), body temperature, blood glucose concentration, heat-sensitive neurons in the hypothalamus, and the initiation and termination of feeding.[44] The initiation of feeding is attributed to a decrease in body core temperature, which increases heat generation in brown adipose tissue, creating a demand for substrate (glucose) and thereby causing a decrease in blood glucose concentration. Termination of feeding is hypothesized to occur when body temperature increases as a result of heat production by brown adipose tissue.

Although it seems reasonable to expect that energy release after the ingestion of food plays a role in satiation and the duration of satiety, the role of DIT in regulating feeding in humans remains to be established. Whether or not this release of energy as heat would be enough to contribute to signals for terminating a meal is difficult to ascertain. In the first half hour or so after initiation of a normal meal, DIT accounts for only 1–2% of the energy of the meal, perhaps in the range of 25–75 kJ (6–18 kcal). In preliminary studies we have found that food intake of young male adults at lunch is inversely related to their DIT in the 20 minutes immediately preceding the meal, suggesting that DIT not only influences meal termination, but may also affect meal interval and the amount of the next meal.[45]

Preabsorptive signals. Preabsorptive signals arise from the presence of food in the gastrointestinal tract. These signals are most likely transmitted to the brain by the vagus nerve and may arise from physical, chemical, osmotic, or hormonal responses.[10]

The rate of gastric emptying has been implicated in the regulation of energy intake, with higher gastric emptying rates associated with greater appetite.[46] The mechanism proposed for this response depends in part on monitoring the change in stomach volume (using stretch receptors), and in part on delivery of calories to the duodenum. Release of food to the small intestine leads to the release of several peptide hormones that may contribute to the process of satiation.[10,37] The most studied of these hormones is cholecystokinin. Cholecystokinin slows gastric emptying by contracting the pyloric sphincter. In addition, release of this hormone may play a more direct role in satiation through interaction with neural inputs to feeding centers in the brain.[10] Digestion releases the components of macronutrients and provides signals to the brain via the vagus nerve through chemoreceptors in the wall of the small intestine. Thus, mechanical, secretory, and receptive elements within the gastrointestinal system contribute to the regulation of feeding behavior.[10]

Postabsorptive signals. Postabsorptive signals arise after the absorption of digested food components. Signals can be initiated by the entry of nutrients into the portal vein of the liver, or by fluctuations of nutrient concentrations in plasma or the brain.[2]

The liver is the first organ that nutrients enter after absorption. It is believed to play an important role in the control of feeding by integrating information from peripheral glucose and fatty acid metabolism and by relaying this information to the brain via the vagus nerve.[47,48] The specific metabolic signals remain unidentified, however.[48]

Plasma transports nutrients to the brain and tissues, and therefore much work has been done to determine the roles of plasma hormone and metabolite concentrations in regulating feeding behavior. Glucose, insulin, and amino acids have also received considerable attention.

Mayer proposed that blood glucose plays a regulatory role in food intake behaviour because it is the primary source of cellular energy for the central nervous system.[49] His glucostatic theory of feeding proposes that blood glucose reflects the availability of energy to the brain and other tissues, and that glucose levels are closely monitored. Evidence in support of the glucostatic theory has been slow to emerge, and indeed, in 1980, Mayer wrote that blood glucose may not be as central to the control of food intake as originally thought.[50] More recently, however, the hypothesis is again receiving considerable attention. In the rat, small ($\approx12\%$), transient declines in blood glucose, lasting ≈18 minutes, have been associated with the initiation of feeding.[51] Similarly, humans isolated from time cues show an association between declines in blood glucose and increased hunger ratings and meal requests.[52]

Insulin response to a meal has been hypothesized to be a regulatory signal to the central nervous system, either indirectly through its effect on metabolism or by direct influence on the brain. It is not clear which action is the primary regulator of food intake.

Peripheral to the CNS, insulin is an anabolic hormone, promoting the uptake and metabolism of glucose and amino acids in target tissues.[53] Perhaps for this reason, hyperinsulinemia is associated with increased hunger, food intake, and obesity.[54]

Although the origin of cerebral insulin remains uncertain, insulin action in the CNS leads to suppression of food intake.[55,56] In the arcuate nucleus insulin is believed to inhibit synthesis of neuropeptide Y (NPY), a potent stimulator of feeding.[53] Because central insulin infusions reduce levels of NPY mRNA in the arcuate nucleus, and levels of NPY in the paraventricular nucleus, it has been proposed that caloric deprivation, which reduces circulating and brain insulin, permits the increased production of NPY, which in turn stimulates feeding.[53]

The concept that plasma amino acids may influence feeding began with the observation of an inverse relationship between plasma amino acid concentrations and subjective appetite in humans.[57] This observation led to the aminostatic theory that appetite is controlled through the ability of the brain to monitor fluctuations in plasma amino acid concentrations.[2,30]

In support of the aminostatic theory, the anorexia caused by an imbalanced diet is preceded by abnormal plasma and brain concentrations of the amino acids and involves neural mechanisms in the prepyriform cortex.[58,59] Suppression of food intake and increased concentrations of amino acids in the plasma and brain also occur in rats after the ingestion of high-protein diets.[60,61] However, plasma and whole-brain concentrations of amino acids do not change in any direction that might predict a similarly mechanistic explanation for the effect of balanced proteins or amino acid mixtures on food intake.[62] One mechanistic hypothesis depends upon the precursor roles of the amino acids tryptophan, tyrosine, and histidine on the synthesis of the neurotransmitters serotonin, the catecholamines, and histamine, respectively.[30,31] However, this hypothesis remains controversial, and the relationship of amino acid neurotransmitter precursors to the control of either food intake or selection remains unestablished.[3,62]

Although recent advances in genetics and the neurosciences hold considerable promise for the future, a skeptical attitude is appropriate toward any report of a unitary system for the control of food intake. For example, the mouse obese gene and human analogue have been cloned recently, and the injection of the protein product of this gene causes overweight mice to lose weight through neuronal mechanisms.[64-66] Although this discovery appears to have great potential, one must remember that regulatory systems in experimental animals are not necessarily the same as in humans. This point is emphasized by the observation that fat cells from morbidly obese subjects produce as much of the obesity gene protein as cells from normal weight subjects.[67] Possibly the defect in humans is in sensitivity of the central nervous system receptor, but that remains to be established. More likely obesity is a multigene disorder mediated by environmental exposures, as has been proposed by others, and it remains to be determined how genes regulate food intake.[68] Clearly, considerable research effort can be expected in this area.

In summary, the regulation of food intake is a complex process that remains to be understood. The increasing incidence of obesity in some human populations and its negative health consequences provide an impetus to understand the process and find practical means of prevention and treatment.

References

1. Castonguay TW, Stern JS (1990) Hunger and appetite. In Brown M (ed), Present knowledge in nutrition, 6th ed. International Life Sciences Institute, Washington, DC, pp 13–22
2. Anderson GH (1994) Regulation of food intake. In Shils ME, Olson JA, Shike M (eds), Modern nutrition in health and disease, 8th ed. Lea & Febiger, Malvern, pp 524–536
3. Anderson GH, Black RM, Li ETS (1992) Physiologic determinants of food selection: association with protein and carbohydrate. In Anderson GH, Kennedy SH (eds), The biology of feast and famine: relevance to eating disorders. Academic Press, Toronto, pp 73–91
4. Rozin P, Vollmecke TA (1986) Food likes and dislikes. Annu Rev Nutr 6:433–456
5. Leibowitz SF (1994) Specificity of hypothalamic peptides in the control of behavioral and physiological processes. Ann N Y Acad Sci 739:12–35
6. Akabayashi A, Koenig JI, Watanabe Y, et al (1994) Galanin-containing neurons in the paraventricular nucleus: a neurochemical marker for fat ingestion and body weight gain. Proc Natl Acad Sci USA 91:10375–10379
7. Drewnowski A (1994) Human preferences for sugar and fat. In Fernstrom JD, Miller GD (eds), Appetite and body weight regulation. CRC Press, Boca Raton, pp 137–147
8. Flatt J-P (1995) Use and storage of fat and carbohydrate. Am J Clin Nutr 61(suppl):952S–959S
9. Friedman MI (1990) Body fat and the metabolic control of food intake. Int J Obes 14(suppl)3:53–67
10. Read N, French S, Cunningham K (1994) The role of the gut in regulating food intake in man. Nutr Rev 52:1–10
11. Flatt J-P (1993) Dietary fat, carbohydrate balance and weight maintenance. Ann N Y Acad Sci 683:122–140
12. Horton TJ, Drougas H, Brachey A, et al (1995) Fat and carbohydrate overfeeding in humans: different effects on energy storage. Am Soc Clin Nutr 62:19–29
13. Rolls BJ, Kim-Harris S, Fischman MW, et al (1994) Satiety after preloads with different amounts of fat and carbohydrate: implications for obesity. Am J Clin Nutr 60:476–487
14. Lissner L, Heitmann BL (1995) Dietary fat and obesity: evidence from epidemiology. Eur J Clin Nutr 49:79–90
15. McGee CD (1992) Effect of dietary fat composition on macronutrient selection [PhD dissertation]. University of Toronto, Toronto
16. McGee CD, Greenwood CE (1990) Protein and carbohydrate selection respond to changes in dietary saturated fatty acids but not to changes in essential fatty acids. Life Sci 47:67–76
17. Mullen BJ, Martin RJ (1992) The effect of dietary fat on diet selection may involve central serotonin. Am J Physiol 263:R559–R563
18. Wurtman JRW, Mark S, Tsay R, et al (1985) D-fenfluramine selectively suppresses snack intake among carbohydrate cravers but not among noncarbohydrate cravers. Int J Eat Disord 6:687–699
19. Booth DA (1972) Conditioned satiety in the rat. J Comp Physiol Psych 81:457–471
20. Luo S, Trigazis L, Pang MB, et al (1994) The effect of carbohydrate on short-term food intake in rats. Int J Obes 18(suppl 2):519
21. Geliebter AA (1979) Effects of equicaloric loads of protein, fat, and carbohydrate on food intake in the rat and man. Physiol Behav 22:267–273
22. Blundell JE, Green S, Burley V (1994) Carbohydrates and human appetite. Am J Clin Nutr 59(suppl):728S–734S
23. Rodin J, Reed D, Jamner L (1988) Metabolic effects of fructose and glucose: implications for food intake. Am J Clin Nutr 47:683–689
24. Raben A, Christensen NJ, Madsen J, et al (1994) Decreased postprandial thermogenesis and fat oxidation but increased fullness after a high-fiber meal compared with a low-fiber meal. Am J Clin Nutr 59:1386–1394
25. Anderson GH (1995) Sugars, sweetness, and food intake. Am J Clin Nutr 62(suppl):195S–202S
26. Black R, Anderson GH (1994) Sweeteners, food intake and

selection. In Fernstrom JD, Miller G (eds), Appetite and body weight regulation: sugar, fat and macronutrient substitutes. CRC Press, Boca Raton, pp 125–136

27. Hill JO, Prentice AM (1995) Sugar and body weight regulation. Am J Clin Nutr 62(suppl):264S–274S

28. Van Zeggeren A, Li ETS (1990) Food intake and choice in lean and obese Zucker rats after intragastric carbohydrate preloads. J Nutr 120:309–316

29. Wurtman JJ, Moses PL, Wurtman RJ (1983) Prior carbohydrate consumption affects the amount of carbohydrate that rats choose to eat. J Nutr 113:70–78

30. Anderson GH (1979) Control of protein and energy intake: role of plasma amino acids and neurotransmitters. Can J Physiol Phamacol 57:1043–1057

31. Anderson GH, Li ETS, Glanville NT (1984) Brain mechanisms and the quantitative and qualitative aspects of food intake. Brain Res Bull 12:167–173

32. Li ETS, Anderson GH (1982) Meal composition influences subsequent food selection in the young rat. Physiol Behav 29:779–783

33. Booth DA, Chase A, Campbell AT (1970) Relative effectiveness of protein in the late stages of appetite suppression in man. Physiol Behav 5:1299–1302

34. Barkeling BS, Rossner S, Bjorvell H (1990) Effects of a high-protein meal (meat) and a high-carbohydrate meal (vegetarian) on satiety measured by automated computerized monitoring of subsequent food intake, motivation to eat and food preferences. Int J Obes 14:743–751

35. Hetherington AW, Rausen SW (1940) Hypothalamic lesions and adiposity in the rat. Anat Rec 78:149–172

36. Anand BK, Brobeck JR (1951) Hypothalamic control of food intake in rats and cats. Yale J Biol Med 24:123–133

37. Bray G (1992) Peptides affect the intake of specific nutrients and the sympathetic nervous system. Am J Clin Nutr 55:265S–271S

38. Leibowitz SF (1992) Neurochemical-neuroendocrine systems in the brain controlling macronutrient intake and metabolism. Trends Neurosci 15:491–197

39. Horton ES (1983) An overview of the assessment and regulation of energy balance in humans. Am J Clin Nutr 38:972–977

40. Landsberg L (1994) Pathophysiology of obesity-related hypertension: role of insulin and the sympathetic nervous system. J Cardiovasc Pharmacol 23(suppl)1:S1–S8

41. Strominger JL, Brobeck JR (1953) A mechanism of regulation of food intake. Yale J Biol Med 25:383–390

42. Rampone AJ, Reynolds PJ (1991) Food intake regulation by diet-induced thermogenesis. Med Hypotheses 34:7–12

43. Leibowitz SF, Hammer NJ, Chang K (1981) Hypothalamic paraventricular nucleus lesions produce overeating and obesity in the rat. Physiol Behav 27:1031–1040

44. Himms-Hagen J (1995) Does thermoregulatory feeding occur in newborn infants? A novel view of the role of brown adipose tissue thermogenesis in control of food intake. Obes Res 3:361–369

45. Biernacka M, (1995) Sugars, diet induced thermogenesis, and subsequent food intake in normal weight males. (MSc dissertation) University of Toronto, Toronto

46. McHugh PR, Moran TH (1985) The stomach: a conception of its dynamic role in satiety. Prog Psychobiol Physiol Psychol 11:197–232

47. Novin D, Robinson K, Culbreth LA, et al (1985) Is there a role for the liver in the control of food intake? Am J Clin Nutr 42:1050–1062

48. Friedman MI, Rawson NE (1994) Fuel metabolism and appetite control. In Fernstrom JD, Miller GD (eds), Appetite and body weight regulation: sugar, fat and macronutrient substitutes. CRC Press, Boca Raton, pp 63–76

49. Mayer J (1955) Regulation of energy intake and the body weight, the glucostatic theory and the lipostatic hypothesis. Ann NY Acad Sci 63:15–43

50. Mayer J (1980) Physiology of hunger and satiety. In Goodhart RS, Schils ME (eds), Modern nutrition and disease, 6th ed. Lea & Febiger, Philadelphia, pp 560–577

51. Campfield LA, Smith FJ (1990) Transient declines in blood glucose signal meal initiation. Int J Obes 14(suppl)3:15–33

52. Campfield LA, Smith FJ, Rosenbaum M, et al (1992) Human hunger: is there a role for blood glucose dynamics? Appetite 18:244

53. Schwartz MW, Figlewicz DP, Woods SC, et al (1993) Insulin, neuropeptide Y, and food intake. Ann NY Acad Sci 692:60–71

54. Heller RF, Heller RF (1994) Hyperinsulinemic obesity and carbohydrate addiction: the missing link is the carbohydrate frequency factor. Med Hypotheses 42:307–312

55. Gerozissis M, Orosco M, Rouch C, et al (1993) Basal and hyperinsulinemia-induced immunoreactive hypothalamic insulin changes in lean and genetically obese Zucker rats revealed by microdialysis. Brain Res 611:258–263

56. McGowan MK, Andrews KM, Grossman SB (1992) Chronic intrahypothalamic infusions of insulin or insulin antibodies alter body weight and food intake in rats. Physiol Behav 51:753–756

57. Mellinkoff SM, Frankland M, Boyle D, et al (1956) Relationship between serum amino acid concentration and fluctuations in appetite. J Appl Physiol 8:535–538

58. Gietzen DW (1986) Time course of food intake and plasma and brain amino acid concentrations in rats fed amino acid-imbalanced or -deficient diets. In Morley JE, Kave R, Brand JG (eds), Interaction of the chemical senses with nutrition. Academic Press, New York, pp 415–456

59. Geitzen DW (1993) Neural mechanisms in the responses to amino acid deficiency. J Nutr 1223:610–625

60. Glanville NT, Anderson GH (1985) The effect of insulin deficiency, dietary protein intake, and plasma amino acid concentrations on brain amino acid levels in rats. Can J Physiol Pharmacol 63:487–494

61. Anderson HL, Benevanga NJ, Harper AE (1969) Associations among food and protein intake, serine dehydratase, and plasma amino acids. Am J Physiol 214:1008–1013

62. Anderson GH, Li ETS, Anthony SP, et al (1994) Dissociation between plasma and brain amino acid profiles and short-term food intake in the rat. Am J Physiol 266:R1675–R1686

63. Fernstrom JD (1987) Food-induced changes in brain serotonin synthesis: is there a relationship to appetite for specific macronutrients? Appetite 8:163–182

64. Zhang Y, Proenca R, Maffei M, et al (1994) Positional cloning of the mouse obese gene and its human analogue. Nature 372:425–432

65. Halaas JL, Gajiwala KS, Maffei M, et al (1995) Weight-reducing effects of the plasma protein encoded by the obese gene. Science 269:543–546

66. Campfield LA, Smith FJ, Guisez Y, et al (1995) Recombinant mouse OB protein: evidence for a peripheral signal linking adiposity and central neural networks. Science 269546–549

67. Hamilton BS, Paglia D, Kwan AYM, et al (1995) Increased obese mRNA expression in omental fat cells from massively obese humans. Nature Med 1:953–956

68. Burns TL, Moll PP, Lauer RM (1993) Genetic models of human obesity-family studies. Crit Rev Food Sci Nutr 33:339–343

Chapter 4

Obesity

George A. Bray

This chapter will focus on the physiological and nutritional aspects of being overweight and will point out that the location of body fat may be more significant than the total amount of fat itself in the health risks associated with obesity. The role of increased food intake, reduced physical activity, and altered thermogenesis as mechanisms for the development of excessive fat deposits will be reviewed. Finally, an approach to treatment for obesity will be discussed using a risk-benefit approach. For more detailed information about various facets of obesity, especially treatment, the reader is referred to several recent monographs.[1–6]

Definition and Measurement of Body Fat and Its Distribution

Because both overweight and fat distribution may be useful predictors of health risks associated with obesity, we need to have a clear definition of these terms. Overweight is an increase of body weight above a standard defined in relation to height. Obesity, on the other hand, is an abnormally high percentage of body fat, which may be generalized or localized. To determine whether an individual is obese or simply overweight because of increased muscle mass, one needs techniques and standards for quantitating body weight, body fat, and distribution of body fat. Several approaches to determining this are listed in Table 1, which also includes an estimate of the cost, ease of use, and accuracy of these methods. (Also see Chapter 2, "Body Composition.")

Anthropometric Measurements

Anthropometric measurements include height and weight; circumferences of the chest, waist, hips, or extremities; and skinfold thickness[3] (see Table 1).

Height and weight can be related in several ways. Of these, the ratio called the body mass index (BMI) or Quetelet index (kg/m^2) is most useful. The correlation of BMI with body fat as measured from body density is between 0.7 and 0.8.[7] Figure 1 is a nomogram for determining BMI. The desirable range for BMI for each height may increase slightly with age for women but not

for men.[8] Based on these observations, tables of good weight for men and women have been published by the US Department of Agriculture and the Department of Health and Human Services. The BMI also can be used to assess health risks associated with overweight and may also be used as a guide to therapy (see the following discussion).

The degree of body fat or obesity can be assessed from the thickness of skinfolds.[3] One difficulty with skinfold measurements is that the equations used to estimate body fat vary with age, sex, and ethnic background. Body fat increases with age even though the sum of the skinfold measurements remains constant.[3] This finding implies that, with aging, fat accumulates at other than subcutaneous sites.

The ratio of waist or abdominal circumference to the hip or gluteal circumference provides an index of the regional fat distribution and has proven valuable as a guide to health risks in epidemiologic studies. A more practical individual guide is provided by the waist circumference.[9] Men and women in the top quintile for waist circumference, i.e., the top 20%, have a substantially increased risk of heart disease and diabetes.

Isotopic, Chemical, and Other Methods to Measure Body Compartments

Both chemical and isotopic markers can be used to estimate body water, body fat, or potassium.[3,10] Measurement of body density provides a valuable quantitative technique for measuring body fat and fat-free mass (see Table 1). Density is determined from the weight of the body after submersion and out of water using the principle of Archimedes.[3,7] The technique is relatively easy if appropriate facilities are available, but it remains primarily a research method.

Total body electrical conductivity also can be used to quantitate lean tissue and fat because of differences in the ability of these components to conduct electromagnetic waves.[11] However, the instrument used for this test is expensive.[11] A relatively inexpensive instrument for measuring body fat uses electrical impedance (bioelectric impedance analysis).[12] Electrodes are applied to one

Table 1. Methods of estimating body fat and its distribution

Method	Cost	Ease of use	Accuracy	Regional fat
Height and weight	$	Easy	High	No
Skinfold thicknesses	$	Easy	Low	Yes
Circumferences	$	Easy	Moderate	Yes
Ultrasound	$$	Moderate	Moderate	Yes
Density				
Immersion	$	Moderate	High	No
Plethysmograph	$$$	Difficult	High	No
Heavy water				
Tritiated	$$	Moderate	High	No
Deuterium oxide or heavy oxygen	$$$	Moderate	High	No
Potassium isotope (^{40}K)	$$$$	Difficult	High	No
Total body electrical conductivity	$$$	Moderate	High	No
Bioelectric impedance	$$	Easy	High	No
Fat-soluble gas	$$	Difficult	High	No
Absorptiometry (dual energy x-ray absorptiometry, dual photon absorptiometry)	$$$	Easy	High	No
Computed tomography (CT)	$$$$	Difficult	High	Yes
Magnetic resonance imaging (MRI)	$$$$	Difficult	High	Yes
Neutron activation	$$$$	Difficult	High	No

$, low cost; $$, moderate cost; $$$, high cost; $$$$, very high cost.

arm and leg, and the impedance is measured. Because impedance is related to the aqueous portion of the body, formulas are used to estimate the percentage of fat in the

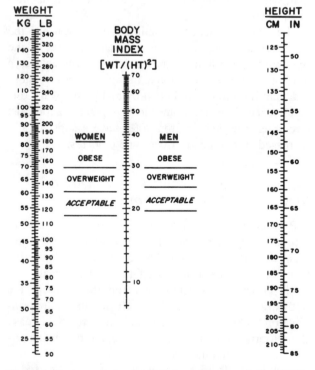

Figure 1. Nomogram for determining body mass index (BMI). To use this nomogram, place a ruler or other straight edge between the body weight in kilograms or pounds (without clothes) located on the left-hand line and the height in centimeters or in inches (without shoes) located on the right-hand line. The BMI is read from the middle of the scale and is in metric units. (Copyright 1978, George A. Bray. Used with permission.)

body; there is concern about the validity of this method. Dual-energy x-ray or dual photon absorptiometry appears to be the best method for estimating total body fat.[10]

Computerized tomographic scans and nuclear magnetic resonance scans (see Table 1) can provide quantitative estimates of regional fat and give a ratio of intra-abdominal to extraabdominal fat.[13] Ultrasonic waves applied to the skin will be reflected by the fat, muscle, and other interfaces and can also provide a measure of fat thickness in regional locations.[14] Finally, neutron activation of the whole body can be used to identify chemical components by their emission spectra.[10,15] This procedure is expensive and available only in a few centers.

In summary, body fat can be estimated in several ways. From a practical point of view, three methods are most useful. Measurements of height and weight, preferably expressed as the BMI, provide an estimate of the degree of overweight. When available, dual-energy x-ray absorptiometry provides the best index of total body fat. For estimating regional fat distribution, measurement of the circumference of the waist is a practical measure; the thickness of the subscapular skinfold may also be used.

The proportions of fat and nonfat components are depicted for a normal-weight (70 kg) and an obese (100 kg) male as well as a normal-weight (55 kg) and an obese (85 kg) female. The extra 30 kg of weight adds ≈50% to body weight but increases body energy stored as fat by 200% (Figure 2).

Prevalence of Obesity

At birth, the human body contains approximately 12% fat. This amount is higher than that for any other mam-

BODY COMPOSITION   ENERGY CONTENT

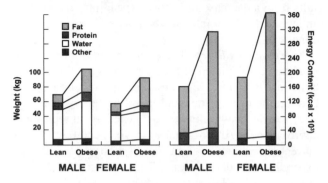

Figure 2. Body composition in obesity. The percentage of fat, protein, water, and other components for a normal 70 kg man and 55 kg woman are shown at the left of each group along with the data for an obese individual who is 30 kg heavier (data are in the middle). The contribution of the fat and protein to body energy stores is also indicated in the bar to the right of the one for weight. (Copyright 1987, George A. Bray. Used with permission.)

mal except the whale. In the newborn period, body fat rises rapidly to reach a peak of about 25% by age 6 months and then declines to 15–18% in the prepubertal years.[6] At puberty there is a significant increase in the percentage of fat in females and a significant decrease in males. By age 18, males have approximately 15–18% body fat and females have 20–25%. Fat increases in both sexes after puberty, and during adult life it rises to between 30% and 40% of body weight. Between ages 20 and 50, fat content of males approximately doubles and that of females increases by approximately 50%. Total body weight, however, rises by only 10–15%, indicating that there is a reduction in lean body mass.[3]

The prevalence of obesity in Americans is now estimated by the National Center for Health Statistics to be 35%.[16] The percentage of overweight black and Hispanic women is substantially higher than that of white women, but these racial differences are much less obvious in men. In both sexes, the prevalence of overweight increases with age and has risen sharply in the past decade (Figure 3).[16]

The percentage of body fat is influenced by the level of physical activity.[17] During physical training, body fat usually decreases and lean tissue increases. After training ends, however, the process is reversed. These shifts between body fat and lean tissue can occur without a change in body weight, but if regular activity is maintained throughout adult life, the increase in body fat may be prevented. The value of exercise is most easily seen after weight loss.[18] Figure 4 shows the results of a study on the relationship between weight loss and exercise[18]: adding exercise to a diet did not have a significant effect on weight loss. However, at the 18-month followup, the men who had continued to be active kept off almost all of the weight they had lost, while the men who had stopped exercising gained weight.

Socioeconomic conditions also play an important role in the development of obesity. Excess body weight is 7 to 12 times more frequent in women from lower social classes than in women from upper social classes. In men, social class and race have a much less pronounced relationship to overweight.

Americans are among the fattest people in the world. There are at least three possible explanations for the high prevalence of obesity in North America. First, the high proportion of automobiles and large amounts of time spent watching television may significantly reduce energy expenditure more than in other countries. Second, there may be differences in quantity or quality of dietary intake. Third, higher rates of smoking may explain the lower rate of obesity outside North America.

Pathogenesis of Obesity

Nutrient imbalance and food intake. Obesity is a problem of nutrient imbalance as more foodstuffs are stored as fat than are used for energy and metabolism. Do obese subjects ingest more food energy than lean ones? The answer to this question is an unequivocal yes. Yet, based on both cross-sectional and longitudinal studies measuring food intake the answer would appear to be no. This apparent discrepancy has been resolved by the use of a new technique to measure energy expenditure, called doubly labeled water, which has shown that both obese and lean persons underreport their food intake.[19] As illustrated in the left side of Figure 5, doubly labeled water ($^2H_2{}^{18}O$) is given to the subject. The right side of Figure 5 illustrates that deuterium ($^2H_2$) can leave the body only as water, but ^{18}O can leave the body as both $C^{18}O_2$ and $H_2{}^{18}O$. Thus, ^{18}O is lost more rapidly than ^2H_2O and the difference in rate of disappearance is proportional to CO_2 production (see the lower line in Figure 5). The

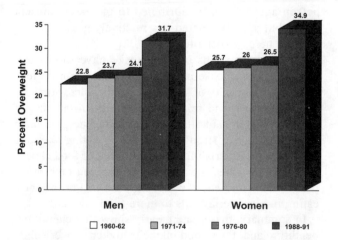

Figure 3. Prevalence of obesity. Data from the National Center for Health Statistics show the rise in prevalence of obesity over the past 30 years, particularly the past 10 years. (Redrawn from Kuczmarski et al.[14])

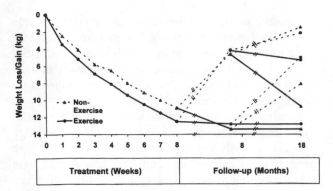

Figure 4. Weight loss and exercise. During the first 8 months, subjects were in groups with diet or diet plus exercise, with little difference in weight loss. Thereafter, the subjects that exercised maintained better weight than those that did not. Subjects who ceased to exercise regained or demonstrated a tendency to return to prestudy weight. During follow-up, those subjects initiating nonsupervised exercises showed weight loss. (Drawn from Pavlou et al.[18])

first measurement of deuterium and [18]O is within a few hours, and the second measurement is 7 to 14 days later (see Figure 5, lower panel). If one knows the respiratory quotient, it is possible to estimate energy expenditure reliably. Data on a group of obese and lean subjects using this technique are shown in Figure 6.[20] In the three groups studied, obese subjects had higher total energy expenditure than lean ones. When compared with food intake, both obese and nonobese subjects underreported energy intake, by 20–50% and 10–30%, respectively.

Energy requirements decline with age. Thus, to maintain body weight, food intake should show a corresponding decrease as a person ages. The values for energy intake from three surveys are presented in Figure 7.[3] The peak values occur in the second decade of life, followed by a gradual decline in successive decades for both sexes. Thus, the increase in body weight and body fat as a person ages cannot be attributed to increased nutrient intake but must be related to a relatively greater reduction in energy expenditure.

Direct observations of food intake have shown that obese persons choose or eat larger meals than do lean persons. In a variety of studies on food choice, Stunkard and Kaplan[21] found relative uniformity in the size of meals chosen in naturalistic settings. The energy content of the meals was strongly affected by eating site, and there was great variability in the amount of food chosen at each site. Thus, the major influence on how much people choose to eat is where they eat it. For instance, eating in a cafeteria leads to more food ingestion.

In summary, these data clearly show that energy expenditure and, thus, food intake is higher in overweight than in lean subjects. Direct observation of obese subjects supports the conclusion that they choose and eat more food and often do so more rapidly than normal-

weight subjects. Weight gain in adult life probably results from a decrease in energy expenditure rather than an increase in food intake, which actually seems to decline with age.[22]

Energy expenditure. The components of energy expenditure are depicted in Figure 8. Basal (resting) metabolic rate is defined as the total energy required by the body in the resting state and is influenced by age, sex, body weight, drugs, climate, and genetics.[23] It represents approximately 70% of total energy expenditure. When corrected for body weight, the highest rate of energy expenditure occurs in infants. There is a gradual decline in this rate in childhood and a further slower decline of approximately 2% per decade in adult life. Metabolic rates for women are usually lower than those for men of comparable height and weight, primarily because of the higher body fat level in women.[24,25] Resting metabolic rate has the best relationship to fat-free body mass, but it is also closely related to surface area and total body weight because heat loss is related to the surface area of the skin. A higher body weight or greater lean body mass has been found to be associated with a higher metabolic rate in studies using both metabolic chambers[26,27] and doubly labeled water techniques.

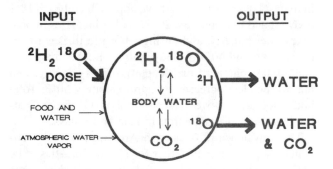

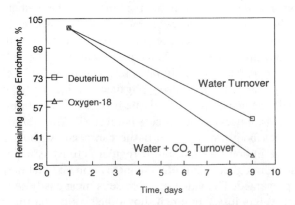

Figure 5. Model of doubly labeled water. Water labeled with [18]O and ^{2}H is given to the subject. After equilibration with body water, a sample of blood, saliva, or urine is taken to determine the ratio of [18]O to [2]H. A second sample, taken 7 to 14 days later, is used for a second ratio determination. From the changing ratios totaled, daily energy expenditure can be calculated.

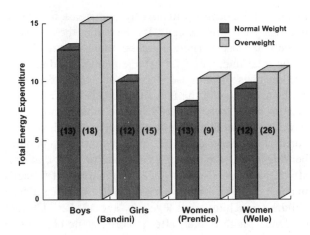

Figure 6. Energy expenditure and food intake. Total daily energy expenditure was measured by the doubly labeled water method and food intake was measured by standard methods. In this group of obese individuals, underreporting of food intake was nearly 50%. USDA, U.S. Department of Agriculture; LRC, Lipid Research Clinics; HANES-1, first Health and Nutrition Examination Survey. (Redrawn from Welle et al.[20])

Metabolic rate clusters in families. If one individual is below the median for energy expenditure, other members of the family also tend to be below the median.[28] A low resting metabolic rate in relation to lean body mass may also be a predictor for lower physical activity, higher body fat, and an increased likelihood of becoming obese.[29]

The relationship of physical activity to obesity can be studied by laboratory observations or by observation in the natural environment. In the laboratory, the treadmill and cycle ergometer have been the main tools used to examine the efficiency of exercising muscle in obese subjects. In both obese and lean individuals, the efficiency for coupling energy release to muscular contraction is approximately 30%.[30] That is, the work of turning the flywheel on a cycle ergometer accounts for 30% of the energy expended during cycling. Thus, there is no evidence to indicate an abnormality in the metabolic coupling of substrate metabolism to the contraction of muscular tissue in moderately or massively obese subjects.[30]

The second approach to studying energy expenditure is observation. Obese individuals often are observed to be less active than normal-weight individuals. A lower level of spontaneous movement, however, does not necessarily imply reduced energy expenditure because the overweight individual uses more energy for any given movement.

In normal-weight individuals, graded increases in physical activity have been reported to increase food intake.[31] In obese individuals, however, changing the level of physical activity has a much smaller effect on food intake.[32] Thus, the level of physical activity may modulate food intake and body fat in lean individuals. A dis-

turbance in this system may play a key role in the development of obesity.

When food is eaten, the metabolic rate increases and then returns toward normal. This process requires several hours, and during this time the increase in energy expenditure can approximate 10–15% of the total energy value of the ingested food. One explanation for this thermogenic response to a meal is that it results from enhanced activity of the sympathetic nervous system, the effects of which are shown in activity of brown adipose tissue or muscle.[33] If this is correct, a reduction in sympathetic activity of obese subjects compared with lean ones might provide a mechanism for enhanced metabolic efficiency that might allow energy to be stored rather than burned. A reduction in sympathetic nervous system activity to brown adipose tissue has been observed in many forms of obese experimental animals and man, and might also explain why increasing physical activity does not significantly reduce food intake in obese subjects.[34]

The concept that an altered thermic response to food may serve as a mechanism for the storage of extra calories that causes human obesity is intriguing and controversial.[35-37] Some studies have shown a difference between obese and lean subjects in energy produced after a meal, but other studies have not. The discrepancy may lie in the size of the meal eaten, in the techniques of recording intake, in the palatability of the food, and in whether subjects had abnormal glucose tolerance.[36] Golay et al.[37] examined 55 subjects with varying degrees of

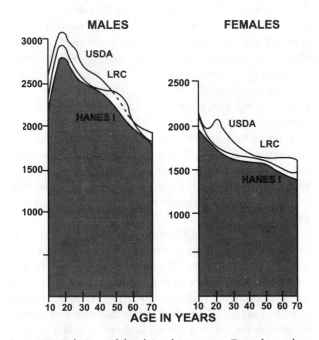

Figure 7. Relation of food intake to age. Data from three studies of food intake in relation to age are plotted for men and women. (Copyright 1987, George A. Bray. Used with permission.)

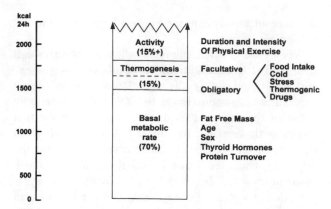

Figure 8. Components of energy expenditure. The energy partition into basal energy needs, thermogenesis, and activity was estimated based on a 2500 kcal/d requirement. The upper end is open, indicating that activity is variable and can be increased for the normal individual. However, this component comprises ≈30% of total daily energy expenditure. (Copyright 1987, George A. Bray. Used with permission.)

obesity and impairment in glucose tolerance, including frank diabetes. The increment in energy expenditure was significantly lower in obese nondiabetic subjects and in those with impaired glucose tolerance than in normal volunteers. In turn, obese diabetic subjects had a smaller response than the normal-weight or obese nondiabetic subjects. There was a negative correlation between the degree of thermic response and circulating insulin. The thermic effect of glucose is partially blocked by propranolol, a drug that blocks β-receptors. This component of diet-induced thermogenesis is called facultative thermogenesis. These data suggest that there is an impairment in the thermic response to a meal in obese subjects and that one mechanism associated with this change is the anticipatory (cephalic phase) secretory response of the pancreatic system of releasing insulin. After weight loss, the thermic effect of a meal in obese subjects is reduced, providing additional evidence for this hypothesis.

Adipose tissue. Over 90% of body energy is stored as triacyglycerol in adipose tissue.[3,38] Protein provides important but smaller quantities of energy. Glycogen stores are minute in comparison, but glycogen provides a critical source of glucose during exercise or short-term fasting.

Adipose tissue has a number of functions, the most obvious one being the storage of fatty acids in triacylglycerols and release of these fatty acids as a source of metabolic fuel. Fat cells may also serve as a source of information about body energy stores. Triacyglycerol is stored in fat cells, which differ in number and size between one region of the body and another. Women generally have more gluteal fat than men. The total number of fat cells is increased in individuals with obesity beginning in childhood.[39] Storage of fat in the first

months of life occurs primarily by an increase in the size of already-existing fat cells. By the end of the first year, fat cell size has nearly doubled but there is little change in the total number of fat cells, either in children who become obese or in those who do not.[39] In children who are lean, the size of the fat cells decreases after the first year of life. Obese children, on the other hand, retain throughout childhood the large fat cells that developed during the first year of life. Fat cells multiply in number throughout the growing years in a process that usually terminates in adolescence. The number of fat cells in obese children increases more rapidly than that in lean children, reaching adult levels by age 10–12.[39] Current evidence suggests that, after puberty, acute changes in body fat stores occur primarily by increasing the size of adipocytes that already exist, with little or no change in their total number. Sudden weight loss is likewise accomplished primarily by a reduction in the size of extant fat cells. However, recent evidence suggests that the number of fat cells also may change in adult life.[40] A long-term increase in body fat may lead to an increase in the number of fat cells; conversely, a prolonged reduction in body fat may possibly lead to a decrease in the number of fat cells.[40] This provocative observation still awaits confirmation.

The size, number, and distribution of fat cells are useful in classifying obesity and in estimating the prognosis with different forms of therapy.[41] Obese individuals who are ≥75% above desirable weight almost always have an increased number of fat cells, whereas those with more modest degrees of extra weight may be hypercellular but are much more likely to have only an increase in fat cell size (hypertrophic obesity). The duration of weight loss that follows successful dietary treatment for obesity is shorter and the rate at which weight is regained is more rapid in individuals with hypercellular obesity than in those with hypertrophic obesity.

Adipose tissue also appears to produce and release a number of substances.[41] The first of these is adipsin, a serine protease that functions as complement D in the alternative pathway of thrombosis. Fat cells also make and secrete cytokines. One of these, tissue necrosis factor-α, has been proposed as a modulator of insulin response.[42] Adipose tissue also makes angiotensinogen. Most recently it has been the primary site to produce the protein involved in at least one form of genetic obesity.

Health Risks Associated with Being Overweight

Overweight and health risk. The effects of overweight on health have been evaluated in both prospective and retrospective studies. Studies involving >750,000 subjects each from the life insurance industry, the American Cancer Society, and Norway yielded similar results,

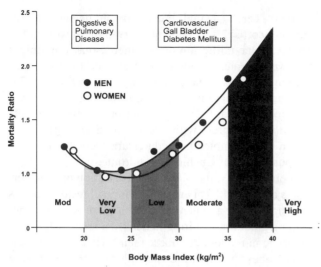

Figure 9. Mortality ratio and BMI. Data from the American Cancer Society study are plotted for men and women to show relationship of BMI to overall mortality. At BMI <20 kg/m² and >25 kg/m² , there is an increase in relative mortality. The major causes for this increased mortality are listed, along with a division of BMI groupings into various levels of risk. (Adapted from reference 44. Copyright 1987, George A. Bray. Used with permission.)

which are consistent with many but not all smaller prospective studies.[43–47] The overall relationship between BMI and excess mortality is shown in Figure 9, which plots relative mortality for various deviations of BMI using the American Cancer Society data.[44] The data show a J-shaped curve, with the minimum mortality for both men and women occurring among individuals with a BMI of 22–25 kg/m². Deviations in BMI above and below this range are associated with an increase in mortality. Individuals with a BMI of 30 kg/m² clearly have increased mortality. As BMI approaches 40 kg/m², the curve becomes progressively steeper. Mortality may also increase when BMI falls below 20 kg/m².

Fat distribution and health risks. One of the most important developments in understanding health risks associated with overweight has come from measurements of body fat distribution. There are two types of fat distribution: 1) the abdominal, android, upper-body, or male type; and 2) the gynoid, lower-body, or female type. In the late 1940s, Vague [48] suggested that a preponderance of abdominal fat might increase the risk for diabetes and cardiovascular disease. More than 30 years later, five prospective studies examining the relation of fat distribution to morbidity and mortality have confirmed this prediction.[49–53] Whether the distribution of fat was measured as the ratio of waist-to-hip circumference or a combination of skinfold thicknesses, all studies found a clear-cut and highly significant increase in the risk of death or an increased risk of diabetes, hypertension, heart attack, and stroke with increased upper-body obesity. Fat distribution was a more important risk factor for mor-

bidity and mortality than overweight per se and had a relative risk ratio of ≥2.

In addition to the prospective data just described, cross-sectional studies have also shown increased prevalence of glucose intolerance, insulin resistance, elevated blood pressure, and elevated blood lipids in both males and females with increased abdominal fat or upper-body obesity.[9,54] Abdominal fatness also predicts the risk of breast cancer in women.[55] It has been suggested that the abdominal or android fat pattern may represent an increase in the size or number, or both, of more metabolically active intraabdominal fat cells. These fat cells release free fatty acids directly into the portal circulation, which might interfere with insulin clearance in the liver and thus affect various metabolic processes. It is interesting in this context that two recent papers, one from Japan and one from the Framingham study, have defined relative morbidity using estimates of risk and found that the optimal BMI of 27 is very close to that from older estimates using mortality.[56,57]

Obesity and organ function: cardiovascular system. The relation of hypertension to obesity has been widely recognized. When measuring blood pressure, it is important to use a cuff that encircles 75% of the arm, because smaller cuffs may artificially elevate blood pressure. However, even with the limitations in the techniques of measuring blood pressure by indirect auscultation, the available data almost uniformly indicate the important relationship between body weight and blood pressure and between fat distribution and blood pressure.[58] Upper-body obesity is associated with further elevations in blood pressure.[59]

Increased blood pressure probably results from increased peripheral arteriolar resistance. During and after weight loss, there is usually a reduction in blood pressure. Obesity also increases the work of the heart even when blood pressure is normal.[60] This, too, can be reversed with weight loss. A cardiomyopathy of obesity has been reported and is associated with congestive heart failure.

Diabetes mellitus. Obesity appears to aggravate the development of diabetes, and weight loss appears to reduce the risk of this disease. The risk of diabetes is worsened with increased abdominal fat and weight gain (Figure 10).[61] With weight loss, glucose tolerance improves, insulin secretion decreases, and insulin resistance is reduced.[62]

Gallbladder disease. The association of obesity with gallbladder disease has been documented in several studies.[3,63] Obese women aged 20–30 had a sixfold increase in the risk of developing gallbladder disease compared with normal-weight women. By age 60, nearly one third of obese women can expect to develop gallbladder disease.[3] The relation of gallbladder disease to fat distribution is also evident. This tendency to gallstones may

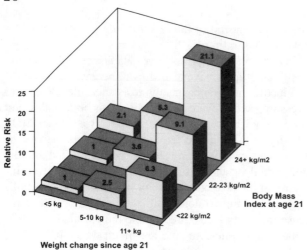

Figure 10. Effect of weight change on risk of diabetes. Both higher BMI and weight gain increased the risk for developing diabetes in the Health Professional Study. (Redrawn from Chan et al.[61])

result from increased cholesterol synthesis that is observed in obesity. Approximately 20 mg/d of cholesterol are synthesized for each extra kilogram of stored fat. This, in turn, results in increased biliary excretion of cholesterol, producing a bile that is more saturated in cholesterol, which increases the risk of gallstone disease.[3]

Pulmonary function. Measurements of pulmonary function are normal in most obese individuals.[64,65] Only with massive obesity are decreased reserve volumes and lowered arterial oxygen saturation obvious. The most important pulmonary problem in the obese patient is obstructive sleep apnea and the obesity-hypoventilation syndrome that, although uncommon, occurs mainly in massively obese individuals. There is increasing evidence in the literature suggesting that sleep apnea in these patients may relate to pharyngeal fat. Treatment includes continuous positive airway pressure and weight loss.

Endocrine and metabolic changes. The basal concentration of growth hormone is normal or reduced in obese subjects, and there is a negative correlation between BMI and the integrated concentration of growth hormone obtained by frequent sampling over 24 hours.[66] The induction of hypoglycemia with insulin normally stimulates an increase in growth hormone, but in obese patients this response is blunted.[6,67]

Nutrition appears to be more important than body weight in determining the circulating concentration of triiodothyronine.[68] During fasting and severe caloric restriction, total thyroxine (T_4) levels remain normal, but the serum concentration of total triiodothyronine (T_3) decreases, and that of reverse T_3 increases. In contrast to starvation, overnutrition is associated with an increase in serum T_3 and a fall in reverse T_3 in both obese and lean subjects.[68]

The diurnal rhythm of cortisol is preserved in patients with simple obesity,[3,66] but afternoon values may be above normal. There is a small but significant negative correlation of cortisol with percent overweight in women but not men. One milligram of dexamethasone at midnight followed by measurement of plasma cortisol the next morning or measurement of urinary-free cortisol in a 24-hour urine collection is the best screening test to separate obesity from Cushing's syndrome. Obese patients who do not suppress with this test are a small group for whom more complex procedures are needed to exclude the possibility of Cushing's syndrome.

In obese males, the plasma concentration of testosterone is decreased.[3] This reduction in total testosterone is accompanied by a reduction in the level of sex hormone-binding globulin, resulting in a normal level of free testosterone in moderately obese men.[69] However, in massively obese men, there may be a decrease in free testosterone as well.

In obese girls, the onset of menarche occurs at a younger age than in normal-weight girls.[3] The observation that menstruation is initiated when body weight reaches critical mass may provide an explanation for this phenomenon. As the rate of growth accelerates in late childhood, the entrance into this critical weight range may initiate puberty. Because obese girls grow faster and enter this critical mass at a younger age than normal-weight girls do, menstruation usually starts at an earlier age. The obese patient often shows a decrease in the regularity of menstrual cycles and an increase in the frequency of menstrual abnormalities. In one study, 43% of women with menstrual disorders were overweight.[70] Menopause may also occur at a younger age in obese women.

Does weight loss improve health? Both the insurance companies and the Framingham study provide data suggesting that weight reduction may be beneficial.[43,71] In both men and women who successfully lose and maintain a lower weight, mortality was reduced to within the normal limits based on sex and age according to life insurance statistics. From the data obtained in Framingham, MA, a 10% reduction in relative weight for men was associated with a decrease in serum glucose of 0.14 mmol/L, a decrease in serum cholesterol of 0.292 mmol/L, a decrease in systolic blood pressure of 6.6 mm Hg, and a decrease in serum uric acid of 19.6 mmol/L.[71] For each 10% reduction in the body weight of men, these data predict that there would be an anticipated 20% decrease in the incidence of coronary artery disease.

Clinical Types of Obesity

Genetic factors in obesity. Genetic transmission of obesity has been well established in animals for over 40 years.[34] The field of study has been given new impetus by cloning of the gene involved in the yellow mouse and in the obese (ob/ob) mouse and by the identification of

Table 2. A comparison of syndromes of obesity—hypogonadism and mental retardation

Feature	Syndrome				
	Prader-Willi	Bardet-Biedl	Ahlstrom	Cohen	Carpenter
Inheritance	Sporadic 2/3 have defective chromosome 15	Autosomal recessive	Autosomal recessive	Probably autosomal recessive	Autosomal recessive
Stature	Short	Normal, infrequently short	Normal, infrequently short	Short or tall	Normal
Obesity	Generalized Moderate to severe Onset 1–3 years	Generalized Early onset 1–2 years	Truncal Early onset 2–5 years	Truncal Mid childhood Age 5	Truncal Gluteal
Cranofacies	Narrow bifrontal diameter Almond-shaped eyes Strabismus V-shaped mouth High-arched palate	Not distinctive	Not distinctive	High nasal bridge Arched palate Open mouth Short philtrum	Acrocephaly Flat nasal bridge High-arched palate
Limbs	Small hands and feet Hypotonia	Polydactyly	No abnormalities	Hypotonia Narrow hands and feet	Polydactyly Syndactyly Genu valgum
Reproductive status	1° Hypogonadism	1° Hypogonadism	Hypogonadism in males but not in females	Normal gonadal function or hypogonadotrophic hypogonadism	2° Hypogonadism
Other features	Enamel hypoplasia Hyperphagia Temper tantrums Nasal speech			Dysplastic ears Delayed puberty	
Mental retardation	Mild to moderate		Normal IQ	Mild	Slight

several other chromosomal locations in which diet and genes interact to produce dietary obesity.[2,72,73]

In human obesity, genetic factors are expressed in two ways. First, there is a group of rare forms of dysmorphic obesity in which genetic factors are of prime importance. Second, there is a genetic substrate upon which environmental factors interact in the development of obesity.

The dysmorphic forms of obesity are listed in Table 2.[74] In most of these forms, obesity is only of moderate degree, but it may be pronounced, particularly in the Prader-Willi syndrome. These forms of obesity are transmitted both by recessive and dominant modes of inheritance. The Prader-Willi syndrome is associated in half or more of the cases with a translocation or deletion on the short arm of chromosome 15.[75]

Family studies show a familial relationship in obesity, but these studies do not critically separate environmental from genetic factors.[2] The distinction can be made in studies using adopted children or twins. In the Danish adoption registry, a sample of 800 adoptees showed no relationship between BMI of the adoptive parents and their children. On the other hand, there was a direct relationship between the BMI of the biological parents and the increasing weight of the children. These data suggest that inheritance plays an important role in the risk of developing obesity, and are consistent with most, but not all other, studies of adopted children.

The most definitive evidence for genetic versus environmental factors in the development of obesity comes from the examination of body weight in twins.[2,76,77,78]

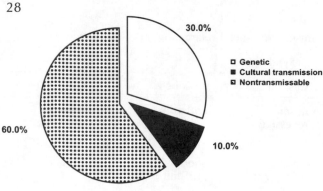

Genetic Factors in Obesity

Figure 11. Genetic factors in obesity. The genetic and non-genetic transmission of fat-free mass and the ratio of subcutaneous fat to fat mass are presented. (Redrawn from Bouchard et al.[76])

Monozygotic twins have identical genetic material whereas dizygotic twins have the genetic diversity of brothers or sisters, or both. However, environmental closeness of monozygotic twins should permit evaluation of these groups of twins along with other siblings and more distant relatives to identify genetic factors in obesity. Using BMI as the criterion for obesity, Stunkard et al.[77] compared 1974 monozygotic and 2097 dizygotic male twins from the National Academy of Sciences twin registry. Monozygotic twins had a higher correlation between their body weights than did dizygotic twins, and calculations of the heritability for obesity suggested that nearly two thirds of the variability in BMI was attributable to genetic factors.

Bouchard and his colleagues[78] measured skinfold thicknesses and total body fat in various groups of individuals with differing degrees of genetic relationship, including monozygotic and dizygotic twins. In adopted siblings, there is a very low order of correlation. Biological siblings, however, showed a higher correlation and, as might be expected, the correlation was highest among monozygotic twins. Biological siblings had a lower order of correlation for all of the variables than did dizygotic twins, although both groups have the same genetic variability, implying that there was an environmental influence operative in the dizygotic twins that was absent in their biological siblings. On the basis of a technique called path analysis, these data on the genetic and nongenetic components for body fat and BMI can be partitioned into transmissible and nontransmissible components (Figure 11). Approximately 60% of the distribution of body fat is nontransmissible and approximately 30% is genetic.

In summary, single and polygenic inheritance are both involved in the transmission of obesity in humans. The best estimates suggest that genetic factors may be of less importance than environmental factors in the determination of total body fat, but genetic factors are of more significance in determining distribution of body fat.

Classification of obesity. Obesity can be classified in at least three ways: by the anatomic characteristics and regional distribution of adipose tissue, by etiologic causes, and by the functional feature of the obesity.

An anatomic classification of obesity is based on the number of adipocytes and on fat distribution. In many obese individuals whose problems began in childhood, the number of adipocytes may be increased by two- to fourfold (normal range = $20–60 \times 10^9$ fat cells). Individuals with increased numbers of fat cells have hypercellular obesity. This is distinguished from other forms of obesity in which the total number of adipocytes is normal, but the size of individual fat cells is increased. In general, all obesity is associated with an increase in the size of adipocytes, but only selected forms have an increase in the total number of fat cells.

Obesity may also be classified according to body fat distribution, which has important genetic determinants.[79] Both males and females with upper-body obesity have an increased risk of cardiovascular disease, hypertension, and diabetes. On the other hand, lower-body obesity appears to carry a much lower health risk.

There are a number of etiologic causes for obesity. Endocrine diseases may cause obesity, but such cases are rare.[3] Moreover, endocrine diseases usually produce only small increases in body fat. Hyperinsulinism, caused by islet cell tumors or by injection of excess quantities of insulin, results in increased food intake and increased fat storage, but the magnitude of this effect is usually modest. A somewhat more substantial obesity is observed with the increased cortisol secretion of Cushing's syndrome. Obesity may also occur with hypothyroidism. Finally, aberrations in the distribution of body fat are also observed with hypogonadism.

Hypothalamic obesity is a rare syndrome in humans[80] but can be regularly produced in animals by injury to the ventromedial region of the hypothalamus. This region is responsible for integrating information about energy stores and regulating the function of the autonomic nervous system. Hypothalamic obesity has been reported in human subjects under a variety of circumstances. The major factors producing hypothalamic damage are trauma, malignancy, and inflammatory disease. Symptoms and signs that accompany the syndrome include those related to intracranial pressure, endocrine alterations, and a variety of neurological and physiological derangements. Treatment of the syndrome requires treating the underlying disease and giving appropriate endocrine support.

Physical inactivity plays an important role in the development of obesity.[18] Gross obesity in rats can be produced by severe restriction of activity. In a modern affluent society, energy-sparing devices also reduce energy expenditure and may enhance the tendency to become fat.[3]

NUTRIENT INTAKE

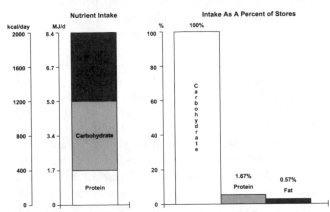

Figure 12. Nutrient intake versus stores. The daily intake of carbohydrate approximates body stores of carbohydrate. Intakes of fat and protein are only a small fraction of the stored quantities of these nutrients.

Diet is another etiologic factor in obesity. This is particularly prominent in experimental animals but also may play a role in the development of human obesity.[81] When rodents eat a high-fat diet, drink sucrose-containing solutions, or eat a cafeteria type of diet, most strains are unable to appropriately regulate energy balance, and ingest more energy than is needed for weight maintenance. To maintain nutrient balance—that is, keep the stores of fat and carbohydrate in the body constant—the ratio of fat to carbohydrate in the diet, a term called food quotient (FQ) by Flatt,[81] must equal the respiratory quotient (RQ):

$$FQ = RQ \quad \text{Fat balance} = 0$$
$$FQ > RQ \quad \text{Fat balance negative}$$
$$FQ < RQ \quad \text{Fat balance positive}$$

If the FQ is higher than the RQ, that is, the body is burning more fat than is being eaten, body fat will be reduced. On the contrary, if FQ is less than the RQ, fat balance will be positive, with a gain in body fat. One corollary of this is what we tend to eat for carbohydrate. The relation of carbohydrate, fat, and protein in the diet is shown in Figure 12. The daily intake of carbohydrate is nearly equal to body stores. On the other hand, fat and protein intakes are only a small fraction of body stores. Thus, regulation of carbohydrate stores is more drastically influenced by diet than are fat or protein stores. Recent epidemiologic data show that overweight is more likely when the diet is high in fat.

Goals and realities of treatment. Treating individuals with weight problems has many similarities to treating other chronic diseases (Table 3). Hypertension, for example, can be effectively treated by current medications. Yet, the side effects of treatment and the need to treat individuals who may have no overt symptoms from hypertension lead to high levels of therapeutic failure, including unwillingness of such individuals to seek medical help, unwillingness to maintain treatment once prescribed, and termination of treatment because of some of the side effects of medication. Treatment of obesity has similar problems.

In addition, treatments for overweight individuals are almost always palliative and not curative. With current knowledge, we are usually unable to cure obesity; that is, most treatments for obesity, when terminated, do not produce a permanent remission. A simple analogy is appendectomy, where the patient is cured by surgical removal of the diseased appendix. Comparable results with treatment of overweight patients are rare. One example would be effective treatment for Cushing's syndrome, where the primary initial symptom is obesity. For most cases of obesity, however, we are seeking palliation and alleviation of symptoms associated with the condition, not a cure.

Recidivism, or regaining lost weight, is a third reality of treatment for obesity. Of those patients who lose weight on any treatment program, a significant percentage will fail to maintain this weight loss. Identification of those individuals who will be successful in losing weight is at best an inexact procedure. Some suggested techniques for identifying those who are likely to succeed include the initial 1-week weight loss, frequency and regularity of attendance at a weight-loss program, and the belief that persons can control their own weight. However, additional insight is needed before we will be able to identify successful individuals at the beginning of treatment.

The fourth reality of treatment for obesity is its cost. Each year, more than $30 billion is spent on efforts to control weight gain or induce weight loss. More than 50% of the expenditure is for diet foods ($20 billion), with the remainder distributed into several other categories. In the

Table 3. Realities of obesity

Obesity is a chronic disease whose prevalence is increasing

It has many causes, but cure is rare

Increasing weight produces increasing health risk

Visceral upper-body fat carries more risk than lower-body fat

Obesity is a stigmatized condition

Drug treatment struggles under the negative amphetamine halo

Treatments work as long as they are continued

Recidivism is common because drug and other treatments do not work when discontinued

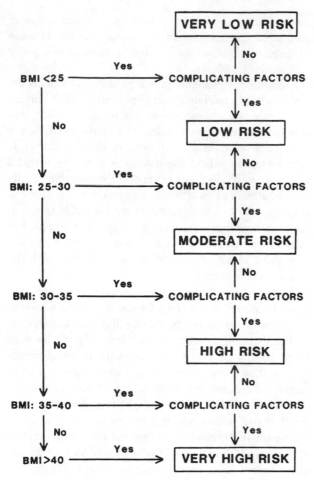

Figure 13. Risk classification algorithm. The patient is first placed into a category based on BMI. The presence or absence of complicating factors determines the degree of health risk. Complicating factors include elevated abdominal-gluteal ratio (male, 0.95; female, 0.85), diabetes mellitus, hypertension, hyperlipidemia, male sex, and age <40. (Copyright 1987, George A. Bray. Used with permission.)

following discussion we will try to evaluate the cost and effectiveness of various methods of weight control.

Evaluation of risk associated with obesity. Because all treatments entail some risk, the first essential in deciding whether treatment is appropriate for obesity and what that treatment should be is the assessment of the risk associated with adiposity. Two independent variables can be used to assess this risk. The first is the risk associated with the degree of deviation in body weight from normal. Underweight individuals have increased risk for respiratory disease, tuberculosis, digestive disease, and some cancers (see Figure 9). Overweight individuals, on the other hand, are more prone to cardiovascular disease, gallbladder disease, high blood pressure, and diabetes. Body weights associated with a BMI of 20–25 kg/m² have no increased risk from body weight. When BMI is <20 kg/m² or >25 kg/m², risk increases in a curvilinear fashion. Individuals with a BMI of 25–30 kg/m² have

low risk, those with a BMI between 30 and 35 kg/m² have moderate risk, those with a BMI between 35 and 40 kg/m² have high risk, and those with a BMI >40 kg/m² have very high risk from their degree of excess weight.

The distribution of body fat is also a useful guide to risks. The larger the abdominal circumference, the greater the risk. The algorithm in Figure 13 provides a means of including both total body fat, as estimated from the BMI, and the distribution of body fat in making decisions about relative risk from adiposity.[82] At any given level of BMI, the risk to health is increased with abdominal fat. Other factors included in Figure 13 that increase risk from overweight are the presence of medical problems such as diabetes mellitus, hypertension, or hyperlipidemia; age <40 years with increasing weight; and male sex.

A risk-benefit assessment of treatment. Treatments for obesity can be grouped by their relative risk (Figure 14). They can be further divided by whether they influence nutrient intake or energy loss. In a quantitative sense, treatments that reduce energy intake have a greater potential for sudden weight loss than those that increase energy expenditure. Because all of our nutrient energy comes from food, we can reduce energy intake to zero (starvation). Energy expenditure, on the other hand, has a minimum level associated with the energy required to maintain body temperature and to repair tissues and maintain function of the heart and other organs. Thus, simply staying in bed and engaging in no physical activity reduces energy expenditure to ≈0.8 kcal/min (1150 kcal/d) for a normal-weight adult. High levels of physical activity can increase this by two- to fourfold over 24 hours. Thus, for initial weight loss, decreasing food intake is the most effective action, whereas increasing energy expenditure through physical activity appears to

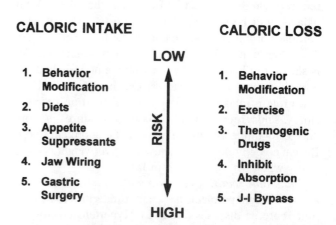

Figure 14. Treatments for obesity in relation to risk. On the left are treatments that affect energy intake and on the right are treatments that increase energy expenditure or loss. They are ranked in estimated overall order for risk, with lowest risk at the top and highest risk at the bottom. J-I, jejunoileal.

have a particular attractiveness in efforts at long-term maintenance of a lower body weight.

Acknowledgment

Supported in part by grants DK 32089 and 31988 from the National Institutes of Health.

References

1. Blackburn GL, Kanders BS, eds (1994) Obesity. Pathophysiology, psychology and treatment. Chapman and Hall, New York

2. Bouchard C, ed (1993) The genetics of obesity. CRC Press, Boca Raton, FL

3. Bray GA (1989) Overweight and fat distribution—Basic consideration and clinical approaches. Dis Mon 7:451–537

4. Perri MG, Nezu AM, Viegener BJ (1992) Improving long-term management of obesity. Theory, research, and clinical guidelines. John Wiley & Sons, New York

5. Stunkard AJ, Wadden TA, eds (1992) Obesity. Theory and therapy, 2nd ed. Raven Press, New York

6. Bray GA (1976) The obese patient: major problems in internal medicine, 9th ed. WB Saunders, Philadelphia

7. Keys A, Fidanza F, Karvonen MJ, Kimuro N, Taylor HL (1972) Indices of relative weight and obesity. J Chronic Dis 25:329–343

8. National Research Council. Committee on Diet and Health (1989) Calories: total macronutrient intake, energy expenditure, and net energy stores. In Diet and health; implications for reducing chronic disease risk. National Academy Press, Washington, DC, pp 139–158

9. Pouliot MC, Despres JP, Lemieux S, et al (1994) Waist circumference and abdominal sagittal diameter: best simple anthropometric indexes of abdominal visceral adipose tissue accumulation and related cardiovascular risk in men and women. Am J Cardiol 73:460–468

10. Wang ZM, Pierson RN, Heymsfield SB (1992) The 5-level model—a new approach to organizing body-composition research. Am J Clin Nutr 56:19–28

11. Lukaski HC (1987) Methods for the assessment of human body composition: traditional and new. Am J Clin Nutr 46:537–556

12. Segal KR, Van Loan M, Fitzgerald PI, Hodgdon JA, Van Itallie TB (1988) Lean body mass estimation by bioelectrical impedance analysis: a four-site cross-validation study. Am J Clin Nutr 47:7–14

13. Sjostrom L, Kvist H, Cederblad A, Tyler V (1986) Determination of total adipose tissue and body fat in women by computed tomography, 40 K and tritium. Am J Physiol 250:E736–E745

14. Kuczmarski RJ, Fanelli MT, Koch GG (1987) Ultrasonic assessment of body composition in obese adults: overcoming the limitations of the skinfold caliper. Am J Clin Nutr 45:717–724

15. Cohn SH, Vartsky D, Yasumura S, et al (1980) Compartmental body composition based on total-body nitrogen, potassium, and calcium. Am J Physiol 239:E524–E530

16. Kuczmarski RJ, Flegal KM, Campbell SM, Johnson CL (1994) Increasing prevalence of overweight among US adults: The National Health and Nutrition Examination Surveys, 1960 to 1991. JAMA 272:205–211

17. Ballor DL, Keesey RE (1991) A meta-analysis of the factors affecting exercise-induced changes in body-mass, fat mass and fat-free mass in males and females. Int J Obes 15:717–726

18. Pavlou KN, Steffee WP, Lerman RH, Burrows BA (1985) Effects of dieting and exercise on lean body mass, oxygen uptake and strength. Med Sci Sports Exerc 17:466–471

19. Lichtman SW, Pisarska K, Berman ER, et al (1992) Discrepancy between self-reported and actual caloric intake and exercise in obese subjects. N Engl J Med 327:1893–1898

20. Welle S, Forbes GB, Statt M, Barnard RR, Amatruda JM (1992) Energy expenditure under free-living conditions in normal-weight and overweight women. Am J Clin Nutr 55:14–21

21. Stunkard AJ, Kaplan D (1977) Eating in public places: a review of reports of the direct observation of eating behavior. Int J Obes 1:89–101

22. Kromhout D (1983) Changes in energy and macronutrients in 871 middle-aged men during 10 years of follow-up (the Zutphen Study). Am J Clin Nutr 37:287–294

23. Ravussin E, Swinburn BA (1992) Pathophysiology of obesity. Lancet 340:404–408

24. Owen OE, Kavle E, Owen RS, et al (1986) A reappraisal of caloric requirements of healthy women. Am J Clin Nutr 44:1–19

25. Owen OE, Holup JL, D'Alessio DA, et al (1987) A reappraisal of the caloric requirements of men. Am J Clin Nutr 46:875–885

26. Jequier E, Schutz Y (1983) Long-term measurements of energy expenditure in humans using a respiration chamber. Am J Clin Nutr 38:989–998

27. de Boer JO, van Es AJ, van Raaij JM, Hautvast JG (1987) Energy requirements and energy expenditure of lean and overweight women, measured by indirect calorimetry. Am J Clin Nutr 46:13–21

28. Bogardus C, Lillioja S, Ravussin E, et al (1986) Familial dependence of the resting metabolic rate. N Engl J Med 315:96–100

29. Ravussin E, Lillioja S, Knowler WC, et al (1988) Reduced rate of energy expenditure as a risk factor for body-weight gain. N Engl J Med 318:467–472

30. Bray GA (1983) The energetics of obesity. Med Sci Sports Exerc 15:32–40

31. Woo R, Garrow JS, Pi-Sunyer FX (1985) Effect on exercise on spontaneous calorie intake in obesity. Am J Clin Nutr 36:470–477

32. Woo R, Daniels-Kush R, Horton ES (1985) Regulation of energy balance. Annu Rev Nutr 5:411–433

33. Glick Z, Teague RJ, Bray GA (1981) Brown adipose tissue: thermic response increased by a single low protein meal. Science 213:1125–1127

34. Bray GA (1991) Obesity, a disorder of nutrient partitioning: The MONA LISA hypothesis. J Nutr 121:1146–1162

35. Segal KR, Albu J, Chun A, et al (1992) Independent effects of obesity and insulin resistance on postprandial thermogenesis in men. J Clin Invest 89:824–833

36. LeBlanc J, Brondel L (1985) Role of palatability on meal induced thermogenesis in human subjects. Am J Physiol 248:E333–E336

37. Golay A, Jallut D, Schutz Y, Felber JP, Jequier E (1991) Evolution of glucose induced thermogenesis in obese subjects with and without diabetes: a six-year follow-up study. Int J Obes 15:601–607

38. Ailhaud G, Grimaldi P, Negrel R (1992) A molecular view of adipose tissue. [review]. Int J Obes 16 (suppl 2):S17–S21

39. Knittle JL, Timmers K, Ginsberg-Fellner F, Brown RE, Katz DP (1979) The growth of adipose tissue in children and adolescents: cross-sectional and longitudinal studies of adipose cell number and size. J Clin Invest 63:239–246

40. Sjostrom L, William-Olsson T (1981) Prospective studies on adipose tissue development in man. Int J Obes 5:597–604

41. Flier JS (1995) The adipocyte: storage depot or node on the energy information superhighway. Cell 80:15–18

42. Hotamisligil GS, Shargill NS, Spiegelman BM (1993) Adipose expression of tumor necrosis factor-α: direct role of obesity-linked insulin resistance. Science 259:87–91

43. Society of Actuaries. Build Study of 1979 (1980): Society of Actuaries/Association of Life Insurance Medical Directors of America, Chicago

44. Lew EA, Garfinkel L (1979) Variations in mortality by weight among 750,000 men and women. J Chronic Dis 32:563–576

45. Waaler HT (1984) Height, weight and mortality: the Norwegian experience. Acta Med Scand 679:1–56

46. Sjostrom LV (1992) Morbidity of severely obese subjects. Am J Clin Nutr 55(suppl 2):508S–515S

47. Sjostrom LV (1992) Mortality of severely obese subjects. Am J Clin Nutr 55(suppl 2):516S–523S

48. Vague J (1956) Degree of masculine differentiation of obesities: factor determining predisposition to diabetes, atherosclerosis, gout, and uric calculous disease. Am J Clin Nutr 4:20–34

49. Lapidus L, Bengtsson C, Larsson B, et al (1984) Distribution of adipose tissue and risk of cardiovascular disease and death: a 12 year follow-up of participants in the population study of women in Gothenburg, Sweden. BMJ 289:1257–1261

50. Larsson B, Svardsudd K, Welin L, et al (1984) Abdominal adipose tissue distribution, obesity, and risk of cardiovascular disease and death: 13 year follow-up of participants in the study of men born in 1913. BMJ 288:1401–1404

51. Stokes J III, Garrison RJ, Kannel WB (1985) The independent contributions of various indices of obesity to the 22-year incidence of coronary heart disease: the Framingham Heart Study. In Vague J, Bjorntorp P, Guy-Grand B, Rebuffe-Scrive M, Vague P (eds), Metabolic complications of human obesities. Excerpta Medica, Amsterdam, pp 49–57

52. Ducimetiere P, Richard J, Cambien F (1986) The pattern of subcutaneous fat distribution in middle-aged men and the risk of coronary heart disease: the Paris Prospective Study. Int J Obes 10:229–240

53. Donahue RP, Abbott RD, Bloom E, Reed DM, Yano K (1987) Central obesity and coronary heart disease in men. Lancet 1:821–824

54. Folsom AR, Kaye SA, Sellers TA, et al (1993) Body fat distribution and 5-year risk of death in older women. JAMA 269:483–487

55. Schapira DV, Clark RA, Wolff P, et al (1994) Visceral obesity and breast cancer risk. Cancer 74:632–639

56. Tokunaga K, Matsuzaw Y, Kotani K, et al (1991) Ideal body weight estimated from the body mass index with the lowest morbidity. Int J Obes 15:1–5

57. Garrison RJ, Kannel WB (1993) A new approach to estimating healthy body weights. Int J Obes 17:417–423

58. Blair D, Habicht JP, Sims EA, Sylvester D, Abraham S (1984) Evidence for an increased risk for hypertension with centrally located body fat and the effect of race and sex on this risk. Am J Epidemiol 119:526–540

59. Hartz AJ, Rupley CC, Rimm AA (1984) The association of girth measurements with disease in 32,856 women. Am J Epidemiol 119:71–80

60. Drenick EJ, Fisler JS (1992) Myocardial mass in morbidly obese patients and changes with weight reduction. Obes Surg 2:19–27

61. Chan JM, Rimm EB, Colditz GA, Stampfer MJ, Willett WC (1994) Obesity, fat distribution, and weight gain as risk factors for clinical diabetes in men. Diabetes Care 17:961–969

62. Long SD, O'Brien K, MacDonald KG, et al (1994) Weight loss in severely obese subjects prevents the progression of impaired glucose tolerance to Type II diabetes. Diabetes Care 17:372–375

63. Maclure KM, Hayes KC, Coldiz GA, et al (1989) Weight diet, and the risk of symptomatic gallstones in middle-aged women. N Engl J Med 321:563–569

64. Jenkins SC, Moxham J (1991) The effects of mild obesity on lung function. Respir Med 85:309–311

65. Ray CS, Sue DY, Bray GA, Hansen JE, Wasserman K (1983) Effects of obesity on respiratory function. Am Rev Respir Dis 128:501–506

66. Chalew S, Nagel H, Shore S (1995) The hypothalamic pituitary adrenal axis in obesity. A review. Obes Res 3:371–382

67. Zelissen PMJ, Koppeschaar HPF, Thijssen JH, Erkelens DW (1992) Growth hormone secretion in obese patients with non-insulin dependent diabetes mellitus: effect of weight reduction and of fluoxetine treatment. Diabetes Nutr Metab 5:131–135

68. Danforth E Jr, Horton ES, O'Connell M (1969) Dietary-induced alterations in thyroid hormone metabolism during overnutrition. J Clin Invest 64:1336–1347

69. Zumoff B, Strain GW, Miller LK, et al (1990) Plasma free and non-sex-hormone-binding-globulin-bound testosterone are decreased in obese men in proportion to their degree of obesity. J Clin Endocrinol Metab 71:929–931

70. Frisch RE (1991) Body weight, body fat, and ovulation. Trends Endocrinol Metab 2:191–197

71. Ashley FW, Kannel WB (1974) Relation of weight change to changes in atherogenic traits: the Framingham Study. J Chronic Dis 27:103–114

72. Lu D, Willard D, Patel IR, et al (1994) Agouti protein is an antagonist of the melanocyte-stimulating-hormone receptor. Nature 371:799–802

73. Zhang YY, Proenca R, Maffei M, et al (1994) Positional cloning of the mouse obese gene and its human homolog. Nature 372:425–432

74. Bray GA (1992) Obesity. In King RA, Rotter JI, Motulsky AG (eds), The Genetic Basis of Common Diseases. Oxford University Press, New York, pp 507–528

75. Nicholls RD, Glenn CC, Jong MTC, et al (1995) Molecular pathogenesis of Prader-Willi syndrome. In Bray GA, Ryan DH (eds), Molecular and Genetic Aspects of Obesity: Volume V of the Pennington Nutrition Series. Louisiana State University Press, Baton Rouge

76. Stunkard AJ, Thorkild IA, Sorensen TIA, et al (1986) An adoption study of human obesity. N Engl J Med 314:193–198

77. Stunkard AJ, Foch TT, Hrubec Z (1986) A twin study of human obesity. JAMA 256:51–54

78. Bouchard Cm Oerysse L, Leblanc C, et al (1988) Inheritance of the amount and distribution of human body fat. Int J Obes 12:205–215

79. Bouchard C, Despres J, Mauriege P (1993) Genetic and nongenetic determinants of regional fat distribution [review]. Endocr Rev 14:72–93

80. Bray GA (1984) Syndromes of hypothalamic obesity in man. Pediatr Ann 13:525–536

81. Flatt JP (1987) Dietary fat, carbohydrate balance, and weight maintenance: effects of exercise. Am J Clin Nutr 45:296–306

82. Bray GA (1988) Obesity. Part II - Treatment. West J Med 149:555–571

5

Carbohydrates

Béla Szepesi

Our basic knowledge of carbohydrate nutrition has changed somewhat since publication of the sixth edition of *Present Knowledge in Nutrition.*[1] The controversies concerning the alleged health effects of sucrose and fructose have ended and the issues have been resolved. The interaction of dietary fructose with copper nutrition and its effect on heart function was shown not to apply to human beings. And finally, the emergence of ketohexoses (D-sorbose, D-tagatose) as strong antidiabetic agents, and the fact that D-tagatose contributes no useful energy while metabolized, opens a new chapter in carbohydrate nutrition.

Carbohydrate Intake and Disposition

Type and amount. Carbohydrates constitute the majority of living matter on our planet, so it is not surprising that carbohydrates constitute the majority of our diet: 50–70% of the total calories ingested. Depending upon cultural and dietary choices, the composition of indigenous dietary carbohydrate can vary, but generally includes starch, simple sugars, complex polymers known as "dietary fibers," and minor components. A number of other carbohydrates are added in quantity: hydrolyzed cornstarch, fructose syrups made from corn starch, modified starches, gums, mucilages, sugar alcohols, and other industrial products. These are added to change texture, mouth feel, shelf life, color, viscosity, and taste. Since carbohydrate is the most abundant food energy source for human beings, the food industry has begun to look in earnest at carbohydrates as a means of reducing the energy content of food. Reduced caloric starches, sugar alcohols, and a ketohexose (D-tagatose, which has very interesting properties) are under active consideration by the food industry.[2] Research is also underway to increase the amylose:amylopectin ratio of food starches. Amylose (the straight-chain starch) causes a smaller rise in blood glucose than amylopectin (the branched starch).[3] Complex carbohydrates in cruciferous vegetables and modified pectin are believed to reduce cancer risk and may be added to food in the future. Carbohydrate nutrition is once again becoming an area of intense scientific interest.

Requirement. It is generally believed that human beings have no short-term requirement for carbohydrate in food. That is to say, one cannot demonstrate deficiency symptoms by feeding a carbohydrate-free diet. However, disturbances in metabolism and intestinal function can appear. And in the long term, the lack of dietary fiber and its beneficial effects can lead to serious health risks such as diverticulitis in the aged and increased possibility of cancer. The scope of this chapter does not include the voluminous and well-documented area of research on dietary fiber.

Digestion, absorption, transport, and regulation. The most impressive property of living things is their ability to adapt to differing external or internal conditions. Human beings can survive on diets with different levels and types of fats, carbohydrates, and total energy content and can gain or lose weight and even survive periods of total starvation. All this is possible because of built-in regulation. Regulation is built into the organism at all levels and involves diverse but interacting functions.

Keeping blood glucose constant and increasing glucose production at times of increased need are the most important biological imperatives of carbohydrate disposition in humans. Part of the task of keeping blood glucose constant is accomplished by regulating the intake of carbohydrate and the rate at which it is absorbed into the blood stream. In the average person appetite is regulated so that the normal adult remains in energy balance while energy intake and energy expenditure fluctuate from hour to hour and day to day. The average human is designed to sustain heavy physical labor and comes equipped with a sensory apparatus to prefer an appropriate energy-dense diet. Given this sensory predilection for high-energy diets, it is nothing short of remarkable that most people remain lean. We have heard people who are lean saying, "I can eat anything I want and still stay thin." It turns out that such people regulate their energy intake unconsciously but with remarkable effectiveness. Those who do not have such an acute energy-sensing control mechanism to regulate appetite become fat to various degrees.

The ingestion, digestion, absorption, and transport of carbohydrates are highly regulated and interactive processes. Visual and olfactory cues of impending food ingestion stimulate the release of saliva (and salivary amylase) and also insulin. Insulin prepares the intestine for increased nutrient transport, and recruits inactive glucose transporters (those that are insulin sensitive) and brings them to the cell surface where they are active. The presence of food in the stomach releases hormones that decrease (or suppress) feeding and activate intestinal processes that speed absorption. As food reaches the intestine, it activates receptors, which in turn release hormones from the intestine. These hormones cause a further release of insulin. The presence of carbohydrates in the intestine exaggerates the insulinogenic response.

The effect of interactive controls is a "rolling" activation of tissues and processes ensuring that the process of breaking down food is spaced out, rather than dumped all at once into the intestine; the absorption of the end products of digestion is spaced out; and the internal organs are prepared to receive the nutrient inflow and are primed to alter metabolism to maintain a constant internal environment (homeostasis).

In terms of carbohydrates, the digestive and transport systems need to minimize the fluctuation of glucose inflow while the individual takes in food in meals which may be rather short and far apart. The biological imperative of maintaining a steady inflow of nutrients, which requires a slow and even emptying of the stomach and the intestine, is weighed against the biological cost of carrying the weight of the stomach and intestines. Thus, birds that fly must have very fast intestinal emptying, must eat small, frequent meals, and cannot have multiple (heavy) stomachs. All these mechanisms allow adaptation, both acute and long term, to dietary changes that can be severe at times. Thus, a human is able to consume, digest, and absorb carbohydrate from small, short meals, from a few large (even gargantuan) meals, and from liquids.

Finally, the human organism must also metabolize not only glucose (the end product of starch digestion), but fructose, galactose, and some mannose, all of which occur naturally in food.

The special role of the large intestine. We now know that the majority of complex carbohydrates, other than starch, are digested to a variable extent in the large intestine. Even some of the ingested starch, referred to as limit dextrins, can escape digestion in the small intestine and end up (along with unabsorbed sugar alcohols) in the large intestine.[2] The bacterial flora of the large intestine then metabolizes these compounds and produces short-chain fatty acids: butyric, isobutyric, propionic, and acetic acids. Cellulose is largely undigested. Butyric and isobutyric acids are believed to be important nutrient sources for the gut cells and to reduce the risk of carcinogenic changes to these cells. It is believed that part of the anticancer properties of dietary fibers is due to events subsequent to their digestion in the large intestine. Another possible result of the functioning of the large intestinal microflora is the production of a large bacterial mass, the retention of moisture, and the production of soft stools. This helps to prevent diverticulitis, the entrapment of pieces of hard fecal matter in intestinal folds. Bacterial metabolism reduces the energy available (an energy cost) from carbohydrate fermented in the large intestine.[2] As our population becomes nutritionally more sophisticated, a warning should be issued about self-medication with dietary fiber. If too much fiber, or the wrong type, is ingested excessive loss of minerals and diarrhea may ensue. Nutritionists need to transfer the results of their research into practical recommendations that can be easily understood and followed by the average person.

Digestive enzymes and carbohydrate transporters. Carbohydrate is ingested in three basic forms: 1) raw or processed vegetables, fruits, or grains (cooked, boiled, ground etc.), 2) purified carbohydrates added to foods, and 3) carbohydrates dissolved in various drinks. The first step in digestion of carbohydrates is mastication of food by the teeth. During mastication, starch granules are exposed or broken open, and surface area is increased by reducing particle size. Food in the mouth is mixed with salivary α-amylase that begins to break down starch immediately. Hydrolysis of starch slows or stops in the stomach (because of the change in pH) and resumes again in the duodenum, where pancreatic α-amylase is secreted. The cumulative action of the two amylases is to produce maltose and maltotriose from amylose; and maltotriose, maltose, some glucose plus limit dextrin (three to five glucose units [1,4-α] and one glucose unit [1,6-α] from amylopectin).[4] Digestion of starch remnants is then completed by the intestinal brush-border enzymes. Polysaccharides that are not digested in the small intestine may undergo at least partial digestion by bacteria in the large intestine.

Progress in our knowledge of the enzymes of the small intestine has been rapid and has completely altered our conception of how these enzymes work. Maltotriose, maltose, limit dextrins (molecules left after amylopectin is acted on by α-amylase), and the major disaccharides (sucrose, lactose) are split to monosaccharide constituents in the small intestine. The small intestine is covered with microvilli that give a total absorptive surface many times the area of the planar intestinal surface. The extended intestinal surface may be as large as 200 m[2] in the average man.[4] The microvilli extend into the so-called unstirred water layer (UWL) phase of the intestinal lumen. The enzymes that complete the hydrolysis of starch are anchored to the brush-border membrane. If a limit dextrin, trisaccharide, or disaccharide enters the UWL, it is rapidly hydrolyzed by these enzymes. With the exception of trehalase, a minor component (MW 75,000), the other saccharidases of the small intestine share a number of common characteristics: MW of 200,000–300,000, a membrane-spanning hydrophobic portion that acts as an anchor in the brush border, two separate catalytic sites each on a separate domain, and heavy glycosylation. They also undergo extensive posttranslational processing by intracellular and extracellular (pancreatic) hydrolases.[4]

The sucrase-isomaltase complex is anchored to the brush border at its N terminal, and it is split into two peptides by pancreatic hydrolases.[5-7] The anchor peptide complex (isomaltase [maltase]) is held together with the terminal peptide complex (sucrase [maltase]) by noncovalent forces.[4-7] The maltase of this complex also is known as the heat-labile maltase. Isomaltase is the enzyme that splits the 1,6-α glycosidic linkage.[4] The glucoamylase complex contains the heat-stable maltase and glucoamylase (both 1 and 2), which has two active sites. The two domains are held together covalently, and the glucoamylase is anchored to the brush border by its N-terminal.[4,8] The β-glucosidase complex contains lactase and another peptide domain that is referred to as either glycosylceramidase or phlorizin hydrolase. This enzyme complex contains one peptide and is anchored in the brush border at its C terminal.[4] In the brush border of healthy rats and humans, enzyme activity is believed to be more than adequate to take care of all substrate that gets into the UWL.[4]

Regulation of digestion. Digestion is regulated in part by the emptying of stomach and the motility of intestine. The combined result of this regulation is to reduce fluctuations in nutrient inflow and to minimize osmotic shock.[9] Because the half-lives of intestinal brush-border enzymes are shorter than the life span of the intestinal cells, the activities of these enzymes can be regulated, and they are known to be adaptive.[4] In the rat, sucrase and lactase concentrations may be increased by feeding either sucrose or lactose.[10,11] Sucrase activity is decreased by both starvation and starch intake.[12,13] Earlier studies indicated that changes in rates of synthesis were responsible for changes in sucrase activity.[14] However, another report indicates that at least in short-term experiments, sucrose and fructose depress the expression of the sucrase-isomaltase complex by a leupeptin-sensitive degradation process possibly through alteration in glycosylation.[15]

Diabetes produces very large changes in intestinal function.[4] Concentrations of intestinal enzymes and intestinal transport are increased.[16-20] The UWL becomes less a barrier to absorption, and the sodium gradient between intestinal lumen and intestinal cells increases.[21,22] The adaptation of intestinal function to diabetes speeds up digestion and increases the rate of transport of carbohydrate into the blood stream.

Absorption and transport of carbohydrates. Carbohydrates, which are polyols and polar, cannot pass through nonpolar membranes without some type of transport system. There are four known types of carbohydrate transport: bacterial permease mediated, the dolichol system, Na[+]-dependent active transport, and the facilitated carrier.[23]

Dolichol is used to transport oligosaccharides and monosaccharides into the endoplasmic reticulum and the Golgi membrane system for use in glycosylation. Dolichol has a long nonpolar portion that easily inserts into the membrane.

Even before the carbohydrate-transporting proteins were isolated, their existence and a number of their properties were deduced and described by Crane.[24-26] Intestinal glucose transport was shown to be active (requiring energy), to be Na[+]-dependent, and to have stereospecificity for glucose and galactose.[25,26] It was deduced that the brush-border enzymes not only provide transportable monosaccharides but somehow enhance their transport as well.[27] It is believed that this enhancing effect on transport is due to adjacent location and is particularly effective for disaccharides.[26,27]

Animal cells have two basic types of glucose carriers: one that is Na[+] dependent and one that is not.[4,23] The Na[+]-dependent carriers are found in intestinal wall and in kidney.[23] The intestinal cell wall carrier and one of the kidney carriers have stoichiometry of one Na[+] ion per carrier, whereas the second kidney transporter works with two Na[+] ions per carrier.[23] The rest of the glucose carriers also can be divided into two groups: muscle and adipose tissue carriers are insulin-dependent, and the others are not.[4,23]

The essential features of the Na[+]-dependent glucose carrier have been described.[19,28] Sodium is pumped from the cell to create a sodium gradient between the intestinal lumen and the interior of the cell. The sodium pump requires ATP hydrolysis, and the resultant sodium gradient drives the cotransporter so that one molecule of sodium and one molecule of glucose are cotransported by a "gated-pore" mechanism.[23,27] The carriers that do not require sodium are thought to work like an enzyme except that no bonds are broken or formed. The driving force for this carrier is the glucose gradient and the entropy change that occurs when highly organized water is replaced on the carrier by glucose. The resultant change in electric fields (set up by the movement of electrons) then alters the local magnetic fields, which in turn move the part of the carrier that has glucose bound to it. Thus, glucose is moved across the membrane where it leaves the carrier. Much of this explanation is conjecture, but the kinetics of carrier action resemble enzyme kinetics.[29] The fructose carrier is also driven by a concentration gradient, and like the Na[+]-independent glucose carrier, requires no ATP. This type of transport is referred to as facilitated transport.[28-29]

Glucose transporters from many tissues have been isolated. The best known is the erythrocyte carrier that has 12 hydrophobic helical loops spanning the membrane and one external and one internal loop.[30] A number of other transporters have been cloned.[31-34]

Malabsorption and intolerance. Carbohydrate malabsorption is failure to absorb a carbohydrate in the appropriate manner at the appropriate site. This can occur because of enzyme or carrier (transporter) deficiency (primary deficiency), or a deficiency induced by a disease (secondary deficiency).[1] In some cases malabsorption is due to exceeding the absorptive capacity, e.g., a very high fructose diet in man. An increase in breath hydrogen is an indication of malabsorption and can be detected by feeding a large dose of test carbohydrate.[1,2] The hydrogen is a by-product of large intestinal metabolism.

Disaccharidase deficiency is a congenital deficiency of intestinal sucrase and/or isomaltase. Adult onset hypolactasia is probably the most commonly occurring form of disaccharidase deficiency and is most common among populations of non-European origin.[10] In such people lactase declines after weaning, so that while children can consume milk, consumption of milk or even some partially fermented milk products by adults causes abdominal distress. In the United States, the food industry has solved the problem by marketing lactase-treated milk.

Effects of molecular size. Glucose administered intravenously elicits a smaller insulin response than glucose taken by mouth because peptides released by the intestine potentiate insulin release.[35] Indications that there might be some special phenomena associated with the ingestion of disaccharides were found during the first decade of this century.[36] Consumption of sucrose or maltose was found to result in a faster rise in blood glucose, expired CO_2, and heat production than can be seen after the ingestion of monosaccharide equivalents. These effects were observed 30–60 minutes after the ingestion of a disaccharide. The work of Crane[24–26] showed that the transport of disaccharides across the gut is somehow faster than the transport of monosaccharides, implying that the monosaccharides produced by the disaccharidases were somehow more accessible for transport. Such would occur if the disaccharidases transferred the carbohydrate from the stirred to the unstirred region of the villi and thus speeded absorption. However, in a starvation-refeeding experiment (2 days starved, 2 days refed) the level of some liver enzymes "overshot" normal levels during the second day of refeeding.[37] This response was larger with sucrose and maltose and cannot be attributed to a differential rate of absorption of monosaccharides.[38] That is, the earlier observed effects on CO_2 and heat production could have been explained by faster initial rates of monosaccharide absorption from the gut, since these effects were observed shortly after a meal.[36] But the starve-refeed response required 2 days, over which time the original kinetic advantage at refeeding disaccharide is expected to be lost. Szepesi and Michaelis[36] advanced the hypothesis that the "disaccharide effect" observed in the starved-refed response was generated by the presence of the disaccharide in the gut.

An effect of molecule size was also demonstrated on the rate of gluconeogenesis in liver cells from animals adapted to a diet containing maltose, glucose, or starch as the sole carbohydrate.[39] A number of other studies indicate that the molecular size of ingested carbohydrate has a metabolic effect that may be tied to carbohydrates binding to receptors.[38] For example, there are different taste receptors for glucose, maltose, and the octaglucose oligosaccharide.[40] The oligosaccharides in human milk protect infants from some intestinal and urinary infections by acting as "soluble receptors."[41] When these oligosaccharides bind bacteria, the pathogens cannot adhere to intestinal or urinary tract wall, the first step in infection, and infection is prevented.

The concept of glycemic index. Glycemic index is the relative ability of a carbohydrate to raise the level of blood glucose.[42] A carbohydrate with a high glycemic index elevates blood glucose faster and to a higher level than a carbohydrate with a low glycemic index. This appeared to be a straightforward concept at first. However, it was later emphasized that uncontrolled variables in the complex control of blood glucose render the determination of the glycemic index difficult.[43] Nonetheless, it is true that carbohydrates fall into more than two categories with respect to their ability to raise blood glucose. That the rise in blood glucose is influenced by meal size, amount of dietary fat, and health does not invalidate the concept of a glycemic index, but it is not as simple and precise as originally believed.

Trying to use the glycemic index to explain the responses to amylose versus amylopectin in human beings shows that many gaps remain in our understanding of metabolism.[3] Amylose starch elicits a relatively slow and comparatively small response in blood glucose and insulin, while amylopectin elicits a large increase in blood glucose, insulin, and glucagon.[3] While the branched structure of amylopectin allows more attack sites for amylase and, consequently, a faster production of glucose, a larger than expected response of glucagon to amylopectin remains unexplained. Some scientists are hoping to produce varieties of corn and other grains with higher percentages of amylose than is now available. Presumably this would produce a healthier diet by moderating glucose inflow and reducing blood glucose.

Intracellular Carbohydrate Utilization

Disposition of glucose. In monogastric mammals, glucose is the primary fuel used by most of the cells. Some intestinal cells use short-chain fatty acids and in some species sperm cells use fructose but these are the exceptions. The regulation of blood glucose is important because extreme conditions (hyper- and hypoglycemia) are a problem for the organism. Since the principal fuel for the central nervous system is glucose, hypoglycemia can be incapacitating. Hyperglycemia can produce another set of problems associated with diabetes.

In the muscle glucose can be metabolized anaerobically (glycolysis) to pyruvate. Depending on muscle activity and how much O_2 is available, the muscle can metabolize pyruvate to CO_2 or send it into the blood stream to liver. The NADH produced in muscle glycolysis must be reoxidized and this is done by converting pyruvate (the end product of glycolysis) to lactate. During heavy muscle contraction, there is not enough oxygen to burn all the pyruvate to CO_2, so the excess reducing power produced in glycolysis is sent into the blood stream as lactate. This is known as the oxygen debt and is responsible for muscle pain in running. Ultimately, liver converts most of the pyruvate to glucose. The flux of blood from muscle (glucose to pyruvate) to liver (pyruvate to glucose) to blood is known as the Cori cycle. Liver functions as the key organ in maintaining normal blood glucose levels by coordinating glycolysis, gluconeogenesis, and lipogenesis. For a detailed description of how these processes are regulated, see relevant chapters in Voet and Voet.[44]

In liver, glycolysis and gluconeogenesis (synthesis of glucose) take place in the same compartment (cytosol), except the conversion of pyruvate to oxaloacetate, which takes place in the mitochondrion.[44] Glycolysis and gluconeogenesis use the same enzymes except at three regulated sites: hexokinase (glucokinase)/glucose-6-phosphatase; phosphofructokinase (PFK1)/fructose-1,6-bisphosphatase; pyruvate kinase/pyruvate carboxylase + phosphoenol carboxykinase. Control of the pathways resides in controlling the regulatory enzymes. Under glycolytic conditions, hexokinase, phosphofructokinase, and pyruvate kinase are turned on and the opposing enzymes are turned off. During gluconeogenic conditions the opposite is true. The existence of two enzymes that catalyze the opposite reaction in the same compartment (such as hexokinase and glucose-6-phosphatase) has two important consequences: it results in a net hydrolysis of ATP and release of energy (futile cycle) as a source of body heat, and it allows a change in the glycolytic flux by a factor of 90.[44] That is, if the regulatory enzymes were segregated by function into separate compartments, the glycolysis rate could be increased by a factor of 10 by allosteric activators. But, because the two sets of enzymes are in the same compartment, the glycolytic rate can be increased 90-fold by activating the glycolytic enzymes and inhibiting the gluconeogenic enzymes. Such changes are accomplished by local controls (allosteric effectors) and external controls (insulin, glucagon, epinephrine). These controls allow muscle to greatly vary its workload, while the same controls allow liver to rapidly dispose of or make glucose.

Thus, during the absorption of a large, carbohydrate-laden meal, liver glycolysis is activated and gluconeogenesis is inhibited, while during fasting, gluconeogenesis is activated and glycolysis is suppressed. It is easy to see how these controls would result in maintaining normal levels of blood glucose. In diabetes and obesity, these controls break down and both pathways are turned on. The result is some degree of hyperglycemia, depending on the ability of the tissues to respond to insulin. In obesity and diabetes (type II), the response to insulin is reduced, so it takes greater amounts of insulin to maintain normal levels of blood glucose. When the pancreas becomes exhausted after years of overstimulation, diabetic conditions can ensue.

The functioning of glycolysis, the TCA cycle, electron transport, and oxidative phosphorylation are controlled like a precision watch.[44] There are several built-in local controls as well as external controls. Electron transport is controlled by the availability of the fuel (H and electrons) and the O_2 to burn (at body temperature) the hydrogen to H_2O. The energy gained from burning hydrogen atoms (from NADH and $FADH_2$) to water is recovered by pumping hydrogen ions from inside mitochondria into the space between their double membranes. The tremendous potential difference between the intermembrane space and the inside of the mitochondrion drives the process of resynthesizing ATP from ADP and Pi. The adenine nucleotides act as important local control messengers in coordinating the four pathways. High levels of ATP slow the entry of pyruvate to the TCA cycle, the TCA cycle itself, and glycolysis (at PFK1). High levels of ADP and AMP speed glycolysis, the TCA cycle, and ultimately, ATP production. Thus, the cell precisely governs energy production by using the components of the adenine nucleotide family to speed/slow the process. The TCA cycle, in turn, is regulated by its by-products: NADH, citrate, and succinate (in addition to controls by ADP and ATP). This local control is built into the very structure of the key regulatory enzymes, which are also called allosteric enzymes. In addition to local controls, there are external controls over the pathways which are exercised by hormones. These agents activate/slow enzymes by first activating receptors, kinases, or dephosphorylases and then phosphorylating/desphosphorylating regulatory enzymes.[44] Some hormones can raise Ca^{2+} levels, which is important in controlling the TCA cycle.

In sum, carbohydrate (glucose) is metabolized in such a way as to maintain a relatively constant blood concentration of glucose. Excess carbohydrate is stored as glycogen and ultimately as fats. The metabolic controls are geared to minimize change in blood glucose. As will be explained later, excess blood glucose can cause serious organ damage as in diabetes. Overweight and obesity, in fact, are mechanisms by which the organism avoids diabetes-like conditions. Let us take the case of a gargantuan meal containing a great deal of carbohydrate.

Although the stomach and the intestine can somewhat space the inflow of glucose to the bloodstream, the influx of glucose will soon reach maximum. The "rolling" control of carbohydrate disposition primes muscles to produce more glycogen, and this will take out some, but not nearly enough, of the excess blood glucose. The same external controls also increase liver glycogen storage. The inflow of glucose into the blood goes on unabated. This turns on glycolysis, the TCA cycle, electron transport, and oxidative phosphorylation. ATP rises and excess citrate is transported from mitochondria to cytosol. Elevated ATP and citrate actually inhibit PFK1. This causes a rapid rise of F6P (since it cannot be phosphorylated to F1,6BP). This in turn will activate a bifunctional protein that converts some F6P to F2,6BP, which in turn negates the allosteric effects of ATP and citrate on PFK1.[1] These changes truly open the floodgates (the "feed forward" control), and ATP and citrate levels rise rapidly in cytosol leading to an increased splitting of citrate (to OAA and acetyl CoA), the activation of CoA carboxylase, and an increase in fatty acid synthesis. The overall effect is overweight, which can be seen as the price for avoiding diabetes.

Intracellular glycosylation and its biological role. Many proteins that are exported from cytosol acquire carbohydrate sequences during posttranslational modification.[44] Such proteins have a leader sequence that inserts into the endoplasmic reticulum and draws the protein into a membranous structure that later matures into Golgi bodies.[44] During the maturation of the Golgi bodies, carbohydrate is added either on the hydroxyl group of an amino acid such as serine, or on the amino group of asparagine.[44] Glycosylation is complex, but it may be summarized as follows. After a protein enters the endoplasmic reticulum, a carbohydrate sequence is added at either an O or an N site. Such a carbohydrate sequence may be graphically represented as a tuning fork with attachment to the protein by the end of the handle. Carbohydrate sequences enter the membranes by their dolichol attachment.[44] Attachment of the carbohydrate sequence in the endoplasmic reticulum depends on the structure of the protein, the specific glycosyl transferases present, and the specific carbohydrate structures available for glycosylation.[45] As the membrane structure matures, one or both sides of the tuning fork structure may be shortened or added to, or both. These processes are highly specific, but the basis of specificity is just beginning to be understood.[45] The final carbohydrate sequences may be as short as a disaccharide on the glomerular basement membrane or may constitute the major part of some proteins, such as keratins.[44,46] Recent work indicates that not only plasma and cytoplasmic proteins but some nucleoproteins, chromatin, and the cytoskeleton also are glycosylated.[47]

Once the glycosylation process is complete, the carbohydrate moieties impart diverse capabilities to the protein.[44] The first role of the carbohydrate attachments is to serve as "postal codes" that set the destination of proteins.[44] The carbohydrate moieties act as recognition sites enabling a protein to be anchored to the membrane.[47] Carbohydrates act as recognition sites on receptors and antigens and play a crucial role in cellular adhesion.[44] The terminal sialic acid may protect some serum proteins from degradation and may serve to keep albumin in the glomerulus.[48,49] Because most of this work has been done by molecular biologists, little is known about the effect of dietary carbohydrate on glycosylation. The possible effect of fructose on the glycosylation of intestinal disaccharidases was previously mentioned.[40]

Nonenzymatic glycosylation (glycation). Nonenzymatic glycosylation is the addition of glucose, fructose, or their phosphates to a protein (or perhaps even DNA).[50] The reaction occurs between the aldehyde oxygen or keto oxygen and an exposed amino group such as the ε-amino group of lysine or hydroxylysine.[50] The resultant Schiff base then undergoes a number of chemical reactions (rearrangements) leading to the cross-linking of proteins.

Blood glucose can be elevated to three to five times normal levels in insulin-dependent diabetes mellitus (IDDM) or non-insulin-dependent diabetes mellitus (NIDDM). Therefore, proteins that are in contact with the blood of diabetics are the most vulnerable to glycation. Proteins of the smaller blood vessels, such as those of basement membrane, which have a long replacement time (>100 days) are especially vulnerable.[50] The glomerular basement membrane is in reality a net, composed of peptides with frequent helical portions, some heteropolysaccharides, disaccharides (glucose-galactose), and sporadic cross-links.[50] Eye lens capsules and arteries have similar structures and are equally vulnerable.[51,52]

Glycation is a process that occurs throughout life even in the absence of diabetes, but is greatly accelerated during hyperglycemia.[53] Continuous remodeling of biological structures in general, as well as a specific repair mechanism, is enough to maintain normal functions of basement membranes well into middle age.[54] However, with aging, glucose tolerance deteriorates. Some scientists believe that if human lifespan reaches 100 years, diabetes will be a nearly universal malady in the absence of preventive measures.

There are indications that the glycation rates of aldehydic phosphates, keto phosphates, and fructose are 10 times higher than the glycation rate of glucose.[55] Fortunately, cell membranes are not permeable to phosphate esters, which is why these compounds are confined to the intracellular environment composed of mostly short-lived proteins. Also, fructose is metabolized rather rapidly in liver, and thus its potential to cause damage to basement membranes by glycation is minimized. Another ketohexose, D-tagatose, has a glycation rate of only one half that of glucose, and it is being tested as a bulk sweetener that may actually retard aging.

Glycation may be reduced by aminoguanidine.[56] Arginine is the body's guanidine compound, and it was logical to test its effectiveness as an antiglycation agent.[57] It was found that L-arginine reduced both the amount of glucose that reacted with human serum albumin (HSA) in vitro and the amount of HSA cross-linked (unpublished data).[57] Since kidney has been proposed as the major source of circulating L-arginine in blood, and blood arginine was shown to be lower in obese rats, it is reasonable to propose that arginine levels may also be lower in kidney in obesity.[58,59] If arginine in kidney had a protective function against glycation, a lower level of kidney arginine would account for the special vulnerability of kidney to glycation in diabetics, and also provide part of a possible mechanism for obesity acting as a risk factor for diabetes. According to this hypothesis, diabetic damage is caused by low levels of blood arginine and high levels of blood glucose.

The metabolism of simple sugars other than glucose. Fructose, galactose, and mannose are also part of the diet and are disposed of internally in the normal course of events.[44] Mannose is converted to M6P and then to F6P, while galactose is phosphorylated at the C-1 position, uridinylated, and an epimerase then converts UDP-galactose to UDP-glucose. Fructose is also phosphorylated at the C-1 position, but is then split to trioses. This circumvents the PFK controls and fructose can thus flood the TCA cycle causing increased lipid synthesis in liver.[44,60] Fortunately, humans cannot absorb enough fructose to cause fatty liver. Also, the metabolism of fructose from the diet is rapid and it does not accumulate in blood. Even at high levels of dietary fructose, the blood level of fructose is only 10% of the level of glucose.[61] However, since its glycation index is 10 times that of glucose, dietary fructose may add significantly to the normal glycation that occurs with aging. Fructose can cause marginal increases in blood lipids, uric acid, blood insulin, and blood glucose, and impair already impaired glucose tolerance under conditions maximizing the effects of dietary manipulations.[61]

The metabolism of D-tagatose poses a scientific puzzle as well as an opportunity to alter nutritional practices in a healthy way. D-Tagatose is a ketohexose that looks and tastes like sucrose, except that, like fructose, it browns more easily than sucrose during cooking. Its glycosylation power is only one half that of glucose. Of more importance is the ability of D-tagatose to reduce diabetic symptoms and food efficiency.

The use of D-tagatose as a reduced-calorie sweetener and a hypoglycemic agent has been patented by Biospherics, Inc. of Beltsville, Maryland. According to data obtained by Biospherics, most of the carbon atoms ingested as D-tagatose eventually are exhaled as CO_2, in-

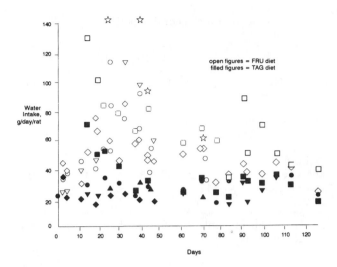

Figure 1. Water intake of rats consuming TAG or FRU diet.

dicating that this sugar is absorbed and metabolized. Szepesi has conducted two pilot studies with D-tagatose. In the first study, SHR/N-cp corpulent rats were fed a diet containing 16% fat, 34% fructose, 10% glucose, 10% lactalbumin, 10% casein and alphacell, salt mix, and vitamins (controls). In the test diet, 10% of the fructose was replaced by D-tagatose. Two rats (□ and ■) were started on the feeding regimen after they had become severely diabetic eating a chow diet. The balance of the rats were given the purified diets immediately after weaning. Figure 1 shows the antidiabetic effect of D-tagatose on water intake. Each symbol represents a single rat.

It is clear that when fed D-tagatose from weaning (filled symbols), rats did not develop polydipsia, and if D-tagatose feeding was delayed until diabetes was severe (■), tagatose feeding was effective in eliminating polydipsia after about 2 weeks. Urine glucose levels were not obtained regularly, but generally tagatose-fed animals had greatly reduced urine glucose levels. Food efficiencies were calculated for 2-month intervals. The control (fructose) versus experimental (tagatose) values were: 10.3 versus 14.7 (first 2 months); 7.5 versus 7.6 (second 2 months); and 7.9 versus 5.0 (last 2 months). Figures represent weight gain (in grams) as the percentage of food eaten (in grams). During the severe diabetic phase (first 2 months), tagatose actually increased food efficiency, possibly by reducing the energy wastage (urine glucose excretion, which can be nearly 2 g/day, the cost of polydipsia, etc.). Once diabetes receded (last 2 months), tagatose food efficiency decreased.

In a second experiment, five lean and five obese SHR/N-cp rats were fed the above diets for 2-week intervals in sequence. The results on urine glucose and food efficiency are shown in Table 1.

Tagatose reduced food efficiency in the lean SHR/N-cp rats and there appeared to be an adaptation so that the tagatose effect was far greater after feeding it the

Table 1. Results of the second experiment with SHA/N-cp rats

Animals	Diet fed			
	Control	Tagatose	Control	Tagatose
Lean				
Food efficiency	4.6	3.9	4.3	1.4
Urine glucose, mg/4h	<0.5	<0.5	<0.5	<0.5
Obese				
Food efficiency	4.2	6.8	4.1	3.0
Urine glucose, mg/4h	117	43	95	6[a]

[a]From four rats only. The fifth rat had an erroneously large value: 340.

second time. In the obese rats, tagatose increased food efficiency during the first feeding and reduced food efficiency during the second feeding. A dramatic reduction in urine glucose occurred during the second feeding of the obese animals.

It is apparent, therefore, that D-tagatose is a strongly antidiabetic sugar. Unpublished studies of Geoffrey Livesey (AFRC Institute of Food Research, Norwich Laboratory, Norwich, UK) and those conducted by Biospherics Inc. show that the caloric utilization of D-tagatose may be 0–50%. In a paper submitted for publication, Livesey and Brown show that the energy value of D-tagatose is zero (personal communication).

Health Issues and Carbohydrate Nutrition

Simple sugars and health. The sugar controversies began with the publications of Yudkin and associates. In 1968, Yudkin claimed that diabetes and arteriosclerosis were caused solely by the intake of sugar.[62] In articles too numerous to review here, scientists in Europe, the United States, and Japan have shown that Yudkin's premises were wrong and his methodology faulty. His results could not be duplicated.

The diabetic rat model of Cohen. Some of the claims of Yudkin were adopted by Cohen, whose epidemiologic studies dealt with the migration of Yemenite Jews to Israel and the increase in the incidence of diabetes among this group as they became acculturated to their new society. Cohen concluded that the incidence of diabetes among Yemenite Jews increased because of their increased sugar intake. He and his associates then set out to demonstrate the diabetic effect of sugar (sucrose) in an animal model.[63] They reported that an animal model was developed by feeding rats a diet that contained >60% sucrose by weight and selecting male and female rats with impaired glucose tolerance and breeding these "upwardly selected rats" while feeding them a high-sucrose diet. It was claimed that after the third generation, this selec-

tion procedure produced rats that developed the classical symptoms of diabetes when fed sucrose, but not if they were fed starch.[63] These studies led to the hypothesis that diabetes in humans is produced by heredity and the intake of sugar. This hypothesis was accepted by many scientists since it was so well supported by Cohen's studies. Doubts, however, soon began to surface when the findings could not be duplicated. At the Second International Workshop on Lessons from Animal Diabetes, Cohen acknowledged that his rats became diabetic when fed practically any simple carbohydrate including sucrose, fructose, glucose, glycerol, and sorbitol.

Studies with sucrose in "carbohydrate sensitive" people. As the claims of Yudkin and Cohen (that consumption of sucrose posed a serious health hazard) failed to gain acceptance, other claims were being advanced by S. Reiser and coworkers from the USDA Laboratories in Beltsville, Maryland.[64–66] Since the physiological effects of dietary sucrose in the average human were relatively small, Reiser selected individuals for his studies who were more sensitive to the consumption of sugar than the average person. Such persons had a higher than normal insulin, cholesterol, and triacylglycerol response to carbohydrate intake and became known as "carbohydrate sensitive" individuals. Reiser hypothesized that "carbohydrate sensitive" individuals were more prone to heart disease and diabetes because of a larger response to sugar in terms of blood triacylglycerols and cholesterol than the average person. Studies in other laboratories noted that the differences between sucrose and starch-fed individuals were highly variable. It was also observed that the response to dietary sucrose was dependent upon the type and amount of fat in the diet. A 1986 report of the FDA concluded that sucrose was not an independent risk factor for either diabetes or heart disease.[67] The FDA report was essentially endorsed by another report from the National Research Council (NRC) three years later.[68]

The fructose-copper interaction. Low levels of trace elements in the blood have been reported to cause impaired glucose tolerance.[69] Both Cohen et al.[70] and Fields et al.[71] have reported that copper deficiency can cause impaired glucose tolerance. To interpret this finding, however, it must be remembered that copper is involved in a number of important biological processes and that each process may be sensitive to other factors.[72] For example, Cu/Zn superoxide dismutase is decreased in copper deficiency and is susceptible to the Cu/Zn ratio. Erythrocyte damage in copper deficiency interacts with dietary iron and some antioxidants, such as ascorbic acid and others.[73,74] From studies conducted with copper-deficient subjects the following has been learned of these interactions: iron and sucrose can increase copper deficiency symptoms,[74] zinc and sucrose can increase copper deficiency symptoms[74] and zinc also decreases copper absorption,[75] sucrose decreases copper absorption unless iron is deficient,[76] copper deficiency anemia is improved by raising iron levels to 25–120 mg/kg but is worsened if iron intake is further increased,[77] and severity of copper deficiency is also influenced by the type of dietary protein ingested.[78]

From these complex interactions it should be apparent that the effectiveness of a single factor (such as dietary fructose) on copper deficiency can be enhanced by manipulating other variables such as dietary zinc, iron, protein, and possibly other parts of the diet, or the duration of the feeding. Thus it is possible for the same nutrient to have different effects in various laboratories.[79]

O'Dell concluded that the effect of fructose on copper deficiency was due to a reduction of copper bioavailability in the intestine of rats.[79] There was no apparent fructose effect on copper bioavailability in pigs. Ultrastructural studies of hearts from copper-deficient SHHS/Mcc-cp rats showed heart hypertrophy in both male and female rats, though hypertrophy was greater in males.[80] Finally, it was shown that copper-depleted rats developed heart pathology in the absence of anemia and hypertrophy.[81] When postweaning copper-deficient rats were repleted with copper, the rats developed heart hypertrophy without ever developing anemia.[81]

The relevance of fructose-copper interaction to human beings. There are two reports of possible fructose-copper interaction in human adults.[82,83] From review of these publications, O'Dell[79] noted that human subjects on a fructose-containing diet absorbed more copper than subjects on a starch diet. These results are contrary to those obtained in rats.

Conclusions

Much has been learned about the nutritional value and fate of dietary carbohydrates. The major metabolic pathways and their controls are largely known. Digestion, absorption, and metabolism of dietary carbohydrate has received a large amount of attention. The effect of carbohydrates on the intestinal absorption of minerals will continue to be a topic of interest. While some carbohydrates can slow the absorption of trace minerals, others, such as lactose, can speed it or slow it depending on circumstances.[84] The next five years will undoubtedly increase our knowledge of some novel fibers and their effects, and see new low-calorie sugar substitutes such as D-tagatose. The great debate over the nutritional toxicity of sucrose and fructose is over. The overwhelming majority of nutritionists view the issues on their merits, and extreme points of view have been rejected.

References

1. Szepesi B (1990) Carbohydrates. In Brown ML (ed), Present knowledge in nutrition. International Life Sciences Institute, Washington, DC, pp 47–55
2. Life Sciences Research Office (1994) The evaluation of the energy of certain sugar alcohols used as food ingredients. Federation of American Societies for Experimental Biology, Bethesda, MD
3. Behall KM, Scholfield DI, Yuhaniak I, Canary J (1989) Diets containing high amylose vs amylopectin starch: effects of metabolic variables in human subjects. Am J Clin Nutr 49:337–344
4. Semanza GS, Auricchio S (1989) Small intestinal disaccharidases. In Scriver CR, Beauset AL, Sly WS, Valle D (eds), The metabolic basis of inherited disease, 6th ed. McGraw-Hill, New York, pp 2975–2997
5. Conklin KA, Vamashiro KM, Gray GM (1975) Human intestinal sucrase-isomaltase: identification of free sucrase and isomaltase and cleavage of the hybrid into active distinct subunits. J Biol Chem 250:5735–5741
6. Riby JE, Kretchmer N (1985) Participation of pancreatic enzymes in the degradation of intestinal sucrase-isomaltase. J Pediatr Gastroenterol Nutr 4:971–979
7. Hauri HP, Quaroni A, Isselbacher KJ (1979) Biogenesis of intestinal plasma membrane: post-translational route and cleavage of sucrose-isomaltase. Proc Natl Acad Sci USA 76:5183–5186
8. Naim HY, Sterchi EE, Lentze MJ (1988) Structure, biosynthesis, and glycosylation of human small intestinal maltase-glucoamylase. J Biol Chem 263:19709–19717
9. Burks TF, Galligan JJ, Porreca F, Barber WD (1985) Regulation of gastric emptying. Fed Proc 44:2897–2901
10. Goda T, Bustamente S, Koldovsky O (1985) Dietary regulation of intestinal lactase and sucrase in adult rats: quantitative comparison of effect of lactose and sucrose. J Pediatr Gastroenterol Nutr 4:998–1008
11. Morrill JS, Kwong LK, Sunshine P, et al (1989) Dietary CHO and stimulation of carbohydrates along villus column of fasted rat jejunum. Am J Physiol 256:G158–G165
12. Yamada K, Goda T, Bustamente S, Koldovsky O (1983) Different effect of starvation on activity of sucrase and lactase in rat jejunoileum. Am J Physiol 245:G449–G455
13. Goda T, Yamada K, Bustamente S, Koldovsky O (1983) Dietary-induced rapid decrease in microvillar carbohydrase activity in rat jejunoileum. Am J Physiol 245:G418–G423
14. Riby JE, Kretchmer N (1984) Effect of dietary sucrose on synthesis and degradation of intestinal sucrase. Am J Physiol 246:G757–G763
15. Danielson EM (1989) Post-translational suppression of expression of intestinal brush border enzymes by fructose. J Biol Chem 264:13726–13729
16. Nakabou Y, Ishikawa Y, Misake A, Hagihira H (1980) Effect of food intake on intestinal absorption and mucosal hydrolases in alloxan diabetic rats. Metabolism 29:181–185
17. Schedl HP, Al-Jurf AS, Wilson HD (1983) Elevated intestinal disaccharidase activity in the streptozotocin-diabetic rat is independent of enteral feeding. Diabetes 32:265–270
18. Gourley GR, Korsmo HA, Olsen WA (1983) Intestinal mucosa in diabetic rats: studies of microvillus membrane composition and microviscosity. Metabolism 30:1053–1058
19. Wen D, Henning SJ, Hazelwood RL (1988) Effect of diabetes on development of small intestinal enzymes of infant rats. Proc Soc Exp Biol Med 187:51–57
20. Morton AP, Hanson PJ (1984) Monosaccharide transport by the intestine of lean and genetically obese (ob/ob) mice. Q J Exp Physiol 69:117–126
21. Thomson ABR (1983) Experimental diabetes and intestinal barriers to absorption. Am J Physiol 244:G151–G159
22. Debnam ES, Karasov WH, Thompson CS (1988) Nutrient uptake by rat enterocytes during diabetes mellitus: evidence

for an increased sodium electrochemical gradient. J Physiol 397:503–512

23. Baly DL, Horuk R (1988) The biology and chemistry of the glucose transporter. Biochim Biophys Acta 947:571–590

24. Crane RK (1960) Intestinal absorption of sugars. Physiol Rev 40:789–825

25. Crane RK (1962) Hypothesis for mechanism of intestinal active transport of sugars. Fed Proc 21:891–895

26. Crane RK (1968) Absorption of sugars. In Code CF, Heidel W (eds), Handbook of physiology, section 6, vol 3. Waverly Press, Baltimore, pp 1323–1351

27. Gray GM (1975) Carbohydrate digestion and absorption: role of the small intestine. Physiol Med 292:1225–1230

28. Gray GM (1981) Carbohydrate absorption and malabsorption. In Johnson LR (ed), Physiology of the gastrointestinal tract. Raven Press, New York, pp 1063–1072

29. Brot-Laroche E, Alvarado F (1983) Mechanism of sugar transport across the intestinal brush border membrane. In Gilles-Baillien M, Gilles R (eds), Intestinal transport. Springer-Verlag, Berlin, pp 147–169

30. Walmsley AR (1988) The dynamics of the glucose transporter. Trends Biochem Sci 13:226–231

31. Fedorak RN, Chang EB, Madara JL, Field M (1987) Intestinal adaptation to diabetes: altered Na-dependent nutrient absorption in streptozotocin-treated chronically diabetic rats. J Clin Invest 79:1571–1578

32. Hediger MA, Coady MJ, Ikeda TS, Wright EM (1987) Expression cloning and cDNA sequencing of the NA+/glucose cotransporter. Nature 330:379–381

33. Thorens B, Sarker HK, Kaback HR, Lodish HF (1988) Cloning and functional expression in bacteria of a novel glucose transporter present in liver, intestine, kidney and B-pancreatic islet cells. Cell 55:281–290

34. Fukumoto H, Kayano T, Buse J, et al (1989) Cloning and characterization of the major insulin-responsive glucose transporter expressed in human skeletal muscle and other insulin-responsive tissue. J Biol Chem 264:7776–7779

35. McIntyre N, Holdworth CD, Turner DS (1965) Intestinal factors in the control of insulin secretion. J Clin Edocrinol 25:1317–1324

36. Szepesi B, Michaelis OE IV (1986) "Disaccharide effect": comparison of metabolic effects of the intake of disaccharides and of their monosaccharide equivalents. In Macdonald I, Vrana A (eds), Metabolic effects of dietary carbohydrates. S Karger, Basel, Switzerland, pp 192–219

37. Michaelis OE IV, Nace CS, Szepesi B (1975) Demonstration of a specific metabolic effect of dietary disaccharides in the rat. J Nutr 105:1186–1191

38. Michaelis OE IV, Szepesi B (1977) Specificity of the disaccharide effect in the rat. Nutr Metab 21:329–340

39. Park JHY, Berdanier CD, Deaver OE Jr, Szepesi B (1986) Effects of dietary carbohydrate on hepatic gluconeogenesis in BHE rats. J Nutr 116:1193–1203

40. Sciafani A, Mann S (1987) Carbohydrate taste preferences in rats: glucose, sucrose, maltose, fructose and polyose compared. Physiol Behav 40:563–568

41. Kunz C, Rudloff S (1993) Biological functions of oligosaccharides in human milk. Acta Paediatr 82:903–912

42. Jenkins DJA, Wolever TMS, Taylor RH, et al (1981) Glycemic index of foods: a physiological basis for carbohydrate exchange. Am J Clin Nutr 34:362–366

43. Hollenbeck CB, Coulston AM, Reaven GM (1988) Comparison of plasma glucose and insulin responses to mixed meals of high-, intermediate-, and low-glycemic potential. Diabetes Care 11:323–329

44. Voet D, Voet JG (1990) Biochemistry. John Wiley and Sons, New York, NY

45. Paulson JC, Colley KJ (1989) Glycosyltransferases. J Biol Chem 264:17615–17618

46. Spiro RG (1967) The structure of the disaccharide unit of the renal glomerular basement membrane. J Biol Chem 242:4813–4823

47. Hart GW, Holt GW, Haltiwanger RS (1988) Nuclear and cytoplasmic glycosylation: novel saccharide linkages in unexpected places. Trends Biochem 13:380–384

48. Sharon N, Lis H (1981) Glycoproteins: research booming on long-ignored, ubiquitous compounds. Chem Eng News 59:21–24

49. Brown DM, Andres GA, Hostetter TH, et al (1982) Kidney complications. Diabetes 31(suppl 1):71–81

50. Brownlee M, Vlassara H, Cerami A (1984) Nonenzymic glycosylation and the pathogenesis of diabetic complications. Ann Intern Med 101:527–537

51. Fukushi S, Spiro RG (1969) The lens capsule: sugar and amino acid composition. J Biol Chem 244:2041–2048

52. Brownlee M, Vlassara H, Cerami A (1988) Advanced products of nonenzymatic glycosylation and the pathogenesis of diabetic vascular disease. Diabetes Metab Rev 4:437–451

53. Vlassara H, Valinsky J, Brownlee M, et al (1987) Advanced glycosylation endproducts on erythrocyte cell surface induce receptor-mediated phagocytosis by macrophages: a model for turnover of aging cells. J Exp Med 166:539–549

54. Vlassara H, Brownlee M, Monogue K, et al (1988) Cachetin/TNF and IL-1 induced by glucose-modified proteins: role in normal tissue remodeling. Science 240:1546–1548

55. McPhearson JD, Shilton BH, Walton DJ (1988) Role of fructose in glycosylation and cross-linking of proteins. Biochemistry 27:1901–1907

56. Brownlee M, Vlassara H, Kooney A, et al (1986) Aminoguanidine prevents diabetes-induced arterial wall protein cross-linking. Science 232:1629–1632

57. Servetnick DA, Wiesenfeld PL, Szepesi B (1990) Evidence that L-arginine inhibits glycation of human serum albumin (HSA) in vitro [abstract]. FASEB J 4(3):A2576

58. Featherston WR, Rogers QR, Freedland RA (1973) Relative importance of kidney and liver in synthesis of arginine by the rat. Am J Physiol 224:127–129

59. Yamini S, Staples R, Szepesi B (1989) Effect of obesity and dietary carbohydrate on liver and kidney urea cycle enzyme activities and plasma amino acids in the rat [abstract]. FASEB J 3(3, pt 1):A352

60. Szepesi B, Freedland RA (1968) Time-course of enzyme adaptation. I. Effects of substituting dietary glucose and fructose at constant concentrations of dietary protein. Can J Biochem 46:1459–1470

61. Reiser S, Hallfrish J (1987) Metabolic effects of dietary fructose. CRC Press, Boca Raton, FL

62. Yudkin J (1968) Dietary intake of carbohydrate in relation to diabetes and atherosclerosis. In Dickens F, Randle PJ, Whelan WJ (eds), Carbohydrate metabolism and its disorders, vol 2. Academic Press, London, pp 169–183

63. Cohen AM, Teitelbaum A, Briller S, et al (1974) Experimental models of diabetes. In Sipple HL, McNutt KW (eds), Sugars in nutrition. Academic Press, New York, pp 483–511

64. Reiser S (1982) Health implications of food carbohydrates: heart disease and diabetes. In Lineback D, Englett (eds), Food carbohydrates. AVI Publishing, Westport, CT, pp 170–205

65. Reiser S (1982) Metabolic risk factors associated with heart disease and diabetes in carbohydrate-sensitive humans when

consuming sucrose as compared to starch. In: Metabolic effects of utilizable dietary carbohydrates. Marcel Dekker, New York

66. Reiser S (1983) Physiological differences between starches and sugars. In Bland (ed), The medical applications of clinical nutrition. Keats Publishing, New Canaan, CT, pp 133–177

67. Sugars Task Force (1986) Evaluation of health aspects of sugars contained in carbohydrate sweeteners. Health and Human Services, Food and Drug Administration. US Government Printing Office, Washington, DC

68. Committee on Diet and Health (1989) Implications for reducing chronic disease risk. Food and Nutrition Board, National Research Council. National Academy Press, Washington, DC

69. Armstrong VW, Buschmann U, Ebert R, et al (1980) Biochemical investigations of CAPD: plasma levels of trace elements and amino acids and impaired glucose tolerance during the course of treatment. Int J Artif Organs 3(4):237–241

70. Cohen AM, Teitelbaum A, Miller E, et al (1982) Effect of copper on carbohydrate metabolism in rats. Isr J Med Sci 18(8):840–844

71. Fields M, Ferretti M, Smith RJ, Reiser S (1984) Impairment of glucose tolerance in copper-deficient rats: dependency on the type of carbohydrate. J Nutr 114(2):393–397

72. Johnson MA, Fischer JG (1992) Is copper an antioxidant nutrient? Crit Rev Food Sci Nutr 32(1):1–31

73. Johnson MA, Murphy CL (1988) Adverse effects of high dietary iron and ascorbic acid on copper status in copper-deficient and copper-adequate rats. Am J Clin Nutr 47:96–101

74. Johnson MA, Hove SS (1986) Development of anemia in copper-deficient rats fed high levels of dietary iron and sucrose. J Nutr 116:1225–1238

75. Johnson MA, Flagg EW (1986) Effects of sucrose and cornstarch on the development of copper deficiency in rats fed high levels of zinc. Nutr Res 6:1307–1319

76. Johnson MA, Gratzek JM (1986) Influence of sucrose and starch on the development of anemia in copper- and iron-deficient rats. J Nutr 116(12):2443–2452

77. Johnson MA (1990) Influence of ascorbic acid, zinc, iron, sucrose and fructose on copper status. In Kies C (ed), Copper bioavailability and metabolism. Plenum, New York, pp 29–43

78. Fields M, Lewis CG, Lure MD (1993) Copper deficiency in rats: the effect of type of dietary protein. J Am Coll Nutr 12(3):303–306

79. O'Dell BL (1993) Fructose and mineral metabolism. Am J Clin Nutr 58(suppl):7715–7785

80. Medeiros DM, Liao Z, Hamlin RL (1991) Copper deficiency in genetically hypertensive cardiomyopathic rat: electrocardiogram, functional and ultrastructural aspects. J Nutr 121:1026–1034

81. Davidson J, Medeiros DM, Hamlin RL (1992) Cardiac ultrastructural and electrophysiological abnormalities in postweaning copper-restricted and copper-repleted rats in the absence of hypertrophy. J Nutr 122:1566–1575

82. Reiser S, Smith JC Jr, Mertz W, et al (1985) Indices of copper status in humans consuming a typical American diet containing either fructose or starch. Am J Clin Nutr 42:424–251

83. Holbrook JT, Smith JC, Reiser S (1989) Dietary fructose or starch: effects on copper, zinc, iron, manganese, calcium and magnesium balances in humans. Am J Clin Nutr 49:1290–1294

84. Wirth FH Jr, Numerof B, Pleban P, Neylan MJ (1990) Effect of lactose on mineral absorption in preterm infants. J Pediatr 117(2, pt 1):283–287

Chapter 6

Dietary Fat

Scott M. Grundy

Dietary fat consists mainly of a heterogeneous mixture of triacylglycerols (triglycerides) and makes up a substantial but variable portion of total energy intake. In many European countries, fat accounts for 40–45% of total energy in the diet. In the United States, fat intakes are somewhat lower, ranging between 30% and 40% of total energy; in other populations, particularly in Asia and Africa, fat provides only 15–25% of energy. A widely held belief is that excess dietary fat contributes importantly to several chronic diseases, such as coronary heart disease (CHD), stroke, diabetes mellitus, cancer, and obesity. This belief has fostered the recommendation that dietary fat should be kept relatively low, that is, <30% of total energy.[1] This recommendation has the virtue of simplicity; but one can question whether it is realistic, necessary, or strongly based on scientific data. The overall issue of dietary fat is not simple. Fat is a major nutrient and an important source of body fuel, and fat consists of a complex mixture of triacylglycerol molecules that can differ greatly from one another in their chemical and physical properties. Consequently, data related to the different kinds of triacylglycerols and their constituent fatty acids must be taken into account before general dietary recommendations are made.

Triacylglycerols are composed of three molecules of fatty acids esterified with one molecule of glycerol. Dietary triacylglycerols are derived either unmodified from natural sources (animal and plant fats) or modified industrially for special purposes in foods. Dietary fatty acids differ considerably in their carbon chain length and number of double bonds between carbon atoms. Through various combinations of different kinds of fatty acids, a myriad of different species of triacylglycerols occur in nature and are consumed in the diet.

Table 1 lists the different categories of dietary fatty acids. Typically the fatty acids are divided into three groups: saturated, monounsaturated, and polyunsaturated. Saturated fatty acids are straight-chain acids of variable carbon chain length having no double bonds between carbon atoms. Chain lengths vary from 8 to 18 carbon atoms; increments in chain length occur by two. The most prevalent saturated fatty acids in the American diet are palmitic acid (16:0) and stearic acid (18:0). The first number in parentheses designates the number of carbon atoms in the fatty acid, and the second, the number of double bonds. The predominant monounsaturated fatty acid is oleic acid (*cis*-18:1n–9). The term *"cis"* indicates that the double bond is in the *cis* configuration, and the term "n–9" means that the double bond is located nine carbon atoms from the terminal carbon. Another monounsaturated fatty acid is elaidic acid (*trans*-18:1n–9). The *trans* configuration of the double bond forms during the catalytic hydrogenation of polyunsaturated fatty acids. Other *trans* monounsaturates having double bonds at other locations along the carbon chain are also produced by hydrogenation. Finally, polyunsaturated fatty acids have two or more double bonds. There are two classes of polyunsaturates: n–6 and n–3. The predominant polyunsaturated fatty acid in the diet is linoleic acid (18:2n–6); it occurs mainly in plant oils. Linolenic acid (18:3n–3) is the parent n–3 fatty acid, and it can be elongated to longer-chain polyunsaturates: eicosapentaenoic acid (EPA; 20:5n–3) and docosahexaenoic acid (DHA; 22:6n–3). Linoleic acid can be elongated in the body to arachidonic acid (20:4n–6); the latter is a precursor to products of high biological activity: prostaglandins, thromboxanes, and prostacyclins.

The saturated fatty acids comprise 11–12% of total energy in the American diet.[2] They are derived from both animal and plant fats. The fatty acid patterns of several fats rich in saturated fatty acids are shown in Table 2.

Table 1. Dietary fatty acids

Saturated fatty acids
  Stearic acid (18:0)
  Palmitic acid (16:0)
  Myristic acid (14:0)
  Lauric acid (12:0)
  Medium-chain fatty acids (8:0 and 10:0)
Monounsaturated fatty acids
  Oleic acid (*cis*-18:1)
  Elaidic acid (*trans*-18:1)
Polyunsaturated fatty acids
  n–6 fatty acids
    Linoleic acid (18:2)
  n–3 fatty acids
    Linolenic acid (18:3)
    Eicosapentaenoic acid (EPA) (20:5)
    Docosahexaenoic acid (DHA) (22:6)

The first number indicates the number of carbon atoms; the second denotes the number of double bonds per molecule.

Table 2. Fatty acid compositions of several fats high in saturated fatty acids

Fat	4–10:0*	12:0	14:0	16:0	16:1	18:0	18:1	18:2	18:3	Other
				% of total fatty acids						
Butter fat	9.2	3.1	11.7	6.2	1.9	12.5	28.2	2.9	0.5	3.8
Palm kernel oil	8.2	49.6	16.0	8.0		2.4	13.7	2.0		0.1
Coconut oil	14.9	48.5	17.6	8.4		2.5	6.5	1.5		0.1
Palm oil		0.3	1.1	45.1	0.1	4.7	38.8	9.4		0.5
Beef fat	0.1	0.1	3.3	25.5	3.4	21.6	38.7	2.2	0.6	4.6
Pork fat (lard)	0.1	0.1	1.5	24.8	3.1	12.3	45.1	9.9	1.1	3.0
Chicken fat		0.2	1.3	23.2	6.5	6.4	41.6	18.9	1.3	0.6
Mutton fat	0.2	0.3	5.2	23.6	2.5	24.5	33.3	4.0	1.3	5.1
Cocoa butter			0.1	25.8	0.3	34.5	35.3	2.9		1.1

These fats vary considerably in their overall composition, and many differ in their predominant saturated fatty acid. For example, palm oil is very high in palmitic acid; cocoa butter is richest in stearic acid; and two tropical oils, palm kernel oil and coconut oil, are highest in lauric acid (12:0). Butter fat is high in several saturated fatty acids, whereas beef fat has about equal amounts of palmitic and stearic acids.

Several fats and oils are rich in oleic acid, the predominant monounsaturated fatty acid in the diet. Oleic acid is synthesized by both animals and plants. Table 2 shows that many of the fats high in saturated fatty acids are even higher in oleic acid. Other oils likewise have oleic acid as the predominant fatty acid (Table 3). Among these, canola oil (low-erucic-acid rapeseed oil) is an important high-oleic oil used in American and Northern European diets; olive oil, another high-oleic oil, is the major source of fat in Southern Europe.

Other plant oils contain predominantly polyunsaturated fatty acids (Table 4). Most have linoleic acid as the principal fatty acid, but one of them, linseed oil, is high in linolenic acid. In the American diet, intakes of polyunsaturated fatty acids, mostly linoleic acid, average ≈6% of total energy.[2] This percentage is higher than in the first half of the 20th century, before commercial vegetable oils were widely used. The fish oils are another type of highly polyunsaturated oil, and they are unique in that they are rich in very-long-chain n–3 fatty acids (Table 5). Their contribution to the American diet, however, is quite small.

Trans unsaturated fatty acids are produced through hydrogenation of polyunsaturated oils. Small amounts also are present in butter fat and are produced by hydrogenation of plant oils in the rumen of cattle.[3,4] *Trans* fatty acids are consumed from a variety of sources. About one-third of the American intake of *trans* fatty acids comes from household shortenings, margarines, spreads, and dressings; another third is derived from fats and oils used in food products (snacks, cookies, crackers, bread, cake, potato chips, and french fries); and the final third comes from food-service fats and oils and meat and dairy products.[5] The actual intake of *trans* fatty acids varies considerably among individuals but on average is ≈3% of total energy.[5,6]

Digestion of Dietary Fats

Dietary triacylglycerols enter the gastrointestinal tract, where they come into contact with gastric and intestinal lipases. The latter is the major lipase, and it hydrolyzes the fat into free fatty acids and monoacylglycerols. Fatty acids in positions sn–1 and sn–3 are removed, whereas that at position sn–2 remains attached to glycerol. The solubilization of fatty acids in the gut is enhanced by the polar lipids of bile: bile acids and phospholipids, which promote the formation of expanded, mixed micelles that solubilize fatty acids and monoacylglycerols. These lipid products then pass by monomolecular diffusion into the mucosal cells of the small intestine.

Table 3. Fatty acid composition of oils high in oleic acid

Oil	14:0	16:0	18:0	18:1	18:2	18:3	Other
			% of total fatty acids				
Olive oil		13.7	2.5	71.1	10.0	0.6	2.1
Peanut oil	0.1	11.6	3.1	46.5	31.4	1.5	5.8
Canola oil (LEAR oil)[a]		3.9	1.9	64.1	18.7	9.2	2.2
Rice bran oil	0.5	16.4	2.1	43.8	34.0	1.1	2.1
Sunflower (high oleate)	0.1	5.5	2.2	79.7	12.0	0.2	0.3

[a]LEAR oil, low erucic acid rapeseed oil.

Table 4. Fatty acid composition of oils high in linoleic acid

Oil	14:0	16:0	18:0	18:1	18:2	18:3	Other
				% of total fatty acids			
Corn oil		12.2	2.2	27.5	57.0	0.9	0.2
Cottonseed oil	0.9	24.7	2.3	17.6	53.3	0.3	0.9
Oat oil	0.2	17.1	1.4	33.4	44.8	0.2	2.9
Safflower oil (high linoleate)	0.1	6.5	2.4	13.1	77.7		0.2
Sesame seed oil		9.9	5.2	41.2	43.2	0.2	0.3
Soybean oil	0.1	11.0	4.0	23.4	53.2	7.8	0.5
Sunflower seed oil	0.2	6.8	4.7	18.6	68.2	0.5	1.0

In normal individuals, dietary fat is almost completely absorbed. However, small amounts of saturated fatty acids pass throughout the gastrointestinal tract unabsorbed. Triacylglycerol molecules that contain three saturated fatty acids are poor substrates for pancreatic lipase and may not be digested or absorbed. Some workers have suggested that stearic acid is poorly absorbed, but our studies in humans indicate that ≈90% of stearic acid is absorbed.[7,8] In the absence of bile (e.g., biliary tract obstruction), fat absorption is reduced although not absent. In the absence of pancreatic lipase (e.g., with pancreatic disease), hydrolysis of triacylglycerols is reduced and fat absorption is severely curtailed. In the latter instance, triacylglycerols are excreted intact in the feces. In some forms of intestinal mucosal disease (e.g., sprue), triacylglycerols are hydrolyzed but fatty acids and monoacylglycerols are not absorbed; in this case, excess fatty acids, and not intact triacylglycerols, are excreted in feces.

Absorption and Transport of Exogenous Fat

In the intestinal mucosa cell, monoacylglycerols and fatty acids are recombined into triacylglycerols. The triacylglycerols are incorporated into lipoproteins called chylomicrons, which are secreted into the lymph. Lipoproteins are lipid-rich particles containing a surface coat of proteins (apolipoproteins), polar lipids (phospholipids and unesterified cholesterol), and a nonpolar lipid core consisting of triacylglycerols and cholesterol esters.[9] Chylomicrons are large lipoproteins containing mainly triacylglycerols in their cores. The principal apolipoprotein on the surface coat of chylomicrons is apolipoprotein (apo) B-48, which is a large, hydrophobic protein.[10] Recent investigations have shown that a particular protein, microsomal triacylglycerol transfer protein (MTP), is responsible for transporting and inserting triacylglycerol into the chylomicron core.[11,12] In the congenital absence of MTP, normal chylomicrons are not formed and fat absorption is severely curtailed.[13] Normally, chylomicrons are secreted into the intestinal lymph, where they pass through the thoracic duct into the systemic circulation.

The surface coat contains not only apo B-48, but other apoproteins as well: apo Cs (C-II and C-III), apo Es, and apo As (A-I and A-IV).[9] When chylomicrons pass into the peripheral circulation, they come into contact with lipoprotein lipase (LPL), an enzyme that is located on the endothelial surface of capillaries.[14] LPL is synthesized in adipose tissue and skeletal muscle, and it migrates to the capillaries supplying these organs. This enzyme hydrolyzes the triacylglycerols of chylomicrons, and free fatty acids are released. Most of those fatty acids released in the adipose-tissue bed are taken up by adipocytes, where they are resynthesized into triacylglycerols and are stored. Those released in capillaries of skeletal muscle are taken up and used for energy. Some of the free fatty acids bind to albumin and reenter the systemic circulation. LPL is activated by apo C-II. The role of apo C-II is demonstrated by a rare genetic disease in which apo C-II is absent; in this condition, LPL lacks the cofactor required for activation, and excessive quantities of chylomicrons accumulate in plasma.[15,16] In another rare disorder, LPL is genetically absent, and again chylomicrons accumulate in plasma.[17] Recent investigations have revealed a series of genetic defects in the LPL gene that are responsible for a reduced or absent function.[18]

In the presence of normal LPL function, most of the triacylglycerols of chylomicrons are hydrolyzed. However, the lipoprotein particle remains intact and is released

Table 5. Fatty acid composition of menhaden fish oil

Fatty acid	Percent	Fatty acid	Percent
14:0	8.35	19:0	0.11
15:0	0.86	20:0	0.15
16:0	15.17	20:1	1.32
16:1	11.62	20:2	0.31
16:2	2.37	20:3	0.40
16:3	1.96	20:4	2.30
16:4	1.73	20:5	16.03
17:0	0.76	21:5	0.79
18:0	2.67	22:0	0.10
18:1	9.50	22:1	0.31
18:2	1.81	22:4	0.33
18:3	1.82	22:5	3.92
18:4	3.47	22:6	10.83

back into the circulation as a smaller particle called a chylomicron remnant. These particles retain all of their cholesterol esters and some triacylglycerols in their core. They are taken up directly by liver. According to current concepts, the apo B-48 of remnants binds to a proteoglycan on the surface of a liver cell, and by a process involving apo E, the particles are internalized.[19] A specific chylomicron remnant receptor has never been identified, and no congenital absence of such a remnant receptor has been recognized. However, two hepatic receptors have been implicated in remnant uptake: the low-density-lipoprotein (LDL) receptor[20] and the LDL-receptor-like protein (LRP).[21] Abnormalities in apo E, which binds to LDL receptors, lead to an accumulation of chylomicron remnants in the circulation.[19] There are two common forms of apo E—apo E_3 and apo E_4—that bind avidly to LDL receptors and one less-common form—apo E_2—that binds poorly to LDL receptors.[19] People who inherit two copies of E_2 are devoid of other forms of apo Es; in these people, chylomicron remnants are cleared slowly from the circulation.[19] This implies that apo E is needed for remnant removal, and most likely, it binds to hepatic receptors.

Adipose Tissue Metabolism of Triacylglycerol

Any excess of fat that is ingested in the diet is stored in adipose tissue. Most of the fat present in adipose tissue is derived from dietary fat; adipose tissue has limited capacity to synthesize fatty acids.[22] Also, only small amounts are obtained from fatty acids synthesized in liver from glucose. Fatty acids entering adipose tissue cells are derived from hydrolysis of triacylglycerol-rich lipoproteins (chylomicrons and very-low-density lipoprotein [VLDL]) by LPL located in capillaries in the adipose tissue bed.[23] These fatty acids are activated by forming coenzyme A (CoA) derivatives and in turn are transferred to glycerol-3-phosphate to form triacylglycerol. Glycerol-3-phosphate is derived from the catabolism of glucose through the glycolytic pathway. Adipose tissue lacks the kinase required to phosphorylate glycerol, and thus all glycerol-3-phosphate must be derived from glycolysis.

Adipose tissue is an important reservoir of metabolic fuel. Triacylglycerols are stored in adipose tissue as globules of fat. The fatty acid composition of adipose tissue is a fairly good indicator of the long-term composition of dietary fat.[5,6] Adipose tissue is an important buffer between dietary intake of fat and fatty acid metabolism in various organs. The importance of adipose tissue is illustrated by the rare disorder called generalized lipodystrophy;[24] in this condition, adipose tissue is genetically absent. As a result, fat accumulates in liver, and patients have severe hypertriacylglycerolemia and develop diabetes mellitus relatively early in life.

Fatty acids are released from adipose tissues by a hormone-sensitive lipase,[25] a specialized lipase that is activated by epinephrine, norepinephrine, glucagon, and adrenocorticotropic hormone.[26] These hormones stimulate adenylate cyclase and increase cellular levels of cyclic adenosine monophosphate. The latter stimulates protein kinase, which phosphorylates the lipase and activates it. In opposition to the above-mentioned hormones, insulin inhibits hormone-sensitive lipase activity and decreases hydrolysis of adipose tissue triacylglycerols.[27,28] Fatty acids and glycerol released during lipolysis are released into the circulation. Glycerol cannot be reused by adipose tissue for triacylglycerol synthesis.

When fatty acids are released from adipose tissue, they bind to albumin for transport in the circulation.[29] Here they are in the unesterified (or free) form and hence are called free fatty acids. Adipose tissue release of free fatty acids, and hence plasma free fatty acid levels, are not regulated as exquisitely as is the plasma level of glucose. Although adipose tissue lipase is regulated by hormones, there is a basal level of free fatty acid release that depends on the total amount of adipose tissue present.[30] Consequently, obese people have a greater release than do nonobese people, and they have higher fasting levels.[31,32] The metabolic consequences of this will be discussed later. Of interest and importance, all adipose tissue stores in the body do not have equal propensity to release free fatty acids. Seemingly, adipose tissue located in the trunk is less suppressible by insulin (at a given insulin level it releases more free fatty acids into the circulation).[33] Thus, a predominance of truncal obesity appears to accentuate the metabolic consequences of obesity.[34]

Liver Utilization of Fatty Acids

Liver is one organ that utilizes circulating free fatty acids; seemingly, the higher the concentration, the greater the hepatic uptake. Free fatty acids in liver can have two fates. They can be converted into glycerolipids (triacylglycerols and phospholipids). Hepatic fatty acids can be oxidized completely to carbon dioxide and water or they can be partially oxidized to ketone bodies (acetoacetic acid and β-hydroxybutyric acid). The oxidation process of fatty acids can be considered first.

Fatty acids in liver are oxidized in mitochondria.[35] They are activated by CoA in preparation for entrance into mitochondria. Formation of acyl CoA is a two-step process with acyl adenylate as an intermediate product. An additional mechanism is required for transfer of fatty acids across the mitochondrial membrane.[36,37] First, the CoA group is replaced by carnitine, a zwitterionic compound derived from lysine. This replacement is catalyzed by carnitine acyl(palmityol)transferase I.[38] Acyl carnitine passes through the mitochondrial membrane with the assistance of a translocase, and on the inner membrane, carnitine is replaced by CoA under the influence of carnitine acyl(palmityol)transferase II. Within the mitochondria, fatty acids are oxidized by a process called beta-oxidation. Two-carbon fragments are progressively removed, and at each step, one molecule of acetyl CoA is produced. This acetyl CoA can enter the Krebs cycle for oxidation to carbon dioxide and water. Alternatively, two molecules of acetyl CoA can condense to form acetoacetate and β-hydroxybutyrate. The major site of formation of the latter two four-carbon acids is liver.[36] These acids can exit liver and enter other tissues, where they are used as a fuel source. For example, they are readily used by heart muscle and kidney. Although the brain prefers glucose as an energy source, during long-term fasting, brain can convert to utilization of four-carbon acids as a fuel.

Normally, only small amounts of fatty acids are synthesized in liver in humans, although in many animal species that subsist largely on carbohydrate, hepatic fatty acid synthesis can be appreciable. Fatty acid synthesis occurs in liver cytosol, in contrast to oxidation, which occurs in mitochondria. The enzymes required for fatty acid synthesis exist in a complex called fatty acid synthase.[39] Intermediates in fatty acid synthesis are not activated by CoA, but rather by acyl carrier protein.[40] The two-carbon fragments required for elongation of the fatty acid chain are supplied by malonyl-ACP, and carbon dioxide is released in the transfer. The final step in the elongation of fatty acids is palmitic acid.

Fatty acids that are not oxidized in liver cells are incorporated into triacylglycerols.[41] In the first step of triacylglycerol synthesis, activated fatty acid molecules (acyl CoA) are added to glycerol-3-phosphate. Saturated fatty acids usually are added to the sn–1 position, whereas unsaturated fatty acids are preferentially added to the sn–2 position. The phosphate group is removed next, and a final acyl CoA is added to the resulting diacylglycerol to form a triacylglycerol molecule. Triacylglycerols normally are incorporated into lipoproteins for secretion into the circulation.[9] However, if triacylglycerol synthesis exceeds the capacity of lipoprotein formation, the excess triacylglycerol is stored in fat droplets; the result will be a fatty liver.

Muscle Utilization of Fatty Acids

Skeletal muscle is the major site of utilization of both glucose and fatty acids. Glucose is the preferred substrate during acute muscle activity, whereas fatty acids are the major fuel of resting muscle. Muscle has a large capacity to store glucose as glycogen, and it also can store some fatty acids as triacylglycerol.[42] Fatty acids in muscle are oxidized by mechanisms virtually identical to those described for liver. To some extent there is a competi-

tion between glucose and fatty acid for utilization by muscle.[43,44] If free fatty acid levels are high, muscle uptake and oxidation of free fatty acid is increased; this leads to a reduced utilization of glucose. The result is a condition called insulin resistance (i.e., muscle uptake of glucose for a given plasma insulin is decreased). Many investigators believe that insulin resistance is an important contributing cause of adult-onset diabetes mellitus.[45] Obesity leads to increased plasma free fatty acid levels, and the common association between obesity and adult-onset diabetes may be explained in part by an increased resistance to the action of insulin in muscle.

Transport of Endogenous Triacylglycerols

Liver, like gut, makes and secretes a triacylglycerol-rich lipoprotein: VLDL. The major apolipoprotein of VLDL, apo B-100, is synthesized in ribosomes and is transferred to the Golgi, where it is combined with triacylglycerol.[9] Again MTP is responsible for transfer of triacylglycerol into the lipoprotein particle.[11,12] Current evidence suggests that a proportion of newly synthesized apo B-100 is degraded before incorporation into VLDL;[46] the precise amount degraded in humans, however, is not known. VLDL particles are smaller than chylomicrons, which means that they contain less triacylglycerol. Even so, amounts of triacylglycerol in VLDL particles are variable, and when the hepatic content of triacylglycerol increases, VLDL particles have more triacylglycerol. The extent to which the number of VLDL particles secreted by liver varies from one individual to another is not certain. However, the number of newly secreted particles appears to be increased in obesity and the lipoprotein disorder familial combined hyperlipidemia, but measurement of the number of particles secreted in humans has proven difficult.[47–49]

The metabolism of VLDL in the circulation resembles that of chylomicrons. VLDL particles contain some apo E as they are secreted by liver, and they acquire more apo E from high-density lipoprotein (HDL). VLDL also gets apo Cs from HDL. Interaction of VLDL with LPL results in lipolysis of triacylglycerols leaving a VLDL remnant in the plasma.[14] VLDL remnants can have two fates; they can be taken up by liver or be converted to LDL. Normally, about half of the VLDL pool follows each pathway. Hepatic uptake of VLDL remnants may occur similarly to that of chylomicron remnants, but LDL receptors may play a larger role.[19] Conversion of VLDL remnants to LDL may involve interaction with another lipase, hepatic triacylglycerol lipase. This lipase hydrolyzes both triacylglycerols and phospholipids; it may degrade some of the surface coat phospholipids of VLDL remnants as well as remove most of the remaining core triacylglycerols in the conversion to LDL.

Conversion of VLDL remnants to LDL removes all of the apo Cs and apo Es; LDL contains only apo B-100. Its core is composed almost entirely of cholesterol esters. Therefore, LDL seemingly plays little role in triacylglycerol transport. Instead, it is a residual product of endogenous triacylglycerol transport. Although LDL can deliver cholesterol to peripheral tissues, most circulating LDL particles are removed by liver.[50] Hepatic uptake occurs primarily via LDL receptors, which are located on the surface of the liver cell.[20] These receptors bind to the apo B-100 of LDL, and the receptor-LDL complex is taken into the cell. This complex dissociates within the cell; the receptor returns to the cell surface for reuse whereas the LDL enters lysosomes for degradation. LDL receptors are deficient in the disease called familial hypercholesterolemia; hence removal of LDL from plasma is retarded and circulating levels of LDL are increased markedly.[50] In another condition, familial defective apolipoprotein B, the apo B-100 is defective and binds poorly;[51,52] this too leads to a retention of LDL in the circulation. LDL receptors have the capability of binding to apo E, and hence they also are able to remove a portion of VLDL remnants.

HDLs consitute another class of lipoproteins. These are small lipoprotein particles that principally contain apo As (apo A-I and apo A-II).[53] They mainly have cholesterol esters in their cores, but they play an important role in triacylglycerol metabolism. During the catabolism of triacylglycerol-rich lipoproteins, the surface coat components of these lipoproteins (unesterified cholesterol, apo Cs, and apo Es) are transferred to HDL. Apo A-II and most apo A-I come from liver. A portion of HDL apo A-I, however, is derived from chylomicrons. Apo Cs and apo Es are held in reserve in HDL, and they can be transferred back to newly secreted triacylglycerol-rich lipoproteins to assist in their catabolism.[54] HDLs consist of two types: those having both apo A-I and apo A-II and those having apo A-I only.[55] These two forms of HDL may have two different functions, although the differences have not been fully defined.

HDL not only is important for catabolism of triacylglycerol-rich lipoproteins, but also promotes reverse cholesterol transport (transport of cholesterol synthesized in peripheral tissues to liver for excretion).[56] About half of the cholesterol produced by the body appears to be made in peripheral tissues. This excess cholesterol seemingly is picked off the surface of peripheral cells by HDL particles. It is removed from cells in the unesterified form, and it is esterified in HDL through interaction with an enzyme, lecithin-cholesterol acyl transferase;[57] at this time it becomes incorporated into the core of HDL particles. HDL cholesterol esters are then transferred to triacylglycerol-rich lipoproteins by another protein, cholesterol ester transfer protein.[58] This transfer is achieved by exchange of cholesterol ester with triacylglycerols. The resulting HDL triacylglycerols then are hydrolyzed by hepatic triacylglycerol lipase.

Influence of Dietary Fat on Serum Lipid and Lipoproteins

There has been a great interest in the influence of dietary fats on serum lipids and lipoproteins because of the role of the latter in the development of atherosclerosis and CHD. The following discussion reviews the influence of dietary fats on three serum lipid variables: triacylglycerols, LDL, and HDL. The three major categories of fatty acids—saturated, monounsaturated, and polyunsaturated—will be considered. The subclasses of these three major categories of fatty acids also will be examined. The effects of dietary fats further will be compared with carbohydrates, the other major nutrient in the diet. First, however, let us briefly review the relation between serum lipids (and lipoproteins) and CHD; this review may help to put the health impact of different classes of fatty acids into perspective.

Serum lipids, lipoproteins, and atherosclerotic CHD. The major atherogenic lipoprotein is LDL.[59] Evidence of several types indicates that increase in levels of serum LDL is accompanied by increased risk for developing CHD.[59] In large populations, LDL-cholesterol levels are closely correlated with total cholesterol concentrations, and epidemiologic studies demonstrating a positive relationship between total cholesterol levels and CHD risk mainly reflect the influence of LDL-cholesterol levels on CHD risk.[60-63] Further, in genetic forms of elevated LDL (familial hypercholesterolemia[64] and familial defective apo B-100)[51,52], risk for CHD is markedly increased. In support of this relationship, animal models of hypercholesterolemia are accompanied by enhanced rates of atherogenesis.[65-67] Finally, in human clinical trials in which LDL-cholesterol levels were therapeutically lowered, the risk for CHD was significantly reduced.[68-70] All of this evidence combines to establish the atherogenic potential of high levels of circulating LDL levels. Epidemiologic data allow for a quantitative estimate of the relationship between cholesterol levels and CHD risk. According to available data, for every 0.026 mmol/L (1 mg/dL) increase in LDL cholesterol, the risk for CHD is increased by 1–2%.[71] Moreover, a therapeutic reduction of LDL-cholesterol levels produces a reversal of risk of the same size.[68-70]

The mechanisms whereby high LDL levels promote atherosclerosis are relatively straightforward, although many of the fine details are lacking. Circulating LDLs filter through the arterial intima and into the subintimal space, where they initiate the atherosclerotic process. Current concepts suggest that LDL is trapped and modified in this space, and modified LDL becomes a toxic agent that begins atherogenesis. One important modification may be the oxidation of LDL by oxygen free radicals.[72] Some of the modified LDL is taken up by macrophages in the subintimal space; the macrophages become engorged with cholesterol and are transformed into foam cells. In addition, oxidized LDL acts both as an injurious agent and as a chemoattractant that promotes the cellular reactions of plaque development. If there is a single pathogenic agent in the formation of atherosclerosis, it is LDL. Severe atherosclerosis can develop in the presence of markedly elevated LDL cholesterol (e.g., in familial hypercholesterolemia) even in the absence of other risk factors.[64] In contrast, other risk factors (e.g., cigarette smoking, high blood pressure, and diabetes) seemingly produce little atherosclerosis in the absence of a "threshold" elevation of LDL.[73]

In the fasting state, triacylglycerols are transported mainly in VLDL, and triacylglycerol levels reflect VLDL concentrations. Triacylglycerol levels, like cholesterol levels, are positively correlated with risk for CHD.[74] However, the relation between triacylglycerol levels and development of CHD is much more complex than that for LDL cholesterol. This relation apparently is mediated through other factors, which makes it questionable whether high triacylglycerol levels should be considered an independent risk factor for atherosclerosis.[75] Triacylglycerols themselves do not appear in atherosclerotic lesions the way cholesterol does. Nonetheless, smaller, more cholesterol-enriched VLDL seemingly have an atherogenic potential;[76,77] larger, triacylglycerol-laden VLDL are less atherogenic. Even so, all lipoproteins containing apo B-100 (i.e., VLDL, VLDL remnants, and LDL) probably have some atherogenic potential.

High triacylglycerol levels may promote atherosclerosis in other ways.[75] For example, they can induce atherogenic changes in other lipoprotein fractions. High triacylglycerol levels lead to the formation of small, dense LDL particles[78]; data have been reported showing that an excess of these particles increases risk for CHD.[79] Moreover, high triacylglycerols often accompany low HDL levels[75], and as will be discussed below, a low HDL level also is a risk factor for CHD. Finally, high triacylglycerols may induce a thrombogenic state, which increases the likelihood of coronary thrombosis.[75] Although these changes are the more immediate effectors of enhanced risk, they nonetheless have their origins in an elevation of triacylglycerols. Thus, the view about the significance of high triacylglycerols as a risk factor for CHD has moved in a much more positive direction in the past few years, and we have a better understanding of the role of triacylglycerols than we previously had.

A low serum level of HDL is a major risk factor for CHD.[80,81] As for triacylglycerols, the relation between HDL and atherosclerosis appears to be multifactorial: a high serum concentration of HDL may protect against the development of atherosclerosis in several ways. One concept is that HDL may promote reverse cholesterol transport (i.e., the removal of cholesterol from tissues).[56] If so, a high HDL level could reduce cholesterol accumulation within the arterial wall; conversely, a low HDL level might allow for a greater cholesterol accumulation. HDL may have other effects as well. It may retard the oxidation of LDL or prevent the self-aggregation of LDL, both within the arterial wall;[82,83] these effects also could slow down atherogenesis. Thus, HDL appears to be an antiatherogenic lipoprotein, although at present the mechanisms for this action remain somewhat speculative. This lack of understanding of detail, however, does not take away from the fact that low HDL levels are strongly correlated with the occurrence of CHD.

Saturated fatty acids have been indicted as being the major serum cholesterol-raising fatty acids in the diet, and hence the most atherogenic class of fatty acids. The early reports of Ahrens et al.,[84] Keys et al.,[85] and Hegsted et al.,[86] indicating that saturated fatty acids as a class raise serum total cholesterol concentrations have been amply confirmed by other investigators. However, as suggested by reports in the 1960s and confirmed subsequently by other studies, not all saturated fatty acids have the same effects on serum cholesterol levels. In the development of diet–serum cholesterol equations, Keys et al.[85] and Hegsted et al.[86] arbitrarily assigned oleic acid (cis-18:1n–9) to the neutral position (i.e., they assumed that it neither raised nor lowered total cholesterol levels); the responses of other fatty acids were then compared with oleic acid and so rated. It so happens that total cholesterol responses to oleic acid and carbohydrates are almost identical, and this identity justifies the designation of oleic acid as neutral. Saturated fatty acids as a group raise total cholesterol levels relative to oleic acid and thus can be designated cholesterol-raising.[85,86] Later investigations demonstrated that saturated fatty acids raise LDL-cholesterol levels in parallel with increases in total cholesterol, compared with oleic acid,[87] and it is convenient to call oleic acid "neutral" with respect to LDL-cholesterol levels also. In this review, the convention of calling oleic acid a neutral fatty acid will be followed, and the various saturated fatty acids in the diet will be compared with oleic acid for their effects on cholesterol levels.

Palmitic acid is the principal saturated fatty acid in the American diet. It constitutes ≈60% of saturated fatty acids and is present in meat fats, butter fat, and tropical oils. The earlier research of Keys et al.[85] and Hegsted et al.[86] assigned a cholesterol-raising property to palmitic acid, and ensuing investigations confirmed that palmitic acid increases LDL-cholesterol concentrations in parallel with total cholesterol levels.[88–90] Palmitic acid does not raise serum triacylglycerol compared with oleic acid. It may, however, modestly increase HDL-cholesterol levels in some people. Even so, by far the major difference in total cholesterol levels between palmitic acid and oleic acid resides in the LDL-cholesterol concentration.

Two other cholesterol-raising saturated acids are myristic acid (14:0) and lauric acid. These two fatty acids are relatively high in two tropical oils, coconut oil and palm kernel oil. Butter fat also is high in myristic acid. Lauric and myristic acids have not been examined as thoroughly for their effects on cholesterol levels as has palmitic acid. Keys et al.[85] proposed that these two other fatty acids increased cholesterol concentrations to the same extent as did palmitic acid; Hegsted et al.,[86] however, judged that myristic acid is more hypercholesterolemic than palmitic acid whereas lauric acid is less so. In a study in our laboratory, lauric acid was found to raise cholesterol levels relative to oleic acid, but only about two-thirds as much as does palmitic acid.[91] Another study confirmed that myristic acid increases cholesterol levels at least as much as does palmitic acid.[92] Thus, lauric and myristic acids must be added to the list of cholesterol-raising fatty acids.

Stearic acid makes up ≈25% of the saturated fatty acids in the diet. It is particularly high in beef fat and is present in moderate amounts in butter fat. Many studies extending over a period of many years support the impression that stearic acid, in contrast to 12:0–16:0 saturated acids, does not raise serum cholesterol levels. Earlier investigations noted that cocoa butter and beef fat, which are enriched in stearic acid, increase serum cholesterol levels less than would be predicted from their total content of saturated fatty acids.[85,86] A more recent study from our laboratory used a chemically randomized fat that resembled palm oil in composition except that stearic acid replaced palmitic acid.[93] This fat was compared with palm oil and a high-oleic oil in human feeding studies. The high-stearic fat did not raise total cholesterol (or LDL cholesterol) levels compared with the high-oleic oil, whereas palm oil had the expected cholesterol-raising property. Subsequent investigations have provided additional support for stearic acid not being a cholesterol-raising fatty acid.[94,95]

Whether medium-chain (8:0 and 10:0) saturated fatty acids increase cholesterol levels is uncertain. Butter fat is relatively rich in medium-chain fatty acids, and because butter fat is quite hypercholesterolemic, these fatty acids could contribute to this action.[84] However, several studies have failed to confirm that medium-chain fatty acids increase total cholesterol or LDL cholesterol. However, a recent preliminary investigation indicates that medium-chain fatty acids do in fact raise cholesterol levels.[96]

A question of enduring interest concerns how the 12:0–16:0 saturates raise the total cholesterol level or, more specifically, the LDL-cholesterol level. In a broad sense, three possibilities exist: first, these fatty acids could stimulate the secretion of lipoproteins containing apo B-100 into the circulation; second, they could retard the removal of these lipoproteins from plasma; or third, they could lead to the packing of excess cholesterol into each LDL particle. Various studies have postulated each of these mechanisms. It is true that in some individual cases LDL particles may be enriched with cholesterol,[97] but even though this mechanism was once proposed to be an action, more recent studies indicate that it is a minor mechanism, if one at all.[98,99] A few studies in laboratory animals raise the possibility that saturated fatty acids stimulate the secretion of lipoproteins by the liver, but the stronger evidence indicates that they interfere with the clearance of LDL from the circulation.[100] Most likely this effect is the result of suppression of the activity of LDL receptors.

Exactly how 12:0–16:0 saturates can suppress LDL-receptor reactivity remains to be explained. Some researchers have theorized that high intakes of saturates adjusts the physical-chemical organization of hepatic cell-surface phospholipids in a way that impedes the normal cycling of LDL receptors and thus makes them less active. This enticing conjecture, however, is difficult to probe experimentally. Another, and perhaps more likely, theory is that 12:0–16:0 saturates interfere with the synthesis of LDL receptors. One factor that controls the synthesis of LDL receptors is the cellular content of unesterified cholesterol. This cholesterol, acting through sterol regulatory-element binding proteins, suppresses transcription of LDL receptors.[101] Therefore, any agent that augments the accumulation of hepatic unesterified cholesterol should repress LDL-receptor activity. One regulator of unesterified cholesterol content is the rate of formation of cholesterol esters in liver cells. The cholesterol-ester content of liver is boosted by feeding unsaturated fatty acids, whereas it is reduced by saturated fatty acids.[100] The serum cholesterol-raising saturates thus could hinder the esterification of cholesterol and thereby swell the pool of unesterified cholesterol; if so, the synthesis of LDL receptors should be reduced. This mechanism is provocative and attractive and seems to conform best with the experimental data. However, even if this mechanism appertains, it is not necessarily the only way in which 12:0–16:0 saturates increase LDL-cholesterol levels.

Of similar interest is why stearic acid does not elevate LDL-cholesterol concentrations. Several possible mechanisms have been suggested, but again they are difficult to establish. Measurements in laboratory animals have alluded to a reduction in absorption of stearic acid as being the mechanism. If stearic acid were to fail to enter the body, it of course could not heighten serum cholesterol concentrations. Although this mechanism is plausible, our studies indicate that dietary stearic acid is well absorbed in humans.[7,8] If so, another reason must be sought for its failure to lift the serum cholesterol. Another possible basis could be that stearic acid is rapidly converted into oleic acid in the body. Experimental data in both laboratory animals and in humans hint that a substantial portion of newly absorbed stearic acid is in fact transformed into oleic acid once it enters the body.[7] This transformation merely requires the desaturation of stearic acid at the n–9 position. Conversion of palmitic acid to oleic acid, in contrast, is a two-step process: elongation and desaturation. Accessible data suggest that elongation is a slow process whereas desaturation is rapid. In our view, the most likely reason for the failure of stearic acid to increase LDL-cholesterol concentrations is its modification into oleic acid, but other mechanisms also could be at play.

Although 12:0–16:0 saturates boost levels of LDL cholesterol in most people, the degree of response is variable. Some individuals seem to be unusually sensitive to saturated fatty acids and show a marked response, whereas others are relatively resistant and have only a small rise in serum LDL levels.[88] An issue of considerable interest is the basis for this variability, that is, whether it is genetic, environmental, hormonal, or age determined. This question requires further investigation. In some studies, variability in responsiveness within one individual has been found when repeated challenges are carried out;[102–104] this observation suggests that environmental factors are important, although these factors have not been identified. One factor that may affect responsiveness is the baseline level of LDL cholesterol; people having relatively low levels of LDL often demonstrate only a modest increase in serum amounts of LDL when saturates are added to the diet.[105] A few studies suggest that women are less responsive to saturated fatty acids than are men, although this point has not been rigorously proven. In some laboratory animals, increasing cholesterol in the diet will enhance the serum cholesterol response to dietary saturates, and the same may be true to a lesser extent in humans.[106] Finally, some of the variability in responsiveness to 12:0–16:0 saturates may be genetically determined, although the genetic basis for this diversity is yet to be elucidated.

N–6 polyunsaturates. The major fatty acid in this category is linoleic acid, an n–6 polyunsaturate. This fatty acid is derived entirely from plant sources, mainly plant oils. For many years, linoleic acid was classified as a cholesterol-lowering fatty acid. The original studies suggesting this property were those of Kinsell et al.[107–109] and Ahrens et al.[84,110] These workers observed that vegetable oils, which are rich in linoleic acid, reduce serum cholesterol concentrations when compared with animal fats, which are abundant in saturated fatty acids. Other investigators extended these studies, and on the basis of comparisons of various fat sources concluded that linoleic acid lowers cholesterol levels not only relative to saturated fatty acids but also relative to oleic acid.[85,86] These observations reinforced the concept that linoleic acid lowers serum cholesterol levels relative to oleic acid, which is neutral. For many years thereafter, this concept was widely accepted. It led to the notion that the only two significant determinants of serum cholesterol levels are saturates and polyunsaturates (linoleic acid). The polyunsaturate-to-saturate ratio (P/S) was a standard way of predicting the effects of a given diet on cholesterol levels. As a general rule, it was postulated that saturated fatty acids raise cholesterol concentrations about twice as much as polyunsaturates lower them, both relative to the neutral oleic acid.

In more recent years the effects of linoleic acid on plasma lipids and lipoproteins have been reassessed and many studies have been done. These newer investigations have examined effects of linoleic acid on all of the lipoprotein fractions, not just on total cholesterol levels. The results have led to some important new views about the actions of linoleic acid that go beyond the earlier and simple diet equations for the relative effects of saturated fatty acids and linoleic acid. One interesting result of this more recent research has been that both saturated fatty acids and linoleic acid produce a lesser difference relative to oleic acid than was originally thought. The difference is considerably less for linoleic acid.[99] Some recent studies have noted that linoleic acid does in fact have a small cholesterol-lowering effect relative to oleic acid, but others have found little or no difference.[111] If there is a difference, it is relatively small; moreover, the difference is not limited to LDL cholesterol, but extends to all of the lipoprotein fractions.

For example, relative to oleic acid, dietary linoleic acid also reduces the HDL-cholesterol level.[98,99] This difference, however, becomes manifest only when there is a fairly large substitution of linoleic acid for oleic acid in the diet.[111] Finally, in some individuals, high intakes of linoleic acid lead to a reduction in triacylglycerol concentrations. This is an inconsistent effect, and it tends to be more striking in those who have hypertriglyceridemia.[112]

There is no question that dietary linoleic acid lowers LDL-cholesterol concentrations relative to 12:0–16:0 saturates. If the latter were to be arbitrarily taken as baseline, linoleic acid could be considered to have a strong cholesterol-reducing action. In this case, the possible mechanisms of action would be the opposite of those proposed to explain the cholesterol-increasing property of 12:0–16:0 saturates, namely, a reduction in cholesterol content of LDL particles, a decreased secretion of apo B–containing lipoproteins, and an increased activity of LDL receptor activity. Early claims[113] that linoleic acid reduces the cholesterol content of LDL particles but does not reduce the total number of LDL particles in the circulation were not borne out by subsequent experiments.[98,99] Compared with saturated fatty acids, linoleic acid does lower the number of LDL particles in the circulation.[98,99] The possibility exists that linoleic acid limits the secretion of apo B–containing lipoproteins to some extent, because in some people it lowers triacylglycerol levels. The strongest evidence indicates that linoleic acid increases the clearance of LDL from the circulation, most likely via an enhanced LDL-receptor activity.[101] The possible mechanisms for this effect were discussed above under the action of saturated fatty acids and are essentially the opposite for linoleic acid.

An additional question is whether dietary linoleic acid lowers LDL-cholesterol levels relative to oleic acid. Available evidence suggests that it may slightly reduce LDL levels, compared with oleic acid[111], at least in some individuals. Studies in some laboratory animals suggest that linoleic acid does not enhance LDL receptor activity any more than does oleic acid, although the relative effects of the two unsaturated acids seem to differ from one species to another.[100] If linoleic acid reduces the secretion of apo B–containing lipoproteins, whereas oleic acid does not, this could explain the small difference in response found in some studies. Further studies, therefore, are needed to evaluate the relative effects of different types of fatty acids on the secretion of apo B–containing lipoproteins. Finally, the mechanism whereby linoleic acid lowers HDL cholesterol is uncertain; one study, however, suggested that it decreases the synthesis of apo A-I.[114]

N–3 polyunsaturated fatty acids. The parent n–3 polyunsaturated fatty acid is linolenic acid. Common sources of linolenic acid in the diet are soybean oil and rapeseed oil, but the richest source is linseed oil, which is rarely found in the diet. Another source of n–3 polyunsaturates is fish oil. These oils contain the very-long-chain fatty acids EPA and DHA, which are produced by the elongation of linolenic acid. The fish oils come mainly from deep-sea ocean fish. The n–3 polyunsaturates constitute ≈25% of the fatty acids in fish oils.

The major action of n–3 fatty acids on plasma lipoproteins is to lower triacylglycerol levels.[115] They interfere with the incorporation of triacylglycerols into VLDL particles in liver. This leads to a reduction in the amounts of triacylglycerols secreted into the circulation. Apparently, the total number of lipoproteins secreted into plasma is not reduced, only the amount of triacylglycerol in each particle. In patients with hypertriglyceridemia, ingestion of fish oils reduces triacylglycerol levels but does not decrease plasma levels of apo B.[116] This finding suggests that the total number of lipoprotein particles secreted into plasma is not decreased. When fish oils are substituted for saturated fatty acids in the diets of normotriacylglycerolemic individuals, LDL-cholesterol levels fall, just as they do with linoleic acid. Seemingly n–3 fatty acids do not have any unique effects on LDL metabolism or on HDL metabolism.

Trans *monounsaturated fatty acids.* For many years the *trans* monounsaturated fatty acids were considered to be neutral with respect to cholesterol levels, similar to oleic acid. However, in recent years, their actions have been reevaluated. Recent investigations show that the feeding of *trans* fatty acids increases LDL-cholesterol concentrations.[117–120] The rise of LDL appears to be somewhat less than that produced by palmitic acid, but these fatty acids seemingly reduce HDL-cholesterol levels as well. These new findings raise important questions about the safety of *trans* fatty acids. At the least they indicate that the *trans* fatty acids belong among the cholesterol-raising fatty acids.

Cis *monounsaturated fatty acids (oleic acid).* As indicated before, oleic acid can be considered neutral in its effect on the plasma lipoproteins. It was also noted that carbohydrate has an effect on total cholesterol and LDL-cholesterol levels similar to that of oleic acid.[121] However, here the similarity ends. In contrast to dietary oleic acid, carbohydrates raise triacylglycerol levels and lower HDL cholesterol.[121–123] The mechanisms for these differences are not completely understood. High carbohydrate intakes probably increase hepatic output of triacylglycerols, apparently by enriching VLDL particles with triacylglycerols. Oleic acid does not have this effect. In addition, low-fat, high-carbohydrate diets may reduce the activity of LPL, which should retard VLDL-triacylglycerol lipolysis. The cause of the lowering of HDL cholesterol by low-fat, high-carbohydrate diets is not known. Part of this effect could be through the increase in triacylglycerols, but other mechanisms may be present. For example, it has been reported that a high-carbohydrate diet reduces the production of apo A-I, the major apolipoprotein of HDL.[124]

Summary

Dietary fat is an important fuel source for humans, and in the United States and Northern Europe, fat contributes 30–40% of total energy. In many other countries, fat intake is in the range of 15–25% of energy. Because there is a relatively high prevalence of cardiovascular disease in the United States and Northern Europe, high intakes of dietary fat have been implicated as an important causative factor. Many investigators believe that high-fat diets promote the development of obesity and its complications and that they raise serum cholesterol levels. However, the role of percentage fat intake in the causation of obesity remains uncertain. On the other hand, certain fatty acids in the dietary fat mix definitely raise serum cholesterol levels.

The cholesterol-raising fatty acids include three saturated fatty acids (lauric, myristic, and palmitic acid) and the *trans* fatty acids. The recommendation to reduce intakes of cholesterol-raising fatty acids seems prudent.

Serum cholesterol levels will fall as will the risk for cardiovascular disease. Unsaturated fatty acids, whether monounsaturated or polyunsaturated, in contrast, do not raise cholesterol levels. However, there currently is a dispute among authorities whether unsaturated fatty acids in the American diet should be reduced in favor of dietary carbohydrate. Higher intakes of unsaturated fatty acids may promote obesity, whereas high intakes of carbohydrate may reduce HDL-cholesterol levels and raise triacylglycerols. Thus, more research is needed to determine the desirable mix of unsaturated fatty acids and carbohydrate in the American diet.

References

1. National Cholesterol Education Program (1991) Report of the Expert Panel on Population Strategies for Blood Cholesterol Reduction. Circulation 83:2154–2232
2. Nestle M, Woteki CE (1995) Trends in American dietary patterns: research issues and policy implications. In Bronner F (ed), Modern nutrition: topics and controversies. CRC Press, Boca Raton, FL, pp 1–44
3. Craig-Schmidt MD (1992) Fatty acid isomers in foods. In Chow CK (ed), Fatty acids in foods and their health implications. Marcel Decker, New York, pp 365–398
4. Sommerfield M (1983) *Trans* unsaturated fatty acids in natural products and processed foods. Prog Lipid Res 22:221–233
5. Hunter JE, Applewhite TH (1991) Reassessment of *trans* fatty acid availability in the US diet. Am J Clin Nutr 54:363–369
6. Hunter JE, Applewhite TH (1986) Isomeric fatty acids in the US diet: levels and health perspectives. Am J Clin Nutr 44:707–717
7. Bonanome A, Grundy SM (1988) Effect of dietary stearic acid on plasma cholesterol and lipoprotein levels. N Engl J Med 318:1244–1248
8. Bonanome A, Grundy SM (1989) Intestinal absorption of stearic acid after consumption of high fat meals in humans. J Nutr 119:1556–1560
9. Havel RJ, Kane JP (1995) Structure and metabolism of plasma lipoproteins. In Scriver CR, Beaudet AL, Sly WS, Valle D (eds), The metabolic basis of inherited disease, 7th ed. McGraw-Hill, New York, pp 1841–1851
10. Kane JP, Hardman DA, Paulus HE (1980) Heterogeneity of apolipoprotein B: isolation of a new species from human chylomicrons. Proc Natl Acad Sci USA 77:2465–2469
11. Gordon DA, Jamil H, Sharp D, et al (1994) Secretion of apolipoprotein B-containing lipoproteins from HeLa cells is dependent on expression of the microsomal triglyceride transfer protein and is regulated by lipid availability. Proc Natl Acad Sci USA 91:7628–7632
12. Wetterau JR, Aggerbeck LP, Bouma ME, et al (1992) Absence of microsomal triglyceride transfer protein in individuals with abetalipoproteinemia. Science 258:999–1001
13. Isselbacher KJ, Scheig R, Plotkin GR, Caufield JB (1964) Congenital beta lipoprotein deficiency: a hereditary disorder involving a defect in the absorption and transport of lipids. Medicine 43:347–361
14. Olivecrona T, Bengtsson-Olivecrona G (1987) Lipoprotein lipase from milk—the model enzyme in lipoprotein lipase research. In Borensztajn J (ed), Lipoprotein lipase. Evener Publishers, Chicago, p 15
15. Breckenridge WC, Little JA, Steiner G, et al (1978) Hypertri-

16. Rosseneu M, Labeur C (1995) Physiological significance of apolipoprotein mutants. FASEB J 9:768–776
17. Brunzell JD (1989) Familial lipoprotein lipase deficiency and other causes of the chylomicronemia syndrome. In Scriver CR, Beaudet AL, Sly WS, Valle D (eds), The metabolic basis of inherited disease, 6th ed. McGraw-Hill, New York, pp 1165–1180
18. Santamarina-Fojo S, Dugi KA (1994) Structure, function and role of lipoprotein lipase in lipoprotein metabolism. Curr Opin Lipidol 5:117–125
19. Mahley RW, Rall SC Jr (1995) Type III hyperlipoprotein (dysbetalipoproteinemia): the role of apolipoprotein E in normal and abnormal lipoprotein metabolism. In Scriver CR, Beaudet AL, Sly WS, Valle D (eds), The metabolic basis of inherited disease, 7th ed. McGraw-Hill, New York, pp 1953–1980
20. Goldstein JL, Brown MS (1992) Lipoprotein receptors and control of plasma LDL cholesterol levels. Eur Heart J 13(suppl B):34–36
21. Kowal RC, Herz J, Goldstein JL, et al (1989) Low density lipoprotein receptor-related protein mediates uptake of cholesterol esters derived from apoprotein E-enriched lipoproteins. Proc Natl Acad Sci USA 86:5810–5814
22. Shargo E, Spennetta T, Gordon E (1969) Fatty acid synthesis in human adipose tissue. J Biol Chem 244:2761–2766
23. Nestel PJ, Havel RJ, Bezman A (1962) Sites of initial removal of chylomicron triglyceride fatty acids from the blood. J Clin Invest 41:1915–1921
24. Garg A, Fleckstein JL, Peshock RM, Grundy SM (1992) Peculiar distribution of adipose tissue in patients with congenital generalized lipodystrophy. J Clin Endocrinal Metab 75:358–361
25. Steinberg P (1976) Interconvertible enzymes in adipose tissue regulated by cyclic AMP-dependent proteinkinases. Adv Cyclic Nucleotide Res 1:157–198
26. Khoo JC, Steinberg D (1983) Hormone-sensitive lipase of adipose tissue. The enzymes, vol 16, pp 183–204
27. Fain JN, Kovacev VP, Scow RO (1966) Antilipolytic effect of insulin in isolated fat cells of the rat. Endocrinology 78:773–778
28. Strålfors P, Björsell P, Belfrage P (1984) Hormonal regulation of hormone-sensitive lipase in intact adipocytes: identification of phosphorylated sites and effects on the phosphorylation by lipolytic hormones and insulin. Proc Natl Acad Sci USA 81:3317–3321
29. Spector AA (1975) Fatty acid binding to plasma albumin. J Lipid Res 16:165–179
30. Coppack SW, Jensen MD, Miles JM (1994) In vivo regulation of lipolysis in humans. J Lipid Res 35:177–193
31. Gordon RS Jr (1960) Nonesterified fatty acid in blood of obese and lean subjects. Am J Clin Nutr 8:740–747
32. Björntorp P, Bergman H, Varnauskas E (1969) Plasma free fatty acid turnover in obesity. Acta Med Scand 185:351–356
33. Jensen MD, Haymound MW, Rizza RA, et al (1989) Influence of body fat distribution on free fatty acid metabolism in obesity. J Clin Invest 83:1168–1173
34. Abate N, Garg A, Peshock RM, et al (1995) Relationships of generalized and regional adiposity to insulin sensitivity in men. J Clin Invest 96:88–98
35. Sugen MC, Holmes MJ (1994) Interactive regulation of pyruvate dehydrogenase complex and the carnitine palmitoyltransferase system. FASEB J 8:54–61
36. McGarry JD, Foster DW (1980) Regulation of hepatic fatty acid oxidation and ketone body production. Annu Rev Biochem 49:395–420

glyceridemia associated with deficiency of apolipoprotein CII. N Engl J Med 298:1265–1273

37. Murthy MSR, Pande SV (1987) Malmyl-GA binding sites and overt carnitine palmitoyl transferase activity reside on the opposite sides of the outer mitochondrial membrane. Proc Natl Acad Sci USA 84:378–382

38. McGarry JD, Sen A, Esser V, et al (1991) New insights into the mitochondrial carnitine palmitoyltransferase enzyme system. Biochimie 73:77–84

39. Wakil SJ, Stoops JK, Joshi VC (1983) Fatty acid synthesis and its regulation. Annu Rev Biochem 52:537–579

40. Vagelos PR (1973) Acyl group transfer (acyl carrier protein). In Boyer PD (ed), The enzymes, 3rd ed, vol 8, pp 155–199

41. Tijburg LB, Geelem MJ, van Golde LM (1989) Regulation of the biosynthesis of triacylglycerol, phosphatidylcholine and phosphatidylethanolamine in the liver. Biochim Biophys Acta 1004:1–19

42. Gorski J (1992) Muscle triglyceride metabolism during exercise. Can J Physiol Pharmacol 70:123–131

43. Randle PJ, Garland PB, Hales CN, Newsholme EA (1963) The glucose-fatty acid cycle: its role in insulin sensitivity and the metabolic disturbances of diabetes mellitus. Lancet 1:785–789

44. Randle PJ, Priestman DA, Mistry S, Halsall A (1994) Mechanisms modifying glucose oxidation in diabetes mellitus. Diabetalogia 37:5135–5161

45. DeFronzo RA (1988) The triumvirate: B-cell, muscle, liver: a collusion responsible for NIDDM. Diabetes 37:667–687

46. Olofsson S-O, Bostrom K, Carlsson P, et al (1987) Structure and biosynthesis of apolipoprotein B. Am Heart J 113:446–452

47. Kesaniemi YA, Beltz WF, Grundy SM (1985) Comparisons of metabolism of apolipoprotein B in normal subjects, obese patients, and patients with coronary heart disease. J Clin Invest 76:586–595

48. Egusa G, Beltz WF, Grundy SM, Howard BV (1985) Influence of obesity on the metabolism of apolipoprotein B in man. J Clin Invest 76:596–603

49. Chait A, Albers JJ, Brunzell JD (1980) Very low density lipoprotein overproduction in genetic forms of hypertriglyceridaemia. Eur J Clin Invest 10:17–22

50. Brown MS, Goldstein JL (1986) A receptor-mediated pathway for cholesterol homeostasis. Science 232:34–47

51. Vega GL, Grundy SM (1986) In vivo evidence for reduced binding of low density lipoproteins to receptors as a cause of primary moderate hypercholesterolemia. J Clin Invest 78:1410–1414

52. Innerarity TL, Mahley RW, Weisgraber KH, et al (1990) Familial defective apolipoprotein B-100: a mutation of apolipoprotein B that causes hypercholesterolemia. J Lipid Res 31:1337–1349

53. Puchois P, Kandoussi A, Fievet P, et al (1987) Apolipoprotein AI containing lipoproteins in coronary artery disease. Atherosclerosis 68:35–40

54. Eisenberg S (1984) High density lipoprotein metabolism. J Lipid Res 25:1017–1058

55. Montali A, Vega GL, Grundy SM (1994) Concentrations of apolipoprotein AI-containing particles in patients with hypoalphalipoproteinemia. Arterioscler Thromb 14:511–517

56. Von Eckardstein A, Hyong Y, Assman G (1994) Physiological role and chemical relevance of high-density lipoprotein subclasses. Curr Opin Lipidol 5:404–416

57. Glomset JA (1968) The plasma lecithin: cholesterol acyltransferase reaction. J Lipid Res 9:155–167

58. Tall AR (1993) Plasma cholesterol ester transfer protein. J Lipid Res 34:1255–1274

59. Expert Panel on Detection, Evaluation, and Treatment of High Blood Cholesterol in Adults (1994) The second report of the National Cholesterol Education Program (NCEP) expert panel on detection, evaluation, and treatment of high blood cholesterol in adults (Adult Treatment Panel II). Circulation 89:1239–1445

60. Gordon T, Kannel WB, Castelli WP, et al (1981) Lipoproteins, cardiovascular disease and death: the Framingham study. Arch Intern Med 141:1128–1131

61. Stamler J, Wentworth D, Neaton JD (1986) Is the relationship between serum cholesterol and risk of premature death from coronary heart disease continuous and graded? findings in 356,222 primary screens of the Multiple Factor Intervention Trial (MRFIT). JAMA 256:2823–2828

62. Keys A, Aravanis C, Blackburn H, et al (1980) Seven countries: a multivariate analysis of death and coronary heart disease. Harvard University Press, Cambridge, MA

63. Kagan A, Harris BR, Winkelstein W Jr, et al (1974) Epidemiologic studies of coronary heart disease and stroke in Japanese men living in Japan, Hawaii and California: demographic, physical, dietary and biochemical characteristics. J Chronic Dis 27:345–364

64. Goldstein JL, Hobbs HH, Brown MS (1995) Familial hypercholesterolemia. In Scriver CR, Beaudet AL, Sly WS, Valle D (eds), The metabolic basis of inherited disease, 7th ed. McGraw Hill, New York, pp 1981–2030

65. McGill HC Jr, McMahan CA, Kruski AW, et al (1981) Relationship of lipoprotein cholesterol concentrations to experimental atherosclerosis in baboons. Arteriosclerosis 1:3–12

66. Armstrong ML, Warner ED, Connor WE (1970) Regression of coronary atheromatosis in rhesus monkeys. Circ Res 27:59–67

67. Clarkson TB, Bond MG, Bullock BC, et al (1981) A study of atherosclerosis regression in Macaca mulatta. IV. Changes in coronary arteries from animals with atherosclerosis induced for 19 months and then regressed for 24 or 48 months at plasma cholesterol concentrations of 300 or 200 mg/dl. Exp Mol Pathol 34:345–368

68. Lipid Research Clinics Program (1984) The Lipid Research Clinics coronary primary prevention trial results. I. Reduction in the incidence of coronary heart disease. JAMA 251:351–364

69. Scandinavian Simvastatin Survival Study Group (1994) Randomised trial of cholesterol lowering in 4444 patients with coronary heart disease: the Scandinavian Simvastatin Survival Study (4S). Lancet 344:1383–1389

70. Sheperd J, Cobbe SM, Ford I, et al (1995) Prevention of coronary heart disease with pravastatin in men with hypercholesterolemia. N Engl J Med 333:1301–1307

71. Davis C, Rifkind B, Brenner H, Gordon D (1990) A single cholesterol measurement underestimates the risk of CHD: an empirical example from the Lipid Research Clinics mortality follow-up study. JAMA 264:3044–3046

72. Steinberg D, Parthasarathy S, Carew TE, et al (1989) Beyond cholesterol: modifications of low-density lipoproteins that increase its atherogenicity. N Engl J Med 320:915–923

73. Grundy SM, Wilhelmsen L, Rose G, et al (1990) Coronary heart disease in high-risk populations: lessons from Finland. Eur Heart J 11:462–471

74. Austin MA (1991) Plasma triglyceride and coronary heart disease. Arterioscler Thromb 11:2–14

75. Grundy SM, Vega GL (1992) Two different views of the relationship of hypertriglyceridemia to coronary heart disease: implications for treatment. Arch Intern Med 152:28–34

76. Tatami R, Mabuchi H, Ueda K, et al (1981) Intermediate-density lipoprotein and cholesterol-rich very low density lipoprotein in angiographically determined coronary artery disease. Circulation 64:1174–1184

77. Krauss RM, Williams PT, Brensike J, et al (1987) Intermediate-density lipoproteins and progression of coronary artery disease in hypercholesterolemic men. Lancet 2:62–66

78. Austin MA, Breslow JL, Hennekens CH, et al (1988) Low-density lipoprotein subclass patterns and risk of myocardial infarction. JAMA 260:1917–1921

79. Austin MA, King MC, Vranizan KM, Krauss RM (1990) Atherogenic lipoprotein phenotype: a proposed genetic marker for coronary heart disease risk. Circulation 82:495–506

80. Miller GJ, Miller NE (1975) Plasma high density lipoprotein concentration and development of ischaemic heart disease. Lancet 1:16–19

81. Gordon DJ, Probstfeld JL, Garrison RJ (1989) High-density lipoprotein cholesterol and cardiovascular disease: four prospective American series. Circulation 79:8–15

82. Parthasarathy S, Barnett J, Fong LG (1990) High density lipoprotein inhibits the oxidative modification of low density lipoprotein. Biochim Biophys Acta 1044:275–283

83. Khoo JC, Miller E, McLoughlin P, Steinberg D (1990) Prevention of low density lipoprotein aggregation by high density lipoprotein or apolipoprotein A-I. J Lipid Res 31:645–658

84. Ahrens EH, Hirsch J, Insull W, et al (1957) The influence of dietary fats on serum-lipid levels in man. Lancet 1:943–953

85. Keys A, Anderson JT, Grande F (1965) Serum cholesterol response to changes in the diet. IV. Particular saturated fatty acids in the diet. Metabolism 14:776–787

86. Hegsted DM, McGandy RB, Myers ML, Stare FJ (1965) Quantitative effects of dietary fat on serum cholesterol in man. Am J Clin Nutr 17:281–295

87. Grundy SM, Denke MA (1990) Dietary influences on serum lipids and lipoproteins. J Lipid Res 31:1149–1172

88. Grundy SM, Vega GL (1988) Plasma cholesterol responsiveness to saturated fatty acids. Am J Clin Nutr 47:822–824

89. Mensink RP, Katan MB (1989) Effect of a diet enriched with monounsaturated or polyunsaturated fatty acids on levels of low-density and high-density lipoprotein cholesterol in healthy women and men. N Engl J Med 321:436–441

90. Grundy SM, Florentin L, Nix D, Whelan MF (1988) Comparison of monounsaturated fatty acids and carbohydrates for reducing raised levels of plasma cholesterol in man. Am J Clin Nutr 47:965–969

91. Denke MA, Grundy SM (1992) Comparison of effects of lauric acid and palmitic acid on plasma lipids and lipoproteins. Am J Clin Nutr 56:895–898

92. Zock PL, de Vries JHM, Katan MB (1994) Impact of myristic acid versus palmitic acid on serum lipid and lipoprotein levels in healthy women and men. Arterioscler Thromb 14:567–575

93. Bonanome A, Grundy SM (1988) Effect of dietary stearic acid on plasma cholesterol and lipoprotein levels. N Engl J Med 318:1244–1248

94. Denke MA, Grundy SM (1991) Effects of fats high in stearic acid on lipid and lipoprotein concentrations in men. Am J Clin Nutr 54:1036–1040

95. Kris-Etherton PM, Derr J, Mitchell DC (1993) The role of fatty acid saturation on plasma lipids, lipoproteins, and apolipoprotein. I. Effects of whole food diets high in cocoa butter, olive oil, soybean oil, dairy butter, and milk chocolate on the plasma lipids of young men. Metabolism 42:121–129

96. Cater NB, Heller HJ, Denke MA (1995) Effects of medium-chain triglycerides on lipids and lipoproteins. Circulation 92(suppl 1):I–351

97. Abate N, Vega GL, Grundy SM (1993) Variability in cholesterol content and physical properties of lipoproteins containing apolipoprotein B-100. Atherosclerosis 104:159–171

98. Vega GL, Groszek E, Wolf R, Grundy SM (1982) Influence of polyunsaturated fats on plasma lipoprotein composition apolipoprotein. J Lipid Res 23:811–822

99. Mattson FH, Grundy SM (1985) Comparison of effects of dietary saturated, monounsaturated, and polyunsaturated fatty acids on plasma lipids and lipoproteins in man. J Lipid Res 26:194–202

100. Dietschy JM, Turley SD, Spady DK (1993) Role of liver in the maintenance of cholesterol and low density lipoprotein homeostasis in different animal species, including humans. J Lipid Res 34:1637–1659

101. Briggs MR, Yokoyama C, Wang X, et al (1993) Nuclear protein that binds sterol regulatory element of low density lipoprotein receptor promoterm. I. Identification of the protein and delineation of its target nucleotide sequence. J Biol Chem 268:14490–14496

102. Beynen AC, Katan MB, van Zutphen LFM (1987) Hypo- and hyperresponders: individual differences in the response of serum cholesterol concentrations to changes in diet. Adv Lipid Res 22:115–171

103. Katan MB, van Gastel AC, de Rover CM, et al (1988) Differences in individual responsiveness of serum cholesterol to fat-modified diets in man. Eur J Clin Invest 18:644–647

104. Katan MB, Burns MAM, Glatz JFC, et al (1988) Congruence of individual responsiveness to dietary cholesterol and to saturated fat in man. J Lipid Res 29:883–892

105. Hayes KC, Khosla P (1992) Dietary fatty acid thresholds and cholesterolemia. FASEB J 6:2600–2607

106. Fielding CJ, Havel RJ, Todd KM, et al (1995) Effects of dietary cholesterol and fat saturation on plasma lipoproteins in an ethnically diverse population of healthy young men. J Clin Invest 95:611–618

107. Kinsell LW, Partridge J, Boling L, et al (1952) Dietary modification of serum cholesterol and phopholipid levels. J Clin Endocrinol 12:909–913

108. Kinsell LW, Michaels GD, Partridge JW, et al (1953) Effect upon serum cholesterol and phospholipids of diets containing large amounts of vegetable fat. J Clin Nutr 1:231–244

109. Kinsell LW, GD Michael (1955) Letter to the editor. Am J Clin Nutr 3:247–253

110. Ahrens EH Jr, Blankenhorn DH, Tsaltas TT (1954) Effect on human serum lipids of substituting plant for animal fat in diet. Proc Soc Exp Biol Med 86:872–878

111. Mensink RP, Katan MB (1992) Effects of dietary fatty acids on serum lipids and lipoproteins: a meta-analysis of 27 trials. Arteriosclerosis 12:911–919

112. Grundy SM (1975) Effects of polyunsaturated fats on lipid metabolism in patients with hypertriglyceridemia. J Clin Invest 55:269–282

113. Spritz N, Mishkel MA (1969) Effects of dietary fats on plasma lipids and lipoproteins: a hypothesis for the lipid-lowering effect of unsaturated fatty acids. J Clin Invest 48:78–86

114. Shepherd J, Packard CJ, Patsch JR (1978) Effects of dietary polyunsaturated and saturated fat on the properties of high density lipoproteins and the metabolism of apolipoprotein A-I. J Clin Invest 1582–1592

115. Connor WE (1986) Hypolipidemic effects of dietary omega-3 fatty acids in normal and hyperlipidemic humans: effectiveness and mechanisms. In Simopoulos AP, Kifer RR, Martin RE (eds), Health effects of polyunsaturated fatty acids in seafoods. Academic Press, Orlando, FL, pp 173–210

116. Failor RA, Childs MT, Bierman EL (1988) The effects of w3 and w6 fatty acid-enriched diets on plasma lipoproteins and apoproteins in familial combined hyperlipidemia. Metabolism 37:1021–1028

117. Mensink RP, Katan MB (1990) Effect of dietary *trans* fatty acids on high-density and low-density lipoprotein cholesterol levels in healthy subjects. N Engl J Med 323:439–445

118. Zock PL, Katan MB (1992) Hydrogenation alternatives: effects of *trans* fatty acids and stearic acid versus linoleic acid on serum lipids and lipoproteins in humans. J Lipid Res 33:399–410

119. Lichtenstein AH, Ausman LM, Carrasco W, et al (1993) Effects of canola, corn and olive oils on fasting and postprandial plasma lipoproteins in humans as part of a National Cholesterol Education Program Step 2 diet. Arterioscler Thromb 13:1533–1542

120. Judd JT, Clevidence BA, Meusing RA, et al (1994) Dietary trans fatty acid: effects on plasma lipids and lipoproteins of healthy men and women. Am J Clin Nutr 59:861–868

121. Grundy SM (1986) Comparison of monounsaturated fatty acids and carbohydrates for lowering plasma cholesterol. N Engl J Med 314:745–748

122. Mensink RP, Katan MB (1987) Effect of monounsaturated fatty acids versus complex carbohydrates on high-density lipoproteins in healthy men and women. Lancet 1:122–125

123. Mensink RP, de Groot MJM, van den Broeke LT, et al (1989) Effects of monounsaturated fatty acids v complex carbohydrates on serum lipoproteins and apoproteins in healthy men and women. Metabolism 38:172–178

124. Brinton EA, Eisenberg S, Breslow JL (1990) A low fat diet decreases high density lipoprotein (HDL) cholesterol levels by decreasing HDL apolipoprotein transport rates. J Clin Invest 85:144–151

Chapter 7

Essential Dietary Lipids

Sheila M. Innis

Fat, together with protein and carbohydrate, was recognized as an essential component of the diet about 170 years ago. Still, as late as 1920 it was believed that dietary fat fulfilled no essential role, provided sufficient quantities of fruits and vegetables to supply vitamins and minerals were eaten daily.[1] Later that decade, advances in the use of semipurified diets containing sucrose rather than starch allowed Evans and Burr[2-4] to demonstrate impaired growth and reproductive failure in animals fed fat-free diets. They suggested the possibility of a new vitamin, "vitamine F," and in classic papers, Burr and Burr[5,6] introduced the concept of essential fatty acids, specifically linoleic acid as a fatty acid that cannot be made by the body. Deficiency symptoms, which included scaliness of the skin and increased water consumption without increased urine output, that could be reversed by linoleic acid were described. Hansen in 1933 reported on the use of oils to treat eczema in infants, and in 1958 and 1963, through studies with infants fed skim milks, he and his coworkers were able to show that humans required a dietary source of fat.[7-9] The importance of essential fatty acids in clinical nutrition became widely accepted with the advent of intravenous feeding with eucaloric or hypercaloric solutions of glucose and amino acids for patients unable to receive enteral nutrition. The high insulin levels caused by nutrient infusions led to inhibition of adipose tissue lipase activity and fatty acid release, resulting in clinical symptoms of essential fatty acid deficiency despite large tissue reserves.

Reports linking a dietary deficiency of n–3 fatty acids to abnormal electroretinographic recordings in animals were published in the early 1970s.[10,11] The essentiality of n–3 fatty acids in human nutrition, however, has been more difficult to establish because of the small amounts required and because brain and retina avidly retain n–3 fatty acids even during long-term deficiency.[12-16] The optimum amount of n–3 fatty acids in the diet, and the biochemical explanation for the crucial role these fatty acids play in the central nervous system, are areas of intensive research. There is, however, no longer any doubt that a dietary source of n–3 fatty acids is essential for optimum tissue function.[17]

The presence in tissue of substances with vasodilating properties was recognized as early as 1913, and in 1930 the effect of semen in causing relaxation and contraction of the uterus was described.[18,19] Shortly thereafter, the active factor was identified as lipid-soluble and named prostaglandin by von Euler, but it was not until the early 1960s that the structure of prostaglandin E_1 (PGE_1) was identified, and the middle 1970s that thromboxane A_2 (TXA_2) and prostacyclin (PGI_2) were discovered. The term "eicosanoids" was introduced in 1980 to describe substances with 20 carbon atoms derived from n–6 and n–3 fatty acids. Although the importance of several of the eicosanoids in normal physiological processes and in certain disease states is understood, the effects of many metabolites have yet to be determined.[18-22] The roles of dietary n–6 and n–3 fatty acids can now be considered to include the specific roles of certain n–6 and n–3 fatty acids related to their positions in membrane phospholipids and to maintaining the precursor pool of n–6 fatty acids used for synthesis of eicosanoids.

Fatty Acid Nomenclature

Fatty acids are commonly referred to using a shorthand notation in which the first number denotes the number of carbon atoms in the acyl chain, followed by a colon, then a number to indicate the number of unsaturated bonds, and a symbol n– (or ω) followed by the number of carbon atoms from the methyl end of the acyl chain to the first double bond (Figure 1). Common names and the shorthand notation for several of the more usual fatty acids are in Table 1. Note that in the systematic nomenclature, the carbons are numbered from the carboxy end of the chain.

Fatty Acid Metabolism

Mammalian cells are able to synthesize saturated and n–9 and n–7 series unsaturated fatty acids de novo from acetyl CoA, but lack the delta (Δ) 12 and 15 desaturase enzymes necessary for insertion of a double bond at the n–6 and n–3 positions, respectively, of the fatty acid carbon chain.[17,23] The dietary essential fatty acids are li-

Saturated

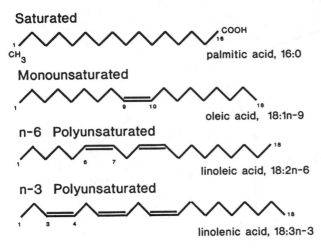

Figure 1. Saturated, n–9 monounsaturated, and n–6 and n–3 polyunsaturated fatty acids.

noleic acid (18:2n–6) and linolenic acid (18:3n–3). Longer-chain, more unsaturated n–6 and n–3 fatty acids, including arachidonic acid (20:4n–6), eicosapentaenoic acid (20:5n–3), and docosahexaenoic acid (22:6n–3), are synthesized from 18:2n–6 and 18:3n–3 by alternating desaturation and elongation (Figure 2). The enzymes responsible for desaturation are named by the position in the fatty acid carbon chain, counting from the carboxy terminal, at which the double bond is inserted (Figure 1). The synthesis of 20:4n–6 from 18:2n–6, and of 20:5n–3 from 18:3n–3, is accomplished by Δ6 desaturation, elongation, and Δ5 desaturation. These desaturases are membrane-bound enzymes that occur in the endoplasmic reticulum of many tissues, for example, liver, intestinal mucosa, brain, and retina.[17,23–27] They require an electron transport chain from the reduced form of nicotinamide adenine dinucleotide (NADH) or the reduced form of nicotinamide adenine dinucleotide phosphate (NADPH) catalyzed by cytochrome b_5. The activity of the Δ6 desaturase is altered by a variety of hormonal and dietary factors. For example, insulin and essential fatty

acid–deficient diets increase, whereas glucose, epinephrine, and glucagon decrease, desaturase enzyme activity.[28] In vitro, there is preferential desaturation in order 18:3n–3 > 18:2n–6 > 8:1n–9. High dietary intakes of 20:5n–3 and 22:6n–3, most usually from fish and fish oils, increase the amounts of 20:5n–3 and 22:6n–3 in plasma and tissue phospholipids and also reduce 20:4n–6. The decrease in 20:4n–6 is explained by inhibition of the Δ6 and Δ5 desaturases, reducing synthesis of 20:4n–6 from 18:2n–6, and by competition between 20:4n–6 and 20:5n–3 for acylation into phospholipids.

The final steps involved in the synthesis of 22:6–3 were only recently elucidated.[23,29] These are now known to occur by elongation of 20:5n–3→ 22:5n–3→ 24:5n–3, then Δ6 desaturation to 24:6n–3, and partial β-oxidation to 22:6n–3. The synthesis of 22:5n–6 occurs by a similar pathway; that is, 22:4n–6→ 24:4n–6→ 24:5n–6 to 22:5n–6.[30] The evidence for chain length–specific Δ6 desaturases (i.e., for 18:2n–6 and 18:3n–3, and 24:4n–6 and 24:5n–3) is not yet conclusive. However, the desaturation of 24:5n–3 is inhibited in a dose-dependent manner by 18:3n–3.[23]

The oxidation of 20:4n–6, 20:5n–3, and 22:6n–3, unlike that of shorter-chain polyunsaturated fatty acids, e.g., 18:2n–6 and 18:3n–3, involves peroxisomal metabolism. Chain shortening of 22:6n–3 to 20:5n–3 requires saturation of the double bond by 2-*trans*-4 *cis*-dienylo-reductase and rearrangement of the double-bond structure by Δ3-*cis*-Δ2-*trans*-enoyl-CoA isomerase, both of which occur in peroxisomes.[23] The conversion of 24:6n–3 to 22:6n–3, and presumably 24:5n–6 to 22:5n–6, involves one cycle of β-oxidation without elimination of double bonds, and occurs in some site other than the endoplasmic reticulum.[30] What controls continued catabolism via oxidation and generation of energy, as opposed to acylation into membrane lipids, is not yet known.[23] Inborn errors of metabolism leading to absence of, or abnormality in, peroxisomal metabolism often include problems in the synthesis and oxidation of long-chain fatty

Table 1. Common and systematic names of some dietary fatty acids

Systematic name	Common name	Symbol
Octanoic	Caprylic	8:0
Decanoic	Capric	10:0
Dodecanoic	Lauric	12:0
Tetradecanoic	Myristic	14:0
Hexadecanoic	Palmitic	16:0
Octadecanoic	Stearic	18:0
9-Octadecaenoic	Oleic	18:1n–9
9,12-Octadecadienoic	Linoleic	18:2n–6
6,9,12-Octadecatrienoic	γ-Linolenic	18:3n–6
9,12,15-Octadecatrienoic	α-Linolenic	18:3n–3
5,8,11,14-Eicosatetraenoic	Arachidonic	20:4n–6
5,8,11,14,17-Eicosapentaenoic	EPA	20:5n–3
4,7,10,13,16,19-Docosahexaenoic	DHA	22:6n–3

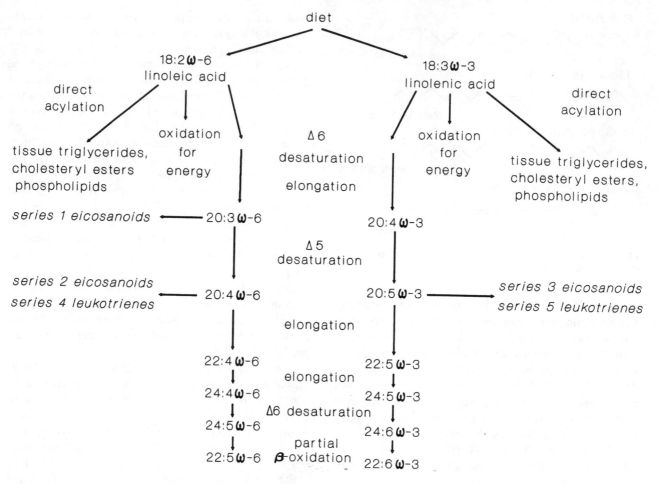

Figure 2. Potential pathways of n–6 and n–3 acid metabolism.

acids.[31] An example is the inability of fibroblasts from patients with Zellweger syndrome (an inborn error of metabolism with an absence of peroxisomes) to convert (retroconversion) 22:6n–3 to 20:5n–3.[32]

Dietary Sources of Essential Fatty Acids

The major dietary sources of 18:2n–6 and 18:3n–3 are polyunsaturated fatty acid–rich vegetable oils. The relative proportions and amounts of 18:2n–6 and 18:3n–3 differ widely among different oils. The composition of some common oils is presented in Table 2. For example, 18:2n–6 is particularly high in sunflower, safflower, corn, and soybean oils. Soybean, linseed, and canola oils are all high in 18:3n–3. In contrast, corn, sunflower, and safflower oils all contain very low amounts of 18:3n–3 (<1% fatty acids), and when fed as the single dietary source of polyunsaturated fat,

Table 2. Typical fatty acid composition of some vegetable oils (% of fatty acids)

Oil	14:0	16:0	18:0	18:1	18:2n–6	18:3n–3	20:0	20:1
Soybean		10	4	25	54	7		
Safflower		7	2	14	76	0.5		
Sunflower		7	5	19	68	1		
Corn		11	4	24	54	1		
Olive		13	3	71	10	1	1	1
Canola		4	2	62	22	10		
Palm	1	45	4	40	10	1		
Cottonseed	1	22	3	19	54	1		
Peanut		11	2	48	32		1	2
Linseed		5	4	21	16	54		

these oils result in n–3 fatty acid deficiency. Some oils, such as olive and canola oils, contain high amounts of the monounsaturated fatty acid oleic acid (18:1n–9). Some more unusual oils, including evening primrose, borage, and blackcurrant seed oils, contain relatively high levels of γ-linolenic acid (18:3n–6), which is the Δ6 desaturation product of 18:2n–6. Vegetable oils and fats do not contain C20 or 22 n–6 or n–3 fatty acids. Foods of animal origin, particularly egg yolk and meat, liver, and other organ meats, contain 20:4n–6 and 22:6n–3. The longer-chain n–3 fatty acids, 20:5n–3 and 22:6n–3, are found in highest amounts in high-fat fish and in marine mammals.

Dietary n–6 and n–3 Fatty Acid Requirements

Dietary requirements for 18:2n–6 and 18:3n–3 have been estimated from the intake required to prevent or reverse deficiency symptoms in animals and humans and to achieve maximum tissue levels of 20:4n–6 and 22:6n–3 in animals. Intakes of about 2.4% of dietary energy as 18:2n–6 support maximum tissue levels of 20:4n–6 in rodents and prevent the appearance of signs of n–6 fatty acid deficiency in human infants and adults.[8,9,17,33] Recommended dietary intakes of linoleic acid are usually about 3–5% of dietary energy.[34] A dietary intake of 0.5–1.0% of energy from 18:3n–3 gives maximum tissue levels of 22:6n–3 and also avoids any apparent deficiency symptoms.[35–39] A potential need for dietary 20:4n–6 and 22:6n–3 in some groups, particularly newborn infants, is a major area of current study.[40] With the possible exception of the Felinae, no mammalian species has yet been found to require dietary 20:4n–6 and 22:6n–3.[17] It is not yet clear why some studies have found lower visual acuity in infants fed formulas without 22:6n–3 than in breast-fed infants,[41] while the studies in North America have not found differences.[37] Possibly, differences in the 18:3n–3 content of the formula, or some inherent environmental or genetic differences between the breast-fed and formula-fed infants, may explain the discrepancies. Very premature infants have special nutrient needs, which often exceed the needs of healthy term infants. The essential fatty acid requirements of very premature infants (infants with a birthweight below 1500 g), including the possibility of a need for dietary 20:4n–6 and 22:6n–3, is an area of intense clinical research.[40,42] One study has reported higher visual acuity in premature infants fed 22:6n–3 than in infants fed 18:3n–3 as the only dietary n–3 fatty acid.[43] This potential benefit in visual function was no longer evident after 6 months of age; thus, the long-term significance of dietary 22:6n–3 is still unclear.

Deficiency of 18:2n–6 and 18:3n–3 due to inadequate intake or malabsorption results in increased desaturation of 16:0 and 18:1 to 16:1n–7 and 20:3n–9, respectively. Under normal circumstances the preference of Δ6 desaturase for 18:3n–3 and 18:2n–6 prevents accumulation of 16:1n–7 and 20:3n–9.[28] Usually a ratio of 20:3n–9 to 20:4n–6 (known as the triene-tetraene ratio) of >0.2 is taken to indicate deficiency of n–6 and n–3 fatty acids. Deficiency of 18:3n–3 in the presence of adequate 18:2n–6 leads to increased synthesis of 22:5n–6.[17] Thus, calculation of the 22:5n–6:22:6n–3 ratio in tissue phospholipids can be a sensitive index of n–3 fatty acid deficiency.[35] Typical North American diets provide 7% of energy as linoleic acid (18:2n–6), much more than needed to prevent deficiency.[44] However, high intakes of 18:2n–6 with low intakes of 18:3n–3 (because of hydrogenation of polyunsaturated oils) and relatively low intakes of 20:5n–3 and 22:6n–3 could result in competitive pressure against n–3 fatty acids. Whether this has any undesirable physiological effects, for example, in increasing the risk of certain diseases, is not known.[44]

Metabolic Roles of Essential Fatty Acids

The enzymes that incorporate fatty acids into glycerolipids place saturated fatty acids at the sn-1 position and C16 and C18 unsaturated fatty acids at the sn-2 position.[44] Remodeling enzymes involved in phospholipid metabolism then place C20 and 22 n–6 and n–3 fatty acids at the sn-2 position.[45] These enzyme selectivities result in phospholipids with about 41–46% saturated fatty acids, 32–35% C16 and 18 unsaturated fatty acids, and 20–25% C20 and 22 n–6 and n–3 fatty acids, and triacylglycerols with about 30% saturated fatty acids, 60% C16 and 18 unsaturated fatty acids, and 2–5% C20 and 22 n–6 and n–3 fatty acids.

Phospholipids (for example, phosphatidylethanolamine, phosphatidylserine, phosphatidylcholine, and phosphatidylinositol) are a crucial component of the structural matrix of all cell and subcellular membranes. The fatty acid composition of membrane phospholipids is in part determined by the n–6 and n–3 fatty acid composition of the diet. As a result, dietary fat composition can influence several membrane-related functions, such as hormone binding and associated enzyme and transporter activities. The n–6 and n–3 fatty acids, however, are not irreplaceable components of membrane phospholipids, and it is difficult to consider their essentiality from this perspective.

Essential Fatty Acids as Precursors of Eicosanoids

Enzymatic metabolism of 20:3n–6, 20:4n–6, and 20:5n–3 fatty acids by cyclooxygenase and lipoxygenase produces a wide range of oxidized products, collectively known as eicosanoids.[19-21] These eicosanoids are important and potent mediators of many biochemical processes and play a critical role in the coordinating physiological interactions among cells. Oxidized products of 20:4n-6 are also formed by cytochrome P450 through omega hydroxygenation and epoxygenation.[46] Nonenzymatic peroxidation produces a variety of products with prostaglandin-like structures known as isoprostanes.[47] The physiological effects of many of these compounds are not yet known. Although the discovery of eicosanoids as products of n-6 and n-3 fatty acid metabolism is relatively recent, it now seems likely that many of the signs of essential fatty acid deficiency may be due to changes in eicosanoid metabolism. For example, some of the problems with growth and reproduction may involve the role of eicosanoids in hypothalamic and pituitary hormone release and in enhancing the response of the thyroid to thyroid-stimulating hormone.[44] Either of the n-6 or n-3 fatty acids can support growth, development, and gestation, but dermal and renal integrity and parturition depend specifically on n-6 fatty acids.[44] The role of n-6 fatty acids in parturition seems to involve n-6 fatty acid–derived eicosanoids. The essentiality of n-6 fatty acids for normal dermal integrity, however, relates to a specific role of linoleic acid (18:2n-6) in the o-linoleoyl-ceramides, which form part of the lipid bilayers (lamellae) that fill the intercellular spaces in the upper part of the epidermis (stratum corneum).[47-49] In essential fatty acid deficiency, 18:1n-9 (oleic acid) replaces 18:2n-6, and this is accompanied by changes in the epidermal water barrier function and epidermal hyperproliferation. The biochemical explanation for these defects is not clear, but it is known that the changes are more effectively reversed by 18:2n-6 than 20:4n-6, and that the n-3 fatty acids, 18:3n-3, 20:5n-3, and 22:6n-3, are ineffective. Other specific roles for various n-6 fatty acids also are still being discovered. For example, 1-O-alkyl-2-arachidonyl phosphatidylcholine is the precursor of platelet-activating factor, a potent chemoattractant and chemical mediator. Another recent and exciting area of research in lipids is the effect of n-6 and n-3 fatty acids on gene expression. Several studies have shown that n-6 and n-3 fatty acids influence the expression of genes involved in regulation of cell growth and genes for a variety of enzymes.[50,51] The application of this to further understanding of the role of dietary lipids in human health and disease is likely to generate much interest in future years.

The nutritional essentiality of n-6 and n-3 fatty acids can now be considered to include the roles as precursors for formation of eicosanoids, as well as specific roles of 18:2n-6, 20:4n-6, and 22:6n-3 in a variety in normal physiological processes. No essential metabolic role for 18:3n-3, other than as a precursor for synthesis of 20:5n-3 and 22:6n-3, has yet been identified.

Eicosanoids derived from 20:4n-6 seem to be most important under normal circumstances. This is explained by the higher content of 20:4n-6 than of 20:3n-6 or 20:5n-3 in most membrane phospholipids, and a lower specificity of cycloxygenase for 20:3n-6 and 20:5n-3 than for 20:4n-6. Prostaglandins derived from 20:3n-6, 20:4n-6, and 20:5n-3 are known as the series 1, series 2, and series 3, respectively (for example, PGE_1, PGI_2, and PGI_3 are derived from 20:3n-6, 20:4n-6, or 20:5n-3, respectively), and series 4 leukotrienes and series 5 leukotrienes are formed from 20:4n-6 or 20:5n-3, respectively (Figure 2). In many cases, the eicosanoids formed from 20:5n-3 oppose or have weaker effects than the eicosanoids formed from 20:4n-6. For example, platelet aggregation is supported more actively with eicosanoids from 20:4n-6 than from 20:5n-3, and this may be a reason for the lower mortality from acute thrombosis in individuals with high intakes of 20:5n-3.[44] Changes in the synthesis of the eicosanoids may be involved in a variety of pathophysiological conditions.[18-20,22,44] For example, the cyclooxygenase products, thromboxane and prostacyclin, regulate thrombosis; the leukotrienes produced by the lipoxygenase pathway are powerful chemotactic agents and play a major role in inflammation and smooth muscle contraction. Production of eicosanoids may also be important in atherosclerosis and other vascular disorders.

Synthesis of eicosanoids is initiated by generation of free 20:4n-6 and the availability of various cofactors. The major substrate pool is generally considered to be phospholipids with 20:4n-6 at the sn-2 position, and tissue levels of unesterified 20:4n-6 are generally very low.[21] Dietary fat composition can, therefore, influence eicosanoid synthesis by influencing the substrate pool of n-6 and n-3 fatty acids available. High dietary intakes of 20:5n-3 increase tissue concentration of 20:5n-3 and reduce that of 20:4n-6. As a result, manipulation of dietary fat, or supplementation with 20:5n-3, can be used to modify physiological processes that involve eicosanoid action. Eicosanoid formation, in response to some specific stimulus, is initiated following transmembrane signaling, which results in activation of phospholipases and release of 20:4n-6 from its usual position in phospholipids.[26,44] Once formed, eicosanoids leave the cell, possibly by facilitated diffusion, then act on the parent or neighboring cells in an autocrine or paracrine manner via interaction with specific G-protein–linked receptors. These receptors then signal inhibition or stimulation of second messengers.[21] Distinct receptors for thromboxane (TX) A_2, PGE_1, $EGF_{2\alpha}$, and the leukotrienes (LT) LTB_4, and LTD_4, have been found in various tissues. The molecular biology of these receptors is still being explored.[20-22] The first committed step in the synthesis of eicosanoids is an enzymatic oxygenation of unesterified 20:4n-6 in an initial reaction catalyzed by

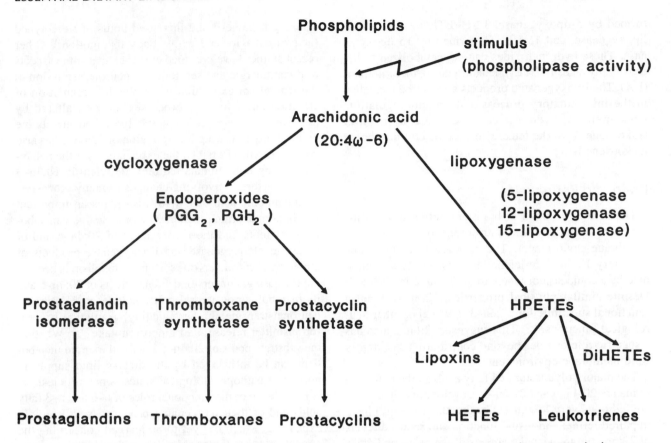

Figure 3. Major pathways of synthesis of eicosanoids from arachidonic acid. PG, prostaglandin; HPETE, hydroperoxy eicosatrienoic acid; HETE, hydroxy fatty acid; diHETE, dihydroxy eicosapentaenoic acid.

cyclooxygenase (prostaglandin G/H synthase) or lipoxygenases (Figure 3). The biological roles of some of the eicosanoids such as TXA_2, prostacyclins, and leukotrienes are quite well understood, but the functional roles of others, such as lipoxins and hydroxyeicosatetraenoic acids (HETEs), are still being found. The initial enzyme of the prostaglandin sequence, cyclooxygenase, oxygenates 20:4n–6 to intermediate endoperoxides, PGG_2 and PGH_2.[18,20–22] This enzyme is the main site of inhibition of aspirin and the nonsteroidal anti-inflammatory drugs. The endoperoxides are unstable under physiological conditions and are quickly converted to the more stable PGE_2, PGD_2, and $PGF_{2\alpha}$, depending on the cell and tissue. For example, PGD_2 is synthesized from PGH_2 by prostaglandin D synthase in brain, platelets, alveolar macrophages, mast cells, uterus, skin, renal medulla, and skeletal muscle. Prostaglandin D_2 is a major metabolite of arachidonic acid in brain, where it is involved in functions related to sleep, thermoregulation, and pain response.[18,20] Prostaglandin F synthase is an aldoketo reductase and converts PGH_2 to $PGF_{2\alpha}$, and PGD_2 to 9a,11b-PGF_2. The PGE_2 synthesis occurs in many tissues including vasculature, renal medulla, gastrointestinal tract, reproductive system, prostate gland, ovarian tube, and uterus. Prostaglandin $F_{2\alpha}$ is synthesized in the lung, where it elevates pulmonary vascular resistance and constricts bronchial airways, brain, and semen.[18] Thromboxane A synthase catalyses the conversion of PGH_2 to TXA_2, which is a major product in platelets.[19,22] Thromboxane A_2 is very short-lived with a half-life of 30 seconds and is a potent platelet aggregator and vasoconstrictor of vascular and respiratory smooth muscle. Thromboxane A_2 has been implicated in the pathophysiology of atherosclerosis, myocardial infarction, and stroke.[19,20,22] Prostaglandin I_2 is formed in aorta and is a potent vasodilator and platelet antiaggregatory agent with a half-life of 5 to 10 minutes. Prostaglandin D_2 synthesis also occurs in platelets, alveolar macrophages, mast cells, uterus, skin, renal medulla, and skeletal muscle.

There are three major forms of lipoxygenases in mammalian tissues, the 5-, 12-, and 15-lipoxygenases, which catalyze the incorporation of dioxygen into positions 5, 12, and 15, respectively, of 20:4n–6.[20] The lipoxygenases contain a nonheme iron atom and are widely distributed in tissues. The major products of 20:4n–6 formed by the three major lipoxygenases are known as hydroperoxy eicosatrienoic acids (HPETEs) and include 5-HPETE formed by 5-lipoxygenase, 12-HPETE formed by 12-lipoxygenase, and 15-HPETE formed by 15 lipoxygenase. These hydroperoxides can be metabolized to hydroxy fatty acids (HETEs), leukotrienes (LT), or lipoxins (LX). The lipoxygenated products seem to be mediators in the inflammatory process and immunoregulation. Leukotriene Δ_4 hydrolase catalyzes the conversion of leukotriene A_4 to the leukocyte chemotactic metabolite leukotriene B_4.

Brain and Retina

The role of 22:6n–3 in brain and retina is often assumed to be structural, contributing to a highly fluid membrane environment. The decrease in 22:6n–3 due to dietary 18:3n–3 deficiency is consistently accompanied by a compensatory increase in 22:5n–6.[10,17,35,36,38,39,52] Despite similar physical properties, 22:5n–6 is not a functional substitute for 22:6n–3 in visual or other neurological functions.[36-39] This suggests 22:6n–3 also has a specific role or roles beyond contributing to a highly fluid membrane environment.

The major polyunsaturated fatty acids in the brain and retina are 20:4n–6 and 22:6n–3. Developing animals that are fed diets very low in 18:3n–3 (<0.1% energy) have impaired retinal and visual function and reduced levels of 22:6n–3 in the visual elements of the retina and other regions of the brain.[17,35,36,38,39,52] The precise role of 22:6n–3 in the visual processes is not well understood; however, 22:6n–3 seems to be essential for the normal function of rhodopsin.[53] Dietary 18:3n–3 fatty acid deficiency has been associated with rod outer segment disk disruptions, reduced light-stimulated disk shedding, and light-induced photoreceptor cell death in rats.[54] A reduced ability to catch photons appeared to be due to a slower rate of rhodopsin regeneration, indicating a defect in the visual cycle.

Evidence that dietary 18:3n–3 deficiency alters learning behaviors or ability, even when the deficiency is extreme and prolonged, is more contentious.[55] Several studies have reported lower performance on visually cued learning tasks by rats fed diets deficient in 18:3n–3 for two or more generations. The problems could involve changes in sensory functions, motivation, activity, other aspects of learning and cognition, or disturbances in the visual system. Fundamentally important work on the role of n–3 fatty acids in the central nervous system has come from studies with monkeys fed diets profoundly deficient in 18:3n–3. These diets contained safflower oil as the only fat (0.09% of dietary energy from 18:3n–3), and when compared with monkeys fed diets with 2.3% of energy as 18:3n–3 (from soybean oil), the deficient diets resulted in an 85% decrease in cerebral cortex 22:6n–3.[38,39] Recent studies have shown that monkeys fed similar 18:3n–3-deficient diets also have increased

drinking behavior[56] and increased bouts of stereotyped (active) behavior and whole-body locomotion.[57] Other recent studies have provided evidence that some aspects of dopaminergic and serotonergic neurotransmission in the frontal cortex, which is involved in regulation of attention and cognitive processes, may be altered by prolonged 18:3n–3 deficiency.[58] Increased membrane permeability following incorporation of 22:6n–3 has also been reported.[59] Possibly, the explanation for the behavioral changes in animals fed diets deficient in 18:3n–3 is multifactorial, involving changes in many processes.

Arachidonic acid (20:4n–6) also plays an important role in normal brain function. The brain actively metabolizes 20:4n–6, and the involvement of 20:4n–6 and of several cyclooxygenase and lipoxygenase products of 20:4n–6 in central nervous system metabolism is becoming increasingly understood.[60] The effects of 20:4n–6 and its metabolites on neural cells include modulation of neuronal transmembrane signaling, regulation of neurotransmitter release, and glucose uptake.[61-64] Whether the substrate pools of 20:4n–6 involved in brain metabolism can be influenced by the dietary lipid supply in normal or pathophysiological states is not yet clear.

Knowledge of the functional roles of n–6 and n–3 fatty acids and of their oxygenated products is still rapidly expanding. Much has yet to be learned concerning the crucial role that fatty acids play in the central nervous system, and of the various pathways that regulate fatty acid metabolism. Similarly, the role fatty acids play in influencing gene expression and many aspects of eicosanoid biology have yet to be explored. As knowledge accumulates, this will be translated into recommendations for dietary fatty acids to prevent deficiency and to reduce the incidence and severity of certain chronic diseases. New applications for n–6 and n–3 fatty acids based on modulation of eicosanoid precursor pools and in treating various inborn errors of fatty acid metabolism can also be expected.

References

1. Sinclair HM (1990) History of essential fatty acids. In Omega-6 essential fatty acids. Pathophysiology and roles in clinical medicine. AR Liss, New York, pp 1–20
2. Evans HM, Burr GO (1927) A new dietary deficiency with highly purified diets. Proc Soc Exp Biol Med 24:740–743
3. Evans HM, Burr GO (1927) New dietary deficiency with highly purified diets. II. Supplementary requirement of diet of pure casein, sucrose, and salt. Proc Soc Exp Biol Med 25:41–48
4. Evans HM, Burr GO (1928) A new dietary deficiency with highly purified diets. III. The beneficial effect of fat in the diet. Proc Soc Exp Biol Med 25:390–397
5. Burr GO, Burr MM (1929) A new deficiency disease produced by the rigid exclusion of fat from the diet. J Biol Chem 82:345–367
6. Burr GO, Burr MM (1930) On the nature and the role of fatty acids essential in nutrition. J Biol Chem 86:587–621

7. Hansen AE (1933) Serum lipid changes and therapeutic effect of various oils in infantile eczema. Pro Soc Exp Biol Med 31:160–161

8. Hansen AE, Wiese HF, Boelsche AN, et al (1963) Role of linoleic acid in infant nutrition. Clinical and chemical study of 428 infants fed on milk mixtures varying in kind and amount of fat. Pediatrics 31(suppl 1):171–192

9. Adam DJD, Hansen AE, Wiese HF (1958) Essential fatty acids in infant nutrition. J Nutr 66:555–564

10. Futterman S, Downer John L, Hendrickson A (1971) Effect of essential fatty acid deficiency on the fatty acid composition, morphology, and electroretinographic response of the retina. Invest Opthalmol 10:151–156

11. Wheeler TG, Benolken RM, Anderson RE (1975) Visual membranes: Specificity of fatty acid precursors for the electrical response to illumination. Science 188:1312–1314

12. Bazan NG, Rodriguez de Turco EB, Gordon WC (1993) Pathways for the conservation of docosahexaenoic acid in photoreceptors and synapses: biochemical and autoradiographic analysis. Can J Physiol Pharmacol 79:690–698

13. Bourre JM, Dumont OS, Piciotti MJ, et al (1992) Dietary α-linolenic acid deficiency in adult rats for 7 months does not alter brain docosahexaenoic acid content, in contrast to liver, heart and testes. Biochim Biophys Acta 1124:119–122

14. Tinoco J, Miljanich P, Medwadowski B (1977) Depletion of docosahexaenoic acid in retinal lipids of rats fed a linolenic acid-deficient, linoleic acid containing diet. Biochim Biophys Acta 486:575–578

15. Tinoco J, Babcock R, Hincenbergs, et al (1978) Linolenic acid deficiency: changes in fatty acid patterns in female and male rats raised on a linolenic acid-deficient diet for two generations. Lipids 13:6–17

16. Wiegand RD, Koutz CA, Sinson AM, Anderson RE (1991) Conservation of docosahexaenoic acid in rod outer segments of rat retina during ω-3 and ω-6 fatty acid deficiency. J Neurochem 57:1690–1699

17. Innis SM (1991) Essential fatty acids in growth and development. Prog Lipid Res 30:39–103

18. Sinzinger H, Virgolini I, Gazso A, O'Grady JO (1991) Eicosanoids in atherosclerosis. Exp Pathol 43:2–19

19. Makheja AN (1992) Atherosclerosis: the eicosanoid connection. Mol Cell Biochem 111:137–142

20. Funk CD (1993) Molecular biology in the eicosanoid field. Prog Nucleic Acid Res Mol Biol 45:67–98

21. Smith WL (1992) Prostanoid biosynthesis and mechanism of action. Am J Physiol 263:F181–F191

22. Reilly M, Fitzgerald GA (1993) Cellular activation by thromboxane A2 and other eicosanoids. Eur Heart J 14:88–93

23. Sprecher H (1992) Interconversions between 20- and 22-carbon ω-3 and ω-6 fatty acids via 4-desaturase independent pathways. In Sinclair A, Gibson R (eds), Essential fatty acids and eicosanoids. American Oil Chemists' Society, Campaign, IL, pp 18–22

24. Moore SA, Yoderk L, Spector AA (1990) Role of the blood-brain barrier in the formation of long-chain ω-3 and ω-6 fatty acids from essential fatty acid precursors. J Neurochem 55:391–402

25. Moore SA, Yoder E, Murphy S, et al (1991) Astrocytes, not neurons, produce docosahexaenoic acid (22:6ω-3) and arachidonic acid (20:4ω-6). J Neurochem 56:518–524

26. Wang N, Anderson RE (1993) Synthesis of docosahexaenoic acid by retina and retinal pigment epithelium. Biochemistry 32:13703–13709

27. Wetzel MG, Li J, Alvarez RA, et al (1991) Metabolism of linolenic acid and docosahexaenoic acid in rat retinas and rod outer segments. Exp Eye Res 53:437–446

28. Brenner RR (1981) Nutritional and hormonal factors influencing fatty acid desaturation of essential fatty acids. Prog Lipid Res 20:41–47

29. Voss A, Reinhart M, Sankarappa S, Sprecher H (1991) The metabolism of 7,10,13,16,19-docosapentaenoic acid to 4,7,10,13,16,19-docosahexaenoic acid in rat liver is independent of a 4-desaturase. J Biol Chem 266:19995–20000

30. Mohammed BS, Sankarappa S, Geiger M, Sprecher H (1995) Reevaluation of the pathway for the metabolism of 7,10,13,16-docosatetraenoic acid to 4,7,10,13,16-docosapentaenoic acid in rat liver. Arch Biochem Biophys 317:179–18

31. Martinez M, Mougan I, Roig M, Ballabriga A (1994) Blood polyunsaturated fatty acids in patients with peroxisomal disorders. A multicenter study. Lipids 29:273–280

32. Gronn M, Christensen E, Hagve T-A, Christophersen BO (1990) The Zellweger syndrome: deficient conversion of docosahexaenoic acid (22:(n-3)) to eicosapentaenoic acid (20:5(n-3)) and normal Δ⁴-desaturase activity in cultured skin fibroblasts. Biochim Biophys Acta 1044:249–254

33. Bourre J-M, Piciotti M, Dumont O, et al (1990) Dietary linoleic acid and polyunsaturated fatty acids in rat brain and other organs. Minimal requirements of linoleic acid. Lipids 25:465–472

34. Food and Agriculture Organization/World Health Organization (1993) Fat in human nutrition. Report of an expert consultation. Publications Division, FAO, Rome

35. Arbuckle LD, MacKinnon MJ, Innis SM (1994) Formula 18:2ω(ω-6) and 18:3(ω-3) content and ratio influence long-chain polyunsaturated fatty acids in the developing piglet liver and central nervous system. J Nutr 124:289–298

36. Bourre JM, Francois M, Youyou A, et al (1989) The effects of dietary α-linolenic acid on the composition of nerve membranes, enzymatic activity, amplitude of electrophysiological parameters, resistance to poisons and performance of learning tasks in rats. J Nutr 119:1880–1892

37. Innis SM, Nelson CM, Rioux FM, King DJ (1994) Development of visual acuity in relation to plasma and erythrocyte ω-6 and ω-3 fatty acids in healthy term gestation infants. Am J Clin Nutr 60:347–352

38. Neuringer M, Connor WE, Van Petten C, Barstad L (1984) Dietary omega-3 fatty acid deficiency and visual loss in infant rhesus monkeys. J Clin Invest 73:272–276

39. Neuringer M, Connor WE, Lin DS, et al (1986) Biochemical and functional effects of prenatal and postnatal omega 3 fatty acid deficiency on retina and brain in rhesus monkeys. Proc Natl Acad Sci USA 83:4021–4025

40. Innis SM, Lupton BA, Nelson CM (1994) Biochemical and functional approaches to study of fatty acid requirements of very premature infants. Nutrition 10:72–76

41. Makrides M, Simmer K, Goggin M, Gibson RA (1993) Erythrocyte docosahexaenoic acid correlates with the visual response of healthy, term infants. Pediatr Res 34:425–427

42. Innis SM (1992) In Tsang RC, Lucas A, Uauy R, Zlotkin S (eds), Nutritional needs of the preterm infant. Scientific basis and practical guidelines. Williams & Wilkins, Baltimore, pp 65–86

43. Carlson SE, Werkman SH, Rhodes PG, Tolley EA (1993) Visual-acuity development in healthy preterm infants: effect of marine-oil supplementation. Am J Clin Nutr 58:35–42

44. Lands WEM (1991) Biosynthesis of prostaglandins. Annu Rev Nutr 11:41–60

45. MacDonald JIS, Sprecher H (1991) Phospholipid fatty acid remodelling in mammalian cells. Biochim Biophys Acta 1084:105–121

46. Capdevilla JH, Falck JR, Estabrook RW (1992) Cytochrome

P450 and the arachidonate cascade. FASEB J 6:731–736

47. Hansen HS (1994) New biological and clinical roles for the n-6 and n-3 fatty acids. Nutr Rev 52:162–167

48. Ziboh VA, Miller CC (1990) Essential fatty acids and polyunsaturated fatty acids: significance in cutaneous biology. Annu Rev Nutr 10:433–50

49. Ziboh VA (1994) Essential fatty acids/eicosanoid biosynthesis in the skin: biological significance. Proc Soc Exp Biol Med 205:1–11

50. Clark SD, Jump DB (1993) Regulation of gene transcription by polyunsaturated fatty acids. Prog Lipid Res 32:139–149

51. Glauert HP (1993) Dietary fat, gene expression, and carcinogenesis. In Berdanier CD, Hargrove JL (eds), Nutrition and gene expression. CRC Press, Boca Raton, FL, pp 247–268

52. Hrboticky N, Mackinnon MJ, Puterman ML, Innis SM (1989) Effect of linoleic acid-rich infant formula on brain synaptosomal lipid accretion and enzyme thermotropic behaviour in the piglet. J Lipid Res 30:1173–1184

53. Weidmann TS, Pates RD, Beach JM, et al (1988) Lipid-protein interactions mediate the photochemical function of rhodopsin. Biochemistry 27:64–69

54. Bush RA, Malnoe, A, Reme CE, Williams TP (1994) Dietary deficiency of ω-3 fatty acids alters rhodopsin content and function in rat retina. Invest Ophthalmol Vis Sci 35:91–100

55. Wainwright PE (1992) Do essential fatty acids play a role in brain and behavioral development. Neurosci Biobehav Rev 16:193–205

56. Reisbick S, Neuringer M, Hasnain R, Connor WE (1992) Polydipsia in rhesus monkeys deficient in omega-3 fatty acids. Physiol Behav 47:315–323

57. Reisbick S, Neuringer M, Hasnain R, Connor WE (1994) Home cage behaviour of rhesus monkeys with long-term deficiency of omega-3 fatty acids. Physiol Behav 55:231–239

58. Delion S, Chalon S, Herault J, et al (1994) Chronic dietary α-linolenic acid deficiency alters dopaminergic and serotoninergic neurotransmission in rats. J Nutr 124:2466–2476

59. Stillwell W, Ehringer W, Jenski LJ (1993) Docosahexaenoic acid increases permeability of lipid vesicles and tumor cells. Lipids 28:103–108

60. Adesuyi SA, Cockrell DA, Gamache DA, Ellis EF (1985) Lipoxygenase metabolism of arachidonic acid in brain. J Neurochem 45:770–776

61. Piomelli D, Greengard P (1990) Lipoxygenase metabolites of arachidonic acid in neuronal transmembrane signalling. Trends Pharmacol Sci 11:367–373

62. Schweitzer P, Madamba S, Champagnat J, Siggins GR (1993) Somatostatin inhibition of hippocampal CA 1 pyramidal neurons: meditation by arachidonic acid and its metabolites. J Neurosci 13:2033–2049

63. Fraser DD, Hoehn K, Weiss S, MacVicar BA (1993) Arachidonic acid inhibits sodium currents and synaptic transmission in cultured striatal neurons. Neuron 11:633–644

64. Yu N, Martin J-L, Stella N, Magistretti PJ (1993) Arachidonic acid stimulates glucose uptake in cerebral cortical astrocytes. Proc Natl Acad Sci USA 1993, 90:4042–4046

Chapter 8

Protein and Amino Acids

Peter J. Reeds and Phillip R. Beckett

Proteins form the major cellular structural elements, are biochemical catalysts, and are important regulators of gene expression. As such, any discussion of protein and amino acid nutrition necessarily involves virtually every element of mammalian biochemistry and physiology. In this chapter we will concentrate as far as possible on advances that have occurred since the sixth edition of this book.[1] We will try to balance nutritional, metabolic, and mechanistic aspects of protein science, provide information that we believe is necessary for the development of flexible dietary recommendations, and focus on aspects of the subject that bear on human nutrition.

General Comments on Terminology

The controversies concerning the subject of human amino acid requirements are still unresolved.[1-6] Failure to resolve these difficulties stems in part from the word "requirement," which is used in different ways by different authors. It may be useful to define our understanding of the terms.

Metabolic need. This is a direct reflection of rates of metabolic pathways (e.g., protein deposition) that consume the nutrient in question and is fundamentally a function of genotype as well as the developmental and physiological state of the individual.

Dietary requirement. This is the quantity of the nutrient that must be supplied in the diet in order to satisfy the metabolic need; it includes factors associated with digestion, absorption, and cellular bioavailability.

Recommended dietary allowance (RDA). This is the practical expression of nutritional recommendations. An RDA is designed explicitly to be applicable to populations rather than to individuals and thus attempts to account for variability among subjects in need and dietary requirement. RDAs are intended to prevent nutrient deficiency, and are often expressed as "safe levels." An RDA, so defined, is the intake that reduces the prevalence of nutrient deficiency to some desired proportion of the population while avoiding excessive intakes.

Metabolic need < dietary requirement < RDA. Thus the daily basal nitrogen excretion of adults, analogous to the minimal metabolic need, is ≈50 mgN/kg. This formed the basis for the 1965 recommendation by the Food and Agriculture Organization (FAO).[7] The mean nitrogen intake necessary to maintain nitrogen equilibrium is ≈75 mg N/kg and is equivalent to the dietary requirement. This was the basis for the proposals by the National Research Council (NRC) and FAO for 1974 and 1985, respectively.[8,9] Finally, current RDAs or "safe levels" of intake of high-quality protein for adults are 96–125 mg N/kg (600–800 mg/kg protein).

High-quality protein. The use of the term "high-quality protein" in the RDA indicates that dietary proteins differ in their nutritional quality. This reflects the differences in amino acid composition of proteins and the fact that the protein need is, in many respects, a surrogate for the sum of the needs for each amino acid. In theory, the term "high quality" should reflect how closely the amino acid composition of dietary protein and the individual's needs for different amino acids match one another. This has led those concerned with farm animal nutrition to develop the concept of the "ideal protein," an ideal protein being defined as one with an amino acid composition that maximizes its productive utilization by the recipient animal.[10,11]

In human nutrition, the term "high quality" is often taken to be synonymous with proteins of animal origin, usually milk or whole egg. However, assessment of the quality of a given dietary protein should start with a consideration of the amino acid needs of the individuals to whom it will be fed. The equation of "high quality" and "animal origin" is not necessarily correct for any stage of life other than perhaps early infancy. For example, it has been shown that relative requirements for different amino acids of preschool children are not the same as relative quantities of amino acids in egg and milk.[12,13] The requirements of this population can be readily satisfied with mixtures of foods of vegetable origin. Indeed it is possible to prepare mixtures of proteins of plant origin (e.g., a cereal and a legume) that, for school-age children, have a higher biological value than mixed egg and milk diets.[14,15] The authors of these papers commented explicitly on the fact that defining protein quality in formal terms, e.g., as a chemical score, would confer some objectivity on estimates of the adequacy or otherwise of the amino acid patterns in common staple diets.[12–15] Unfortunately, definition of the most appropriate scoring method continues to generate argument.[16,17]

Nutritional and Metabolic Classification of Amino Acids

The distinction between dispensable (nonessential) and indispensable (essential) amino adds is strictly nutritional, inasmuch as an indispensable amino acid *must* be part of the diet, while a dispensable amino acid *need not necessarily* be present in food. However, the nutritional terms indispensable and dispensable become blurred once interest shifts to the metabolic level.[1,18] By definition, an indispensable amino acid cannot be synthesized by the organism in question. In the strictest sense, lysine and perhaps threonine are the only metabolically indispensable amino acids, because they are not transaminated to any nutritionally significant extent. This is a crucial point, because lysine and threonine are generally the first and second limiting amino acids in cereal protein sources. Lysine also appears to be the first limiting amino acid in human milk.[6]

It can be argued in reverse that glutamic acid and possibly serine are the only truly dispensable amino acids, because they are the only amino acids that can be synthesized by mammals via reductive amination of the appropriate keto acid. Other dispensable amino acids derive from transamination reactions, and require either glutamate or serine as nitrogen or carbon donors. A recent study[19] suggests that the contribution of endogenous synthesis to glutamate and serine turnover is greater than the contribution of endogenous synthesis to the metabolism of other "dispensable" amino acids.

There is, moreover, a third group of amino acids for which the term "conditionally essential" has been coined.[20–23] This group is characterized by two features.

First, their synthesis uses other amino acids as carbon precursors and may be confined to specific organs.[24,25] This is an important metabolic distinction from the dispensable amino acids. For some conditionally essential amino acids (e.g., tyrosine) the precursor is an indispensable amino acid (phenylalanine); for others (e.g., arginine, proline, and glycine) the precursor is a dispensable amino acid; while for yet others (e.g., cysteine) both an essential (methionine as sulfur donor) and a nonessential (serine) amino acid are required. At the metabolic level, the organism's ability to synthesize a conditionally essential amino acid could be constrained by availability of a suitable amino acid precursor.

Second, the maximum rate at which their synthesis can proceed may be limited and potentially constrained by developmental or pathophysiological factors. Thus very low-birth-weight infants are apparently unable to synthesize cysteine and proline and may lack the ability to synthesize *adequate* quantities of glycine.[26,27] The latter is important because human milk proteins have a very low glycine content.[28]

Functional and Metabolic Basis for Amino Acid Needs

Minimal needs for growth. At the simplest level, the optimum pattern of amino acids required for protein deposition is the product of the amino acid composition of proteins deposited and the rate at which they are deposited. That being so, the composition of body protein should provide a firm basis for defining the quantities of individual indispensable amino acids obligatorily needed for protein deposition.[10,29–31] The relative "requirements" of different essential amino acids, as measured by nitrogen balance trials, show a commonality among species and are similar to the composition of body protein.[28,29]

While there is no reason to suppose that the human infant will greatly differ from this general mammalian pattern, all current amino acid RDAs for infants[5,6,9] use the amino acid pattern of human milk as the standard. Indeed, Beaton and Chery[30] have gone further by taking the "typical" protein—and hence amino acid—intake of breast-fed children as the upper limit of protein *requirement* of infants. This is a useful line of reasoning for predicting prevalence of protein undernutrition in populations of breast-fed infants. However, it is important to note that the "safe level" of amino acid intake as defined by the amino acid composition of milk does not directly reflect the amino acid needs of infants.[6] In fact, the mixed proteins of human milk have a biological value of only 0.75.[31] The dissimilarity between the amino acid needs for protein deposition and the amino acid composition of mixed milk protein is not unique to human infants. The milk of different species contains remarkably similar relative quantities of amino acids despite the wide range of postnatal protein deposition rates among mammals.[28]

Minimal needs for maintenance of body nitrogen equilibrium. The other major "process" that demands continual provision of amino acids in the diet is maintenance of the existing body protein mass. Basal nitrogen loss is a function of body weight and, when normalized to body weight $(kg)^{0.75}$, varies little with age.[32] The contribution of maintenance to total amino acid needs is inversely proportional to the fractional rate of growth (g protein deposited/g body protein). Because human beings have a remarkably slow rate of postnatal protein deposition, even at 1 month of age the maintenance amino acid needs of infants account for ≈50% of total need.[6,32] While there is consensus regarding the quantity of protein required for maintenance, the optimal pattern of amino acids within this protein requirement is very controversial.[2,3,33,34]

The pioneering work on nitrogen balance in men by Rose[35] and in women by Leverton[36] suggested that the pattern of indispensable amino acids that optimizes protein utilization at body protein equilibrium is substantially different from the mixture that optimizes protein deposition. Similar results have been obtained in other mammals by nitrogen balance trials.[10] The specific features of maintenance amino acid pattern defined from measurements of nitrogen balance are a much lower total essential amino acid contribution (≈20% of total compared with >40% for growth), particularly low needs for lysine and branched-chain amino acids, and relatively high needs for sulfur amino acids and threonine.

These features were widely accepted as the standard for more than two decades,[9] but in the early 1980s Young and his coworkers[33,34] initiated a stable-isotope approach in which they measured the carbon catabolism of specific indispensable amino acids and used this number as the basis for determining the dietary requirement of adult males. The idea was that amino acids are nutritionally essential because we cannot synthesize their respective carbon chains. In their earliest studies, the authors based their estimates on measurements of the intake of a limiting indispensable amino acid at which its oxidation rose above a basal value—the so-called break-point method. The results of these studies implied that the dietary requirements for leucine and lysine were at least twice the values defined in Rose's studies.[37,38]

Young et al. then measured the intake of a given essential amino acid at which body protein synthesis, measured from kinetics of the labeled amino acid in plasma, was maximized.[33] This approach was an important conceptual advance because it was based on a *functional* index of amino acid adequacy, i.e., body protein turnover. Moreover, the results obtained by this method suggested an even higher leucine need than was calculated by the oxidation break-point analysis.

Commenting on these results, Young[33,34] criticized two aspects of Rose's studies on the basis that 1) there are systematic errors in nitrogen balance measurements that lead to consistent false-positive balances[4] and 2) the feeding design used by Rose inevitably led to low estimates of amino acid requirements because (a) subjects were studied after a period of very low amino acid intake and (b) their intake of nonprotein energy was very high in relation to protein intake. Young argued that the subjects of Rose's studies were adapted to low amino

acid intakes, and that aspects of amino acid catabolism related to energy and carbohydrate metabolism were maximally suppressed. In Young's view, the values measured by Rose were at best absolute minima, and hence not useful in developing dietary recommendations for safe intakes, and at worst substantially underestimated even the basal amino acid needs.

More recently Young and his group have explored two other approaches. First, they based their calculations on the assumption that maintenance amino acid needs are largely set by the product of protein loss under nitrogen-free feeding conditions and composition of body protein.[39] This approach inevitably generated an amino acid pattern that resembled the growth pattern—and incidentally the FAO 1985 preschool pattern[9]—more closely than the maintenance pattern defined from nitrogen balance trials. In a second set of experiments, the authors determined the 24-hour carbon balance of a given amino acid by measuring its rate of oxidation in both fed and fasting states.[40,41] This latter approach generally substantiated the group's earlier conclusions.

Differences between the FAO 1985 recommendations and Young's are substantial. The new values have important implications for food policy, especially in assessing the adequacy of amino acid intakes of populations consuming various staple diets.[42] It is still not obvious why the two values differ so greatly, and discussion on this point has centered largely on technical matters. It can be argued that the data are generated in young active males and might not be generally applicable.[33,34,39–41] It has also been pointed out that the studies involved subjects ingesting abundant quantities of other essential amino acids, so that amino acid catabolism in general might be increased.[3,43–45] A particularly useful discussion of these matters has been published recently and another is in press.[4,6]

Nonprotein aspects of maintenance amino acid needs. The continuing need for protein in the diet ultimately reflects the continuing catabolism of indispensable amino acids. This fact underlies the carbon-balance approach to determining indispensable amino acid requirements. Although there are mechanisms that allow almost complete suppression of catabolism of some indispensable amino acids,[46] these mechanisms are apparently not fully active in individuals who are close to nitrogen equilibrium or who are receiving no dietary protein. We would argue that this reflects consumption of specific amino acids in support of physiological functions that are separate from tissue protein metabolism, and that these demands assume a great importance at limiting protein intakes. In this context, maintenance of host defenses and neural and muscular function seems to be crucial, and a case can be made for the importance to these functions of amino acids in general and of nonessential or conditionally essential amino acids specifically.

Two factors influence the individual's ability to withstand bacterial or viral infection: maintenance of a barrier to prevent invasion by pathogenic organisms and maintenance of all the elements of immune protection. An important part of the barrier function at the two most vulnerable surfaces, the lungs and small intestine, is continuous secretion of mucus glycoproteins. Approximately 90% of the mass of these glycoproteins consists of complex carbohydrate side chains. These side chains are attached to a core protein with extensive cysteine-sulfur cross-links via O-glycosidic linkages to threonine. Threonine contributes 22% of the core protein's mass.[47] Secretion of these proteins continues irrespective of current protein intake and places a persistent drain on threonine supply. Recent measurements of amino acid losses in ileostomy effluents imply that 61% of maintenance threonine needs of adults can be ascribed to threonine loss from small intestine.[48] At very low threonine intakes, subjects remain in apparent negative threonine carbon balance, which is the predictable result of a persistent and unquantified loss of threonine into the gastrointestinal tract.[49]

Protein-depleted individuals have impaired immunocompetence.[50] Part of this impairment can be ascribed to limited availability of amino acids for synthesis of cellular proteins of the immune system and to support the hepatic acute-phase protein response.[51] The acute-phase response is clearly suboptimal in malnourished laboratory animals and infants.[52,53] Amino acids are also involved in other aspects of the defense mechanism. Glutathione, a key free radical scavenger, is synthesized from glutamate (glutamine), glycine, and cysteine. Hepatic and intestinal mucosal glutathione is depleted in protein-restricted animals.[54,55] In rats, low levels can be restored merely by providing cysteine in diet.[54] Of particular note are observations that glutathione concentration in the erythrocytes of infants suffering from kwashiorkor is markedly reduced, and that low-birth-weight infants also have low circulating levels of reduced glutathione.[56,57] In each case this may be due to limited intake of cysteine or inability to synthesize cysteine.[26]

Glutamine, an amino acid that is strongly concentrated in skeletal muscle, appears to play a specific role in maintaining function of rapidly proliferating cells such as lymphocytes and mucosal enterocytes.[58–60] Glutamine may also regulate muscle protein turnover,[61,62] and it is noteworthy that under conditions of infection and trauma, muscle concentrations of glutamine fall.[63] Recent work also suggests that provision of glutamine to tissues of the splanchnic bed plays a specific role in maintaining glutathione synthesis under traumatic conditions.[64,65]

Other amino acid metabolites may play important physiological roles in both the immune and neural systems. Taurine, a β-amino sulfonic acid derived from cysteine, appears to be an effective scavenger of peroxidation products (particularly those containing the oxychloride groups[66]) and acts as a neuromodulatory agent.[67] Taurine is specifically concentrated in skeletal musculature and in the central nervous system.

Creatine, a compound that is crucial for energy flow within skeletal muscle, is synthesized from glycine, arginine, and a suitable source of methyl groups.[68] Creatine is concentrated in skeletal muscle and brain. Infection and trauma lead to a specific loss of creatine in addition to causing loss of muscle protein, glutamine, and taurine.[69] These conditions are accompanied by derangements of muscle contractile function.[70] Finally, glutamine, creatine, and taurine are maintained at substantial concentrations in the free amino acid fraction of milk,[71,72] implying an important role of all three compounds in supporting postnatal development.

A particularly important development has been identification of nitric oxide, a product of arginine metabolism, as a key regulator of a variety of physiological processes. These include regulation of blood vessel tone and hence blood pressure and flow, development of higher cognitive functions, and neural regulation of intestinal motility and pancreatic secretion.[73–76] Nitric oxide has also been implicated in regulating hepatic protein and urea metabolism.[77–79] Arginine appears to play an important role in the immune system, and while the exact mechanism underlying these observations is not known with any certainty, nitric oxide production from arginine appears to be involved in macrophage killer function and in regulating interactions between macrophages and lymphocyte adhesion and activation.[80–83]

These are crucial new findings, the nutritional significance of which is still a subject of intense investigation. Unfortunately, with the exception of some recent studies, neither the quantitative impact of nitric oxide synthesis on the body's need for arginine nor the impact of arginine status on nitric oxide–mediated responses has been studied extensively.[84,85]

From the foregoing we wish to emphasize the following key points.

- The metabolic end products of specific amino acids are crucial intermediates in maintaining a variety of physiological functions.
- These functions bear only an indirect relationship to protein metabolism.
- Precursors for synthesis of these compounds are often nonessential (e.g., glutamate, glutamine) or conditionally essential amino acids (e.g., glycine, arginine, and cysteine).

The fact that these amino acids appear to be particularly important in individuals who are close to nitrogen equilibrium may reflect their role in these key "nonprotein" pathways of disposal. Despite research extending over a number of years, details of nonessential and conditionally essential amino acid synthesis and metabolism in vivo remain fragmentary.[86-88] Advances in this area remain important in understanding amino acid requirements in general.

Factors Affecting the Link Between Minimal Needs and Dietary Requirements

Digestibility and forms of amino acid absorption. As emphasized above, the minimal metabolic need for amino acids is not the same as the dietary requirement. The first link between these two "requirements" is protein digestion and absorption. Protein digestion is covered in all standard texts and will not be considered here, and amino acid transport from lumen into hepatic portal circulation is discussed extensively by Webb.[91] Amino acids are transported from lumen by passive and facilitated diffusion and by Na^+-dependent, active transport. The relative contribution of these systems is highly dependent on amino acid concentration, with sodium-independent systems predominating at substrate concentrations >1.0 mM. The exact number of Na^+-dependent transport systems in the mucosal brush border membrane is unknown, but on the basis of cross-inhibition studies, they appear to be generally similar to the well-defined transporters in nonepithelial cells.[92] Overlap exists in the substrate specificity of the transporters, and there is competition and synergism between amino acids for transport across the brush border.

The fact that considerable quantities of di- and tripeptides are removed from the intestinal lumen without luminal hydrolysis has been known for many years.[93,94] Peptides are transported by separate systems and are removed more rapidly from lumen. Peptide transport is electrogenic and driven by a basolateral-apical pH gradient maintained by a Na^+/H^+ exchange at the apical membrane and a Na^+/K^+ exchange at the basolateral membrane.[91,95] It seems unlikely that there are separate transporters for each peptide, as the number of di- and tripeptides that could arise as a result of proteolysis is very large. Even though di- and tripeptides are transported by different membrane proteins, the literature generally implies that the number of carrier proteins is limited. Earlier studies discussed at length the possibility that peptide transport might avoid the competition phenomena noted in amino acid transport, yet competition for transport between different dipeptides has now been demonstrated in a number of systems.[96,97]

The ability of mammalian cells to use extracellular oligopeptides has received considerable attention, particularly in relation to the potential use of peptides in total parenteral nutrition.[98] There is little doubt that nitrogen balance can be maintained in animals sustained entirely with intravenous peptides,[69] and most tissues are able to utilize circulating peptides, either by hydrolyz-

ing the peptides at the plasma membrane—as is the case with the intestinal[91] and renal brush border[97] membranes—or by peptide uptake and intracellular hydrolysis.[99,100] However, while the removal of peptides from the intestinal contents undoubtedly occurs, whether these peptides enter the portal circulation in nutritionally significant amounts is less certain. Similarly, although cells are capable of using extracellular peptides, the question whether oligopeptides play a significant role in interorgan amino acid transport remains unanswered.[101] It appears from the limited literature on this subject that the apparent contribution of oligopeptides derived from the diet to the hepatic portal outflow varies considerably among species. Even so, we must interpret this literature with caution because there is insufficient documentation for the absence of contaminating low molecular proteins from "peptide-containing" extracts.

It should be emphasized that a significant proportion of peptides could arise either because they contain proline or hydroxyproline (and hence are not hydrolyzed by the brush border exopeptidases) or because they limit peptides containing D-amino acids. Nevertheless, intact absorption of oligopeptides from the diet may make a substantial contribution to the portal outflow of amino acids in ruminants, while in nonruminant species the contribution is 30% or less.[102-104] It is noteworthy that in at least one study the overall concentration of oligopeptides was slightly lower in the portal circulation than in the arterial plasma.[104] This suggests the intriguing possibility that the small (<2000 Da) peptides that can be detected in blood plasma arise from endogenous proteolysis.[91,104] An important unanswered question is whether circulating oligopeptides play a role in mammalian amino acid nutrition.

Contribution of endogenous sources of nitrogen to the intestinal protein pool. Traditionally, assessment of the availability of dietary proteins and amino acids under practical conditions has been based on "apparent digestibility"—i.e., nitrogen intake–fecal nitrogen output. This method obscures two important points, however. First, fecal nitrogen consists largely of bacterial protein, and as such its amino acid composition gives very little information on the digestibility of different amino acids. Second, fecal nitrogen derives from at least three sources: undigested dietary protein, proteins from the intestinal mucosa, and urea nitrogen that has diffused from the blood into the intestinal lumen.

The availability of ^{15}N-labeled edible proteins has allowed human studies of the disappearance of the isotope from intestinal contents, leading to formulation of values for "true" digestibility.[105,106] A number of studies in pigs have infused ^{15}N-amino acids intravenously for prolonged periods to measure the endogenous nitrogen outflow.[107-109] A similar study in infants used prolonged feedings of ^{15}N-glycine for the same purpose.[110] By and large, the results of these studies lead to the following conclusions:

- Provided the dietary protein has not been grossly damaged by food processing, its true digestibility is 90%, and differences in apparent digestibility are largely reflections of differences in endogenous contribution to luminal nitrogen pool.
- 80% of protein outflow from ileum consists of endogenous nitrogenous secretions, but this represents only ≈30% of the total protein secreted into small intestine.
- 50–90% of fecal nitrogen derives from endogenous nitrogen sources.

Urea nitrogen circulating in the blood can enter the intestinal tract, where it is hydrolyzed by resident flora and becomes fixed in bacterial protein. In ruminants, a crucial part of regulation of nitrogen flow and metabolism is urea nitrogen cycling and metabolism in the rumen. It is now recognized that urea nitrogen cycling, presumably in the large bowel but also potentially in the distal ileum, is also an important component of nonruminant nitrogen metabolism. The appearance of urea nitrogen in fecal protein has been demonstrated repeatedly since the early 1950s,[111,112] but recent work suggests not only that this host–bacterial urea nitrogen recycling is regulated, but that fixation of urea nitrogen into indispensable amino acids can occur—i.e., true nutritional benefit can accrue from the process.[113] This is a provocative and controversial idea, and to date studies of retention of oral ^{15}N-urea in infants have given conflicting results.[114,115]

Jackson[116] argues that the degree to which urea cycles between body and gut is a sensitive measure of the degree to which the dietary supply of amino acids satisfies the metabolic demand for amino acids. He and his coworkers have demonstrated increased urea nitrogen cycling under conditions of restricted protein intake or enhanced demand, e.g., during pregnancy.[113,116,117]

Recent evidence in animals suggests that systemic essential amino acids do become labeled with ^{15}N-when ^{15}N-urea is administered.[118] It is critically important that this work has identified labeling of lysine, which is not transaminated by mammals and is the first limiting indispensable amino acid in many cereal proteins. The availability to the host of an indispensable amino acid synthesized by intestinal microflora, if confirmed, will have an important bearing on estimates of dietary amino acid requirements derived from nitrogen- and carbon-balance methods. By conserving nitrogen in a beneficial way, the process leads to a systematic underestimation of true amino acid uptake, and would contribute to underestimating amino acid need by nitrogen-balance method. Estimates of requirements of individual indispensable amino acids derived from carbon-balance method should not be materially affected, because these figures reflect losses of individual amino acids.[33,34]

Absorption of protein components of milk. Native—i.e., newly secreted and unprocessed—milk is a complex mixture of proteins. Although in quantitative terms a relatively limited number of proteins contribute the bulk of total milk protein, milk contains a wide range of growth factors and hormones as well as immunoglobulins and proteins with specific metal ion–binding properties.[119–124]

The newborn mammal's intestine is temporarily permeable to proteins.[125] In altricial species such as rats and mice, this permeability may extend into the third week of life. In a number of species this phenomenon relates to acquisition of passive immunity from absorption of colostral IgG and secretory IgA.[126,127] Recent work has established that newborn infants, especially low-birth-weight infants, absorb lactoferrin from maternal milk, and it has been argued that absorption of proteins such as lactoferrin confers a functional benefit to breast-fed infants.[128]

Similar proposals concern potential effects of growth factors in milk. In a variety of species the ingestion of colostrum stimulates a rapid increase in gut mass, although much of this growth represents the pinocytosis of colostral immunoglobulins. Ingestion of colostrum by newborn pigs has specific stimulatory effects on jejunal and muscle protein synthesis that cannot be reproduced by ingestion of an isonitrogenous, isoenergetic formula.[129] Unfortunately, with the exception of epidermal growth factor in rodents, which may be highly specific, the identity of the precise stimulatory factor(s) remains unknown.[119,130] A number of authors have speculated on the potential role of insulin-like growth factors.[121,122,131–133] This aspect of infant nutrition may have important implications for the development of infant formulas.

Intestinal and hepatic utilization of dietary amino acids. Despite continuing debate regarding the systemic appearance of dietary peptides, substantial quantities of free amino acids are released into portal vein for subsequent utilization by other tissues. However, a considerable amount of amino acid metabolism occurs in tissues of splanchnic bed in general, and in intestinal mucosa and liver in particular. Quantitative information continues to accumulate on the proportion of luminal amino acids that are metabolized in the first pass by tissues of splanchnic bed.[134–138]

In considering the nutritional and functional significance of this first-pass metabolism, it is important to separate protein synthesis from amino acid catabolism.[138,139] The rate of protein synthesis in intestinal mucosa is very high.[140] A considerable proportion of this protein synthesis, however, is destined for export to intestinal lumen, and from a metabolic perspective this secretion is part of the amino acid needs of the individual. A luminal supply of amino acids is necessary for normal mucosal cell function and turnover, and the deleterious effects of total parenteral nutrition on mucosal mass are well known. In one sense, then, the first-pass utilization of dietary indispensable amino acids for protein synthesis could be regarded as beneficial to the organism.[141]

It is presumed that most portal amino acids removed by the liver are catabolized and that only a small proportion are used for hepatic protein synthesis. However, isotopic studies in humans and in pigs suggest that extracellular amino acids supply ≈70% of the hepatic protein synthetic precursor pool and that ≈50% of this is derived from portal amino acids.[142–145] The quantitative significance of stimulation of plasma albumin synthesis following ingestion of protein has been highlighted recently, reviving the old idea of a labile protein reserve.[146,147] These experiments may lead to a reappraisal of the overall physiological and nutritional significance of hepatic first-pass amino acid metabolism.

Amino Acid Catabolism

Although protein turnover has the greatest quantitative impact on circulating amino acid dynamics, protein turnover alone does not lead to loss of amino acids from the body. Aside from loss of proteins from the skin and intestine, net body amino acid (N) loss is largely a function of the irrevocable catabolism of carbon skeletons of indispensable amino acids.[48] For kinetic reasons, the catabolism of many amino acids is a function of their concentration in the free amino acid pool of the body.[37,38,49,148] The need to keep amino acid concentrations at levels sufficient to maintain cellular protein synthesis is accompanied by some degree of inevitable amino acid catabolism. Studies of amino acid catabolism in animals receiving very limited intakes of specific amino acids suggest that this inevitable amino acid catabolism may account for 10% of maintenance amino acid need.[46] It follows from this that the rate at which dietary amino acids are utilized in protein synthesis and the minimum amino acid concentration at which protein synthesis is maintained will both have an indirect effect on overall rate of amino acid catabolism.

It has been argued that protein synthesis is the primary factor regulating overall amino acid catabolism.[149] If so, then lowering the concentration of amino acids to the minimum needed to maintain protein synthesis could have a marked effect on the efficiency with which amino acids are used for protein deposition.

General nutritional factors regulating amino acid catabolism. Indispensable amino acid catabolism is primarily influenced by the following four nutritional factors:

1. The degree to which the pattern of amino acids in dietary protein matches amino acid need. This is reflected directly in the efficiency with which a given dietary protein is utilized in productive processes (e.g., growth, lactation) and is the principal factor underlying differences in biological value of dietary proteins. Adaptation to this nutritional variable demands that the organism regulate the catabolism of individual indispensable amino acids independently of the total.

2. The degree to which total nitrogen intake approximates total nitrogen needs of the individual. This factor affects amino acid catabolism in general and is reflected in adaptations in urea synthesis.

3. The balance between essential and nonessential amino acids. As emphasized earlier, dietary indispensable amino acids represent 45% of total amino acid needs for protein deposition and 30% of total for maintenance; the rest consists of dispensable amino acids.[150] Although nonessential amino acids do not have to be supplied in the diet, the organism still has a metabolic need for these nutrients, and if the diet fails to provide them, dispensable amino acids must be synthesized endogenously. An imbalance between indispensable and dispensable amino acids in food demands catabolism of essential amino acids to supply nitrogen for nonessential amino acid synthesis.

4. The degree to which energy intake matches energy needs. Because ultimately the organism must maintain ATP synthesis, amino acid catabolism is also part of the body's energy supply. The most obvious expression of this is the difference between nitrogen balance of a fasting individual (≈ –150 mg N/kg/day) and an individual receiving a zero-protein diet (≈ –50 mg N/kg/day). Furthermore, variations in nonprotein energy intake can have rapid and marked effects on overall amino acid catabolism.[151] Once again, this nutritional variable affects overall amino acid catabolism and is reflected in changes in urea synthesis.[152]

Tissue specificity of amino acid metabolism. The principal sites of amino acid catabolism are small intestine, liver, muscle, and kidney. There are some features of amino acid metabolism that are organ-specific, and amino acid degradation at each site could be regarded as serving different functions.

Of all amino acids, systemic glutamine and enteral (dietary) glutamate appear to be the most extensively metabolized by small intestine, with ≈25% of total plasma glutamine metabolized during each pass through mucosal tissue bed.[153] Recent data from humans suggest that tissues of splanchnic bed remove 80–95% of dietary glutamate supply.[137] Studies in pigs show essentially no portal appearance of enterally administered glutamate.[154,155] Parallel isotopic data show essentially complete catabolism of enteral glutamate by small intestinal mucosa.[156] In terms of carbon flow, the metabolism of enteral glutamate by mucosa greatly exceeds that of arterial glutamine.

The precise fate of glutamate and glutamine metabolized by portal-drained viscera has not been quantified in vivo. The now-classic studies of Windmueller and Spaeth[157] have been interpreted to imply that most of the glutamine—and, by implication, glutamate—carbon is oxidized to CO_2. This oxidation is incomplete, however, and a substantial portion of glutamine carbon and nitrogen may appear as alanine or lactate.[158] There is also increasing evidence that systemic glutamine, and probably dietary glutamate, functions as an important biosynthetic precursor in intestinal cells by supporting synthesis of glutathione, proline, and arginine.[55,65,89,90,137,157,159]

Liver plays a primary role in modifying the quantities and proportions of amino acids from portal blood that are distributed to the rest of the body. The liver is the only organ capable of catabolizing all amino acids, although hepatic catabolism of branched-chain amino acids is slow compared with catabolism of other indispensable amino acids.[160] Only ≈25% of hepatic portal inflow of amino acids appears to exit liver, and a nutritionally significant proportion of portal amino acids removed by liver is directed toward catabolism.[161] This is particularly marked for alanine, which is an important end product of intestinal glutamate and glutamine catabolism.[161,162] There is, moreover, selectivity in hepatic amino acid uptake with regard to level of protein intake and to specific amino acids. For example, ≈25% of portal alanine is removed by liver in rats fed a diet containing a modest amount of protein, whereas 50% is removed by liver in rats fed high-protein diets.[162] Other amino acids such as glycine, serine, tyrosine, phenylalanine, and threonine show similar patterns of response to protein intake.

Skeletal muscle metabolizes the bulk of branched-chain amino acids, whose nitrogen is exported as glutamine and alanine.[160,163] The carbon skeletons then enter the citric acid cycle and are either oxidized completely to CO_2 or are used in glutamine and alanine synthesis. The catabolism of branched amino acids by skeletal muscle is under particularly complex regulation.

Together with liver, kidney maintains acid-base balance by converting glutamine to glutamate (and thence to glucose) or by converting glycine to serine.[164] Both mechanisms generate ammonium ions and bicarbonate. Ammonium ions are excreted in urine whereas bicarbonate is retained in the body and increases extracellular pH. Kidney is also the main site of D-amino acid deamination.

Mechanisms regulating amino acid catabolism: disposal of amino acids provided in excess of metabolic need. For each amino acid, the activity of one enzyme in its catabolic pathway—the rate-limiting or flux-generating enzyme—is less than the activity of other enzymes, and its K_m is usually similar to the plasma concentration of the amino acid in question. The rates of catabolism of specific amino acids are largely influenced by their tissue concentrations, which in turn reflect the balance between dietary supply and metabolic need. Thus the low rate at which the nutritionally limiting amino acid is catabolized is often accompanied by a substantially lower circulating concentration.[37,38,49]

Catabolism of individual amino acids is not simply a function of their ambient concentrations, however. Two further mechanisms, substrate activation and covalent enzyme modification, are used to regulate catabolic pathways in the short term. For example, phenylalanine hydroxylase, the enzyme catalyzing the rate-limiting step of phenylalanine catabolism, not only is activated by binding of phenylalanine to a regulatory site but is also controlled by reversible phosphorylation and dephosphorylation.[165,166] Furthermore, it appears that activation of the hydroxylase by phenylalanine and by phosphorylation is synergistic, such that phosphorylation of the enzyme enhances phenylalanine binding and the presence of phenylalanine facilitates phosphorylation of the hydroxylase.

The catabolic pathway for branched-chain amino acids is another excellent example of regulation via covalent modification of rate-limiting (or flux-generating) enzyme.[167] This pathway is regulated by activity of mitochondrial dehydrogenase, branched-chain keto acid dehydrogenase (BCKADH).[160,167] This enzyme is structurally and functionally similar to pyruvate dehydrogenase. Both multienzyme complexes are regulated by reversible phosphorylation, and in each case phosphorylation inactivates the enzyme. The kinases and phosphatases responsible for catalyzing these reactions are specific to each dehydrogenase complex.[168] The branched-chain keto acids (especially α-ketoisocaproic acid, the transamination product of leucine) inhibit the BCKADH kinase and hence activate BCKADH.[169] This mechanism is of critical importance because it allows persistent activation of the complex by high-protein diets without increasing the overall level of expression, and hence synthesis, of BCKADH.

Relationship between protein intake and protein need. Amino acid catabolism changes rapidly after protein intake.[45,170] Even in the fed state, amino acid catabolism changes within hours in response to a change in overall level of dietary protein.[147] An important factor in the immediate response to protein intake is the concentration of amino acids. The quantitative relationship between circulating amino acid concentrations and their rate of catabolism is not uniform, either between individuals or between diets. A persistently high or low intake of protein leads to an overall increase or decrease in rate of amino acid catabolism that is partially independent of circulating amino acid concentrations.[3,45]

Both short- and long-term changes in protein intake alter the levels of insulin, glucagon, and glucocorticoids, all of which are capable of altering the function of amino acid catabolic enzymes. Glucagon, for example, both activates and induces a wide range of amino acid catabolic enzymes.[171,172] The positive relationship between glucocorticoid level and hepatic amino acid catabolism has been known for many years,[173] but there is now evidence for direct regulation of catabolic enzyme synthesis by amino acids that is independent of hormonal effects.[174,175]

Changes in urea synthesis must accompany changes in catabolism of individual amino acids in relation to protein intake. To some extent, the long half-life (6–8 hours) of the plasma urea pool obscures the short-term responsiveness of urea synthesis to protein intake.[151] The initial enzyme of the urea cycle, carbamoyl-phosphate synthase, has a K_m greatly in excess of hepatic concentration of ammonia, so it is immediately responsive to changes in ammonia production via activity of glutaminase, which is in turn activated by ammonia. In addition, carbamoyl-phosphate synthase is activated by acetyl glutamate, a product of hepatic glutamate-glutamine metabolism that is rapidly sensitive to protein intake.[176]

Long-term regulation of urea synthesis by habitual protein intake is achieved by a coordinate increase in enzyme levels of the complete urea cycle. This occurs largely in response to concomitant changes in glucagon and glucocorticoid hormones.[177] Changes in amounts of enzymes are regulated by different mechanisms, illustrating the multiple levels of control available to mammals. Thus mRNA levels for arginase and carbamoyl-phosphate synthase rise as a result of increased gene transcription and mRNA stability. The mRNAs for arginosuccinate lyase and synthase increase as a result of enhanced mRNA stability, while increase in ornithine transcarbamylase appears to result from stabilization of the enzyme.

Relationship between amino acid and glucose metabolism. Amino acid catabolism provides an important energy source via intermediate products of glycolytic pathways and the citric acid cycle. The urea cycle and the citric acid cycle are linked at the metabolic level by the fact that both effectively involve interconversion of oxaloacetate and fumarate. Channeling of substrates and tight control over concentrations of intermediates of both pathways emphasize the point that amino acid catabolism is not independent of other metabolic processes, but an integral part of homeostasis in the whole organism.[178] A specific relationship exists between dietary carbohydrate and amino acid metabolism because, with the exception of leucine, amino acids—particularly those that lead to synthesis of succinate and fumarate—are precursors of glucose synthesis.[151] Hepatic metabolism of alanine and glutamine to glucose may account for 30% of

hepatic glucose synthesis, but because much of the carbon for peripheral alanine and glutamine synthesis derives from glucose metabolism, hepatic gluconeogenesis from these amino acids is, in effect, a recycling phenomenon akin to the Cori cycle.[179]

There is increasing evidence that carbon skeletons generated by hepatic amino acid catabolism may be specifically channeled toward glucose production. For example, during hyperinsulinemic-euglycemic clamps, coinfusion of a complete mixture of amino acids lowers the rate of glucose infusion necessary to achieve euglycemia.[180] While part of this effect is related to suppression of peripheral glucose utilization, Tappy et al.[180] calculated that close to 100% of carbon derived from catabolism of the amino acid infusion had passed through the gluconeogenic pathway. This occurred despite the fact that hyperinsulinemia had apparently inhibited hepatic glucose output. Jungas et al.[181] reached a similar conclusion from comparisons of the rate of amino acid catabolism and the metabolic rate of liver. They point out that if all carbon derived from hepatic amino acid metabolism were catabolized completely to CO_2 within the liver, then the liver's capacity for disposal of reducing equivalents via ATP synthesis would be exceeded. They concluded that a substantial proportion of hepatic amino acid catabolism *must* be directed toward glucose synthesis. This pathway of amino acid carbon disposal does not affect outcome—either production of ATP or storage of amino acid carbon in body triglyceride—but has an important bearing on efficiency with which amino acids are used as energy sources, and may well underlie the fact that the thermic effect of amino acid catabolism exceeds that calculated from simple oxidative stoichiometry.

Nitrogen metabolism and acid-base balance. Liver has two methods for disposal of nitrogen (ammonium ions), as urea or by forming glutamine from glutamate. The two systems are separated in liver, with ureagenesis occurring in periportal hepatocytes and glutamine synthesis in perivenous compartment.[182] This division enables liver to incorporate most ammonia into urea, but liver maintains the potential for glutamine synthesis if the rate of urea synthesis becomes inadequate for removing hepatic ammonia. Regulation of ammonia disposal in liver provides a particularly interesting example of the regulatory consequences of the kinetic properties of enzymes.

Carbamoyl-phosphate synthase is functionally linked to glutaminase, so in effect there is direct metabolic channeling from glutamine (synthesized in the periphery) and incorporation of amide-N into carbamoyl phosphate. Furthermore, carbamoyl-phosphate synthase has a K_m for ammonia higher by an order of magnitude than typical hepatic ammonia concentrations, while glutamine synthase has a low K_m.[182] In general, carbamoyl phosphate synthesis is directly proportional to prevailing ammonia concentration while glutamine synthesis is maintained at low ammonia concentrations. Glutaminase, on the other hand, is activated by ammonia and strongly inhibited by hydrogen ions.[183] Thus, increased hepatic acidity simultaneously lowers the synthesis of carbamoyl phosphate (hence lowers fixation of NH^{3+} and HCO_3^-) and increases glutamine synthesis. Glutamine is then released and metabolized in kidney, leading to release of urinary ammonia.[164] Both chronic renal failure and liver cirrhosis lead to metabolic acidosis, illustrating the importance of regulation of the urea cycle and interorgan regulation of glutamine metabolism for acid-base balance.

Protein Turnover

From a quantitative standpoint, by far the greatest influence on amino acid turnover and metabolism is the "protein turnover cycle" in which proteins are continuously degraded and resynthesized.[184,185] Coregulation of synthetic and degradative arms of the cycle is crucial to maintaining cellular viability, to regulation of growth and cellular protein mass, and to control of enzyme levels. At least 20% of basal energy expenditure is used in maintaining whole-body protein synthesis.[186,187] Protein synthesis and degradation therefore are of critical importance to the body's physiology. Measurement of protein synthesis and degradation in vivo relies almost exclusively on the use of isotopically labeled amino acids. The best approach continues to be a matter of active and unresolved debate, and comments on the effect of nutritional, hormonal, or other physiological influences on protein turnover must be tempered by the possibility of measurement artifacts.[188-194] Central to the problem is a definition of isotopic enrichment of amino acid pool feeding protein synthesis. Intracellular amino acid pools of cells are compartmentalized, and the isotopic enrichment of tRNA-bound amino acids is not the same as that of the extracellular and intracellular amino acid pools.[143,194] Furthermore, labeling relationships may vary with nutritional and physiological states.[141,195]

Because it is extremely difficult to measure labeling of amino acyl tRNA, and essentially impossible in humans, a variety of indirect approaches have been used in an attempt to circumvent the problem. A frequently used approach in animal studies is to administer a large dose of the amino acid being traced along with the isotopic tracer.[196,197] Opinions differ as to validity of this method and specifically whether large quantities of a single amino acid (leucine, phenylalanine, or valine) acutely alter protein synthesis.[192,193]

Clinical studies have used other indirect indices of intracellular amino acid labeling. Labeling of α-ketoisocaproic acid, the leucine transamination product, has been used to infer the isotopic enrichment of the intracellular leucine pool.[190,198,199] This seems a very useful method for studying muscle protein metabolism, but may be less applicable to other tissues. Equilibrium labeling of apolipoprotein B-100 has also been used to measure isotopic enrichment of hepatic amino acids.[142,143,200,201]

Quantification of protein degradation is even more problematical. Isotopic approaches to determining proteolysis suffer the same problems of intracellular amino acid pool heterogeneity as those of synthesis. A recent report measured whole-body 3-methyl histidine kinetics to determine whole-body myofibrillar protein degradation.[202] Release of this posttranslationally modified amino acid has been used to measure myofibrillar protein degradation in vitro.[203-207]

A particularly useful method has been applied extensively in clinical studies. This method combines measurements of concentrations and isotopic enrichments of tracer amino acids across specific tissues like leg or forearm.[208,209] This is an important advance because, in principle at least, it allows simultaneous determination of protein synthesis and degradation. In a recent report the tracer balance approach was combined with measurements of 3-methylhistidine release to show the selective effect of insulin on nonmyofibrillar protein degradation.[210]

A second advance, made possible by improvements in mass spectrometric sensitivity, involves using stable isotopic methods in combination with immunological or chemical techniques of protein purification to study regulation of turnover of specific proteins.[197,200,201,211-214] Reports on the use of stable isotopes to study synthesis of specific proteins in tissues are also now appearing.[215]

Tracers labeled in specific positions with either ^{13}C or ^2H are being used with greater frequency to study amino acid synthesis and interconversion. Data are now available regarding metabolic relationships between methionine and cysteine, phenylalanine and tyrosine, arginine and its precursors and products, and glutamate and proline synthesis.[84,85,137,159,216-218]

Factors regulating overall protein synthesis and degradation. Protein mass and rates of protein gain or loss in a cell are entirely dependent on the balance—i.e., the relative rates—of protein synthesis and degradation. The two processes are mechanistically distinct. Although both are influenced by protein and energy nutritional status and by the same hormones (e.g., insulin, growth factors, growth hormone, and glucocorticoids), direction and magnitude of a response of either process are not easily predicted.[219-228] Furthermore, nutritional status—especially amino acid intake—and the response of protein turnover to endocrinological changes interact in a complex way.[229-232]

As a result of these complexities it has proved difficult to identify a common response even when the same outcome variable (e.g., increased protein deposition) is achieved. For example, stimulation of proliferative growth involves a simultaneous increase in protein synthesis and decrease in protein degradation, while hypertrophic growth (e.g., of a muscle in response to increased workload) involves simultaneous increases in both protein synthesis and degradation.[233–236] Similarly, increases in whole-body protein retention brought about by either increased intake of energy, limiting amino acid, or insulin infusion appear to involve primary changes in whole-body protein degradation.[221,237,238] On the other hand, separate evidence implies that changes associated with total protein intake or following growth hormone administration involve primarily protein synthesis.[225,226,230,237,239] Furthermore, the magnitude of changes in whole-body protein turnover, even in response to a common nutritional manipulation, can depend on the prior nutritional status of the individual.[219]

Rates of protein turnover also vary systematically between tissues, and the relative importance of protein synthesis and degradation in the control of cellular protein mass may be tissue-specific.[240–243] Failure to recognize tissue-specific effects can lead to confusion in interpreting studies of whole-body protein turnover because failure to find a change in the body as a whole can merely reflect equal but opposite changes at different sites. Such may be the case with respect to changes in protein turnover accompanying lactation in humans, whose increases in protein turnover in visceral compartments are balanced by lower rates of peripheral protein turnover.[244,245] The reverse appears to be the case with regard to growth hormone administration in humans, who show no effect on a whole-body basis but a stimulation of muscle protein synthesis.[226]

Developmental factors influence regulation of protein turnover as it relates to protein deposition. Protein synthesis appears to be of particular importance to nutritional regulation of growth of immature tissues, but the response of protein synthesis to protein intake becomes progressively smaller as subjects approach adulthood.[243,246–248] In adults, protein degradation seems to be the critical factor regulating protein balance in the short term. Clearly much still needs to be learned about the nutritional, physiological, and hormonal regulation of this major metabolic process.

Potential mechanisms for the regulation of protein synthesis. Regulation of protein synthesis—i.e., mRNA translation—is almost necessarily complex. Because enzymes responsible for synthesis of amino acyl tRNAs have very low K_ms, they are fully saturated with their substrate amino acids under all but the most extreme circumstances of amino acid depletion. Thus, although severe amino acid deprivation will inhibit protein synthesis via substrate limitation, it is unlikely that amino acid concentrations normally regulate protein synthesis

via a kinetic mechanism. This finding stands in marked contrast to the regulation of amino acid catabolism. Translation of mRNA is regulated by enzyme activity—i.e., the concentration and translational activity of ribosomes. Both of these aspects are under developmental, nutritional, and hormonal control.

Considerable progress in our understanding of the biochemical steps and regulation of translation was made in the past decade, and comprehensive reviews appeared in the 1980s.[249,250] Further advances have taken place recently, particularly with regard to the nature and roles of the multiple accessory factors that regulate the selection of mRNA for translation. Two recent reviews are particularly useful sources of information on these mechanistic matters.[251,252]

Protein synthesis is regulated in both the long and short term. Long-term regulation of protein synthesis, such as that associated with postnatal development and with tissue differences in protein synthesis, is largely a function of the concentration of ribosomes—i.e., the capacity for protein synthesis. Cellular ribosome concentrations are affected by nutrient status, increased functional demand, and hormones such as insulin, thyroid, growth hormone, and the glucocorticoids.[253–258] The ribosome is an extremely complex organelle that contains at least 85 proteins in addition to the rRNA species.[251] Control of ribosome biosynthesis involves the coregulation of synthesis of both RNA and protein moieties. Although there have been considerable advances in understanding rRNA synthesis and processing, less is known about factors regulating ribosomal protein synthesis.[259,260] There is, however, evidence that insulin, a hormone that appears to stimulate protein anabolism in virtually all cells, has specific effects on both synthesis and degradation of ribosomal proteins.[261]

Regarding the short-term regulation of translation, most evidence suggests that primary regulation by insulin, glucocorticoids, and amino acids is exerted at the initiation stage, although other factors such as cellular ATP supply may act at other steps.[252,262,263] Activation of initiation and hence translation as a whole can occur very rapidly, and it can be argued that the rapidity of this response has a very important effect on the efficiency with which dietary amino acids are stored in protein, as opposed to being irrevocably catabolized.[229,243,245,264] It is less certain which factors are responsible for the short-term regulation of initiation, particularly as it relates to nutritional effects. It seems increasingly likely that different factors may be important in different organs or with regard to different regulatory influences.[262,265,266]

Protein degradation and its regulation. Degradation of cellular protein is also an ongoing process. Among other functions, protein degradation serves to remove "error" proteins and provides cells with a supply of free amino adds during periods of nutrient deprivation.[267,268]

Two factors must be taken into account when considering protein degradation and its regulation. First, the half-lives of different proteins vary widely (by at least three orders of magnitude) even within cells, and these differences are maintained even when overall proteolysis changes markedly. Amino acid sequences that either increase or decrease susceptibility to proteolytic attack by a specific proteolytic system have been identified,[269–272] but these sequences appear to influence degradation of only a restricted set of proteins, and the molecular basis for the specificity of protein degradation remains largely unknown. Second, proteins do not exist in free solution within cells but are organized either in distinct organelles or in other structures such as myofilaments and multienzyme complexes. If functional integrity of these structures is to be maintained, the degradation of each component of the structure must be coregulated. There is good evidence for independent regulation of the degradation of myofibrillar and nonmyofibrillar protein in skeletal muscle.

Our understanding of protein degradation at the mechanistic level has progressed to the point where we now know not only that there are at least three major proteolytic systems, but that these systems have protein substrate specificities and may well play different roles within the cell.[273–275]

The *lysosomal-autophagic system* involves primarily cathepsins and is important to the degradation of proteins that have entered cells via endocytosis. The system involves the formation of distinct vacuolar structures capable of engulfing and degrading complete organelles.[276] Although most evidence suggests that this pathway of degradation is unselective, there is some evidence for the involvement of specific peptide sequences in targeting proteins to the lysosomal compartment.[271] This system may also be involved in hepatic RNA turnover.[277] At the physiological level the lysosomal system appears to be of special importance under conditions in which cellular proteolysis is maximally activated, e.g., extreme deprivation of nutrients and anabolic hormonal or growth factors.[268,278] The role of macroautophagy in amino acid and insulin regulation of hepatic proteolysis has been studied extensively, and leucine and alanine have been identified as key amino acids that interact with one another and with insulin in regulating the pathway.[278,279] Recent research has made significant inroads into identifying cell-surface amino acid receptors involved in hepatic proteolysis.[280]

The *calpain-calpastatin system* is the major calcium-activated pathway of protein degradation, and consists of a complex of papain-like cysteine protease and a smaller-molecular-weight, calmodulin-like, calcium-binding regulatory subunit.[281] At least two main calpain isoforms have been identified on the basis of calcium concentrations (micromolar and millimolar) at which they are activated. The system is also subject to inhibition by the protein calpastatin. Paradoxically calpastatin activity seems to be greater than calpain activity, and in some cases coactivation of gene expression for both components has been demonstrated.[282,283] A characteristic of calpain-catalyzed proteolysis is that it is incomplete. It is generally held that these proteases play an important role in proteolysis of cellular membrane and microfilamentous structures. The calpains probably play a key role in muscle myofibrillar protein turnover by catalyzing initial disruption of the structure via proteolysis at the Z-disc.[284] There is also evidence to suggest that nutritional regulation of muscle proteolysis may involve changes in calpain activity that are modulated both by changes in gene expression and by enhanced translational selection of mRNA at the ribosomal level.[285]

The *ubiquitin-proteasome system* has received considerable attention since its identification in the 1980s, and its proteolytic mechanisms and their regulation are perhaps better understood than those involved in other proteolytic pathways.[273] There are four key features of this pathway: 1) it is widely distributed among tissues; 2) it has a relatively broad protein specificity; 3) it catalyzes the complete hydrolysis of protein substrates; and 4) it is ATP-dependent.

The ubiquitin-proteasome pathway consists of two components, a recognition system involving the protein ubiquitin, which is responsible for targeting the protein substrates toward degradation, and a large-molecular-weight, multifunctional protease now generally termed the proteasome.[286] Targeting of proteins for degradation by this system is via ATP-dependent formation of an isopeptide bond between the ε-amino group on lysine residues of substrate proteins and the carboxyterminal glycine of ubiquitin. Formation of the isopeptide bond is catalyzed by a family of four proteins collectively termed E3; these proteins may confer substrate specificity to the pathway. Although each of the E3 isoforms recognizes somewhat different amino acid sequences at the N-termini of target proteins, polypeptides that do not bear these sequences are also ubiquitinated.

Once proteins have been targeted by formation of a polyubiquitin complex, they are degraded by the proteolytic multienzyme complex, the proteasome. There is still controversy regarding the exact structure of the complex, and two apparently closely related particles with sedimentation coefficients of 20 and 26S have been identified. Although these are generally held to be closely related, their precise relationship is still the subject of research. In an ATP-dependent process, the 20S multicatalytic protease is thought to be incorporated into the 26S "proteasome," which requires participation of three other protein factors, CF-1, -2, and -3. Formation of this complex is an important part of regulation of the system as a whole.[274]

The precise role of this complex pathway of proteolysis, and specifically whether it is responsible for the bulk of physiological protein turnover, remains unclear. A strong case has been made for its involvement in the initial proteolytic steps of antigen processing and in the rapid turnover of oncogenic products and abnormal proteins.[287,288] Although the ubiquitin pathway is activated in skeletal muscle during fasting or glucocorticoid treatment and in diabetes, both lysosomal and calcium-activated proteolysis are activated under the same conditions. The only circumstance in which ubiquitin may be specifically involved is in denervation atrophy.[274,289-291]

Even less is known about regulation of proteolysis than about protein synthesis; nevertheless, long-term changes in proteolysis associated with frank catabolic states probably involve an overall increase in all components of the proteolytic system. The level of expression of mRNAs for key protein components has been elucidated for a number of different circumstances,[292,293] yet virtually nothing is known about the mechanisms underlying the rapid responses of protein degradation.

Conclusion

Our knowledge, if not our understanding, of many aspects of protein and amino acid metabolism, function, and nutrition continues to expand. Studies involving combinations of molecular and kinetic techniques are beginning to unravel the complex multicellular organization of these integral parts of mammalian physiology. Completely new roles for amino acids, such as arginine as precursor of nitric oxide synthesis, are emerging. As Harper[294] points out, we may be entering a period of research into amino acid metabolism. This developing information will not only resolve nutritional controversies, but will also provide the basis for flexible recommendations about protein and amino acid intake.

Acknowledgment

This work is a publication of the USDA/ARS Children's Nutrition Research Center, Department of Pediatrics, Baylor College of Medicine and Texas Children's Hospital, Houston, TX. Funding has been provided from the USDA/ARS under Cooperative Agreement No. 5862-5-01003. The contents of this publication do not necessarily reflect the views or policies of the USDA, nor does mention of trade names, commercial products, or organizations imply endorsement by the U.S. government.

References

1. Steele RD, Harper AE (1990) Proteins and amino acids. In Brown, ML (ed), Present knowledge in nutrition, 6th ed. ILSI Press, Washington, DC, pp 67–79

2. Young VR (1994) Adult amino acid requirements: the case for a major revision in current recommendations. J Nutr 126:1517S–1523S

3. Millward DJ (1994) Can we define indispensable amino acid requirements and assess protein quality in adults? J Nutr 126:1509S–1516S

4. Fuller MF, Garlick PJ (1994) Human amino acid requirements: can the controversy be resolved? Annu Rev Nutr 14:217–241

5. Food and Agricultural Organization and World Health Organization (1991) Assessment of protein quality. Food and Agricultural Organization, Rome, Italy

6. International Dietary Energy Consultancy Group (1995) Reappraisal of energy and protein requirements of human beings. Eur J Clin Nutr, in press

7. Food and Agriculture Organization and World Health Organization (1965) Protein requirements. World Health Organization Technical Report Series 301. Geneva, Switzerland

8. Committee on Dietary Allowances, Food and Nutrition Board, National Research Council (1974) Recommended dietary allowances. National Academy of Sciences, Washington, DC

9. Food and Agriculture Organization, World Health Organization and United Nations University (1985) Energy and protein requirements. World Health Organization Technical Report Series 724, Geneva, Switzerland

10. Fuller MF, McWilliam R, Wang TC, Giles LR (1989) The optimum dietary amino acid pattern for growing pigs. Br J Nutr 64:255–267

11. Chung TK, Baker DA (1992) Ideal amino acid pattern for 10 kg pigs. J Anim Sci 70:3102–3111

12. Pineda O, Torun B, Viteri FE, Arroyave G (1981) Protein quality in relation to estimates of essential amino acid requirements. In Bodwell CE, Adkins JS, Hopkins DT (eds), Protein quality in humans. AVI Publishing, Westport, CT, pp 374–393

13. Torun B (1989) Current concepts on requirements of essential amino acids. In Kim WY, Lee YC, Lee, KY, et al (eds), Proceedings of the 14th international congress of nutrition. Ehwa Women's University Press, Seoul, Korea, pp 87–91

14. Gattas V, Barrera GA, Riumallo JS, Uauy R (1990) Protein-energy requirements of prepubertal school-age boys determined by using the nitrogen-balance response to a mixed protein diet. Am J Clin Nutr 52:1037–1042

15. Gattas V, Barrera GA, Riumallo JS, Uauy R (1992) Protein-energy requirements of boys 12–14 years old determined by using the nitrogen-balance response to a mixed protein diet. Am J Clin Nutr 56:499–503

16. Young VR (1995) Protein quality of enteral nutritionals. J Nutr 127:1363–1364

17. Sarwar G, Peace RW (1995) Protein quality of enteral nutritionals: a response to Young. J Nutr 127:1365–1366

18. Womack M, Rose WC (1947) The role of proline, hydroxyproline and glutamic acid in growth. J Biol Chem 171:37–50

19. Berthold HK, Hachey DL, Reeds PJ, et al (1991) Uniformly labelled algal protein used to determine amino acid essentiality in vivo. Proc Natl Acad Sci USA 88:8091–8095

20. Chipponi JX, Bleier JC, Sanb MT, Rudman D (1982) Deficiencies of essential and conditionally essential nutrients. Am J Clin Nutr 35:1112–1116

21. Visek WJ (1984) An update of concepts of essential amino acids. Annu Rev Nutr 4:137–155

22. Jackson AA (1983) Amino acids: essential or non-essential? Lancet 1:1034–1039

23. Laidlaw SA, Kopple JD (1987) Newer concepts of the indispensable amino acid. Am J Clin Nutr 46:593–605

24. Featherstone WR, Rogers QR, Freedland RA (1973) Relative importance of kidney and liver in the synthesis of arginine by the rat. Am J Physiol 224:G127–G129

25. Wakabayashi Y, Yamada E, Yoshida T, Takahashi H (1994) Arginine becomes an essential amino acid after massive resection of the rat small intestine. J Biol Chem 269:32667–32671

26. Jaksic T, Jahoor F, Reeds PJ, Heird WC (1993) The determination of amino acid synthesis in human neonates with a glucose stable isotope. Surg Forum 44:642–686

27. Jackson AA, Shaw JCL, Barber A, Golden MHN (1981) Nitrogen metabolism in pre-term infants fed human donor breast milk: the possible essentiality of glycine. Pediatr Res 15:1454–1461

28. Davis TA, Nguyen HV, Garcia-Bravo R, et al (1994) The amino acid composition of human milk is not unique. J Nutr 124:1128–1134

29. Reeds PJ, Hutchens TW (1994) Protein requirements: from nitrogen balance to functional impact. J Nutr 126:1754S–1764S

30. Beaton GA, Chery A (1988) Protein requirements of infants: a reexamination of concepts and approaches. Am J Clin Nutr 48:1403–1412

31. Stack T, Reeds PJ, Preston T, et al (1989) 15N-tracer studies of protein metabolism in low birth weight infants. Pediatr Res 25:167–172

32. Reeds PJ (1988) Nitrogen metabolism and protein requirements. In Blaxter KL, Macdonald I (eds), Comparative nutrition. John Libbey, London, pp 55–72

33. Young VR (1987) Kinetics of human amino acid metabolism: nutritional implications and some lessons. Am J Clin Nutr 46:709–725

34. Young VR, Bier DM, Pellett PL (1989) A theoretical basis for increasing current estimates of the amino acid requirements in adult man, with experimental support. Am J Clin Nutr 50:80–92

35. Rose WC (1957) The amino acid requirements of adult man. Nutrition Abstr Rev 27. Commonwealth Agricultural Bureau, Wallingford, UK, pp 631–647

36. Leverton RM (1959) Amino acid requirements of young adults. In Albanese AA (ed), Protein and amino acid nutrition. Academic Press, New York, pp 477–506

37. Meguid MM, Matthews DE, Bier DM, et al (1986) Leucine kinetics at graded leucine intakes in young men. Am J Clin Nutr 43:770–780

38. Meredith CN, Wen Z-M, Bier DM, et al (1986) Lysine kinetics at graded lysine intakes in young men. Am J Clin Nutr 43:787–794

39. Young VR, Khoury AE (1995) Can amino acid requirements for nutritional maintenance in adult humans be approximated from the amino acid composition of body mixed proteins? Proc Natl Acad Sci USA 92:300–304

40. Khoury AE, Fukagawa NK, S'anchez M, et al (1994) The 24-hour pattern and rate of leucine oxidation, with particular reference to tracer estimates of leucine requirements in healthy adults. Am J Clin Nutr 59:1012–1020

41. Khoury AE, Fukagawa NK, S'anchez M, et al (1994) Validation of the tracer-balance concept with reference to leucine: 24-h intravenous tracer studies with L-[1-13C]-leucine and [15N-15N]-urea. Am J Clin Nutr 59:1000–1011

42. Young VR, Pellett PL (1994) Plant proteins in relation to human protein and amino acid nutrition. Am J Clin Nutr 59:1203S–1212S

43. Millward DJ, Rivers JPW (1988) The nutritional role of indispensable amino acids and the metabolic basis for their requirements. Eur J Clin Nutr 42:367–393

44. Millward DJ, Jackson AA, Price G, Rivers JPW (1989) Human amino acid requirements: current dilemmas and uncertainties. Nutr Rev Lett 2:109–132

45. Pacy PJ, Price GM, Halliday D, et al (1994) Nitrogen homeostasis in man: diurnal responses of protein synthesis and degradation and amino acid oxidation to diets with increasing protein intakes. Clin Sci 86:103–118

46. Beckett PR, Fuller MF, Cadenhead A, et al (1987) Whole body flux and degradation of amino acids measured with [3H]- and [14C]-labels in pigs given diets deficient in histidine, phenylalanine or leucine. In Bergner A (ed), Proceedings of the 5th International Symposium on Protein Metabolism and Nutrition, September 1987. European Association for Animal Production, Rostock, Germany, pp 7–12

47. Roberton AM, Rabe B, Harding CA, et al (1991) Use of the ileal conduit as a model for studying human small intestinal mucus glycoprotein secretion. Am J Physiol 261:G728–G734

48. Fuller MF, Milne A, Harris CI, et al (1993) Amino acid losses in ileostomy fluid on a protein-free diet. Am J Clin Nutr 59:70–73

49. Zhao X-H, Wen Z-M, Meredith CN, et al (1986) Threonine kinetics at graded threonine intakes in young men. Am J Clin Nutr 43:795–803

50. Chandra RK (1991) Nutrition and immunity: lessons from the past and new insights into the future. Am J Clin Nutr 53:1089–1101

51. Colley CM, Fleck A, Goode AW, et al (1983) Early time course of the acute phase protein response in man. J Clin Pathol 36:203–207

52. Jennings G, Bourgeois C, Elia M (1992) The magnitude of the acute phase protein response is attenuated by protein deficiency in rats. J Nutr 122:1325–1331

53. Doherty JF, Golden MHN, Rayned JG, et al (1993) Acute phase protein response is impaired in severely malnourished children. Clin Sci 84:169–175

54. Grimble RF, Jackson AA, Persaud C, et al (1992) Cysteine and glycine supplementation modulate the metabolic response to tumor necrosis factor A in rats fed a low protein diet. J Nutr 122:2066–2073

55. Jahoor F, Wykes LJ, Heird WC, et al (1995) Protein-deficient pigs cannot maintain reduced glutathione homeostasis when subjected to the stress of inflammation. J Nutr 125:1462–1472

56. Jackson AA (1986) Blood glutathione in severe malnutrition in childhood. Trans R Soc Trop Med Hyg 80:911–913

57. Hansen TN, Smith CV, Martin NE, et al (1990) Oxidant stress responses in ventilated newborn infants [abstract]. Pediatr Res 27:208A

58. Newsholme EA, Crabtree B, Ardawi MSM (1985) Glutamine metabolism in lymphocytes: its biochemical, physiological and clinical importance. Q J Exp Physiol 70:473–489

59. Souba WW, Herskowitz K, Salloum RM, et al (1990) Gut glutamine metabolism. J Parenter Enter Nutr 14:456–463

60. Scheppach W, Loges C, Bartram P, et al (1994) Effect of free glutamine and alanyl-glutamine dipeptide on mucosal proliferation of the human ileum and colon. Gastroenterology 107:429–434

61. McLennan PA, Brown RA, Rennie MJ (1987) A positive relationship between protein synthetic rate and intracellular glutamine concentration in perfused rat skeletal muscle. FEBS Lett 215:187–191

62. McLennan PA, Smith K, Weryk B, et al (1988) Inhibition of protein breakdown by glutamine in perfused skeletal muscle. FEBS Lett 237:133–136

63. Rennie MJ, Babij P, Taylor PM, et al (1986) Characteristics

of a glutamine carrier in skeletal muscle have important consequences for nitrogen loss in injury, infection and chronic disease. Lancet 2:1008–1012

64. Welbourne TC, King AB, Horton K (1993) Enteral glutamine supports hepatic glutathione efflux during inflammation. J Nutr Biochem 4:236–242

65. Harward TR, Coe D, Souba WW, et al (1994) Glutamine preserves gut glutathione during intestinal ischemia/reperfusion. J Surg Res 56:351–355

66. Weiss SJ, Klein R, Slivka A, Wei M (1982) Chlorination of taurine by human neutrophils. Evidence for hypochlorous acid generation. J Clin Invest 70:598–607

67. Schmieden V, Kuhse J, Betz H (1992) Agonist pharmacology of neonatal and adult glycine receptor a subunits; identification of amino acid residues involved in taurine activation. Eur Mol Biol Org J 11:2025–2032

68. Reeds PJ. (1981) Creatine and creatinine metabolism. In Waterlow JC, Stephen JML, (eds), Nitrogen metabolism in man. Applied Science Publishers, London, pp 263–269

69. Vazquez JA, Paleos GA, Steinhard HJ, et al (1986) Protein nutrition and amino acid metabolism after 4 weeks of total parenteral nutrition with a mixture of 14 dipeptides: serendipitous observations on effects of sepsis in baboons. Am J Clin Nutr 44:24–32

70. Brough W, Horne G, Blount A, et al (1986) Effects of nutrient intake, surgery, sepsis and long term administration of steroids on muscle function. Br Med J 293:983–988

71. Rassin DK, Sturman JA, Gaull GE (1978) Taurine and other free amino acids in milk of man and other mammals. Early Hum Devel 2:1–13

72. Wu G, Knabe DA (1994) Free and protein-bound amino acids in sow's colostrum and milk. J Nutr 124:415–424

73. Rees DD, Palmer RMJ, Moncada S (1989) Role of endothelium-derived nitric oxide in the regulation of blood pressure. Proc Natl Acad Sci USA 86:3375–3378

74. Bredt DS, Hwang PM, Snyder SH (1990) Localization of nitric oxide synthase indicating a neural role for nitric oxide. Nature 347:768–770

75. O'Dell TJ, Hawkins RD, Kandel ER, Arancio O (1991) Tests for the roles of two diffusible substances in long-term potentiation: evidence for nitric oxide as a possible early retrograde messenger. Proc Natl Acad Sci USA 88:11285–11289

76. Ekblad E, Alm P, Sundler F (1994) Distribution, origin and projections of nitric oxide synthase-containing neurons in gut and pancreas. Neuroscience 63:233–248

77. Curran RD, Ferrari FK, Kisbert PH, et al (1991) Nitric oxide and nitric oxide-generating compounds inhibit hepatocyte protein synthesis. FASEB J 5:2085–2092

78. Frederick JA, Hasselgren PO, Davis S, et al (1993) Nitric oxide may upregulate in vivo hepatic protein synthesis during endotoxemia. Arch Surg 130:152–156

79. Stadler J, Barton D, Beil-Moeller M, et al (1995) Hepatocyte nitric oxide biosynthesis inhibits glucose output and competes with urea synthesis for L-arginine. Am J Physiol 268:G183–G188

80. Kirk SJ, Regan MC, Wasserkrug HL, et al (1992) Arginine enhances T-cell responses in athymic nude mice. J Parenter Enter Nutr 16:429–432

81. Liew FY, Millott S, Parkinson C, et al (1990) Macrophage killing of Leishmania parasite in vivo is mediated by nitric oxide from L-arginine. J Immunol 144:4794–4797

82. Denham S, Rowland IJ (1992) Inhibition of the reactive proliferation of lymphocytes by activated macrophages: the role of nitric oxide. Clin Exp Immunol 87:157–162

83. Kubes P, Suzuki M, Granger DN (1991) Nitric oxide: an endogenous modulator of leukocyte adhesion. Proc Natl Acad Sci USA 88:4651–4655

84. Castillo L, deRojas TC, Chapman TE, et al (1993) Splanchnic metabolism of dietary arginine in relation to nitric oxide synthesis in normal adult man. Proc Natl Acad Sci USA 90:193–197

85. Castillo L, S'anchez M, Vogt J, et al (1995) Plasma arginine, citrulline and ornithine kinetics in adults, with observations on nitric oxide synthesis. Am J Physiol 268:E360–E367

86. Robert J-J, Bier DM, Zhao XH, et al (1982) Glucose and insulin effects on de novo amino acid synthesis in young men: studies with stable isotope labelled alanine, leucine and lysine. Metabolism 31:1210–1218

87. Hoffer LJ, Yang RD, Matthews DE, et al (1985) Effects of meal consumption on whole body leucine and alanine kinetics in young adult men. Br J Nutr 53:31–38

88. Darmaun D, Matthews DE, Bier DM (1986) Glutamine and glutamate kinetics in humans. Am J Physiol 251:E117–E126

89. Berthold HK, Reeds PJ, Klein PD (1995) Isotopic evidence for the differential regulation of arginine and proline synthesis in man. Metabolism 44:466–473

90. Wu G, Knabe DA, Yan W, Flynn NE (1995) Glutamine and glucose metabolism in the enterocytes of the neonatal pig. Am J Physiol 268:R334–R342

91. Webb KE Jr (1990) Intestinal absorption of protein hydrolysis products: a review. J Anim Sci 68:3011–3022

92. Kilberg MS, Stevens BR, Novak DA (1993) Recent advances in mammalian amino acid transport. Annu Rev Nutr 13:137–165

93. Matthews DM, Adibi SA (1976) Peptide absorption. Gastroenterology 7:151–161

94. Silk DBA (1974) Progress report: peptide absorption in man. Gut 14:494–501

95. Daniel H, Morse EL, Adibi SA (1992) Determinants of substrate affinity of the oligopeptide H+ symporter in the renal brush border membrane. J Biol Chem 267:9565–9573

96. Thwaites DT, Hirst BH, Simmons NL (1994) Substrate specificity of the di/tri transporter in human intestinal epithelia (Caco-2): identification of substrates that undergo H+-coupled absorption. Br J Pharmacol 113:1050–1056

97. Minami H, Daniel H, Adibi SA (1992) Oligopeptides: mechanism of renal clearance depends on molecular structure. Am J Physiol 263:F109–F115

98. Grimble GK (1994) The significance of peptides in clinical nutrition. Annu Rev Nutr 14:419–447

99. Adibi SA, Krzysik BA (1977) Cytoplasmic dipeptidase activities of kidney, ileum, jejunum, liver, muscle and blood. Am J Physiol 233:E450–E456

100. Raghunath M, Morese EL, Adibi SA (1990) Mechanism of clearance of dipeptides by perfused hindquarters: sarcolemmal hydrolysis of peptides. Am J Physiol 259:E463–E469

101. Backwell FRC (1994) Peptide utilization by tissues: current status and applications of stable isotopic procedures. Proc Nutr Soc 53:457–464

102. Koeln L, Schlagheck TG, Webb KE (1993) Amino acid flux across the gastrointestinal tract and liver of calves. J Dairy Sci 76:2275–2285

103. Gardner MLG, Lindblad BS, Burton D, Matthews DM (1983) Transmucosal passage of intact peptides in the guinea-pig small intestine in vivo: a reappraisal. Clin Sci 64:433–439

104. Seal CJ, Parker DS (1991) Isolation and characterization of circulating low molecular weight peptides in steer, sheep and rat portal and peripheral blood. Comp Biochem Physiol [B] 99:679–685

105. Mahe S, Roos N, Benamouzig R, et al (1994) True exogenous and endogenous nitrogen fractions in the human small

jejunum after ingestion of small amounts of ^{15}N-labeled casein. J Nutr 124:548–555

106. Roos N, Mahe S, Benamouzig RM, et al (1995) ^{15}N-labeled immunoglobulins from bovine colostrum are partially resistant to digestion in human intestine. J Nutr 125:1238–1244

107. de Lange CFM, Souffrant WB, Sauer WC (1990) Real ileal and amino acid digestibilities in feedstuffs for growing pigs as determined with the ^{15}N-isotope dilution technique. J Anim Sci 68:409–418

108. Huisman J, Heinz T, van der Poel AF, et al (1992) True protein digestibility and amounts of endogenous protein measured with the ^{15}N-dilution technique in piglets fed on peas and common beans. Br J Nutr 68:101–110

109. Souffrant WB, Rerat A, Laplace JP, et al (1993) Exogenous and endogenous contributions to nitrogen fluxes in the digestive tract of pigs fed a casein diet. III: recycling of endogenous nitrogen. Reprod Nutr Dev 33:373–382

110. Shulman RJ, Gannon NG, Reeds PJ (1995) Cereal feeding and the nitrogen economy of the infant. Am J Clin Nutr 62:969–972

111. Liu CH, Hays VW, Svec HJ, et al (1955) The fate of urea in growing pigs. J Nutr 57:241–247

112. Wrong OM, Vinci AJ, Waterlow JC (1985) The contribution of endogenous urea to fecal ammonia in man determined with ^{15}N-labelling of plasma urea. Clin Sci 68:193–199

113. Jackson AA, Doherty J, de Benoist MH, et al (1990) The effect of the level of dietary protein, carbohydrate and fat on urea kinetics in young during rapid catch-up weight gain. Br J Nutr 64:371–385

114. Fomon SJ, Matthews DE, Bier DM, et al (1987) Bioavailability of dietary urea nitrogen in the infant. J Pediatr 111:221–224

115. Heine W, Tiess M, Wutzke KD (1986) ^{15}N-tracer investigations of the physiological availability of urea nitrogen in mother's milk. Acta Pediatr Scand 75:439–443

116. Danielson M, Jackson AA (1992) Limits of adaptation to a diet low in protein in normal man: urea kinetics. Clin Sci 83:103–108

117. Forrester T, Badaloo AV, Persaud C, Jackson AA (1994) Urea production and salvage during pregnancy in normal Jamaican women. Am J Clin Nutr 60:341–346

118. Torrallardona D, Harris CI, Milne E, Fuller MF (1993) Contribution of intestinal microflora to lysine requirements in nonruminants [abstract]. Proc Nutr Soc 52:153A

119. Berseth CL (1987) Enhancement of intestinal growth in neonatal rats by epidermal growth factor in milk. Am J Physiol 253:G662–G665

120. Klagsbrun M (1978) Human milk stimulates DNA synthesis and cellular proliferation in cultured fibroblasts. Proc Natl Acad Sci USA 75:5057–5061

121. Grosvener CE, Picciano MF, Baumrucker CR (1993) Hormones and growth factors in milk. Endocr Rev 14:710–728

122. Donovan SM, Ode J (1994) Growth factors in milk as mediators of infant development. Annu Rev Nutr 14:147–167

123. Lonnedal B (1985) Biochemistry and physiological function of human milk proteins. Am J Clin Nutr 42:1299–1317

124. Hutchens TW, Yip T-T, Morgan WT (1992) Identification of histidine-rich glycoprotein in human colostrum and milk. Pediatr Res 31:239–246

125. Gardner MLG (1988) Gastrointestinal absorption of intact proteins. Annu Rev Nutr 8:329–350

126. Kumoves LG, Heath JP (1992) Uptake of maternal immunoglobulins in the enterocytes of suckling piglets: improved detection with a streptavidin-biotin bridge gold technique. J Histochem Cytochem 40:1637–1646

127. Goldblum RM, Schanler RJ, Garza C, Goldman AS (1989) Human milk feeding enhances the excretion of immuno-

128. Hutchens TW, Henry JF, Yip T-T, et al (1991) Origin of intact lactoferrin and its DNA binding fragments found in the urine of human milk-fed infants: evaluation by stable isotopic enrichments. Pediat Res 29:243–250

129. Burrin DG, Davis TA, Ebner S, et al (1995) Stimulation of skeletal muscle protein synthesis in colostrum-fed newborn pigs by nutrient-independent factors. Pediatr Res 37:593–599

130. Kanda Y, Yamamoto N, Abe Y (1994) Growth factor from human milk: purification and characterization. Life Sci 55:1509–1520

131. Xu RJ, Mellor DJ, Birtles MJ, et al (1994) Effects of oral IGF-I or IGF-II on digestive organ growth in newborn piglets. Biol Neonate 66:280–287

132. Schams D (1994) Growth factors in milk. Endocrine Regul 28:3–8

133. Koldovsky O, Kong W, Phillips AF, Rao RK (1993) Studies on milk-borne insulin-like growth factor-1 and -2 (IGF-1 and IGF-2) and epidermal growth factor (EGF) in suckling rats. Endocrine Regul 27:149–153

134. Hoerr RA, Matthews DE, Bier DM, Young VR (1991) Leucine kinetics of ^{2}H$_3$- and ^{13}C-leucine infused simultaneously by gut and vein. Am J Physiol 260:E111–E117

135. Biolo GM, Tessari P, Inchiostro S, et al (1992) Leucine and phenylalanine kinetics during a mixed meal ingestion: a multiple tracer approach. Am J Physiol 262:E445–E463

136. Hoerr RA, Matthews DE, Bier DM, Young VR (1993) Effects of protein restriction and acute refeeding on leucine and lysine kinetics in young men. Am J Physiol 264:E567–E575

137. Matthews DE, Mariano MA, Campbell RG (1993) Splanchnic bed utilization of glutamine and glutamate in humans. Am J Physiol 264:E848–E854

138. Beaufrere B, Fournier V, Salle B, Putet G (1992) Leucine kinetics in fed low-birth-weight infants: importance of splanchnic tissues. Am J Physiol 263:E214–E220

139. Collin-Vidal C, Cayol M, Obled C, et al (1994) Leucine kinetics are different during feeding with whole protein or oligopeptides. Am J Physiol 267:E907–E914

140. McNurlan MA, Tomkins AM, Garlick PJ (1979) The effect of starvation on the rate of protein synthesis in rat liver and small intestine. Biochem J 178:373–379

141. Dudley MA, Nichols BL, Rosenberger J, et al (1992) Feeding status affects in vivo prosucrase-isomaltase processing in rat jejunum. J Nutr 122:528–534

142. Reeds PJ, Hachey DL, Patterson BW, et al (1992) VLDL apolipoprotein B-102, a potential indicator of the isotopic labeling of the hepatic protein synthetic precursor pool in humans: studies with multiple stable isotopically labeled amino acids. J Nutr 122:457–467

143. Lichtenstein AH, Cohn JS, Hachey DL, et al (1990) Comparison of deuterated leucine, valine and lysine in the measurement of human apolipoprotein A-I and B-102 kinetics. J Lipid Res 31:1693–1701

144. Baumann PQ, Stirewalt WS, O'Rourke BD, et al (1994) Precursor pools of protein synthesis: a stable isotope study in a swine model. Am J Physiol 267:E203–E209

145. Berthold HK, Jahoor F, Klein PD, Reeds PJ (1995) Estimates of the effect of feeding on whole-body protein degradation in women vary with the amino acid used as tracer. J Nutr 125:2516–2527

146. De Feo P, Horber HF, Haymond MW (1993) Meal stimulation of albumin synthesis: a significant contributor to whole body protein synthesis in humans. Am J Physiol 263:E794–E799

147. Hunter KA, Ballmer PE, Anderson SE, et al (1995) Acute

stimulation of albumin synthesis rate with oral meal feeding in healthy subjects measured with [ring-^{2}H$_5$]phenylalanine. Clin Sci 88:235–242

148. Motil KJ, Opekun AR, Montandon CM, et al (1994) Leucine oxidation changes rapidly after dietary protein intake is altered in adult women but lysine flux is unchanged as is lysine incorporation into VLDL-apolipoprotein B-102. J Nutr 124:41–51

149. Benevenga NJ, Gahl MJ, Blemings KP (1993) Role of protein synthesis in amino acid catabolism. J Nutr 123:332S–336S

150. Hiramatsu T, Cortiella J, Marchini JS, et al (1994) Source and amount of dietary nonspecific nitrogen in relation to whole-body leucine, phenylalanine, and tyrosine kinetics in young men. Am J Clin Nutr 59:1347–1355

151. Munro HN (1951) Carbohydrate and fat as factors in protein utilization and metabolism. Physiol Rev 31:449–488

152. Reeds PJ, Fuller MF, Cadenhead A, Hay SM (1987) Urea synthesis and leucine turnover in growing pigs: changes over a two day period after supplementation of the diet with carbohydrate or fat. Br J Nutr 58:301–311

153. Windmueller HG (1982) Glutamine utilization by the small intestine. Adv Enzymol Relat Areas Mol Biol 53:201–237

154. Rerat A, Simoes-Nunes C, Mendy F, et al (1992) Splanchnic fluxes of amino acids after duodenal infusion of carbohydrate solutions containing free amino acids or oligopeptides in the non-anesthetized pig. Br J Nutr 68:111–138

155. Ebner S, Schoknecht P, Reeds PJ, Burrin DG (1994) Growth and metabolism of gastrointestinal and skeletal muscle tissues in protein-malnourished neonatal pigs. Am J Physiol 266:R1736–R1743

156. Reeds PJ, Burrin DG, Jahoor F, et al (1995) Portal drained viscera dominate the splanchnic metabolism of enteral glutamate [abstract]. FASEB J 9:A3257

157. Windmueller HG, Spaeth AE (1980) Respiratory fuels and nitrogen metabolism in vivo in small intestine of fed rats: quantitative importance of glutamine, glutamate, and aspartate. J Biol Chem 255:107–112

158. Watford M (1994) Glutamine metabolism in rat small intestine: synthesis of three carbon products in isolated enterocytes. Biochim Biophys Acta 1200:73–78

159. Jones ME (1985) conversion of glutamate to ornithine and proline. J Nutr 115:509–515

160. Harper AE, Miller RH, Block KP (1984) Branched-chain amino acid metabolism. Annu Rev Nutr 4:409–454

161. Elwynn DH (1970) The role of the liver in regulation of amino acid and protein metabolism. In Munro HN (ed), Mammalian protein metabolism, Vol 4. Academic Press, New York, pp 523–557

162. Remesy C, Demigne C, Aufrere J (1978) Inter-organ relationships between glucose, lactate and amino acids in rats fed on high-carbohydrate or high-protein diets. Biochem J 170:321–329

163. Darmaun D, Dechelote P (1991) Role of leucine as a precursor of glutamine alpha-amino nitrogen in vivo in humans. Am J Physiol 260:E326–329

164. Curthoys NP, Watford M (1995) Regulation of glutaminase activity and glutamine metabolism. Annu Rev Nutr 15:134–159

165. Kaufman S (1986) Regulation of the activity of hepatic phenylalanine hydroxylase. Adv Enzyme Regul 25:37–64

166. Pogson CI, Dickson AJ, Knowles RG, et al (1986) Control of phenylalanine and tyrosine metabolism by phosphorylation mechanisms. Adv Enzyme Regul 25:309–327

167. Harris RA, Popov KM, Zhao Y, Shimomura Y (1994) Regulation of branched-chain amino acid catabolism J Nutr 124:1499S–1502S

168. Popov KM, Shimomura Y, Harris RA (1991) Purification and comparative study of the kinase specific for branched-chain α-ketoacid dehydrogenase and pyruvate dehydrogenase. Protein Expression Purif 2:278–286

169. Lau KS, Fatania HR, Randle PJ (1982) Regulation of the branch-chain 2-oxoacid dehydrogenase kinase reaction. FEBS Lett 144:57–62

170. Quevado MR, Price GM, Halliday DH, et al (1994) Nitrogen homeostasis in man: diurnal changes in nitrogen excretion, leucine oxidation and whole body leucine kinetics during a reduction from a high to a moderate protein intake. Clin Sci 86:185–193

171. Fisher MJ, Pogson CI (1984) The determination of flux through phenylalanine hydroxylase and homogentisate oxidase in isolated hepatocytes. Biosci Rep 3:28–40

172. Nagao M, Nakamura T, Ichihara A (1986) Developmental control of gene expression of tryptophan 2,3-dioxygenase in neonatal rat liver. Biochim Biophys Acta 867:179–186

173. Berlin CM, Schimke RT (1965) Influence of turnover rates on the responses of enzymes to cortisone. Mol Pharmacol 1:149–156

174. Ogawa H, Fujioka M, Su Y, Kanamoto R, Pitot HC (1991) Nutritional regulation and tissue-specific expression of the serine dehydratase gene in rat. J Biol Chem 266:20412–20417

175. Chinsky JM, Bohlen LM, Costeas PA (1994) Noncoordinated responses of branched-chain α-ketoacid dehydrogenase subunit genes to dietary protein. FASEB J 8:114–120

176. Stewart PM, Walser M (1980) Short term regulation of ureagenesis. J Biol Chem 255:5270–5280

177. Ulbright C, Snodgrass PJ (1993) Coordinate induction of the urea cycle enzymes by glucagon and dexamethasone is accomplished by three different mechanisms. Arch Biochem Biophys 301:237–243

178. Watford M (1991) The urea cycle: a two-compartment system. Essays Biochem 26:49-58

179. Kaloyianni M, Freedland RA (1990) Contribution of several amino acids and lactate to gluconeogenesis in hepatocytes isolated from rats fed various diets. J Nutr 120:116–122

180. Tappy L, Acheson K, Normand S, et al (1992) Effects of infused amino acids on glucose production and utilization in healthy human subjects. Am J Physiol 262:E826–E833

181. Jungas RL, Halperin ML, Brosnan JT (1992) Quantitative analysis of amino acid oxidation and related gluconeogenesis in humans. Physiol Rev 72:419–448

182. Haussinger D, Lamers WH, Moorman AF (1992) Hepatocyte heterogeneity in the metabolism of amino acids and ammonia. Enzyme 46:72–93

183. Haussinger D. (1990) Nitrogen metabolism in liver: structural and functional organization and physiological relevance. Biochem J 267:281–290

184. Waterlow JC, Garlick PJ, Millward DJ (1978) Protein turnover in mammalian tissues and in the whole body. North Holland, Amsterdam

185. Waterlow JC (1984) Protein turnover with special reference to man. Q J Exp Physiol 69:409–438

186. Reeds PJ, Nicholson BA, Fuller MF(1985) Metabolic basis for energy expenditure with particular reference to protein. In Garrow J, Halliday D (eds), Energy and substrate metabolism in man. John Libbey, London, pp 47–56

187. Welle S, Nair KS (1990) Relationship between metabolic rate to body composition and protein turnover. Am J Physiol 258:E990–E998

188. Bier DM (1989) Intrinsically difficult problems: the kinetics

of body proteins and amino acids. Diabetes Metab Rev 5:111–132

189. Slevin K, Jackson AA, Waterlow JC (1991) A model for the measurement of whole body protein turnover incorporating a protein pool with lifetime kinetics. Proc R Soc Lond [Biol] 243:87–92

190. Cobelli C, Saccomani MP, Tessari P, et al (1991) Compartmental model of leucine kinetics in humans. Am J Physiol 261:E539–E550

191. Reeds PJ (1992). Isotopic measurement of protein synthesis and proteolysis in vivo. In Nissen S (ed), Current methods in protein nutrition and metabolism. Academic Press, New York, pp 249–273

192. Garlick PJ, McNurlan MA, Essen P, Wernerman J (1994) Measurement of tissue protein synthesis rates in vivo: a critical analysis of contrasting methods. Am J Physiol 266:E287–297

193. Rennie MJ, Smith K, Watt PW (1994) Measurement of human tissue protein synthesis: an optimal approach. Am J Physiol 266:E298–E307

194. Samarel AM (1991) In vivo measurements of protein turnover during muscle growth and atrophy. FASEB J 5:2020–2028

195. Vidrich A, Airhart J, Bruno MK, Khairallah EA (1976) Compartmentation of free amino acids in protein biosynthesis. Biochem J 162:257–266

196. Garlick PJ, McNurlan MA, Preedy VR (1980) A rapid and convenient technique for measuring the rate of protein synthesis in tissue by injection of [³H]-phenylalanine. Biochem J 192:719–726

197. Ballmer PE, McNurlan MA, Milne E, et al (1990) Measurement of albumin synthesis in humans: a new approach employing stable isotopes. Am J Physiol 259:E797–E803

198. Schwenk WF, Beaufrere B, Haymond MW (1985) Use of reciprocal pool specific activities to model leucine metabolism in humans. Am J Physiol 249:E646–E650

199. Pacy PJ, Thompson GN, Halliday DH (1991) Measurement of whole-body protein turnover in insulin dependant (type I) diabetic patients during insulin withdrawal and infusion: comparison of [¹³C]leucine and [²H₅]phenylalanine methodologies. Clin Sci 8:345–352

200. Cryer DR, Matsushima T, Marsh JB, et al (1986) Direct measurement of apolipoprotein B synthesis in human very low density lipoprotein using stable isotopes and mass spectrometry. J Lipid Res 27:508–516

201. Parhofer KG, Barrett PHR, Bier DM, Schonfield G (1990) Determination of kinetic parameters of apolipoprotein B metabolism using amino acids labeled with stable isotopes J Lipid Res 32:1311–1323

202. Rathmacher JA, Link G, Nissen S (1993) Measurement of 3-methylhistidine production in lambs by using compartmental analysis Br J Nutr 69:743–755

203. Goodman MN, Gomez MDP (1987) Decreased myofibrillar proteolysis after refeeding requires dietary protein or amino acids. Am J Physiol 253:E52–E58

204. Hasselgren P-O, James J H, Benson DW, et al (1989) Total and myofibrillar protein breakdown in different types of rat skeletal muscle: effects of sepsis and regulation by insulin. Metabolism 38:634–640

205. Benson DW, Foley-Nelson T, Chance WT, et al (1991) Decreased myofibrillar protein breakdown following treatment with clenbuterol. J Surg Res 50:1–5

206. Tiao G, Fagan JM, Samuels N, et al (1994) Sepsis stimulates nonlysosomal, energy-dependent proteolysis and increases ubiquitin mRNA levels in rat skeletal muscle. J Clin Invest 94:2255–2264

207. Reeds PJ, Davis TA (1992) Hormonal regulation of muscle protein synthesis and degradation. In Buttery PJ, Boorman KN, Lindsay DB (eds), Lean and fat deposition. Butterworth-Heineman Scientific, Oxford, pp 1–26

208. Gelfand RA, Barrett EJ (1987) Effect of physiologic hyperinsulinemia on skeletal muscle protein synthesis and breakdown in man. J Clin Invest 80:1–6

209. Thompson GN, Pacy PJ, Merritt H, et al (1989) Rapid measurement of whole body and forearm protein turnover using a [²H₅]-phenylalanine model. Am J Physiol 256:E631–E639

210. Moller-Loswick A-C, Zachrisson H, Hyltander A, et al (1994) Insulin selectively attenuates breakdown of nonmyofibrillar proteins in peripheral tissues of normal men. Am J Physiol 266:E645–E652

211. De Feo P, Volpi E, Lucidi P, et al (1993) Physiological Increments in plasma insulin concentrations have selective and different effects on synthesis of hepatic proteins in normal humans. Diabetes 42:995–1002

212. Cohn JS, Wagner DA, Cohn DS, et al (1990) Measurements of very low density and low density lipoprotein apolipoprotein B-100 and high density lipoprotein production in human subjects using deuterated leucine: effect of feeding and fasting. J Clin Invest 85:804–811

213. Jahoor F, Burrin DG, Reeds PJ, Frazer M (1994) Measurement of plasma protein synthesis rate in the infant pig: an investigation of alternative tracer approaches. Am J Physiol 267:R221–R227

214. Bhattiprolu S, Jahoor F, Burrin DG, et al (1994) Fractional synthetic rates of retinol binding protein (RBP), transthyreitin (TTR) and of a new peptide associated with RBP measured with stable isotopes in neonatal pigs. J Biol Chem 269:26196–26200

215. Dudley MA, Jahoor F, Burrin DG, Reeds PJ (1994) Sucrase isomaltase and lactase phlorizin hydrolase synthesis in infant pigs measured in vivo with ²H₃-leucine. Am J Physiol 267:G1127–G1136

216. Hiramatsu T, Fukagawa NK, Marchini JS, et al (1994) Methionine and cysteine kinetics at different intakes of cystine in healthy adult men. Am J Clin Nutr 60:525–533

217. Marchini JS, Cortiella J, Hiramatsu T, et al (1994) Phenylalanine and tyrosine kinetics for different patterns and indispensable amino acid intakes in adult humans. Am J Clin Nutr 60:79–86

218. Jaksic T, Wagner DA, Burke JF, Young VR (1991) Proline metabolism in adult male burned patients and healthy control subjects. Am J Clin Nutr 54:408–413

219. Garlick PJ, McNurlan MA, Ballmer PE (1991) Influence of dietary protein intake on whole-body protein turnover in humans. Diabetes Care 14:1189–1198

220. Welle S, Matthews DE, Campbell RG, Nair KS (1989) Stimulation of protein turnover by carbohydrate overfeeding in men. Am J Physiol 257:E413–E417

221. Fukagawa NK, Minaker KL, Rowe JW, et al (1985) Insulin-mediated reduction of whole body protein breakdown. J Clin Invest 76:2306–2311

222. Louard RJ, Fryburg DA, Gelfand RA, Barrett EJ (1992) Insulin sensitivity of protein and glucose metabolism in human forearm muscle. J Clin Invest 90:2348–2354

223. Tessari P, Inchiostro S, Biolo G, et al (1991) Effects of acute systemic hyperinsulinemia on forearm muscle proteolysis in healthy man. J Clin Invest 88:27–33

224. Laager R, Ninnis R, Keller U (1993) Comparison of the effects of recombinant human insulin-like growth factor-I and insulin on glucose and leucine kinetics in humans. J Clin Invest 92:1903–1909

225. Fryburg DA, Louard RJ, Gerow KE, et al (1992) Growth hormone stimulates skeletal muscle protein synthesis and antagonizes insulin's antiproteolytic action in humans. Diabetes 41:424–429

226. Fryburg DA, Barrett EJ (1993) Growth hormone acutely stimulates skeletal muscle but not whole-body protein synthesis in humans. Metabolism 42:1223–1227

227. Beaufrere B, Horber FF, Schwenk WF, et al (1989) Glucocorticosteroids increase leucine oxidation and impair leucine balance in humans. Am J Physiol 257:E712–E721

228. Van Goudoever JB, Wattimena JDL, Carnielli VP, et al (1994) Effect of dexamethasone on protein metabolism in infants with bronchopulmonary dysplasia. J Pediatr 124:112–118

229. Garlick PJ, Grant I (1988) Amino acid infusion increases the sensitivity of muscle protein synthesis in vivo to insulin. Effect of branched-chain amino acids. Biochem J 254:579–584

230. Watt PW, Corbett ME, Rennie MJ (1992) Stimulation of protein synthesis in pig skeletal muscle by infusion of amino acids during constant insulin availability. Am J Physiol 263:E453–E460

231. Bennet WM, Connacherm AA, Scrimgeour CM, et al (1990) Euglycemic hyperinsulinemia augments amino acid uptake by human leg tissues during hyperaminoacidemia. Am J Physiol 259:E185–E194

232. Flakoll PJ, Kulaylat K, Frexes-Steed M, et al (1989) Amino acids augment insulin's suppression of whole body proteolysis. Am J Physiol 257:E839–E847

233. Ballard FJ (1982) Regulation of protein accumulation in cultured cells. Biochem J 208:275–287

234. Florini JR (1987) Hormonal control of muscle growth. Muscle Nerve 10:577–598

235. Laurent GJ, Sparrow MP, Millward DJ (1978) Turnover of muscle protein in the fowl. Changes in the rates of protein synthesis and breakdown during hypertrophy of the anterior and posterior latissimus dorsi muscles. Biochem J 176:407–417

236. McMillan DN, Reeds PJ, Lobley GE, Palmer RM (1987) Changes in protein turnover in hypertrophying plantaris muscles of rats. Effect of Fenbufen, an inhibitor of prostaglandin synthesis. Prostaglandins 34:841–852

237. Reeds PJ, Fuller MF, Cadenhead A, et al (1981) Effects of changes in the intakes of protein and non-protein energy on whole-body protein turnover in growing pigs. Br J Nutr 45:539–546

238. Fuller MF, Reeds PJ, Cadenhead AC, et al (1987) Effects of the amount and quality of dietary protein on nitrogen metabolism and protein turnover in growing pigs. Br J Nutr 58:287–300

239. Liu SM, Lobley GE, Macleod NA, et al (1995) Effects of long term excess or deficiency on whole body protein turnover in sheep nourished by the intragastric infusion of nutrients. Br J Nutr 73:829–839

240. Goldspink DF, Kelly FJ (1984) Protein turnover and growth in the whole-body, liver and kidney of the rat from foetus to senility. Biochem J 217:507–516

241. Lewis SEM, Kelly FJ, Goldspink DF (1984) Pre- and postnatal growth and protein turnover in smooth muscle, heart and slow- and fast-twitch muscles of the rat. Biochem J 217:517–526

242. Scornik OA, Botbol V (1976) Role of changes in protein degradation in the growth of regenerating livers. J Biol Chem 251:2891–2896

243. Garlick PJ, Fern M, Preedy VR (1983) The effect of insulin infusion and food intake on muscle protein synthesis in postabsorptive rat. Biochem J 210:669–676

244. Motil KJ, Montandon CM, Hachey DL, et al (1989) Whole body protein metabolism in lactating and nonlactating women. J Appl Physiol 66:370–376

245. Thomas MR, Irving CS, Reeds PJ, et al (1991) Lysine and protein metabolism in the young lactating woman. Eur J Clin Nutr 45:227–242

246. Davis TA, Fiorotto ML, Nguyen HN, Reeds PJ (1993) Enhanced response of muscle protein biosynthesis and plasma insulin to food in suckling rats. Am J Physiol 265:R334–R340

247. Baillie AG, Garlick PJ (1992) Attenuated responses of muscle protein synthesis to fasting and insulin in adult female rats. Am J Physiol 262:E1–E5

248. Mosoni L, Houlier M-L, Patureau-Mirand P, et al (1993) Effect of amino acids alone or with insulin on muscle and liver protein synthesis in adult and old rats. Am J Physiol 264:E614–E620

249. Moldave K (1985) Eukaryotic protein synthesis. Annu Rev Biochem 54:1109–1149

250. Pain VM (1986) Initiation of protein synthesis in mammalian cells. Biochem J 235:625–637

251. Arnstein HRV, Cox RA (1992) Protein biosynthesis. IRL Press, New York

252. Kimball SR, Vary TC, Jefferson LS (1994) Regulation of protein synthesis by insulin. Annu Rev Physiol 56:321–348

253. Seve B, Ballevre O, Ganier P, et al (1993) Recombinant growth hormone and dietary protein enhance protein synthesis in growing pigs. J Nutr 123:529–540

254. Goldspink DF, Cox VM, Smith SK, et al (1995) Muscle growth in response to mechanical stimuli. Am J Physiol 268:E288–E297

255. Pain VM, Albertse EC, Garlick PJ (1983) Protein metabolism in skeletal muscle, diaphragm and heart of diabetic rats. Am J Physiol 245:E604–E610

256. Brown JG, Millward DJ (1983) Dose response of protein turnover in rat skeletal muscle to triiodothyronine treatment. Biochim Biophys Acta 757:182–186

257. Pell JM, Bates PC (1992) Differential actions of growth homrone and insulin-like growth factor-I on tissue protein metabolism in dwarf mice. Endocrinology 130:1942–1950

258. Odedra BR, Bates PC, Millward, DT (1983) Time course of the effect of catabolic doses of corticosterone on protein turnover in rat skeletal muscle and liver. Biochem J 214:616–627

259. Eichler DC, Craig N (1994) Processing of eukaryotic ribosomal RNA. Prog Nucleic Acid Res Mol Biol 49:197–239

260. Larson DE, Zahradka P, Sells BH (1994) Control points in eukaryotic ribosome biogenesis. Biochem Cell Biol 69:5–22

261. Ashford AJ, Pain VM (1986) Insulin stimulation of growth in diabetic rats. Synthesis and degradation of ribosomal and total tissue protein in skeletal muscle and heart. J Biol Chem 261:4066–4071

262. Welsh GI, Proud CG (1992) Regulation of protein synthesis in Swiss 3T3 fibroblasts. Rapid activation of guanine-nucleotide-exchange factor by insulin and growth factors. Biochem J 284:19–23

263. McLennan PA, Rennie MJ (1989) Effects of ischaemia, blood loss and reperfusion on rat muscle protein synthesis, metabolite concentrations and polyribosome profiles in vivo. Biochem J 260:195–200

264. Reeds PJ, Davis TA, Fiorotto ML (1991) Nutrient partitioning: an overview. In Bray GA, Ryan DH (eds), The science of food regulation. LSU Press, Baton Rouge, pp 103–120

265. Kimball SR, Jefferson LS (1994) Mechanisms of translational control in liver and skeletal muscle. Biochimie 76:729–736

266. Ernst V, Levin DH, London IM (1979) In situ phosphorylation of the a-subunit of eukaryotic initiation factor 2 in reticulocyte lysates inhibited by heme deficiency, double-stranded

RNA, oxidized glutathione or the heme regulated protein kinase. Proc Natl Acad Sci USA 76:2118–2122

267. Schimke RT, Bradley MO (1975) Properties of protein turnover in animal cells and a possible role for turnover in "quality" control of proteins. In Reich E (ed), Proteases and biological control. Cold Spring Harbor Laboratory, Cold Spring Harbor, NY, pp 515–530

268. Scornik OA (1984) Role of protein degradation in the regulation of cellular protein content and amino acid pools. Proc Fed Am Soc Exp Biol 43:1283–1288

269. Bachmair A, Finley D, Varsharsky A (1986) In vivo half life of a protein is a function of its amino-terminal residue. Science 234:179–183

270. Rogers S, Wells R, Rechsteiner M (1986) Amino acid sequences common to rapidly degraded proteins: the PEST hypothesis. Science 234:364–369

271. Wing SS, Chiang H-L, Goldberg AL, Dice JF (1991) Proteins containing peptide sequences related to lys-phe-glu-arg-gln are selectively degraded in liver and heart but not skeletal muscle of fasted rats. Biochem J 275:165–169

272. Varshavsky A (1992) The N-end rule. Cell 69:725–735

273. Ciechanover A, Schwartz AL (1994) The ubiquitin-mediated proteolytic pathway: mechanisms of recognition of the proteolytic substrate and involvement in the degradation of native cellular proteins. FASEB J 8:182–191

274. Attaix D, Taillandier D, Temparis S, et al (1994) Regulation of ATP-ubitquitin-dependent proteolysis in muscle wasting. Reprod Nutr Dev 34:583–597

275. Glauman H, Ballard FJ (1987) Lysosomes: their role in protein breakdown. Academic Press, New York

276. Lardeux BR, Mortimore GE (1987) Amino acid and hormonal control of macromolecular turnover in perfused rat liver: evidence for selective autophagy. J Biol Chem 262:14514–14519

277. Heydrick SJ, Lardeux BR, Mortimore GE (1991) Uptake and degradation of cytoplasmic RNA by hepatic lysosomes: quantitative relationship to RNA turnover. J Biol Chem 266:8790–8796

278. Mortimore GE, Poso AR, Kadowaki M, Wert JJ (1987) Multiphasic control of hepatic protein degradation by regulatory amino acids. J Biol Chem 262:16322–16327

279. Venerando R, Miotto G, Kadowaki M, et al (1994) Multiphasic control of proteolysis by leucine and alanine in the isolated rat hepatocyte. Am J Physiol 266:C455–C461

280. Miotto G, Venerado R, Khurana KK, et al (1992) Control of hepatic proteolysis by leucine and isovaleryl-L-carnitine through a common locus. Evidence for a possible mechanism of recognition at the plasma membrane. J Biol Chem 267:22066–22072

281. Melloni E, Pontremoli S (1991) The calpain-calpastatin system: structural and functional properties. J Nutr Biochem 2:467–476

282. Goll DE, Thompson VF, Taylor RG, Zalewska T (1992) Is calpain activity regulated by membranes and autolysis or by calcium and calpastatin? Bioessays 14:549–556

283. Bardsley RG, Allcock SM, Dawson JM, et al (1992) Effect of beta-agonists on expression of calpain and calpastatin activity in skeletal muscle. Biochimie 74:267–273

284. Goll DE, Dayton WR, Singh I, Robson RM (1991) Studies of the alpha actinin/actin interaction in the Z-disc by using calpain. J Biol Chem 266:8501–8510

285. Ilian MA, Forsberg NE (1992) Gene expression of calpains and their specific endogenous inhibitor, calpastatin, in skeletal muscle of fed and fasted rabbits. Biochem J 287:163–171

286. Rivett AJ (1993) Proteasomes: multicatalytic proteinase complexes. Biochem J 291:1–10

287. Goldberg AL, Rock KL (1992) Proteolysis, proteasomes and antigen presentation. Nature 357:375–379

288. Ciechanover A, DiGiuseppe JA, Barcovich B, et al (1991) Degradation of nuclear oncogenes by the ubiquitin system in vitro. Proc Natl Acad Sci U S A 88:139–143

289. Medina R, Wing SS, Haas A, Goldberg Al (1991) Activation of the ubiquitin-ATP-dependent proteolytic system in skeletal muscle during fasting and denervation atrophy. Biomed Biochim Acta 50:347–356

290. Wing SS, Goldberg AL (1993) Glucocorticoids activate the ATP-ubiquitin-dependent proteolytic system in skeletal muscle during fasting Am J Physiol 267:E39–E48

291. Kettelhut IC, Wing SS, Goldberg AL (1988) Endocrine regulation of protein breakdown in skeletal muscle. Diabetes Metab Rev 4:751–772

292. Tawa NE Jr, Kettelhut IC, Goldberg AL (1992) Dietary protein deficiency reduces lysosomal and nonlysosomal ATP dependent proteolysis in muscle. Am J Physiol 263:E326–E334

293. Temparis S, Asensi M, Taillandier D, et al (1994) Increased ATP-ubiquitin-dependent proteolysis in skeletal muscles from tumor-bearing rats. Cancer Res 54:5568–5573

294. Harper AE (1994) Some concluding remarks on emerging aspects of amino acid metabolism. J Nutr 124:1529S–1532S

Chapter 9

Dietary Fiber

Daniel D. Gallaher and Barbara O. Schneeman

An early definition of dietary fiber described it as the remnants of plant cells remaining after hydrolysis by the enzymes of the mammalian digestive system.[1] This "physiological" definition attempts to characterize fiber relative to the process of digestion within the gastrointestinal tract. This definition was understood to include both plant cell wall material, such as cellulose, hemicelluloses, pectin, and lignin, as well as intracellular polysaccharides such as gums and mucilages. A "chemical" definition has been suggested describing fiber as plant nonstarch polysaccharides plus lignin.[2] In practice, both definitions encompass essentially the same heterogeneous mixture of plant components.

Through the years a number of other indigestible materials have been proposed for inclusion in the group of materials that compose dietary fiber. Some of these, such as waxes, cutins, and indigestible cell wall proteins, are found associated with the plant cell wall. Other noncell wall compounds include resistant starch (starch that is resistant to digestion by mammalian enzymes), Maillard reaction products, and animal-derived materials that resist digestion (e.g., aminopolysaccharides). Although these are minor components of most foods consumed by humans, they may have physiological activities that are difficult to separate from the activities of the substances traditionally considered as dietary fiber. This points to a basic, unresolved dilemma in the study of the physiological effects of dietary fiber, which is the difficulty of separating the responses due to fiber from those due to other materials found in fiber-rich foods. One frequently used approach to this problem is to use purified fibers to study the effect of fiber in isolation. However, purification may alter the physical form and properties of the fiber and therefore its physiological effect. There is evidence, for example, that fermentation of plant cell wall material differs from that of the same fibers in purified form.[3] Consequently, it seems necessary that both approaches—use of isolated fibers and fiber-rich foods—will continue to be employed.

The major components of dietary fiber are the nonstarch polysaccharides, which include cellulose, mixed-linkage β-glucans, hemicelluloses, pectins, and gums.[4] Each of these fractions is characterized by its sugar residues and the linkages among them. Cellulose and mixed-linkage β-glucans are glucose polymers with β 1→4 linkages; in the mixed-linkage β-glucans these linkages are interspersed with β 1→3 bonds. Cellulose is found in all plant cell walls, and oats and barley are particularly rich sources of mixed-linkage β-glucans. The hemicelluloses are a diverse group of polysaccharides with varying degrees of branching. These can be classified according to the monosaccharide in the backbone (e.g., xylans, galactans, and mannans) and in the side chains (e.g., arabinose, galactose). The major backbone sugar for pectins is galacturonic acid, and side chains typically include galactose and arabinose. The degree of methoxylation on the uronic acid residues varies. The structural features of gums vary according to the source. Typically, these are a minor polysaccharide constituent in most foods; however, certain gums are used frequently in research studies (e.g., guar gum and locust bean gum, which are classified as galactomannans). The structure of a starch and several types of dietary fiber is shown in Figure 1. The noncarbohydrate constituent that is included in most definitions of fiber is lignin, which has a highly complex three-dimensional structure and contains phenylpropane units. Lignin is usually not an important component of human foods because it is generally associated with tough or woody tissue. The one exception is foods that contain intact seeds consumed with the food. Sources of dietary fiber have been classified as providing soluble or insoluble fiber. The reference to solubility indicates polysaccharides that are dispersible in water rather than true chemical solubility. Insoluble polysaccharides are poorly dispersible in water. Originally it was thought that this categorization of fiber type might provide a simple prediction of physiological function, which has not been the case. Given the diversity in chemical and physical properties among fiber sources, finding a simple predictive index will be difficult.

The interest in fiber as an important component of the diet has remained high as a result of epidemiological associations of a high fiber intake with a lower incidence of certain chronic disorders, such as cardiovascular disease and large bowel cancer. However, the epidemiological

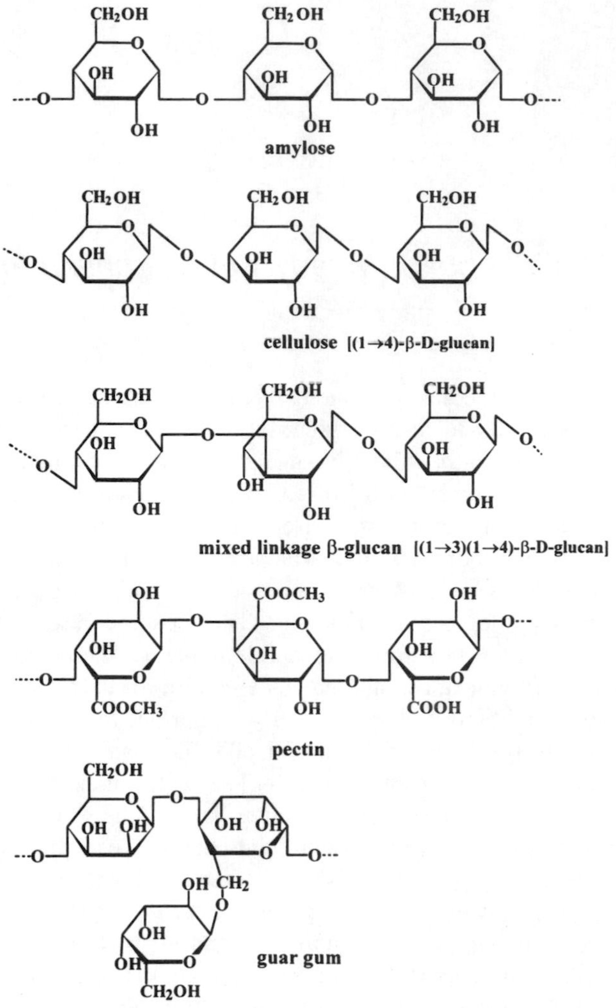

Figure 1. Structure of amylose (starch) and several types of dietary fiber.

data linking a reduced risk of chronic disease with a high fiber intake are inconsistent and complex to evaluate, partly because of the difficulty in determining fiber intake in populations. The majority of epidemiological studies examining the relationship between fiber intake and chronic disease have focused on colon cancer. In a critical review and meta-analysis of the epidemiological evidence, Trock et al.[5] reported that, overall, there was support for the hypothesis that a fiber-rich diet reduces colon cancer risk. However, the data did not allow the effect caused by fiber to be separated from nonfiber effects caused by vegetables. As previously mentioned, separation of the effect of fiber from independent effects due to compounds present in its food matrix remains an unsolved problem. It has been estimated that 45% of total fiber intake in the United States comes from vegetables.[6] As pointed out by Block et al.,[7] consumption of fruits and vegetables is associated with a reduced risk of colon cancer. Less support exists for a reduction in risk by grains and legumes. However, since the types of fiber differ between fruits and

vegetables and grains and legumes, it remains unclear whether differences in risk reduction are due to differences in the types of fiber or to nonfiber components of fruits and vegetables. Another confounding factor is that total energy intake may have an important role in determining colon cancer risk in a population, and a high fiber intake may lead to a decrease in energy intake.[8] Clearly, associations between disease risk and dietary factors are multifactorial and our present knowledge indicates that fiber cannot be isolated as a single factor affecting risk but must be evaluated in the context of the total dietary pattern.

Methods of Analysis

Methods of dietary fiber analysis fall into one of two categories: gravimetric or component (or chemical) analysis. Gravimetric methods are simpler and faster, but are limited to estimates of total fiber or soluble and insoluble fiber. Component analysis yields the quantity of individual neutral sugars and the total quantity of acidic sugars (i.e., uronic acids). The total fiber content is then calculated as the sum of the individual sugars. When desired, lignin can be estimated separately and added to the sum of the individual sugars. Component analysis, however, is more involved in terms of both expertise and equipment and consequently is less suitable for routine dietary fiber analysis. A number of methods of analysis are summarized in Table 1.

Gravimetric procedures. The oldest and first official method of dietary fiber analysis was "crude fiber." This method measures the weight of the residue after extraction with organic solvents and digestion with dilute acid and alkali, with a correction for ash. Although an official Association of Official Analytical Chemists (AOAC) method since 1955, the method does not accurately measure dietary fiber. All soluble fiber is lost, along with variable amounts of insoluble fiber, thus underestimating the true fiber content of the food. As the losses are variable, crude fiber values do not correlate with other measures of total dietary fiber.[13]

Highly reproducible values for insoluble fiber are obtained by the neutral detergent method.[14] Food samples are boiled with a detergent at neutral pH and the residue collected by filtration. However, as soluble fibers are lost in the neutral detergent method procedures, the fiber content of many foods, in particular fruits and vegetables, is underestimated.

The growing awareness of the potential importance of soluble fiber and the desire for a simple and reliable measure of dietary fiber led to the development of the present official AOAC method, commonly referred to as Total Dietary Fiber.[11] Duplicate samples are subjected to enzymatic hydrolysis of starch and protein and the fiber precipitated with ethanol. The precipitate is collected on a filter, dried, and weighed. The residue from one set

Table 1. Dietary fiber methods of analysis

Method	Materials measured	Comments	Reference
Crude Fiber	Lignins, variable amounts of cellulose and hemicelluloses	Does not correlate with other methods of fiber measurement	9
Neutral Detergent Fiber	Cellulose, insoluble hemicelluloses, lignins	Soluble fibers are lost	10
Acid Detergent Fiber	Cellulose and lignin	Soluble fibers are lost	10
Total Dietary Fiber	Nonstarch polysaccharides, lignin, some retrograded starch, Maillard reaction products	AOAC-approved method; can be modified to give soluble and insoluble fiber	11
Englyst procedure	Nonstarch polysaccharides	Can be modified to give cellulose and non-cellulosic polysaccharides separately	12

of duplicates is incinerated to correct for ash and the other is analyzed for nitrogen to correct for protein contamination. Since its original publication, several modifications of the Total Dietary Fiber procedure have been developed to both simplify and reduce the variability of the method.

Gravimetric procedures that measure total fiber can be modified to give estimates of soluble and insoluble fiber.[15] This is accomplished by filtering the fiber digest before precipitation with ethanol; the filter residue contains the insoluble fraction ,whereas the filtrate contains the soluble fraction. The soluble fraction is then precipitated with ethanol, collected by filtration, dried, and weighed. Marlett[16] has pointed out that variations in sample handling and food preparation result in variability in the soluble fiber content.

Component analysis procedures. The primary difference between component analysis and the gravimetric methods is in the manner of quantitating the fiber residue obtained after digestion and collection of the fiber residue. Component analysis involves hydrolyzing the residue with strong acids, usually sulfuric acid, and quantitation of the monomeric sugars.[12] Neutral sugars can be determined by high-performance liquid chromatography, colorimetrically, or, more commonly, by gas chromatography after derivitization. Acidic sugars can be quantitated colorimetrically. Summation of the monomeric sugars then yields a value for total dietary fiber. Minor modifications allow estimates of cellulose, soluble and insoluble fiber, and noncellulosic polysaccharides (essentially hemicellulose).

The demonstration that some starch in foods, particularly thermally processed foods, escapes digestion within the small intestine led to the concept of resistant starch.[17] Resistant starch is formed during retrogradation of amylose and consequently is formed in large amounts in foods high in amylose such as potatoes.[18] Being resistant to the action of amylolytic enzymes, resistant starch is not removed in enzymatic-gravimetric procedures such as the Total Dietary Fiber method and consequently is measured as dietary fiber in these procedures. There are

opposing views as to whether resistant starch should be considered as dietary fiber or as a separate entity.[19,20]

Results with the newer methods of component analysis, such as those of Englyst and Hudson,[21] correlate well with the AOAC Total Dietary Fiber procedure, but are generally lower. The difference appears to be largely due to residual (resistant) starch and, to a lesser extent, lignin, which contribute to the fiber fraction in the Total Dietary Fiber procedure but are not measured in the method of Englyst and Hudson.

Physical Properties of Dietary Fiber

Knowledge of the chemical composition of dietary fibers, such as the monomeric sugar content, has provided little insight into their physiological effects. Progress in understanding the action of different types of dietary fiber in the intestinal tract has come primarily from the characterization of their physical properties. Therefore, determining such characteristics as the water-holding capacity, viscosity, susceptibility to fermentation, inhibition of digestive enzymes, bile acid binding capacity, and cation exchange capacity is more likely to be useful in understanding the physiological effects of dietary fiber than the detailed chemical composition provided by component analysis.

Water-holding capacity. The water-holding capacity of a fiber source refers to its ability to retain water within its matrix. Interest in the water-holding capacity of fiber preparations stems from the suggestion that fibers with a large water-holding capacity will increase stool weight.[22] Water-holding capacity can be measured by saturating the fiber with water and then removing unretained water, either by centrifugation, filtration,[23] or osmotic suction.[24] Soluble fibers, such as pectin and the gums, have a much higher water-holding capacity than do insoluble fibers such as cellulose and wheat bran. Vegetable fibers have intermediate values. Unfortunately, the water-holding capacity determined in vitro does not predict the fecal bulking ability of a fiber source,[25] because of fermentation of the fiber and the increase in microbial mass in the colon. The potential water-holding capacity of a fiber source is a measure developed to take these factors into account.[26] The potential water-holding capacity is essentially the water-holding capacity of the fiber source residue and microbial mass after in vitro fermentation as determined by osmotic suction. Using fiber sources with a broad range of water-holding capacity and fermentability, the potential water-holding capacity ranked the fibers in the same order as their fecal bulking ability. Although the potential water-holding capacity is more difficult to determine than the water-holding capacity, it appears to be a physiologically meaningful measure.

Viscosity. Certain groups of dietary fiber can form highly viscous solutions. These include pectins, various gums, mixed-linkage β-glucans, and algal polysaccharides such as agar and carrageenan. Within a group, the actual viscosity is highly dependent upon the chemical structure of the compound. For example, the viscosity of pectin depends on both the molecular weight and methyl ester content; a reduction in either will reduce its viscosity. Soluble fibers exhibit pseudoplastic (shear thinning) behavior; i.e., as the shear rate increases, the apparent viscosity decreases. Because the shear rate within the small intestine is unknown, the viscosity of the contents within the small intestinal lumen after consumption of a viscous fiber cannot be determined exactly. Guar gum consumption, however, clearly increases the viscosity of intestinal contents.[27] Another factor likely to influence the viscosity of the intestinal content is the rate of stomach emptying. A slower rate of emptying would likely lead to a lower concentration of fiber within the contents, thus decreasing viscosity, possibly drastically, as viscosity is related to concentration of a viscous material by a power curve: small changes in concentration can lead to large changes in viscosity.

Susceptibility to fermentation. Dietary fibers, although resistant to digestion by mammalian enzymes, are readily fermented by the microflora of the large intestine. The degree and rate of fermentation will be influenced by the type of fiber, the physical form or context (e.g., within a food or isolated, particle size), and the microflora present in the host. In general, isolated fibers are fermented more readily than those found within a food matrix. Fiber sources fed in large particle size lead to a less complete fermentation than the same sources fed in small particle size. The insoluble fiber cellulose is the most resistant to fermentation, whereas soluble fiber types such as pectins and guar gum are completely fermented. However, solubility is not the sole guide to fermentability. For example, several soluble fiber types, such as psyllium, xanthan gum, and the modified celluloses (e.g., methylcellulose), are either incompletely fermented or totally nonfermentable. Regardless of the fiber type, fermentation leads to the production of short-chain fatty acids, principally acetate, propionate, and butyrate, as well as hydrogen gas. Methane is also produced in some individuals.

Bile acid binding. Dietary fiber is capable of binding bile acids both in vitro[28,29] and in vivo.[30] In general, cellulose binds very little, wheat bran and alfalfa somewhat more, pectin and guar gum in moderate amounts, and lignin binds a great deal. Caution should be exercised in regard to lignin binding, however, as lignin preparations most often used in these studies are isolated from wood using harsh procedures and may bear little resemblance to lignins in food. Bile acid binding is greatest at acid pH and declines as the pH rises.[31,32] The nature of the binding was first proposed to be a hydrophobic attraction of bile acids to the lignin component of the fiber sources,[32] based on the decrease in binding after delignification. Binding due to the presence of saponins has also been proposed,[33] although this finding could not be confirmed.[34] On the other hand, Selvendran et al.[4] reported that in cell wall material from runner bean pods, bile acid binding was reduced in depectinated material and in material in the hydrogenated form. Their results suggest that bile acid binding is hydrophilic in nature and that pectin is the component responsible. The reason for these disparate results is not apparent, although the two types of binding are not mutually exclusive. Differences in the conditions used for measuring binding and in the fiber preparation may account for the lack of agreement.

Cation exchange capacity. Many fiber sources have a demonstrable cation exchange capacity in vitro and thus may bind minerals within the gastrointestinal tract. For example, McBurney et al.[35] have examined the cation exchange capacity of a number of neutral detergent fibers and found that copper was retained by an ion-exchange mechanism. Carboxyl, hydroxyl, and amino groups were all related to the cation exchange capacity. As would be expected from the presence of uronic acids, pectins demonstrate in vitro the capacity to bind divalent minerals such as iron, calcium, copper, and zinc.[36,37] Highly esterified pectins (high methoxy) have a lower cation exchange capacity than do less esterified pectins (low methoxy).

Physiological Response to Sources of Dietary Fiber

Several physiological responses, such as lowering of plasma cholesterol levels, modification of the glycemic response, improving large bowel function, and lowering nutrient availability, have been associated with isolated fiber fractions or diets rich in fiber-containing foods. In mediating these responses it is clear that the physical properties of dietary fibers affect the functioning of the gastrointestinal tract and influence the rate and site of nutrient absorption. Hence, our discussion of the current understanding of these physiological responses will be done in the context of the physical properties of dietary fiber and the effects on gastrointestinal function.

Plasma cholesterol lowering. A tremendous number of studies in both humans and experimental animals have been conducted examining the ability of different types of dietary fiber to lower plasma cholesterol concentrations. From these studies certain generalities can be deduced. Most isolated fibers that are water soluble will lower plasma cholesterol in humans and plasma and liver cholesterol in animals. These include pectins, psyllium, and various gums such as guar gum, locust bean gum, and modified celluloses such as carboxymethylcellulose. Consumption of fiber-rich sources containing water-soluble fibers, such as oat bran and barley (sources of mixed-linkage β-glucans), legumes, and vegetables, usually results in a lowering of plasma cholesterol. Reductions in total plasma cholesterol up to 25% have been reported, but most studies find reductions in the range of 5–10%. Almost invariably the reductions occur in the low-density lipoprotein fraction, with little or no change in high-density lipoprotein cholesterol. In contrast, isolated fibers or fiber sources that are not water soluble have rarely been found to alter plasma cholesterol. These fibers include cellulose, lignin, corn bran, and wheat bran.

How cholesterol-lowering dietary fibers mediate their action remains a subject of controversy. One hypothesis is that a fiber-induced increase in bile acid excretion leads to an increased demand for bile acid synthesis, resulting in an increased rate of conversion of cholesterol to bile acids.[38] If cholesterol synthesis rates do not increase sufficiently to compensate for the loss of cholesterol to bile acids, then cholesterol concentrations will decrease. However, not all fibers that lower cholesterol increase bile acid excretion.[39] A corollary to this hypothesis is that cholesterol-lowering fibers alter the bile acid profile by differential binding to bile acids, which could lead to decreases in absorption or synthesis of cholesterol.[40] Changes in the profile of the bile acid pool with feeding of cholesterol-lowering fibers have been noted in several studies.[41,42] Future studies with additional fiber types will be necessary to establish the importance of this correlation. Many water-soluble fibers form a viscous matrix within the small intestine,[43] which could interfere with cholesterol or bile acid absorption in the small intestine. Guar gum has been found to delay cholesterol disappearance from the small intestine in one study,[44] but to have no effect on absorption in another.[45] Likewise, pectin has been found to reduce cholesterol absorption in one study[46] but not in another.[47] Using a highly viscous but nonfermentable modified cellulose, hydroxypropyl methylcellulose, it has been shown that cholesterol absorption decreases linearly with the logarithm of intestinal contents viscosity.[48] Another hypothesis is that sources of fiber will modify cholesterol synthesis. Cholesterol synthesis as measured by ^{14}C-acetate incorporation into cholesterol[49] or hepatic 3-OH-3-methyl glutaryl coenzyme A activity[50] is elevated in rats fed pectin, a hypocholesterolemic fiber source.[51] This elevation is undoubtedly due to reduced cholesterol absorption or enhanced bile acid excretion in pectin-fed rats. Studies with isolated hepatocytes have demonstrated that propionate, which can be produced by fermentation of soluble fiber, inhibits fatty acid synthesis and ^{14}C-acetate incorporation into cholesterol but does not inhibit total cholesterol synthesis.[52] A preliminary report indicates that in humans in vivo lipogenesis may be suppressed in subjects fed a high-carbohydrate diet that is rich in complex carbohydrates, including starch and dietary fiber.[53] These results suggest that the effect of fermentable fibers on hepatic fatty acid synthesis and secretion should be investigated further, especially since hepatic-derived triglyceride-rich lipoproteins are the precursors of the low-density lipoprotein fraction. Overall, the evidence suggests that more than one mechanism contributes to the cholesterol-lowering effect of dietary fiber. The physical properties of fiber that seem most likely to be responsible are bile acid binding (or entrapment) and viscosity.

Modification of the glycemic response. Numerous studies have demonstrated that consumption of certain water-soluble fibers will reduce the postprandial glycemic and insulinemic responses.[54] This effect occurs when the fiber is coadministered with a glucose load or as part of a meal, in both normal and diabetic individuals. The effect of fiber on the rate of gastric emptying has been associated with its ability to blunt the glycemic response to a glucose load and to slow nutrient absorption. Long-term blood glucose control, as measured by glycated hemoglobin, is also improved with guar feeding in both humans[55] and animals.[56] Further, guar gum has been shown to reduce the renal enlargement associated with the onset of diabetes in animals.[27,56] The renal enlargement of diabetes is highly correlated with blood glucose concentrations.[57]

The postprandial glucose curve flattening ability of various fiber supplements is highly correlated with their viscosity.[58,59] Possible explanations for this effect include a delayed rate of stomach emptying and delayed starch digestion within or a slowing of glucose absorption from the small intestine. These mechanisms are obviously not mutually exclusive. Viscous polysaccharides but not insoluble fiber sources such as cellulose have been reported to delay gastric emptying.[60,61] Comparing oral administration of a guar-containing meal to one that was administered directly into the intestine, Leclère et al.[62] concluded that a slowing of gastric emptying was the main factor in flattening the postprandial glucose curve. Their study also suggested that guar gum slowed the rate of starch digestion, but had no effect on glucose diffusion.

With a steady-state intestinal perfusion technique, guar gum has been shown to slow the rate of glucose uptake in humans.[63] Thus, evidence exists in favor of all the mechanisms described, and the predominant action will depend on numerous factors, such as the type and source of fiber used, its rate of hydration, and its ultimate viscosity.

Improving large bowel function. The presence of fiber in the diet can influence large bowel function by reducing transit time, increasing stool weight and frequency, diluting large intestinal contents, and providing fermentable substrate for microflora normally present in the large intestine. All of these factors are influenced by the source of fiber in the diet as well as other dietary and nondietary factors. Transit time has been shown to decrease because of wheat bran supplementation in 14 studies and decrease because of the addition of fruits and vegetables to the diet. In two studies, cellulose has been reported to decrease transit time and in two other studies to have no effect. Pectin, based on three studies, does not affect transit time.[64] Transit time is related to stool weight, but not in a simple linear manner. By examining population data from healthy subjects, Spiller[65] reported that a low stool weight is associated with delayed transit time; as stool weight increases transit time tends to decrease. However, once a transit time of 20–30 hours is achieved, further increases in stool weight do not shorten transit time significantly.

Stool weight can be increased by sources of fiber in a dose-related manner.[66] The nonstarch polysaccharides and resistant starch are the primary dietary components that increase fecal bulk. Cummings[67] summarized a number of studies by estimating the increase in fecal weight relative to the weight of fiber fed. Fiber sources that contain insoluble fiber components, such as wheat bran, tend to produce the greatest increase in stool weight. Fruits and vegetables and gums and mucilages also produce a moderate increase in fecal output ,whereas legumes and pectin increase stool weight only slightly. An increase in stool weight is typically associated with an increase in the microbial cell mass, in the undigested fecal residue, or the noncellular matrix in the feces. Hence, the fecal bulking ability of a fiber source is related to a change in one or all of these phases. For example, wheat bran is more effective in increasing the amount of undigested residue, whereas the fiber in fruits and vegetables and the soluble polysaccharides can be fermented extensively and are more likely to increase the microbial cell mass of the feces. Differences in particle size of the fiber source have been studied for wheat bran; reducing the particle size reduces fecal weight.[68,69]

The effects of fiber on stool weight and transit time, although inherently variable, are physiological responses important for maintaining large bowel function. A consensus of opinion exists that dietary fiber has an important role in large bowel function.[64,70] Other metabolic consequences of fiber in the large intestine are more poorly understood and, thus, are more difficult to define in terms of their physiological significance. For example, during the fermentation of the polysaccharides associated with dietary fiber, the microflora produce short-chain fatty acids, primarily acetate, propionate, and butyrate. Butyrate can be used by large intestinal cells as an energy source. In vitro, butyrate causes transformed cells to undergo differentiation.[71] Yet, in vivo, all short-chain fatty acids cause large intestinal hypertrophy.[72] Feeding of purified, highly fermentable fibers has been found to stimulate large intestinal cell growth[73] and to promote tumor formation in carcinogen-treated animals in some studies, but not in others. In contrast, other investigators have speculated that production of certain short-chain fatty acids may protect against colon cancer.[74] The production of short-chain fatty acids in the large intestine is obviously an important consequence of consuming fiber sources that are fermentable; however, the metabolic consequences of short-chain fatty acid production remain poorly understood.

Lowering nutrient availability. Within the small intestine the digestible components of the diet are broken down by hydrolysis and nutrients are absorbed through the mucosal cells. In vitro data indicate that various fiber sources can inhibit the activity of pancreatic enzymes that digest carbohydrates, lipids, and proteins.[75] The mechanisms for inhibiting digestive enzyme activity are not clearly established, but in some nonpurified fiber sources, specific enzyme inhibitors exist.[76] It is difficult to assess the physiological importance of this inhibition because an excess of digestive enzyme activity is secreted in response to a meal. However, several lines of evidence indicate that specific fibers may reduce the availability of the enzyme for hydrolyzing triglycerides, starch, and proteins within the intestinal contents. Gallaher and Schneeman[77] reported that a diet high in cellulose (20% by weight) delayed the disappearance of labeled triolein but not labeled cholesterol from the small intestine. The results indicated that the high cellulose content of the diet interfered with triolein breakdown but not with overall lipid absorption. Lairon et al.[78,79] reported that an inhibitor of pancreatic lipase is present in wheat bran and wheat germ. A blunting of the blood plasma increase in triglycerides during the alimentary period has been associated with fiber sources that contain lipase inhibitor.[80] The characteristics of this inhibitor suggest that it may be active in the small intestine and capable of slowing the digestion of triglycerides. Legumes have been reported to contain amylase inhibitors that could slow the hydrolysis of starch in the small intestine.[76] Inhibition of amylase in human pancreatic or duodenal fluid by wheat bran, xylan, cellulose, guar gum, and psyllium has been reported.[75] Many cereals and legumes contain pancreatic protease inhibitors that can decrease protein digestibility. These inhibitors are often inactivated by heat treatment; however, some inhibitor activity can potentially survive normal processing conditions and remain active in the gut. In patients with pancreatic insufficiency the amylase, trypsin, chymotrypsin, and lipase activity available from pancreatic replacement treatment was significantly reduced when the patients were given a meal containing pectin or wheat bran, which suggests that it is possible for these fiber sources to significantly reduce digestive enzyme capacity in the small intestine.[81] In addition to direct inhibition of digestive enzyme activity, the presence of plant cell wall matrix in a food provides a physical barrier to digestion.[82-84] An intact cell wall will slow the penetration of digestive enzymes into plant foods. Consequently, grinding of the fiber source to a very fine particle size may disrupt the cell wall structure sufficiently to make digestible nutrients more available for hydrolysis.

Studies on the effect of dietary fiber on vitamin absorption have been conducted for most vitamins. Although differences in the type and amount of fibers fed and the methods for determining uptake make comparisons across studies difficult, it appears that generally fiber has little if any effect on vitamin absorption.[85] The effect of fiber on mineral absorption is somewhat less clear. Natural sources of fiber, such as cereals and fruits, generally have a depressing effect on absorption of minerals such as calcium, iron, zinc, and copper.[86] However, at least part of this effect is likely to be due to the presence of phytic acid in these foods, which is known to interfere with mineral absorption.[87] When isolated fiber sources are examined, such as cellulose, pectin, and gums, the large majority of studies find no detrimental effect on mineral balance or absorption.[86]

The physical characteristics of the intestinal contents will be changed by the physical properties of the fiber sources in the diet. The bulk or amount of material in the small intestine will increase because the fiber is not digestible and hence remains during the transit of digesta through the small intestine.[88] The volume of the intestinal contents can increase because of the water-holding capacity of the fiber source. Sandberg et al.[89,90] reported that addition of wheat bran or pectin to a low-fiber meal increased the volume of ileostomy fluid by about 20–30%. In addition, animal data indicate that a greater dry and wet weight of intestinal contents is associated with the addition of a fiber supplement to experimental diets.[88] The presence of certain viscous polysaccharides in the fiber source will increase the viscosity of the contents and in particular of the aqueous phase of the intestinal contents from which nutrients are absorbed.[91-93] Greater viscosity of the aqueous phase of the intestinal contents will cause an apparent thickening of the unstirred layer at the epithelial surface, which is the theoretical barrier to lipid absorption in the intestine.[94] An increase in the bulk, volume, or viscosity of the intestinal contents is likely to slow diffusion of enzymes, substrates, and nutrients to the absorptive surface, all of which can lead to a slower appearance of nutrients in the plasma following a meal.

The bile acid and phospholipid binding capacities of various fibers are likely to affect micelle formation in the small intestine and consequently the rate and site of lipid absorption. Vahouny and coworkers[95,96] have demonstrated that addition of fiber supplements to rat diets can slow the appearance of fatty acids and cholesterol in the lymph. The ability of the soluble forms of fiber to slow fatty acid absorption and to interfere with cholesterol absorption undoubtedly contributes to the effect of these fiber sources on plasma lipid levels. Studies in humans have indicated that diets supplemented with oat bran, pectin, or guar gum, but not wheat bran or cellulose, lower plasma cholesterol levels by 5–18%.[64]

The experimental evidence suggests that, through a variety of mechanisms, certain fiber sources, especially those containing viscous polysaccharides, can slow the process of digestion and absorption, although total nutrient absorption is not necessarily reduced. Because of its effect on the rate of absorption, a greater proportion of nutrients from a diet high in fiber will undoubtedly be absorbed from the lower half of the small intestine. This pattern of nutrient absorption is likely to contribute to the physiological responses to various fiber sources. For example, the rate of nutrient absorption will affect the pattern of hormone release in response to diet[97] and the rate of nutrient delivery to the tissues. Evidence also exists that the presence of nutrients in the ileum can influence satiety and food intake, gastric emptying, and the composition and size of chylomicrons.[98,99] The presence of fiber in the gut has an important function in maintaining the gastrointestinal system by regulating the rate and site of nutrient absorption. Sigleo et al.[100] have demonstrated that chronic feeding of fiber supplements will alter the morphology of the small intestine. Both the distribution of nutrient absorption in the small intestine and the influence of bulk in the small intestine on intestinal cell renewal are likely to contribute to this response.[101]

Our current understanding has indicated that the physical-chemical properties of dietary fiber such as viscosity and bile acid binding exert effects within the small intestine and stomach that are important in understanding the mechanisms by which fiber sources lower plasma cholesterol, blunt the glycemic response, and slow nutrient absorption. In addition to these effects within the upper gut, the metabolism of dietary fiber sources within the large intestine is important to understanding the overall physiological response to sources of fiber.

Adequacy of Fiber Intake

Several groups have proposed recommendations for fiber intake in the population. The challenge to nutritionists in making these recommendations has been to evaluate the adequacy of fiber intake given our current knowledge about the physiological responses to sources of fiber in the diet. To assess the adequacy of intake, two approaches are possible. One approach is to determine an optimal intake of dietary fiber based on studying the intake of different population groups that vary in their risk of chronic disorders. The second approach is to use a physiological parameter to assess adequacy. Both approaches have several limitations with respect to recommendations for dietary fiber intakes with our current knowledge.

Bingham[102] has pointed out two systematic biases inherent in comparing the fiber intake of different populations. These are differences in the methods of estimating food consumption and in the methods for estimating dietary fiber content of foods. Additionally, dietary factors other than fiber intake may influence disease risk. For example, the intake of nonstarch polysaccharides is similar in Japan and the United Kingdom, yet Japan is a population at low risk for colon cancer and diverticular disease compared with the United Kingdom.[102,103] Differences in the consumption of meat and fat, variations in the dietary fiber sources, as well as nonnutritional factors could all contribute to the differences in disease risk between these populations. Population data can provide guidance for the range of fiber intakes that are likely to be safe, but are inadequate to determine the fiber intake that is nutritionally adequate.

In this chapter we have reviewed the effects of dietary fiber in the gastrointestinal tract with respect to lowering of plasma cholesterol, blunting the glycemic response, decreasing nutrient bioavailability, and its impact on large bowel function. Use of the first two responses as criteria to assess nutritional adequacy of fiber intake is limited because fasting plasma cholesterol levels or plasma glucose and insulin levels may not change in healthy subjects. Consequently, a wide range in fiber intakes will be associated with similar responses. These parameters may be more useful in monitoring improvement due to dietary intervention for therapeutic management of hyperlipidemia or hyperglycemia. Evaluating mineral status relative to nutrient bioavailability is likely to be useful in setting the maximum amount of fiber or fiber-rich foods to be consumed because excessive fiber intake could compromise mineral status. These three physiological responses are all limited relative to assessment in that the criteria tend to be directed at a disease state rather than normal physiological function.

Dietary fiber clearly has an important physiological role in normal large bowel functioning by providing bulk and

substrates for fermentation. Several recommendations have been made that stool weight and transit time, as indicators of large bowel function, are useful in assessing the adequacy of dietary fiber intake.[64,65,70] In this context the adequacy of fiber intake could be assessed using normal physiological function as the criteria. Cummings et al.[66] demonstrated that a dose-response relationship exists between intake of nonstarch polysaccharides and stool weight up to an intake of 32 g/day. An average stool weight of <150 g/day has been associated with increased disease risk. These facts have been used by the Ministry of Health in the UK to suggest that intakes of 18 g/day of nonstarch polysaccharides are needed in a healthful diet.[104] This value is similar to the estimate of 10 g/1000 kcal of dietary fiber recommended by the Life Sciences Research Office Expert Panel, which also used stool weight as a physiological predictor of adequacy of fiber intake. For consumers it is important that recommendations on fiber intake are expressed in terms of foods that provide fiber, because many benefits associated with fiber are due to many components that provide fiber, not fiber alone. Food selection should be evaluated with respect to meeting the recommendations for consumption of fruits, vegetables, cereals, grains, and legumes in the Food Guide Pyramid and the Dietary Guidelines. The recommendation to select items high in fiber (e.g., fruit versus fruit juice, whole-grain versus milled grains) encourages the use of fiber-containing foods in the diet.[105]

References

1. Trowell HC (1973) Dietary fibre, ischemic heart disease and diabetes mellitus. Proc Nutr Soc 32:151–157
2. Spiller GA (1993) Definition of dietary fiber. In Spiller GA (ed), Dietary fiber in human nutrition, 2nd ed. CRC Press, Boca Raton, FL, pp 15–18
3. Bourquin LD, Titgemeyer EC, Garleb KA, Fahey GC Jr (1992) Short-chain fatty acid production and fiber degradation by human colonic bacteria: effects of substrate and cell wall fractionation procedures. J Nutr 122:1508–1520
4. Selvendran RR, Stevens BJH, Du Pont MS (1987) Dietary fiber: chemistry, analysis and properties. Adv Food Res 31:117–209
5. Trock B, Lanza E, Greenwald P (1990) Dietary fiber, vegetables, and colon cancer: critical review and meta-analysis of the epidemiological evidence. J Natl Cancer Inst 82:650–661
6. Block G, Lanza E (1987) Dietary fiber sources in the United States by demographic group. J Natl Cancer Inst 79:83–91
7. Block G, Patterson B, Subar A (1992) Fruit, vegetables, and cancer prevention: a review of the epidemiological evidence. Nutr Cancer 18:1–19
8. Burley VJ, Blundell JE (1995) Dietary fiber and the pattern of energy intake. In Kritchevsky D, Bonfield C (eds), Dietary fiber in health and disease. Eagan Press, St. Paul, MN, pp 243–256
9. Horwitz W, ed (1980) Official methods of analysis of the Association of Official Analytical Chemists, 13th ed. AOAC, Washington, DC, p 132
10. Robertson JB, Van Soest PJ (1981) The detergent system of

analysis and its application to human foods. In James WPT, Theander O (eds), The analysis of dietary fiber in foods. Marcel Dekker, New York, pp 123–158

11. Prosky L, Asp N-G, Furda I, et al (1984) Determination of total dietary fiber in foods, food products, and total diets: interlaboratory study. J Assoc Off Anal Chem 68:677–679

12. Englyst HN, Quigley ME, Hudson GJ (1994) Determination of dietary fibre as non-starch polysaccharides with gas-liquid chromatographic, high-performance liquid chromatography or spectrophotometric measurement of constituent sugars. Analyst 119:1497–1509

13. Spiller GA (1993) Comparison of analyses of dietary fiber and crude fiber. In Spiller GA (ed), Dietary fiber in human nutrition, 2nd ed. CRC Press, Boca Raton, FL, p 615

14. Goering HK, van Soest PJ (1970) Forage fiber analysis. Handbook no. 379, US Department of Agriculture. US Government Printing Office, Washington, DC, p 1

15. Prosky L, Asp N-G, Schweizer TF, et al (1988) Determination of insoluble, soluble, and total dietary fiber in foods and food products: interlaboratory study. J Assoc Off Anal Chem 71:1017–1023

16. Marlett JA (1990) Analysis of dietary fiber in human foods. In Kritchevsky D, Bonfield C, Anderson JW (eds), Dietary fiber: chemistry, physiology, and health effects. Plenum Press, New York, pp 31–48

17. Englyst HN, Cummings JH (1987) Digestion of polysaccharides of potato in the small intestine of man. Am J Clin Nutr 45:423–431

18. Berry CS (1986) Resistant starch: formation and measurement of starch that survives exhaustive digestion with amylolytic enzymes during the determination of dietary fibre. J Cereal Sci 4:301–314

19. Englyst HN, Trowell H, Southgate DAT, et al (1987) Dietary fiber and resistant starch. Am J Clin Nutr 46:873–874

20. Asp N-G, Furda I, Schweizer TF, Prosky L (1988) Dietary fiber definition and analysis. Am J Clin Nutr 48:688–690

21. Englyst HN, Hudson GJ (1993) Dietary fiber and starch: classification and measurement. In Spiller GA (ed), Dietary fiber in human nutrition, 2nd ed. CRC Press, Boca Raton, FL, pp 53–71

22. McConnell AA, Eastwood MA, Mitchell WD (1974) Physical characteristics of vegetable foodstuffs that could influence bowel function. J Sci Food Agric 25:1457–1464

23. Robertson JA, Eastwood MA, Yeoman MM (1980) An investigation into the physical properties of fibre prepared from several carrot varieties at different stages of development. J Sci Food Agric 31:633–638

24. Robertson JA, Eastwood MA (1981) A method to measure the water-holding properties of dietary fibre using suction pressure. Br J Nutr 46:247–255

25. Stephen AM, Cummings JH (1979) Water-holding by dietary fibre in vitro and its relationship to faecal output in man. Gut 20:722–729

26. McBurney MI, Horvath PJ, Jeraci JL, van Soest PJ (1985) Effect of in vitro fermentation using human faecal inoculum on the water-holding capacity of dietary fibre. Br J Nutr 53:17–24

27. Gallaher DD, Schaubert D (1990) The effect of dietary fiber type on glycated hemoglobin and renal hypertrophy in the diabetic rat. Nutr Res 10:1311–1323

28. Kritchevsky D, Story JA (1974) Binding of bile salts in vitro by nonnutritive fiber. J Nutr 104:458–462

29. Vahouny GV, Tombes R, Cassidy MM, et al (1980) Dietary fibers, V: Binding of bile salts, phospholipids and cholesterol from mixed micelles by bile acid sequestrants and dietary fibers. Lipids 15:1012–1018

30. Gallaher DD, Schneeman BO (1986) Intestinal interaction of bile acids, phospholipids, dietary fibers and cholestyramine. Am J Physiol 250:G420–G-426

31. Eastwood MA, Hamilton D (1968) Studies on the adsorption of bile salts to non-absorbed components of diet. Biochim Biophys Acta 152:165–173

32. Eastwood MA, Mowbray L (1976) The binding of the components of mixed micelle to dietary fiber. Am J Clin Nutr 29:1461–1467

33. Oakenfull DG, Fenwick DE (1978) Adsorption of bile salts from aqueous solution by plant fibre and cholestyramine. Br J Nutr 40:299–309

34. Calvert GD, Yeates RA (1982) Adsorption of bile salts by soya-bean flour, wheat bran, lucerne (Medicago sativa), sawdust and lignin: the effect of saponins and other plant constituents. Br J Nutr 47:45–52

35. McBurney MI, Allen MS, van Soest PJ (1986) Praseodimium and copper-exchange capacities of neutral detergent fibers relative to composition and fermentation kinetics. J Sci Food Agric 50:666–672

36. Nair BM, Asp N-G, Nyman M, Persson H (1987) Binding of mineral elements by some dietary fibre components—in vitro(I). Food Chem 23:295–303

37. Schlemmer U (1989) Studies of the binding of copper, zinc and calcium to pectin, alginate, carrageenan and guar gum in HCO_3–CO_2 buffer. Food Chem 32:223–234

38. Story JA, Kritchevsky, D (1976) Dietary fiber and lipid metabolism. In Spiller GA, Amen RJ (eds), Fiber in human nutrition. Plenum Press, New York, pp 171–184

39. Anderson JW, Deakins DA, Floore TL, et al (1990) Dietary fiber and coronary heart disease. Crit Rev Food Sci Nutr 29:95–147

40. Story JA, Thomas JN (1982) Modification of bile acid spectrum by dietary fiber. In Vahouny GV, Kritchevsky D (eds), Dietary fiber in health and disease. Plenum Press, New York, pp 193–201

41. Everson GT, Daggy BP, McKinley C, et al (1992) Effects of psyllium hydrophilic mucilloid on LDL-cholesterol and bile acid synthesis in hypercholesterolemic men. J Lipid Res 33:1183–1192

42. Marlett JA, Hosig KB, Vollendorf NW, et al (1994) Mechanism of serum cholesterol reduction by oat bran. Hepatology 20:1450–1457

43. Eastwood MA, Morris ER (1992) Physical properties of dietary fiber that influence physiological function: a model for polymers along the gastrointestinal tract. Am J Clin Nutr 55:436–442

44. Ebihara K, Schneeman BO (1989) Interaction of bile acids, phospholipids, cholesterol and triglyceride with dietary fibers in the small intestine of rats. J Nutr 119:1100–1106

45. Miettinen TA, Tarpila S (1989) Serum lipids and cholesterol metabolism during guar gum, plantago ovata and high fibre treatments. Clin Chim Acta 183:253–262

46. Kelley JJ, Tsai AC (1978) Effect of pectin, gum arabic and agar on cholesterol absorption, synthesis, and turnover in rats. J Nutr 108:630–639

47. Fernandez ML, Lin EC, Trejo A, et al (1994) Prickly pear (Opuntia sp.) pectin alters hepatic cholesterol metabolism without affecting cholesterol absorption in guinea pigs fed a hypercholesterolemic diet. J Nutr 124:817–824

48. Carr TP, Gallaher DD, Yang C-H, et al (1996) Intestinal contents viscosity and cholesterol absorption efficiency in hamsters fed hydroxypropyl methylcellulose. J Nutr (in press).

49. Mokady S (1974) Effects of dietary pectin and algin on the biosynthesis of hepatic lipids in growing rats. Nutr Metab 16:203–207

50. Nishina PM, Schneeman BO, Freedland RA (1991) Effects of dietary fibers on nonfasting plasma lipoprotein and apolipoprotein levels in rats. J Nutr 121:431–437

51. Tinker L, Davis PA, Schneeman BO (1994) Prune fiber or pectin compared to cellulose lowers plasma and liver lipids in rats with diet-induced hyperlipidemia. J Nutr 124:31–40

52. Nishina PM, Freedland RA (1990) Effects of propionate on lipid biosynthesis in isolated rat hepatocytes. J Nutr 120:668–673

53. Hudgins L, Hellerstein M, Seldman C, et al (1993) Increased de novo lipogenesis on a eucaloric low fat high carbohydrate diet does not alter energy expenditure [abstract]. Obesity Res 1 (suppl 2):92S

54. Wolever TMS, Jenkins DJA (1993) Effect of fiber and foods on carbohydrate metabolism. In Spiller GA (ed), Dietary fiber in human nutrition, 2nd ed. CRC Press, Boca Raton, FL, pp 111–152

55. Peterson DB, Ellis PR, Baylis JM, et al (1987) Low dose guar in a novel food product: improved metabolic control in non-insulin-dependent diabetes. Diab Med 4:111–115

56. Gallaher DD, Olson JM, Larntz K (1992) Guar gum halts further renal enlargement in rats with established diabetes. J Nutr 122:2391–2397

57. Seyer-Hansen K (1977) Renal hypertrophy in experimental diabetes: relation to severity of diabetes. Diabetologia 13:141–143

58. Jenkins DJA, Wolever TMS, Leeds AR, et al (1978) Dietary fibres, fibre analogues, and glucose tolerance: importance of viscosity. Br Med J i:1392–1394

59. Edwards CA, Blackburn NA, Craigen L, et al (1987) Viscosity of food gums determined in vitro related to their hypoglycemic actions. Am J Clin Nutr 46:72–77

60. Schwartz SE, Levine RA, Singh A, et al (1982) Sustained pectin ingestion delays gastric emptying. Gastroenterology 83:812–817

61. Torsdottir I, Alpsten M, Andersson H, et al (1989) Dietary guar gum effects on postprandial blood glucose, insulin and hydroxyproline in humans. J Nutr 119:1925–1931

62. Leclère CJ, Champ M, Boillot J, et al (1994) Role of viscous guar gums in lowering the glycemic response after a solid meal. Am J Clin Nutr 59:914–921

63. Blackburn NA, Redfern JS, Jarjis H, et al (1984) The mechanism of action of guar gum in improving glucose tolerance in man. Clin Sci Molec Med 66:329–336

64. LSRO (Life Sciences Research Office) (1987) In Pilch SM (ed), Physiological effects and health consequences of dietary fiber. Federation of American Societies for Experimental Biology, Bethesda, MD

65. Spiller GA (1993) Suggestions for a basis on which to determine a desirable intake of dietary fiber. In Spiller GA (ed), Dietary fiber in human nutrition, 2nd ed. CRC Press, Boca Raton, FL, pp 351–354

66. Cummings JH, Bingham SA, Heaton KW, Eastwood MA (1992) Fecal weight, colon cancer risk and dietary intake of non-starch polysaccharides (dietary fiber). Gastroenterology 103:1783–1789

67. Cummings JH (1993) The effect of dietary fiber on fecal weight and composition. In Spiller GA (ed), Dietary fiber in human nutrition, 2nd ed. CRC Press, Boca Raton, FL, pp 263–349

68. Brodribb AJM, Groves C (1978) Effect of bran particle size on stool weight. Gut 19:60–63

69. Heller SN, Hackler LR, Rivers JM, et al (1980) Dietary fiber: the effect of particle size of wheat bran on colonic function in young adult men. Am J Clin Nutr 33:1734–1744

70. UK Department of Health (1991) Dietary reference values for food energy and nutrients for the United Kingdom. Her Majesty's Stationery Office, London, pp 61–71

71. Augeron C, Laboisse CL (1984) Emergence of permanently differentiated cell clones in a human colonic cancer cell line in culture after treatment with sodium butyrate. Cancer Res 44:3961–3969

72. Sakata T (1987) Stimulatory effect of short-chain fatty acids on epithelial cell proliferation in the rat intestine: a possible explanation for trophic effects of fermentable fibre, gut microbes and luminal trophic factors. Br J Nutr 58:95–103

73. Jacobs LR, Lupton JR (1984) Effect of dietary fibers on rat large bowel mucosal growth and cell proliferation. Am J Physiol 246:G378–385

74. McIntyre A, Gibson PR, Young GP (1993) Butyrate production from dietary fibre and protection against large bowel cancer in a rat model. Gut 34:386–391

75. Schneeman BO, Gallaher DD (1993) Effects of dietary fiber on digestive enzymes. In Spiller GA (ed), Dietary fiber in human nutrition, 2nd ed. CRC Press, Boca Raton, FL, pp 377–385

76. Gallaher DD, Schneeman BO (1986) Nutritional and metabolic response to plant inhibitors of digestive enzymes. In Friedman M (ed), Advances in experimental medicine and biology, vol 199: Nutritional and toxicological significance of enzyme inhibitors in foods. Plenum Press, New York, pp 167–184

77. Gallaher DD, Schneeman BO (1985) Effect of dietary cellulose on site of lipid absorption. Am J Physiol 249:G184–G191

78. Lairon D, Lafont H, Vigne JL, et al (1985) Effects of dietary fibers and cholestyramine on the activity of pancreatic lipase in vitro. Am J Clin Nutr 42:629–638

79. Lairon D, Borel E, Termine R, et al (1985) Evidence for a proteinic inhibitor of pancreatic lipase in cereals, wheat bran and wheat germ. Nutr Rep Int 32:1107–1113

80. Cara L, Dubois C, Borel P, et al (1992) Effects of oat bran, wheat fiber, and wheat germ on postprandial lipemia in healthy adults. Am J Clin Nutr 55:81–88

81. Isaksson G, Lundquist B, Akesson B, Ihse I (1984) Effects of pectin and wheat bran on intraluminal pancreatic enzyme activities and on fat absorption as examined with the triolein breath test in patients with pancreatic insufficiency. Scand J Gastroenterol 19:467–472

82. Collier G, O'Dea K (1982) Effect of physical form of carbohydrate on the postprandial glucose, insulin and gastric inhibitory polypeptide responses in type 2 diabetes. Am J Clin Nutr 36:10–14

83. Snow P, O'Dea K (1981) Factors affecting the rate of hydrolysis of starch in food. Am J Clin Nutr 34:2721–2727

84. Wong S, O'Dea K (1983) Importance of physical form rather than viscosity in determining the rate of starch hydrolysis in legumes. Am J Clin Nutr 37:66–70

85. Kasper H (1993) Effects of dietary fiber on vitamin metabolism. In Spiller GA (ed), Dietary fiber in human nutrition, 2nd ed. CRC Press, Boca Raton, FL, pp 253–260

86. Torre M, Rodriguez AR, Saura-Calixto F (1991) Effects of dietary fiber and phytic acid on mineral availability. Crit Rev Food Sci Nutr 1(1):1–22

87. Sandström B, Almgren A, Kivistoe B, Cederblad A (1987) Zinc absorption in humans from meals based on rye, barley, oat meal, triticale, and whole wheat. J Nutr 117:1898–1902

88. Schneeman BO (1982) Pancreatic and digestive function. In Vahouny GV, Kritchevsky D (eds), Dietary fiber in health and disease. Plenum Press, New York, pp 73–83

89. Sandberg AS, Ahderinee R, Andersson H, et al (1983) The effect of citrus pectin on the absorption of nutrients in the small intestine. Hum Nutr Clin Nutr 37C:171–183

90. Sandberg AS, Andersson H, Hallgren B, et al (1981) Experimental model for in vivo determination of dietary fibre and its effect on the absorption of nutrients in the small intestine. Br J Nutr 45:283–294

91. Blackburn NA, Johnson IT (1981) The effect of guar gum on the viscosity of the gastrointestinal contents and on glucose uptake from the perfused jejunum in the rat. Br J Nutr 46:239–246

92. Elsenhans B, Sufke U, Blume R, Caspary WF (1980) The influence of carbohydrate gelling agents on rat intestinal transport of monosaccharides and neutral amino acids in vitro. Clin Sci 59:373–380

93. Johnson IT, Gee JM (1981) Effect of gel-forming gums on the intestinal unstirred layer and sugar transport in vitro. Gut 22:398–403

94. Schneeman BO (1994) Carbohydrates: significance for energy balance and gastrointestinal function. J Nutr 124:1747S–1753S

95. Vahouny GV, Satchitanandam S, Chen I, et al (1988) Dietary fiber and intestinal adaptation: effect on lipid absorption and lymphatic transport in the rat. Am J Clin Nutr 47:201–206

96. Vahouny GV (1982) Dietary fibers and intestinal absorption of lipids. In Vahouny GV, Kritchevsky D (eds), Dietary fiber in health and disease. Plenum Press, New York, pp 203–227

97. Jenkins DJA (1978) Action of dietary fiber in lowering fasting serum cholesterol and reducing postprandial glycemia: gastrointestinal mechanisms. In Carlson LA (ed), International conference on atherosclerosis. Raven Press, New York, pp 173–182

98. Wu AL, Clark SB, Holt PR (1980) Composition of lymph chylomicrons from proximal or distal rat small intestine. Am J Clin Nutr 33:582–589

99. Spiller RC, Trotman IF, Adrian TE, et al (1988) Further characterization of the "ileal brake" reflex in man: effect of ileal infusion of partial digests of fat, protein and starch on jejunal motility and release of neurotensin, enteroglucagon and peptide YY. Gut 29:1042–1051

100. Sigleo S, Jackson MJ, Vahouny GV (1984) Effects of dietary fiber constituents on intestinal morphology and nutrient transport. Am J Physiol 246:G34–G39

101. Johnson LR (1988) Regulation of gastrointestinal mucosal growth. Physiol Rev 68:456–502

102. Bingham S (1987) Definitions and intakes of dietary fiber. Am J Clin Nutr 45:1226–1231

103. Klurfeld DM (1987) The role of dietary fiber in gastrointestinal disease. J Am Diet Assoc 87:1172–1177

104. Cummings JH, Englyst HN (1995) Gastrointestinal effects of food carbohydrates. Am J Clin Nutr 61(suppl):938S–945S

105. Gambera P, Davis PA, Schneeman BO. Use of the Food Guide Pyramid to improve dietary intake and reduce cardiovascular risk in active duty air force members. J Am Diet Assoc. In press

Chapter 10

Water

Eldon Wayne Askew

Water is essential to life. No other substance is as widely involved in as many diverse functions of the human body as water. A water deficiency manifests rapidly, and symptoms occur with as little as 1% hypohydration. With continued dehydration, the cardiovascular, respiratory, and thermoregulatory systems are compromised, and complete water deprivation leads to death in a matter of days. Water plays a key role in maintaining homeostasis of the internal environment for optimum function of cells. This internal environment—body fluid with associated cations and anions—enveloping cells remains relatively constant despite the diversity of cells and cellular functions. The most easily appreciated roles of water in the human body are to provide a medium for transport of blood components, to dissolve and pass nutrients from blood to cells, to provide a medium for intracellular reactions to take place, and to transfer metabolic products to the blood for redistribution or elimination via the urine.

Water is, however, more than just a nutrient: it is a major component of the thermoregulatory system of the body. The body's metabolic apparatus for digestion and processing of nutrients and for muscular contraction is highly endergonic, liberating large quantities of heat that must be dissipated to maintain homeothermy. For example, the thermogenic effect of digestion of food is 10–15% of the caloric content of a mixed meal. Muscular contraction is an even more important contributor to the body's heat burden. The transformation of chemical energy to mechanical energy for muscular contraction is only 25–30% efficient, liberating 70–75% of the energy as heat. Water absorbs heat where it is generated and dissipates it over the fluid compartment of the body, minimizing the risk of localized damage to enzymes or structural proteins by heat. Once the heat of chemical reactions has been transferred to body fluid, it is routed to the surface of the skin where it is dissipated by convection, radiation, conduction, or evaporation.

The evaporation of sweat is a concerted mechanism whereby water plays two simultaneous roles to dissipate heat. Water in blood transfers heat to the skin surface during heat-induced vasodilation; in turn, this heat is transferred to water in sweat released at the skin surface to be evaporated, thus transferring body heat to the surrounding environment. The heat of vaporization of water is 2.452 MJ/L (586 kcal/L) of water evaporated at 20 °C, and humans are capable of sweating up to 10 L of fluid/day. A quick calculation shows that it is theoretically possible to dissipate large quantities of heat/day by this mechanism, provided the relative humidity permits a vapor pressure gradient from the skin to the air. This heat-dissipation process is coordinated by the body's thermoregulatory system. Although the human body is capable of dissipating large quantities of heat, the usual heat burden of a sedentary postabsorptive adult is only 6.276–7.531 MJ/day (1500–1800 kcal/day); this burden can increase dramatically during exercise.

Water is a very broad topic and the subject of numerous reviews. Discussions of water's physiological roles, hormonal aspects regulating fluid volume and acid-base balance, clinical aspects of dehydration and rehydration, fluid homeostasis, and osmotic and renal factors regulating fluid distribution, excretion, and resorption have appeared recently.[1-9] Much of the current interest in fluid physiology focuses on glucose-electrolyte beverages and physical performance, which has engendered a specialized literature. The reader is referred to recent reviews by Coyle and Montain,[10] Gisolfi and Duchman,[11] Puhl and Buskirk,[12] Johnson,[13] and Hawley et al.[14]

The number of publications related to various aspects of fluid homeostasis attests to the considerable body of literature on water, its essential nature, and its many roles. This review will focus on water for maintaining fluid balance and thermoregulation in a variety of environmental extremes (heat, cold, and high altitude), and how these environments influence fluid requirements.

Fluid Homeostasis

By weight, water constitutes ≈60% of the human male body and 50–55% of the female body, which has a higher proportion of fat. The water content of various organs ranges from 83% in blood to only 10% in adipose tissue (Table 1).

Table 1. Water composition of tissues and organs by weight[a]

Tissue	% Water
Blood	83.0
Kidneys	82.7
Heart	79.2
Lungs	79.0
Spleen	75.8
Muscle	75.6
Brain	74.8
Intestine	74.5
Skin	72.0
Liver	68.3
Skeleton (bone)	22.0
Adipose tissue	10.0

[a]Reprinted with permission from Pivarnik and Palmer.[15]

Table 2. Distribution of body water among compartments[a]

Compartment	Male	Female
Body weight (kg)	70	55
Total body water (L)	42	28
Intracellular	26	17
Extracellular	13	9
(interstitial)	(10)	(6.5)
(plasma)	(3)	(2.5)
Transcellular	3	2

[a]Reprinted with permission from Pivarnik and Palmer.[15]

Water is distributed throughout the body but is found primarily in two compartments, one within cells and one between cells (Table 2). The largest pool of water in the body ($\approx 62\%$) is inside cells. Water contained within the erythrocytes is considered part of the intracellular fluid compartment. Extracellular water accounts for $\approx 30\%$ of total body water, and includes fluid located between tissues (interstitial) and in blood plasma ($\approx 7\%$ of total). Roughly three-quarters of extracellular water is contained in the interstitium, a complex gel-like matrix found between tissues throughout the body. Some authors consider a third compartment, a transcellular one, consisting of specialized structures such as joints, eyeballs, and spinal cord. The volume of fluid in this compartment is small ($\approx 10\%$ of total).

Electrolyte Composition of Body Fluids

The vasculature and interstitium are in intimate contact and, as might be expected, plasma and interstitial fluid exhibit similar electrolyte concentrations. Energy-dependent concentration gradients of electrolytes are maintained between interstitial fluid and intracellular fluid: gradients for Na^+ (the major cation of extracellu-lar fluid) and K^+ (the major cation of intracellular fluid) are particularly important to functions like nerve impulse transmission and muscular contraction. Approximately one-third of resting energy expenditure is devoted to ATP-driven pumps to maintain these electrolyte concentration gradients.

While the electrolyte composition may vary between intracellular and extracellular fluid, the distribution of water containing these electrolytes is held relatively constant. The osmolarity of fluid on opposite sides of cellular membranes maintains fluid and electrolyte equilibrium. The osmolarity of body fluid is typically ≈ 290 mosmol/L. Sodium$^+$ and Cl$^-$ are the major contributors to the osmolarity of plasma, while K^+ and Mg^{2+} are key to maintaining intracellular osmolarity. Sweat is hypotonic compared to plasma and tissue. Electrolyte concentrations of plasma, sweat, and muscle cells are given in Table 3.

Avenues of Water Gain and Loss

Typical quantities and sources of daily water output are depicted in Figure 1. Water loss is influenced strongly by activity level and resultant sweat loss. The ambient environment can further influence water loss through sweat, urine, and respiratory routes.

The primary source of daily water intake in humans is fluid consumption. The fluid content of food also contributes greatly to daily water balance, although this fact is probably not universally appreciated. The combined water intake through fluids and foods consumed at meals is the normal route for maintaining fluid balance. Almost 50 years ago, Rothstein et al.[16] first pointed out the importance of eating and drinking at meals to restoring fluid balance. Although it is possible to maintain fluid balance when meals are skipped, it requires a conscious effort to drink fluids at regular intervals,

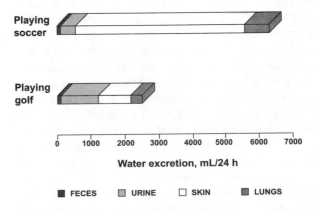

Figure 1. Avenues and approximate magnitudes of fluid loss for light activity in temperate environment versus exercise in a hot humid environment. Modified and used with permission from Katch and McArdle.[1]

Table 3. Electrolyte concentration of plasma, sweat, and muscle[a]

Body fluid	Osmolarity (mosmol/L)	Electrolyte (mEq/L)			
		Na+	Cl-	K+	Mg++
Sweat	80–150	40–60	30–50	3–4	1–5
Plasma	290	140	101	4	1–2
Muscle	290	9	6	162	31

[a]Reprinted with permission from Pivarnik and Palmer.[15]

Table 4. Metabolic water production from the oxidation of carbohydrate, fat, and protein

Substrate and product/mol	g H_2O/g substrate	g H_2O/J substrate (g H_2O/kcal)
Glucose[a] (MW=180) $C_6H_{12}O_6 + 6O_2 \rightarrow 6CO_2 + 6H_2O$	≈0.60	≈35.9(0.15)
Palmitic acid (MW=256) $C_{16}H_{32}O_2 + 23O_2 \rightarrow + 16CO_2 + 16H_2O$	≈1.12	≈31.1(0.13)
Albumin[b,c] (MW=16,954) $C_{720}H_{1134}N_{218}O_{248}S_5 + 723.5O_2 \rightarrow$ $611CO_2 + 5SO_3 + 109CO(NH_2)_2 + 349H_2O$	≈0.37	≈21.5(0.09)

[a]Assumes glucose comes from nonglycogen origin. If glucose oxidized comes from glycogen, an additional 2.7 g H_2O of hydration is liberated per gram glycogen converted to glucose.

[b]The equation for albumin oxidation is based on the molecular structure for crystalline albumin and assumes all nitrogen is converted to urea. The actual production of water from protein oxidation depends upon its molecular structure and the products of metabolism.

[c]McArdle et al.[19] estimated that 15 mL H_2O are required to eliminate 1 g urea through urine. Oh[4] estimated that the oxidation of 1 g of tissue protein results in excretion of 3 g H_2O in urine. Calloway and Spector[20] suggested that ≈50 mL H_2O are required to excrete each gram of urea nitrogen formed. These various rules of thumb suggest that protein oxidation requires 3–8 mL H_2O to excrete urea per gram of protein oxidized, indicating that protein oxidation results in net water loss.

since drinking invariably decreases during busy activities and increases during periods of rest. Activity generally accentuates a gap in fluid balance, whereas leisure reduces it.[16]

The metabolism of energy substrates yields endogenously produced water.[17] The contribution of substrate oxidation to metabolic water production can be examined by considering the theoretical stoichiometry of the reactions involved.[18] Table 4 calculates metabolic water production from typical carbohydrate, fat, and protein substrates. Under similar conditions, the oxidation of 4 mol glucose (≈12.049 MJ [≈2800 kcal]) will produce 24 mol water, while the oxidation of 1 mol of palmitate (≈9.623 MJ [≈2300 kcal]) will produce 16 mol water. Some confusion exists in the literature regarding the amount of water generated from the oxidation of carbohydrate, fat, and protein. In the case of fat, small differences may relate to the source of fat—whether a fatty acid or triacylglycerol (three fatty acids plus glycerol)— or to the chain length and degree of unsaturation of fatty acids. Proteins show a wider range of values for metabolic water production than fats. For example, McArdle et al.[19] list 100 g H_2O/100 g protein, while Janssen[8] and Schmidt-Nielsen[18] report 39 g H_2O/100 g protein. Using albumin as an example of protein oxidation, the equation in Table 4 predicts 37 g H_2O/100 g of albumin; however, the excretion of urea formed during protein oxidation requires water, so there is no net gain of water during protein oxidation.[4,19,20] Lusk[17] gives the following formula for calculating metabolic water production from substrate oxidation:

Grams metabolic water production = 0.41 × g protein oxidized + 0.60 × g CHO oxidized + 1.07 × g fat oxidized.

This formula is in general agreement with the values calculated in Table 4.

When glycogen is the source of carbohydrate oxidized, additional waters of hydration are liberated during the mobilization of glycogen (≈2.7 g H_2O/g glycogen). Furthermore, the immediate production of metabolic water from carbohydrate oxidation depends upon tissue oxygenation. The anaerobic metabolism of 1 mol glucose to lactate generates only 2 mol water, whereas the complete aerobic oxidation of 1 mol glucose provides 6 mol water. This means that less metabolic water will be gen-

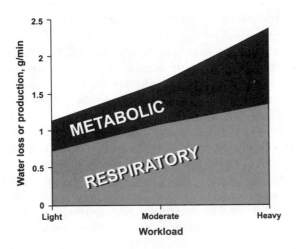

Figure 2. Mean respiratory water loss and metabolic water production for six endurance-trained heat-acclimated male test subjects during 1 hour of treadmill running at three workloads: light, moderate, and heavy (37%, 56%, 74% $\dot{V}O_2$max). Sweat loss was 11.5 g/minute at the light workload and ≈20 g/minute at the higher workloads. Data from Pivarnik et al.[21]

erated during anerobic work at high $\dot{V}O_2$max workloads than during submaximal aerobic $\dot{V}O_2$max efforts.

Although the exact quantity of metabolic water that is produced during exercise depends on a number of variables, it does increase in direct proportion to the workload or amount of substrate oxidized (Figure 2). Pivarnik et al.[21] found that metabolic water production during exercise increased up to 13× the rate of production at rest. However, the contribution of metabolic water was relatively small compared with the total body-water pool. According to Pivarnik et al.,[21] the absolute amount of metabolic water gain would be ≈144 g/hour during exercise at 74% $\dot{V}O_2$max. Assuming an even distribution of water produced in all body fluid compartments, Pivarnik et al.[21] estimated that only 6–10% of the 144 g of metabolic water would be added to the vascular volume, not a sufficient amount to maintain plasma volume during endurance exercise. This amount of water would be of minimal value in replacing water loss through sweating (20.9 g/minute at high work load), but would adequately compensate for respiratory water loss (Figure 2).

Exercise can markedly alter not only the total fluid output, but also the relative contributions of various avenues of water output. Water is lost through the skin from both cutaneous (insensible) and sweat (sensible) losses. Insensible loss is small (≈350 mL/day) compared to potential sweat loss. The amount of water lost from the skin as sweat is proportional to the amount of heat generated (≈30 mL/418.4 kJ [100 kcal] of energy expenditure).[4] Respiratory water losses are usually on the order of ≈13 mL/418.4 kJ (100 kcal) of ex-

penditure. In the absence of fever or hyperventilation, the loss of water via lungs is approximately equal to the amount of water produced by metabolism. Exercise can increase respiratory water loss to 2–5 mL/minute.[21] Respiratory water loss also varies with climate, decreasing in hot, humid weather and rising in cold climates or at high altitudes, where the cold inspired air contains little moisture and the ventilatory rate is faster.[19]

Although feces contain ≈70% water, fecal excretion of water in the absence of diarrhea is relatively small because of the efficient resorption of water from digested matter in the jejunum and colon. Diarrhea or vomiting can increase normal daily water loss from 100 mL/day to 10–50 times that amount.[19]

The most variable and quantitatively most important routes of water loss in humans are the sweat glands and the kidneys. Sweat rates of 1–2 L/hour are common in athletes working at moderate to high rates of energy expenditure[22,23] (Figure 3). The volume of water lost through sweat depends upon several factors, including work load, temperature, relative humidity, hydration status, and degree of prior heat acclimation.[22,23] Total sweat loss is usually 500–700 mL/day, but can be as much as 8–12 L/day.[1] The kidney has the ability to regulate water loss in the urine by increasing the tubular resorption of water (as in exercise or with inadequate water intake). Although water conservation by the kidney is an important homeostatic mechanism, the total quantity of water that can be conserved is relatively small compared to sweat loss during exercise (Figure 4).

Homeostatic Regulation of Body Water

The kidneys (fluid retention) and hypothalamus (fluid intake) are jointly responsible for maintaining body fluid volume homeostasis. Unfortunately the "thirst center" in the brain often seems to be "asleep at the switch," remaining inactive until >2% of the body fluid has been

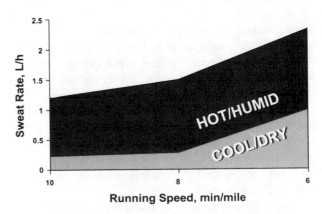

Figure 3. Effect of heat, humidity, and work load on sweat rate. After Sawka and Pandolf.[22]

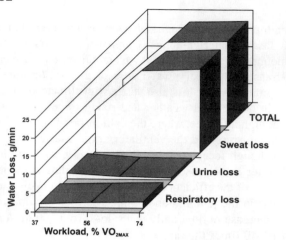

Figure 4. Mean water losses at three workloads for six endurance-trained heat-acclimated male subjects during 1 hour of treadmill running. Ambient temperature was 23.8 °C, relative humidity 74.5%. Adapted from Pivarnik et al.[21]

lost.[24] The kidney responds more rapidly than the hypothalamus to changes in plasma volume. Alterations in extracellular fluid osmolarity and intravascular distensions trigger receptors that stimulate the hypothalamus to release antidiuretic hormone (ADH), which in turn stimulates tubular resorption of water from the glomerular filtrate of kidney. The renin-angiotensin-aldosterone system is simultaneously activated, and this causes aldosterone to be released from the adrenal cortex. Aldosterone increases renal tubular absorption of Na^+ ions, which indirectly stimulates ADH release via the rise in extracellular fluid osmolarity. Eventually the thirst center in the brain responds to decreased blood volume and increased extracellular fluid osmolarity by increasing the thirst drive and thus fluid intake.

Hypohydration

Before the effects of lack of water or hypohydration on physiological function are discussed, some terms used by thermal physiologists should be defined.[22] Euhydration refers to normal body water content. Dehydration and hypohydration are often used interchangeably, but hypohydration (the condition of body water deficit) properly denotes the condition resulting from dehydration (the process of losing body water).[23] Acclimation refers to heat adaptation occurring in response to repeated bouts of heat exposure in an environmental chamber, whereas acclimatization refers to heat adaptation occurring during exposure to heat in a natural environment. For all practical purposes, however, once the body has acclimated or acclimatized, the resulting states are physiologically indistinguishable.

During dehydration, body water is lost from both the intracellular and extracellular fluid compartments. Were

hypohydration simply a temporary loss of body weight with no physiological consequences, merely to be tolerated until the next opportunity to drink, it would be of little concern. Unfortunately, water deficiency leading to hypohydration rapidly results in a number of adverse thermoregulatory and performance decrements (Figure 5).

The impact of hypohydration on exercise performance has been reviewed by Sawka[22,23] and Pandolf.[22] Dehydration leads to reductions in anaerobic capacity, muscular endurance, physical work capacity, and maximal aerobic power. Total body fluid losses of only 1–2%, while of little immediate consequence to a sedentary person in a thermoneutral environment, can reduce the work capacity of an exercising individual who is generating a thermal load. With or without a thermal load, 4% dehydration can result in a serious 20–30% decrement in work capacity.[23] During exercise in the hypohydrated state, skin blood flow and the onset of sweating are delayed and reduced until the body temperature rises, thus contributing to a thermoregulatory disadvantage.[14]

The method used to induce hypohydration can affect the distribution of water between the body fluid spaces.[8] Thermally induced hypohydration results in hyperosmotic plasma from sweat loss. The increased osmolarity of plasma mobilizes fluid from intracellular to extracellular spaces to preserve blood volume. More extracellular water—and therefore plasma water—is lost through diuretic-induced hypohydration than through sweat-induced hypohydration.[22] Exercise- and thermally induced dehydration can cause differences in redistribution of water between fluid compartments,[23] but these differences are not as pronounced as those resulting from diuretic-induced dehydration.

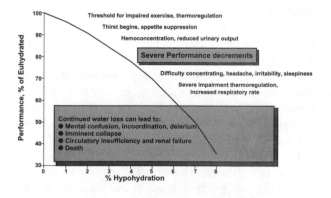

Figure 5. Predicted effects of dehydration on symptomatology and physical performance. This diagram is only semiquantitative, because the onset, severity, and magnitude of the effects depend on the workload, physical fitness level, degree of acclimation, ambient temperature, and relative humidity. Adapted from Frye[6] and Greenleaf.[24]

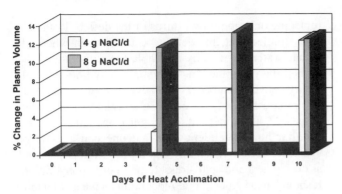

Figure 6. Effect of sodium intake on mean changes in plasma volume of male soldiers during 10 days of heat acclimation (ambient temperature 41°C, 21% relative humidity) while walking on a treadmill for 240 minutes/day. Adapted from Armstrong et al.[26]

Hypovolemia

Except where noted, the following discussion concerns primarily sweat-induced hypovolemia. At low levels of body-water loss, the water deficit occurs mainly in the extracellular space. As water loss increases, a greater proportion of the deficit comes from the intracellular space. During dehydration, water is redistributed from the intracellular and extracellular spaces of muscle and skin to maintain blood volume. The water content of vital organs such as the brain and liver are defended by homeostatic mechanisms at the expense of water in muscle and skin.[22]

The degree to which an individual is acclimated to the heat can alter the magnitude of the hypovolemia associated with hypohydration.[22] This phenomenon is probably related to increased plasma protein and decreased sodium loss that occurs during heat acclimation, even in the face of increased sweat. The net result of heat acclimation is maintenance of a high osmotic gradient in plasma and improved preservation of plasma volume in heat-acclimated, hypohydrated individuals.[22]

A beneficial adaptation to both exercise and heat acclimation is a larger plasma volume, which enables lower heart rates, increases cooling capacity, and provides a more effective buffer against sweat loss. The plasma volume can be expanded acutely in response to exercise or chronically in response to heat acclimation.[25] Sodium plays an important role in the mechanism of plasma volume expansion, perhaps influencing the speed and magnitude of the initial change more than the ultimate value. Armstrong et al.[26,27] studied heat acclimation over a 10-day period with two levels of dietary NaCl (4 g/day and 8 g/day) to determine if heat acclimation could occur at the relatively low dietary intake of 4 g/day. Provided the subjects had adequate fluid consumption to maintain body weight during work

in the heat, similar increases in plasma volume were recorded by 9 days, but the rate of expansion was slower with 4 g/day NaCl than with 8 g/day (Figure 6). In a shorter (3-day) study of cyclists exercising in a thermoneutral environment, Luetkemeier[28] found the magnitude of increase in plasma volume to be directly proportional to dietary sodium intake (Figure 7). Perhaps if Luetkemeier's[28] study had extended to 10 days, the subjects might have had similarly expanded plasma volumes despite different sodium intakes, and the significant correlation between sodium intake and plasma volume might not have been evident.

Sodium is the principal cation of extracellular fluid. As such, sodium helps the body retain water and is intimately related to fluid homeostasis.[29] The gradient established by the Na^+-K^+ pump is maintained at considerable energy cost to the body. The intake of sodium through a normal diet is sufficient to replace sodium lost by sweat and to permit heat acclimation during work in the heat.[25-27] Barr et al[30] could find no significant thermoregulatory or cardiovascular benefit of a saline solution over water during 6 hours of exercise in a thermoneutral environment. Gisolfi and Duchman[11] stated that there is little reason other than palatability to provide sodium in beverages offered to participants in athletic events lasting less than 3 hours.

Fluid Replacement and Exercise

To prevent hypohydration and sustain physical performance, one should begin exercising while in a euhydrated state and drink fluids throughout. Hypohydration increases plasma tonicity by decreasing plasma volume,

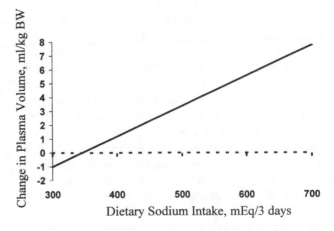

Figure 7. Change in plasma volume in 10 male cyclists who trained for 3 days at 60% $\dot{V}O_2$max for 2 hours/day. Sodium intakes (1 mEq Na^+ = 23 mg Na^+) were estimated from 3-day food records. The prediction equation was $y = 0.022x - 7.62$ and the correlation coeficient was $r = 0.81$. Adapted from Luetkemeier.[28]

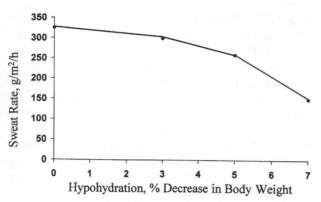

Figure 8. Examples of reduction in sweating rate with increasing levels of hypohydration during exercise in the heat. In these examples, body core temperature increased from 37.4 to 38.1 °C as hypohydration increased. Sweat rate varies at each level of hypohydration depending upon actual core temperature. Adapted from Sawka et al.[31]

which in turn raises the threshold temperature for sweating and skin blood flow.[22] With increasing hypohydration there is a systematic reduction in sweat rate (Figure 8).[31] The relationship between hypohydration and rise in body core temperature during work in the heat has long been appreciated (Figure 9).[32] Barr et al.[30] demonstrated that heart rate and rectal temperature could be maintained within normal ranges during sustained intermittent cycling over a 4-hour period as long as water was consumed to maintain body weight during that time (Figure 10).

Euhydration is especially important to athletes who wish to maintain high levels of work performance. Armstrong et al.[33] found that running velocity in long-distance races was significantly decreased by a pre-exercise 2% body weight hypohydration (Figure 11). The reduction in exercise performance induced by hypohydration is even greater in hot environments than in thermoneutral environments. Sawka et al.[34] found that heat stress alone decreased maximal aerobic power by ≈7% in euhydrated individuals, primarily by shunting blood from core and musculature to skin. A hypohydrated person has a smaller blood volume circulating through peripheral vessels and perfusing contracting skeletal muscles, and this further compromises work output under heat stress. Environmental heat stress and hypohydration act independently to limit cardiac output to the muscle, thereby reducing oxygen delivery during maximal exercise.[22] Dehydration, therefore, negates much of the thermoregulatory advantages gained from prior heat acclimation and aerobic fitness.[22]

Voluntary Dehydration

Pitts et al.[35] reported that during work in the heat, men invariably failed to drink as much water as they lost,

replacing only about two-thirds of the deficit. Rothstein et al.[16] noted that this deficit occurred even when adequate water was readily available for rehydration, and termed the phenomenon "voluntary dehydration." Voluntary dehydration occurs whenever humans experience severe stress,[24] and can occur in cold as well as in hot climates.[36] It is important to recognize and anticipate this peculiar human tendency so that one can encourage "voluntary drinking" before and during exercise, as well as during heat and cold stress, to prevent hypohydration. It should also be noted that older adults have a "blunted" thirst response compared with active young adults, and may need to be especially aware of the need to drink before they are thirsty.[37]

Environmental Influences on Fluid Homeostasis

The ambient environment is a significant impediment to maintaining a fluid balance.[38] Heat, cold, and high altitude all exert strong physiological influences that either increase fluid loss or reduce fluid intake. A hot, dry environment increases sweat loss and fluid requirements, whereas a hot, humid environment increases thermal strain by enhancing fluid loss and reducing evaporative cooling. What is not as apparent is how a cold environment or high altitude can also increase fluid loss. Fluid requirements for work in the cold and at high elevations (which are usually cold in addition to hypoxic) are increased mainly via diuresis and respiratory water loss.[38] Sweating, while a major pathway of water loss during work in a hot environment, may or may not be a significant avenue of fluid loss in the cold, depending on how well clothing and ventilation are managed dur-

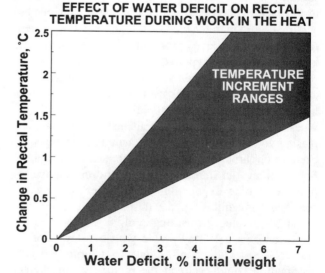

Figure 9. Increments in rectal temperatures at various water deficits in men hiking across rough desert terrain without packs at 4.8–6.4 km/hour for 16–22 kms/day at ambient temperatures of 32–38 °C. Adapted from Rothstein and Towbin.[32]

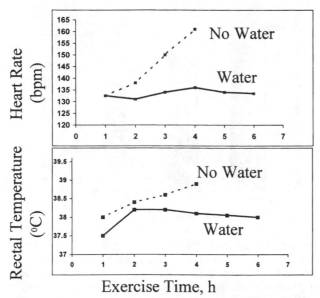

Figure 10. Effect of fluid replacement during exercise at 50% $\dot{V}O_2$max (30 °C ambient temperature, 50% relative humidity) on heart rate and rectal temperature in eight trained cyclists. Subjects drank water every 15 minutes according to weight loss during the same level of exercise in the no-water exercise bout. Exercise was intermittent: 13 minutes exercise, 2 minutes rest for the time period shown. Adapted from Barr et al.[30]

ing periods of work. Freund and Sawka[36] estimated that sweat rates of subjects doing moderate to heavy exercise in the cold and clothed in the equivalent of four CLO can reach 2 L/hour. (One CLO equals the insulation provided by a business suit.) Euhydration in the cold may be compromised by cold-induced diuresis, respiratory water loss, sweating, lack of availability of fluids, and reduced fluid intake.[36]

Although there is some disagreement regarding the mechanism of cold-induced diuresis, displacement of fluid from the skin to the core as a consequence of peripheral vasoconstriction is probably involved. Unlike sweat-induced dehydration, cold-induced diuresis is self-limiting.[36] As fluid loss progresses, diuresis abates, but respiratory water loss does not.

Respiratory water loss is related to both energy expenditure and vapor pressure of water in ambient inspired air. Cold air has a low partial vapor pressure of water. The difference in water vapor pressure between warm saturated air in lung and ambient air determines the amount of respiratory water lost in exhaled air. The relationship between the partial pressure of water vapor in cold inspired and warm expired air is shown in Figure 12. The relationship between ambient temperature and respiratory water loss is shown in Figure 13. Approximately 50% more water is lost during activity at –20°C than during similar activity at +25°C.[36] Total respiratory fluid loss in temperate, cold, and high-altitude environments can range from 200 to 1500 mL/24 hours,

and depends on temperature and humidity of inspired air as well as on ventilatory rate. Energy expenditure has a greater influence on respiratory water loss than ambient temperature, since respiratory rate is proportional to energy expenditure.[36]

Hypohydration not only affects physical performance, but also predisposes to frostbite in the cold because of decreased skin blood flow.[39] In addition, decreased blood flow to the skin impairs the cold-induced vasodilation (CIV) response that permits periodic warming of the extremities under normal conditions. Roberts and Berbrich[40] found that the extremities of a hypohydrated person exposed to the cold were colder than those of a euhydrated person, indicating that dehydration blunted CIV.

Hoyt and Honig[41] reviewed the literature on altitude-induced diuresis and concluded that it is more than just another form of cold diuresis. Baroreceptor response to reduced atmospheric pressure or chemoreceptor response to reduced partial pressure of oxygen in inspired air may be involved in initiating diuresis on rapid ascent to altitude. Bartsch et al.[42] measured high-altitude diuresis and found that it could not be overcome by fluid intake. In fact, subjects who had strong diuresis at altitude remained well, whereas those who became ill with altitude sickness experienced fluid retention. Hoyt and Honig[41] proposed that diuresis may be a physiological response to hypoxemia, with the resulting loss of total body water and decreased plasma volume a beneficial adaptation that led to increased concentration of hemoglobin in blood and improved oxygen delivery to peripheral tissues.[43] Whatever the reason, acute high-altitude diuresis contributes to hypohydration.

Sweating during work at high altitudes can contribute to fluid loss similar to that experienced during work in cold. High-altitude environments usually lack cloud cover and are exposed to direct and reflected sunlight, which can lead to an appreciable heat burden during work

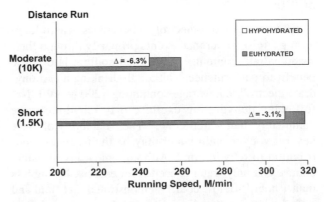

Figure 11. Mean running velocity for short and moderate distances of subjects when euhydrated or hypohydrated by furosemide: ≈2% decrease in body weight and ≈11% decrease in plasma volume. Adapted from Armstrong et al.[33]

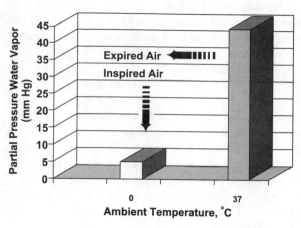

Figure 12. Example of water required to humidify inspired cold air. Cold air holds less water vapor than does warm air. When cold air is inhaled it is saturated with water vapor as it is warmed to body temperature before exhalation. Adapted from Freund and Sawka.[36]

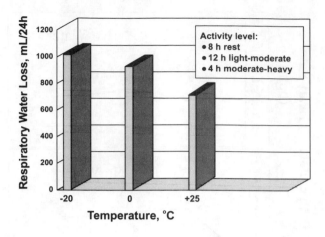

Figure 13. Estimation of respiratory water loss at –20, 0, and +25°C ambient temperatures assuming 24-hour activity levels of 8 hours rest, 12 hours light to moderate activity, and 4 hours of moderate to heavy activity. Adapted from Freund and Sawka.[36]

even at low ambient temperatures. Although work rate at high altitude may be limited by the hypoxic nature of the atmosphere, an immediate adaptation to high-altitude exposure is an increased ventilatory rate to assist in the hypoxic drive to oxygenate the tissues.[44] A faster respiratory rate means that a greater volume of cold dry air is moved through the lungs, which in turn leads to more insensible water loss through the lungs.[45,46] Comparative respiratory water loss at sea level and 4300 m is shown in Figure 14 as a function of energy expenditure. Note that metabolic water production is slightly less than respiratory water loss at sea level and considerably less than respiratory water loss at an elevation of 4300 m. At this altitude, an inappropriate thirst response coupled with a transient diuresis and increased respiratory water loss can result in rapid dehydration if adequate fluid is either unavailable or neglected.[38]

Alternatives to Water: Glucose-Electrolyte Solution

In general, glucose-electrolyte beverages benefit long-term exercise endurance events primarily through their carbohydrate content.[12] Additional sodium is of little benefit to performance,[30] although drinking a carbohydrate-electrolyte beverage containing ≈200 mmol/L Na+ following dehydrating exercise may rehydrate more completely than water alone.[47] The palatability of these beverages over plain water may be their greatest contribution to rehydration.[11] Although most investigators believe that only water is needed for exercise lasting less than 1 hour,[14] Below et al.[48] demonstrated that fluid and carbohydrate ingested simultaneously over a period of high-intensity exercise maintained plasma volume better than equivalent amounts of either fluid or carbohydrate alone. The test subjects were endurance-trained

cyclists working at high rates of energy expenditure for 50 minutes. It is not known whether a similar effect on plasma volume would be evident for lower-intensity work conducted over a similar or longer period or if a combination of carbohydrate and fluid would be more effective than just fluid alone during periods of severe thermal dehydration.

Hyperhydration

It has long been a desire of man to carry a reserve of body water as a hedge against dehydration during periods of intense exercise or heat exposure or in situations where water is not readily available. Unfortunately, overhydration results in rapid excretion of excess water as urine, and euhydration was the best man could hope for—until recently. Research into the ingestion of glycerol solutions as a mechanism to hyperhydrate the body[49–51] has shown some practical potential for preventing or

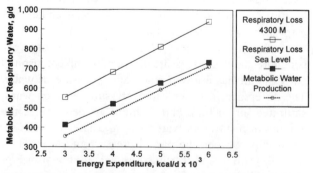

Figure 14. Predicted respiratory water loss and metabolic water production at sea level and at 4300 m elevation as a function of energy expenditure. Predictions based on the regression equations developed by Hoyt and Honig.[42] Sea level respiratory water loss: $y = 0.107x + 92.2$; 4300 m water loss: $y = 0.129x + 166.6$; metabolic water production: $y = 0.0119x - 2.25$.

delaying hypohydration. Glycerol increases the osmolarity of blood and most other body water compartments, which are then temporarily able to retain substantial quantities (1.25–1.75 kg) of fluid, with a corresponding decrease in urine production.[49] Glycerol as a hyperhydrating agent may someday be useful in preparing for ultraendurance events in heat, where sweat loss is great, or in cold or high altitude, where water may be in short supply. Its value during short-term events is doubtful because of the time necessary for glycerol to distribute throughout the body compartments.[47] Although not yet proved experimentally, glycerol ingestion before work in cold may help avoid cold-related injuries by helping prevent hypohydration. It is premature to say how effective glycerol solutions will be in assisting fluid balance in cold, hot, or high-altitude environments, but initial reports are encouraging.[36,47,52]

Summary

Water is a macronutrient that is more critical to the maintenance of life than food. Although humans can live without food for weeks and even months, without water death occurs within days. Water serves as a mechanism to transport nutrients and waste products between body tissues and organs. Moist surfaces in lungs permit diffusion of oxygen and carbon dioxide between inspired air and capillaries in alveoli. Water dissolves waste products in urine and feces and serves as a vehicle for their excretion. Water lubricates and gives structural support to tissues and joints. Water's most important function, however, is in thermoregulation. The body generates a considerable heat burden through metabolism and muscular contraction, and water helps dissipate this load by absorbing large quantities of heat while undergoing only small changes in temperature.

Body heat is continually transferred to the environment as water vaporizes from lung and skin surfaces. For each liter of sweat or respiratory water that the human body vaporizes, it dissipates ≈ 2427 kJ (580 kcal) of heat. An adequate water intake is critical to sustained exercise performance, where large quantities of heat are generated and large quantities of oxygen must be delivered to working muscles. Hypohydration raises body core temperature, makes the cardiovascular system work harder, impairs thermoregulation, and decreases physical performance. Hypohydration compromises thermoregulation in cold as well as in heat. Fluid intake becomes even more important during work in extreme heat, cold, or high altitude, where heat strain, sweating, and respiratory water losses are increased. Environmental factors acting in concert with voluntary or involuntary dehydration can result in severe hypohydration.

Water is much more than just a nutrient: it is the physiological river upon which vital nutrients navigate the pathways of metabolism. Without water, all other nutrients are as parched silt and sand at the bottom of a dry river bed.

Acknowledgment

The author gratefully acknowledges the assistance of Sharon L. Askew in the preparation of this manuscript.

References

1. Katch FI, McArdle WD, eds (1993) Introduction to nutrition, exercise and health, 4th ed. Lea & Febiger, Philadelphia, pp 129–135
2. Berdanier, CD, ed (1995) Advanced nutrition: macronutrients. CRC Press, Boca Raton, FL, pp 19–40
3. Franci CR (1994) Aspects of neural and hormonal control of water and sodium balance. Braz J Med Biol Res 27: 885–903
4. Oh MS (1994) Water, electrolyte, and acid-base balance. In Shils ME, Olson JA, Shike M (eds), Modern nutrition in health and disease, 8th ed. Lea & Febiger, Philadelphia, pp 112–143
5. Wilmore JH, Costill DL, eds (1994) Physiology of sport and exercise. Human Kinetics, Champaign, IL, pp 362–368
6. Frye S (1995) Fluids, hydration, and performance concerns of all recreational athletes. In Jackson CGR (ed), Nutrition for the recreational athlete. CRC Press, Boca Raton, FL, pp 137–152
7. Groff JL, Gropper SS, Hunt SM, eds (1995) Advanced nutrition and human metabolism, 2nd ed. West Publishing, St Paul, MN, pp 423–438
8. Janssen HF (1990) Water. In Brown ML (ed), Present knowledge in nutrition, 6th ed. ILSI Press, Washington, DC, pp 88–95
9. Vokes T (1987) Water homeostasis. Annu Rev Nutr 7:383–406
10. Coyle EF, Montain SJ (1992) Benefits of fluid replacement with carbohydrate during exercise. Med Sci Sports Exerc 24:S324–S330
11. Gisolfi CV, Duchman SM (1992) Guidelines for optimal replacement beverages for different athletic events. Med Sci Sports Exerc 24:679–687
12. Puhl SM, Buskirk ER (1994) Nutrient beverages for exercise and sport. In Wolinsly I, Hickson JF (eds), Nutrition in exercise and sport. CRC Press, Boca Raton, FL, pp 263–294
13. Johnson HL (1995) The requirements for fluid replacement during heavy sweating and the benefits of carbohydrates and minerals. In Kies CV, Driskell JA (eds), Sports nutrition. Minerals and electrolytes. CRC Press, Boca Raton, FL, pp 215–233
14. Hawley JA, Dennis SC, Noakes TD (1995) Carbohydrate, fluid, and electrolyte requirements during prolonged exercise. In Kies CV, Driskell JA (eds), Sports nutrition. Minerals and electrolytes. CRC Press, Boca Raton, FL, pp 235–265
15. Pivarnik JM, Palmer RA (1994) Water and electrolyte balance during rest and exercise. In Wolinsly I, Hickson JF (eds), Nutrition in exercise and sport. CRC Press, Boca Raton, FL, pp 245–262
16. Rothstein A, Adolph EF, Wills JH (1947) Voluntary dehydration. In Adolph EF et al (eds), Physiology of man in the desert. Interscience, New York, pp 254–270
17. Lusk G (1928) The elements of the science of nutrition, 4th ed. Academic Press, New York. Reprinted in 1976 by Johnson Reprint Corp, New York

18. Schmidt-Nielsen K (1979) Animal physiology: adaptation and the environment, 2nd ed. Cambridge University Press, New York, pp 314–336

19. McArdle WD, Katch FI, Katch VL, eds (1991) Exercise physiology. Energy, nutrition and human performance, 3rd ed. Lea & Febiger, Philadelphia, pp 60–64, 151, 551

20. Calloway DH, Spector H (1954) Nitrogen balance as related to caloric and protein intake in active young men. Am J Clin Nutr 2:405–412

21. Pivarnik JM, Leeds EM, Wilkerson JE (1984) Effects of endurance exercise on metabolic water production and plasma volume. J Appl Physiol 56:613–618

22. Sawka MN, Pandolf KB (1990) Effects of body water loss on physiological function and exercise performance. In Gisolfi CV, Lamb DR (eds), Perspectives in exercise science and sports medicine. Volume 3, Fluid homeostasis during exercise. Benchmark Press, Carmel, IN, pp 1–38

23. Sawka MN (1992) Physiological consequences of hypohydration: exercise performance and thermoregulation. Med Sci Sports Exerc 24:657–670

24. Greenleaf JE (1992) Problem: thirst, drinking behavior, and involuntary dehydration. Med Sci Sports Exerc 24:645–656

25. Wenger CB (1987) Human heat acclimation. In Pandolf KB, Sawka MN, Gonzalez RR (eds), Human performance physiology and environmental medicine at terrestrial extremes. Cooper Publishing, Carmel, IN, pp 153–197

26. Armstrong LE, Hubbard RW, Askew EW, Francesconi RP (1993) Responses of soldiers to 4-gram and 8-gram NaCl diets during 10 days of heat acclimation. In Marriott BM (ed), Nutritional needs in hot environments. National Academy Press, Washington, DC, pp 247–228

27. Armstrong LE, Hubbard RW, Askew EW, et al (1993) Responses to moderate and low sodium diets during exercise-heat acclimation. Int J Sports Nutr 3:207–221

28. Luetkemeier MJ (1995) Dietary sodium intake and changes in plasma volume during short-term exercise training. Int J Sports Med 16:435–438

29. Hubbard RW, Szlyk PC, Armstrong LE (1990) Influence of thirst and fluid palatability on fluid ingestion during exercise. In Gisolfi CV, Lamb DR (eds), Perspectives in exercise science and sports medicine. Volume 3, Fluid homeostasis during exercise. Benchmark Press, Carmel, IN, pp 39–95

30. Barr SI, Costill DL, Fink WJ (1991) Fluid replacement during prolonged exercise: effects of water, saline, or no fluid. Med Sci Sports Exerc 23:811–817

31. Sawka MN, Young AJ, Francesconi RP, et al (1985) Thermoregulatory and blood responses during exercise at graded hypohydration levels. J Appl Physiol 59:1394–1401

32. Rothstein A, Towbin EJ (1947) Blood circulation and temperature of men dehydrating in the heat. In Adolph EF et al (eds), Physiology of man in the desert. Interscience, New York, pp 172–196

33. Armstrong LE, Costill DE, Fink WJ (1985) Influence of diuretic-induced dehydration on competitive running performance. Med Sci Sports Exerc 9:159–163

34. Sawka MN, Young AJ, Cadarette BS, et al (1985) Influence of heat stress and acclimation on maximal aerobic power. Eur J Appl Physiol 53:294–298

35. Pitts GC, Johnson RE, Consolazio FC (1944) Work in the heat as affected by intake of water, salt and glucose. Am J Physiol 142:253–259

36. Freund BJ, Sawka MN (1996) Influence of cold stress on human fluid balance. In Marriott B (ed), Nutrient requirements for work in cold and high altitude environments. National Academy Press, Washington, DC, in press

37. Chernoff R (1994) Nutritional requirements and physiological changes in aging: thirst and fluid requirements. Nutr Rev 52:S3–S5

38. Askew EW (1994) Nutrition and performance at environmental extremes. In Wolinsly I, Hickson JF (eds), Nutrition in exercise and sport. CRC Press, Boca Raton, FL, pp 455–474

39. Gamble WB (1994) Perspectives in frostbite and cold weather injuries. Adv Plast Surg 10:21–71

40. Roberts DE, Berberich JJ (1988) The role of hydration on peripheral response to cold. Mil Med 12:605–608

41. Hoyt RW, Honig A (1996) Environmental influences on body fluid balance during exercise: altitude. In Buskirk ER, Puhl SM (eds), Body fluid balance in exercise and sport. CRC Press, Boca Raton, FL, in press

42. Bartsch P (1991) Effects of slow ascent to 4559 m on fluid homeostasis. Aviat Space Environ Med 62:105–110

43. Hoyt RW, Honig A (1996) Body fluid and energy metabolism at high altitude. In Blatteis CM, Fregley MJ (eds), Handbook of physiology: adaptation to the environment. Oxford University Press, New York, 1277-1289

44. Schoene RB (1988) Ventilatory adaptation to extreme hypoxia. In Sutton JR, Houston CS, Coates G (eds), Hypoxia, the tolerable limits. Benchmark Press, Carmel, IN, pp 153–159

45. Ferrus L, Commenges D, Gire G, Varene P (1984) Respiratory water loss as a function of ventilatory or environmental factors. Respir Physiol 56:11–20

46. Millege J (1992) Respiratory waterloss at altitude. Newsletter Int Soc Mount Med 2:5

47. Murray RH (1995) Fluid needs in hot and cold environments. Int J Sports Nutr 5:S62–S73

48. Below PR, Mora-Rodriguez R, Gonzalez-Alonso J, Coyle EF (1995) Fluid and carbohydrate ingestion independently improve performance during 1 h of intense exercise. Med Sci Sports Exerc 27:200–210

49. Lyons TP, Riedesel ML, Meuli LE, Chick TW (1990) Effects of glycerol-induced hyperhydration prior to exercise in the heat on sweating and core temperatures. Med Sci Sports Exerc 22:447–483

50. Murray R, Eddy DE, Paul GL, et al (1991) Physiological responses to glycerol ingestion during exercise. J Appl Physiol 71:144–149

51. Freund BJ, McKay JM, Roberts DE, et al (1994) Glycerol hyperhydration reduces the diuresis induced by water alone during cold air exposure. Med Sci Sports Exer 26:S5

52. Askew EW (1993) Hydration for top physical performance. Olympic Coach 3:12–13

Chapter 11

Vitamin A

James Allen Olson

Night blindness and some eye disorders, which were well recognized in ancient Egypt, were treated by the topical application of juice squeezed from cooked liver or by prescribing liver in the diet. This medical lore was lost over the centuries, and night blindness, called "this curious and obscure disease" by R.J. Hicks, a surgeon serving with the Confederate army in the American Civil War, plagued armies throughout the world in the nineteenth century.[1] The active principle of liver in treating eye disease was vitamin A, which was identified as a necessary fat-soluble factor for rat growth in 1914 and was structurally elucidated in 1930. The biological conversion of β-carotene to vitamin A was shown the same year. These early studies on vitamin A are well reviewed in Moore's fine treatise.[2]

Chemistry and Nomenclature

The parent compound in the vitamin A group is called all-*trans* retinol (Figure 1A).[3] Its aldehyde and acid forms are retinal (Figure 1B) and retinoic acid (Figure 1C). The active form of vitamin A in vision is 11-*cis* retinal (Figure 1D), and a therapeutically useful form (Accutane, isotretinoin) is 13-*cis* retinoic acid (Figure 1E). Retinyl palmitate (Figure 1F) is a major storage form, and retinoyl β-glucuronide is a biologically active, water-soluble metabolite (Figure 1G). A synthetic aromatic analog (etretin), which has therapeutic usefulness, is depicted in Figure 1H. Finally, β-carotene, a major provitamin A carotenoid, is shown in Figure 1I.

In a nutritional sense the vitamin A family includes all naturally occurring compounds with the biological activity of retinol. Because provitamin A carotenoids are nutritionally active, they are included in the vitamin A family. Only 50 of ≈600 carotenoids found in nature are converted to vitamin A, but most carotenoids, including those with provitamin A activity, also can serve as singlet oxygen quenchers and as antioxidants under certain conditions. These characteristics are not possessed by retinol. (Symposia that deal with various aspects of carotenoids in health and disease have recently been published.[4,5]) Thus, in considering the biological actions of carotenoids, it is important to differentiate between provitamin A activity and other possible effects.

Methods of Analysis

Because of its conjugated system of double bonds, vitamin A absorbs blue light very well. The maximal absorption wavelengths and molecular extinction coefficients (ε) in ethanol are, respectively, 325 nm and 52,480 for all-*trans* retinol, 381 nm and 43,400 for all-*trans* retinal, and 350 nm and 45,200 for all-*trans* retinoic acid.[6] *Cis* isomers absorb less strongly at somewhat lower wavelengths. Carotenoids tend to show triple maxima, e.g., all-*trans* β-carotene shows maximal absorption in ethanol at 453 nm (ε = 140,700) with a shoulder at 427 nm and a secondary peak at 477 nm.[7] These spectroscopic properties primarily are used in quantitating vitamin A and carotenoids in tissues and in pharmaceutical preparations. Although many chromatographic systems are available for separating vitamin A and carotenoids, the most commonly used procedure is high-pressure liquid chromatography (HPLC). Straight-phase, reverse-phase, isocratic, and gradient HPLC systems are used for specific needs.[6,7]

The analysis of vitamin A and carotenoids in serum can be conducted without extraction with organic solvents,[8] although most procedures for serum, other body fluids, and tissues involve extraction techniques.[6] With the increasing use of deuterated and ^{13}C-labeled vitamin A and carotenoids in human studies, both conventional and isotope-ratio mass spectrometry techniques have been developed.[9,10]

In the assessment of vitamin A status in humans, a variety of biochemical, physiological, histological, and clinical methods are used.[11]

Absorption, Transport, and Storage

Preformed vitamin A in foods is present largely as retinyl ester. During proteolytic digestion in the stomach, retinyl ester and provitamin A carotenoids are released from foods and aggregate together with other lipids. In the small intestine, because of the combined action

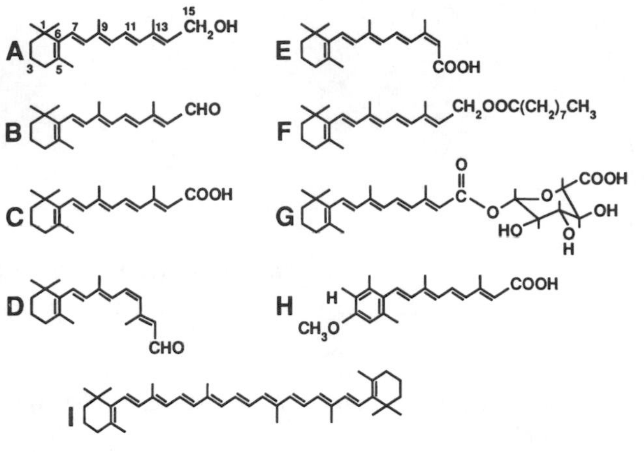

Figure 1. Formulas of major retinoids and of β-carotene. A, all-*trans* retinol; B, all-*trans* retinal; C, all-*trans* retinoic acid; D, 11-*cis* retinal; E, 13-*cis* retinoic acid; F, all-*trans* retinyl palmitate; G, all-*trans* retinoyl β-glucuronide; H, the trimethyl methoxyphenol analog of all-*trans* retinoic acid (etretin, acitretin); I, all-*trans* β-carotene.

of bile and pancreatic esterases, esters of retinol and carotenols (xanthopylls) are hydrolyzed. Together with hydrocarbon carotenoids, retinol and carotenols are transported in micellar form across the plasmalemma of the absorptive epithelial cells of the intestinal villus.[12]

The absorption efficiency of dietary vitamin A in healthy people who ingest significant amounts of fat (>10 g/day) is >80%. Dietary carotenoids (in the range of 1–3 mg) are absorbed approximately half as well as vitamin A. As the amount of carotenoids in the diet increases, however, the absorption efficiency decreases.[13] The intestinal absorption of carotenoids is much more critically dependent on the presence of bile salts than is that of vitamin A.[14]

A major pathway for the conversion of all-*trans* β-carotene and other provitamin A carotenoids to vitamin A by animals, including humans, is by oxidative cleavage of the central 15,15′ double bond.[15] Beta-carotene can also be cleaved eccentrically to yield β-apocarotenals, one of which can be further degraded to retinal.[16] The central cleavage enzyme also slowly converts 9-*cis* β-carotene to a mixture of 9-*cis* and all-*trans* retinals.[17,18]

Within the intestinal epithelia the retinal produced by carotenoid cleavage is bound to a cellular retinoid-binding protein, CRBP Type II.[19] Bound retinal is then reduced to bound retinol, which is esterified primarily by transacylation from the a-position of lecithin[19] but also from acyl-coenzyme A.[20] The resultant retinyl ester, together with a small amount of unesterified retinol, hydrocarbon carotenoids, and xanthophylls, is incorporated into chylomicra that are released into the lymph. The triacylglycerols of chylomicra are hydrolyzed rapidly by plasma lipoprotein lipase, leaving chylomicron remnants with associated carotenoids and vitamin A. These remnants

are taken up mainly by parenchymal cells of the liver and to some degree by other tissues.[21]

In the fasting state both vitamin A and carotenoids circulate in the plasma. The major form of circulating vitamin A is holo-retinol-binding protein (holo-RBP), which consists of a 1:1 complex of all-*trans* retinol with RBP (molecular weight 21,000). The plasma concentration of holo-RBP, which is synthesized and released from parenchymal cells, is homeostatically controlled by mechanisms that are not well defined. Only when liver reserves of vitamin A are nearly depleted do plasma concentrations of retinol decrease significantly. Other endogenous compounds of vitamin A that circulate in the plasma, albeit at much lower concentrations, are retinyl ester, retinoic acid, retinyl β-glucuronide, and retinoyl β-glucuronide.[20] Little is known about the regulation of these compounds in plasma or about their modes of uptake by cells.

Major plasma carotenoids include zeaxanthin, lutein, lycopene, cryptoxanthin, α-carotene, and β-carotene as well as traces of many other species.[14] The hydrocarbon carotenoids are associated primarily with low-density lipoproteins (LDLs), whereas the xanthophylls are distributed more evenly among LDLs and high-density lipoproteins (HDLs). Beta-carotene usually composes 15–30% of total plasma carotenoids. Unlike the plasma concentration of holo-RBP, both the total carotenoid concentration in plasma and the relative amounts of individual components are dependent on the ingested diet.

Vitamin A is very well stored in the body, with >90% of the total being found in the liver of well-nourished individuals. Two major cell types are involved in storage: the parenchymal cells and the stellate cells. The parenchymal cells, which are the predominant cell type of liver, contain very small amounts of retinol and significant amounts of retinyl ester. These cells take up and process chylomicron remnants as well as synthesize and release plasma RBP.[21] Stellate cells, also termed fat-storing cells, lipocytes, and Ito cells, are distinct, relatively small, nonphagocytic cells of the liver that line the Space of Disse. Stellate cells compose 5–15% of total liver cells. In well-nourished humans and animals, >80% of the total vitamin A of the liver is stored in special vitamin A–containing globules in these cells. Ingested vitamin A is transferred from parenchymal cells to stellate cells in the form of retinol, is reesterified, and is stored there. When used, retinyl ester is hydrolyzed to retinol, which is bound to RBP and is released into the plasma. The nature of the interaction between stellate cells and parenchymal cells in this process is still unclear.[21] Stellate cells are also involved in retinyl ester storage in many tissues other than liver. In a vitamin A–depleted state, the relative amounts of vitamin A in the kidney and in most epithelial tissues increase in relation to that in the liver.

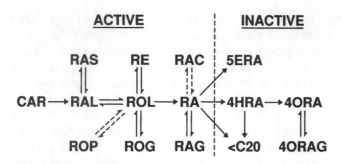

Figure 2. Major metabolic transformations of vitamin A. CAR, provitamin A carotenoids; RAL, retinal; RAS, Schiff base of retinal; ROL, retinol; RE, retinyl ester; ROP, retinyl phosphate; ROG, retinyl β-glucuronide; RA, retinoic acid, RAC, retinoyl coenzyme A; RAG, retinoyl β-glucuronide; 4HRA, 4-hydroxyretinoic acid; 5ERA, 5,6-epoxyretinoic acid; 4ORA, 4-oxoretinoic acid; 4ORAG, 4-oxoretinoyl β-glucuronide; <C20, oxidized metabolites with fewer than 20 carbon atoms. Single arrows denote irreversible reactions; double arrows, interconvertible compounds; dotted arrows, minor or not fully established in vivo reactions.

Metabolism

Vitamin A, although extensively stored in the liver and depleted from its reserves at the relatively low net rate of 0.5%/day,[22,23] is nonetheless in a highly dynamic state within the body. The half-life value for holo-RBP bound to transthyretin in human plasma ≈11 h,[24] and administered vitamin A equilibrates with total body reserves largely within 2 weeks. Retinol recycles rapidly between liver and peripheral tissues.[25] Holo-RBP synthesized in peripheral tissues may well be the major transporter in recycling,[26] although lipoprotein-bound retinyl esters may also perform this role.

Retinoid β-glucuronides, which are released as endogenous components of bile, are reabsorbed from the intestine and also recirculated back to the liver.[21] The leakage of holo-RBP into the urine during the passage of blood through the kidney is extremely small under normal conditions[24] but can become a major route for the loss of vitamin A during severe infections accompanied by fever.[27] Thus a variety of conservation mechanisms exist to minimize the loss of vitamin A from the body. These mechanisms may well have developed to foster survival during evolution because of the crucial functional roles that vitamin A plays in mammalian physiology.

Vitamin A undergoes many enzymatic transformations in mammals.[21] As already indicated, retinyl esters in food are hydrolyzed to retinol by pancreatic esterase in the intestinal lumen, and provitamin A carotenoids are oxidatively cleaved to retinal in the intestinal mucosa as well as in other tissues. Retinal is reversibly reduced to retinol and irreversibly converted to retinoic acid in many tissues. Retinol also is conjugated in several ways; namely, to form retinyl esters by transacylation both from phospholipid and from acyl-coenzyme A and to form retinyl β-glucuronide by interaction with UDP-glucuronic acid. CRBP II plays an important role as a co-ligand in several of these enzymatic reactions in the intestinal mucosa, and CRBP seems to play a similar role in other tissues.[19] Retinal can form Schiff bases with the ε-amino group of lysine in proteins, the most specific and functionally important interaction being between 11-*cis* retinal and opsin in the eye.[28]

Retinoic acid can form retinoyl β-glucuronide by reaction with UDP-glucuronic acid[21] and probably retinoyl coenzyme A via a conventional ATP and coenzyme A activation reaction.[29] Both retinoyl β-glucuronide and retinoyl coenzyme A might transfer the retinoyl moiety to form esters with hydroxyl, amino, and sulfhydryl groups. Conjugated forms of vitamin A, of course, can also be hydrolyzed back to the parent compounds.

Some, if not all, of the biological activity of vitamin A is retained during the above transformations. In contrast, vitamin A is generally inactivated by hydroxylation, epoxidation, dehydration, and oxidative carbon–carbon bond cleavage. Some tumor cells enzymatically dehydrate vitamin A to the inactive product retroanhydroretinol. Although most retro forms of the conjugated double-bond system are inactive, α-14 hydroxyretroretinol strongly stimulates the growth of B lymphoblastoid cells.[30] 3,4-Didehydroretinol, which occurs naturally in freshwater fish, also shows significant biological activity in growth and cellular differentiation. Major metabolic transformations are summarized in Figure 2.

In addition, both biological and chemical isomerization of carotenoids and vitamin A occur. A functionally significant biological isomerization reaction is the conversion of all-*trans* to 11-*cis* retinol in the eye.[31] Interestingly, the enzyme catalyzing this reaction is an isomerohydrolase, in that all-*trans* retinyl palmitate in the pigment epithelium is directly converted to 11-*cis* retinol and palmitic acid. Another important isomerization reaction is the formation of 9-*cis* retinoic acid. All-*trans* retinoic acid can be isomerized to the 9-*cis* isomer chemically and possibly biologically in cells.[31] In addition, as already mentioned, 9-*cis* β-carotene, a common constituent of foods, can be cleaved to yield all-*trans* and 9-*cis* retinals, which then can be oxidized to their respective retinoic acids.[17,18] All-*trans* and 13-*cis* forms of vitamin A are also readily interconvertible.[17] The 13-*cis* isomer is generally much less active than the all-*trans* and 9-*cis* forms in nature.

Retinol, retinal, and retinoic acid are primarily bound to specific retinoid-binding proteins within the plasma, intercellular spaces, and cells.[19,26,32] Retinol is bound in plasma by RBP and in cells by the cellular binding proteins CRBP and CRBP Type II (in the intestine). The retinoid is bound in a β-barrel within the center of the protein and has limited access to the external fluid.[19,32]

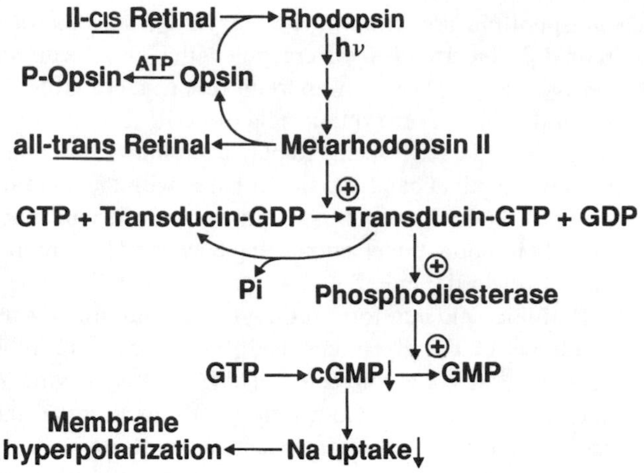

11-cis Retinal ⟶ Rhodopsin
P-Opsin ⟵ATP⟵ Opsin ↓hν
all-trans Retinal ⟵ Metarhodopsin II
GTP + Transducin-GDP ⟶ Transducin-GTP + GDP ⊕
Pi   Phosphodiesterase ⊕
GTP ⟶ cGMP↓ ⟶ GMP ⊕
Membrane hyperpolarization ⟵ Na uptake↓

Figure 3. Visual pathway for transducing light energy into an enhanced membrane potential in the rod outer segment. + denotes stimulated reactions or enzymes.

Retinal is bound in the eye by cellular retinal-binding protein (CRALBP). Retinoic acid is bound by cellular retinoic acid–binding protein (CRABP) in many tissues and in some tissues of the newborn by CRABP Type II. In the interphotoreceptor space of the eye, retinol is bound by an interphotoreceptor (interstitial)-binding protein (IRBP). The three-dimensional structure and ligand-binding site of several of these retinoid-binding proteins have been determined,[32] and nearly all have been cloned and sequenced. Several other retinoid-binding proteins have been partially characterized from specific tissues and selected species. The retinoid-binding proteins are involved in the transport of vitamin A in the body, the biological transformation of vitamin A, its protection from oxidation and nonspecific enzymatic reactions, and the protection of membranes and other lipid structures of cells from the amphophilic surface-active properties of vitamin A.

Functions

The best defined function of vitamin A is in vision. The pathway for the delivery of vitamin A to the eye involves the following steps: 1) interaction of plasma holo-RBP with specific cell-surface receptors on retinal pigment epithelial cells, 2) uptake of retinol by retinal pigment epithelial cells and its enzymatic isomerization to 11-cis retinol, 3) transport by IRBP to the rod outer segment, 4) enzymatic oxidation of the 11-cis retinol to 11-cis retinal, and 5) nonenzymatic association of the latter with a specific lysine group in the membrane-bound protein opsin.[28] The 11-cis retinal in the resultant rhodopsin, when exposed to light, isomerizes to a transoid intermediate, which in turn triggers a series of conformational changes in the protein. An intermediate form, metarhodopsin II, interacts with a complex G protein,

termed transducin, which causes the α unit of the latter to replace bound GDP with GTP.[28] The GTP-α unit complex of transducin activates phosphodiesterase, which in turn hydrolyzes cGMP to GMP. cGMP is involved in keeping the sodium channels of the rod outer segment open. As cGMP decreases, sodium ion entry decreases, thereby hyperpolarizing the rod cell membrane. The change in membrane potential is transmitted through a complex set of synapses to the brain, where the pulses received at a given time are integrated. Events occurring in the rod outer segment are summarized in Figure 3. A similar metabolic sequence seems to occur in the color-sensing cone cells of the retina.

Activated processes of temporal importance must be returned to the basal state. In the visual cascade, metarhodopsin II is converted through other conformational states to opsin and all-trans retinal, neither of which activates transducin. Phosphorylation of opsin also prevents its activation of transducin. Transducin possesses a GTPase activity that converts the active GTP complex to an inactive GDP-binding form. Subsequent activated processes return as well to their basal states. All-trans retinal is reduced, transported to the pigment epithelial cells, and stored as retinyl ester.

A second major function of vitamin A is in cell differentiation. The recent discovery of two sets of retinoic acid receptors, the RAR and RXR, has clarified in large part the molecular action of vitamin A in this process.[33] Each set has three distinct subgroups: α, β, and γ. Each receptor has six domains: an amino-terminal activation domain (A/B), a highly conserved DNA-binding domain (C), a hinge region (D), a ligand-binding domain (E), and a carboxy-terminal tail that is involved in heterodimerization. The RAR receptors bind either all-trans or 9-cis retinoic acid, whereas the RXR set binds only 9-cis retinoic acid. The RXR receptors form heterodimers with themselves as well as with RAR, the vitamin D receptor, and the triiodothyronine receptor. These interactions usually activate gene expression. RAR can also be inhibitory. For example, it interacts with Jun in a nonproductive complex. Jun normally forms a heterodimer with Fos, which binds at the AP-1 site and stimulates cell proliferation.[33] In the absence of the Jun-Fos heterodimer, the AP-1 site is not activated. Thus retinoic acid isomers, in conjunction with their nuclear receptors, can both stimulate and inhibit gene expression.

A variety of synthetic analogs of retinoic acid show specificity of binding towards individual retinoic acid receptors. By their use, as well as by "knock-out" studies with transgenic mice, the functions of specific nuclear receptors and of other retinoid binding proteins are being clarified.[33] The actions of retinoic acid in cell differentiation are summarized in Figure 4.

Another way in which retinoic acid may affect cell differentiation is by the formation of retinoylated pro-

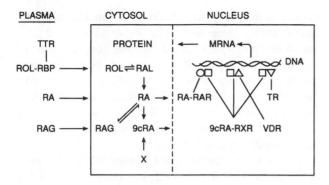

Figure 4. Roles of retinoids in the differentiation of target cells. All retinoids are considered to be all-*trans* isomers unless otherwise specified. ROL, retinol; RAL, retinal; RA, retinoic acid; 9cRA, 9-*cis* retinoic acid; RAG, retinoyl β-glucuronide; RBP, plasma retinol-binding protein; TTR, transthyretin; RAR, retinoic acid receptor; RXR, retinoic acid receptor that specifically binds 9cRA; VDR, vitamin D receptor; TR, thyroxine receptor; DNA, deoxyribonucleic acid; MRNA, messenger ribonucleic acid; X, other precursors including 9-*cis* β-carotene, of 9cRA; O□, □△, and □▽, heterodimers of various nuclear receptors. From reference 39.

teins. Retinoylated proteins that are the same size as nuclear receptors have been identified in the nuclei of several differentiated cells.[34] Because acylation of certain proteins with selected fatty cells or polyisoprenoids markedly affects their function, the possibility that retinoic acid may play a role in such processes is attractive. Although retinoyl β-glucuronide might serve well as a retinoyl group donor, the enzymatic steps involved have not yet been defined.

Retinol and retinoic acid are also essential for embryonic development.[35] Retinoic acid has been implicated in the expression of hox genes, which determine the sequential development of various parts of an organism. The study of these exciting relationships, however, is still in its infancy.

In addition to vision, cell differentiation, and embryonic development, vitamin A has been implicated in many other physiological processes, including spermatogenesis, immune response, taste, hearing, appetite, and growth. Most of these processes depend directly or indirectly on cellular differentiation.

Deficiency

Vitamin A deficiency is a major public health problem in many areas of the less-industrialized world. It was estimated that 500,000 preschool-age children become blind each year because of vitamin A deficiency.[36] Most blind children do not survive. Common clinical signs of vitamin A deficiency are night blindness and xerophthalmia. The most diagnostic clinical signs of vitamin A deficiency in young children are Bitot's spots, which

are foamy white accumulations of sloughed cells that usually appear on the temporal quadrant of the conjunctiva. Bitot's spots are a gross manifestation of the squamous metaplasia of the conjunctival epithelia, in which keratinized cells replace goblet cells and normal epithelial cells. Low concentrations (<0.35 mmol/L) of serum retinol also are closely associated with clinical signs of deficiency.[11]

In addition to clinical deficiency, more than 100 million children suffer from vitamin A inadequacy in the absence of clinical signs of acute deficiency.[36] These children generally show a higher mortality rate and a higher incidence of severe infections than do vitamin A–sufficient children.[37] With the current reduction of severe vitamin A deficiency in much of the world, inadequate vitamin A status and its consequences have become the major focus of public health programs worldwide. An inadequate vitamin A status is commonly associated with protein-calorie malnutrition, a low intake of fat, lipid malabsorption syndromes, and febrile diseases. Among adults, lactating women are most at risk.

Inadequate vitamin A status, which is also termed marginal status or preclinical deficiency, can be measured by several relatively new procedures: the relative-dose-response test, the modified relative-dose-response test, frequency analysis of serum retinol concentrations before and after supplementation, conjunctival impression cytology, and vision restoration time. Of biochemical indicators, the modified relative dose response test is proving to be a highly reliable procedure as performed by different laboratories in many different countries. Isotope dilution methods, which measure total body reserves of vitamin A, currently are being refined.[38] The utility of various indicators[39] for total body reserves of vitamin A is shown in Figure 5.

Requirements and Recommended Intakes

The average daily amount of vitamin A that should be ingested by healthy individuals varies with age, body mass, metabolic activity, and special conditions, e.g., pregnancy and lactation. The operational endpoint also must be defined; namely, whether the objective is just to prevent deficiency or to provide as well for a suitable body reserve. The heterogeneity of the population must be considered if the recommended intake is intended to meet the needs of a specified portion of the population. In general, recommended dietary intakes for population groups have tended to decrease as more information has become available.

Vitamin A status can be classified in five categories: deficient, marginal, satisfactory, excessive, and toxic. The deficient and marginal states were discussed earlier. The satisfactory state implies the absence of clinical signs, full physiological functions that are dependent either

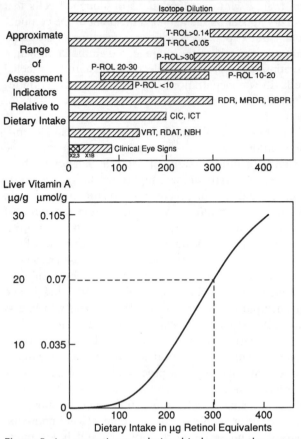

Figure 5. An approximate relationship between the average daily dietary intake of vitamin A and provitamin A carotenoids and the vitamin A concentration in the liver of a preschool child. Nonhepatic stores of vitamin A are ≈10% of the liver reserves when total body stores are high (>30 mg for a 15-kg child) but are proportionally greater (20–50%) when body reserves are low (<6 mg for a 15-kg child). A satisfactory liver vitamin A concentration is considered to be 0.07 mmol (20 μg)/g wet weight. The approximate ranges for the responses of various indicators of vitamin A status, relative to dietary intake, are given above the figure. Thus, clinical signs appear when the average daily intake of vitamin A is very low, which corresponds to negligible liver reserves. Plasma retinol concentrations <0.35 μmol/L (<10 μg/dL) are usually associated with other signs of vitamin A inadequacy, whereas a plasma retinol concentration in the range 0.35–0.70 μmol/L (10–20 μg/dL) may either be associated with Bitot's spots and other signs of deficiency or be found in a vitamin A–sufficient child, albeit often plagued with infections. Isotope dilution, which involves analysis of the dilution in the plasma of endogenous vitamin A by a dose of deuterated vitamin A, provides information about total body reserves. X2, corneal xerosis; X3, corneal ulceration and keratomalacia; X1B, Bitot's spots with conjunctival xerosis; VRT, vision restoration time; RDAT, rapid dark-adaptation test time; NBH, night blindness by history; CIC, conjunctival impression cytology test; ICT, impression cytology with transfer test; RDR, relative-dose-response test; MRDR, modified relative-dose-response test; RBPR, retinol-binding protein response test; P-ROL, plasma (or serum) retinol concentration; and T-ROL, tear fluid retinol concentration, followed by values expressed in μg retinol/dL. 1 μmol retinol = 286 μg retinol; 1 μg retinol = 1 μg retinol equivalents = 0.0035 μmol retinol. From reference 11, with permission of the ILSI Press.

directly or indirectly on vitamin A, and an adequate total body reserve to meet stresses of various kinds and periods of low dietary intake. Mean total body contents of vitamin A that fulfill all functions of the vitamin and provide a 3-month reserve on a low vitamin A intake for a 76-kg male and for a 62-kg female are 0.18 mmol and 0.14 mmol, respectively. These values are derived from a satisfactory liver vitamin A concentration of 0.07 mmol vitamin A/g in both sexes.

Three sets of recommended dietary intakes for vitamin A are presented in Table 1: the 1988 recommended dietary intakes (RDI) of the Food and Agriculture Organization and the World Health Organization (FAO/WHO);[40] the 1989 recommended dietary allowances (RDAs) of the Food and Nutrition Board, National Research Council, U.S. National Academy of Sciences;[41] and the 1991 dietary reference values (DRV) for the United Kingdom.[42] The listed age categories in the table are largely but not entirely concordant. Three different systems have been used: a single value in the RDA (United States), a two-tier system in the RDI (FAO/WHO), and a three-tier system in the DRV (United Kingdom). The higher tier in the FAO/WHO system (safe intake), the top tier in the U.K. system (reference nutrient intake), and the single RDA values in the U.S. system are roughly equivalent conceptually. All presume the presence of an adequate total body reserve of vitamin A for most individuals in society but also include the requirements of "those few members of the community with particularly high needs."[42]

The lowest tiers in the FAO/WHO system and in the DRV system show similar values but are defined differently. The FAO/WHO defines basal requirement as the "(average daily) amount needed to prevent clinically demonstrable impairment of function."[40] The lower reference nutrient intake is defined as the "(average daily) amount of the nutrient that is enough for only the few people in a group who have low needs."[42]

The estimated average requirement in the U.K. system is the average daily amount of a nutrient that meets the needs of 50% of the analyzed group of people. In the U.K. system, the lower reference nutrient intake is two standard deviations below and the reference nutrient intake is two standard deviations above the estimated average requirement. The assigned values for the lower reference nutrient intake in the U.K. system (an inadequate intake for most people) and the basal requirement in the FAO/WHO classification (a minimally adequate intake for most people) being similar is confounding. The explanation may partly be due to different reference standards for weight that are used. The reference weights for adult men and women, respectively, in the FAO/WHO report are 65 and 55 kg, in the U.K. report are 74 and 60 kg, and in the U.S. report are 76 and 62 kg. Despite these differences, the RDA in the United States is still

Table 1. Recommended dietary intakes of vitamin A in retinol equivalents[a]

Group	RDI (FAO/WHO)[40] Basal	RDI (FAO/WHO)[40] Safe	RDA (USA)[41]	DRV (U.K.)[42] Lower reference nutrient intake	DRV (U.K.)[42] Estimated average requirement	DRV (U.K.)[42] Reference nutrient intake
Infants						
0–0.5 years	180	350	375	150	250	350
0.5–1 years	180	350	375	150	250	350
Children						
1–2 years	200	400	400	200	300	400
2–6 years	200	400	500	200	300	400
6–10 years	250	400	700	250	350	500
Males						
10–12 years	300	500	1000	250	400	600
12–70+ years	300	600	1000	300	500	700
Females						
10–70+ years	270	500	800	250	400	600
Pregnancy	+100	+100	0			+100
Lactation						
0–6 months	+180	+350	+500			+350
>6 months	+180	+350	+400			+350

[a]A retinol equivalent is defined as 1 μg retinol, which is considered equal to 6 μg β-carotene or 12 μg of mixed provitamin A carotenoids. RDI, recommended dietary intake; RDA, recommended dietary allowance; DRV, dietary reference value.

very generous relative to those of many other countries.

Recommended nutrient intakes are established for healthy individuals. Sickness, and particularly febrile conditions and lipid malabsorption, can markedly increase needs. Genetic defects in the handling of vitamin A also can significantly affect requirements, but homozygous defects have not been identified, probably because they are inconsistent with survival. Nonetheless, cases of vitamin A intolerance, in which toxic signs appear in some individuals who ingest only moderate amounts of vitamin A, have been reported.[43] These cases, although rare, seem to have a genetic basis.

Sources of Vitamin A

Common dietary sources of preformed vitamin A in the United States are liver; various dairy products, such as milk, cheese, butter, and ice cream; and fish, such as herring, sardines, and tuna. The richest sources of preformed vitamin A, although rarely ingested now in the United States, are liver oils of shark; marine fish, such as cod and halibut; and marine mammals, such as the polar bear.

Common dietary sources of provitamin A carotenoids are carrots, yellow squash, dark-green leafy vegetables, corn, tomatoes, papayas, and oranges. The color of fruits and vegetables is not necessarily an indicator of its concentration of provitamin A; tomatoes, for example, are particularly rich in lycopene, which is nutritionally inactive, and the green color of leafy vegetables is due to chlorophyll, which masks the yellow color of the carotenoids.

Mean and median dietary intakes of vitamin A for adults in the United States are ≈1000 and ≈624 mg retinol equivalents (RE), respectively.[23] In the United States ≈75% of the RE in ingested foods is derived from preformed vitamin A and 25% from provitamin A carotenoids. The bioavailability of carotenoids in foods can vary widely, however, as a function of their specific chemical structures, the matrix in which they exist in foods, food preparation methods, storage procedures, amount ingested, and concomitant presence of fat in the diet. Nonetheless, as a rough general guide, most national and international committees have accepted the convention that 6 μg of all-*trans* β-carotene or 12 μg of other all-*trans* provitamin A carotenoids in food are equivalent nutritionally to 1 μg retinol.

The use of international units (IUs) to express the amount of vitamin A is not encouraged because of the ambiguity that has resulted in unit designations during the historical development of our knowledge about vitamin A. Nonetheless, 1 IU of vitamin A, but not of β-carotene, currently equals 0.3 μg retinol. Thus the RDA values for adult men and women are 3333 IU and 2667 IU, respectively, of preformed vitamin A.

In addition to dietary sources, commercial supplements of vitamin A are used extensively by the American people.[44] In most cases the supplemental intake is 5000 IU, or 1.5 times the RDA of preformed vitamin A, but vitamin A supplements containing ≥10,000 IU are available in health food stores. Thus, some individuals are almost certainly ingesting very large, unneeded, and possibly toxic supplements of vitamin A.

On the opposite tack, significant numbers of children and pregnant women from socioeconomically disadvantaged American families show an inadequate vitamin A status as measured by the modified relative-dose-response test.[45,46] Thus, although most Americans ingest adequate amounts of vitamin A, complacency about the overall vitamin A nutriture of the U.S. population is not warranted.

Toxicity

When ingested in large doses, vitamin A can be toxic.[47-49] There are three categories of toxicity: acute, chronic, and teratogenic. Acute toxicity is produced by one or several closely spaced very large doses of vitamin A, usually >100 times the recommended intake (RDI or RDA) in adults and >20 times the RDI in children. Early signs of acute toxicity include nausea, vomiting, headache, vertigo, blurred vision, muscular incoordination, and, in infants, bulging of the fontanelle. These signs are usually transient and disappear within a few days. When the dose is very large, a second phase, characterized by drowsiness, malaise, inappetence, physical inactivity, itching, skin exfoliation, and recurrent vomiting, follows during the next week.[50] When lethal doses are given to monkeys, the terminal phase includes coma, convulsions, respiratory abnormalities, and then death by respiratory failure or convulsions within 1–16 d.[50] For young monkeys the LD_{50} value (i.e., the single intramuscular dose that killed half of the treated animals) is 168 mg retinol (560,000 IU)/kg body weight. In humans the only comparable case is that of a 1-month-old male infant weighing 2.25 kg who died after receiving 1,000,000 IU of vitamin A during a 11-day period, or a total dose of ≈440,000 IU/kg.[51] Nonetheless, after acute dosing with smaller but still toxic amounts, recovery is usually complete within a few weeks.

Chronic toxicity, which is much more common than acute toxicity, is induced by the recurrent ingestion over a period of weeks to years of excessive doses of vitamin A that are usually ≤10 times the recommended intake (RDI or RDA). Toxic signs commonly include headache, alopecia, cracking of the lips, dry and itchy skin, hepatomegaly, bone and joint pain, as well as many other complaints.[47-49] Most cases of chronic hypervitaminosis were reported in children with daily intakes of 12,000–600,000 IU (2,000–60,000 IU·kg⁻¹·d⁻¹) and in adults with daily intakes of 50,000–1,000,000 IU (700–15,000 IU·kg⁻¹·d⁻¹).[47] As already indicated, signs of chronic toxicity were noted in a very few children and adults who were presumably ingesting much lower amounts of vitamin A daily (i.e., 6000–53,000 IU, or 200–800 IU·kg⁻¹·k⁻¹).[47] These cases of vitamin A intolerance seem to have a genetic basis, although the metabolic defect has not been defined. After dosing is terminated, most patients recover fully from toxicity. Permanent damage to liver, bone, and vision as well as chronic muscular and skeletal pain, however, results in some cases.

Fetal resorption, abortion, birth defects, and permanent learning disabilities in the progeny are the most serious teratogenic effects of vitamin A. Permanent learning disabilities in animals occur at lower doses than those that cause gross abnormalities.[52] Generally, the drugs Accutane (13-*cis* retinoic acid) and etretinate, an aromatic analog of the ethyl ester of all-*trans* retinoic acid, were most implicated in producing human terata.[49,53] In comparison with all-*trans* retinoic acid, both all-*trans* retinol and 13-*cis* retinoic acid were less toxic in several pregnant animal models.[52] Because of differences in the sensitivity of various species to teratogenic doses of retinoids, extrapolation of the toxicity of given doses among species must be done with caution.[54] Interestingly, high doses of all-*trans* retinoyl β-glucuronide and of some retinoylamides are much less teratogenic, if at all, in rodent models.[54,55]

Because of concern about birth defects that might be caused by excessive intakes of vitamin A, the International Vitamin A Consultative Group (IVACG)[56] recommends average daily intakes of 650 RE for pregnant women. IVACG approves the use of daily supplements of 10,000 IU for pregnant women to prevent deficiency-induced fetal abnormalities only in regions of the world where vitamin A deficiency is common. The Teratology Society[57] recommends that women of child-bearing age limit their total daily intake of preformed vitamin A, including food and supplements, to ≤8000 IU and that supplements, if taken, be in the form of provitamin A carotenoids. The Council for Responsible Nutrition,[58] a trade association of the nutritional-supplement industry, advises pregnant women to limit their daily intake of supplements to 10,000 IU. Thus, several groups with different orientations suggest maximal daily intakes of ≤10,000 IU of preformed vitamin A during pregnancy.

Supplements are not needed by healthy people ingesting a balanced diet. In this regard, the American Institute of Nutrition, the American Society for Clinical Nutrition, and the American Dietetic Association[59] issued a formal joint statement that supplements of vitamins and minerals were not needed by well-nourished, healthy individuals except under some specific circumstances, for example, folate and iron for pregnant women and vitamin K for newborns.

Carotenoids in foods are not known to be toxic even when ingested in large amounts. Hypercarotenosis, a benign condition characterized by a jaundice-like yellowing of the skin and high plasma carotenoid concentrations, however, can result when large amounts of carotene-rich foods, i.e., tomato juice, carrot juice, or daily β-carotene supplements (>30 mg), are ingested.[60] The only known toxic manifestation of carotenoid intake is canthaxanthin retinopathy, which may occur in patients treated therapeutically with large daily doses (50–100 mg) of this 4,4′-diketo derivative of β-carotene for long periods.[61] After cessation of intake, however, the crystalline canthaxanthin inclusion bodies in the retina slowly disappear.[61]

As an action independent from their conversion to vitamin A, both nutritionally active and nutritionally inactive carotenoids (e.g., lutein and lycopene) may have protective effects in reducing oxidative stress and some forms of chronic disease.[4,5,62] The extent to which carotenoid ingestion affects the onset of chronic disease in humans, however, is still unclear.

Summary

Vitamin A, ingested either as preformed vitamin A or as provitamin A carotenoids, is required in small amounts for vision, cellular differentiation, and embryonic development. The digestion and absorption of vitamin A is closely associated with lipid absorption. Vitamin A normally is stored in ester form in the liver and is chaperoned in the plasma, across intercellular spaces, and within cells by several specific retinoid-binding proteins. Biologically active, water-soluble retinoid β-glucuronides are formed in several tissues, and retinoic acid receptors in the nucleus serve as transcription regulatory proteins.

Increasingly, two- and three-tier systems of recommended dietary intakes are being promulgated. The advantage is that the needed intakes for various nutritional states are better defined; the disadvantage is that more complicated tables of recommendations confuse the lay public.

Foods containing vitamin A and provitamin A carotenoids, although widespread, usually inexpensive, and available, are not eaten by preschool children in many societies, primarily because of cultural patterns and food aversions. Although acute clinical vitamin A deficiency is becoming less common worldwide, an inadequate (marginal) vitamin A status, which has been associated with increased mortality and severe illness, still plagues over 100 million children, including some in the United States. Several new methods for diagnosing marginal vitamin A status have been developed, of which the modified relative-dose-response test is increasingly being used.

Excessive ingestion of vitamin A, but not of most carotenoids, can cause several forms of toxicity, the most serious of which are birth defects. The dose of vitamin A, as distinct from the retinoid drugs, that can cause abortion or birth defects, is not well defined, although it is probably quite high. Unless there is a clear need for vitamin A supplements, women of child-bearing age should exercise prudence in their use. Indeed, pregnant women should preferentially ingest carotenoid-rich foods.

Acknowledgment. This work was supported in part by grants from the NIH (DK 39733), the USDA (NRICGP 94-37200-0490 and ISU/CDFIN/CSRS 94-34115-0269) and the W.S. Martin Fund. This is publication J-16397 of the Iowa Agriculture and Home Economics Experiment Station, Ames, IA (Project 3035).

References

1. Hicks RJ (1867) Night blindness in the Confederate army. Richmond Med J 3:34–38
2. Moore T (1957) Vitamin A. Elsevier, Amsterdam
3. American Institute of Nutrition (1990) Nomenclature policy: generic descriptors and trivial names for vitamins and related compounds. J Nutr 120:12–19
4. Canfield LM, Krinsky NI, Olson JA, eds (1994) Carotenoids in human health. Ann NY Acad Sci 691:1–300
5. Britton G, ed (1994) Tenth international symposium on carotenoids. Pure Appl Chem 66:931–1076
6. Furr HC, Barua AB, Olson JA (1994) Analytic methods. In Sporn MB, Roberts AB, Goodman DS (eds), The retinoids: biology, chemistry, and medicine. 2nd ed. Raven Press, New York, pp 179–209
7. Britton G, Liaaen-Jensen S, Pfander H, eds (1994) Carotenoids, vol. 1A and 1B. Birkhauser Verlag, Basel, pp 390, 420
8. Barua AB, Kostic D, Olson JA (1993) Simplified procedures for the extraction and simultaneous HPLC analysis of retinol, tocopherols and carotenoids in human serum. J Chromatogr 617:257–264.
9. Novotny JA, Dueker SR, Zech L, Clifford A (1995) Compartmental analysis of the dynamics of β-carotene metabolism in an adult volunteer. J Lipid Res 36:1825–1838
10. Parker RS, Swanson JE, Marmor B, et al (1993) Study of β-carotene metabolism in humans using ^{13}C-β-carotene and high-precision isotope ratio mass spectrometry. Ann NY Acad Sci 671:86–95
11. Underwood BA, Olson JA (eds) (1993) A brief guide to current methods of assessing vitamin A status. International Vitamin A Consultative Group, International Life Science Institute, Washington, DC, pp 1–37
12. Ong DE (1994) Absorption of vitamin A. In Blomhoff R (ed), Vitamin A in health and disease. Marcel Dekker, New York, pp 37–72
13. Brubacher G, Weiser H (1985) The vitamin A activity of beta-carotene. Int J Vitam Nutr Res 55:5–15
14. Olson JA (1994) Absorption, transport and metabolism of carotenoids in humans. Pure Appl Chem 66:1011–1016
15. Devery J, Milborrow BV (1994) β-Carotene-15,15′-dioxygenase (EC 1.13.11.21): isolation, reaction mechanism and an improved assay procedure. Br J Nutr 72:397–414
16. Krinsky NI, Wang X-D, Tang G, Russell RM (1993) Mechanism of carotenoid cleavage to retinoids. Ann NY Acad Sci 691:167–176

17. Nagao A, Olson JA (1994) Enzymatic formation of 9-*cis*, 13-*cis*, and all-*trans* retinals from isomers of β-carotene. FASEB J 8:968–973

18. Wang X-D, Krinsky NI, Benotti PN, Russell RM (1994) Biosynthesis of 9-*cis* retinoic acid from 9-*cis* β-carotene in human intestinal mucosa in vitro. Arch Biochem Biophys 313:150–155

19. Ong D, Newcomer ME, Chytil F (1994) Cellular retinoid-binding proteins. In Sporn MB, Roberts AB, Goodman DS (eds), The retinoids: biology, chemistry, and medicine, 2nd ed. Raven Press, New York, pp 283–317

20. Olson JA (1994) Vitamin A, retinoids and carotenoids. In Shils ME, Olson JA, Shike M (eds), Modern nutrition in health and disease, 8th ed. Lea & Febiger, Philadelphia, pp 287–307

21. Blaner WS, Olson JA (1994) Retinol and retinoic acid metabolism. In Sporn MB, Roberts AB, Goodman DS (eds), The retinoids: biology, chemistry, and medicine, 2nd ed. Raven Press, New York, pp 229–255

22. Sauberlich HE, Hodges RE, Wallace DL (1974) Vitamin A metabolism and requirements in the human studied with the use of labelled retinol. Vitam Horm 32:251–275

23. Olson JA (1987) Recommended dietary intakes (RDI) of vitamin A in humans. Am J Clin Nutr 45:704–716

24. Goodman DS (1984) Plasma retinol-binding protein. In Sporn MB, Roberts AB, Goodman DS (eds), The retinoids, vol 2. Academic Press, Orlando, pp 41–88

25. Green MH, Green JB, Berg T, et al (1993) Vitamin A metabolism in rat liver: a kinetic model. Am J Physiol 264:G509–G521

26. Soprano DR, Blaner WS (1994) Plasma retinol-binding protein. In Sporn MB, Roberts AB, Goodman DS (eds), The retinoids: biology, chemistry, and medicine, 2nd ed. Raven Press, New York, pp 257–281

27. Stephenson CB, Alvarez JO, Kohatsu J, et al (1994) Vitamin A is excreted in the urine during acute infection. Am J Clin Nutr 60:388–392

28. Saari JC (1994) Retinoids in photosensitive systems. In Sporn MB, Roberts AB, Goodman DS (eds), The retinoids: biology, chemistry, and medicine, 2nd ed. Raven Press, New York, pp 351–385

29. Miller DA, De Luca HF (1985) Activation of retinoic acid by coenzyme A for the formation of ethyl retinoate. Proc Natl Acad Sci (USA) 82:6419–6422

30. Ross AC, Hämmerling UG (1994) Retinoids and the immune system. In Sporn MB, Roberts AB, Goodman DS (eds), The retinoids: biology, chemistry, and medicine, 2nd ed. Raven Press, New York, pp 521–543

31. Rando RR (1994) Isomerization reactions of retinoids in the visual system. Pure Appl Chem 66:989–994

32. Banaszak L, Winter N, Xu Z, et al (1993) Lipid binding proteins: a family of fatty acid and retinoid transport proteins. Adv Protein Chem 45:89–149

33. Mangelsdorf DJ, Umesono K, Evans RM (1994) The retinoid receptors. In Sporn MB, Roberts AB, Goodman DS (eds), The retinoids: biology, chemistry, and medicine, 2nd ed. Raven Press, New York, pp 319–349

34. Takahashi N, Breitman TR (1994) Induction of differentiation and covalent binding to proteins by the synthetic retinoids Ch55 and Am 80. Arch Biochem Biophys 314:82–89

35. Hofmann C, Eichele G (1994) Retinoids in development. In Sporn MB, Roberts AB, Goodman DS (eds), The retinoids: biology, chemistry, and medicine, 2nd ed. Raven Press, New York, pp 387–441

36. Underwood BA (1994) Vitamin A in human nutrition: public health considerations. In Sporn MB, Roberts AB, Goodman

DS (eds), The retinoids: biology, chemistry, and medicine, 2nd ed. Raven Press, New York, pp 211–227

37. Beaton GH, Martorell R, L'Abbé KA, et al (1992) Effectiveness of vitamin A supplementation in the control of young child morbidity and mortality in developing countries. Report to the Canadian Agency for International Development, University of Toronto, Toronto, Canada

38. Dueker SR, Jones AD, Clifford AJ (1994) Stable isotope methods for the study of β-carotene d$_8$ metabolism in humans utilizing tandem mass spectrometry and high performance liquid chromatography. Anal Chem 66:4177–4185

39. Olson JA (1995) Biochemistry of vitamin A and carotenoids. In Sommer A, West KP Jr (eds), Vitamin A deficiency: health, survival and vision. Oxford University Press, Oxford UK, in press

40. Food and Agriculture Organization/World Health Organization (1989) Requirements of Vitamin A, iron, folate, and vitamin B$_{12}$. Report of a joint FAO/WHO Expert Committee. FAO Food and Nutrition Series 23, FAO, Rome, pp 1–107

41. National Research Council (1989) Recommended dietary allowances, 10th ed. National Academy Press, Washington DC, pp 1–284

42. Department of Health (1991) Dietary reference values for food energy and nutrients for the United Kingdom. Report No. 41 on health and social subjects. HMSO, London, pp 1–210

43. Olson JA (1989) Upper limits of vitamin A in infant formulas, with some comments on vitamin K. Am J Clin Nutr 119:1820–1824

44. Stewart ML, McDonald JL, Levy AS, et al (1985) Vitamin/mineral supplement use: a telephone survey of adults in the United States. J Am Diet Assoc 85:1585–1590

45. Duitsman PK, Cook LR, Tanumihardjo SA, Olson JA (1995) Vitamin A inadequacy in socioeconomically disadvantaged pregnant Iowan women as assessed by the modified relative dose response (MRDR) test. Nutr Res 15:1263–1276

46. Spannaus-Martin DJ, Tanumihardjo S, Cook L, Olson JA (1994) The vitamin A statuses of young children of several ethnic groups in a socioeconomically disadvantaged urban population. FASEB J 8:A940

47. Bauernfeind JC (1980) The safe use of vitamin A. International Vitamin A Consultative Group, Nutrition Foundation, Washington DC

48. Hathcock JN, Hattan DG, Jenkins MV, et al (1990) Evaluation of vitamin A toxicity. Am J Clin Nutr 52:183–202

49. Armstrong RB, Ashenfelter KO, Eckhoff C, et al (1994) General and reproductive toxicology of retinoids. In Sporn MB, Roberts AB, Goodman DS (eds), The retinoids: biology, chemistry, and medicine, 2nd ed. Raven Press, New York, pp 545–572

50. Macapinlac MP, Olson JA (1981) A lethal hypervitaminosis A syndrome in young monkeys following a single intramuscular dose of a water-miscible preparation containing vitamins A, D$_2$ and E. Int J Vitam Nutr Res 51:331–341

51. Bush ME, Dahms BB (1984) Fatal hypervitaminosis in a neonate. Arch Pathol Lab Med 108:838–842

52. Adams J (1993) Structure-activity and dose-response relationships in the neural and behavioral teratogenesis of retinoids. Neurotoxicol Teratol 15:193–202

53. Lammer EJ, Chen DT, Hoar RM, et al (1985) Retinoic acid embryopathy. N Engl J Med 313:837–841

54. Howard WB, Willhite CC (1986) Toxicity of retinoids in humans and animals. J Toxicol Toxin Rev 5:55–94

55. Gunning DB, Barua AB, Olson JA (1993) Comparative teratogenicity and metabolism of all-*trans* retinoic acid, all-*trans* retinoyl β-glucose, and all-*trans* β-glucuronide in pregnant Sprague-Dawley rats. Teratology 47:29–36

56. Underwood BA (1986) The safe use of vitamin A by women during the reproductive years. International Vitamin A Consultative Group, ILSI-Nutrition Foundation, Washington DC

57. Teratology Society (1987) Recommendations for vitamin A use during pregnancy [position paper]. Teratology 35:269–275

58. Council for Responsible Nutrition (1986) Safety of vitamins and minerals: a summary of findings of key reviews. Council for Responsible Nutrition, Washington, DC

59. American Institute of Nutrition, American Society of Clinical Nutrition, American Dietetic Association (1987) Joint statement on vitamin and mineral supplements. J Nutr 117:1649

60. Micozzi MS, Brown ED, Taylor PR, Wolfe E (1988) Carotenodermia in men with elevated carotenoid intake from foods and β-carotene supplements. Am J Clin Nutr 48:1061–1064

61. Weber U, Goerz G, Baseler H, Michaelis L (1992) Canthaxanthin retinopathy: follow-up of over 6 years. Klin Monatsbl Augenheilkd 201:174–177

62. Bendich A, Olson JA (1989) Biological actions of carotenoids. FASEB J 3:1927–1932

Chapter 12

Vitamin D

Anthony W. Norman

Vitamin D is essential for life in higher animals. It is one of the most important biological regulators of calcium metabolism. Along with the two peptide hormones parathyroid hormone and calcitonin, vitamin D has long been known to be responsible for the minute-by-minute as well as the day-to-day maintenance of calcium and mineral homeostasis. It is now agreed that these important biological effects are achieved as a consequence of the metabolism of vitamin D into a family of daughter metabolites, and that one of these metabolites, namely $1\alpha,25(OH)_2D_3$, is considered to be a steroid hormone. Thus the bulk of the biological responses we attribute to the parent vitamin D occurs through its acting in the fashion of a steroid hormone through its chemical messenger $1\alpha,25(OH)_2D_3$.

It has become increasingly apparent since the 1980s that $1\alpha,25(OH)_2D_3$ also plays an important multidisciplinary role in tissues not primarily related to mineral metabolism; e.g., the hematopoietic system affects cell differentiation and proliferation including interaction with cancer cells, and participates in the process of insulin secretion. The purpose of this chapter is to provide a succinct overview of our current understanding of the important nutritional substance vitamin D and the mechanisms by which its daughter hormone $1\alpha,25(OH)_2D_3$ mediates biological responses. The interested reader is referred to other reviews in the recent scientific literature that provide differing extensive coverages and perspectives.[1-4]

Humans are reported to have been aware since early antiquity of the substance we now know as vitamin D.[5] The first scientific description of a vitamin D deficiency, namely rickets, was provided in the 17th century by both Dr. Daniel Whistler (1645) and Professor Francis Glisson (1650).[4] The major breakthrough in understanding the causative factors of rickets was the development of nutrition as an experimental science and the appreciation of the existence of vitamins. Considering the fact that the biologically active form of vitamin D is a steroid hormone, it is somewhat ironic that vitamin D, through a historical accident, became classified as a vitamin. It was in 1919–1920 that Sir Edward Mellanby,[6] working with dogs raised exclusively indoors (in the absence of sunlight or ultraviolet light), devised a diet that allowed him to unequivocally establish that rickets was caused by a deficiency of a trace component present in the diet. In 1921 he wrote, "The action of fats in rickets is due to a vitamin or accessory food factor which they contain, probably identical with the fat-soluble vitamin." Furthermore he established that cod-liver oil was an excellent antirachitic agent. Shortly thereafter McCollum and associates[7] observed that by bubbling oxygen through a preparation of the "fat soluble vitamin" they were able to distinguish between vitamin A (which was inactivated) and vitamin D (which retained activity). In 1923 Goldblatt and Soames[8] clearly identified that when a precursor of vitamin D in the skin (7-dehydrocholesterol) was irradiated with sunlight or ultraviolet light, a substance equivalent to the fat-soluble vitamin was produced. Hess and Weinstock[9] confirmed the dictum that "light equals vitamin D." They excised a small portion of skin, irradiated it with ultraviolet light, and then fed it to groups of rachitic rats. The skin that had been irradiated provided an absolute protection against rickets, whereas the unirradiated skin provided no protection whatsoever; clearly, these animals possessed endogenous body mechanisms to produce adequate quantities of "the fat-soluble vitamin," suggesting that it was not an essential dietary trace constituent. However, because of the rapid rise of the science of nutrition—and the discovery of the families of water-soluble and fat-soluble vitamins—it rapidly became firmly established that the antirachitic factor was to be classified as a vitamin.

The chemical structures of the vitamins D were determined in the 1930s in the laboratory of Professor A. Windaus at the University of Göttingen in Germany. Vitamin D_2, which could be produced by ultraviolet irradiation of ergosterol, was chemically characterized in 1932.[10] Vitamin D_3 was not chemically characterized until 1936 when it was shown to result from the ultraviolet irradiation of 7-dehydrocholesterol.[11] Virtually simultaneously, the elusive antirachitic component of cod-liver oil was shown to be identical to the newly characterized vitamin D_3.[12] These results clearly established that the antirachitic substance vitamin D was chemically a steroid, more specifically a secosteroid (which will be discussed in the following section).

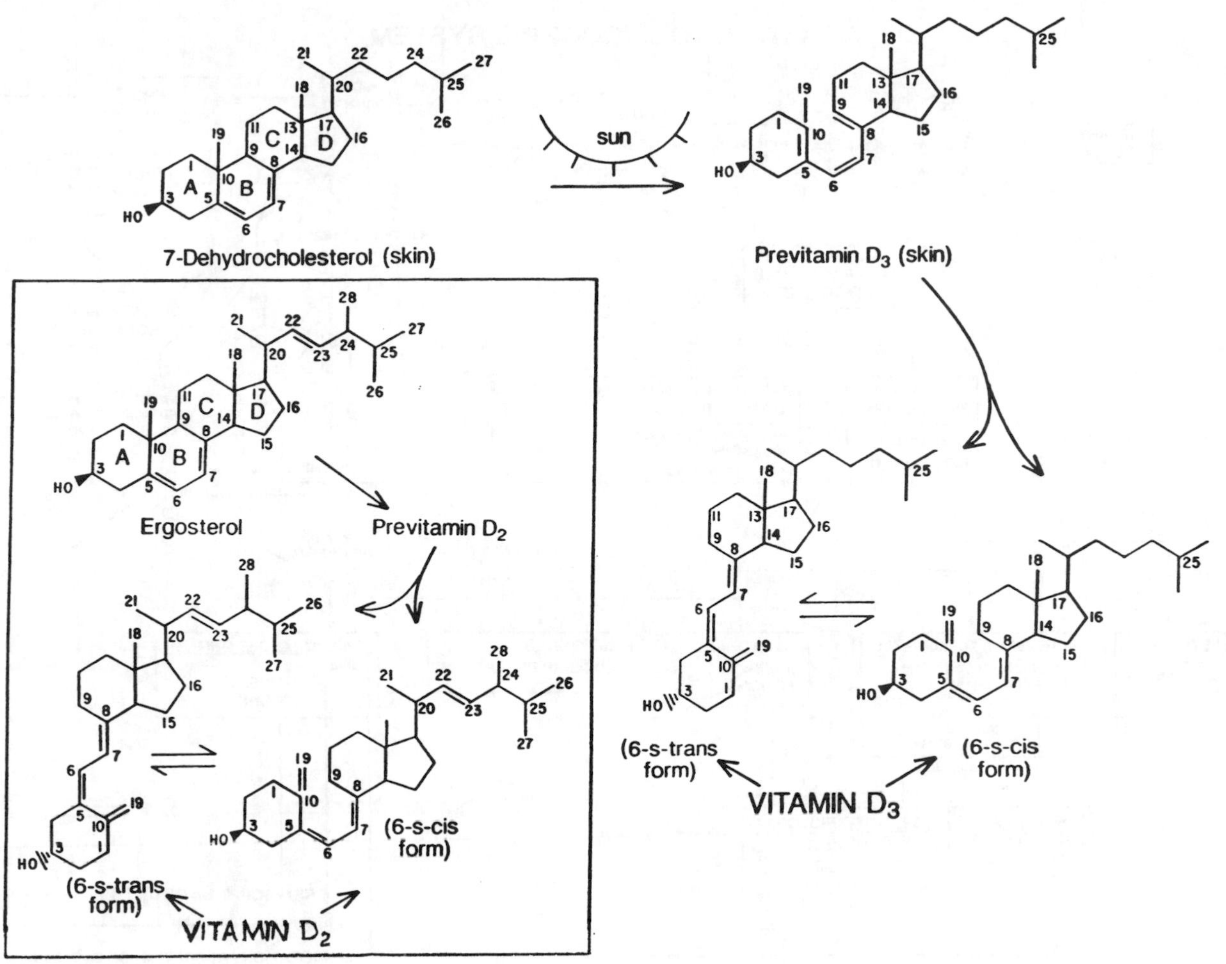

Figure 1. Chemistry and irradiation pathway for production of vitamin D_3 (a natural process) and vitamin D_2 (a commercial process). In each instance the provitamin, which is characterized by the presence in the B ring of a $\Delta 5, 7$ conjugated double-bond system, is converted to the seco-B previtamin steroid, where the 9,10 carbon-carbon bond has been broken. Then the previtamin D, in a process independent of ultraviolet light, thermally isomerizes to the "vitamin" form, which is characterized by a $\Delta 6,7$, $\Delta 8,9$, $\Delta 10,19$ conjugated double-bond system. In solution (and in biological systems), vitamin D is capable of assuming a large number of conformational shapes because of rotation about the 6,7 carbon-carbon single bond of the B ring. Presented for both vitamin D_3 and vitamin D_2 are the 6-s-cis conformer (the steroid-like shape) and the 6-s-trans conformer (the extended shape). These two conformations are in very rapid equilibrium with one another. There are also a wide variety of other conformations that are generated by the conformational flexibility of the side chain[13] and the A ring.[14] There is currently much research being conducted to understand structure-function relationships in the vitamin D endocrine system and their relation to development of new drugs.[15-17] The interested reader should consult the indicated references for a more thorough discussion.

Chemistry of Vitamin D

The structures of vitamin D_2 (ergocalciferol) and vitamin D_3 (cholecalciferol) and their provitamins are presented in Figure 1. (A discussion of the conformational shapes of vitamin D is given in the legend of Figure 1.) Vitamin D is a generic term and indicates a molecule of the general structure shown for rings A, B, C, and D with differing side chain structures. The A, B, C, and D ring structure is derived from the cyclopentanoperhydrophenanthrene ring structure for steroids.[18] Technically, the steroid vitamin D is classified as a secosteroid. Secosteroids are those in which one of the rings has been broken; in vitamin D, the 9,10 carbon-carbon bond of

ring B is broken, and it is indicated by the inclusion of "9,10-seco" in the official nomenclature.

Vitamin D (synonym calciferol) is named according to the revised rules of the International Union of Pure and Applied Chemists.[19] Because vitamin D is derived from a steroid, the structure retains its numbering from the parent compound cholesterol (see Figure 1). Asymmetric centers are designated by using the R,S notation[18]; the configuration of the double bonds is notated E for "eingang" or trans, and Z for "zusammen" or cis. Thus the official name of vitamin D_3 is 9,10-seco(5Z,7E)-5,7,10(19)cholestatriene-3β-ol, and the official name of vitamin D_2 is 9,10-seco(5Z,7E)-5,7,10(19),22-ergostatetraene-3β-ol.

VITAMIN D ENDOCRINE SYSTEM

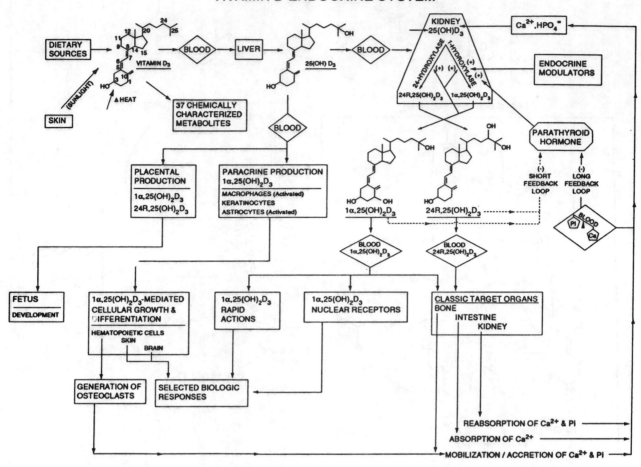

Figure 2. Summary of the vitamin D endocrine system. In this system, the biologically inactive vitamin D_3 is activated, first in the liver, and then converted by the kidney to the hormones $1\alpha,25(OH)_2D_3$ and $24R,25(OH)_2D_3$. Table 1 summarizes those tissues that possess the nuclear receptor for $1\alpha,25(OH)_2D_3$ (nVDR) and also summarizes those tissues that have been shown to be involved in the rapid actions and membrane-initiated signal transduction pathway for $1\alpha,25(OH)_2D_3$ (see Figure 3). Pi, inorganic phosphate.

Vitamin D_3 can be produced photochemically by the action of sunlight or ultraviolet light from the precursor sterol 7-dehydrocholesterol, which is present in the epidermis or skin of most higher animals. The chief structural prerequisite of a provitamin D is that it be a sterol with a 5-7 double bond system in ring B (see Figure 1). The conjugated double bond system in this specific location of the molecule allows the absorption of light quanta at certain wavelengths in the ultraviolet range; this can readily be provided in most geographical locations by natural sunlight. This initiates a complex series of transformations (partially summarized in Figure 1) that ultimately result in the appearance of vitamin D_3. Thus it is important to appreciate that vitamin D_3 can be endogenously produced and that as long as the animal (or human) has access on a regular basis to sunlight there is no dietary requirement for this vitamin.

Vitamin D_2 is a completely synthetic form of vitamin D that is produced by irradiation of the plant steroid

ergosterol. Historically, vitamin D_2 was used in the period 1940–1960 in food supplementation to provide vitamin D activity.

Physiology and Biochemistry

Vitamin D endocrine system. A detailed study of the biochemical mode of action of the fat-soluble vitamin D was not possible until the availability in the 1960s of radioactive vitamin D of high specific activity.[20] As a consequence of efforts in several laboratories, a new model emerged to be used to describe the biological mechanisms of action of vitamin D_3.[21] This model is based on the concept that, in terms of its structure and mode of action, vitamin D is similar to that understood for the classic steroid hormones, e.g., aldosterone, testosterone, estrogen, cortisol, and ecdysterone.[22,23]

As described in Figure 2, the concept of the existence of the vitamin D endocrine system is now firmly

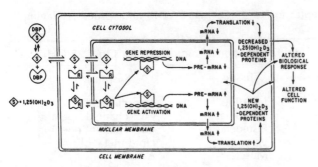

Figure 3. A (above): Proposed model for the mechanism of action of the steroid hormone $1\alpha,25(OH)_2D_3$ in terms of regulation of gene transcription.[37] DBP, the serum vitamin D–binding protein; S, $1\alpha,25(OH)_2D_3$ steroid; R, receptor for $1\alpha,25(OH)_2D_3$; P, phosphorylation; F, transcription factor; DNA, deoxyribonucleic acid; mRNA, messenger ribonucleic acid; POL II, RNA polymerase II. B (right): A working schematic model illustrating the participation of the membrane-initiated signal transduction pathway for $1\alpha,25(OH)_2D_3$ in the process of intestinal Ca^{2+} absorption. The general model of vesicular Ca^{2+} transport includes formation of Ca^{2+}-containing endocytic vesicles at the brush border membrane,[38] fusion of endocytic vesicles with lysosomes, movement of lysosomes along the microtubules, and exocytotic extrusion of Ca^{2+} via fusion of the lysosomes with the basal lateral membrane of the intestinal enterocyte.[38] The binding of $1\alpha,25(OH)_2D_3$ to the membrane receptor results in an increase of several second messengers including IP_3, cAMP, or intracellular Ca^{2+} as well as activation of protein kinase C, one or more of which may result in the transient opening of Ca^{2+} channels. The increased Ca^{2+} concentration may then initiate the exocytosis of the lysosomal vesicles. EV, endocytic vesicle; L2, secondary lysosome; N, nucleus; GA, Golgi apparatus.

established.[15,24–26] The elements of the vitamin D endocrine system include the following: a) in the skin, photoconversion of 7-dehydrocholesterol to vitamin D_3 or dietary intake of vitamin D_3; b) metabolism of vitamin D_3 by the liver to $25(OH)D_3$, which is the major form of vitamin D circulating in the blood compartment; c) conversion of $25(OH)D_3$ by the kidney (functioning as an endocrine gland) to produce the two principal dihydroxylated metabolites, namely $1\alpha,25(OH)_2D_3$ and $24R,25(OH)_2D_3$; d) systemic transport of the dihydroxylated metabolites $24R,25(OH)_2D_3$ and $1\alpha,25(OH)_2D_3$ to distal target organs; and e) binding of the dihydroxylated metabolites, particularly $1,25(OH)_2D_3$, to either a nuclear receptor or membrane receptor at the target organs followed by the subsequent generation of appropriate biological responses. An additional key component in the operation of the vitamin D endocrine system is the plasma vitamin D binding protein that carries vitamin D_3 and all its metabolites to their various target organs.[15,27]

Over the past 25 years, research efforts have largely focused on understanding how $1\alpha,25(OH)_2D_3$ generates biological responses. By comparison, the biological actions of $24R,25(OH)_2D_3$ have been relatively less studied. However, evidence has been presented to support the view that the combined presence of both $1\alpha,25(OH)_2D_3$ and $24R,25(OH)_2D_3$ is required to generate the complete spectrum of biological responses attributable to the parent vitamin D_3.[28–30] The remainder of this chapter, however, will focus on the nutritional and biological aspects of only vitamin D_3 and $1\alpha,25(OH)_2D_3$.

Metabolism of vitamin D. Vitamin D_3 is, in reality, a prohormone and is not known to have any intrinsic biological activity itself. It is only after vitamin D_3 is metabolized first to $25(OH)D_3$ in the liver and then $1\alpha,25(OH)_2D_3$ and $24R,25(OH)_2D_3$ by the kidney that biologically active molecules are produced. In toto some 37 vitamin D_3 metabolites have been isolated and chemically characterized.[31,32]

The key kidney enzymes, the $25(OH)D_3$-1-hydroxylase and the $25(OH)D_3$-24-hydroxylase,[31] as well as the liver vitamin D_3-25-hydroxylase,[33] are all known to be cytochrome P-450 mixed-function oxidases. Both of the renal enzymes are localized in mitochondria of the proximal tubules of the kidney. Mixed-function oxidases use molecular oxygen as the oxygen source instead of water. Mitochondrial mixed-function oxidases are composed

Table 1. Summary of the tissue location of the nuclear receptor for $1\alpha,25(OH)_2D_3$ (nVDR) and tissues displaying "rapid" or membrane-initiated biological responses

Tissue distributions of nuclear $1,25(OH)_2D_3$ receptors			Distribution of rapid responses to $1,25(OH)_2D_3$	
			Tissue	Response
Adipose	Intestine	Pituitary	Intestine	Transcaltachia
Adrenal	Kidney	Placenta	Osteoblast	Ca^{2+} channel opening
Bone	Liver (fetal)	Prostate	Osteoclast	Ca^{2+} channel opening
Bone marrow	Lung	Retina	Liver	Lipid metabolism
Brain	Muscle, cardiac	Skin	Muscle	A variety
Breast	Muscle, embryonic	Stomach		
Cancer cells (many)	Muscle, smooth	Testis		
Cartilage	Osteoblast	Thymus		
Colon	Ovary	Thyroid		
Eggshell gland	Pancreas β cell	Uterus		
Epididymis	Parathyroid	Yolk sac (bird)		
Hair follicle	Parotid			

of three proteins that are integral components of the mitochondrial membrane: renal ferredoxin reductase, renal ferredoxin, and cytochrome P-450.[34]

The most important point of regulation of the vitamin D endocrine system occurs through the stringent control of the activity of the renal 1-hydroxylase. In this way the production of the hormone $1\alpha,25(OH)_2D_3$ can be modulated according to the calcium and other endocrine needs of the organism. The chief regulatory factors are $1\alpha,25(OH)_2D_3$ itself, parathyroid hormone, and the serum concentrations of calcium[31,35] and phosphate.[36] Probably the most important determinant of activity of the 1-hydroxylase is the vitamin D status of the animal.[35] When circulating concentrations of $1\alpha,25(OH)_2D_3$ are low, production of $1\alpha,25(OH)_2D_3$ by the kidney is high, and when circulating concentrations of $1\alpha,25(OH)_2D_3$ are high, the output of $1\alpha,25(OH)_2D_3$ by the kidney is sharply reduced.

Mechanism of action of $1\alpha,25(OH)_2D_3$. The secosteroid $1\alpha,25(OH)_2D_3$ is now known to initiate biological responses via regulation of gene transcription as well as via a separate signal transduction pathway(s) that has been shown to generate biological responses very rapidly. Schematic models describing these actions are summarized in Figure 3. Table 1, left panel, summarizes ≈30 target organs that are known to possess the nuclear vitamin D receptor and for which there is regulation of gene transcription.[39–41] The right panel of Table 1 summarizes tissues where the presence of "rapid" biological actions mediated by $1\alpha,25(OH)_2D_3$ has been reported. In most instances these responses are argued to occur too rapidly to be explained via regulation of gene transcription. These rapid responses have included transcaltachia or the rapid stimulation by $1\alpha,25(OH)_2D_3$ of intestinal Ca^{2+} absorption,[42–45] the opening of voltage-gated Ca^{2+} channels,[46] rapid uptake of $^{45}Ca^{2+}$ into ROS 17/2.8 osteoblast cells,[46–48] phospholipid metabolism in

the intestine[49] and liver,[50] and a variety of responses in muscle cells.[51]

The regulation of gene transcription by $1\alpha,25(OH)_2D_3$ is known to be mediated by interaction of this ligand with a nuclear receptor protein, (nVDR).[37,41,52] As mentioned earlier, the nVDR is known to occur in over 30 different cell types (see Table 1). In addition $1\alpha,25(OH)_2D_3$ and the nVDR are known to regulate the transcription of over 40 different proteins.[41] A number of excellent articles have appeared describing our current understanding of how the nVDR regulates gene transcription.[40,52,53]

The rapid responses mediated by $1\alpha,25(OH)_2D_3$ are postulated to be mediated through interaction of the $1\alpha,25(OH)_2D_3$ with a protein receptor located on the external membrane of the cell[54,55]; this receptor is referred to as the mVDR. The mVDR is believed to be involved in either the opening of voltage-gated Ca^{2+} channels[46] or the activation of protein kinase C or both.[56,57] The ligand-binding preferences of the nVDR and mVDR have been extensively studied.[45,58,59] A key consideration is the position of rotation about the 6,7 single carbon-carbon bond that can be in either the 6-s-*cis* or the 6-s-*trans* orientation (see legend to Figure 1). Each receptor is believed to have specific preferences for the shape of the conformationally flexible $1\alpha,25(OH)_2D_3$, which it uses as an agonist.[60]

Nutritional Aspects

Recommended dietary allowance (RDA). The World Health Organization has responsibility for defining the "International Unit" of vitamin D_3. Their most recent definition, provided in 1950, stated that "the International Unit of vitamin D recommended for adoption is the vitamin D activity of 0.025 μg of the international standard preparation of crystalline vitamin D_3."[4] Thus 1.0 IU of vitamin D_3 is 0.025 μg, which is equivalent to 65.0 pmol.

With the discovery of the metabolism of vitamin D_3 to other active secosteroids, particularly $1\alpha,25(OH)_2D_3$, it was recommended that 1.0 IU of $1\alpha,25(OH)_2D_3$ be set equivalent in molar terms to that of the parent vitamin D_3. Thus 1.0 IU of $1\alpha,25(OH)_2D_3$ has been operationally defined to be equivalent to 65 pmol.[61]

The vitamin D requirement for healthy adults has never been precisely defined. Because vitamin D_3 is produced in the skin after exposure to sunlight, the human does not have a requirement for vitamin D when sufficient sunlight is available. However, vitamin D does become an important nutritional factor in the absence of sunlight. It is known that a substantial proportion of the US population is exposed to quite suboptimal levels of sunlight, especially during the winter months[62,63]; it is likely that during these intervals a regular dietary supply of vitamin D_3 should be provided. In addition to geographical and seasonal factors, ultraviolet light from the sun may also be blocked by air pollution. Man's tendency to wear clothes, to live in cities where tall buildings block adequate sunlight from reaching the ground, to live indoors, to use synthetic sunscreens that block ultraviolet rays, and to live in geographical regions of the world that do not receive adequate sunlight, all contribute to the inability of the skin to biosynthesize sufficient amounts of vitamin D_3.[64] Under extremes of these conditions vitamin D becomes a true vitamin in that it must be supplied in the diet on a regular basis.

Because vitamin D_3 can be endogenously produced by the body and because it is retained for long periods of time by vertebrate tissue, it is difficult to determine with precision the minimum daily requirements for this secosteroid. The requirement for vitamin D is also known to depend on the concentration of calcium and phosphorus in the diet, the physiological stage of development, age, sex, degree of exposure to the sun, and the amount of pigmentation in the skin.[65]

The current allowance of vitamin D recommended in 1989 by the Food and Nutrition Board of the Commission on Life Sciences of the National Research Council is 200 IU/day (5 µg/day) for adults beyond the age of 24.[66] The same Food and Nutrition Board has also made additional RDA recommendations for vitamin D for other physiological circumstances.[66] Thus the RDA of vitamin D for both pregnant and lactating women of all ages is 400 IU (10 µg/day), which reflects their greater calcium needs. For infants from birth to 6 months of age, the RDA is set at 300 IU (7.5 µg/day). Finally, the RDA for children older than 6 months of age to adults of age 24 is 400 IU (10 µg/day).

In the United States, adequate amounts of vitamin D can readily be obtained from the diet and from casual exposure to sunlight. However, in some parts of the world where food is not routinely fortified and sunlight is often limited during some periods of the year, obtaining adequate amounts of vitamin D becomes more of a problem. As a result, the incidence of rickets in these countries is higher than in the United States.

Food sources. Animal products constitute the main source of vitamin D that occurs naturally in unfortified foods. Salt water fish such as herring, salmon, sardines, and fish liver oils are good sources of vitamin D_3. Small quantities of vitamin D_3 are also derived from eggs, veal, beef, butter, and vegetable oils while plants, fruits, and nuts are extremely poor sources of vitamin D. In the United States, artificial fortification of foods such as milk (both fresh and evaporated), margarine and butter, cereals, and chocolate mixes help in meeting the RDA recommendations.[67]

Excess and Toxicity

Vitamin D. Excessive amounts of vitamin D are not normally available from usual dietary sources and thus reports of vitamin D intoxication are rare. However, there is always the possibility that vitamin D intoxication may occur in individuals who are taking excessive amounts of supplemental vitamins. Recently, there was one report of vitamin D intoxication occurring from drinking milk that had been fortified with inappropriately high levels of vitamin D_3.[68] Symptoms of vitamin D intoxication include hypercalcemia, hypercalciuria, anorexia, nausea, vomiting, thirst, polyuria, muscular weakness, joint pains, diffuse demineralization of bones, and general disorientation. If allowed to go unchecked, death will eventually occur.

The biological basis for intoxication resulting from the inappropriate intake of the parent vitamin D_3 is believed to be due to the unrestrained metabolism by the liver of the vitamin D_3 to $25(OH)D_3$; this is a largely unregulated metabolic step.[69] The vitamin D intoxication is thought to occur as a result of high plasma levels of $25(OH)D$ rather than high plasma levels of $1\alpha,25(OH)_2D_3$.[70] Patients suffering from hypervitaminosis D have been shown to exhibit a 15-fold increase in plasma $25(OH)D$ concentration compared with normal individuals; however, their $1\alpha,25(OH)_2D$ levels are not substantially altered.[70] It has also been shown that large concentrations of $25(OH)D_3$ can mimic the actions of $1\alpha,25(OH)_2D_3$ at the level of the nVDR,[71] which can lead to a massive stimulation of intestinal Ca^{2+} absorption and bone Ca^{2+} resorption, and ultimately soft-tissue calcification and kidney stones.[72]

Drug forms of $1\alpha,25(OH)_2D_3$. The potential for vitamin D intoxication, i.e., hypercalcemia and soft-tissue calcification, is much higher when an individual has access to drug formulations of $1\alpha,25(OH)_2D_3$, since the medication effectively bypasses the stringent physiological control point of the vitamin D endocrine system, namely the $25(OH)D_3$-1-hydroxylase of the kidney. Table

Table 2. Drug forms of vitamin D metabolites

Compound name	Commerical name	Pharmaceutical company	Effective daily dose[a] (µg)	Approved use
Dihydrotachysterol$_3$	Hytakerol	Winthrop	200–1000	RO
25(OH)-5,6-*trans* D$_3$	Deklamin	Hoechst	50–600	RO
25(OH)-5,6-*trans* D$_3$		Roussell-UCLAF	50–600	RO
25(OH)D$_3$	Calderol	Organon-USA	50–500	RO
25(OH)D$_3$	Dedrogyl	Roussell-UCLAF-France	50–500	RO
1α-OH-D$_3$	One-alpha	Leo-Denmark	1–2	RO
1α-OH-D$_3$	Alpha-D$_3$	Teva-Israel	0.25 1.0	RO
1α-OH-D$_3$	Onealfa	Teijin Ltd.-Japan	0.25–1.0	RO, O
1α-OH-D$_3$	Onealfa	Ilsung Corp.-Korea	0.25–1.0	RO, O
1α-OH-D$_3$	Onealfa	Chugai-Japan	0.25–1.0	RO, O
1α,25(OH)$_2$D$_3$	Rocaltrol[b]	Hoffmann-La Roche	0.5–1.0	RO, HP, O[b]
1α,25(OH)$_2$D$_3$	Calcijex	Abbott Laboratories	0.5 (i.v.)	HC
1α,24S(OH)$_2$-22-ene-26,27,dehydrovitamin D$_3$	Dovonex	Leo-Denmark	40–80 (topical)	P
1α,24(OH)$_2$D$_3$	Bonalfa	Teijin Ltd.-Japan	40–80 (topical)	P

Drug formulations of the hormonal form of vitamin D$_3$. The key to the approved uses of the vitamin D analogs is as follows: RO = renal osteodystrophy; O = postmenopausal osteoporosis; HP = patients with hypocalcemia, which may frequently be encountered in patients with hypoparathyroidism, pseudohypoparathyroidism, or in circumstances of postoperative hypoparathyroidism; HC = hypocalcemia (frequently present in patients with renal osteodystrophy who are subjected to hemodialysis); P = psoriasis.
[a]Oral dose unless indicated otherwise.
[b]The use of Rocaltrol for osteoporosis is not approved by the U.S. Food and Drug Administration; however, its use for postmenopausal osteoporosis is approved in Argentina, Australia, Austria, Czech Republic, Colombia, India, Ireland, Italy, Japan, Malaysia, Mexico, New Zealand, Peru, Philippines, South Korea, South Africa, Switzerland, Turkey, and the United Kingdom.

2 lists the drug forms of 1α,25(OH)$_2$D$_3$ that are currently available for treatment of several disease states including hypoparathyroidism, vitamin D–resistant rickets, renal osteodystrophy, osteoporosis, and psoriasis.

Vitamin D–related Disease States in Man

Figure 4 presents a schematic diagram of the metabolic processing of vitamin D via its endocrine system. Listed under each of the substeps of the various metabolic or regulatory steps are disease states that are known to be clinically focused at that particular locus. Conceptually, human clinical disorders related to vitamin D can be considered as those arising because of a) altered availability of vitamin D, b) altered conversion of vitamin D$_3$ to 25(OH)D$_3$, c) altered conversion of 25(OH)D$_3$ to 1α,25(OH)$_2$D$_3$ or 24R,25(OH)$_2$D$_3$ or both, d) variations in end-organ responsiveness to 1α,25(OH)$_2$D$_3$ or possibly 24R,25(OH)$_2$D$_3$, and e) other conditions of uncertain relation to vitamin D. Thus the clinician and nutritionist and biochemist are faced with a problem, in a diagnostic sense, of identifying parameters of hypersensitivity, antagonism, or resistance (including genetic aberrations) to vitamin D or one of its metabolites as well as identifying perturbations of metabolism that result in problems in production or delivery (or both) of the hormonally active form, 1α,25(OH)$_2$D$_3$. A detailed consideration of this area is beyond the scope of this presentation; the interested reader should consult other sources.[16,25,73]

Summary

Current evidence supports the concept that the classical biological actions of the nutritionally important fat-soluble vitamin D in mediating calcium homeostasis are supported by a complex vitamin D endocrine system, which coordinates the metabolism of vitamin D$_3$ into 1α,25(OH)$_2$D$_3$ and 24R,25(OH)$_2$D$_3$. It is now clear that the vitamin D endocrine system embraces many more target tissues than simply the intestine, bone, and kidney. Notable additions to this list include the pancreas, pituitary gland, breast tissue, placenta, hematopoietic cells, skin, and cancer cells of various origins. Key advances in understanding the mode of action of the 1α,25(OH)$_2$D$_3$ have been made by a thorough study of nuclear receptors as well as emerging studies describing a membrane receptor for this steroid hormone. Integral to these observations are efforts to define the signal transduction systems that are subservient to the nuclear and membrane receptors for 1α,25(OH)$_2$D$_3$ and to obtain a thorough study of the tissue distribution and subcellular localization of the gene products induced by this steroid hormone. There are clinical applications for 1α,25(OH)$_2$D$_3$ or related analogs for treatment of the bone diseases of renal osteodystrophy and osteoporosis,

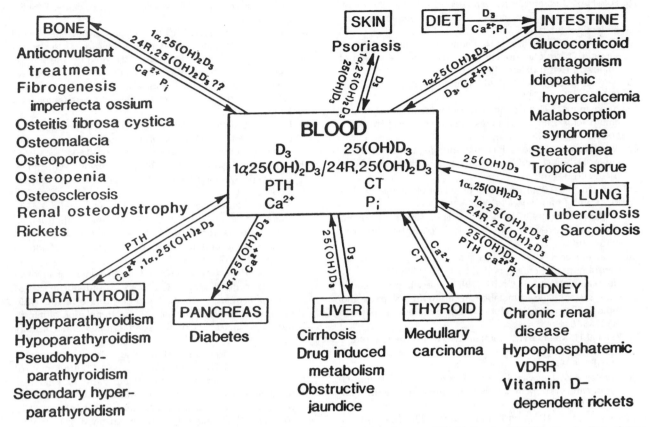

Figure 4. Human disease states related to vitamin D. PTH, parathyroid hormone; CT, calcitonin; VDRR, vitamin D–resistant rickets; Pi, inorganic phosphate; Ca²⁺, calcium.

psoriasis, and hypoparathyroidism; other clinical targets for $1\alpha,25(OH)_2D_3$ currently under investigation include its use in leukemia, breast, prostate, and colon cancer as well as its use as an immunosuppressive agent.

Acknowledgments

Work in the laboratory of the author was supported by National Institutes of Health grants DK-09012-30 (National Institute of Diabetes and Digestive and Kidney Diseases) and CA-43,277-08 (National Cancer Institute).

References

1. Norman AW, Bouillon R, Thomasset M, eds (1994) Vitamin D, a pluripotent steroid hormone: structural studies, molecular endocrinology and clinical applications. Walter de Gruyter, Berlin
2. Norman AW, Bouillon R, Thomasset M, eds (1991) Vitamin D: gene regulation, structure function analysis and clinical application. Walter de Gruyter, Berlin
3. Fraser DR (1980) Regulation of the metabolism of vitamin D. Physiol Rev 60:551–613
4. Norman AW (1979) Vitamin D: the calcium homeostatic steroid hormone. Academic Press, New York
5. Soleki RS (1971) Shanidar: the humanity of Neanderthal man. Knopf, New York, pp 1–220
6. Mellanby E (1921) Experimental rickets. Medical Research Council of Great Britain, Special Report Series 61:4–78.
7. McCollum EV, Simmonds N, Becker JE, Shipley PG (1922) Studies on experimental rickets. XXI. An experimental demonstration of the existence of a vitamin which promotes calcium deposition. J Biol Chem 53:293–312
8. Goldblatt H, Soames KN (1923) A study of rats on a normal diet irradiated daily by the mercury vapor quartz lamp or kept in darkness. Biochem J 17:294–297
9. Hess AF, Weinstock M (1925) The antirachitic value of irradiated cholesterol and phytosterol. II. Further evidence of change in biological activity. Methods Enzymol 64:181–191
10. Windaus A, Linsert O, Luttringhaus A, Weidlich G (1932) Über das Krystallisierte Vitamin D_2. Justus Liebigs Ann Chem 492:226–231
11. Windaus A, Schenck F, Werder vF (1936) Über das antirachitisch wirksame Bestrahlungsprodukt aus 7-Dehydrocholesterin. Hoppe Seylers Z Physiol Chem 241:100–103
12. Brockmann H (1936) Die Isolierung des Antirachitischen Vitamins aus Thunfischleberöl. Hoppe Seylers Z Physiol Chem 245:96–102
13. Midland MM, Plumet J, Okamura WH (1993) Effect of C20 stereochemistry on the conformational profile of the side chains of vitamin D analogs. Bioorg Med Chem Lett 3:1799–1804
14. Wing RM, Okamura WH, Pirio MR, et al (1974) Vitamin D_3: conformations of vitamin D_3, $1\alpha,25$-dihydroxyvitamin D_3, and dihydrotachysterol₃. Science 186:939–941
15. Bouillon R, Okamura WH, Norman AW (1995) Structure-function relationships in the vitamin D endocrine system. Endocr Rev 16:200–257

16. Pols HAP, Birkenhäger JC, van Leeuwen JPTM (1994) Vitamin D analogues: from molecule to clinical application. Clin Endocrinol (Oxf) 40:285–292

17. Okamura WH, Palenzuela JA, Plumet J, Midland MM (1992) Vitamin D: structure-function analyses and the design of analogs. J Cell Biochem 49:10–18

18. Norman AW, Litwack G (1987) Hormones. Academic Press, Orlando, FL, pp 355–396

19. Anonymous (1960) Definitive rules for the nomenclature of amino acids, steroids, vitamins and carotenoids. J Am Chem Soc 82:5575–5586

20. Norman AW, DeLuca HF (1963) The preparation of ^{3}H-vitamins D_2 and D_3 and their localization in the rat. Biochemistry 2:1160–1168

21. Norman AW (1968) The mode of action of vitamin D. Biol Rev Camb Philos Soc 43:97–137

22. O'Malley BW (1990) The steroid receptor superfamily: more excitement predicted for the future. Mol Endocrinol 4:363–369

23. Gronemeyer H (1992) Control of transcription activation by steroid hormone receptors. FASEB J 6:2524–2529

24. Norman AW, Roth J, Orci L (1982) The vitamin D endocrine system: steroid metabolism, hormone receptors and biological response (calcium binding proteins). Endocr Rev 3:331–366

25. Reichel H, Koeffler HP, Norman AW (1989) The role of the vitamin D endocrine system in health and disease. N Engl J Med 320:980–991

26. Norman AW, Hurwitz S (1993) The role of the vitamin D endocrine system in avian bone biology. J Nutr 123 (suppl):310–316

27. VanBaelen H, Allewaert K, Bouillon R (1988) New aspects of the plasma carrier protein for 25-hydroxycholecalciferol in vertebrates. Ann N Y Acad Sci 538:60–68

28. Henry HL, Norman AW (1978) Vitamin D: two dihydroxylated metabolites are required for normal chicken egg hatchability. Science 201:835–837

29. Norman AW, Henry HL, Malluche HH (1980) 24R,25-Dihydroxyvitamin D_3 and 1α,25-dihydroxyvitamin D_3 are both indispensable for calcium and phosphorus homeostasis. Life Sci 27:229–237

30. Norman AW, Leathers VL, Bishop JE (1983) Studies on the mode of action of calciferol (XLVIII) Normal egg hatchability requires the simultaneous administration to the hen of 1α,25-dihydroxyvitamin D_3 and 24R,25-dihydroxyvitamin D_3. J Nutr 113:2505–2515

31. Henry HL, Norman AW (1984) Vitamin D: metabolism and biological action. Annu Rev Nutr 4:493–520

32. Norman AW, Henry HL (1993) Vitamin D: metabolism and mechanism of action. In Favus MJ (ed), Primer on the metabolic bone diseases and disorders of mineral metabolism. Raven Press, New York, pp 63–70

33. Kawauchi H, Sasaki J, Adachi T, et al (1994) Cloning and nucleotide sequence of a bacterial cytochrome P-450$_{VD25}$ gene encoding vitamin D_3-25-hydroxylase. Biochim Biophys Acta 1219:179–183

34. Henry HL, Dutta C, Cunningham N, et al (1992) The cellular and molecular regulation of $1,25(OH)_2D_3$ production. J Steroid Biochem Mol Biol 41:401–407

35. Henry HL, Midgett RJ, Norman AW (1974) Studies on calciferol metabolism X: regulation of 25-hydroxyvitamin D_3-1-hydroxylase, in vivo. J Biol Chem 249:7584–7592

36. Baxter LA, DeLuca HF (1976) Stimulation of 25-hydroxyvitamin D_3-1alpha-hydroxylase by phosphate depletion. J Biol Chem 251:3158–3161

37. Minghetti PP, Norman AW (1988) $1,25(OH)_2$-vitamin D_3 receptors: gene regulation and genetic circuitry. FASEB J 2:3043–3053

38. Nemere I, Norman AW (1991) Transport of calcium. In Field M, Frizzel RA (eds), Handbook of physiology. American Physiological Society, Bethesda, MD, pp 337–360.

39. Freedman LP, Arce V, Perez-Fernandez R (1994) DNA sequences that act as high affinity targets for the vitamin D_3 receptor in the absence of the retinoid X receptor. Mol Endocrinol 8:265–273

40. Liu M, Freedman LP (1994) Transcriptional synergism between the vitamin D_3 receptor and other nonreceptor transcription factors. Mol Endocrinol 8:1593–1604

41. Hannah SS, Norman AW (1994) 1,25-Dihydroxyvitamin D_3 regulated expression of the eukaryotic genome. Nutr Rev 52:376–382

42. Nemere I, Yoshimoto Y, Norman AW (1984) Studies on the mode of action of calciferol. LIV. Calcium transport in perfused duodena from normal chicks: enhancement with 14 minutes of exposure to 1,25-dihydroxyvitamin D_3. Endocrinology 115:1476–1483

43. de Boland AR, Norman AW (1990) Evidence for involvement of protein kinase C and cyclic adenosine 3′, 5′ monophosphate-dependent protein kinase in the 1,25-dihydroxyvitamin D_3-mediated rapid stimulation of intestinal calcium transport (transcaltachia). Endocrinology 127:39–45

44. Norman AW, Nemere I, Muralidharan RK, Okamura WH (1992) 1β,25(OH)$_2$-vitamin D_3 is an antagonist of 1α,25(OH)$_2$-vitamin D_3 stimulated transcaltachia (the rapid hormonal stimulation of intestinal calcium transport). Biochem Biophys Res Commun 189:1450–1456

45. Norman AW, Okamura WH, Farach-Carson MC, et al (1993) Structure-function studies of 1,25-dihydroxyvitamin D_3 and the vitamin D endocrine system: 1,25-dihydroxy-pentadeuterio-previtamin D_3 (as a 6-s-cis analog) stimulates nongenomic but not genomic biological responses. J Biol Chem 268:13811–13819

46. Caffrey JM, Farach-Carson MC (1989) Vitamin D_3 metabolites modulate dihydropyridine-sensitive calcium currents in clonal rat osteosarcoma cells. J Biol Chem 264:20265–20274

47. Baran DT, Sorensen AM, Shalhoub V, et al (1991) 1,25-Dihydroxyvitamin D_3 rapidly increases cytosolic calcium in clonal rat osteosarcoma cells lacking the vitamin D receptor. J Bone Miner Res 6:1269–1275

48. Farach-Carson MC, Sergeev IN, Norman AW (1991) Nongenomic actions of 1,25-dihydroxyvitamin D_3 in rat osteosarcoma cells: structure-function studies using ligand analogs. Endocrinology 129:1876–1884

49. Lieberherr M, Grosse B, Duchambon P, Drüeke T (1989) A functional cell surface type receptor is required for the early action of 1,25-dihydroxyvitamin D_3 on the phosphoinositide metabolism in rat enterocytes. J Biol Chem 264:20403–20406

50. Baran DT, Sorensen AM, Honeyman RW, et al (1990) 1α,25-Dihydroxyvitamin D_3-induced increments in hepatocyte cytosolic calcium and lysophosphatidylinositol: inhibition by pertussis toxin and 1β,25-dihydroxyvitamin D_3. J Bone Miner Res 5:517–524

51. Drittant L, de Boland AR, Boland RL (1987) Changes in muscle lipid-metabolism induced in vitro by 1,25-dihydroxyvitamin-D_3. Biochim Biophys Acta 918:83–92

52. Lowe KE, Maiyar AC, Norman AW (1992) Vitamin D-mediated gene expression. Crit Rev Eukaryot Gene Exp 2:65–109

53. Pike JW (1991) Vitamin D_3 receptors: structure and function in transcription. Annu Rev Nutr 11:189–216

54. Nemere I, Dormanen MC, Hammond MW, et al (1994) Identification of a specific binding protein for 1α,25-

dihydroxyvitamin D_3 in basal-lateral membranes of chick intestinal epithelium and relationship to transcaltachia. J Biol Chem 269:23750–23756

55. Baran DT, Ray R, Sorensen AM, et al (1994) Binding characteristics of a membrane receptor that recognizes $1\alpha,25$-dihydroxyvitamin D_3 and its epimer, $1\beta,25$-dihydroxyvitamin D_3. J Cell Biochem 56:510–517

56. Khare S, Tien X-Y, Wilson D, et al (1994) The role of protein kinase-$C\alpha$ in the activation of particulate guanylate cyclase by $1\alpha,25$-dihydroxyvitamin D_3 in CaCo-2 cells. Endocrinology 135:277–283

57. Bissonnette M, Tien X-Y, Niedziela SM, et al (1994) $1,25(OH)_2$ vitamin D_3 activates PKC-α in Caco-2 cells: a mechanism to limit seco-steroid-induced rise in $[Ca^{2+}]_i$. Am J Physiol 267:G465–475

58. Norman AW, Bouillon R, Farach-Carson MC, et al (1993) Demonstration that $1\beta,25$-dihydroxyvitamin D_3 is an antagonist of the nongenomic but not genomic biological responses and biological profile of the three A-ring diastereomers of $1\alpha,25$-dihydroxyvitamin D_3. J Biol Chem 268:20022–20030

59. Dormanen MC, Bishop JE, Hammond MW, et al (1994) Nonnuclear effects of the steroid hormone $1\alpha,25(OH)_2$-vitamin D_3: analogs are able to functionally differentiate between nuclear and membrane receptors. Biochem Biophys Res Commun 201:394–401

60. Okamura WH, Midland MM, Hammond MW, et al (1994) Conformation and related topological features of vitamin D: structure-function relationships. In Norman AW, Bouillon R, Thomasset M (eds), Vitamin D, a pluripotent steroid hormone: structural studies, molecular endocrinology and clinical applications. Walter de Gruyter, Berlin, pp 12–20.

61. Norman AW (1972) Problems relating to the definition of an international unit for vitamin D and its metabolites. J Nutr 102:1243–1246

62. Webb AR, Holick MF (1988) The role of sunlight in the cutaneous production of vitamin D_3. Annu Rev Nutr 8:375–399

63. Webb AR, Pilbeam C, Hanafin N, Holick MF (1990) An evaluation of the relative contributions of exposure to sunlight and of diet to the circulating concentrations of 25-hydroxyvitamin D in an elderly nursing home population in Boston. Am J Clin Nutr 51:1075–1081

64. Holick MF (1995) Environmental factors that influence the cutaneous production of vitamin D. Am J Clin Nutr 61(suppl):638S–645S

65. Yendt ER (1970) Vitamin D, part II. XIII. Pharmacological activities of vitamin D. Int Encyclop Pharm 1 section 51:139–195

66. Subcommittee on the Tenth Edition of the RDAs, Food and Nutrition Board (1989) Recommended dietary allowances. National Academy Press, Washington, DC

67. Collins ED, Norman AW (1990) Vitamin D. In Machlin LJ (ed), Handbook of vitamins. Marcel Dekker, New York, pp 59–98

68. Jacobus CH, Holick MF, Shao Q, et al (1992) Hypervitaminosis D associated with drinking milk. N Engl J Med 326:1173–1177

69. Bhattacharyya MH, DeLuca HF (1973) The regulation of rat liver calciferol-25-hydroxylase. J Biol Chem 248:2969–2973

70. Hughes MR, Baylink DJ, Jones PG, Haussler MR (1976) Radioligand receptor assay for 25-hydroxyvitamin D_2/D_3 and $1alpha,25$-dihydroxyvitamin D_2/D_3. J Clin Invest 58:61–70

71. Brumbaugh PF, Haussler MR (1973) 1Alpha,25-dihydroxyvitamin D_3 receptor: competitive binding of vitamin D analogs. Life Sci 13:1737–1746

72. Hartenbower DL, Stanley TM, Coburn JW, Norman AW (1977) Serum and renal histologic changes in the rat following administration of toxic amounts of 1,25-dihydroxyvitamin D_3. In Norman AW, Schaeferk, Coburn JW, et al (eds), Vitamin D: biochemical, chemical and clinical aspects related to calcium metabolism. Walter de Gruyter, Berlin, pp 587–589

73. Bikle DD (1992) Clinical counterpoint: vitamin D: new actions, new analogs, new therapeutic potential. Endocr Rev 13:765–784

Chapter 13

Vitamin E

Ronald J. Sokol

The term vitamin E applies to a family of eight related compounds, the tocopherols and the tocotrienols, which consist of substituted hydroxylated ring systems (chromanol ring) linked to a phytyl side chain. Evans[1] proposed the name tocopherol, which means to carry (*pherein*) to birth (*tocos*), because this vitamin was necessary for pregnant dam rats to reproduce and bear young.

The four major forms of vitamin E are designated alpha, beta, delta, and gamma, on the basis of the number and position of methyl groups on the chromanol ring (Figure 1). The tocotrienols have three double bonds in the phytyl side chain but otherwise resemble the tocopherols. The tocotrienols are less widely distributed in nature than the tocopherols, although they are present in palm oil. Tocotrienols may have biological activity comparable with that of the tocopherols but are generally considered of less nutritional importance.

Esterification of the phenol group on the chromanol ring with acetate, succinate, or nicotinate protects the tocopherol molecule from oxidation. However, because this phenol group is the active site for the antioxidant activity of vitamin E, hydrolysis of tocopheryl esters is necessary before the compound can become bioactive.

Tocopherols contain three asymmetric chiral centers at the number 2 position of the chromanol ring and the number 4' and 8' positions on the phytyl side chain. Therefore, there are eight possible stereoisomers of each tocopherol. Only one of these stereoisomers is abundant in nature, the *RRR* isomer, which is also known as *d*-α-tocopherol. The R rotation at the number 2 position confers greater bioactivity to the molecule than does the S rotation. When vitamin E is synthesized, an equal mixture of the eight stereoisomers is obtained, the product being designated all-racemic α-tocopherol (previously called *dl*-α-tocopherol).[2] The *RRR* isomer is frequently called the natural form of α-tocopherol because it is the predominant form in nature.

Current methods for analysis of plasma or tissues for tocopherol are based on high-performance liquid chromatography (HPLC).[3,4] This technique permits very rapid analysis of plasma and other tissue extracts; α-, γ-, and δ-tocopherol can be separated easily, with simultaneous measurements of retinol and β-carotene also possible. This methodology can also be used to determine the vitamin E content of foods, oils, and other substances. Gas chromatography methods have also been described but are not routinely used.

Absorption, Transport, Storage, and Turnover

Absorption. Dietary vitamin E is primarily composed of α- and γ-tocopherol, of which ≈20–50% is normally absorbed. Because of its hydrophobic nature, vitamin E is absorbed similarly to dietary fat.[5-7] It must be solubilized by bile acids secreted from the liver so that it can traverse the aqueous environment in the intestinal lumen to reach the surface of absorptive intestinal cells. Esters of vitamin E are hydrolyzed before absorption by pancreatic esterases and intestinal mucosal esterases. Vitamin E is absorbed into the intestinal mucosal cell by a nonsaturable, non-carrier-mediated, passive diffusion process. Vitamin E may also be absorbed with intact micelles that penetrate mucosal cells.

Once inside the enterocyte, the free α- and γ-tocopherol are incorporated with other products of dietary lipid digestion and apolipoproteins produced by intestinal cells into chylomicrons, which are transported via mesenteric lymphatics and the thoracic duct into the systemic circulation (Figure 2). Thus, any pathologic process that impairs digestion and absorption of dietary fat can lead to poor absorption and possible deficiency of vitamin E.

Because pancreatic secretions are required for the digestion of dietary fat, any problem in the pancreas that reduces pancreatic enzyme output (e.g., cystic fibrosis) can result in vitamin E malabsorption.[8] The requirement for bile acids is absolute, so that cholestatic liver diseases will result in vitamin E malabsorption as well.[9] Any disease that decreases the surface area of intestinal cells (e.g., celiac disease) or the total length of the intestine (e.g., surgical resection of intestine) can also result in vitamin E malabsorption.[10] Defects in the synthesis or assembly of chylomicrons in intestinal cells will cause vitamin E malabsorption, as will blockage or abnormal formation of intestinal lymphatic channels.[11]

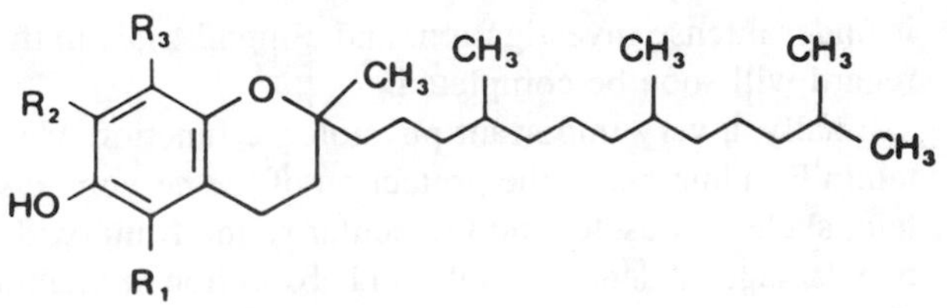

R₃, R₂, HO, R₁, CH₃, O, CH₃, CH₃, CH₃, CH₃, CH₃

COMPOUND	R₁	R₂	R₃
α-tocopherol	CH₃	CH₃	CH₃
β-tocopherol	CH₃	H	CH₃
γ-tocopherol	H	CH₃	CH₃
δ-tocopherol	H	H	CH₃

Figure 1. Chemical structure of the four tocopherols.

Transport. Vitamin E is initially transported in chylomicrons, but as these are hydrolyzed by lipoprotein lipase in the circulation, vitamin E may be released to tissues or transferred to high-density lipoproteins (HDL).[6,7] Most of the absorbed vitamin E (both α- and γ-tocopherol), however, returns to the liver in chylomicron remnants as they are taken up by hepatocytes.

In the hepatocyte, the vitamin E is released from these lipoproteins and is bound to the hepatic tocopherol transfer protein, a 30-kDa cytosolic protein.[12,13] This protein putatively discriminates between the various forms of vitamin E that enter the hepatocyte,[12] with preferential secretion into very-low-density lipoproteins (VLDLs) of the *RRR* stereoisomer of α-tocopherol.[14] Gamma-tocopherol and other stereoisomers of α-tocopherol do not appear in substantial amounts in VLDL. Thus, tocopherol entering the hepatocyte in chylomicrons remnants first appears in the hepatocyte lysosomes, then appears bound to tocopherol transfer protein in cytosol, where it is transferred to endoplasmic reticulum or the Golgi for packaging into VLDL.[7]

Once in circulating VLDL, the α-tocopherol can be transferred to HDL during lipolysis of VLDL in the circulation, can travel with the VLDL core during conversion to LDL in the circulation, or can return to the liver in VLDL remnants. A small amount of α- and γ-tocopherol entering the liver can also appear in bile, presumably as excretory products.[14] During a fasting state, most α-tocopherol is carried by LDL in males and by HDL in females.[15] Tocopherol transfer from lipoproteins to tissues may occur during lipolysis of chylomicrons and VLDL by lipoprotein lipase and hepatic triacylglycerol lipase, by receptor binding of LDL to target tissues, and by nonspecific binding of LDL to various cells.[6]

Because of its high lipid solubility and transport in lipoproteins, there is a strong correlation between plasma tocopherol concentrations and the plasma total lipid concentration.[16] The correlation with total plasma cholesterol is less strong. For this reason, it has been proposed that serum vitamin E levels be normalized to the total plasma lipid level to determine tocopherol status.[16,17] This is of particular importance when patients have either high or low plasma lipid values.[12]

In normal adults, plasma α-tocopherol concentration ranges from ≈11.5 to 46 μmol/L (5 to 20 μg/mL) if plasma lipid values are normal. Children and infants have slightly lower values than do adults, particularly preterm infants, who have low circulating levels of serum lipids, approximately half the serum α-tocopherol levels found in adults.[18] The lower limit of normal for adults is 18.6 μmol tocopherol/g total lipid (0.8 mg/g).[16] In children under the age of 12 years, 14.0 μg/g (0.6 mg/g) may indicate vitamin E adequacy.[19] This value is particularly important in assessing vitamin E status in children and adults with chronic cholestatic liver disease in whom serum lipid levels may be elevated two- to threefold. In these patients, a serum vitamin E level may be in the normal range despite the presence of deficiency, but the ratio of vitamin E to total lipid will be low and indicate deficiency.[17]

Storage. The liver functions as a rapid turnover store of vitamin E, never accumulating large amounts because of the function of the tocopherol transfer protein. Adipose tissue is clearly a long-term store of vitamin E; however, vitamin E accumulates slowly and is released slowly from adipose tissue. Muscle accounts for much of the body stores of tocopherol. Vitamin E is found almost exclusively in the adipose cell fat droplet, all cell membranes, and circulating lipoproteins.

Turnover. Recent studies showed that the apparent half-life in plasma of the *RRR*-α-tocopherol form of vitamin E is ≈48 hours. Approximately 40–50% of the pool of vitamin E is turned over in plasma each day.[20] In animal studies the turnover of vitamin E in brain, spinal cord, heart, testes, and muscle is slow (in the range of 20–80 days), whereas plasma, liver, lung, and kidney have turnover rates of 5–20 days.[21]

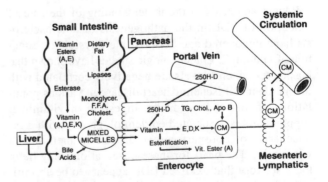

Figure 2. Intestinal absorption of vitamin E (E) and how it compares with absorption of other fat-soluble vitamins [vitamin A (A), vitamin D (D), and vitamin K (K)]. TG, triacylglycerols; CM, chylomicrons; ApoB, apolipoprotein B.

Physiologic Function

The physiologic function of vitamin E is its role as a scavenger of free radicals, thus preventing free radical, or oxidant, damage to polyunsaturated fatty acids in cell membranes, thiol-rich protein constituents of membranes and the cytoskeleton, and nucleic acids.[22,23] Reactive oxygen species and other free radicals are normally formed by numerous cellular enzyme systems, mitochondrial electron transport, and the exposure to various environmental factors, so a complex system of enzymatic and nonenzymatic antioxidants to detoxify free radicals has evolved. Vitamin E is one of the primary factors in this defense system because it is lipid soluble and therefore can directly protect cell membranes. Other antioxidants are vitamin C, β-carotene, and selenium. By reacting with a free radical, the tocopherol molecule is converted into the tocopheroxyl radical, which can be reduced back to tocopherol by either vitamin C or glutathione and possibly by ubiquinone.

The potential physiologic effects of vitamin E are related to its antioxidant activity. In animal models, vitamin E protects against heavy metals, hepatotoxins generating free radicals, and various drugs that cause oxidant injury.[24] Vitamin E can also protect against environmental pollutants such as ozone.[25,26] However, there is no convincing evidence that vitamin E supplements protect human populations against environmental pollutants, although this is being investigated.[26]

Vitamin E is important for normal immune function, particularly the function of T lymphocytes. This has been demonstrated in animal models[27] and in elderly populations in the United States.[28,29] Epidemiologic data suggest that people with low vitamin E intake and plasma levels are at increased risk for certain types of cancer, particularly in lung and breast;[30] however, no studies of vitamin E supplementation in Western populations have yet to show a reduction in cancer risk. Over the next decade many such studies in progress will have been completed.

Recent advances in the understanding of the role of oxidation of LDL in the pathogenesis of atherosclerosis have uncovered another possible physiologic function of vitamin E. Epidemiologic studies have shown that plasma tocopherol levels are negatively correlated with the incidence of ischemic heart disease in various populations of men.[31] In addition, ingestion of vitamin E supplements is associated epidemiologically with a reduced risk of coronary artery disease in men and in women.[32,33] The basis for these observations may lie in the discovery that oxidized LDL appears to be an initiating factor in atherosclerosis.[34] Vitamin E supplementation clearly protects LDL from oxidation by preventing the propagation initiated by free radical attack.[35,36] Whether vitamin E will protect against atherosclerosis

is under intense investigation, and clinical trials in this regard will soon be completed.

Finally, a very important physiologic function of vitamin E in humans is the protection of the nervous system, skeletal muscle, and the ocular retina from oxidative damage.[5] Adequate intake and absorption of vitamin E are necessary for normal development of the human neuromuscular systems and proper functioning of the retina. The production of neurotransmitters in the nervous system is accompanied by generation of large amounts of free radicals, thus vitamin E appears to be essential in preventing damage to mitochondria and axonal membranes of the nervous system caused by free radicals.

Deficiency

At the cellular level. Deficiency of vitamin E at the cellular level is generally accompanied by an increase of lipid peroxidation of cellular membranes. This may lead to decreased energy production by mitochondria, oxidation and mutation of DNA, and alterations of normal transport processes of the plasma membrane. In particular, cells that are exposed to an oxidant stress will show more rapid injury and necrosis when rendered vitamin E deficient. The lipid peroxide by-products produced by vitamin E deficiency may be released from cells and attract white blood cells, activate macrophages, and increase the synthesis of collagen by other cells.

Animal models. Vitamin E deficiency affects many tissues in mammalian and bird models.[37] Impaired male and female fertility occurs in rodents, many animal species develop a necrotizing muscle disease as well as central nervous system and peripheral nerve degeneration, a cardiomyopathy develops in several mammalian species, and hemolysis of red blood cells is also common. The effect of concomitant selenium deficiency magnifies some of these changes. The neuromuscular degeneration described in rhesus monkeys rendered vitamin E deficient closely resembles that observed in vitamin E–deficient humans.[38]

Human vitamin E deficiency. Symptomatic deficiency of vitamin E in humans rarely, if ever, occurs because of inadequate oral intake of this vitamin, probably because of its ubiquitous distribution in nature. However, individuals who have alterations in intestinal absorption of dietary fat are predisposed to malabsorption of vitamin E and subsequent deficiency.[39]

The most common disorders associated with low plasma levels of vitamin E are cystic fibrosis,[8,40] abetalipoproteinemia,[11] chronic cholestatic liver diseases,[39,41] celiac disease, short bowel syndrome,[42] and other forms of chronic diarrhea. The most severe malabsorption of vitamin E occurs when bile flow is impaired or when intestinal lipoprotein synthesis is defective. When malabsorption of vitamin E occurs in adults, it takes several years before plasma vitamin E levels decrease to a deficient range because of the presence of body stores. The mature nervous system of the adult is relatively resistant to vitamin E deficiency, so that it may take 5–10 years before neurologic abnormalities may appear.[5] In contrast, children who have vitamin E malabsorption from infancy, such as those with biliary atresia or other cholestatic liver diseases, develop profound vitamin E deficiency early on in life and rapidly develop neurologic symptoms if the vitamin E deficiency is untreated.[41] Thus, the developing nervous system appears to be much more susceptible to the effects of vitamin E deficiency.

Vitamin E deficiency primarily affects the posterior columns of the spinal cord, the third and fourth cranial nerve nuclei, large caliber myelinated axons of peripheral nerves, the nucleus gracillus and cuneatus of the brain stem, and eventually muscle and retina. Thus, the typical neurologic findings in vitamin E deficiency include loss of deep tendon reflexes, impaired vibratory and position sensation, alterations in balance and coordination, impaired movement of the eyes (ophthalmoplegia), muscle weakness, and visual field disturbances.[5,41]

If the vitamin E deficiency is corrected before the first few years of life, all symptoms can be reversed or prevented.[43,44] If the vitamin E deficiency is not detected until the neurologic damage is advanced, limited improvement can be expected with repletional therapy. There is some evidence that vitamin E deficiency can adversely affect the cognitive as well as motor development of young children.

Hemolytic anemia (breakdown of red blood cells) has been described in preterm infants who received diets rich in polyunsaturated fatty acids (the substrate for lipid peroxidation) and supplementary iron (a pro-oxidant).[45] Subsequently, infant formulas have been modified to prevent this problem. Mild hemolysis without anemia has also been observed in patients with cystic fibrosis and vitamin E deficiency.

Preterm infants are born with low tissue levels of tocopherol and have impaired intestinal absorption of vitamin E. Because preterm infants are exposed to many oxidant stresses, it was proposed that many of the problems unique to this population might benefit from vitamin E supplementation. Treatment with large doses of vitamin E failed to significantly alter the course of the respiratory distress syndrome, hyperbilirubinemia, and retinopathy of prematurity. In preterm infants with intracranial hemorrhage (a relatively common, serious complication in very-low-birth-weight infants <1500 g), several studies suggest a benefit of intramuscular injections of vitamin E given shortly after birth.[46,47] However, this has not been adopted as standard practice, in part because of possible toxicity of vitamin E in preterm infants.[48]

Plasma levels of vitamin E are relatively low in patients with several inherited hematologic disorders in which hemolytic anemia occurs because of defective hemoglobin structure, abnormal red blood cell structure, or deficient antioxidant defenses in red blood cells.[49,50] These disorders include thalassemia, sickle cell anemia, and glucose-6-phosphate dehydrogenase deficiency. A possible overutilization of vitamin E exists in these conditions caused by the breakdown of red blood cells or the deficiency of other antioxidant pathways. Vitamin E supplements have slowed down the rate of hemolysis in some of these patients.[50]

There has been recent interest in the effects of low-normal vitamin E status and the risk for atherosclerosis, cancer, the formation of cataracts, and other degenerative processes involved with aging. Epidemiologic studies suggest that people with lower vitamin E and other antioxidant intake and plasma levels may be at increased risk for certain types of cancer and for atherosclerosis.[30–33] Conversely, studies suggest that supplementation with antioxidants may decrease the risk of these and other degenerative processes.[51] Large controlled studies in progress will help shed light on the utility of vitamin E and other antioxidants for these disorders. Until more conclusive studies have been reported, antioxidants and vitamin E cannot be recommended to prevent these disorders.

Requirements

The recommended intake of forms of vitamin E depends, to some extent, on the bioactivity of each form. Alpha-tocopherol is the most bioactive of all forms, with β-tocopherol having 25–50% bioactivity, γ-tocopherol having 10–35%, and α-tocotrienol having ≈30%.[52]

One international unit of vitamin E is defined as the activity of 1 mg of all-racemic α-tocopheryl acetate. One α-tocopherol equivalent is the activity of 1 mg of *RRR*-α-tocopherol. To estimate α-tocopherol equivalents of other forms of vitamin E, milligrams of β-tocopherol should be multiplied by 0.5, milligrams of γ-tocopherol by 0.1, milligrams of α-tocotrienol by 0.3, and milligrams of all-racemic α-tocopherol by 0.74.

The current recommended dietary allowance in the 1989 revised National Research Council recommendations is 10 mg of α-tocopherol equivalents for adult males, 8 mg for adult females, 10 mg for pregnant females, 12 mg for lactating females, and 3 mg for infants increasing progressively to 7 mg for children aged 7–10 years.[53] Another factor that needs to be considered in recommending vitamin E intake is the amount of polyunsaturated fatty acids in the diet. Increasing amounts of polyunsaturated fatty acids increase the vitamin E requirement because of the propensity of polyunsaturated fatty acids to undergo lipid peroxidation. Approximately

0.4 mg of α-tocopherol equivalents for each gram of polyunsaturated fatty acid has been suggested to be adequate in adult humans. Infant formulas should have a similar balance of α-tocopherol and polyunsaturated fatty acids.

Food and Other Sources

The richest sources of vitamin E in the U.S. diet are vegetable oils (soy bean, corn, cottonseed, and safflower), products made from these oils (such as margarine, shortening, and mayonnaise), wheat germ, nuts, and other grains. Meats, fish, animal fat, and most fruits and vegetables contain little vitamin E; green leafy vegetables supply appreciable amounts. Some of the oil products contain more γ- than α-tocopherol. Considerable losses of the tocopherol content of food may occur during processing, storage, and preparation.

Excess Toxicity

Compared with the other fat-soluble vitamins, vitamin E is relatively nontoxic when taken orally. Most of the reports of adverse symptoms are subjective and have not been upheld in large controlled series.[54,55] Large intakes of vitamin E might interfere with absorption of vitamin A and vitamin K. More importantly, intakes of vitamin E >1200 mg of tocopherol equivalents per day can interfere with metabolism of vitamin K, thus potentiating the anticoagulation effect of drugs such as Coumadin.[56]

Large intravenous doses of vitamin E have caused an increased risk of sepsis (both bacterial and fungal) in premature infants, most likely because of inhibition of normal neutrophil bacterial and fungal killing.[48] Oral preparations of vitamin E with high osmolality have been associated with an increased risk of necrotizing enterocolitis in preterm infants, which is probably due to the osmolality of the formulation.[57] An intravenous form of vitamin E caused many preterm infant deaths in 1983, which may have had more to do with the solubilizing agent (polysorbate) than with the vitamin E.[58] This preparation was taken off the market.

In adults, 200–800 mg of tocopherol equivalents per day are well tolerated without adverse effects. Occasionally, gastrointestinal upset of short duration may occur, but it also occurs in patients taking the placebo in controlled trials.[54] Large doses (>800–1200 mg/day) of vitamin E may decrease platelet adhesion to some extent, and therefore might lead to postsurgery bleeding.[56] It is therefore advisable to discourage large doses of vitamin E supplements for the 2 weeks before and after surgery. Despite this decrease in platelet function, no increased risk of hemorrhagic stroke or other bleeding problems has been identified in large trials in adults.[54]

Summary

Vitamin E is the major lipid-soluble, membrane-localized antioxidant in humans. Deficiency states in humans have been well described, and the possible use of vitamin E and other antioxidants to retard the aging process and various degenerative diseases is under investigation. Although there is no current justification for recommending routine supplementation with more than standard doses of vitamin E, larger doses are generally well tolerated.

Acknowledgment

Supported in part by NIH grants RR00069, RR00123, R01DK38446, and IP30AM34914, and the Abbey Bennett Liver Research Fund.

References

1. Evans HM (1963) The pioneer history of vitamin E. Vitam Horm 20:379–387
2. Kasparek S (1980) Chemistry of tocopherols and tocotrienols. In Machlin LJ (ed), Vitamin E, a comprehensive treatise. Marcel Dekker, Inc., New York, pp 7–66
3. Bieri JG, Tolliver TJ, Catignani GL (1979) Simultaneous determination of alpha-tocopherol and retinol in plasma or red cells by high pressure liquid chromatography. Am J Clin Nutr 32:2143-2149
4. Lang JK, Gohil K, Packer L (1986) Simultaneous determination of tocopherols, ubiquinols, and ubiquinones in blood, plasma, tissue homogenates, and subcellular fractions. Anal Biochem 157:106–116
5. Sokol RJ (1993) Vitamin E deficiency and neurological disorders. In Packer L, Fuchs J (eds), Vitamin E in health and disease. Marcel Dekker, New York, pp 815–850
6. Traber MG, Cohn W, Muller DPR (1993) Absorption, transport and delivery to tissues. In Packer L, Fuchs J (eds), Vitamin E in health and disease. Marcel Dekker, New York, pp 35–51
7. Kayden HJ, Traber MG (1993) Absorption, lipoprotein transport, and regulation of plasma concentrations of vitamin E in humans. J Lipid Res 34:343–358
8. Sokol RJ, Reardon MC, Accurso FJ, et al (1989) Fat-soluble vitamin status during the first year of life in infants with cystic fibrosis identified by screening of newborns. Am J Clin Nutr 50:1064–1071
9. Sokol RJ, Heubi JE, Iannaccone S, et al (1983) Mechanism causing vitamin E deficiency in children with chronic cholestasis. Gastroenterology 85:1172–1182
10. Muller DPR, Harries JT, Lloyd JK (1974) The relative importance of the factors involved in the absorption of vitamin E in children. Gut 15:966
11. Rader DJ, Brewer HB Jr (1993) Abetalipoproteinemia—new insights into lipoprotein assembly and vitamin E metabolism from a rare genetic disease. JAMA 270:865–869
12. Sato Y, Hagiwara K, Arai H, Inoue K (1991) Purification and characterization of the α-tocopherol transfer protein from rat liver. FEBS Lett 288:41–45
13. Arita M, Sato Y, Miyata A, et al (1995) Human α-tocopherol transfer protein: cDNA cloning, expression and chromosomal localization. Biochem J 306:437–443

14. Traber MG, Kayden HJ (1989) Preferential incorporation of α-tocopherol vs. γ-tocopherol in human lipoproteins. Am J Clin Nutr 49:517–526

15. Behrens WA, Thompson JN, Madere R (1982) Distribution of alpha-tocopherol in human plasma lipoproteins. Am J Clin Nutr 35:691–696

16. Horwitt MK, Harvey CC, Dahm CH Jr, Searcy MT (1972) Relationship between tocopherol and serum lipid levels for determination of nutritional adequacy. Ann NY Acad Sci 203:223–236

17. Sokol RJ, Heubi JE, Iannaccone ST, et al (1984) Vitamin E deficiency with normal serum vitamin E concentrations in children with chronic cholestasis. N Engl J Med 310:1209–1212

18. Mino K, Kitagawa M, Nakagawa S (1985) Red blood cell tocopherol concentrations in a normal population of Japanese children and premature infants in relation to assessment of vitamin E status. Am J Clin Nutr 41:631–638

19. Farrell PM (1980) Deficiency states, pharmacological effects, and nutrient requirements. In Machlin LJ (ed), Vitamin E, a comprehensive treatise. Marcel Dekker, New York, pp 520–620

20. Traber MG, Ramakrishnan R, Kayden HJ (1994) Human plasma vitamin E kinetics demonstrate rapid recycling of plasma RRR α-tocopherol. Proc Natl Acad Sci USA 91:10005–10008

21. Burton GW, Ingold KU (1993) Biokinetics of vitamin E using deuterated tocopherols. In Packer L, Fuchs J (eds), Vitamin E in health and disease. Marcel Dekker, New York, pp 329–344

22. Packer L, Kagan VE (1993) Vitamin E: the antioxidant harvesting center of membranes and lipoproteins. In Packer L, Fuchs J (eds), Vitamin E in health and disease. Marcel Dekker, New York, pp 179–192

23. Tappel AL (1962) Vitamin E as a biological antioxidant. Vitam Horm 20:493–510

24. Pascoe GA, Reed DJ (1987) Vitamin E protection against chemical-induced cell injury. II. Evidence for a threshold effect of cellular alpha-tocopherol in prevention of adriamycin toxicity. Arch Biochem Biophys 256:159–166

25. Konings AWT (1986) Mechanism of ozone toxicity in cultured cells. 1. Reduced clonogenic ability of polyunsaturated fatty acid-supplemented fibroblasts. Effect of vitamin E. J Toxicol Environ Health 18:491–497

26. Pryor WA (1991) Can vitamin E protect humans against the pathological effects of ozone in smog? Am J Clin Nutr 53:702–722

27. Gogu SR, Blumberg JB (1992) Vitamin E enhances murine natural killer cell cytotoxicity against YAC-1 tumor cells. J Nutr Immunol 1:31–38

28. Meydani SN, Barklund PM, Liu S, et al (1990) Vitamin E supplementation enhances cell-mediated immunity in healthy elderly subjects. Am J Clin Nutr 1990; 52:557–563

29. Penn ND, Purkins L, Kelleher J, et al (1991) The effect of dietary supplementation with vitamins A, C and E on cell-mediated immune function in elderly long-stay patients: a randomized controlled trial. Age Ageing 20:169–174

30. Knekt P (1993) Epidemiology of vitamin E: evidence for anticancer effects in humans. In Packer L, Fuchs J (eds), Vitamin E in health and disease. Marcel Dekker, New York, pp 513–527

31. Gey KF, Puska P, Jordan P, Moser UK (1991) Inverse correlation between plasma vitamin E and mortality from ischemic heart disease in cross-cultural epidemiology. Am J Clin Nutr 53: 326S–334S.

32. Rimm EB, Stampfer MJ, Ascherio A, et al (1993) Vitamin E consumption and the risk of coronary heart disease in men. N Engl J Med 328:1450–1456

33. Stampfer MJ, Hennekens CH, Manson JE, et al (1993) Vitamin E consumption and the risk of coronary heart disease in women. N Engl J Med 328:1444–1449

34. Steinberg D, Parthasarathy S, Carew TE, et al (1989) Beyond cholesterol: modifications of low-density lipoprotein that increase its atherogenicity. N Engl J Med 320:915–924

35. Esterbauer H, Dieber-Rotheneder M, Striegl G, Waeg G (1991) Role of vitamin E in preventing the oxidation of low density lipoprotein. Am J Clin Nutr 53:314S–321S

36. Jialal I, Grundy SM (1992) Effect of dietary supplementation with alpha-tocopherol on the oxidative modification of low density lipoprotein. J Lipid Res 33:899–906

37. Nelson JS (1980) Pathology of vitamin E deficiency. In Machlin LJ (ed), Vitamin E, a comprehensive treatise. Marcel Dekker, New York, pp 397–428

38. Nelson JS (1983) Neuropathological studies of chronic vitamin E deficiency in mammals including humans. Ciba Found Symp 101:92–105

39. Sokol RJ (1994) Fat soluble vitamins and their importance in patients with cholestatic liver diseases. Gastroenterol Clin North Am 23:673–705

40. Elias E, Muller DPR, Scott J (1981) Association of spino-cerebellar disorders with cystic fibrosis or chronic childhood cholestasis and very low serum vitamin E. Lancet 2:1319–1321

41. Sokol RJ, Guggenheim MA, Heubi JE, et al (1985) Frequency and clinical progression of the vitamin E deficiency neurologic disorder in children with prolonged neonatal cholestasis. Am J Dis Child 139:1211–1215

42. Satya-Murtl S, Howard L, Krohel G, Wolf B (1986) The spectrum of neurological disorder from vitamin E deficiency. Neurology 36:917–921

43. Sokol RJ, Guggenheim MA, Iannaccone ST, et al (1985) Improved neurologic function following long-term correction of vitamin E deficiency in children with chronic cholestasis. N Engl J Med 313:1580–1586

44. Sokol RJ, Butler-Simon N, Conner C, et al (1993) Multicenter trial of d-alpha tocopherol polyethylene glycol-1000 succinate for treatment of vitamin E deficiency in children with chronic cholestasis. Gastroenterology 104:1727–1735

45. Oski FA, Barness LA (1967) Vitamin E deficiency: a previously unrecognized cause of hemolytic anemia in the premature infant. J Pediatr 70:211–220

46. Speer ME, Blifeld C, Rudolph AJ, et al (1984) Intraventricular hemorrhage and vitamin E in the very low-birth-weight infant: evidence for efficacy of early intramuscular vitamin E administration. Pediatrics 74:1107–1112

47. Sinha S, Davies J, Toner N, et al (1987) Vitamin E supplementation reduces frequency of periventricular haemorrhage in very preterm babies. Lancet 1:466–471

48. Johnson L, Bowen FW, Abbasi S, et al (1985) Relationship of prolonged pharmacologic serum levels of vitamin E to incidence of sepsis and necrotizing enterocolitis in infants with birth weight 1500 grams or less. Pediatrics 75:619–638

49. Natta C, Machlin LJ (1979) Plasma levels of tocopherol in sickle cell anemia subjects. Am J Clin Nutr 32:1359–1362

50. Rachmilewitz EA, Shifter A, Kakane I (1979) Vitamin E deficiency in beta-thalassemia major: changes in hematological and biochemical parameters after a therapeutic trial with alpha-tocopherol. Am J Clin Nutr 32:1850–1858

51. Blot WJ, Li J-Y, Taylor PR, et al (1993) Nutrition intervention trials in Linxian, China: supplementation with specific vitamin/mineral combinations, cancer incidence, and disease-specific mortality in the general population. J Natl Cancer Inst 85:1483–1492

52. Dillard CJ, Gavino VC, Tappel AL (1983) Relative antioxidant effectiveness of α-tocopherol and γ-tocopherol in iron-loaded rats. J Nutr 131:2266–2273

53. National Research Council (1989) Recommended dietary allowances, 10th ed. National Academy Press, Washington, DC, pp 99–107

54. Bendich A, Machlin L (1988) Safety of oral intake of vitamin E. Am J Clin Nutr 48:612–619

55. Farrell PM, Bieri JG (1975) Megavitamin E supplementation in man. Am J Clin Nutr 28:1381-1386

56. Corrigan JJ Jr (1979) Coagulation problems relating to vitamin E. Am J Pediatr Hematol Oncol 1:169–173

57. Finer NN, Peters KL, Hayek Z, Merkel CL (1984) Vitamin E and necrotizing enterocolitis. Pediatrics 73:387–393

58. Alade SL, Brown RE, Paquet A Jr (1986) Polysorbate 80 and E-ferol toxicity. Pediatrics 77:593–597

Chapter 14

Vitamin K

John W. Suttie

Vitamin K was discovered in the early 1930s when Dam noted a hemorrhagic syndrome in chicks fed a lipid-free diet. This condition could be cured by the addition of alfalfa meal to the diet or by the administration of a lipid extract of green plants. By 1939 a series of investigations led by Dam in Denmark, Almquist at Berkeley, and Doisy at St. Louis University had established that the form of the vitamin in alfalfa, now called vitamin K₁ or phylloquinone, was 2-methyl-3-phytyl-1,4-naphthoquinone. Bacterial forms of the vitamin, a series of multiprenyl menaquinones with an unsaturated side chain that were originally called vitamin K₂, were subsequently characterized. The hemorrhagic condition that resulted from the dietary lack of vitamin K was originally thought to be due solely to a lowered concentration of plasma prothrombin (factor II), but it was later shown that the synthesis of clotting factors VII, IX, and X was also depressed in the deficient state. This early history of vitamin K research has been adequately reviewed.[1,2]

Knowledge of the biochemical events involved in the production of the vitamin K–dependent proteins has been developed during the past 30 years. The 4-hydroxycoumarins were identified in the 1940s as vitamin K antagonists and were used to experimentally regulate the production of these proteins. However, the lack of a general understanding of the mechanism of protein biosynthesis prevented serious experimental approaches to the cellular and molecular mechanisms involved in the synthesis of vitamin K–dependent proteins until the mid 1960s. By the early 1970s it was possible to demonstrate that the vitamin was a substrate for a microsomal enzyme involved in the conversion of inactive precursors of the vitamin K–dependent proteins to their active forms, and by the early 1990s this enzyme had been isolated and characterized.

Chemistry

Natural compounds with vitamin K activity are 2-methyl-1,4-naphthoquinones with a hydrophobic substituent at the 3-position (Figure 1). Phylloquinone (vitamin K₁), the form isolated from green plants, has a phytyl group, whereas the bacterially synthesized forms of the vitamin (menaquinones) have an unsaturated multiprenyl group at this position. Although a wide range of menaquinones are synthesized by bacteria, menaquinones with 6–10 isoprenoid groups in the side chain (MK-6 to MK-10) are the most common.[3,4] The synthetic compound, menadione (2-methyl-1,4-naphthoquinone), is commonly used as a source of the vitamin in animal feeds and is known to be alkylated to MK-4 by mammalian liver.[5]

Vitamin K is extracted from plant and animal tissues with nonpolar solvents, and the small amounts of vitamin K present in the crude complex lipid extract has made quantitation difficult. Advances in high-performance liquid chromatography (HPLC) separations and development of new methods of detection in column effluents have now made this possible,[6] and reproducible measurements of both phylloquinone and menaquinones in plasma and tissues are now obtainable.

Absorption, Transport, Storage, and Turnover

Absorption of phylloquinone from the gut is via the lymphatic system, and conditions that result in a general impairment of lipid absorption also adversely influence vitamin K absorption.[7] After being absorbed from the duodenum and jejunum, the vitamin is transported in chylomicrons to target tissues. The concentration of circulating phylloquinone is increased in a hyperlipidemic state,[8,9] and apolipoprotein E (apo E) genotype has been demonstrated to influence circulating concentrations.[10] Concentrations of phylloquinone in plasma are low, and a normal range of 0.3–2.6 nmol/L (0.14–1.17 ng/mL) was reported.[9] Early studies did not detect circulating menaquinones in plasma, but more recent reports indicate that significant concentrations of some long-chain menaquinones, mainly MK-7 and MK-8, are present.[11–13] Some measurements of human liver vitamin K content are now also available. Values reported have been in the range of 2–20 ng phylloquinone/g liver.[13–15] A spectrum of bacterially produced menaquinones is also found in liver, and the total menaquinone concentration appears to be ≈10-fold higher than that of phylloquinone. Both forms of the vitamin are rapidly concentrated in liver, but in contrast to the other fat-soluble

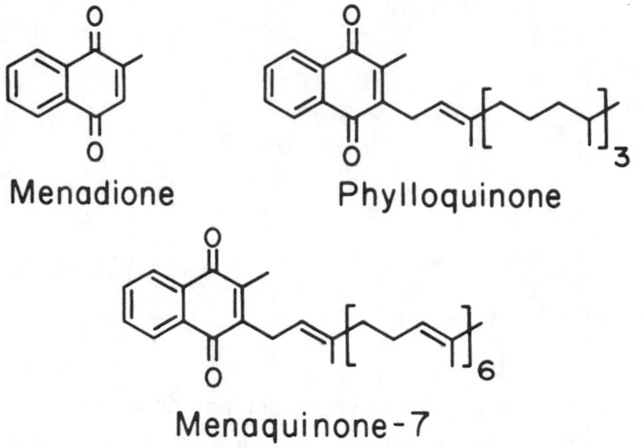

Menadione   Phylloquinone

Menaquinone-7

Figure 1. Structures of the biologically active forms of vitamin K.

vitamins, phylloquinone has a very rapid turnover in this organ. The relatively high concentration of menaquinone found in human liver may reflect the slower turnover of long-chain menaquinones relative to phylloquinone, which has been demonstrated in an animal model.[16]

Excretion of phylloquinone occurs predominantly in feces via the bile, but significant amounts are also excreted in the urine. Very little dietary phylloquinone is excreted unmetabolized; the major metabolites appear to represent the stepwise oxidation of the side chain at the 3-position followed by glucuronide conjugation.[8] The utilization of the vitamin as a substrate for the liver microsomal γ-glutamyl-carboxylase results in the production of the 2,3-epoxide of the vitamin, and this metabolite appears to be subject to the same oxidative degradation as the parent vitamin.[17] The limited information available suggests that the pathway of degradative metabolism of menaquinones is similar to that of phylloquinone.

Intestinal anaerobes such as *Escherichia coli* and *Bacillus fragilis* produce menaquinones, and early studies with germ-free animals indicated that they had an increased vitamin K requirement.[18] The human gut also contains large quantities of bacterially produced menaquinones, but the nutritional significance of this potential source of vitamin K is not yet clear.[19] The extent and mechanism of absorption of these menaquinones from the lower bowel has not been clearly established, although it has been demonstrated that human liver does contain significant quantities of menaquinones. Limited data[20] from a rat model suggest that MK-9, when present in liver at concentrations similar to those of phylloquinone, is not as effectively utilized as is phylloquinone. The current data, therefore, suggest that menaquinones provide only a minor portion of the vitamin K needed to satisfy the human requirement.

Biochemical Function

Vitamin K–dependent proteins and γ-carboxyglutamic acid. From the time of their discovery until the early 1970s, it was assumed that the classical vitamin K–dependent clotting factors were the only proteins requiring the vitamin for their synthesis, and studies of the biosynthesis of prothrombin were used to determine the vitamin's role. Indirect studies in the mid 1960s strongly suggested that vitamin K was involved in converting an inactive cellular precursor of prothrombin to biologically active prothrombin. This hypothesis was strengthened by the observation of immunochemically similar but biologically inactive prothrombin molecules that increased in the plasma of anticoagulant-treated patients. Characterization of the bovine form of this abnormal prothrombin revealed that it lacked the specific calcium-binding sites present in normal prothrombin and did not demonstrate a calcium-dependent association with phospholipid surfaces.

The lack of calcium-binding ability of the abnormal plasma prothrombin suggested that the function of vitamin K was to modify a liver precursor of this plasma protein to facilitate this binding. Acidic peptides obtained by enzymatic digestion of prothrombin were subsequently shown to contain γ-carboxyglutamic acid (Gla), a previously unrecognized acidic amino acid (Figure 2). All 10 of the glutamic acid residues in the first 42 residues of bovine prothrombin were subsequently shown to be γ-carboxylated in a posttranslational vitamin K–dependent reaction to form the effective calcium-binding groups.[21]

Plasma clotting factors VII, IX, and X also depend on vitamin K for their synthesis and contain Gla residues. The amino-terminal regions of these proteins are very homologous,[22] and the Gla residues are in essentially the same position in all of these clotting factors. Two more homologous, Gla-containing, plasma proteins, protein C

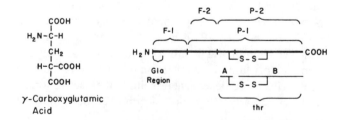

Figure 2. Structure of γ-carboxyglutamic acid (Gla) and a representation of the prothrombin molecule. Specific proteolysis of prothrombin by thrombin and factor Xa will cleave prothrombin into the specific large peptides shown: fragment-1 (F-1), fragment-2 (F-2), prethrombin-1 (P-1), prethrombin-2 (P-2), and thrombin (thr). The Gla residues in bovine prothrombin are located at residues 7, 8, 15, 17, 20, 21, 26, 27, 30, and 33, and they occupy homologous positions in the other vitamin K–dependent plasma proteins.

and protein S, play an anticoagulant rather than a procoagulant role in normal hemostasis. Another Gla-containing bovine plasma protein (protein Z) has been described, but its function is not yet known. These proteins play a critical role in hemostasis; the cDNA and genomic organization of each of these proteins was recently reviewed.[23]

A protein containing three Gla residues, called osteocalcin or bone Gla protein, was isolated from bone. There is little structural homology between this protein and the vitamin K–dependent plasma proteins and its function is not known, but it is most likely involved in some aspect of the control of tissue mineralization or skeletal turnover.[24,25] The demonstration that the level of this protein in plasma varies in some metabolic bone diseases has opened possible clinical implications as has the demonstration that the synthesis of this protein is to some extent regulated by vitamin D.[26,27] A second protein isolated from bone and structurally related to osteocalcin (matrix Gla protein) is also present in other tissues, but its physiological role is also unclear. The vitamin K–dependent carboxylation is present in most tissues, and a reasonably large number of proteins are subjected to this posttranslational modification. Other than the well-established role of the plasma clotting factors, the physiological role of these proteins has not been established.

Vitamin K–dependent metabolic reactions. The reactions shown in Figure 3 summarize the known major metabolic transformation of vitamin K in rat liver microsomes.[28] At least in in vitro incubations, three forms of vitamin K (the quinone, hydroquinone, and 2,3-epoxide) can feed into this liver vitamin K cycle. The quinone and hydroquinone forms are interconverted by a number of NAD(P)H-linked reductases including one that appears to be a microsomal-bound form of the extensively studied liver DT-diaphorase activity and also by a dithiol-dependent reductase. The reduced form, vitamin KH_2, serves as a substrate for the microsomal γ-glutamyl carboxylase-epoxidase that converts the vitamin to its 2,3-epoxide and carboxylates glutamyl to γ-carboxyglutamyl residues. The epoxide formed in this reaction is reduced and recycled by the microsomal epoxide reductase.

The discovery of Gla residues in prothrombin led to the demonstration that crude rat liver microsomal preparations contain an enzymatic activity that promotes a vitamin K–dependent incorporation of $H^{14}CO_3^-$ into specific Glu residues within microsomal precursors of these vitamin K–dependent proteins to form Gla residues.[29–31] The enzyme activity was soon shown to be active in a number of detergent-solubilized systems, and the pentapeptide Phe-Leu-Glu-Glu-Val was found to be a substrate for this enzyme.[32] Most subsequent studies have used this or similar peptide substrates, rather than the endogenous substrates, to study enzyme activity. The

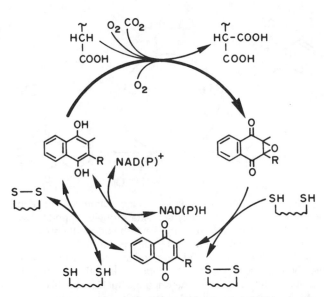

Figure 3. Vitamin K–dependent reactions catalyzed by crude liver microsomes. Evidence suggests that the carboxylation and epoxidation activities are catalyzed by the same enzyme. The dithiol-dependent reductions of the epoxide and of vitamin K quinone are extremely sensitive to the action of coumarin anticoagulants such as warfarin.

rough microsomal fraction of liver is highly enriched in carboxylase activity, and lower but significant levels are found in smooth microsomes. Mitochondria, nuclei, and cytosol have negligible activities.[33] The data obtained from protease sensitivity studies are consistent with the hypothesis that the carboxylation event occurs on the lumen side of the rough endoplasmic reticulum.

Early studies also demonstrated that this carboxylation reaction does not require ATP,[34] and the available data are consistent with the view that the energy to drive this carboxylation reaction is derived from the reoxidation of the reduced form of vitamin K. This unique carboxylase requires O_2; the involvement of biotin in the system has been ruled out. These findings and a direct study of the CO_2 and HCO_3^- requirement indicate that CO_2 rather than HCO_3^- is the active species in the reaction. The vitamin K antagonist, 2-chloro-3-phytyl-1,4-naphthoquinone, is an effective inhibitor of the carboxylase, and the reduced form of this analog has been shown to be competitive versus the reduced vitamin site. Polychlorinated phenols are strong inhibitors; substitution of a trifluoromethyl group, a hydroxymethyl group, or a methoxymethyl group at the 2-position also results in inhibitory compounds.[35]

Review of studies of substrate specificity at the vitamin site suggests that the only important structural features of this substrate in a detergent-solubilized system are a 2-methyl-1,4-naphthoquinone substituted at the 3-position with a rather hydrophobic group. Methyl substitution of the benzenoid ring has little effect or

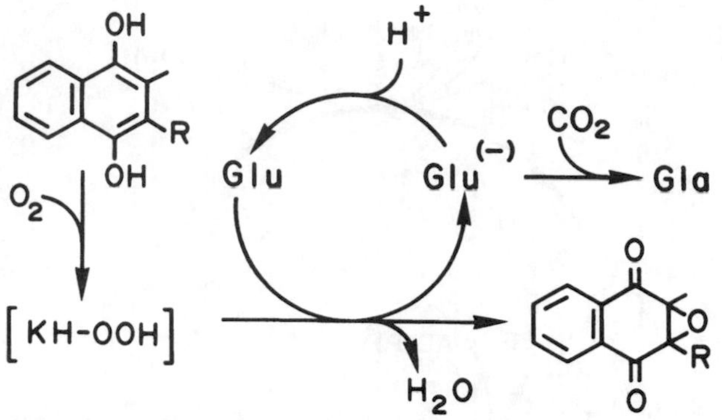

Figure 4. Generalized mechanism of the vitamin K–dependent carboxylase-epoxidase enzyme. Data strongly support the vitamin K–dependent formation of a carbanion at the γ-carbon of the Glu residue followed by carboxylation in a step not involving the vitamin. The intermediate shown as KH-OOH is not meant to represent a hydroperoxide of the vitamin, but rather some oxygenated intermediate such as the alkoxide, which has been postulated to be the strong base needed to abstract the γ-carbon hydrogen.

decreases binding. Synthesis and assay of a large number of low-molecular-weight peptide substrates of the enzyme failed to reveal any unique sequence needed as a signal for carboxylation. In general, peptides with Glu-Glu sequences are better substrates than those with single Glu residues. Gln, D-Glu, or homo-Glu residues have been demonstrated to be noncarboxylated residues whereas Asp residues are poorly carboxylated. Why only the first of the two adjacent Glu residues in these substrates is carboxylated by the enzyme is not yet apparent. A consensus sequence within the Gla region that may be important for efficient carboxylation has been identified, but its significance is not known.[36] Details of the current understanding of the specificity of the various substrates for the carboxylase have been reviewed.[34,35,37,38]

Vitamin K 2,3-epoxide was discovered as a major liver metabolite of the vitamin before it was known to be a product of the carboxylase,[39] and it is the substrate for another microsomal enzyme, the 2,3-epoxide reductase. This enzyme uses a sulfhydryl compound as a reductant and is the site of the physiological action of the 4-hydroxycoumarins as anticoagulants.[40,41] In in vitro systems dithiothreitol will also reduce vitamin K to vitamin KH_2 in a 4-hydroxycoumarin–sensitive reaction; this step may be of physiological importance in the action of these anticoagulants.[42] Whether this reduction is catalyzed by the same enzyme that reduces the epoxide is not known, but evidence suggests that the quinone is the initial product of the reduction of vitamin K 2,3-epoxide and that this product is then further reduced. The physiological reductant for the enzyme that catalyzes the reduction of vitamin K epoxide to vitamin KH_2 has not yet been established.

Mechanism of action of carboxylation. Early studies of the mechanism of action of the carboxylation reaction indicated that vitamin K was a cofactor used to abstract the hydrogen on the γ-position of the glutamyl residue to allow attack of CO_2 at this position.[37] Use of the substrate Phe-Leu-Glu-Glu-Leu, tritiated at the γ-carbon of each Glu residue, demonstrated that the enzyme catalyzed a vitamin KH_2–dependent, O_2-dependent, and CO_2-independent release of tritium from this substrate, establishing the role of the vitamin in removing the γ-hydrogen of the Glu substrate.[37] The 2,3-epoxide of the vitamin is a coproduct of Gla formation; at saturating concentrations of CO_2 there is an apparent equivalent stoichiometry between epoxide formation and Gla formation. At lower CO_2 concentrations a large excess of vitamin K epoxide is produced. The degree to which these two reactions are coupled in routine incubations is therefore strongly dependent on incubation conditions.

How epoxide formation is coupled to γ-hydrogen abstraction has not been established, but one possibility is through the action of an oxygenated intermediate, such as hydroperoxide, that would be a logical intermediate on the pathway to epoxide formation. Hydrogen abstraction is stereospecific, and the pro S hydrogen at the γ-position is removed.[43] The enzyme will catalyze a vitamin KH_2– and oxygen-dependent exchange of ^3H from ^3H_2O into the γ-position of a Glu residue in the substrate Boc-Glu-Glu-Leu-OMe. Exchange of ^3H with the γ-carbon hydrogen is decreased as the concentration of HCO_3^- in the media is increased. The fate of the activated Glu residue in the absence of CO_2 is to protonate rather than form an adduct with some other component of the incubation that would result in an altered Glu residue. More recent studies using γ-^3H–labeled Glu substrates demonstrated a close association among epoxide formation, Gla formation, and γ-C-H bond cleavage.[44] The efficiency of the carboxylation reaction (ratio of Gla formed to γ-C-H bonds cleaved) was found to be independent of Glu substrate concentration, and the data suggest that this ratio approaches unity at high CO_2 concentrations. The available data are consistent with the model shown in Figure 4, which indicates that the role of vitamin K is to abstract the γ-methyl hydrogen to leave a carbanion.

A major gap in an understanding of the mechanism of action of this enzyme has been the assumption that abstraction of the γ-methyl hydrogen would require a strong base (presumably formed from the vitamin) and the lack of evidence for such an intermediate. An initial attack of O_2 at the carbonyl carbon adjacent to the methyl group was suggested to result in the formation of a dioxetane ring, which generates an alkoxide intermediate.[45,46] This intermediate is hypothesized to be the strong base that abstracts the γ-methyl hydrogen. This pathway leads to the possibility that a second atom of molecular oxygen can be incorporated into the carbonyl group of the epoxide product and that this activity can be followed by use of $^{18}O_2$ in the reaction. This partial dioxygenase activity was verified by a second group.[47] Although this general scheme is consistent with all of the available data, the mechanism remains a hypothesis.

Role of the propeptide domain of carboxylase substrates. Normal functioning of the vitamin K–dependent carboxylase poses an interesting question about enzyme-substrate recognition. This microsomal enzyme recognizes a small fraction of the total hepatic secretory protein pool and then carboxylates 9–12 Glu sites in the first 45 residues of these proteins. Cloning of the vitamin K–dependent proteins has revealed that the primary gene products contain a very homologous propeptide between the amino terminus of the mature protein and the signal peptide.[23] This region appears from both early in vitro and in vivo lines of evidence to be a docking or recognition site for the enzyme.[22] This domain of the carboxylase substrates was also shown to be a modulator of the activity of the enzyme by decreasing the apparent K_m of the Glu site substrate.[48] The structural features of the propeptide domain that are important in stimulating the activity of the enzyme are the same as those involved in targeting these proteins for carboxylation.[49] The propeptide domain is undoubtedly of major importance in directing the efficient carboxylation of the multiple Glu sites in these substrates. Whether the enzyme starts at one end of the Gla region and sequentially carboxylates all Glu sites or carboxylates randomly within this region is not known. Interference with an adequate amount of vitamin K (anticoagulant therapy) results in the production of a complex mixture of partially carboxylated forms of prothrombin,[50] and some prothrombin genetic variants are also partially carboxylated.[51] The available data suggest that the most amino-terminal residue is preferentially carboxylated, but other sites of increased carboxylation appear to be present.[52] A recent study showed that in contrast to the data obtained from a study of under-γ-carboxylated plasma prothrombin, the enzyme preferentially carboxylates the most carboxy terminal potential Gla site when des-γ-carboxy BGP (dBGP) is used as an in vitro substrate.[53] This pattern is not altered when dproBGP, which contains the covalently bound propeptide, is the substrate, although the proportion of mono- to di- to tri-Gla product is shifted to more complete carboxylation.

Purification of the vitamin K–dependent carboxylase. Significant progress toward a detailed understanding of the properties of the enzyme has been limited by the lack of a pure enzyme. A preparation that has 500–1000 times the specific activity of microsomes and can be routinely prepared in 2 days has been available for a number of years.[54] The first report of purification of the enzyme to homogeneity was of a 77-kDa protein that was subsequently acknowledged to represent the purification of the endoplasmic reticulum heat-shock protein BiP or GRP78.[55,56] Two microsomal proteins of 94 kDa[57,58] and 98 kDa[59] were purified and claimed to be the carboxylase. The subsequent expression, by using a baculovirus expression system, of the 94-kDa protein in an insect cell line that lacks any endogenous carboxylase activity established that this protein was previously associated with crude preparations of the carboxylase.[60] The role of the 98-kDa protein in the overall carboxylase mechanism, if any, is not known.

Vitamin K Deficiency in Animals

The classical sign of a vitamin K deficiency is an increase in the one-stage prothrombin time brought about by a failure to produce normal amounts of essential clotting factors. Largely on the basis of this response, the requirements for rat, dog, and pig have been established to be 50–150 µg phylloquinone/kg diet.[1] More recent data suggest that >500 µg/kg may be needed to prevent the appearance of more sensitive signs of the deficiency in rats.[61] Vitamin K was discovered in chicks, a species in which a deficiency is easily produced. The basis for this high vitamin K requirement is related to a decreased activity of the vitamin K–epoxide reductase, resulting in a less efficient recycling of vitamin K epoxide to biologically active forms of the vitamin.[62]

Vitamin K Deficiency in Humans

Primary vitamin K deficiency is uncommon in healthy humans. The hemorrhagic disease of newborns is, however, a long-recognized syndrome that is at least partly responsive to vitamin K.[63] Vitamin K stores are low at birth because of poor placental transfer, and the sterile gut precludes any possible use of menaquinones during early life. The condition is complicated by a general hypoprothrombinemia in infants caused by the inability of immature liver to synthesize normal levels of clotting factors.[64] The low vitamin K content of breast milk and low milk intake are contributing factors to vitamin K deficiency in newborns.[65-67] Commercial formulas are now routinely supplemented with vitamin K, and the American Academy of Pediatrics[68] has recommended intramuscular administration of phylloquinone at birth as routine prophylaxis.

The most common condition known to result in a vitamin K–responsive hemorrhagic event in adults occurs in the patient who has a low dietary intake of vitamin K and is also receiving antibiotics.[69,70] These cases are numerous and have been reviewed.[7] The prevalence of this condition suggests that patients with restricted food intake or those on total parenteral nutrition who are also receiving antibiotics should be closely observed for signs of vitamin K deficiency. These episodes have historically been attributed to an interference with the synthesis of menaquinones in the gut, but evidence to substantiate the effect is lacking. The second and third generation cephalosporins have been implicated in many episodes of hypoprothrombinemia; although it has been suggested that these drugs directly affect the vitamin K–dependent carboxylase,[71] it is more likely that they are exerting a weak coumarin-like response in patients with low vitamin K status.[72]

Vitamin K deficiency was reported in patients subjected to long-term total parenteral nutrition, and supplementation of the vitamin is advised under these circumstances.[73] Supplementation in the case of biliary obstruction is also advisable, as the impairment of lipid absorption resulting from the lack of bile salts will also adversely affect vitamin K absorption. Depression of the vitamin K–dependent coagulation factors has frequently been found in malabsorption syndromes and in other gastrointestinal disorders (e.g., cystic fibrosis, sprue, celiac disease, ulcerative colitis, regional ileitis, ascaris infection, and short-bowel syndrome) and has usually responded to vitamin administration.[7]

The low requirement and the relatively large amounts of vitamin K found in most diets prevented an accurate assessment of the requirement until recent years. In an early study, starved intravenously fed debilitated patients were given antibiotics to decrease intestinal vitamin K synthesis; 0.1 μg phylloquinone·kg^{-1}·day^{-1} was not sufficient to maintain normal prothrombin levels and 1.5 μg·kg^{-1}·day^{-1} was sufficient to prevent any decreases in clotting factor synthesis.[74] Two other studies with very limited numbers of subjects did successfully decrease vitamin K intake to the extent that clotting factor activities were decreased and also suggested that the vitamin requirement of humans is in the range of 0.5–1.0 μg vitamin K·kg^{-1}·day^{-1}.[75,76] A major problem in determining a dietary requirement for vitamin K has been the relative insensitivity of the commonly used prothrombin time measurement.[77] A more recent study modifying the vitamin K intake of young adults by restriction of foods with a high phylloquinone content resulted in two symptoms of a mild deficiency: increased circulating under-γ-carboxylated prothrombin and decreased Gla excretion.[78] These responses were reversed by additional dietary vitamin, and the data obtained are consistent with a requirement in the range previously suggested. A more carefully controlled metabolic-ward study found alterations in the same two sensitive measures of deficiency in subjects consuming 10 μg phylloquinone/day,[79] and increased circulating under-γ-carboxylated prothrombin was observed in a second controlled study.[80]

Recent advances in methodology have made it possible to routinely measure circulating concentrations of phylloquinone, but the factors influencing these concentrations and their relationship to dietary intake have not yet been clarified. Alteration of plasma phylloquinone by dietary restriction of the vitamin was reported in studies of limited scope,[78–80] and plasma phylloquinone concentration was shown to be low in debilitated patient populations.[72,81] However, because of the close relationship of plasma phylloquinone to recent intakes, these measurements lack utility for assessing vitamin K status. Assessment of adequacy by use of the rather insensitive one-stage prothrombin time has meant that a rather large decrease in vitamin K–dependent clotting factor synthesis was needed to produce an apparent deficiency. More sensitive clotting assays and the ability to immunochemically detect circulating des-γ-carboxy prothrombin permit the monitoring of much milder forms of vitamin K deficiency.[77,82] Vitamin K status may be important in maintaining skeletal health,[83] and the extent of under-γ-carboxylation of circulating osteocalcin is a very sensitive criterion of vitamin K sufficiency.[84,85] This method will likely become increasingly important in future studies defining vitamin K status.

Vitamin K Requirement

The 10th edition of the National Research Council's *Recommended Dietary Allowances* was the first to include a recommendation for vitamin K.[86] The intake recommended was 1 μg phylloquinone/kg body weight for adults. Intakes of 5 μg phylloquinone/day for infants during the first 6 months and 10 μg/day from 6 to 12 months were also recommended. In the absence of any specific information about a unique vitamin K requirement for children, the 1 μg/kg body intake was also applied to children.

Food and Other Sources of Vitamin K

Methodology for the analysis of foods for their vitamin K content by lipid extraction and HPLC separation are now available.[87] Data summarized in standard nutrition texts and reviews that were obtained from chick biological assays before a suitable standard was available should be used with a great deal of caution.[1,88] Analyses of many foods and edible oils by modern methods are now available.[89,90] In general, green vegetables are the major source of phylloquinone in the diet, and such foods as spinach, broccoli, Brussels sprouts, kale, and turnip greens are excellent sources of the vitamin. These contain a few hundred micrograms of phylloquinone per 100 g of fresh weight, whereas the more commonly consumed green vegetables such as peas, green beans, cabbage, and lettuce furnish 10–100 μg/100 g fresh weight. Some cooking oils, chiefly soybean, rapeseed, and to a lesser extent olive oil, are also major contributors to the total daily intake. The usual intake of the vitamin in the human diet has been assumed to be 300–500 µg/day,[88] but at least one study showed that this is a rather high estimate and that the intake of young adults is only ≈100 µg/day.[78] Liver provides a significant dietary intake of menaquinones, but except for a few specialized fermented food and cheese products, the major source of vitamin in the diet is phylloquinone of plant origin.

Toxicity

There is no known toxicity associated with the administration of high doses of phylloquinone, a natural form of the vitamin.[91] Administration of menadione to infants is associated with hemolytic anemia and liver toxicity, and phylloquinone is now prescribed to prevent hemorrhagic disease of newborns. The toxicity of dietary menadione is, however, relatively low, and animals have been fed as much as 1000 times the daily requirement with no adverse effects.

References

1. Suttie, JW (1984) Vitamin K. In Machlin LJ (ed), Handbook of vitamins: nutritional, biochemical, and clinical aspects. Marcel Dekker, New York, pp 147–198
2. Olson RE, Suttie JW (1978) Vitamin K and γ-carboxyglutamate biosynthesis. Vitam Horm 35:59–108
3. Ramotar K, Conly JM, Chubb H, Louie TJ (1984) Production of menaquinones by intestinal anaerobes. J Infect Dis 150:213–218
4. Fernandez F, Collins MD (1987) Vitamin K composition of anaerobic gut bacteria. FEMS Microbiol Lett 41:175–180
5. Taggart WV, Matschiner JT (1969) Metabolism of menadione-6,7-^{3}H in the rat. Biochemistry 8:1141–1146
6. Shearer MJ (1983) High-performance liquid chromatography of K vitamins and their antagonists. In Giddings JC, Grushka E, Cazes J, Brown PR (eds), Advances in chromatography, vol. 21. Marcel Dekker, New York, pp 243–301
7. Savage D, Lindenbaum J (1983) Clinical and experimental human vitamin K deficiency. In Lindenbaum J (ed), Nutrition in hematology. Churchill Livingstone, New York, pp 271–320
8. Shearer MJ, McBurney A, Barkhan P (1974) Studies on the absorption and metabolism of phylloquinone (vitamin K$_1$) in man. Vitam Horm 32:513–542
9. Sadowski JA, Hood SJ, Dallal GE, Garry PJ (1989) Phylloquinone in plasma from elderly and young adults: factors influencing its concentration. Am J Clin Nutr 50:100–108
10. Saupe J, Shearer MJ, Kohlmeier M (1993) Phylloquinone transport and its influence on γ-carboxyglutamate residues of osteocalcin in patients on maintenance hemodialysis. Am J Clin Nutr 58:204–208
11. Hodges SJ, Pilkington MJ, Shearer MJ, et al (1990) Age-related changes in the circulating levels of congeners of vitamin K$_2$, menaquinone-7 and menaquinone-8. Clin Sci 78:63–66
12. Hodges SJ, Pilkington MJ, Stamp TCB, et al (1991) Depressed levels of circulating menaquinones in patients with osteoporotic fractures of the spine and femoral neck. Bone 12:387–389
13. Usui Y, Tanimura H, Nishimura N, et al (1990) Vitamin K concentrations in the plasma and liver of surgical patients. Am J Clin Nutr 51:846–852
14. Shearer MJ, McCarthy PT, Crampton OE, Mattock MB (1988) The assessment of human vitamin K status from tissue measurements. In Suttie JW (ed), Current advances in vitamin K research. Elsevier Science, New York, pp 437–452
15. Uchida K, Komeno T (1988) Relationships between dietary and intestinal vitamin K, clotting factor levels, plasma vitamin K and urinary Gla. In Suttie JW (ed), Current advances in vitamin K research. Elsevier Science, New York, pp 477–492
16. Will BH, Suttie JW (1992) Comparative metabolism of phylloquinone and menaquinone-9 in rat liver. J Nutr 122:953–958
17. Shearer MJ, McBurney A, Breckenridge AM, Barkhan P (1977) Effect of warfarin on the metabolism of phylloquinone (vitamin K$_1$): dose-response relationships in man. Clin Sci Mol Med 52:621–630
18. Gustafson BE (1959) Vitamin K deficiency in germfree rats. Ann NY Acad Sci 78:166–174
19. Suttie JW (1995) The importance of menaquinones in human nutrition. Annu Rev Nutr 15:399–417
20. Reedstrom CK, Suttie JW (1995) Comparative distribution, metabolism, and utilization of phylloquinone and menaquinone-9 in rat liver. Proc Soc Exp Biol Med 209:403–409
21. Stenflo J, Suttie JW (1977) Vitamin K-dependent formation of γ-carboxyglutamic acid. Annu Rev Biochem 46:157–172
22. Furie B, Furie BC (1992) Molecular and cellular biology of blood coagulation. N Engl J Med 326:800–806
23. Ichinose A, Davie EW (1994) The blood coagulation factors: their cDNAs, genes, and expression. In Colman RW, Hirsh J, Marder VJ, Salzman EW (eds), Hemostasis and thrombosis: basic principles and clinical practice, 3rd ed. Lippincott, Philadelphia, pp 19–54
24. Price PA (1988) Role of vitamin K-dependent proteins in bone metabolism. Annu Rev Nutr 8:565–583
25. Vermeer C, Knapen MHJ, Jie K-SG, Grobbee DE (1992) Physiological importance of extra-hepatic vitamin K-dependent carboxylation reactions. Ann NY Acad Sci 669:21–33
26. Brown JP, Delmas PD, Edouard C, et al (1984) Serum bone Gla protein: a specific marker for bone formation in postmenopausal osteoporosis. Lancet i:1091–1093
27. Price PA, Baukol SK (1980) 1,25-Dihydroxyvitamin D$_3$ increases synthesis of the vitamin K-dependent bone protein by osteosarcoma cells. J Biol Chem 255:11660–11663
28. Suttie JW (1987) Recent advances in hepatic vitamin K metabolism and function. Hepatology 7:367–376
29. Nelsestuen GL, Zytkovicz TH, Howard JB (1974) The mode of action of vitamin K identification of γ-carboxyglutamic acid as a component of prothrombin. J Biol Chem 249:6347–6350
30. Stenflo J, Fernlund P, Egan W, Roepstorff P (1974) Vitamin K-dependent modifications of glutamic acid residues in prothrombin. Proc Natl Acad Sci USA 71:2730–2733
31. Esmon CT, Sadowski JA, Suttie JW (1975) A new carboxylation reaction. The vitamin K-dependent incorporation of H^{14}CO$_3^-$ into prothrombin. J Biol Chem 250:4744–4748
32. Suttie JW, Hageman JM, Lehrman SR, Rich DH (1976) Vitamin K-dependent carboxylase: development of a peptide substrate. J Biol Chem 251:5827–5830
33. Carlisle TL, JW Suttie (1980) Vitamin K-dependent carboxylase: subcellular location of the carboxylase and enzymes involved in vitamin K metabolism in rat liver. Biochemistry 19:1161–1167
34. Suttie JW (1985) Vitamin K-dependent carboxylase. Annu Rev Biochem 54:459–477

35. Suttie JW (1993) Synthesis of vitamin K-dependent proteins. FASEB J 7:445–452

36. Price PA, Fraser JD, Metz-Virca G (1987) Molecular cloning of matrix Gla protein: implications for substrate recognition by the vitamin K-dependent γ-carboxylase. Proc Natl Acad Sci USA 84:8335–8339

37. Suttie JW (1988) Vitamin K-dependent carboxylation of glutamyl residues in proteins. BioFactors 1:55–60

38. Vermeer C (1990) γ-Carboxyglutamate-containing proteins and the vitamin K-dependent carboxylase. Biochem J 266:625–636

39. Matschiner JT, Bell RG, Amelotti JM, Knauer TE (1970) Isolation and characterization of a new metabolite of phylloquinone in the rat. Biochim Biophys Acta 201:309–315

40. Whitlon DS, Sadowski JA, Suttie JW (1978) Mechanism of coumarin action: significance of vitamin K epoxide reductase inhibition. Biochemistry 17:1371–1377

41. Hildebrandt EF, Suttie JW (1982) Mechanism of coumarin action: sensitivity of vitamin K metabolizing enzymes of normal and warfarin-resistant rat liver. Biochemistry 21:2406–2411

42. Fasco, MJ, Hildebrandt EF, Suttie JW (1982) Evidence that warfarin anticoagulant action involves two distinct reductase activities. J Biol Chem 257:11210–11212

43. Dubois J, Gaudry M, Bory S, et al (1983) Vitamin K-dependent carboxylation: study of the hydrogen abstraction stereochemistry with γ-fluoroglutamic acid-containing peptides. J Biol Chem 258:7897–7899

44. Wood GM, Suttie JW (1988) Vitamin K-dependent carboxylase: stoichiometry of vitamin K epoxide formation, γ-carboxyglutamyl formation, and γ-glutamyl-^{3}H cleavage. J Biol Chem 263:3234–3239

45. Dowd P, Ham SW, Geib SJ (1991) Mechanism of action of vitamin K. J Am Chem Soc 113:7734–7743

46. Dowd P, Ham S-W, Hershline R (1992) Role of oxygen in the vitamin K-dependent carboxylation reaction: incorporation of a second atom of ^{18}O from molecular oxygen-^{18}O$_2$ into vitamin K oxide during carboxylase activity. J Am Chem Soc 114:7613–7617

47. Kuliopulos A, Hubbard BR, Lam Z, et al (1992) Dioxygen transfer during vitamin K-dependent carboxylase catalysis. Biochemistry 31:7722–7728

48. Knobloch JE, Suttie JW (1987) Vitamin K-dependent carboxylase: control of enzyme activity by the "propeptide" region of factor X. J Biol Chem 262:15334–15337

49. Cheung A, Suttie JW, Bernatowicz M (1990) Vitamin K-dependent carboxylase: structural requirements for peptide activation. Biochim Biophys Acta 1039:90–93

50. Malhotra OP (1981) Dicoumarol-induced prothrombins. Ann NY Acad Sci 370:426–437

51. Borowski M, Furie BC, Furie B (1986) Distribution of γ-carboxyglutamic acid residues in partially carboxylated human prothrombins. J Biol Chem 261:1624–1628

52. Liska DJ, Suttie JW (1988) Location of γ-carboxyglutamyl residues in partially carboxylated prothrombin preparations. Biochemistry 27:8636–8641

53. Benton ME, Price PA, Suttie JW (1995) Multi-site specificity of the vitamin K-dependent carboxylase: in vitro carboxylation of des-γ-carboxylated bone Gla protein and des-γ-carboxylated pro bone Gla protein. Biochemistry 34:9541–9551

54. Harbeck MC, Cheung AY, Suttie JW (1989) Vitamin K-dependent carboxylase: partial purification of the enzyme by antibody affinity techniques. Thromb Res 56:317–323

55. Hubbard BR, Ulrich MMW, Jacobs M, et al (1989) Vitamin K-dependent carboxylase: affinity purification from bovine liver by using a synthetic propeptide containing the γ-carboxylation recognition site. Proc Natl Acad Sci USA 86:6893–6897

56. Kuliopulos A, Cieurzo CE, Furie B, et al (1992) N-bromoacetyl-peptide substrate affinity labeling of vitamin K-dependent carboxylase. Biochemistry 31:9436–9444

57. Wu S-M, Morris DP, Stafford DW (1991) Identification and purification to near homogeneity of the vitamin K-dependent carboxylase. Proc Natl Acad Sci USA 88:2236–2240

58. Wu S-M, Cheung W-F, Frazier D, Stafford D (1991) Cloning and expression of the cDNA for human γ-glutamyl carboxylase. Science 254:1634–1636

59. Berkner KL, Harbeck M, Lingenfelter S, et al (1992) Purification and identification of bovine liver γ-carboxylase. Proc Natl Acad Sci USA 89:6242–6246

60. Roth DA, Rehemtulla A, Kaufman RJ, et al (1993) Expression of bovine vitamin K-dependent carboxylase activity in baculovirus infected cells. Proc Natl Acad Sci USA 90:8372–8376

61. Kindberg CG, Suttie JW (1989) Effect of various intakes of phylloquinone on signs of vitamin K deficiency and serum and liver phylloquinone concentrations in the rat. J Nutr 119:175–180

62. Will BH, Usui Y, Suttie JW (1992) Comparative metabolism and requirement of vitamin K in chicks and rats. J Nutr 122:2354–2360

63. Lane PA, Hathaway WE (1985) Vitamin K in infancy. J Pediatr 106:351–359

64. Andrew M, Paes B, Milner R, et al (1987) Development of the human coagulation system in the full-term infant. Blood 70:165–172

65. Canfield LM, Hopkinson JM (1989) State of the art vitamin K in human milk. J Pediatr Gastroenterol Nutr 8:430–441

66. Kries RV, Becker A, Gobel U (1987) Vitamin K in the newborn: influence of nutritional factors on acarboxy-prothrombin detectability and factor II and VII clotting activity. Eur J Pediatr 146:123–127

67. Motohara K, Matsukura M, Matsuda I, et al (1984) Severe vitamin K-deficiency in breast-fed infants. J Pediatr 105:943–945

68. American Academy of Pediatrics, Committee on Nutrition (1971) Vitamin K supplementation for infants receiving milk substitute infant formulas and for those with fat malabsorption. Pediatrics 48:483–487

69. Ansell JE, Kumar R, Deykin D (1977) The spectrum of vitamin K deficiency. JAMA 238:40–42

70. Alperin JB (1987) Coagulopathy caused by vitamin K deficiency in critically ill, hospitalized patients. JAMA 258:1916–1919

71. Lipsky JJ (1988) Antibiotic-associated hypoprothrombinaemia. J Antimicrob Chemother 21:281–300

72. Shearer MJ, Bechtold H, Andrassy K, et al (1988) Mechanism of cephalosporin-induced hypoprothrombinemia: relation to cephalosporin side chain, vitamin K metabolism, and vitamin K status. J Clin Pharmacol 28:88–95

73. Dudrick SJ, Wilmore DW, Vars HM, Rhoads JE (1968) Long-term total parenteral nutrition with growth, development and positive nitrogen balance. Surgery 64:134–142

74. Frick PG, Riedler G, Brogli H (1967) Dose response and minimal daily requirement for vitamin K in man. J Appl Physiol 23:387–389

75. Doisy EA (1971) The biochemistry, assay and nutritional value of vitamin K and related compounds. Association of Vitamin Chemists, Chicago, pp 79–92

76. O'Reilly RA (1971) Vitamin K in hereditary resistance to oral anticoagulant drugs. Am J Physiol 221:1327–1330

77. Suttie JW (1992) Vitamin K and human nutrition. J Am Diet Assoc 92:585–590

78. Suttie JW, Mummah-Schendel LL, Shah DV, et al (1988) Vitamin K deficiency from dietary vitamin K restriction in humans. Am J Clin Nutr 47:475–480

79. Ferland G, Sadowski JA, O'Brien ME (1993) Dietary induced subclinical vitamin K deficiency in normal human subjects. J Clin Invest 91:1761–1768

80. Allison PM, Mummah-Schendel LL, Kindberg CG, et al (1987) Effects of a vitamin K-deficient diet and antibotics in normal human volunteers. J Lab Clin Med 110:180–188

81. Cohen H, Scott SD, Mackie IJ, et al (1988) The development of hypoprothrombinaemia following antibiotic therapy in malnourished patients with low serum vitamin K_1 levels. Br J Haematol 68:63–66

82. Blanchard RA, Furie BC, Jorgensen M, et al (1981) Acquired vitamin K-dependent carboxylation deficiency in liver disease. N Engl J Med 305:242–248

83. Binkley NC, Suttie JW (1995) Vitamin K nutrition and osteoporosis. J Nutr 125:1812–1821

84. Knapen MHJ, Hamulyak K, Vermeer C (1989) The effect of vitamin K supplementation on circulating osteocalcin (bone Gla protein) and urinary calcium excretion. Ann Intern Med 111:1001–1005

85. Jie KG, Hamulyak K, Gisjsbers BLMG, et al (1992) Serum osteocalcin as a marker for vitamin K-status in pregnant women and their newborn babies. Thromb Haemostas 68:388–391

86. National Research Council (1989) Recommended dietary allowances, 10th ed. National Academy Press, Washington, DC

87. Booth SL, Davidson KW, Sadowski JA (1994) Evaluation of an HPLC method for the determination of phylloquinone (vitamin K_1) in various food matrices. J Agric Food Chem 42:295–300

88. Olson RE (1988) Vitamin K. In Shils ME, Young VR (eds), Modern nutrition in health and disease, 7th ed. Lea & Febiger, Philadelphia, pp 328–339

89. Booth SL, Sadowski JA, Weihrauch JL, Ferland G (1993) Vitamin K_1 (phylloquinone) content of foods: a provisional table. J Food Comp Anal 6:109–120

90. Ferland G, Sadowski JA (1992) Vitamin K_1 (phylloquinone) content of edible oils: effects of heating and light exposure. J Agric Food Chem 40:1869–1873

91. National Research Council (1987) Vitamin tolerance of animals. National Academy Press, Washington, DC

Chapter 15

Vitamin C

Mark Levine, Steven Rumsey, Yaohui Wang,
Jae Park, Oran Kwon, Wei Xu, and Nobuyuki Amano

The best recommendations for nutrient intake would describe ideal intake as well as intake to prevent deficiency. Unfortunately, determining ideal ingestion for any nutrient is very difficult. Perhaps no other nutrient has generated as much controversy as vitamin C. In contrast to ideal ingestion, it is clinically obvious when the deficiency disease scurvy occurs and when replacement is effective. Thus, determining the amount that prevents deficiency is straightforward.

A disease that probably was scurvy was described by ancient Egyptians, Greeks, and Romans.[1,2] Members of Jacque Cartier's exploration team who had scurvy were cured when they ingested a tree extract as recommended by Native North Americans.[3] Scurvy and its treatment were described in Europe by Sir Richard Hawkins and Urban Hiaerne, and it is likely that others found cures that were later forgotten because they were unrecorded.[4,5] James Lind systematically studied the deficiency disease and its prevention in British sailors in his work *Treatise of the Scurvy* published in 1753.[6] Unfortunately, vitamin C was no stranger to controversy even then. It took more than 40 years and countless deaths for the British Admiralty to provide sailors with lemon juice, accounting for the naval nickname "limey."

From 1928 to 1932 the laboratories of Albert Szent-Gyorgyi and C.C. King independently isolated vitamin C and showed that it had antiscorbutic activity, although only the former scientist received the Nobel Prize for this work.[7,8] Experiments soon after indicated that the amount of vitamin C that prevented deficiency could be less than that needed for other physiologic functions.[9,10] Other experiments implied that vitamin C was involved in response to stress and to infections.[11,12]

It was a short leap from these experiments to experiments in patients. In 1942 the incidence of colds was measured in patients who were given either 200 mg vitamin C or a placebo.[13] Although the investigators concluded that vitamin C had no effect, 30 years later the data were revisited and the conclusions were challenged. Great controversy ensued when Linus Pauling and others recommended that gram doses of vitamin C could prevent and treat colds.[14,15] Controversy was inevitable because doses as low as 10 mg daily were re-ported to prevent scurvy in human volunteers, and the recommended dietary allowance (RDA) at that time—45 mg—was based on providing a margin of safety against scurvy.[16-20] Because the current RDA is 60 mg, it is not surprising that further controversy erupted when gram doses of vitamin C were suggested by some to be useful in preventing atherosclerosis, cancer, cataracts, and aging and in treating cancer, schizophrenia, acquired immune deficiency syndrome (AIDS), and idiopathic thrombocytopenic purpura.[21-28] The controversies remain heated today, and their very mention often induces strong emotional responses.

These controversies are indicative of the fundamental issue raised more than 50 years ago, that optimal vitamin ingestion might be different than vitamin ingestion to prevent deficiency.[9,10,29] We will explore this concept and related ones in the following sections, with the goal of making recommendations for vitamin C intake.

Chemistry, Catabolism, and Biosynthesis

Vitamin C is also known as ascorbic acid, ascorbate, or ascorbate monoanion. Ascorbic acid is a six-carbon α-ketolactone weak acid with a pK of 4.2 (Figure 1). Ascorbate is reversibly oxidized and forms the free radical called semidehydroascorbic acid, ascorbate$^{\bullet-}$, or ascorbate free radical. Ascorbate$^{\bullet-}$ is a relatively stable free radical, although the rate constant for its decay is approximately 10^5 M^{-1} second^{-1}.[31] Ascorbate$^{\bullet-}$ is oxidized to dehydroascorbic acid, which probably exists in vivo in multiple forms (and thus acid is a misnomer).[32] Dehydroascorbic acid can be reduced back to the intermediate free radical and then to vitamin C, and it is unstable in aqueous solutions. Its ring structure is easily ruptured by hydrolysis to yield diketogulonic acid. Dehydroascorbic acid hydrolysis is irreversible. Although diketogulonic acid metabolism is not well characterized, metabolic products are believed to include oxalate, threonate, xylose, xylonic acid, and lynxonic acid.[33]

Because ascorbic acid loses electrons easily, it is a good reducing agent. Values for the standard redox potential of the dehydroascorbic acid–ascorbic acid (DHA/AA)

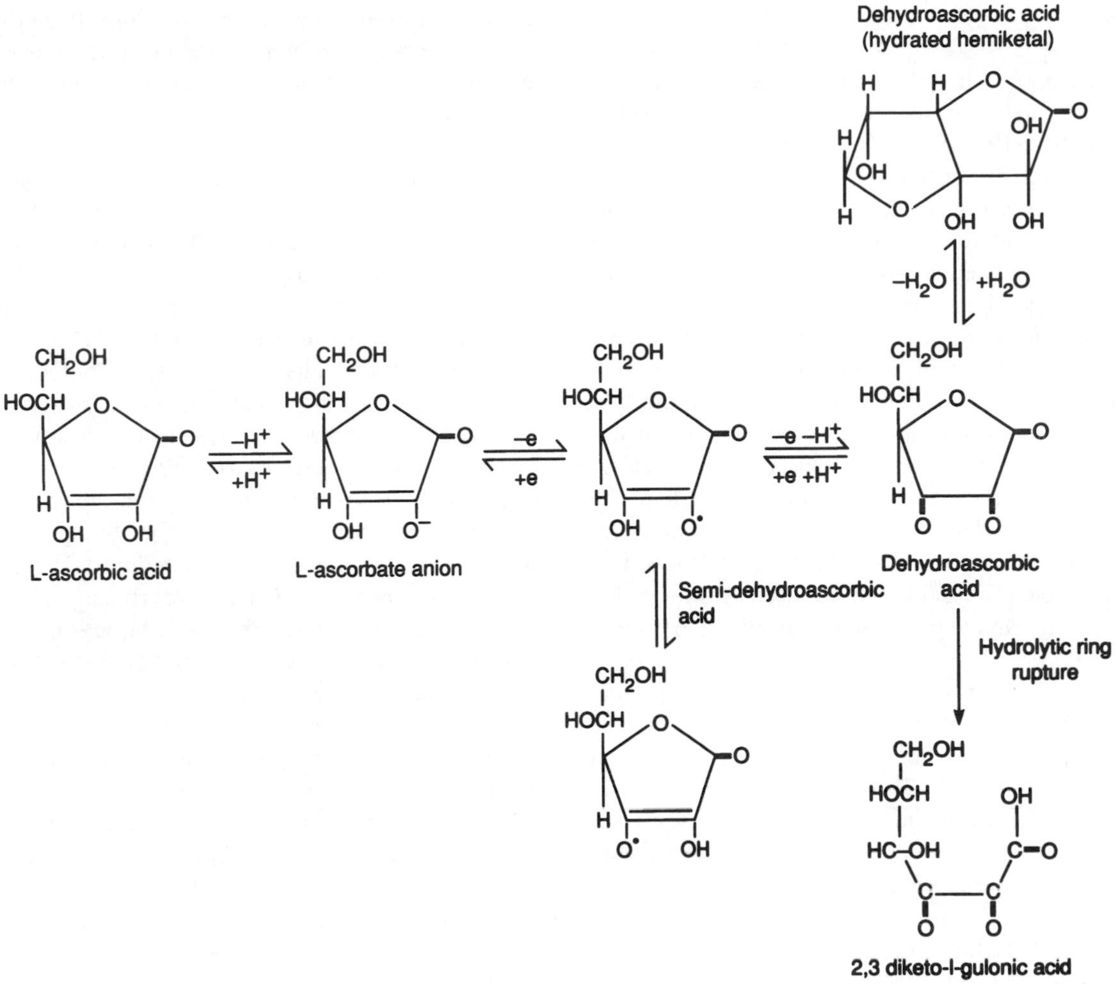

Figure 1. Ascorbic acid and its oxidation products. Only two forms of dehydroascorbic acid are shown. Reprinted with permission from reference 30.

couple are $\approx$0.06–0.1 volts.[33,34] However, these numbers by themselves underestimate ascorbate's value as a reducing agent. Ascorbate almost certainly acts as an electron donor via its free radical form. The redox potential for semidehydroascorbic acid–ascorbic acid (SDA/AA) is $\approx$0.28 and for dehydroascorbic acid–semidehydro-ascorbic acid (DHA/SDA) is –0.17.[34] On the basis of these potentials, ascorbate is an outstanding electron donor for several reasons. In comparison with many other compounds, the SDA/AA and DHA/SDA redox potentials result in reduction of many oxidizing compounds. The radical intermediate ascorbate$^{\cdot-}$ is relatively harmless because it is neither strongly oxidizing nor reducing. Ascorbate$^{\cdot-}$ reacts poorly with oxygen, producing little if any superoxide. Only a tiny amount of ascorbate$^{\cdot-}$ is necessary under physiologic conditions because of its kinetic properties and redox potential. In addition, another property of ascorbate that makes it an excellent electron donor is that the oxidized product dehydro-ascorbic acid is rereduced and available for reuse, as discussed below.

Ascorbate is often called an outstanding antioxidant. In chemical terms this is simply a reflection of the redox properties of SDA/AA and DHA/SDA. In physiologic terms this means that ascorbate provides electrons for enzymes or chemical compounds that are oxidants. In either case, biochemical action of ascorbate is mediated by its properties as an electron donor.

Most mammals synthesize ascorbate from glucose. Humans and other primates lack the terminal enzyme, gulonolactone oxidase, in the ascorbate biosynthetic pathway. The gene is present but the coding sequence has so many mutations that there is no gene product.[35] The mutations were estimated to have occurred millions of years ago. Because humans do not synthesize ascorbate, we must ingest ascorbate to survive. Ascorbate ingestion by our paleolithic ancestors was estimated to be $\approx$350–400 mg/day.[36]

Assays

There are approximately a dozen types of assays for ascorbate and dehydroascorbic acid. Detection systems usually are based on one of the following: oxidation of ascorbate to dehydroascorbic acid, reduction of dehydroascorbic acid to ascorbate, hydrolysis of dehydroascorbic acid to diketogulonic acid, or ultraviolet absorption of either ascorbate or dehydroascorbic acid. Sometimes the detected compound is a chemical derivative of ascorbate, dehydroascorbic acid, or diketogulonic acid. Ascorbate and dehydroascorbic acid assays must take into account four factors: sensitivity, specificity, stability of the substance being measured, and substance interference.[30] Inattention to these factors has caused a great deal of confusion about vitamin C and its function. Perhaps the most vexing measurement problem is a consequence of inadvertent oxidation of ascorbate or hydrolysis of dehydroascorbic acid. Both of these substances can easily degrade during sample procurement, handling, or preparation for assay.

For ascorbate, high-pressure liquid chromatography (HPLC) with electrochemical detection is the assay type of choice. With this method ascorbate is separated from other substances by HPLC and is detected by oxidizing electrodes that produce a measurable current. The electrodes are either flow through (coulometric) or flow by (amperometric). These assays have many variations because different columns and mobile phases can be used, depending on the choice of detector. The best of these assays accounts for sensitivity, specificity, ascorbate stability at all times, and substance interference.[30,37,38] The advantages of these assays far outweigh the disadvantages, which are that they need experienced operators, require dedicated instruments, can sometimes be difficult to operate and maintain, and have a relatively high initial cost.

Other HPLC assays for ascorbate depend on HPLC for separation but use other detectors to detect ascorbate derivatives. The most common of these assays use HPLC coupled to an ultraviolet detector, which detects ascorbate because of its absorption of ultraviolet light between 254 and 266 nm.[30,33] The advantage of these assays is that they are much simpler to run and maintain than an electrochemical system. The disadvantage is that there is incomplete characterization of ascorbate stability during sample preparation, storage, and assay. If the stability problems can be solved, this type of assay would be ideal for clinical chemistry use.

Another common assay type is based on ascorbic acid oxidation by the plant enzyme ascorbate oxidase.[30] Detection is based on the interaction of oxidized and unoxidized samples with a reagent, whose absorbance of ultraviolet light depends on ascorbate concentration. Again, information is incomplete regarding sample stability at different steps of the procedure. Because other reducing samples are not separated from ascorbate, detection of low ascorbate concentrations is limited because of interference.

Older assays for ascorbate use dipyridyl or ferrozine; 2,6 dichlorophenol-indophenol; dinitrophenylhydrazine; or o-phenylenediamine.[30] These assays are nonspecific, are insensitive, give falsely high readings at low ascorbate concentrations, are subject to interference by other biological substances, or may produce unintentional oxidation of ascorbate. They should not be used for biological samples because of the many problems associated with them and the availability of better alternatives.[30]

Dehydroascorbic acid assays are not as advanced as ascorbate assays.[30] Dehydroascorbic acid assays using HPLC with electrochemical detection are indirect and are based on ascorbate measurement. Samples are first analyzed for ascorbate and then reduced for measurement of ascorbate plus dehydroascorbic acid. Dehydroascorbic acid is determined by subtraction, which is problematic when dehydroascorbic acid is < 5% of the total. To our knowledge direct electrochemical detection of dehydroascorbic acid is not yet possible. Despite these problems, the best assay type for dehydroascorbic acid is HPLC with electrochemical detection.

Other assays for dehydroascorbic acid are plagued by disadvantages. HPLC with ultraviolet detection is so insensitive that its use is limited. Non-HPLC methods are worse. They are insensitive, nonspecific, and subject to interference and should be used only when there is no alternative.

Analysis of dehydroascorbic acid will be greatly advanced when it can be detected as such, without modification. HPLC would be used to separate other substances from dehydroascorbic acid, and it would then be detected directly.

Biochemical and Molecular Function

Ascorbate is the biochemically active form of the vitamin. Semidehydroascorbic acid may be biochemically active, but it is more likely that its activity is based on its reduction to ascorbate.[34,39] Likewise, dehydroascorbic acid action is indirect in that its activity is based on reduction to ascorbate[40,41] Dehydroascorbic acid has no definite biochemical function of its own. Recent proposals of direct dehydroascorbic acid action await more definitive evidence, especially from in vivo experiments.[42]

Ascorbate is a cofactor or cosubstrate for eight isolated enzymes (Table 1). Three enzymes require ascorbate for proline or lysine hydroxylation in collagen biosynthesis, depending on whether proline or lysine is hydroxylated and where hydroxylation occurs on the amino acid.[43–45] Two enzymes require ascorbate in the

Table 1. Ascorbic acid and enzyme function

Proline hydroxylase (EC 1.14.11.2)	Collagen synthesis
Procollagen-proline 2 oxoglutarate-3-dioxygenase (EC 1.14.11.7)	Collagen synthesis
Lysine hydroxylase (EC 1.14.11.4)	Collagen synthesis
Gamma-butyrobetaine 2-oxoglutarate 4-dioxygenase (EC 1.14.11.1)	Carnitine synthesis
Trimethyllysine 2-oxoglutarate dioxygenase (EC 1.14.11.8)	Carnitine synthesis
Dopamine beta-monooxygenase (EC 1.14.17.3)	Catecholamine synthesis
Peptidyl glycine alpha amidating monooxygenase (EC 1.14.17.3)	Peptide amidation
4-Hydroxylaphenylpyruvate dioxygenase (EC 1.13.11.27)	Tyrosine metabolism

biosynthetic pathway for carnitine, which in turn is used by mitochondria for transmembrane electron transfer in ATP synthesis.[46,47] Two enzymes, dopamine β-monooxygenase and peptidyl-glycine α-monooxygenase, contain an active-site copper moiety and require ascorbate for hormone biosynthesis. The former enzyme is necessary for norepinephrine synthesis from dopamine.[48,49] The latter enzyme mediates amidation at the carboxy terminus of peptide hormones, thereby conferring stability to hormones such as thyrotropin-releasing hormone, adrenocorticotropic hormone, vasopressin, oxytocin, and cholecystokinin.[50-52] Ascorbate is also required for enzymatic metabolism of tyrosine.[53] The role of ascorbate with purified enzymes has been better characterized than for the enzymes in situ,[29,54] but the role of ascorbate with enzymes in situ provides the best information for making recommendations about vitamin intake.[29,54]

Ascorbate is an electron donor (or reducing agent) for intra- and extracellular chemical reactions. As discussed above, ascorbate is often called an antioxidant vitamin for these reactions. Ascorbate reduces superoxide, hydroxyl radicals, hypochlorous acid, and other reactive oxidants. Because these oxidants may affect DNA transcription or could damage DNA, proteins, or membrane structures, ascorbate may have a central role in cellular oxidant defense.[55,56] Ascorbate within cells is used as an electron donor as part of the interaction between iron and ferritin.[57] Ascorbate outside of cells may prevent low-density lipoprotein (LDL) oxidation.[58,59] Extracellular ascorbate may also transfer electrons to tocopherol radicals in lipid particles or membranes.[60] For many of these reactions there is strong in vitro but not in vivo evidence, and in some cases in vivo data contradict in vitro findings.

By keeping iron in its reduced form, ascorbate enhances intestinal iron absorption.[61-64] This observation is applied clinically to enhance iron absorption in patients with iron deficiency.

Recent data suggest that ascorbate might regulate protein translation, although the mechanism is uncertain.[65] Ascorbate could possibly regulate gene transcription other than by quenching oxidants, but this possibility is still theoretical.

Ascorbate is also accumulated by tissues where its function is uncertain, such as endocrine tissues (e.g., adrenal cortex, ovaries, testis, and pancreas) and cells of host defense (B lymphocytes, T lymphocytes, and platelets).[29,54,66]

Ascorbate and Dehydroascorbic Acid Transport

Ascorbate is transported into many cells and accumulated against a concentration gradient. Ascorbate concentrations in plasma in people without scurvy vary nearly 10-fold, from 10 to 90 μM.[67,68] Because it is water soluble and not protein bound, ascorbate is appropriately assumed to be at similar concentrations extracellularly.[68,69] Ascorbate is found in millimolar concentrations in neutrophils and other cells of host defense, many endocrine tissues, liver, fibroblasts, lens, retina, brain and neuronal tissue, bone-forming cells, and parotid glands.[66,70-78]

Although data for dehydroascorbic acid are more controversial, dehydroascorbic acid is probably not found in plasma.[68,79] Dehydroascorbic acid is not detected within cells under physiologic conditions.[40,41] Some assays may provide artifactual evidence for the presence of dehydroascorbic acid because of inadvertent oxidation of ascorbate. Dehydroascorbic acid may form transiently outside of cells locally because of ascorbate oxidation resulting from oxidants in the extracellular milieu.[40,80]

Ascorbate accumulation occurs by at least two distinct mechanisms.[40] By the first mechanism, ascorbate is accumulated as such by active transport.[66,72-78] The transporter is concentration, sodium, and energy dependent and displays saturation kinetics. The transporter protein has not yet been isolated but is known to exist in a cDNA library and to be expressible from injected mRNA in *Xenopus laevis* oocytes.[81] Ascorbate transport has a K_m of 5–10 μM in human cells and achieves Vmax at ≈70–80 μM.[66,70,75,82-84]

The second mechanism of ascorbate accumulation is based on dehydroascorbic acid transport and intracellular reduction.[40,41] Dehydroascorbic acid is transported by one or more glucose transporters and immediately reduced intracellularly to ascorbate.[40,41,85,86] Dehydroascorbic acid reduction is most likely mediated by glutaredoxin (thioltransferase) in many tissues, although in some tissues a slower rate of dehydroascorbic acid reduction may be chemically mediated by glutathione or by other proteins.[87,88] Kinetics of dehydroascorbic acid transport are complex and difficult to determine accurately because they can be calculated only when there is complete reduction of dehydroascorbic acid to ascorbate.[40]

Because dehydroascorbic acid is reduced as soon as it is transported, no dehydroascorbic acid is usually found intracellularly.[40,41,85] Dehydroascorbic acid is transported at least 10-fold faster than ascorbate,[40] but transport is limited by availability. Dehydroascorbic acid transport occurs only when dehydroascorbic acid forms from ascorbate. By contrast, ascorbate is always present in plasma and the extracellular milieu except in severe scurvy. On the basis of substrate availability, ascorbate transport can be considered constitutive substrate transport and dehydroascorbic acid transport considered induced substrate transport. Because separate transport proteins are required for each process, it remains possible that the transport proteins are also inducible.

Ascorbate appears to be absorbed by active transport in the human gut by an intestinal transporter, although this protein has not been isolated.[89–93] Intestinal absorption of dehydroascorbic acid has not been well characterized.[94] The available data suggest that dehydroascorbic acid is also transported, but by a different mechanism from that for ascorbate, and then reduced to ascorbate. Although one candidate for dehydroascorbic acid reduction in intestinal mucosa is glutaredoxin, there are other possibilities and the mechanism is not known.

It is not clear whether the reduced substrate (ascorbate), oxidized substrate (dehydroascorbic acid), or both are found in the gut lumen. The form present in foodstuffs and supplements is predominately ascorbate.[95] Dehydroascorbic acid could also be formed by oxidation and absorbed, but because it is easily hydrolyzed it would be expected to have a much shorter half-life in the gut than that for ascorbate. In the gut lumen, it is therefore logical to assume that the primary substrate is ascorbate.

Availability for Ingestion

Ascorbate is found in many fruits and vegetables.[96] Rich fruit sources include cantaloupe, grapefruit, honeydew, kiwi, mango, orange, papaya, strawberries, tangelo, tangerine, and watermelon. Fruit juices rich in vitamin C include grapefruit and orange juices. Some fruit juices are fortified with vitamin C, including apple, cranberry, and grape juices. Rich vegetable sources of vitamin C include asparagus, broccoli, brussels sprouts, cabbage, cauliflower, kale, mustard greens, pepper (red or green), plantains, potatoes, snow peas, sweet potato, and tomatoes and tomato juices. Estimates of food content for vitamin C are affected by season, food trans-

port, time in market before purchase, and storage and cooking practices.

Ascorbate is available in vitamin tablets, and many multivitamin supplements contain ascorbate. Ascorbate is also available by itself across a very wide dose range and in supplements that have other selected vitamins, commonly in tablets sold as antioxidant supplements.

As indicated by its many sources, vitamin C is readily available for consumption. Vitamin C ingestion is governed by food selection. U.S. Department of Agriculture (USDA) and National Cancer Institute (NCI) guidelines are similar, with recommendations for eating at least five fruits and vegetables daily.[97] If these recommendations are followed, vitamin C ingestion will be at least 210 mg and quite possibly closer to 300 mg.

The most recent data from the third National Health and Nutrition Examination Survey (NHANES III Part 1, 1988–1991) suggest that median vitamin C consumption from foods in U.S. males excluding children is 84 mg/day and for females is 73 mg/day.[98] However, approximately one-fourth of females and one-third of men ingested <2.5 servings of fruits and vegetables daily. Data are available on mean dietary intake from more recent surveys but are limited in scope. For example, a study of 9- and 10-year-old girls indicated that approximately one-fourth had vitamin C ingestion below the RDA (45 mg) for this age group.[99] A survey of Latino children indicated that <15% consumed the recommended intake of fruits and vegetables.[100] Older data from the second National Health and Nutrition Examination Survey (NHANES II) were examined more extensively and indicated that 20–30% of U.S. adults ingested <60 mg/day of vitamin C.[101–103] Unfortunately, the most recent ingestion data do not include vitamin C consumption from supplements.[104] It is a reasonable estimate that at least 50% of the U.S. population do not ingest supplements,[101,104,105] and it is not clear whether supplement ingestion substantially changes total vitamin C consumption.[104] The most recent NHANES III data indicate that vitamin C ingestion from foods is increasing. Nevertheless, a substantial number of people in the United States ingest vitamin C at or below the present RDA.

Pharmacokinetics

Steady-state concentrations in plasma. Until recently, steady-state plasma ascorbate concentrations as a function of dose were unknown. Prior inpatient investigations of vitamin C metabolism were not designed to address this issue. These studies, performed on male subects in Iowa, are the basis of the current RDA for adults.[17–21] Subjects were given ≤66.5 mg of ascorbate daily, except for one who received 130.5 mg daily. Not enough doses were given to determine a dose-concentration relationship. Samples were analyzed by the imprecise dinitrophenylhydrazine assay. The investigators themselves realized that this colorometric assay produced falsely elevated results, especially at the lowest ascorbate doses.[106] Other inpatient studies were limited because only one dose was given above 60 mg/day or because only three vitamin C doses were given and the samples were measured by an imprecise technique.[107,108]

Outpatient studies also investigated the relationship between dose and achieved concentration.[109–112] Outpatient studies have the strong disadvantage of not being able to control dietary ascorbate and ascorbate ingestion and are based on dietary recall surveys. Because many people do not know the vitamin content of what they actually eat or have difficulty remembering food choices, surveys result in misleading information and underreporting, especially over narrow dose ranges.[113] Similar to inpatient studies, outpatient studies used narrow dose ranges or assay techniques subject to artifact.

We recently published new pharmacokinetic data about vitamin C, some of which characterize the relationship between ascorbate dose and steady-state plasma concentration.[67] The data are based on studies of seven men who were inpatients for 4–6 months at the National Institutes of Health (NIH). Vitamin C ingestion from foods was <5 mg/day. Ascorbate was measured by HPLC with coulometric electrochemical detection. When subjects achieved plasma concentrations <10 μM ascorbate, each of seven ascorbate repletion doses from 30 to 2500 mg/day were administered in succession. Volunteers reached a steady-state plasma value for each dose before the next dose was administered. These data showed that there was a sigmoid relationship between ascorbate dose and steady-state plasma concentration. The concentration produced by the present RDA was on the bottom third of the steep portion of the curve, the 200-mg dose was beyond the steep portion of the curve and produced >80% plasma saturation, and plasma was completely saturated at the 1000-mg dose.

Steady-state concentrations in cells and tissues.
Little information was available until recently about steady-state concentrations in tissues as a function of ascorbate dose. The limited information available was compromised by being based on few doses.[107,108,114] One study providing information about ascorbate in seminal fluid had only one dose above 60 mg/day.[114]

Data from the NIH volunteer study included vitamin C content of neutrophils, monocytes, and lymphocytes at each dose from 30 to 2500 mg/day.[67] All cell types became saturated at the 100-mg dose. The difference between cell saturation and plasma saturation was most likely due to ascorbate accumulation in cells by active transport and to a renal threshold for ascorbate excretion (see below).

Bioavailability.
Until recently, true bioavailability of ascorbate was unknown. True bioavailability is determined by measuring the increase in the amount of a substance after an oral dose and comparing this with the increase after the same dose is given intravenously.[115,116] For the dose under study, subjects must be at steady state. Before administration of an oral dose, baseline plasma values are obtained. Once the dose is given, plasma values rise and then return to baseline. When the data are displayed, there is an area under the curve and above baseline that represents the increase from the oral dose (AUC_{po}). When values return to baseline, the same dose is given intravenously. Plasma values usually rise much faster, because the gastrointestinal system is bypassed, and then return to baseline. When the data are displayed, the area under the curve and above baseline represents the increase from the intravenous dose (AUC_{iv}). True bioavailability is defined pharmacologically as AUC_{po}/AUC_{iv}. Bioavailability is often displayed as a percentage, with 100% bioavailability representing complete absorption. Studies of true bioavailability are difficult to perform because subjects must be at steady state for the tested dose, the substance must be administered intravenously, and many samples must be analyzed for each tested dose. Ideally, several different doses should be studied and true bioavailability calculated for each.

Because of these difficulties most investigators estimated ascorbate bioavailability indirectly. In some studies oral absorption was compared with urinary excretion;[112,117–119] in other studies absorption of one form of vitamin C (e.g., in foods) was compared with another form (e.g., in a supplement).[120,121] Although these data provide comparative results about vitamin C absorption, they cannot be used to make conclusions about true bioavailability.

One earlier study of true bioavailability was seriously compromised by measuring ascorbate in whole blood instead of plasma with a nonspecific assay and by using a capsule preparation with unclear absorptive properties.[122] The first data to provide detailed information about true bioavailability were recently presented in the NIH volunteer study.[67] Ascorbate bioavailability at steady state for each dose was 100% for 200 mg, 73% for 500 mg, and 49% for 1250 mg. Although it is likely that bioavailability at doses <200 mg was complete, precise calculations could not be made.[67] Bioavailability calculations using AUC ratios are made on the assumptions that there is a constant volume of distribution and constant clearance for the test substance.[115,116] At ascorbate doses <200 mg these assumptions were not valid, most likely because of multicompartmental distribution. Methods to determine bioavailability at ascorbate doses <200 mg depend on models that account for nonlinearity in clearance and volume of distribution. Such models are now being developed.

The data for true bioavailability of vitamin C were based on vitamin C administration alone, with the vitamin given either in the fasting state or at least 90 minutes before meals. There are no data for true bioavailability of vitamin C administered with foods or with compounds found in foods.

Urinary excretion of ascorbate. Ascorbate undergoes renal reabsorption and excretion.[123] Ascorbate probably passes unchanged through glomeruli and is actively reabsorbed in tubules in a concentration-dependent manner by an ascorbate transport protein, which has not been isolated. Once the transport protein reaches saturation, or achieves Vmax, remaining ascorbate is presumed to be excreted. It is not clear whether there is also active secretion of ascorbate into renal tubules distal to the reabsorption site. Ascorbate concentrations in renal tubules are not known. Because there is no dehydroascorbic acid in human plasma, there is no known renal mechanism for dehydroascorbic acid filtration and reabsorption.

Because ascorbate is not protein bound, ascorbate is freely dialyzed in patients undergoing dialysis.[69] These patients require ascorbate replacement, usually ≤500 mg/day, and if ascorbate is not replaced they can develop scurvy. In renal disease short of renal failure requiring dialysis, it is not known whether ascorbate filtration, reabsorption, or both are compromised and whether ascorbate consumption is otherwise altered as a consequence of metabolic abnormalities induced by renal insufficiency.

Until recently, there have been few data concerning urinary excretion of ascorbate at steady state for a given dose. Early clinical investigations, indicating that vitamin C was reabsorbed by a saturable tubular reabsorption mechanism, did not account for achieving steady state.[123] In the Iowa inpatient studies, urinary excretion was stated to occur at ingestion of 60 mg/day, but no data were given.[17–20,124] As already noted, the assays used for vitamin C detection were not specific. In another inpatient study only one dose above 60 mg was given, and there was a wide range in vitamin C excretion.[107] An outpatient study that used excretion of radiolabeled vitamin C as an endpoint did not control for vitamin C ingestion before administration of radiolabeled material.[109] Analysis of the excreted radiolabel, to detect whether the radiolabel was unchanged or metabolized, may also have been flawed. Other outpatient studies used limited doses ≥500 mg.

In the NIH volunteer study, urinary excretion of vitamin C was measured at the steady state of each dose. In six of seven volunteers, no urinary excretion occurred for vitamin C doses <100 mg. At 100 mg approximately one-fourth of the dose was excreted and at 200 mg approximately one-half of the dose was excreted. At the higher doses of 500 mg and 1250 mg, bioavailability was not complete but virtually all of the absorbed dose was excreted. Thus, at steady state, ascorbate doses of ≥500 mg have no effect on ascorbate body stores.[67]

Deficiency

Vitamin C deficiency was described extensively in the Iowa studies. The earliest signs were reported to be small ecchymoses and petechiae.[18,20] Because scurvy can be overlooked at this stage, the differential diagnosis of ecchymoses should always include scurvy.[122] As ecchymoses became more prominent, follicular hyperkeratosis developed, especially on the buttocks and lower extremities. One of the most specific signs was the hyperkeratotic hair follicle with a hemorrhagic halo. These signs were followed by swollen and bleeding gums and ocular hemorrhages in the bulbar conjunctiva. Signs similar to connective tissue disorders included arthralgias, joint effusions, and Sjogren's syndrome (keratoconjunctivitis sicca: dry eyes and dry mouth).[125] Mild anemia was reported but there was incomplete information about its pathogenesis and whether the anemia was microcytic, normochromic, or macrocytic.[18,20] Prominent symptoms were psychologic abnormalities including hypochondriasis, depression, and hysteria. Fatigue and lethargy were reported as relatively late symptoms. Remember that in the Iowa studies, patients developed profound scurvy, with development of signs including femoral neuropathy, hair loss, and edema. These patients were kept vitamin C deficient for as long as 3 months. (A simple mnemonic for the signs and symptoms of scurvy is hemorrhage, hyperkeratosis, hypochondriasis, and hematologic abnormalities—the four Hs.)

In the NIH volunteer study plasma concentrations of ascorbate were brought to very low levels, but no volunteers developed scurvy. In contrast to the Iowa studies, mild fatigue and lethargy were consistently noted by volunteers without any other symptom or sign of scurvy.[67] Despite extensive testing, there were no associated clinical laboratory abnormalities associated with fatigue and no abnormalities on psychologic testing. We believe that mild fatigue is the earliest symptom of vitamin C deficiency. Because there are no other associated signs or symptoms of early vitamin C deficiency and because fatigue is such a common chief complaint of patients in the United States, we advise physicians to include mild vitamin C deficiency in their differential diagnosis of fatigue. A simple, rapid, and inexpensive screening tool is to ask patients whether they consume fruits, vegetables, or vitamin supplements.

Toxicity

Vitamin C has little frank toxicity. Adverse effects do occur and are dose dependent (Table 2).[54] Diarrhea, abdominal bloating, or both can occur when several grams

Table 2. Adverse effects of vitamin C

Diarrhea, abdominal bloating with gram doses
False-negative results for occult blood in stool
Iron overabsorption: thalassemia major, sideroblastic
   anemia, and hemochromatosis
Hyperoxaluria in some patients
?Hyperuricosuria
Hyperoxalemia in dialysis patients
Hemolysis in patients with glucose-6-phosphate
   dehydrogenase deficiency

are taken at once, although there should be no need for ingestion of these large doses. False negative results for detection of occult blood occur with ingestion of ≤ 250 mg of vitamin C.[126] Manufacturers recommend that ingestion of vitamin C, especially in supplement form, should be stopped for several days before testing stool for occult blood.

Because ascorbate maintains iron in its reduced form, iron absorption is facilitated by ascorbate. Patients who are iron overloaded may have hemochromatosis, thalassemia major, sideroblastic anemia, or other diseases requiring multiple red blood cell transfusions.[127,128] Ascorbate may enhance iron overload in these subjects or be otherwise harmful.[127–129] It is not known whether ascorbate induces iron overabsorption in normal people. Ferritin concentrations were stable when 2 g of vitamin C was ingested for as long as 2 years by normal volunteers.[130] Iron absorption was most affected by 25–50 mg of ascorbate per meal,[131] which suggests that it is not likely that higher doses of ascorbate will cause iron overload. Patients with hemochromatosis are homozygous for the disease-causing gene. It is not known whether subjects who are heterozygous for the gene have enhanced iron absorption from vitamin C. The amount of ascorbate in foods is similar to the amount that most enhances iron absorption. Iron overload is very uncommon, and if heterozygous subjects were at risk for iron overload from ascorbate, a higher incidence and prevalence of iron overload would be observed than is actually found. Although there are no definitive answers, the data imply that vitamin C does not cause iron overabsorption in normal people and that subjects who are heterozygous for hemochromatosis are also probably not at risk for iron overload from ascorbate.

Data are conflicting concerning the effect of ascorbate on urate and oxalate excretion. For urate, hyperuricosuria was reported when some subjects received a large dose of ascorbate intravenously,[132] although these findings were contradicted by others.[133] Transient hyperuricosuria occurred when 3 g of vitamin was given.[134] The conflicting findings may be due to the lack of a steady state for vitamin C, differences in plasma concentrations, or the duration of vitamin administration. In the NIH volunteer study uric acid excretion was increased at the 1-g

dose of vitamin C compared with lower doses.[67] There were fewer subjects whose urine was available for measurement at the 1-g dose and the hyperuricosuria may have been transient. It is not clear whether hyperuricosuria would persist if these doses were administered for longer periods. Although these data are not consistent, in all of the experiments hyperuricosuria did not occur with doses of ascorbate <1 g.

A metabolite of ascorbate catabolism is oxalate, and its excretion in relation to ascorbate ingestion has been controversial for many years. Some of the confusing information was due to difficulty in measuring oxalate accurately. In oxalate assays commonly used more than 10 years ago, ascorbate produced false elevation of oxalate.[135] The data are still contradictory despite the use of better assays;[136–138] the best explanation of the data is that subsets of patients may have enhanced oxalate excretion from ascorbate. In particular, patients who form oxalate stones may have enhanced oxalate excretion associated with ascorbate ingestion ≥ 500 mg, and for these patients megadoses of ascorbate could be harmful.[138]

Hyperoxalemia is associated with vitamin C, but only when it is administered intravenously to dialysis patients in repetitive doses of 1 g.[139] We know of no clinical indication for this therapy, so that ascorbate-induced hyperoxalemia is an experimental curiosity rather than a clinical problem.

Although the practice has no clear justification, some health care practitioners administer ascorbate in doses of many grams. In patients with glucose-6-phosphate dehydrogenase deficiency, hemolysis occurred after ascorbate was administered intravenously.[140,141] There is also one case report of hemolysis in patients with glucose-6-phosphate dehydrogenase deficiency who received ≥ 6 g of ascorbate as a single oral dose.[142] We know of no clinical situation where such massive single oral doses are indicated. If there is an indication to administer ascorbate intravenously, patients should first be screened for glucose-6-phosphate dehydrogenase deficiency.

Harmful effects have been mistakenly attributed to ascorbate ingestion, especially at doses >1 g. These misconceptions include hypoglycemia, rebound scurvy, infertility, mutagenesis, and destruction of vitamin B-12. It is erroneous to conclude that gram doses of vitamin C produce these effects.

Epidemiology

Epidemiologic data describe the association of vitamin C consumption with health maintenance and disease outcome. The data are not conclusive and the observations are sometimes contradictory. Diets with high vitamin C content from fruits and vegetables are associated with lower cancer risk, especially for cancers of the oral cavity, esophagus, stomach, colon, and lung.[143] In contrast, consumption of vitamin C as a supplement in experimental trials had no effect on development of colorectal adenoma and stomach cancer.[144,145] The effects of ascorbate ingestion on coronary heart disease and cataract development are also contradictory.[25,146–157]

These differences may have several experimental explanations. Fruit and vegetable ingestion may be associated with lower cancer risk not because of vitamin C alone but because of complex interactions between ascorbate and multiple bioactive compounds in these foods.[143] Another problem is related to a steep relationship between vitamin C plasma concentration and vitamin C daily doses ≤100 mg.[67] Thus patients who served as controls in at least one study were already close to saturation for vitamin C.[145] Additional vitamin C doses would not cause vitamin C concentrations to rise much more and an effect of vitamin C would not be expected. To test future potential benefits of vitamin C, control patients must have lower plasma and tissue vitamin C concentrations than supplemented patients. Unfortunately, most information about vitamin C nutriture in epidemiologic studies is from food surveys and not from plasma measurements. Because food surveys are often inaccurate, it might not be possible to detect these small differences in ingestion by using food surveys.[113] Unfortunately, small differences in vitamin C consumption <100 mg have great consequences for plasma levels.[67]

Ascorbate has been studied for its effects on stroke, overall mortality, and time to development of AIDS. Low plasma vitamin C concentrations were reported to be associated with increased risk of stroke.[149] The vitamin C effect occurred only when there were concomitant low β-carotene concentrations and not when ascorbate alone was low. A widely publicized study in which overall mortality was reduced by vitamin C had several serious flaws. Mortality was reduced in supplement users who ingested >700 mg/day, but vitamin C plasma concentrations were not measured.[25] Data from normal men show that vitamin C ingestion ≥500 mg produced no changes in plasma and tissue concentrations compared with vitamin C ingestion of 400 mg/day.[67] Thus, the effect of prolonging life attributed to vitamin C in supplements was probably due to something else. For example, other important variables such as blood pressure were not measured.[25] A similar study of a similar population found that vitamin C ingestion had no effect on mortality.[150] The effect of vitamin C on development of AIDS in patients positive for human immunodeficiency virus involved small numbers of patients and had several internal inconsistencies.[158]

The contradictions regarding effects of ascorbate in epidemiologic studies may have other explanations. Some inconsistencies may be inherent in observational epidemiologic studies. Observational studies cannot exclude the possibility that another factor accounts for the observed event. Randomized trials might provide clearer answers if they are large enough and long enough and account for the steep dose-concentration relationship at low ascorbate doses. However, if observed effects of ascorbate are due to its interaction with other compounds in fruits and vegetables, interventional epidemiologic studies may be very difficult to conduct.

The RDA for Vitamin C

Present RDA criteria. The current RDA for vitamin C, 60 mg/day for adults, is based on preventing signs and symptoms of scurvy for at least 4 weeks if vitamin C ingestion ceased, estimates of catabolic rates of vitamin C metabolism, and the dose at which urinary excretion occurs.[21] The RDA was chosen to provide enough vitamin C to prevent or cure scurvy and to provide adequate reserves. The RDA is based in part on the concept that urinary excretion of vitamin C indicates that body stores are near saturation.

The RDA is based on these criteria because of limited data available at the time of its formulation and is predominantly based on depletion-repletion studies in inpatient subjects in Iowa.[17–21] These experiments were initially performed with four subjects.[17,18] However, their controlled diet may have had multiple vitamin and mineral deficiencies. The diet was revised and the study was repeated with five subjects.[19,20] The current RDA is based to a large degree on these later data.

Despite their intent, the Iowa studies are flawed. The vitamin C assay overestimated true vitamin concentration, especially at lower values; the authors noted several patients had obvious scurvy despite blood measurements suggesting otherwise.[106] Because of the need for relatively large sample volumes, frequent sampling and true bioavailability sampling were not possible. Urinary excretion data were not presented despite their importance for estimating the RDA. The vitamin C dose range was very narrow. Few other inpatient studies were available, and they suffered from similar problems.[107,108]

Data from some outpatient studies were also used for determining the current RDA.[109–112,159] As discussed earlier, a key problem in these studies is the lack of control for ascorbate ingestion. Unfortunately, these studies also share many of the flaws of the inpatient studies just discussed.

New RDA criteria. The Food and Nutrition Board has recognized that future RDAs should have a broader basis.[160] Evidence to be used in determining ideal RDAs includes availability of the nutrient in the diet, steady-state concentrations of vitamin in relation to dose for plasma and tissues, vitamin distribution in plasma and tissues in relation to dose, true bioavailability as a function of dose, urinary excretion, toxicity, biochemical and molecular function in relation to vitamin concentration, and epidemiologic observations.[54,160]

The Food and Nutrition Board also suggested several new categories for intake recommendations.[160] A requirement is defined as the minimum intake that will maintain normal function and health. Operationally, nutrient requirement is the amount that will maintain body weight and prevent depletion. In contrast, the RDA is the amount that will meet the known nutritional needs of practically all healthy people and for which the risk of inadequacy is very low. Upper safe ingestion indicates the upper limit of intake that is safe for most healthy people and beyond which there is a possibility of toxicity.

Recommendations for Vitamin C Intake: Recommendations Based on the New RDA Criteria

Since the last RDA for vitamin C was published, new data have become available. For the first time, the new broader-based RDA criteria can be applied to recommendations for vitamin C. We suggest the following reference points:

- RDA: a new RDA for adults for vitamin C of 200 mg/day.
- Upper safe: a new upper-safe recommendation for vitamin C ingestion of <1000 mg/day.
- Deficient: deficiency signs and symptoms in adults are prevented by 60 mg/day, which provides a margin of safety of several weeks if vitamin C intake is stopped.

These guidelines are supported by new data as follows:

Availability. Ascorbate is available in the diet if we choose to consume it. Following USDA and NCI recommendations for fruit and vegetable consumption will result in vitamin C intake of ≥210 mg/day.[97]

Steady-state concentrations and distribution in relation to dose. As a function of dose, steady-state plasma concentrations display steep sigmoid kinetics.[67] The first dose beyond the steep portion of the curve is 200 mg/day. At this dose, plasma is ≈80% saturated. Plasma saturates at 1000 mg/day; cells saturate at 100 mg/day.[67] Data for plasma and cells are based on administration of pure vitamin C alone at least 1.5 hours before meals. Because glucose inhibits vitamin C transport in some cells and because vitamin C in foods is present with glucose, it is possible that vitamin C in foods will not be absorbed as well as vitamin C alone.[75,82,161] Thus, the doses that produce near saturation of plasma and saturation of cells may be minimum estimates. Doses ≤100 mg are on the steep portion of the absorption curve, where small changes in dose produce large changes in concentration.

Bioavailability. Bioavailability of 200 mg of ascorbate is 100%. Higher doses have lower bioavailability.[67]

Urinary excretion. When the dose of ascorbate is <100 mg, no ascorbate is excreted in urine. By contrast, at steady-state for doses ≥500 mg, all of the absorbed dose is excreted in urine.[67]

Toxicity. Doses <500 mg have no apparent adverse effects in healthy people.[54,67] Doses of ≥500 mg may increase urinary oxalate excretion in patients with prior history of oxalate kidney stones.[136,138] Doses of 1000 mg can produce hyperuricosuria and hyperoxaluria in healthy people.[67]

Biochemical and molecular function in relation to vitamin concentration. Only indirect information is available regarding function in relation to dose. The plasma concentration achieved at the current RDA of 60 mg/day is close to K_m for vitamin C transport.[66,70,75,82,84] By contrast, vitamin C transport is close to Vmax at the plasma concentration achieved at 200 mg/day.[66,70,75,82,84] This dose may prevent formation of harmful nitrosamines in the gastrointestinal tract and produces a plasma concentration that may inhibit LDL oxidation.[59,162] Much more work, however, is needed to correlate molecular function in situ to vitamin concentration.

Epidemiologic observations. The most powerful epidemiologic observations show that ingestion of five or more fruits and vegetables per day is associated with lower risk for cancers of the gastrointestinal and respiratory tracts.[143] This would result in vitamin C ingestion of >210 mg/day. Vitamin C supplements alone have not yet been shown to confer similar protection.[143–145]

Prevention of deficiency. Fatigue is probably the first symptom of vitamin C deficiency, without any corresponding signs; 60 mg/day will probably alleviate this early symptom of vitamin C deficiency in most people[67] and 60 mg/day will protect against scurvy for several weeks if vitamin C ingestion ceases.[17–21]

References

1. Bourne GH (1944) Records in the older literature of tissue changes in scurvy. Proc R Soc Med 37:512–516
2. Hippocrates (1945) The genuine works of Hippocrates ca 600 B.C. In Major RH (ed), Classic descriptions of disease with biographical sketches of the authors. Charles C. Thomas, Springfield, IL
3. Cartier J (1953) "La Grosse Maladie." Reproduction photographique de son 'Brief Recit et Succincte Narration, 1545, suive d'une traduction en langue anglaise du chapitre traitant des aventures de Cartier aux prises avec le scorbut et d'une nouvelle analyse du Mystere de l'Anneda. Ronald Printing Co., Ltd, Montreal
4. Encyclopaedia Britanica (1771) pp 106–110
5. Aberg F (1950) J Chem Educ 27:334
6. Lind J (1753) A treatise on the scurvy. A. Millar, London
7. Svirbely JL, Szent-Gyorgyi A (1932) The chemical nature of vitamin C. Biochem J 26:865–870
8. King CC, Waugh WA (1932) The chemical nature of vitamin C. Science 75:357–358
9. Perla D, Marmorston J (1937) The role of vitamin C in resistance. Arch Pathol 23:543–575

10. Perla D, Marmorston J (1941) Natural resistance and clinical medicine. Little Brown & Co, Boston, pp 1038–1091

11. Kryzhanovskaya LI, London ES, Rivosh FI (1938) The effect of intravenous administration of ascorbic acid upon adrenalin secretion and upon the role of the suprarenal glands in glutathione and vitamin C metabolism. J Physiol 24:212

12. Torrance CC (1940) Diphtherial intoxication and vitamin C content of the suprarenals of guinea pigs. J Biol Chem 132:575–584

13. Cowan RW, Diehl HS, Baker AB (1942) Vitamins for the prevention of colds. JAMA 120:1268–1271

14. Pauling L (1974) Are recommended daily allowances for vitamin C adequate? Proc Natl Acad Sci USA 71:4442–4446

15. Pauling L (1976) Vitamin C, the common cold and the flu. WH Freeman and Co, San Francisco

16. Food and Nutrition Board, National Academy of Sciences (1974) Recommended dietary allowances. National Academy Press, Washington, DC

17. Baker EM, Hodges RE, Hood J, et al (1969) Metabolism of ascorbic-1-¹⁴C acid in experimental human scurvy. Am J Clin Nutr 22:549–558

18. Hodges RE, Baker EM, Hood J, et al (1969) Experimental scurvy in man. Am J Clin Nutr 22:535–548

19. Baker EM, Hodges RE, Hood J, et al (1971) Metabolism of ¹⁴C- and ³H-labeled L-ascorbic acid in human scurvy. Am J Clin Nutr 24:444–454

20. Hodges RE, Hood J, Canham JE, et al (1971) Clinical manifestations of ascorbic acid deficiency in man. Am J Clin Nutr 24:432–443

21. Food and Nutrition Board, National Academy of Sciences (1989) Recommended dietary allowances, 10th ed. National Academy Press, Washington, DC

22. Jialal I, Grundy SM (1992) Influence of antioxidant vitamins on LDL oxidation. Ann NY Acad Sci 669:237–247

23. Cameron E, Pauling L (1993) Cancer and vitamin C. Camino Books, Philadelphia

24. Taylor A, Jacques PF, Nadler D, et al (1991) Relationship in humans between ascorbic acid consumption and levels of total and reduced ascorbic acid in lens, aqueous humor, and plasma. Curr Eye Res 10:751–759

25. Enstrom JE, Kanim LE, Klein MA (1992) Vitamin C intake and mortality among a sample of the United States population. Epidemiology 3:194–202

26. Suboticanec K, Folnegovic-Smalc V, Korbar M, et al (1990) Vitamin C status in chronic schizophrenia. Biol Psychiatry 28:959–966

27. Harakeh S, Jariwalla RJ (1991) Comparative study of the anti-HIV activities of ascorbate and thiol-containing reducing agents in chronically HIV-infected cells. Am J Clin Nutr 54:1231S–1235S

28. Brox AG, Howson-Jan K, Fauser AA (1988) Treatment of idiopathic thrombocytopenic purpura with ascorbate. Br J Haematol 70:341–344

29. Levine M (1986) New concepts in the biology and biochemistry of ascorbic acid. N Engl J Med 314:892–902

30. Washko PW, Welch RW, Dhariwal KR, et al (1992) Ascorbic acid and dehydroascorbic acid analyses in biological samples. Anal Biochem 204:1–14

31. Bielski BH, Richter HW, Chan PC (1975) Some properties of the ascorbate free radical. Ann NY Acad Sci 258:231–237

32. Tolbert BM, Ward JB (1982) Dehydroascorbic acid. In Seib PA, Tolbert BM (eds), Ascorbic acid: chemistry, metabolism, and uses. American Chemical Society, Washington, DC, pp 101–123

33. Lewin S (1976) Vitamin C: its molecular biology and medical potential. Academic Press, London, pp 5–62

34. Buettner GR (1993) The pecking order of free radicals and antioxidants: lipid peroxidation, alpha-tocopherol, and ascorbate. Arch Biochem Biophys 300:535–543

35. Nishikimi M, Fukuyama R, Minoshima S, et al (1994) Cloning and chromosomal mapping of the human nonfunctional gene for L-gulono-gamma-lactone oxidase, the enzyme for L-ascorbic acid biosynthesis missing in man. J Biol Chem 269:13685–13688

36. Eaton SB, Konner M (1985) Paleolithic nutrition: a consideration of its nature and current implications. N Engl J Med 312:283–289

37. Dhariwal KR, Washko PW, Levine M (1990) Determination of dehydroascorbic acid using high-performance liquid chromatography with coulometric electrochemical detection. Anal Biochem 189:18–23

38. Washko PW, Hartzell WO, Levine M (1989) Ascorbic acid analysis using high-performance liquid chromatography with coulometric electrochemical detection. Anal Biochem 181:276–282

39. Dhariwal KR, Black CD, Levine M (1991) Semidehydroascorbic acid as an intermediate in norepinephrine biosynthesis in chromaffin granules. J Biol Chem 266:12908–12914

40. Welch RW, Wang Y, Crossman A Jr, et al (1995) Accumulation of vitamin C (ascorbate) and its oxidized metabolite dehydroascorbic acid occurs by separate mechanisms. J Biol Chem 270:12584–12592

41. Washko PW, Wang Y, Levine M (1993) Ascorbic acid recycling in human neutrophils. J Biol Chem 268:15531–15535

42. Retsky KL, Freeman MW, Frei B (1993) Ascorbic acid oxidation product(s) protect human low density lipoprotein against atherogenic modification: anti- rather than prooxidant activity of vitamin C in the presence of transition metal ions. J Biol Chem 268:1304–1309

43. Peterkoshy B, Udenfriend S (1965) Enzymatic hydroxylation of proline microsomal polypeptide leading to formation of collagen. Proc Natl Acad Sci USA 53:335–342

44. Puistola U, Turpeenniemi-Hujanen TM, Myllyla R, Kivirikko KI (1980) Studies on the lysyl hydroxylase reaction. I. Initial velocity kinetics and related aspects. Biochim Biophys Acta 611:40–50

45. Kivirikko KO, Myllyla R, Pihlajaniemi T (1989) Protein hydroxylation: prolyl 4-hydroxylase, an enzyme with four cosubstrates and a multifunctional subunit. FASEB J 3:1609–1617

46. Lindblad B, Lindstedt G, Lindstedt S, Rundgren M (1977) Purification and some properties of human 4-hydroxyphenylpyruvate dioxygenase (I). J Biol Chem 252:5073–5084

47. Dunn WA, Rettura G, Seifter E, England S (1984) Carnitine biosynthesis from gamma-butyrobetaine and from exogenous protein-bound 6-N-trimethyl-L-lysine by the perfused guinea pig liver: effect of ascorbate deficiency on the in situ activity of gamma-butyrobetaine hydroxylase. J Biol Chem 259:10764–10770

48. Friedman S, Kaufman S (1965) 3,4-Dihydroxyphenylethylamine beta-hydroxylase: physical properties, copper content, and role of copper in the catalytic acttivity. J Biol Chem 240:4763–4773

49. Levine M (1986) Ascorbic acid specifically enhances dopamine beta-monooxygenase activity in resting and stimulated chromaffin cells. J Biol Chem 261:7347–7356

50. Wand GS, Ney RL, Baylin S, et al (1985) Characterization of a peptide alpha-amidation activity in human plasma and tissues. Metabolism 34:1044–1052

51. Eipper BA, Mains RE (1991) The role of ascorbate in the biosynthesis of neuroendocrine peptides. Am J Clin Nutr 54:1153S–1156S

52. Eipper BA, Perkins SN, Husten EJ, et al (1991) Peptidyl-alpha-hydroxyglycine alpha-amidating lyase purification, characterization and expression. J Biol Chem 266:7827–7833

53. La Du BN, Zannoni VG (1961) The role of ascorbic acid in tyrosine metabolism. Ann NY Acad Sci 92:175–191

54. Levine M, Dhariwal KR, Welch RW, et al (1995) Determination of optimal vitamin C requirements in humans. Am J Clin Nutr 62(suppl):1347S–1356S

55. Frei B, England L, Ames BN (1989) Ascorbate is an outstanding antioxidant in human blood plasma. Proc Natl Acad Sci USA 86:6377–6381

56. Halliwell B (1994) Free radicals and antioxidants: a personal view. Nutr Rev 52:253–265

57. Hoffman KE, Yanelli K, Bridges KR (1991) Ascorbic acid and iron metabolism: alterations in lysosomal function. Am J Clin Nutr 54:1188S–1192S

58. Jialal I, Grundy SM (1993) Effect of combined supplementation with alpha-tocopherol, ascorbate, and beta carotene on low-density lipoprotein oxidation. Circulation 88:2780–2786

59. Jialal I, Vega GL, Grundy SM (1990) Physiologic levels of ascorbate inhibit the oxidative modification of low density lipoprotein. Atherosclerosis 82:185–191

60. Niki E, Noguchi N, Tsuchihashi G, Gotoh N (1995) Interaction among vitamin C, vitamin E and β-carotene. Am J Clin Nutr 62:1322S–1326S

61. Hunt JR, Gallagher SK, Johnson LK (1994) Effect of ascorbic acid on apparent iron absorption by women with low iron stores. Am J Clin Nutr 59:1381–1385

62. Hunt JR, Mullen LM, Lykken GI, et al (1990) Ascorbic acid: effect on ongoing iron absorption and status in iron-depleted young women. Am J Clin Nutr 51:649–655

63. Hallberg L, Brune M, Rossander L (1989) Iron absorption in man: ascorbic acid and dose-dependent inhibition by phytate. Am J Clin Nutr 49:140–144

64. Hallberg L, Brune M, Rossander L (1989) The role of vitamin C in iron absorption. Int J Vitam Nutr Res Suppl 30:103–108

65. Toth I, Rogers JT, McPhee JA, et al (1995) Ascorbic acid enhances iron-induced ferritin translation in human leukemia and hepatoma cells. J Biol Chem 270:2846–2852

66. Bergsten P, Yu R, Kehrl J, Levine M (1995) Ascorbic acid transport and distribution in human B lymphocytes. Arch Biochem Biophys 317:208–214

67. Levine M, Conry-Cantilena C, Wang Y, et al (1996) Vitamin C pharmacokinetics in healthy volunteers: evidence for a recommended dietary allowance. Proc Natl Acad Sci USA (in press)

68. Dhariwal KR, Hartzell WO, Levine M (1991) Ascorbic acid and dehydroascorbic acid measurements in human plasma and serum. Am J Clin Nutr 54:712–716

69. Sullivan JF, Eisenstein AB (1970) Ascorbic acid depletion in patients undergoing chronic hemodialysis. Am J Clin Nutr 23:1339–1346

70. Goldenberg H, Schweinzer E (1994) Transport of vitamin C in animal and human cells. J Bioenerg Biomembr 26:359–367

71. Levine M, Dhariwal KR, Washko PW, et al (1993) Cellular functions of ascorbic acid: a means to determine vitamin C requirements. Asia Pac J Clin Nutr 2:5–13

72. Bergsten P, Moura AS, Atwater I, Levine M (1994) Ascorbic acid and insulin secretion in pancreatic islets. J Biol Chem 269:1041–1045

73. Franceschi RT, Wilson JX, Dixon SJ (1995) Requirement for Na(+)-dependent ascorbic acid transport in osteoblast function. Am J Physiol 268:C1430–C1439

74. Cornu MC, Moore GA, Nakagawa Y, Moldeus P (1993) Ascorbic acid uptake by isolated rat hepatocytes: stimulatory effect of diquat, a redox cycling compound. Biochem Pharmacol 46:1333–1338

75. Welch RW, Bergsten P, Butler JD, Levine M (1993) Ascorbic acid accumulation and transport in human fibroblasts. Biochem J 294:505–510

76. Bode AM, Vanderpool SS, Carlson EC, et al (1991) Ascorbic acid uptake and metabolism by corneal endothelium. Invest Ophthalmol Vis Sci 32:2266–2271

77. Garland DL (1991) Ascorbic acid and the eye. Am J Clin Nutr 54:1198S–1202S

78. Washko P, Rotrosen D, Levine M (1991) Ascorbic acid in human neutrophils. Am J Clin Nutr 54:1221S–1227S

79. Vanderslice JT, Higgs DJ, Beecher GR, et al (1992) On the presence of dehydroascorbic acid in human plasma. Int J Vitam Nutr Res 62:101–102

80. Van den Berg GJ, Lemmens AG, Beynen AC (1993) Copper status in rats fed diets supplemented with either vitamin E, vitamin A, or beta-carotene. Biol Trace Elem Res 37:253–259

81. Dyer DL, Kanai Y, Hediger MA, et al (1994) Expression of a rabbit renal ascorbic acid transporter in Xenopus laevis oocytes. Am J Physiol 267:C301–C306

82. Washko P, Levine M (1992) Inhibition of ascorbic acid transport in human neutrophils by glucose. J Biol Chem 267:23568–23574

83. Zhou A, Nielsen JH, Farver O, Thorn NA (1991) Transport of ascorbic acid and dehydroascorbic acid by pancreatic islet cells from neonatal rats. Biochem J 274:739–744

84. Washko P, Rotrosen D, Levine M (1989) Ascorbic acid transport and accumulation in human neutrophils. J Biol Chem 264:18996–19002

85. Levine M, Dhariwal KR, Wang Y, et al (1994) Ascorbic acid in neutrophils. In Frei B (ed), Natural antioxidants in human health and disease. Academic Press, San Diego, pp 469–488

86. Vera JC, Rivas CI, Fischbarg J, Golde DW (1993) Mammalian facilitative hexose transporters mediate the transport of dehydroascorbic acid. Nature 364:79–82

87. Park JB, Levine M (1996) Purification, cloning, and expression of dehydroascorbic acid reduction activity from human neutrophils: identification as glutaredoxin. Biochem J (in press)

88. Winkler BS, Orselli SM, Rex TS (1994) The redox couple between glutathione and ascorbic acid: a chemical and physiological perspective. Free Radic Biol Med 17:333–349

89. Rose RC, McCormick DB, Li TK, et al (1986) Transport and metabolism of vitamins. Fed Proc 45:30–39

90. Patterson LT, Nahrwold DL, Rose RC (1982) Ascorbic acid uptake in guinea pig intestinal mucosa. Life Sci 31:2783–2791

91. Siliprandi L, Vanni P, Kessler M, Semenza G (1979) Na+-dependent, electroneutral L-ascorbate transport across brush border membrane vesicles from guinea pig small intestine. Biochim Biophys Acta 552:129–142

92. Stevenson NR, Brush MK (1969) Existence and characteristics of Na positive-dependent active transport of ascorbic acid in guinea pig. Am J Clin Nutr 22:318–326

93. Stevenson NR (1974) Active transport of L-ascorbic acid in the human ileum. Gastroenterology 67:952–956

94. Rose RC, Choi JL, Koch MJ (1988) Intestinal transport and metabolism of oxidized ascorbic acid (dehydroascorbic acid). Am J Physiol 254:G824–G828

95. Vanderslice JT, Higgs DJ (1991) Vitamin C content of foods: sample variability. Am J Clin Nutr 54:1323S–1327S

96. Haytowitz D (1995) Information from USDA's nutrient data book. J Nutr 125:1952–1955

97. Lachance P, Langseth L (1994) The RDA concept: time for a change? Nutr Rev 52:266–270

98. Life Sciences Research Office, Federation of American Societies for Experimental Biology, Interagency Board for Nutrition Monitoring and Related Research (1995) Third report on nutrition monitoring in the United States. US Government Printing Office, Washington, DC, pp ES14–ES29, VA102, VA196

99. Simon JA, Schreiber GB, Crawford PB, et al (1993) Dietary vitamin C and serum lipids in black and white girls. Epidemiology 4:537–542

100. Basch CE, Syber P, Shea S (1994) 5-a-day: dietary behavior and the fruit and vegetable intake of Latino children. Am J Public Health 84:814–818

101. Koplan JP, Annest JL, Layde PM, Rubin GL (1986) Nutrient intake and supplementation in the United States (NHANES II). Am J Public Health 76:287–290

102. Murphy SP, Rose D, Hudes M, Viteri FE (1992) Demographic and economic factors associated with dietary quality for adults in the 1987–88 Nationwide Food Consumption Survey. J Am Diet Assoc 92:1352–1357

103. Patterson BH, Block G, Rosenberger WF, et al (1990) Fruit and vegetables in the American diet: data from the NHANES II survey. Am J Public Health 80:1443–1449

104. Block G, Sinha R, Gridley G (1994) Collection of dietary-supplement data and implications for analysis. Am J Clin Nutr 59:232S–239S

105. Dickinson VA, Block G, Russek-Cohen E (1994) Supplement use, other dietary and demographic variables, and serum vitamin C in NHANES II. J Am Coll Nutr 13:22–32

106. Hodges RE (1971) What's new about scurvy? Am J Clin Nutr 24:383–384

107. Jacob RA, Pianalto FS, Agee RE (1992) Cellular ascorbate depletion in healthy men. J Nutr 122:1111–1118

108. Jacob RA, Skala JH, Omaye ST (1987) Biochemical indices of human vitamin C status. Am J Clin Nutr 46:818–826

109. Kallner A, Hartmann D, Hornig D (1979) Steady-state turnover and body pool of ascorbic acid in man. Am J Clin Nutr 32:530–539

110. VanderJagt DJ, Garry PJ, Bhagavan HN (1987) Ascorbic acid intake and plasma levels in healthy elderly people. Am J Clin Nutr 46:290–294

111. Garry PJ, Goodwin JS, Hunt WC, Gilbert BA (1982) Nutritional status in a healthy elderly population: vitamin C. Am J Clin Nutr 36:332–339

112. Kallner A, Hartmann D, Hornig D (1977) On the absorption of ascorbic acid in man. Int J Vitam Nutr Res 47:383–388

113. Hegsted DM (1992) Defining a nutritious diet: need for new dietary standards. J Am Coll Nutr 11:241–245

114. Fraga CG, Motchnik PA, Shigenaga MK, et al (1991) Ascorbic acid protects against endogenous oxidative DNA damage in human sperm. Proc Natl Acad Sci USA 88:11003–11006

115. Gibaldi M, Perrier D (1982) Pharmacokinetics. Marcel Dekker, New York, pp 294–297

116. Rowland M, Tozer TN (1989) Clinical pharmacokinetics: concepts and applications. Lea and Febiger, Philadelphia, pp 459–461

117. Yung S, Mayersohn M, Robinson JB (1982) Ascorbic acid absorption in humans: a comparison among several dosage forms. J Pharm Sci 71:282–285

118. Mayersohn M (1972) Ascorbic acid absorption in man—pharmacokinetic implications. Eur J Pharmacol 19:140–142

119. Melethil SL, Mason WE, Chiang C (1986) Dose dependent absorption and excretion of vitamin C in humans. Int J Pharm 31:83–89

120. Mangels AR, Block G, Frey CM, et al (1993) The bioavailability to humans of ascorbic acid from oranges, orange juice and cooked broccoli is similar to that of synthetic ascorbic acid. J Nutr 123:1054–1061

121. Hartzler ER (1945) The availability of ascorbic acid in papayas and guavas. J Nutr 30:355–365

122. Anonymous (1995) Case records of the Massachusetts General Hospital. Case 39-1955. A 72 year old man with exertional dyspnea, fatigue, and extensive ecchymoses and purpuric lesions. N Engl J Med 333:1695–1702

123. Friedman GJ, Sherry S, Ralli E (1940) The mechanism of excretion of vitamin C by the human kidney at low and normal plasma levels of ascorbic acid. J Clin Invest 19:685–689

124. Baker EM, Saari JC, Tolbert BM (1966) Ascorbic acid metabolism in man. Am J Clin Nutr 19:371–378

125. Hood J, Burns CA, Hodges RE (1970) Sjogren's syndrome in scurvy. N Engl J Med 282:1120–1124

126. Jaffe RM, Kasten B, Young DS, MacLowry JD (1975) False-negative stool occult blood tests caused by ingestion of ascorbic acid (vitamin C). Ann Intern Med 83:824–826

127. Cohen A, Cohen IJ, Schwartz E (1981) Scurvy and altered iron stores in thalassemia major. N Engl J Med 304:158–160

128. Nienhuis AW (1981) Vitamin C and iron [editorial]. N Engl J Med 304:170–171

129. Young IS, Trouton TG, Torney JJ, et al (1994) Antioxidant status and lipid peroxidation in hereditary haemochromatosis. Free Radic Biol Med 16:393–397

130. Cook JD, Monsen ER (1977) Vitamin C, the common cold, and iron absorption. Am J Clin Nutr 30:235–241

131. Hallberg L, Brune M, Rossander-Hulthen L (1987) Is there a physiological role of vitamin C in iron absorption? Ann NY Acad Sci 498:324–332

132. Stein HB, Hasan A, Fox IH (1976) Ascorbic acid-induced uricosuria: a consequence of megavitamin therapy. Ann Intern Med 84:385–388

133. Mitch WE, Johnson MW, Kirshenbaum JM, Lopez RE (1981) Effect of large oral doses of ascorbic acid on uric acid excretion by normal subjects. Clin Pharmacol Ther 29:318–321

134. Sutton JL, Basu TK, Dickerson JW (1983) Effect of large doses of ascorbic acid in man on some nitrogenous components of urine. Hum Nutr Appl Nutr 37:136–140

135. Li MG, Madappally MM (1989) Rapid enzymatic determination of urinary oxalate. Clin Chem 35:2330–2333

136. Wandzilak TR, D'Andre SD, Davis PA, Williams HE (1994) Effect of high dose vitamin C on urinary oxalate levels. J Urol 151:834–837

137. Tinchieri A, Mandressi A, Luongo P, et al (1991) The influence of diet on urinary risk factors for stones in healthy subjects and idiopathic renal calcium stone formers. Br J Urol 67:230–236

138. Urivetzky M, Kessaris D, Smith AD (1992) Ascorbic acid overdosing: a risk factor for calcium oxalate nephrolithiasis. J Urol 147:1215–1218

139. Balcke P, Schmidt P, Zazgornik J, et al (1984) Ascorbic acid aggravates secondary hyperoxalemia in patients on chronic hemodialysis. Ann Intern Med 101:344–345

140. Campbell GD Jr, Steinberg MH, Bower JD (1975) Ascorbic acid-induced hemolysis in G-6-PD deficiency [letter]. Ann Intern Med 82:810

141. Mehta JB, Singhal SB, Mehta BC (1990) Ascorbic-acid-induced haemolysis in G-6-PD deficiency [letter]. Lancet 336:944

142. Rees DC, Kelsey H, Richards JD (1993) Acute haemolysis induced by high dose ascorbic acid in glucose-6-phosphate dehydrogenase deficiency. Br Med J 306:841–842

143. Byers T, Guerrero N (1995) Epidemiologic evidence for vitamin C and vitamin E in cancer prevention. Am J Clin Nutr 62:1385S–1392S

144. Blot WJ, Li J, Taylor PR, et al (1993) Nutrition intervention trials in Linxian, China: supplementation with specific vitamin/mineral combinations, cancer incidence, and disease-specific mortality in the general population. J Natl Cancer Inst 85:1483–1492

145. Greenberg ER, Baron JA, Tosteson TD, et al (1994) A clinical trial of antioxidant vitamins to prevent colorectal adenoma: Polyp Prevention Study Group. N Engl J Med 331:141–147

146. Rimm EB, Stampfer MJ, Ascherio A, et al (1993) Vitamin E consumption and the risk of coronary heart disease in men. N Engl J Med 328:1450–1456

147. Seddon JM, Christen WG, Manson JE, et al (1994) The use of vitamin supplements and the risk of cataract among US male physicians. Am J Public Health 84:788–792

148. Riemersma RA, Wood DA, Macintyre CC, et al (1991) Risk of angina pectoris and plasma concentrations of vitamins A, C, and E and carotene. Lancet 337:1–5

149. Gey KF, Stahelin HB, Eichholzer M (1993) Poor plasma status of carotene and vitamin C is associated with higher mortality from ischemic heart disease and stroke: Basel Prospective Study. Clin Invest 71:3–6

150. Enstrom JE, Kanim LE, Breslow L (1986) The relationship between vitamin C intake, general health practices, and mortality in Alameda County, California. Am J Public Health 76:1124–1130

151. Jacques PF, Chylack LT Jr, McGandy RB, Hartz SC (1988) Antioxidant status in persons with and without senile cataract. Arch Ophthalmol 106:337–340

152. Robertson JM, Donner AP, Trevithick JR (1991) A possible role for vitamins C and E in cataract prevention. Am J Clin Nutr 53:346S–351S

153. Leske MC, Chylack LT, Wu S (1991) The lens opacities case/control study: risk factors for cataract. Arch Opthalmol 109:244–251

154. Italian-American Cataract Study Group (1991) Risk factors for age-related cortical, nuclear, and posterior sub-capsular cataracts. Am J Epidemiol 133:541–553

155. Goldberg J, Flowerdew G, Smith E, et al (1988) Factors associated with age-related macular degeneration: an analysis of data from the first National Health and Nutrition Examination Survey. Am J Epidemiol 128:700–710

156. Vitale S, West S, Hallfrisch J, et al (1993) Plasma antioxidants and risk of cortical and nuclear cataract. Epidemiology 4:195–203

157. Hankinson SE, Stampfer MJ, Seddon JM, et al (1992) Nutrient intake and cataract extraction in women: a prospective study. Br Med J 305:335–339

158. Tang AM, Graham NMH, Kirby AJ, et al (1993) Dietary micronutrient intake and risk of progression to acquired immunodeficiency syndrome (AIDS) in human immunodeficiency virus type 1 (HIV-1)-infected homosexual men. Am J Epidemiol 138:937–951

159. Garry PJ, VanderJagt DJ, Hunt WC (1987) Ascorbic acid intakes and plasma levels in healthy elderly. Ann N Y Acad Sci 498:90–99

160. Food and Nutrition Board (1994) How should the recommended dietary allowances be revised? National Academy Press, Washington, DC

161. Bigley R, Wirth M, Layman D, et al (1983) Interaction between glucose and dehydroascorbate transport in human neutrophils and fibroblasts. Diabetes 32:545–548

162. Helser MA, Hotchkiss JH, Roe DA (1992) Influence of fruit and vegetable juices on the endogenous formation of N-nitrosoproline and N-nitrosothiazolidine-4-carboxylic acid in humans on controlled diets. Carcinogenesis 13:2277–2280

Chapter 16

Thiamin

Gianguido Rindi

Beriberi, the typical disease resulting from thiamin deficiency, was described for the first time in 1630 by Bontius, a Dutch physician in Java. According to ancient Chinese literature, however, beriberi existed as far back as 2600 B.C. The term beriberi, as reported by Bontius, means sheep, because "those whom this same disease attacks, with their knees shaking and the legs raised up, walk like sheep." In 1882, Admiral Takaki of the Japanese Naval Bureau observed that many sailors were affected by beriberi and noted that the quality of food had an important role in the disease. After the addition of meat, vegetables, and bread to the sailors' daily ration of polished rice, the number of subjects developing the disease was greatly reduced.

In 1897, Eijkman, a Dutch physician stationed in Java, observed that chickens developed polyneuritis, a disease similar to beriberi, if they were fed only polished rice. The disease could be prevented completely if unpolished rice or rice bran were added to the chickens' diets.[1,2] In 1911, Funk,[3] who coined the term "vitamin," and Suzuki et al.[4] isolated from rice polishings a crystalline compound with biological activity. In 1936 Williams[5] published the correct structure of thiamin, which was finally synthesized by Williams and Cline.[6] Peters[7] was probably the first to recognize, in the 1930s, the role of thiamin as an essential factor in the metabolism of pyruvate.

Chemistry

Thiamin, also called vitamin B-1 and aneurin, is one of the earliest-recognized vitamins. The thiamin molecule consists of one pyrimidine and one thiazole ring, linked by a methylene bridge (Figure 1). The commercial forms of thiamin are chloride-hydrochloride (usually called hydrochloride) and mononitrate. Both are stable in dry form and in acid solution, but are rapidly destroyed in alkaline solution, especially by heating. Thiamin is particularly sensitive to sulfites, which are used frequently in the production and processing of food, and which split the molecule into the pyrimidine and thiazole moieties, thus destroying its biological activity.

Phosphorylated forms of thiamin (Figure 1) include thiamin monophosphate (TMP), thiamin pyrophosphate (TPP), and thiamin triphosphate (TTP). In animal tissues free thiamin and its phosphorylated forms are present in different amounts, TPP being the most abundant

($\approx$80% of total thiamin). Five to ten percent of total thiamin is accounted for by TTP; the remainder is in the form of thiamin and TMP.[8] In the animal body, the four forms of thiamin are interconvertible by intervention of various enzyme systems as shown in Figure 2.

Absorption and Transport

After a meal, thiamin is found in the intestinal lumen in free form, its phosphoesters being completely hydrolyzed by different intestinal phosphatases. In humans and in rats the intraluminal concentration of thiamin has been estimated to be <2 µmol/L.[10,11] At these very low concentrations, active transport occurs. In all animal species, including man, the pattern of in vivo intestinal absorption of thiamin suggests the presence of a saturable transmucosal transport.[12] In humans, single oral doses of thiamin above 2.5–5 mg are largely unabsorbed, and intestinal uptake in vivo follows saturation kinetics.[13–15] The process of thiamin absorption, as studied in vitro in human tissues, involves two mechanisms.[16–18] At concentrations <1 µmol/L, thiamin is absorbed mainly by an active, carrier-mediated system that involves phosphorylation of the vitamin and is age-related.[19,20] At higher concentrations, passive diffusion prevails. Absorption takes place primarily in the jejunum.

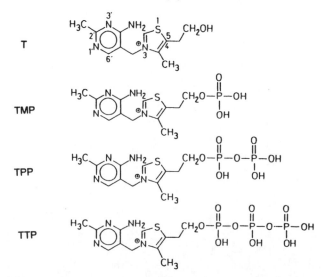

Figure 1. Thiamin and its phosphate esters. T, thiamin (free base); TMP, thiamin monophosphate; TPP, thiamin pyrophosphate; TTP, thiamin triphosphate.

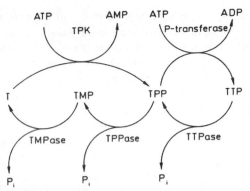

Figure 2. Enzymatic interconversion of thiamin compounds.[9] T, free thiamin; TMP, thiamin monophosphate; TPP, thiamin pyrophosphate; TTP, thiamin triphosphate; Pi, inorganic phosphate; TPK, thiamin pyrophosphokinase; P-transferase, thiamin pyrophosphate kinase; TMPase, thiamin monophosphatase; TPPase, thiamin pyrophosphatase; TTPase, thiamin triphosphatase.

In blood, thiamin is transported in erythrocytes, which contain free thiamin and its phosphorylated forms, and in plasma, which contains only free thiamin and TMP.[21] As in plasma, only free thiamin and TMP are present in the cerebrospinal fluid.[22] In adult humans, total thiamin content is estimated to be $\approx$30 mg and its biological half-life is $\approx$9.5–18.5 days.[23,24] Thiamin levels in tissues and organs vary from one species to another and, in general, are lower in humans than in other mammals. The rank order of total thiamin content (mostly TPP) in different organs (in rats) is as follows: liver > heart > kidney > skeletal muscle > brain > small intestine.[25,26]

Functions

Coenzyme function. TPP is the major coenzymatic form of thiamin, and its enzymatic synthesis requires ATP, Mg^{2+}, and thiaminpyrophosphokinase (Figure 2). TPP is involved in several enzymes that catalyze reactions such as the nonoxidative decarboxylation of α-ketoacids:

$$RCOCOOH \rightarrow RCHO + CO_2. \qquad (1)$$

Nonoxidative decarboxylation of pyruvate is catalyzed by pyruvate decarboxylase, which is widely distributed in plants and yeasts, and which catalyzes the first step of alcoholic fermentation.

TPP is also involved in the oxidative decarboxylation of α-ketoacids:

$$RCOCOOH + HSCoA + NAD^+ \rightarrow RC\text{-}S\text{-}CoA$$
$$+ CO_2 + NADH + H^+. \qquad (2)$$

The oxidative decarboxylation of pyruvate, α-ketoglutarate, and α-ketoacids derived from branched-chain amino acids (leucine, isoleucine, and valine) requires three separate multienzyme complexes: pyruvate dehydrogenase, α-ketoglutarate dehydrogenase, and branched-chain dehydrogenase. All are intramitochondrial enzymes, and produce, respectively, acetyl-coenzyme A (CoA),

succinyl-CoA, and appropriate derivatives of branched-chain amino acids, all of which play important roles in carbohydrate and lipid metabolism.

TPP is also involved in transketolation, an important reaction of the pentose phosphate pathway, which is catalyzed by the cytosolic enzyme transketolase and allows the reversible interconversion of three-, four-, five-, six-, and seven-carbon sugars by transfer of either two or three carbon moieties:

$$
\begin{array}{ccccccc}
R_1 & & & & R_2 & & \\
| & & & & | & & \\
HO\text{-}C\text{-}H & & R_2 & & HO\text{-}C\text{-}H & & R_2 \\
| & & | & & | & & | \\
\cdots & + & \cdots & \rightleftarrows & \cdots & + & \cdots \quad (3)\\
| & & | & & | & & | \\
C=O & & CHO & & C=O & & CHO \\
| & & & & | & & \\
CH_2\text{-}OH & & & & CH_2\text{-}OH & &
\end{array}
$$

Transketolation is not a direct pathway of the main glycolytic cycle for carbohydrate metabolism, but is a major source of pentoses for nucleic acid synthesis and of NADPH for fatty acid synthesis. Because transketolase activity decreases early in thiamin deficiency, its determination in erythrocytes is used as a reliable tool to assess thiamin nutritional status.

Noncoenzyme function. A specific noncoenzymatic role of thiamin in nervous tissue was proposed by Cooper and Pincus[27] and investigated extensively by Bettendorff.[28] Probably, TTP is the compound involved in this role. In fact, TTP is concentrated in neuronal cells and other excitable tissues like skeletal muscle and the electric organs of some fishes; it is hydrolyzed faster during nerve stimulation, it modulates rat brain chloride channels, and its content correlates with chloride permeability of rat brain membranes. Moreover, TTP activates maxi-Cl⁻ channels of neuroblastoma cells in vitro by controlling the number of functional channels, possibly by phosphorylation.[29] This effect represents the first demonstrated action of TTP on ion channels.

Thiamin Antagonists

Two types of thiamin antagonists are known: synthetic structural analogs and natural antithiamin compounds.[30] Several structural analogs of thiamin have been synthesized, and they generally act as competitive inhibitors of the vitamin.[31] Pyrithiamin, an isoster of thiamin possessing a CH=CH group instead of the sulfur atom in the thiamin molecule, and oxythiamin, which possesses a hydroxyl group replacing an amino group, have been used extensively in experiments both in vivo and in vitro. In mammals and birds, pyrithiamin induces anorexia, weight loss, and neurological signs typical of thiamin deficiency (convulsions, ataxia, and opisthotonos), so that it is used to reproduce a mammalian model of Wernicke-like encephalopathy. Pyrithiamin, which accumulates in rat brain, is a strong inhibitor of thiamin phosphorylation and leads to rapid urinary excretion of thiamin, leading to tissue depletion of the vitamin.[32,33] Oxythiamin also induces anorexia and weight loss, but it causes no neurological signs: it cannot cross the blood-brain barrier and is phosphorylated to oxythiamin pyrophosphate, resulting in competition with TPP.[34] Amprolium, a 2-*n* propylpyrimidine, and chloroethylthiamin, another structural analog of thiamin, are used in the treatment of coccidiosis in chickens and exhibit weak antithiamin activity in mammals. Both compounds inhibit the intestinal absorption of thiamin, but only chloroethylthiamin is a strong inhibitor of thiamin phosphorylation in the intestine.[35-37]

Antithiamin natural compounds act by modifying the thiamin structure and are found in plant and animal tissues. Two enzymes causing thiamin degradation are known. Thiaminase I, present in the intestine of carp and some other fishes, fern (*Pteridium aquilinum*), and *Bacillus thiaminolyticus,* catalyzes the cleavage of thiamin by an exchange reaction with a nitrogen base or a thiol compound. The reaction involves displacement of the methylene group as in the case of sulfite. Thiaminase II, present chiefly in intestinal bacteria (*B. thiaminolyticus, B. aneurinelyticus,* and *Chlostridium thiaminolyticus*), catalyzes the simple hydrolysis of thiamin to pyrimidine and thiazole rings.

Ferns and some other vegetables (especially blueberry, red chicory, blackcurrant, red beet root, Brussels sprouts, and red cabbage) contain certain polyhydroxyphenols (caffeic acid, chlorogenic acid, and tannins) that inactivate thiamin by an oxyreductive process. The antithiamin natural factors, especially thiaminase I, can induce severe thiamin deficiency resulting in neurological signs and even death in oxen, horses, sheep, and pigs feeding on the leaves and rhizomes of fern, a plant widely diffused in pastures. In oxen and sheep, the disease is known as cerebrocortical necrosis or polyoencephalomalacia. Ingestion of fish-based feeds containing antithiamin factors is a frequent cause of neurological signs of thiamin deficiency in breedings of silver foxes (Chastek paralysis), minks, and also in domestic cats. Tea leaves and tea infusions, because of their high content of polyhydroxyphenols, can impair thiamin body stores in humans.

Analysis

Several methods for thiamin determination have been described based on the use of experimental animals, microorganisms, physicochemical principles, and enzymatic reactions. The most frequently used method is the fluorimetric thiochrome assay. In alkaline solution, thiamin is oxidized by potassium ferricyanide or other oxidants to the intensely blue fluorescent thiochrome. The amount of phosphorylated thiamin can be evaluated by comparing the assay results before and after treatment with a phosphatase. Interfering substances can be removed through use of an ion-exchange resin. More recently, solid-phase chromatography, electrophoresis, and high-performance liquid chromatography have been used to separate and quantitate very low concentrations of thiamin and its phosphoesters in blood and other animal tissues and in foods.[8,25,26,38-40]

Metabolites

The normal urinary excretion of thiamin in adults is ≥66 µg/g creatinine, and values below 27 µg/g creatinine are indicative of thiamin deficiency.[41] The relationship between thiamin stores and urinary excretion has been used to determine thiamin status and requirements.[42] Free thiamin, TMP, and small amounts of TPP are excreted in urine. Different thiamin catabolites, including the pyrimidine and thiazole moieties and some 20–30 breakdown products, are also found in urine.[43,44]

Thiamin Status

Three main biochemical and functional tests are used for the assessment of thiamin status. These include determination of erythrocyte transketolase activity (ETK), urinary thiamin excretion before or after a thiamin load, and blood thiamin levels.[45] ETK activity is measured in hemolyzed erythrocytes by determining the rate of disappearance of pentose or the appearance of hexose. Usually, ETK activity is determined without (basal) and with (stimulated) addition of TPP in vitro and is expressed as basal activity (ETKA) or as the difference between stimulated and basal activity as a percentage of the basal activity (ETK-AC activation coefficient or TPP effect). Thiamin deficiency is associated with decreased ETKA and increased ETK-AC: the higher the value of ETK-AC, the greater the degree of thiamin deficiency.[45]

The urinary excretion of thiamin is an index of recent dietary intake of the vitamin. Only small changes in urinary excretion occur during intake of low, physiological amounts of the vitamin; the interpretation of excretion values is improved with the use of 24-hour urine samples. Because there is a relationship between the requirement for thiamin and its urinary excretion, a thiamin-loading test can be used to determine thiamin status. The test involves measurement of the amount of thiamin excreted in urine 4 hours after a 5-mg dose of the vitamin: an excretion value <20 µg is indicative of thiamin deficiency.[45]

The measurement of thiamin levels in whole blood and erythrocytes as an index of thiamin status has not been used widely in the past because of the difficulties in quantitating low concentrations of free thiamin and its phosphoesters in blood. However, with the recent development of sensitive high-performance liquid chromatography methods and the ease of standardization of these methods, determination of thiamin levels in blood will probably become the method of choice because of its simplicity and reliability.[38,39,46,47]

Thiamin Deficiency

Inadequate intake is the main cause of human thiamin deficiency in underdeveloped countries. In industrialized countries, however, alcoholism is the most common cause of deficiency.

Beriberi is the ultimate consequence of inadequate intake of thiamin in humans and in various animal species. The main manifestations of the disease affect the cardiovascular and the nervous systems. Cardiovascular manifestations include heart hypertrophy and dilatation (particularly of the right ventricle), tachycardia (bradycardia in rats), respiratory distress, and edema of the legs. Neurological signs include exaggeration of tendon reflexes; polyneuritis (sometimes associated with paralysis), which typically affects the lower extremities and, in a subsequent stage, the upper extremities; muscle weakness and pain; and convulsions. The "burning-feet syndrome" may also be a manifestation of thiamin deficiency and it appears early in the course of the polyneuropathy.[48] In severe thiamin deficiency, neurological and cardiovascular symptoms may be present simultaneously, and may be fatal. In subclinical thiamin deficiency, which may be fairly common in developed countries, symptoms are less prominent and may include tiredness, headache, and reduced productivity.

In the human central nervous system, thiamin deficiency may lead to Wernicke encephalopathy and Korsakoff psychosis. Both conditions are typical for alcoholics and may manifest as Wernicke-Korsakoff syndrome. Wernicke encephalopathy may be characterized by confusion, ataxia, ophthalmoplegia, psychosis, confabulation (pseudomemories), and coma.[49] It is a rather frequent but often undiagnosed disease in chronic alcoholics, but it may also occur in other conditions associated with thiamin deficiency.[50] Korsakoff psychosis is an amnesiac disorder, considered to be the psychotic component of Wernicke disease. Autopsy findings in this disease show abnormalities mainly in the midbrain and lower brain regions. Administration of thiamin results in dramatic clinical improvement.

An encephalopathy associated with severe thiamin deficiency can be produced in rats by pyrithiamin treatment. In these animals, selective changes in the function of neurotransmitters are reported.[51] There is primarily an impairment of cholinergic neurotransmission, but serotonin metabolism is also affected, especially in the cerebellum, a brain region with the highest thiamin turnover rate in rats.[9] In addition, recent studies have shown region-selective reductions of three TPP-dependent enzymes.[52–54]

The loss of neurons observed in severely thiamin-deficient brain is probably due to multiple causes, including impaired energy metabolism, focal acidosis, loss of transketolase activity, and excitotoxic damage from regional increase of extracellular glutamate.[55] In developed countries, clinical and subclinical thiamin deficiency is frequently related to chronic alcoholism. Most of the peripheral and central nervous system abnormalities observed in alcoholism are considered to be a consequence of thiamin deficiency. In particular, Wernicke encephalopathy is clearly induced by lack of thiamin, although the disease is not confined to alcoholism.[49] Alcoholics are deficient in thiamin as a result of low thiamin intake, impaired thiamin absorption and utilization, and possibly increased thiamin excretion. In addition, alcoholics are often affected by liver disease, which worsens the situation and may be an additional cause of cognitive dysfunction and astrocyte alterations. These multifactorial injuries contribute to the so-called alcoholic brain damage, which differs in its sensitivity to thiamin treatment.[56,57] Thiamin deficiency is also probably the cause of fetal alcohol syndrome, which has been described in children born to alcoholic mothers.[58] This syndrome is characterized by intrauterine growth retardation, psychomotor abnormalities, and congenital malformations.

Congenital Defects

Different inherited diseases associated with congenital defects in thiamin metabolism have been described. These include maple syrup urine disease (branched-chain disease), lactate acidosis, Leigh disease, and thiamin-responsive megaloblastic anemia. The cause of maple syrup urine disease is a lack of the enzyme branched-chain α-ketoacid dehydrogenase complex. In patients with this disease, the corresponding α-ketoacids cannot be degraded by oxidative decarboxylation and are found at high concentrations in serum and urine together with the related branched-chain amino acids. The urine of these patients smells like maple syrup. The disease affects neonates, is autosomal recessive, and is partially sensitive to high oral doses of thiamin.[40]

Congenital lactate acidosis is a group of several congenital defects observed primarily in children and characterized by lactic and pyruvic acidosis, neurological abnormalities, and developmental delay.[59] The most important cause is probably a defect in the pyruvate dehydrogenase complex. Patients with lactic acidemia improve after administration of high doses of thiamin.[60]

Leigh disease (or subacute necrotizing encephalomyelopathy) is a fatal disease that develops in infancy and early childhood, and is associated with weakness, anorexia, difficulties in speech and eye motion, and cessation of growth. Necrosis of the brain stem and of the spinal cord are findings at autopsy. The disease is familial and, probably, autosomal recessive. Neuropathological findings and clinical symptoms are similar to those observed in Wernicke encephalopathy. Successful treatment with high oral doses of thiamin or, preferably, its lipophilic forms has been reported.[40]

Thiamin-responsive megaloblastic anemia is a rare disease of infancy and childhood, characterized by megaloblastic anemia associated with sensorineural deafness and diabetes mellitus. Cardiac abnormalities may be also present, as well as optic subatrophy.[61] Patients respond to thiamin therapy, but hearing is only partially recovered. The disease is associated with a state of thiamin deficiency secondary to reduced thiamin cellular transport and absorption (due to a lack of a membrane-specific carrier), and impaired thiamin intracellular pyrophosphorylation.

Requirements and Allowances

Body stores of thiamin are relatively small and regular intake is necessary, especially because large single doses are absorbed poorly. Thiamin requirements are related to energy consumption. The recommended dietary allowance of 0.5 mg/4200 kJ (1000 kcal) is consistent with good health.[62] Assuming that an adult consumes ≈8400 kJ/day (≈2000 kcal/day) and that thiamin losses from cooking are ≈20%, the recommended daily allowances are 1.4 and 1 mg for adult men and women, respectively.[40] In pregnancy and lactation thiamin intake should be 1.6–1.8 mg/day.

Sources

Grain products are the most important dietary sources for humans and provide ≈40% of the vitamin requirement. Because most of the thiamin content is lost in the production of white flour and polished rice, in some developed countries rice and white flour are enriched with vitamins. A significant contribution to thiamin intake can be provided by meat products (27.1%), especially pork muscle, vegetables (11.7%), milk and milk products (8.1%), legumes (5.4%), fruits (4.4%), and eggs (2.0%).[63]

Toxicity

In humans, even very high oral doses of thiamin have been found to have no toxic effects, except for possible gastric upset. Large parenteral doses (100–500 mg) are also generally well tolerated. Only after several injections, by different routes, of doses exceeding by more than 100–200-fold the recommended daily intake have few, if any, toxic effects ascribed to allergic reactions been reported.[48]

Summary

The thiamin molecule consists of a pyrimidine structure linked to a thiazole ring by a methylene group. In animal tissues thiamin is present mainly in its phosphorylated form, TPP being the most abundant form. TPP is a coenzyme of four enzymes (three dehydrogenases and one transketolase) involved in carbohydrate and lipid metabolism. TTP is probably involved also in anion channel modulation in nervous tissue. Thiamin is absorbed from the small intestine by a specific mechanism, the efficiency of which can be impaired by alcohol and by synthetic or natural antagonists present in food. Urine contains small amounts of thiamin, its phosphates, and several catabolites, including the cleavage products pyrimidine and thiazole. Thiamin status can be assessed by measuring transketolase in erythrocytes, by determining the concentration of thiamin and its phosphate esters in blood or serum by high-performance liquid chromatography, and by assessing urinary thiamin excretion.

Severe thiamin deficiency causes beriberi disease, which is associated with extensive neurological and cardiovascular damage. In developed countries, beriberi is a rare disease, but clinical (Wernicke-Korsakoff syndrome) or subclinical manifestations of thiamin deficiency can be induced by chronic alcoholism. Congenital disorders of thiamin metabolism may lead to serious and potentially fatal diseases.

Acknowledgment. The author is grateful to Professor E. Perucca (Clinical Pharmacology Unit, University of Pavia) for revising the English and to Dr. U. Laforenza for assistance in preparing the manuscript.

References

1. Eijkman C (1897) Eine beriberi-ähnliche Krankheit der Huhner. Virchows Arch Pathol Anat Physiol 148:523–532
2. Eijkman C (1906) Uber Ernahrungspolyneuritis. Arch Hyg 58:150–170
3. Funk C (1911) On the chemical nature of the substance which cures polyneuritis in birds induced by a diet of polished rice. J Physiol (Lond) 43:395–400
4. Suzuki V, Shimamura T, Okade S (1912) Uber Oryzanin, ein Bestandteil der Reiskleie und seine physiologische Bedeutung. Biochem Z 43:89–153
5. Williams RR (1936) Structure of vitamin B1. J Am Chem Soc 58:1063–1064
6. Williams RR, Cline JK (1936) Synthesis of vitamin B1. J Am Chem Soc 58:1504–1505
7. Peters RA (1967) The biochemical lesion in thiamine deficiency. In Wolstenholme GEW (ed), Thiamine deficiency: biochemical lesions and their clinical significance. Churchill, London, pp 1–8
8. Rindi G, de Giuseppe L (1961) A new chromatographic method for the determination of thiamin and its mono-, di- and tri-phosphates in animal tissues. Biochem J 78:602–606

9. Rindi G, Comincioli V, Reggiani C, Patrini C (1984) Nervous tissue thiamine metabolism in vivo. II. Thiamine and its phosphoesters dynamics in different brain regions and sciatic nerve of the rat. Brain Res 293:329–342

10. Hoyumpa AM Jr, Middleton HM III, Wlilson FA, Schenker S (1975) Thiamine transport across the rat intestine. I. Normal characteristics. Gastroenterology 68:1218–1227

11. Sklan D, Trostler N (1977) Site and extent of thiamine absorption in the rat. J Nutr 107:353–356

12. Rindi G, Ventura U (1972) Thiamine intestinal transport. Physiol Rev 52:821–827

13. Friedemann TE, KumeciaK TC, Keegan PK, Sheft BB (1948) The absorption, destruction and excretion of orally administered thiamine by human subjects. Gastroenterology 11:100–114

14. Morrison AB, Campbell JA (1960) Vitamin absorption studies. I. Factors influencing the excretion of oral test doses of thiamine and riboflavin by human subjects. J Nutr 72:435–440

15. Thomson AD, Leevy CM (1972) Observation on the mechanism of thiamine hydrochloride absorption in man. Clin Sci 43:153–163

16. Hoyumpa AM Jr, Strickland R, Sheehan JJ, et al (1982) Dual system of intestinal thiamine transport in humans. J Lab Clin Med 99:701–708

17. Rindi G (1984) Thiamin absorption by small intestine. Acta Vitaminol Enzymol 6:47–55

18. Rindi G (1992) Some aspects of thiamin transport in mammals. In Kobayashi T (ed), Proceedings of the International Congress on Vitamin Biofactors in Life Science, Kobe 1991. Center for Academic Publications of Japan, Tokyo, pp 379–382

19. Rindi G, Ferrari G (1977) Thiamine transport by human intestine in vitro. Experientia 33:211–213

20. Gastaldi G, Laforenza U, Ferrari G, et al (1992) Age related thiamin transport by small intestinal microvillous vesicles of rat. Biochim Biophys Acta 1105:271–277

21. Rindi G, de Giuseppe L, Sciorelli G (1968) Thiamine monophosphate, a normal constituent of rat plasma. J Nutr 94:447–454

22. Rindi G, Patrini C, Poloni M (1981) Monophosphate, the only phosphate ester of thiamin in the cerebro-spinal fluid. Experientia 33:211–213

23. Takeda J (1947) Distribution of thiamine in human organs. Niigata Igakukai Zasshi 61:478, 529 [cited in Shimazono N (1965) Metabolism of thiamine in animal body. In Shimazono N, Katsura E (eds), Review of Japanese literature on beriberi and thiamine. Igaku Shoin Ltd., Tokyo, pp 150–178]

24. Ariaey-Nejad MR, Balaghi M, Baker EM, Sauberlich E (1970) Thiamin metabolism in man. Am J Clin Nutr 23:764–778

25. Ishii K, Sarai K, Sanemori H, Kawasaki T (1979) Concentration of thiamine and its phosphate esters in rat tissues determined by high performance liquid chromatography. J Nutr Sci Vitaminol 25:517–523

26. Patrini C, Rindi G (1980) An improved method for the electrophoretic separation and fluorometric determination of thiamine and its phosphates in animal tissues. Int J Vitam Nutr Res 50:10–18

27. Cooper JR, Pincus H (1979) The role of thiamine in the nervous tissue. Neurochem Res 4:223–239

28. Bettendorff L (1994) Thiamine in excitable tissue: reflections on a non-cofactor role. Metab Brain Dis 9:183–209

29. Bettendorff L, Kolb HA, Schoffeniels E (1993) Thiamine triphosphate activated an anion channel of large unit conductance in neuroblastoma cells. J Membr Biol 136:281–288

30. Somogyi JC (1966) Biochemical aspects of the antimetabolites of thiamine. Bibl Nutr Diet 8:74–96

31. Rogers EF (1962) Thiamine antagonists. Ann NY Acad Sci 98:412–429

32. Rindi G, Perri V (1961) Uptake of Pyrithiamine by tissues of rats. Biochem J 80:214–216

33. Steyn-Parvé EP (1967) The mode of action of some thiamine analogues with antivitamin activity. In Wolstenholme GEW (ed), Thiamine deficiency: biochemical lesions and their clinical significance. Churchill, London, pp 26–42

34. Rindi G, de Giuseppe L, Ventura U (1963) Distribution and phosphorylation of oxythiamine in rat tissues. J Nutr 81:147–154

35. Polin D, Wynosky ER, Porter CC (1963) Amprolium. XI. Studies on the absorption of Amprolium and thiamine in laying hens. Poultry Sci 42:1057–1061

36. Komai T, Shindo H (1972) Metabolic fate and mechanism of action of chloroethylthiamine. III. Active transport of thiamine from chick intestine and competitive inhibition by chloroethylthiamine. J Vitaminol 18:55–62

37. Basilico V, Ferrari G, Rindi G, D'Andrea G (1979) Thiamine intestinal transport and phosphorylation: a study in vitro of potential inhibitors of small intestinal thiamine-pyrophosphokinase using a crude enzymatic preparation. Arch Int Physiol Biochim 87:981–995

38. Kimura M, Itokawa Y (1985) Determination of thiamine and its phosphate esters in human and rat blood by high-performance liquid chromatography with post-column derivatization. J Chromatogr 332:181–188

39. Bettendorff L, Grandfils C, De Rycker C, Schoffeniels E (1986) Determination of thiamine and its phosphate esters in human blood serum at femtomole levels. J Chromatogr Biomed Appl 382:297–302

40. Bötticher B, Bötticher D (1986) Simple rapid determination of thiamin by a HPLC method in foods, body fluids, urine and faeces. Int J Vitam Nutr Res 56:155–159

41. Friedrich W (1988) Thiamin, vitamin B1, aneurin. In: Vitamins. W de Gruyter, Berlin pp 341–401

42. Bayliss RM, Brookes R, Mc Culloch J, et al (1984) Urinary thiamine excretion after oral physiological doses of the vitamin. Int J Vitam Nutr Res 54:161–164

43. Ziporin ZZ, Nunes WT, Powell RC, et al (1965) Excretion of thiamine and its metabolites in the urine of young adult males receiving restricted intakes of the vitamin. J Nutr 85:287–296

44. Neal RA (1970) Isolation and identification of thiamin catabolites in mammalian urine: isolation and identification of some products of bacterial catabolism of thiamine. In McCormick DB, Wright AD (eds), Methods in enzymology. Academic Press, New York, pp 133–140

45. Finglass PM (1994) Thiamin. Int J Vitam Nutr Res 63:270–274

46. Tallaksen CME, Bohmer T, Bell H (1991) Concomitant determination of thiamin and its phosphate esters in human blood and serum by high-performance liquid chromatography. J Chromat Biomed Appl 564:127–136

47. Herve C, Beyne P, Delacoux E (1994) Determination of thiamine and its phosphate esters in human erythrocytes by high-performance liquid chromatography with isocratic elution. J Chromatogr B 653:217–220

48. Claus D, Eggers R, Warecka K, Neundorfer R (1985) Thiamine deficiency and nervous system function disturbances. Eur Arch Psychiatry Neurol Sci 234:390–394

49. Gubler CJ (1984) Thiamin. In Machlin LJ (ed), Handbook of vitamins. Dekker, New York, pp 245–297

50. Reuler JB, Girard DE, Cooney TG (1985) Wernike's encephalopathy. N Engl J Med 312:1035–1039

51. Butterworth RF (1982) Neurotransmitter function in thiamine deficiency encephalopathy. Neurochem Int 4:449–464

52. Butterworth RF, Giguère JF, Besnard AM (1985) Activities of thiamine-dependent enzymes in two experimental models of thiamine-deficiency encephalopathy. 1. The pyruvate dehydrogenase complex. Neurochem Res 10:1417–1428

53. Butterworth RF, Giguère JF, Besnard AM (1986) Activities of thiamine-dependent enzymes in two experimental models of thiamine-deficiency encephalopathy. 2. α-ketoglutarate dehydrogenase. Neurochem Res 11:567–577

54. Giguère JF, Butterworth RF (1987) Activities of thiamine-dependent enzymes in two experimental models of thiamine-deficiency encephalopathy. 3. Transketolase. Neurochem Res 12:305–310

55. Butterworth RF (1989) Effects of thiamine deficiency in brain metabolism: implications for the pathogenesis of the Wernicke-Korsakoff syndrome. Alcohol Alcohol 24:271–279

56. Butterworth RF (1995) Pathophysiology of alcohol brain damage: synergistic effects of ethanol, thiamine deficiency and alcoholic liver disease. Metab Brain Dis 10:1–8

57. Wood B, Currie J (1995) Presentation of acute Wernicke's encephalopathy and treatment with thiamine. Metab Brain Dis 10:57–71

58. Butterworth RF (1993) Maternal thiamine deficiency: a factor in intrauterine growth retardation. Ann NY Acad Sci 678:325–329

59. Robinson BH (1993) Lactacidemia. Biochim Biophys Acta 1182:231–244

60. Nato E, Ito M, Yokota I, et al (1994) Molecular analysis of abnormal pyruvate dehydrogenase in two patients with thiamine-responsive congenital lactic acidemia [abstract]. Muscle Nerve 1(suppl):s128

61. Rindi G, Patrini C, Laforenza U, et al (1994) Further studies on erythrocyte thiamin transport and phosphorylation in seven patients with thiamin-responsive megaloblastic anaemia. J Inherited Metab Dis 17:667–677

62. National Research Council (1989) Recommended dietary allowances, 10th ed. National Academy Press, Washington, DC

63. Sauberlich HE, Kretsch MJ, Johnson HL, Nelson RA (1982) In Beitz DC, Hansen RG (eds), Animal products in human nutrition. Academic Press, New York, p 339

Chapter 17

Riboflavin

Richard S. Rivlin

The physiological role of riboflavin resides largely in its being the precursor of riboflavin-5'-phosphate (flavin mononucleotide, or FMN) and flavin adenine dinucleotide (FAD), coenzymes for a wide variety of enzymes in intermediary metabolism. Riboflavin is also the precursor of several other flavoenzymes that include forms covalently bound to tissue proteins. Inasmuch as riboflavin itself has little intrinsic activity, the regulation of its conversion into these active coenzyme derivatives by nutritional factors, hormones, drugs, and diseases assumes major significance.

There have been several advances in understanding of the structure and function of the plethora of tissue flavins and their associated proteins, and of their metabolic end products, as reviewed in the previous edition of this volume.[1] Earlier comprehensive reviews of riboflavin metabolism have been updated with emphasis on medical aspects.[2-5] The chemical and nutritional aspects of riboflavin have also been reviewed.[6-8]

Chemistry

Riboflavin, as well as its coenzyme derivatives and indeed all other tissue flavins, are isoalloxazines. The structures of riboflavin and its two major coenzyme derivatives are given in Figure 1. FMN is formed first from riboflavin by the addition of a phosphate group, catalyzed by the enzyme flavokinase. The second biosynthetic step consists of the combination of FMN with a molecule of ATP to form FAD and is catalyzed by FAD synthetase, also designated pyrophosphorylase. FAD can be converted further into forms covalently bound to tissue proteins. Many important mammalian enzymes contain FAD modified at the 8-α position that is covalently bound to the protein: succinic and sarcosine dehydrogenase in the inner mitochondrial membrane, monoamine oxidase in the outer mitochondrial membrane, and L-gulonolactone oxidase, present in liver microsomes of animals capable of making ascorbic acid. Results of measurements performed with radioactive riboflavin suggest that the covalent linkage to tissue proteins occurs subsequently to the synthesis of FAD from riboflavin.[9,10]

Riboflavin is chemically defined as 7,8-dimethyl-10-(1'-D-ribityl) isoalloxazine, and is a planar structure. It is yellow in color and is highly fluorescent. There are many variations in structure in naturally occurring flavins. Riboflavin and its coenzymes are alkali- and acid-sensitive, particularly in the presence of light. Riboflavin is photodegraded under alkaline conditions to yield lumiflavin (7,8,10-trimethylisoalloxazine), which is inactive biologically. In acid conditions, riboflavin is photodegraded to lumichrome (7,8-dimethylalloxazine). Structure-function relationships of derivatives of riboflavin are discussed more fully in the previous edition of this volume.[1] Riboflavin has only limited solubility in aqueous solutions. This point is of practical importance in that therapeutic solutions prepared for intravenous use cannot deliver massive amounts of the vitamin.

Absorption, Transport, Storage, and Turnover

Because dietary sources of riboflavin are largely in the form of coenzyme derivatives, these molecules must be hydrolyzed before absorption. The absorptive process occurs in the upper gastrointestinal tract by specialized transport involving a phosphorylation-dephosphorylation mechanism, rather than by passive diffusion.[11] This process is sodium-dependent and involves an ATPase active transport system that can be saturated. It has been estimated that under normal conditions the upper limit of intestinal absorption of riboflavin at any one time is ≈25 mg. Dietary covalently bound flavins are largely but not entirely inaccessible as nutritional sources.

Diets high in psyllium gum appear to decrease the rate of riboflavin absorption whereas wheat bran has no detectable effect.[12] The time from oral administration to peak urinary excretion of riboflavin is prolonged by the antacids aluminum hydroxide and magnesium hydroxide. Total urinary excretion is unchanged by these drugs, however, and their major effect appears to be on intestinal absorption rather than on urinary excretion.[13] Alcohol intake interferes with both the digestion of food flavins into riboflavin as well as the direct absorption of this vitamin.[14] This observation suggests that the initial rehabilitation of malnourished alcoholic patients

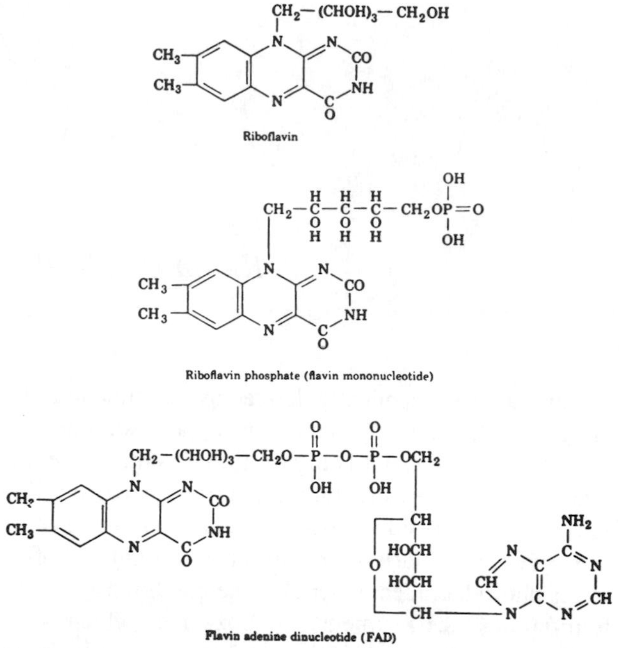

Figure 1. Structural formulas of riboflavin and the two coenzymes derived from riboflavin, riboflavin-5′-phosphate (flavin mononucleotide, FMN) and flavin adenine dinucleotide (FAD). FMN is formed from riboflavin by the addition in the 5′ position of a phosphate group derived from ATP. FAD is formed from FMN after combination with a molecule of ATP.

would be accomplished more efficiently with vitamin supplements containing riboflavin rather than with food sources comprising flavin derivatives.

There is some evidence that the magnitude of riboflavin absorption by the intestine is increased by the presence of food.[11] This effect of food may be due to decreasing the rates of gastric emptying and intestinal transit, thereby permitting more-prolonged contact of dietary riboflavin with the absorptive surface of the intestinal mucosal cells. In general, delaying the rate of gastric emptying tends to increase the intestinal absorption of riboflavin.[15] Bile salts also increase the absorption of both riboflavin and FMN. Several metals and drugs form chelates or complexes with riboflavin and FMN that may affect their bioavailability. Among the agents in this category are the metals copper, zinc, and iron, the drugs caffeine, theophylline, and saccharin, and the vitamins nicotinamide and ascorbic acid, as well as tryptophan and urea.[16] The clinical significance of this binding is not known with certainty in most instances.

In human blood, the transport of flavins involves loose binding to albumin and tight binding to a number of globulins. The major binding of riboflavin and its phosphorylated derivatives in serum is to several classes of immunoglobulins (i.e., IgA, IgG, and IgM).[17–20]

Pregnancy induces the formation of proteins that bind flavins. It has been known for many years that there is an avian riboflavin carrier protein that is genetically

controlled and that determines the amount of riboflavin in chicken eggs.[21] Absence of the protein in autosomal recessive hens results in massive riboflavinuria because there is no mechanism for retaining and binding the vitamin in serum. Eggs become riboflavin-deficient and embryonic death occurs between the 10th and 14th day of incubation.[22,23] Administration of antiserum to the chicken riboflavin-carrier protein leads to termination of the pregnancy.[24]

A new dimension to concepts of protein binding of riboflavin in serum of mammals was provided by the demonstration that riboflavin-binding proteins can also be found in sera from pregnant cows, monkeys, and humans.[25–28] A comprehensive review of riboflavin-binding proteins covers the nature of the binding proteins in various species and provides evidence that, as in birds, these proteins are crucial for successful mammalian reproduction.[29] The pregnancy-specific binding proteins may help transport riboflavin to the fetus. Serum riboflavin-binding proteins also appear to influence placental transfer and fetal-maternal distribution of riboflavin. There are differential rates of uptake of riboflavin at the maternal and fetal surfaces of the human placenta.[30,31] Riboflavin-binding proteins also influence the activity of flavokinase, the first biosynthetic enzyme in the pathway of riboflavin to FAD.[32]

The urinary excretion of flavins occurs predominantly in the form of riboflavin; FMN and FAD are not found in urine. McCormick and his group have been active in identifying many flavins and their derivatives in human urine. Besides the 60–70% of urinary flavins contributed by riboflavin itself, other derivatives include 7-hydroxymethylriboflavin (10–15%), 8-α-sulfonylriboflavin (5–10%), 8-hydroxymethylriboflavin (4–7%), riboflavinyl peptide ester (5%), and 10-hydroxyethylflavin (1–3%). Traces of lumiflavin and other derivatives have also been found. These findings were described more fully by McCormick[1] in the previous edition of this volume.

Ingestion of boric acid greatly increases the urinary excretion of riboflavin.[33] This agent when consumed forms a complex with riboflavin and other molecules having polyhydroxyl groups, such as glucose and ascorbic acid. In rodents riboflavin treatment greatly ameliorates the toxicity of administered boric acid.[34] This treatment should also be effective in humans suffering from accidental exposure to boric acid, although it may be difficult to provide adequate amounts of riboflavin as the result of its low solubility and limited absorptive capacity.

Urinary excretion of riboflavin in rats is also greatly increased by chlorpromazine. Levels are twice those of age- and sex-matched pair-fed control rats.[35] In addition, chlorpromazine accelerates the urinary excretion of riboflavin during dietary deficiency as shown in Figure

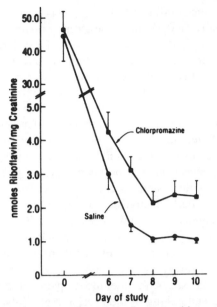

Figure 2. Urinary excretion of riboflavin in chlorpromazine-treated rats and in pair-fed, saline-treated controls during the development of riboflavin deficiency. Data from reference 35.

2. Urinary concentrations of riboflavin are increased within 6 hours of treatment with this drug.

Physiological (Biochemical) Function

As noted, the major function of riboflavin is to serve as the precursor of the coenzymes FMN and FAD and of covalently bound flavins. These coenzymes are widely distributed in metabolism. Riboflavin catalyzes numerous oxidation-reduction reactions. Because FAD is part of the respiratory chain, riboflavin is central to energy production. Other major functions of riboflavin include drug metabolism, in conjunction with the cytochrome P-450 enzymes, and lipid metabolism. The redox functions of flavocoenzymes include one-electron transfers. In addition, two-electron transfers from substrate to flavin are also accomplished.

Flavoproteins catalyze dehydrogenation reactions, as well as hydroxylations, oxidative decarboxylations, dioxygenations, and reductions of oxygen to hydrogen peroxide. Thus, many different kinds of reactions are catalyzed by flavoproteins.[1]

It is not often recognized that riboflavin has powerful antioxidant activity that derives from its role as a precursor to FMN and FAD.[36] Among the FAD-requiring enzymes is glutathione reductase. The glutathione redox cycle provides a major protective role against lipid peroxides. The relationship of the glutathione redox cycle to riboflavin is shown in Figure 3. Glutathione peroxidase, which breaks down lipid peroxides, requires reduced glutathione, which, in turn, is generated by glutathione reductase. Riboflavin deficiency is associated with increased lipid peroxidation; riboflavin can inhibit this process.[37] Riboflavin appears to ameliorate the cardiac damage to rabbit hearts caused by experimental ischemia and reperfusion as well as to reduce damage to rat lungs from toxins and to rat brains from ischemia. This subject is covered more fully in a recent review that also discusses the antimalarial effects of riboflavin deficiency.[5]

Deficiency

At the cellular level. Because the coenzymes derived from riboflavin are distributed widely in intermediary metabolism, the consequences of riboflavin deficiency biochemically may be extensive. In addition, it is important to recall that riboflavin coenzymes are involved in the metabolism of four other vitamins: folic acid, pyridoxine, vitamin K, and niacin.[38] Thus, profound deficiency of riboflavin should have consequences for many enzyme systems in addition to those directly requiring flavin coenzymes.

In riboflavin deficiency, tissue concentrations of FMN and FAD decrease, as does the activity of the biosynthetic enzyme flavokinase, which converts riboflavin to FMN.[39] Concentrations of FMN are decreased proportionately more than are concentrations of FAD. The pattern of liver flavoprotein enzymes is greatly influenced by riboflavin deficiency. Certain enzymes are more sensitive than others to a decrease in availability of their flavin coenzyme. The decrease in activities of enzymes requiring FMN generally parallels the reduction of its tissue concentrations, and activities of FAD-requiring enzymes variably follow the reduction of tissue FAD concentrations.[40]

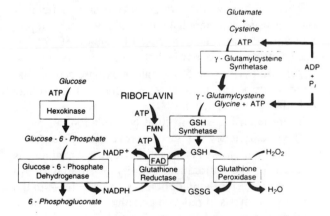

Figure 3. The glutathione redox cycle and its relation to riboflavin and glucose metabolism. Flavin dinucleotide (FAD) formed from riboflavin is utilized by glutathione reductase and its coenzyme and for its structural stabilization. NADPH is generated by glucose-6-phosphate dehydrogenase in the hexose monophosphate shunt. Glutathione reductase converts oxidized glutathione (GSSG) to reduced glutathione (GSH) at the expense of NADPH. GSH, in turn, converts hydrogen peroxide to water.

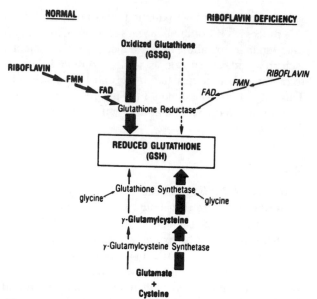

Figure 4. Regeneration of reduced glutathione under normal and riboflavin-deficient conditions. The diagram represents two major pathways for the formation of reduced glutathione in erythrocytes, i.e., reduction of oxidized glutathione (GSSG) via the glutathione reductase pathway and de novo biosynthesis via glutamlycysteine synthetase and glutathione synthetase. Bold arrows emphasize the predominant pathways, thin arrows represent pathways that are operating below maximal levels, and the dotted arrow indicates diminished enzymatic activity.

Hepatic architecture is markedly disrupted in riboflavin deficiency. Mitochondria in riboflavin-deficient mice increase greatly in size and cristae increase in number and size.[41] Hepatic concentrations of RNA and DNA are normal in early riboflavin deficiency but are depressed in later stages.[42]

There are many other effects of riboflavin deficiency on intermediary metabolism, particularly on fat and protein metabolism. The conversion of vitamin B-6 to its coenzyme derivative may be impaired.[43] Decreased FMN-dependent pyridoxine-5'-phosphate oxidase activity has been described in most cases of glucose-6-phosphate dehydrogenase deficiency.[44,45]

There is an increase in lipid peroxidation during riboflavin deficiency that can be prevented by riboflavin supplementation. As discussed previously, glutathione is relevant to the antioxidant activity of riboflavin. An adaptation to riboflavin deficiency is an increase in the de novo synthesis of reduced glutathione from its amino acid precursors, as shown in Figure 4.

In animals. Riboflavin deficiency has been studied in many animal species and has several vital effects, foremost of which is failure to grow. Additional effects include loss of hair, disturbances in the skin, degenerative changes in the nervous system, and impaired reproduction. Congenital malformations occur in the offspring of female rats that are deficient in riboflavin. The conjunc-

tiva becomes inflamed, the cornea is vascularized and eventually opaque, and cataract may result.[46]

Changes in the skin consist of scaliness and incrustation of red-brown material. Alopecia may develop, lips are red and swollen, and filiform papillae on the tongue deteriorate. A decrease in hemoglobin formation during late deficiency leads to anemia. Fatty degeneration of the liver occurs. Important metabolic changes occur so that deficient rats require 15–20% more energy than do control animals to maintain the same body weight. Thus, in all species studied, riboflavin deficiency causes profound structural and functional changes in an ordered sequence. Early changes are very readily reversible.

In humans. The clinical features of human riboflavin deficiency do not have the specificity that may characterize deficits of some other vitamins. Isolated deficiency is rarely encountered. Early symptoms may include weakness, fatigue, mouth pain and tenderness, burning and itching of the eyes, and possibly personality changes. More advanced deficiency may give rise to cheilosis, angular stomatitis, dermatitis, corneal vascularization, anemia, and brain dysfunction. Thus, the syndrome of dietary riboflavin deficiency in humans has many similarities to that in animals, with one notable exception. The spectrum of congenital malformations observed in rodents with maternal riboflavin deficiency has not been clearly identified in humans.[38]

More recently it has been recognized that riboflavin deficiency may result not only from poor dietary intake but also from diseases, drugs, and endocrine abnormalities that may interfere with vitamin utilization. The conversion of riboflavin into its active coenzyme derivatives is inhibited by thyroid and adrenal insufficiency; psychotropic drugs such as chlorpromazine, imipramine, and amitriptyline; the cancer chemotherapeutic drug adriamycin; and antimalarial drugs, such as quinacrine.[35,36,38,39] Alcohol causes riboflavin deficiency by interfering with both its digestion and intestinal absorption.[14] Structural similarities among riboflavin, imipramine, chlorpromazine, and amitriptyline are shown in Figure 5.

The diagnosis of riboflavin deficiency in practice is based first on showing a reduction in the urinary excretion of riboflavin. Although this is a reliable test if the sample is properly collected in a dark bottle and a complete collection is made, the results may be misleading if the subject recently consumed riboflavin. A useful functional test is the activity coefficient of erythrocyte glutathione reductase, an FAD-requiring enzyme. When FAD is added in vitro to an erythrocyte hemolysate, the increase in activity is greater in erythrocytes from riboflavin-deficient than riboflavin-replete individuals, reflecting the lesser degree of saturation of the apoenzyme with its cofactor in deficient compared with normal individuals. Activity coefficients (ratio of activity with FAD in vitro to activity without FAD) greater

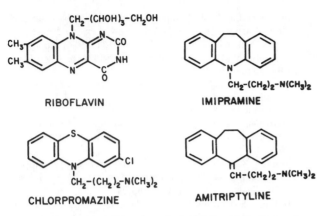

Figure 5. Structural formulas of riboflavin, chlorpromazine, imipramine, and amitriptyline, showing their similarities.

than 1.2–1.3 generally signify some degree of riboflavin deficiency.[38]

Allowances and Requirements

Current recommended dietary allowances (RDAs) for riboflavin from the Food and Nutrition Board do not differ substantially from earlier recommendations.[47] Adult males aged 19–50 y should consume 1.7 mg/day and those aged ≥51 years should consume 1.4 mg daily. Adult females should consume 1.3 mg/day from ages 19 to 50, and 1.2 mg from the age of 51 on. As recommended previously, daily intake should be increased by 0.3 mg during pregnancy to a level of 1.6 mg/day, and by 0.5 mg during lactation to 1.8 mg/day. In the second 6 months of lactation, women should consume 1.7 mg/day.

In a recent study of elderly patients in Guatemala, in which measures of urinary riboflavin excretion and the erythrocyte glutathione reductase activity coefficient were used, it was concluded that the requirements of healthy individuals aged >60 years probably do not differ from those for individuals aged ≤51 years.[48] In a study of elderly residents of nursing homes in the United States, increasing the riboflavin intake through a supplement from 1.7 to 3.4 mg/day doubled riboflavin excretion, showing that this level of intake is clearly above the requirement for the older age group.[49]

On the basis of studies of urinary riboflavin excretion after a test load, it was suggested that the requirement for riboflavin in Chinese may be lower than the figures noted above.[50,51] More research is needed on different populations around the globe to determine more completely the factors that determine riboflavin requirements in various national groups.

Several nutritional and physiological factors may serve to govern riboflavin requirements. Riboflavin excretion is accelerated when there is negative nitrogen balance.[52] Periods of major physical activity in young men and moderate exercise in young women have both been shown to reduce urinary riboflavin excretion.[53,54] These results may be interpreted as suggesting an increased requirement for riboflavin during exercise, particularly because the study in women showed a small increase in the coefficient of erythrocyte glutathione reductase activity. Further research is required to confirm and extend these findings, to determine whether it is physical activity per se that affects metabolism of riboflavin and not some consequence of exercise, such as increased metabolic rate, and to determine what kinds of physical activity may be clinically relevant. Tucker et al.[53] also observed that sleep decreases riboflavin requirements whereas heat stress and prolonged bed rest increase riboflavin excretion.

Food and Other Sources

In the United States the most significant dietary sources of riboflavin are meat and meat products, including poultry, fish, eggs, and milk and dairy products, such as cheese. In developing countries plant sources contribute most of the dietary riboflavin intake. Green vegetables such as broccoli, asparagus, and spinach are fairly good sources of riboflavin. Natural grain products tend to be relatively low in riboflavin, but fortification and enrichment of grains and cereals has led to a great increase in riboflavin intake from these sources.

The food sources of riboflavin are similar to those of other B vitamins. Therefore, it is not surprising that if a given individual's diet has inadequate amounts of riboflavin, it will very likely be inadequate in other vitamins as well.

Several factors in food preparation and processing may influence the amount of riboflavin that is actually consumed. Appreciable amounts may be lost with exposure to light, particularly during cooking and during storage of milk in clear bottles or glasses.[55] Fortunately, most milk is no longer sold in clear bottles. There is some controversy as to whether opaque plastic containers provide greater protection than do cartons. It is highly likely that large amounts of riboflavin are lost during the sun-drying of fruits and vegetables, but the magnitude of the loss is not known precisely. The practice of adding sodium bicarbonate as baking soda to green vegetables to make them appear fresher accelerates the photodegradation of riboflavin.

Excess and Toxicity

There is general agreement that dietary riboflavin intake at many times the RDA is without demonstrable toxicity.[7,8,47,56] Because riboflavin absorption is limited to ≈25 mg as a maximum at any one time, as noted above, consuming megadoses of this vitamin would not be expected to increase the amount absorbed. Furthermore, classical animal investigations showed an apparent upper limit to tissue storage that cannot be exceeded under ordinary circumstances.[40] Thus, several protective mechanisms prevent tissue accumulation of excessive amounts of the vitamin. Because riboflavin also has very low solubility, even intravenous administration of the vitamin would not introduce large amounts into the body. FMN is more water soluble than riboflavin but is not ordinarily available for clinical use.

Nevertheless, the photosensitizing properties of riboflavin raise the possibility of some theoretical, potential risks. Phototherapy in vitro leads to degradation of DNA and increases in lipid peroxidation, which may have implications for carcinogenesis. Irradiation of rat erythrocytes with FMN increases potassium loss.[57] Riboflavin forms an adduct with tryptophan and accelerates the photooxidation of this amino acid.[58] Further research is needed to explore further the full implications of the photosensitivity of riboflavin and its flavin derivatives.

Summary

Knowledge has accumulated rapidly on the structural and functional aspects of riboflavin, its coenzyme derivatives, and a host of tissue flavins. The consequences of riboflavin deficiency are widespread and extend beyond flavin-requiring proteins. Vitamin deficiency results not only from dietary inadequacy but from the effects of drugs, hormones, and diseases and nutritional factors that regulate vitamin utilization. Recent advances have been made in understanding the pathogenesis of riboflavin deficiency and the factors that determine riboflavin requirements. Riboflavin, in its role as a precursor to FAD, is needed for glutathione reductase and has significant antioxidant activity that has not been recognized adequately. Many exciting challenges lie ahead in elucidating new roles for the vitamin in health and disease.

References

1. McCormick DB (1990) Riboflavin. In Brown ML (ed), Present knowledge in nutrition, 6th ed. International Life Sciences Institute, Washington, DC, pp 146–154
2. Rivlin RS (ed) (1975) Riboflavin. Plenum Press, New York
3. Rivlin RS (1970) Medical progress: riboflavin metabolism. N Engl J Med 283:463–472
4. Rivlin RS (1991) Medical aspects of vitamin B₂. In Muller F (ed), Chemistry and biochemistry of flavins, vol 1. CRC Press, Boca Raton, FL, pp 201–214
5. Rivlin RS, Dutta P (1995) Vitamin B₂ (riboflavin): relevance to malaria and antioxidant activity. Nutr Today 30:62–67
6. McCormick DB (1986) Riboflavin. In Tietz NW (ed), Textbook of clinical chemistry. WB Saunders, Philadelphia, pp 927–964
7. McCormick DB (1994). Riboflavin. In Shils ME, Olson JA, Shike M (eds), Modern nutrition in health and disease, 8th ed. Lea and Febiger, Philadelphia, pp 366–375
8. Cooperman JM, Lopez R (1984) Riboflavin. In Machlin LJ (ed), Handbook of vitamins: nutritional, biochemical and clinical aspects. Marcel Dekker, New York, pp 299–327
9. Yagi K, Nakagawa Y, Suzuki O, Ohishi N (1976) Incorporation of riboflavin into covalently-bound flavins in rat liver. J Biochem 79:841–843
10. Pinto J, Rivlin RS (1979) Regulation of formation of covalently bound flavins in liver and cerebrum by thyroid hormones. Arch Biochem Biophys 194:313–320
11. Jusko WJ, Levy G (1967) Absorption, metabolism and excretion of riboflavin-5' phosphate in man. J Pharm Sci 56:58–62
12. Roe DA, Kalkwarf H, Stevens J (1988) Effect of fiber supplements on the apparent absorption of pharmacological doses of riboflavin. J Am Diet Assoc 88:211–213
13. Feldman S, Hedrick W (1983) Antacid effects on the gastrointestinal absorption of riboflavin. J Pharm Sci 72:121–123
14. Pinto JT, Huang YP, Rivlin RS (1987) Mechanisms underlying the differential effects of ethanol upon the bioavailability of riboflavin and flavin adenine dinucleotide. J Clin Invest 79:1343–1348
15. Roe DA (1988) Fiber and riboflavin absorption [letter]. J Am Diet Assoc 88:783
16. Jusko WJ, Levy G (1975). Absorption, protein binding and elimination of riboflavin. In Rivlin RS (ed), Riboflavin. Plenum Press, New York, pp 99–152
17. Merrill AH Jr, Froehlich JA, McCormick DB (1981) Isolation and identification of alternative riboflavin-binding proteins from human plasma. Biochem Med 25:198–206
18. Innis WSA, McCormick DB, Merrill AH Jr (1985) Variations in riboflavin binding by human plasma: identification of immunoglobulins as the major proteins responsible. Biochem Med 34:151–165
19. Innis WS, Nixon DW, Murray DR, McCormick DB, Merrill AH Jr (1986) Immunoglobulins associated with elevated riboflavin binding by plasma from cancer patients. Proc Soc Exp Biol Med 181:237–241
20. Merrill AH Jr, Innis-Whitehouse WSA, McCormick DB (1987) Characterization of human riboflavin-binding immunoglobulins. In Edmondson DE, McCormick DB (eds), Flavins and flavoproteins. de Gruyter, Berlin, pp 445–448
21. Clagett CO (1971) Genetic control of the riboflavin carrier protein. Fed Proc 30:127–129
22. Winter WP, Buss EG, Clagett CO, Boucher RV (1967) The nature of the biochemical lesion in avian renal riboflavinuria. II. The inherited change of a riboflavin-binding protein from blood and eggs. Comp Biochem Physiol 22:897–906
23. Clagett CO, Buss EG, Saylor EM, Girsh SJ (1970) The nature of the biochemical lesion in avian renal riboflavinuria. 6. Hormone induction of the riboflavin-binding protein in roosters and young chicks. Poult Sci 49:1468–1472
24. Natraj U, Kumar AR, Kadam P (1987) Termination of pregnancy in mice with antiserum to chicken riboflavin-carrier protein. Biol Reprod 36:677–685
25. Merrill AH Jr, Froehlich JA, McCormick DB (1979) Purification of riboflavin-binding proteins from bovine plasma and discovery of a pregnancy-specific riboflavin-binding protein. J Biol Chem 254:9362–9364
26. Visweswariah SS, Adiga PR (1987) Purification of a circulatory riboflavin carrier protein from pregnant bonnet monkey (M. radiata): comparison with chicken egg vitamin carrier. Biochim Biophys Acta 915:141–148
27. Murthy CVR, Adiga PR (1982) Isolation and characterization of a riboflavin-carrier protein from human pregnancy serum. Biochem Int 5:289–296
28. Visweswariah SS, Adiga PR (1987) Isolation of riboflavin carrier proteins from pregnant human and umbilical cord

serum: similarities with chicken egg riboflavin carrier protein. Biosci Rep 7:563–571

29. White HB III, Merrill AH Jr (1988) Riboflavin-binding proteins. Annu Rev Nutr 8:279–299

30. Dancis J, Lehanka J, Levitz M (1985) Transfer of riboflavin by the perfused human placenta. Pediatr Res 19:1143–1146

31. Dancis J, Lehanka J, Levitz M (1988) Placental transport of riboflavin: differential rates of uptake at the maternal and fetal surfaces of the perfused human placenta. Am J Obstet Gynecol 158:204–210

32. Slomczynska M, Zak Z (1987) The effect of riboflavin binding protein (RBP) on flavokinase catalytic activity. Comp Biochem Physiol 37B:681–685

33. Pinto J, Huang YP, McConnell RJ, Rivlin RS (1978) Increased urinary riboflavin excretion resulting from boric acid ingestion. J Lab Clin Med 92:126–134

34. Roe DA, McCormick DB, Lin RT (1972) Effects of riboflavin on boric acid toxicity. J Pharm Sci 61:1081–1085

35. Pelliccione N, Pinto J, Huang YP, Rivlin RS (1983) Accelerated development of riboflavin deficiency by treatment with chlorpromazine. Biochem Pharmacol 32:2949–2953

36. Dutta P (1993) Disturbances in glutathione metabolism and resistance to malaria: current understanding and new concepts. J Soc Pharm Chem 2:11–48

37. Dutta P, Serafi J, Halpin D, et al (1995) Acute ethanol exposure alters hepatic glutathione metabolism in riboflavin deficiency. Alcohol 12:43–47

38. Rivlin RS (1991) Disorders of vitamin metabolism: deficiencies, metabolic abnormalities and excesses. In Wyngaarden JH, Smith LH Jr, Bennett JC, Plum F (eds), Cecil textbook of medicine, 19th ed. WB Saunders, Philadelphia, pp 1170–1183

39. Rivlin RS, Menendez C, Langdon RG (1968) Biochemical similarities between hypothyroidism and riboflavin deficiency. Endocrinology 83:461–469

40. Burch HB, Lowry OH, Padilla AM, Combs AM (1956) Effects of riboflavin deficiency and realimentation on flavin enzymes of tissues. J Biol Chem 223:29–45

41. Tandler B, Erlandson RA, Wynder EL (1968) Riboflavin and mouse hepatic cell structure and function. I. Ultrastructural alterations in simple deficiency. Am J Pathol 52:69–95

42. Chatterjee AK, Roy AK, Ghosh BB (1969) Effect of riboflavin deficiency on nucleic acid metabolism of liver in the rat. Br J Nutr 23:657–663

43. McCormick DB (1989) Two interconnected B vitamins: riboflavin and pyridoxine. Physiol Rev 69:1170–1198

44. Powers HJ, Bates CJ (1985) A simple fluorimetric assay for pyridoxamine phosphate oxidase in erythrocyte haemolysates: effects of riboflavin supplementation and of glucose 6-phosphate dehydrogenase deficiency. Hum Nutr Clin Nutr 39:107–115

45. BB Anderson, JE Clements, GM Perry, et al (1987) Glutathione reductase activity in G6PD deficiency. Eur J Haematol 38:12–20

46. Goldsmith GA (1975) Riboflavin deficiency. In Rivlin R (ed), Riboflavin. Plenum Press, New York, pp 221–242

47. Food and Nutrition Board, National Research Council (1989) Recommended dietary allowances, 10th ed. National Academy Press, Washington, DC, pp 132–137

48. Boisvert WA, Mendoza I, Castaneda C, et al (1993) Riboflavin requirement of healthy elderly humans and its relationship to macronutrient composition of the diet. J Nutr 123:915–925

49. Alexander M, Emanuel G, Golin T, et al (1984) Relation of riboflavin nutriture in healthy elderly to intake of calcium and vitamin supplements: evidence against riboflavin supplementation. Am J Clin Nutr 39:540–546

50. Brun TA, Chen J, Campbell TC, et al (1990) Urinary riboflavin excretion after a load test in rural China as a measure of possible riboflavin deficiency. Eur J Clin Nutr 44:195–206

51. Campbell TC, Brun T, Junshi C, et al (1990) Questioning riboflavin recommendations on the basis of a survey in China. Am J Clin Nutr 51:436–445

52. Windmueller HG, Anderson AA, Mickelsen O (1964) Elevated riboflavin levels in urine of fasting human subjects. Am J Clin Nutr 15:73–76

53. Tucker RG, Mickelsen O, Keys A (1960) The influence of sleep, work, diuresis, heat, acute starvation, thiamine intake and bed rest on human riboflavin excretion. J Nutr 72:251–261

54. Belko AZ, Obarzanek E, Kalkwarf HJ, et al (1983) Effects of exercise on riboflavin requirements of young women. Am J Clin Nutr 37:509–517

55. Wanner RL (1960) Effects of commercial processing of milk and milk products on their nutrient content. In Harris RS, Loesecke HV (eds), The nutritional evaluation of food processing. John Wiley, New York, pp 173–196

56. Rivlin RS (1979) Effect of nutrient toxicities (excess) in animals and man: riboflavin. In M Rechcigl (ed), Handbook of nutrition and foods. CRC Press, Cleveland, pp 25–27

57. Ghazy FS, Kimura T, Muranishi S, Sezaki H (1977) The photodynamic action of riboflavin on erythrocytes. Life Sci 21:1703–1708

58. Salim-Hanna M, Edwards AM, Silva E (1987) Obtention of a photo-induced adduct between a vitamin and an essential amino acid: binding of riboflavin to tryptophan. Int J Vitam Nutr Res 57:155–159

Chapter 18

Vitamin B-6

James E. Leklem

Vitamin B-6, a group of nitrogen-containing compounds, occurs naturally in three primary forms: pyridoxine (PN), pyridoxal (PL), and pyridoxamine (PM). Gyorgy's identification of vitamin B-6 in 1934 and the associated research and nomenclature has been reviewed by Snell.[1] Several other reviews and symposia attest to the intriguing and complex nature of vitamin B-6 and to the significant advances made in our understanding of the vitamin's role in metabolism and well-being.[2-9]

Chemistry

Structure. The three B-6 vitamers are 2-methyl-3-hydroxy-5-hydroxy methyl pyridines. When substituted in the 4 position, these occur as the hydroxymethyl (PN), formyl (PL), or aminomethyl (PM) form. Each of these forms can also be phosphorylated at the 5 position (Figure 1). The active coenzyme forms are pyridoxal 5′-phosphate (PLP) and pyridoxamine 5′-phosphate (PMP). Many plant foods contain variable amounts of a glucoside form in which glucose is linked to the 5′-position (5′-0-(β-D-glucopyranosyl) pyridoxine).[10,11] The function of this glucoside in plants is unknown but it may be a storage form of the vitamin.

Chemical properties. The hydrochloride and base forms of the B-6 vitamers are readily soluble in water. The hydrochloride of pyridoxine is the most common commercially sold form of vitamin B-6. The stability of the various forms of vitamin B-6 are of interest to consumers and food producers. In solution the forms are light sensitive but the degree of degradation varies, especially in relation to pH. In an acid medium, PN, PL, and PM are relatively heat stable, but are heat labile in an alkaline medium. The ionic form varies in solution. The aldehyde form PL exists as the hemiacetal of the aldehyde and 5′-hydroxy group. The metabolic end product, 4-pyridoxic acid (4-PA), exists primarily as a lactone. Solutions of PLP and PL will react with free amino groups to form a Schiff base. Pyridoxal 5′-phosphate is especially reactive and readily reacts with amino groups. This Schiff base reaction occurs in most of the enzymatic reactions involving PLP. The structural features of PLP make it well suited for Schiff base formation.[12] The chemistry of vitamin B-6 has been extensively reviewed.[5,6] Data on the fluorescence and ultraviolet characteristics of the B-6 vitamins are available.[13]

Methods of Analysis

Methods of identifying and measuring the forms of vitamin B-6 in biological fluids and foods have been reviewed in several publications.[14,15] Microbiological, enzymatic, and high-performance liquid chromatography (HPLC) assays are utilized in quanitating B-6 vitamers.[14-16] As is true in other areas of nutrition, the use of HPLC is advantageous because several forms of vitamin B-6 can be measured in a single run. However, there are several HPLC methods and not all have been extensively validated against each other. PLP is one of the most commonly measured forms of vitamin B-6.[19,20]

Occurrence in Foods

Any appreciation of the role vitamin B-6 plays in human nutrition includes knowledge of the amounts of the various forms of vitamin B-6 in foods. Pyridoxine

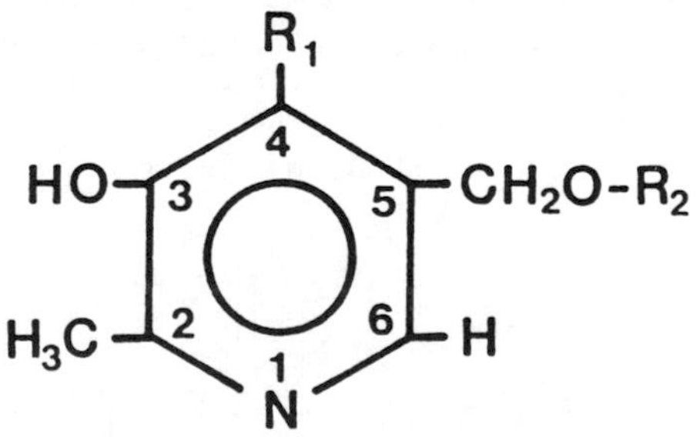

$$PN \; ; \; R_1 = CH_2OH \qquad PNP \; ; \; R_2 = PO_3^=$$
$$PM \; ; \; R_1 = CH_2NH_2 \qquad PMP \; ; \; R_2 = PO_3^=$$
$$PL \; ; \; R_1 = CHO \qquad PLP \; ; \; R_2 = PO_3^=$$

Figure 1. Structure of B-6 vitamers.[9]

and pyridoxamine (along with their phosphorylated forms) are the predominant forms in plant foods. In animal foods the predominant form is pyridoxal (and its phosphorylated form). The glycosylated form was initially identified in rice bran and has been quanitated in

Table 1. Vitamin B-6 and pyridoxine glucoside content of selected foods

Food	Vitamin B-6 (mg/100 g)	Glycosylated vitamin B-6 (mg/100 g)
Vegetables		
Carrots, canned	0.064	0.055
Carrots, raw	0.170	0.087
Cauliflower, frozen	0.084	0.069
Broccoli, frozen	0.119	0.078
Spinach, frozen	0.208	0.104
Cabbage, raw	0.140	0.065
Sprouts, alfalfa	0.250	0.105
Potatoes, cooked	0.394	0.165
Potatoes, dried	0.884	0.286
Yams, canned	0.067	0.007
Beans/legumes		
Soybeans, cooked	0.627	0.357
Beans, navy, cooked	0.381	0.159
Beans, lima, frozen	0.106	0.039
Peas, frozen	0.122	0.018
Peanut butter	0.302	0.054
Beans, garbanzo	0.653	0.111
Lentils	0.289	0.134
Animal products		
Beef, ground, cooked	0.263	n.d.
Tuna, canned	0.316	n.d.
Chicken breast, raw	0.700	n.d.
Milk, skim	0.005	n.d.
Nuts/seeds		
Walnuts	0.535	0.038
Filberts	0.587	0.026
Cashews, raw	0.351	0.046
Sunflower seeds	0.997	0.355
Almonds	0.086	0
Fruits		
Orange juice, frozen concentrate	0.165	0.078
Tomato juice, canned	0.097	0.045
Blueberries, frozen	0.046	0.019
Banana	0.313	0.010
Pineapple, canned	0.079	0.017
Peaches, canned	0.009	0.002
Apricots, dried	0.206	0.036
Avocado	0.443	0.015
Raisins, seedless	0.230	0.154
Cereals/grains		
Wheat bran	0.903	0.326
Shredded wheat, cereal	0.313	0.087
Rice, brown	0.237	0.055
Rice, bran	3.515	0.153
Rice, white	0.076	0.015
Rice cereal, puffed	0.098	0.007
Rice cereal, fortified	3.635	0.382

n.d. = none detected. Sources: Kabir et al.[11] and Leklem and Hardin, unpublished.

several foods.[10,11] Table 1 lists the vitamin B-6 content and glycosylated content of representative foods.

Food processing and storage can affect the vitamin B-6 content of some foods.[21-23] A wide range of loss (10-50%) has been reported for a variety of foods and processing techniques. Heat sterilization of milk can convert pyridoxal to pyridoxamine.[23] As a result of thermal processing and low-moisture storage of certain foods there is reductive binding of PL and PLP to proteins via e-amino groups of their lysyl residues.[24,25] These derivatives possess low- or anti-vitamin B-6 activity.[26]

Absorption, Bioavailability, and Transport

The absorption, transport, and metabolism of vitamin B-6 is shown in Figure 2.

Intestinal uptake. Absorption of the vitamin B-6 vitamers has been examined less in humans than in animals.[9,27,28] From research with rats we conclude that pyridoxine and the other two major forms of vitamin B-6 are absorbed by a nonsaturable, passive process.[27] Included in this process is the simultaneous hydrolysis of the 5'-phosphates by nonspecific phosphatases of the gastrointestinal tract.[28] Absorption occurs primarily in the jejunum. After absorption each of the forms can be phosphorylated and thus retained (a process called metabolic trapping).

The primary forms of vitamin B-6 are readily and efficiently absorbed but the glucoside form is not.[9,29,30] Several studies have found that in humans fed controlled diets the availability of vitamin B-6 is generally >75% for most foods studied.[31-34] There appears to be an inverse relationship between the pyridoxine glucoside (PNG) content of the diet and the bioavailability of vitamin B-6.[35] Some dietary PNG is absorbed intact and is excreted in the urine.[25-36] Gregory and co-workers[37] have found that ≈58% of PNG administered to humans is bioavailable. Other factors may limit the availability, including food processing (formation of ε-pyridoxyllysine), the amount of fiber (incomplete digestion), and presence of other forms of vitamin B-6 (hydroxypyridoxine and pyridoxine glucoside).[9,29,30]

Transport. Vitamin B-6 is transported in the blood both in the plasma and in the red cells. In the plasma PLP is more tightly bound to albumin than PL, and together in plasma PLP and PL account for >90% of the total vitamin B-6.[9,38,39] PN and PL are rapidly taken up by red blood cells where they can be converted to PLP and subsequently bound to hemoglobin, but PLP does not bind as tightly as PL.[40] The precise role the red cell plays in vitamin B-6 transport remains to be determined.

Metabolism. A majority of the absorbed vitamin B-6 is taken up by the liver.[40,41] PLP is not taken up as such but is hydrolyzed by the plasma membrane alkaline phosphatase and the free PL is absorbed. Within the liver the three nonphosphorylated forms are converted to the respective phosphorylated forms by pyridoxine kinase, with zinc and adenosine triphosphate as cofactors.[42] The respective 5'-phosphates can then be converted to PLP via a flavin mononucleotide (FMN) oxidase.[43] The PLP produced is bound by apoenzymes or released in the plasma where it binds to albumin. PLP and the other 5'-phosphates can be hydrolyzed to the free forms by alkaline phosphatases.[42,44] PL is irreversibly converted to 4-pyridoxic acid (4-PA) in an oxidation reaction that probably involves flavin adenine dinucleotide (FAD) and the resultant 4-PA is excreted in the urine.[42]

The metabolism of vitamin B-6 is highly regulated in the liver and probably in other tissues. Studies of the enzymes in human liver indicate that there are similar activities for kinase and phosphatase at physiologic pH. The activity of the FAD oxidase is sufficient to convert excess PL to 4-PA.[42,45] Another important site of regulation of vitamin B-6 metabolism is the product inhibition of the conversion of PMP and PNP to PLP. As a result of regulation at these points, excess PLP does not accumulate in the liver, thus limiting the potentially adverse reactions of highly reactive PLP with other enzymes.

Because levels of PNP and PMP oxidase in most tissues are too low, the liver is considered the main organ responsible for converting diet sources of vitamin B-6 to PLP.[9,41] The liver is also considered the primary organ for catabolism of PL to 4-PA.[42] In humans 40-60% of the daily intake is excreted as 4-PA.[9,46] Of the B-6 intake ≈10% is excreted as other forms of the vitamin, one of which is pyridoxine glucoside.[9,35] The PLP produced in the liver is available for uptake into other tissues but only after hydrolysis of the phosphate group by alkaline phosphatase.[47] While alkaline phosphatase would appear to be important for the availability of PLP for tissues, patients with hypophosphatasia have high circulating levels of PLP and still appear to maintain adequate tissue levels of PLP.[48]

There are numerous body pools of vitamin B-6.[49,50] Of the total body pool, estimated to be 1000 μmol, 80-90% is present in muscle where a majority of the vitamin B-6 is present as PLP bound to glycogen phosphorylase.[49,51] In comparison, the total amount of vitamin B-6 in the circulation is <1 μmol. PLP in plasma is thought to be a two-compartment model, where the slow turnover of the pool is estimated to take 25-33 days.[9]

Several reviews provide additional detail on the metabolism of vitamin B-6, with particular reference to humans.[9,52-54]

Functions

The reactivity of PLP with amino acids and several nitrogen-containing compounds is responsible for the

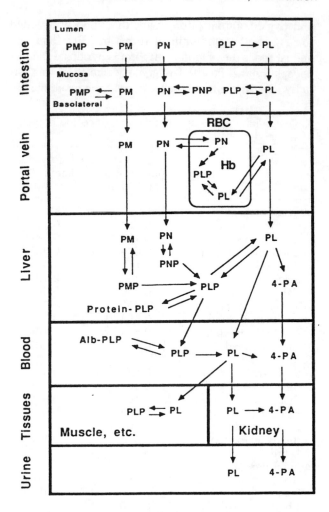

Figure 2. Overview of vitamin B-6 transport and metabolism. Summary of involvement of different organs in the uptake, transport, metabolism, and excretion of vitamin B-6 are summarized. The enzymes involved in these interconversions are pyridoxal (PL) kinase for the phosphorylation of pyridoxine (PN), pyridoxamine (PM), and PL; PNP (PMP) oxidase for pyridoxal 5'-phosphate (PLP) synthesis from pyridoxine 5'-phosphate (PNP) and pyridoxamine 5'-phosphate (PMP) (there is also interconversion of PLP and PMP by aminotransferases not shown); alkaline phosphatase to remove the 5'-phosphates; and PL oxidase and, possibly, PL dehydrogenase to form pyridoxic acid (4-PA). The PL and PLP can be bound by albumin (Alb) and hemoglobin (Hb) in red blood cells (RBC).[128]

≈100 enzymatic reactions in which vitamin B-6 is involved. Details of the complex biochemistry of these enzymes have been reviewed.[5,6]

Table 2 summarizes the six primary types of enzymatic reactions involving PLP. In these reactions the enzyme binds the PLP tightly as a Schiff base with the e-amino group of an active-site lysine. The aminotransferase reactions are especially important to biosynthesis and catabolism of indispensable and dispensable amino acids.

The role PLP plays can also be viewed from a system/cellular perspective. These systems/cellular processes

Table 2. Enzyme reactions catalyzed by pyridoxal 5'-phosphate

Type of reaction	Examples
Aminotransferase	Alanine aminotransferase Aspartate aminotransferase
Decarboxylation	Tryptophan decarboxylase Tyrosine decarboxylase
Decarboxylation with carbon-carbon bond formation	Delta-amino levulinate synthetase Serine palmitoyltransferase
Side chain cleavage	Serine hydroxymethyltransferase Cystathionase
Dehydratase	L-serine dehydratase
Racemization	Interconversion of D and L amino acids (bacteria only)

are depicted in Figure 3. A brief description of each follows.

Gluconeogenesis. PLP is involved in glucose production through its role in transaminase reactions and in the action of glycogen phosphorylase.[51,53,55] However, in humans, a low intake of vitamin B-6 (0.2 mg/day) does not adversely affect fasting plasma glucose levels but does impair glucose tolerance.[56] In rats fed a vitamin B-6–deficient diet glycogen phosphorylase activity decreases in both liver and muscle.[51,57,58] However, the PLP in muscle is not mobilized. During a caloric deficit the glycogen phosphorylase in the muscle decreases and presumably mobilizes the stored PLP.[57] The reservoir of muscle vitamin B-6 appears to be used only when there is an increased need for glucose through gluconeogenesis. In humans this may occur during exercise, a physiologic stress under which plasma PLP levels increase.[59–61]

Niacin formation. There is one enzymatic step (kynureninase) that requires PLP in the conversion of tryptophan to niacin. One would expect, therefore, that a decrease in liver PLP levels would affect niacin formation. However, in humans fed a low intake (<0.2 mg/day) of vitamin B-6 there is only a moderate effect on this conversion.[53,62]

Lipid metabolism. The role PLP plays in lipid metabolism remains fascinating. Early studies in rats have shown that a deficiency of vitamin B-6 results in a decrease in body fat, decreased liver lipid levels, and impaired lysosomal degradation of lipid.[63–65] Sphingolipid biosynthesis (by serine palmitoyltransferase) is a PLP-dependent reaction. The action of this and other PLP-dependent enzymes in phospholipid synthesis may account for the changes seen in the levels of linoleic and arachidonic acids in phospholipids among vitamin B-6–deficient animals.[66,67] A possible mechanism for these changes in phospolipid levels may involve inhibiting methylation of phosphoethanolamine by increased levels of S-adenosylmethionine.[68] Other effects of vitamin B-6 nutrition on lipid metabolism may occur through carnitine synthesis.[69] There is no consensus that vitamin B-6 affects cholesterol levels in humans.[9,70] A deficiency of vitamin B-6 in humans is not associated with a significant change in serum cholesterol.[71]

Nervous system. Several in-depth reviews address vitamin B-6 and nervous system function and biochemistry.[72–74] Numerous enzymatic reactions in which PLP is involved give rise to neurotransmitters, including serotonin, taurine, dopamine, norepinephrine, histamine, and γ-aminobutyric acid.

An unintentional situation in infants provides evidence for vitamin B-6 being involved in brain function. Infants fed a formula in which the vitamin B-6 is destroyed by heat processing develop abnormal electroencephalogram (EEG) tracings and convulsions.[75] Adults fed diets low in vitamin B-6 have also been found to develop abnormal EEG tracings.[76–78]

The progeny of female rats fed low levels of vitamin B-6 develop altered fatty acid levels in the brain.[79] Reduced γ-aminobutyric acid levels are observed in nerve cells of animals fed low levels of vitamin B-6.[80] Other adverse changes have been seen in the nervous system architecture of deficient animals and their offspring.[81–82] Taken together these observations demonstrate the need for adequate amounts of vitamin B-6 during fetal development and after birth.

Nucleic acids and immune system. Vitamin B-6 has an effect on the immune system of both animals and humans.[83–87] In animals made deficient in vitamin B-6 the cell-mediated immune response is impaired.[86] In some cases a rather severe deficiency, characterized by low tissue PLP levels in the spleen (40% of controls), is necessary before changes in lymphocyte proliferation occur.[88] Other animal studies have found that vitamin B-6 nutrition affects tumor formation, but tumor volume is reduced

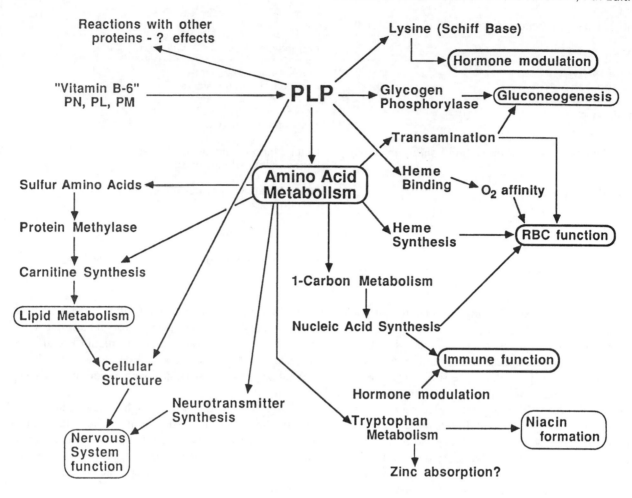

Figure 3. Cellular processes in which pyridoxal 5'-phosphate (PLP) acts as a coenzyme or binds with proteins and modifies the action of the protein. Heme binding refers to PLP binding to hemoglobin.[19]

in animals receiving 0.2 mg/kg of PN compared to animals fed 1.2 mg/kg of PN.[89] In contrast, Ha et al. observed enhanced tumor growth with low intakes (0.0 or 0.1 mg/kg PN) versus higher doses (0.5 or 1.0 mg/kg).[90]

Studies in young and elderly humans demonstrate variable effects of vitamin B-6 nutritional status on immune response.[86] Studies by Talbot et al.[91] and Meydani et al.[87] have found a beneficial effect of PN supplements or PN repletion on lymphocyte proliferation in elderly persons. A significant correlation of EAST activity coefficient and functional parameters of immunity is found in individuals with asymptomatic human immunodeficiency virus type 1 (HIV-1) infection who were studied for vitamin B-6 status and immune function.[92] Other studies have shown that PLP binds to soluble CD4 protein, a protein to which HIV-1 also binds.[93] This suggests PLP may be an effective antiviral agent, but no therapeutic tests have been conducted.

If PLP has an effect on immune function, as many studies indicate, it may be acting by affecting 1-carbon metabolism. Serine transhydroxymethylase is a PLP-dependent enzyme that is involved in 1-carbon metabolism and thus affects synthesis of nucleic acids.[94] PLP also inhibits thymidylate synthase.[95] Through this inhibitory process a deficiency of vitamin B-6 would then impair DNA synthesis, a process important in maintaining immune function.

Hormone modulation. One of the more recently discovered roles for PLP is that of modulating steroid hormone action. Studies by Compton and Cidlowski[96] have shown that PLP binds to steroid receptors. In addition, PLP binds to a second site on the steroid receptor and alters the binding of the steroid receptor to DNA, resulting in decreased action of the steroid. Allgood et al.[97] have reviewed the biochemistry of this hormone modulation by PLP. Oka et al.[98] have found that PLP modulates expression of the cytosolic aspartate aminotransferase gene by inactivating binding of the glucocorticoid receptor to glucocorticoid-responsive elements. Research to date suggests that the action of several steroid hormones are modulated by PLP, and thus vitamin B-6 may have an effect on endocrine-mediated diseases.

Vitamin B-6 Status

A critical part of understanding a person's (or any species') vitamin B-6 nutritional status is applying the proper biochemical tests to evaluate their status. For vitamin B-6 there are several direct and indirect indices which can be used.[99,100] In addition, evaluation of vitamin B-6 and protein intake is important in assessing B-6 status, since increased protein intake decreases plasma PLP concentration and urinary 4-PA excretion.[101]

Direct measures. The metabolites of the B-6 vitamers are measured directly, most commonly in the form of plasma PLP. Both animal and human studies support use of plasma PLP as an indicator.[99,102,103] However, proper interpretation of plasma PLP as a status indicator should take into account the various factors which can affect PLP concentration.[99] For example increased protein intake, increased alkaline phosphatase, smoking, and age are all associated with reduced plasma PLP levels. Other direct measures include urinary 4-PA (short-term indicator) and plasma PL concentration.

Indirect measures. The indirect measures currently used are reflections of metabolic pathways or enzymes that require PLP. It is assumed that these measures are indicators of tissue levels of PLP. Those most commonly used indirect measures are the urinary metabolites of the tryptophan or methionine pathways, and erythrocyte transaminase activity and stimulation.[99,104–106] Assessment of EEG patterns has been used, but less frequently than other indirect measures.[78] Recently measurement of plasma homocysteine has been suggested as an index of vitamin B-6 status. A high plasma concentration of homocysteine has been linked to an increased risk of coronary heart disease.[107] However, current research suggests folic acid is relatively more important than vitamin B-6 in determining the level of plasma homocysteine.[108]

Vitamin B-6 deficiency. Although a frank deficiency of vitamin B-6 is relatively uncommon, marginal deficiencies are more likely. When a deficiency occurs in humans it is probably associated with a deficiency of other nutrients, especially other water-soluble vitamins. Such a multiple deficiency may be of more adverse consequence if there is also a deficiency of riboflavin because riboflavin is involved in the metabolism of vitamin B-6.[109] The signs of severe and chronic vitamin B-6 deficiency are stomatitis, cheilosis, glossitis, irritability, depression, and confusion.

Deficiencies of vitamin B-6 can be induced by certain drugs which form complexes with PLP or PL. Examples of drugs that interfere with vitamin B-6 metabolism are isoniazid, cycloserine, and penicillamine.[110] Patients taking these types of drugs are often given vitamin B-6.

While not a deficiency in a diet-nutrition context, certain genetic defects of PLP-dependent enzymes mimic vitamin B-6 deficiency.[7,8,111] Examples include homocystinuria and cystathionuria (defect of cystathionin B-synthase and cystathionase), xanthurenic aciduria (defect of kynureninase), and a defect in ornithine aminotransferase that produces gyrate atrophy.

Clinical conditions. Several reviews discuss relationships between vitamin B-6 and various disease states for which either altered tryptophan metabolism or decreased plasma PLP have been observed.[4,7,8,52] Given the factors other than vitamin B-6 status that alter tryptophan metabolism, one must be cautious in concluding that vitamin B-6 status per se is adversely affected. Disease states in which decreased plasma PLP concentration has been reported include renal disease, alcoholism, coronary heart disease, breast cancer, Hodgkin's disease, and diabetes.[112–117] In many of these studies PLP was the only B-6 status index measured. Thus the extent to which vitamin B-6 status is truly altered remains open to exploration.

Vitamin B-6 supplementation has been used as a therapeutic agent for several diseases or in an attempt to prevent the disease.[7,8,118] Conditions which have been treated with pyridoxine (of limited benefit) include Down's syndrome, autism, gestational diabetes, premenstrual syndrome, carpal tunnel syndrome, and diabetic neuropathy.[9] The amount of pyridoxine given, the length of time administered, and lack of inclusion of a double-blind placebo control make evaluation of B-6 efficacy difficult.

Toxicity. The use of vitamin B-6 in an attempt to treat conditions such as premenstrual syndrome and related disorders has resulted in a small number of cases of neurotoxicity and photosensitivity.[119,120] These symptoms are usually seen only when daily doses >500 mg are used on a chronic basis. Supplements of <250 mg/day are safe for most individuals.

Requirements

The most recent recommended dietary allowances (RDA)[121] for vitamin B-6 are 2.0 mg/day for males 15 years and older and 1.6 mg/day for females 19 years and older. For infants 3 months and younger, the RDA is 0.3 mg/day and increases to 0.6 mg/day for older infants. For children the RDA increases from 1.0 mg/day at 1 year of age to 1.4 mg at age 7–10 years. For adolescents the RDA is 1.7 mg/day for males and 1.4–1.5 mg/day for females. During pregnancy the RDA is increased 0.6 mg/day above the adult female value of 1.6 mg/day. For lactating women the RDA increases 0.5 mg/day. A comprehensive review discusses the factors which affect vitamin B-6 requirements and other aspects of vitamin B-6 nutrition during pregnancy, lactation, and infancy.[122]

Several factors potentially affect the RDA for vitamin B-6. Of these, the effect of protein intake has been the most extensively studied. In the current RDA for adults for vitamin B-6, this effect is expressed as the ratio 0.016

mg B-6/g of protein.[9,76,101] Whether this relationship between vitamin B-6 and protein holds over a wide range of protein intakes is unknown. In both men and women there is an inverse correlation of plasma PLP concentration and urinary excretion of 4-PA with protein intake.[101,123] No specific studies relating to the effect of bioavailability (and PNG intake) on vitamin B-6 requirement have been done.

The effects of sex and age on vitamin B-6 requirement have received only minor attention.[9] Plasma PLP concentration tends to be lower in females than in males, and vitamin B-6 status appears to decrease with age.[103,124] A higher vitamin B-6 requirement has been suggested for the elderly.[125]

The RDA for vitamin B-6 for adult males and females is based in large part on metabolic studies, intake of vitamin B-6, and protein intakes of selected population groups.[9,126] Given the interrelationship between riboflavin and vitamin B-6, one would expect the status of riboflavin to affect the requirement, but this has not been adequately studied.[109] Other factors such as exercise may also be important.[61] A comprehensive review of vitamin B-6 requirements for growth in several species is available.[127]

Summary

Vitamin B-6 occurs in foods in three forms, pyridoxal, pyridoxamine (mainly as the 5'-phosphates), and pyridoxine (and as the 5'-glucoside). The bioavailability of vitamin B-6 is affected by food processing and the amount of pyridoxine glucoside in foods. After intestinal absorption (a nonsaturable process), the three forms are taken up by the liver and converted to pyridoxal 5'-phosphate in a metabolic process which also involves riboflavin-containing coenzymes. Pyridoxal 5'-phosphate serves as a cofactor for >100 enzymes. Excess amounts of vitamin B-6 are metabolized to 4-pyridoxic acid and excreted in the urine along with the other nonphosphorylated forms. Enzymes that require pyridoxal 5'-phosphate influence several processes, including gluconeogenesis, niacin formation, nervous system function, lipid metabolism, nucleic acid metabolism, and hormone modulation. Supplemental vitamin B-6 (as pyridoxine hydrochloride) has been used to treat or prevent a number of clinical conditions, but with the exception of specific genetic disorders its efficacy is limited. Doses of vitamin B-6 >500 mg/day can be toxic when used chronically. The requirement for vitamin B-6 is affected by pregnancy, lactation, possibly age, protein intake, bioavailability, and exercise.

References

1. Snell EE (1986) Pyridoxal phosphate: history and nomenclature. In Dolphin D, Poulson R, Avramovic O (eds), Pyridoxal phosphate: chemical, biochemical and medical aspects, Part A, vol 1A. John Wiley & Sons, New York, pp 1–12

2. Henderson LM (1984) Vitamin B6. In Olson RE, Broquist HP, Chichester CD, et al (eds), Present knowledge in nutrition, 5th ed. The Nutrition Foundation, Washington, DC, pp 303–317

3. Leklem JE, Reynolds RD, eds (1980) Methods in vitamin B-6 nutrition, analysis and assessment. Plenum Press, New York

4. Reynolds RD, Leklem JE, eds (1985) Vitamin B-6: its role in health and disease. Current Topics in Nutrition and Disease, vol 13. Liss, New York

5. Dolphin D, Poulson R, Avramovic O, eds (1986) Pyridoxal phosphate: chemical, biochemical and medical aspects, parts A and B, vol 1A and 1B. John Wiley & Sons, New York

6. Korpela TK, Christen P, eds (1987) Biochemistry of vitamin B6. Proceedings of the 7th International Congress on Chemical and Biological Aspects of Vitamin B6 Catalysis. Birkhauser Congress Reports, Life Sciences, vol 2. Birkhauser Verlag, Basel

7. Reynolds RD, Leklem JE, eds (1987) Clinical and physiological applications of vitamin B6. Current Topics in Nutrition and Disease, vol 19. Liss, New York

8. McCormick DB (1988) Vitamin B6. In Shils ME, Young VN (eds), Modern nutrition in health and disease. Lea and Febiger, Philadelphia, pp 376–382

9. Leklem JE (1991) Vitamin B-6. In Machlin LJ (ed), Handbook of vitamins, 2nd ed. Dekker, New York, pp. 341–392

10. Yasumoto K, Tsukji H, Iwami K, Metsuda H (1977) Isolation from rice bran of a bound form of vitamin B-6 and its identification as 5'-0-(β-D-glucopyranosyl) pyridoxine. Agric Biol Chem 41:1061–1067

11. Kabir H, Leklem JE, Miller LT (1983) Measurement of glycosylated vitamin B-6 in foods. J Food Sci 48:1422–1425

12. Leussing DL (1986) Model reactions. In Dolphin D, Poulson R, Avramovic O (eds), Coenzymes and cofactors, vol 1, Vitamins B-6 pyridoxal phosphate. John Wiley & Sons, New York, pp 69–115

13. Bridges JW, Davies DS, Williams RT (1966) Fluorescence studies on some hydroxypyridines including compounds of the vitamin B-6 group. Biochem J 98:451–468

14. Gregory JF, III (1988) Methods for determination of vitamin B-6 in foods and other biological materials: a critical review. J Food Comp 1:105–123

15. Polansky MM, Reynolds RD, Vanderslice JT (1985) Vitamin B6. In Augustine J, Klein BP, Becker DA, Venigopal PB (eds), Methods of vitamin assay, 4th ed. John Wiley & Sons, New York, pp 417–443

16. Polansky M (1981) Microbiological assay of vitamin B-6 in foods. In Leklem JE, Reynolds RD (eds), Methods in vitamin B-6 nutrition. Plenum Press, New York, pp 21–44

17. Chabner B, Livington DA (1970) A simple enzymic assay for pyridoxal phosphate. Anal Biochem 34:413–423

18. Mahuren JD, Coburn SP (1990) B-6 vitamers: cation exchange HPLC. J Nutr Biochem 1:659–663

19. Leklem JE, Reynolds RD (1988) Challenges and direction in the search for clinical applications of vitamin B-6. In Leklem JE, Reynolds RD (eds), Clinical and physiological applications of vitamin B-6. Liss, New York, pp 437–454

20. Leklem JE, Reynolds RD (1981) Recommendations for status assessment of vitamin B-6. In Leklem JE, Reynolds RD (eds), Methods in vitamin B-6 nutrition. Plenum Press, New York, pp 389–392

21. Richardson LR, Wilkes S, Ritchey SJ (1961) Comparative vitamin B-6 activity of frozen, irradiated, and heat-processed foods. J Nutr 73:363–368

22. Ang CYW (1981) Comparison of sample storage methods of vitamin B-6 assay in broiler meats. J Food Sci 47:336–337

23. Woodring MJ, Storvick CA (1960) Vitamin B-6 in milk: review of literature. J Assoc Off Agric Chem 43:63–80

24. Gregory JF, Kirk JR (1978) Assessment of roasting effects on vitamin B-6 stability and bioavailability in dehyrated food systems. J Food Sci 43:1585–1589

25. Gregory JF, Kirk JR (1977) Interaction of pyridoxal and pyridoxal phosphate with peptides in a model food system during thermal processing. J Food Sci 42:1554–1561

26. Gregory JF (1980) Effects of ε-pyridoxyllysine bound to dietary protein on the vitamin B-6 status of rats. J Nutr 110:995–1005

27. Henderson LM (1985) Intestinal absorption of B-6 vitamers. In Reynolds RD, Leklem JE (eds), Vitamin B-6: its role in health and disease. Liss, New York, pp 22–33

28. Mehansho H, Hamm MW, Henderson LM (1979) Transport and metabolism of pyridoxal and pyridoxal phosphate in the small intestine of the rat. J Nutr 109:1542–1551

29. Gregory JF, Ink SL (1985) The bioavailability of vitamin B-6. In Reynolds RD, Leklem JE (eds), Vitamin B-6: its role in health and disease. Liss, New York, pp 3–23

30. Leklem JE (1986) Bioavailability of vitamins: application of human nutrition. In Dobernz AR, Milner JA, Schweigert BS (eds), Food and agricultural research opportunities to improve human nutrition. University of Delaware, Newark, pp A56–A73

31. Leklem JE, Miller LT, Perera AD, Peffers DE (1980) Bioavailability of vitamin B-6 from wheat bread in humans. J Nutr 110:1819–1928

32. Lindberg AS, Leklem JE, Miller LT (1983) The effect of wheat bran on the bioavailability of vitamin B-6 in young men. J Nutr 113:2578–2586

33. Kies C, Kan S, Fox HM (1984) Vitamin B-6 availability from wheat, rice, corn brans for humans. Nutr Rep Int 30:483–491

34. Kabir H, Leklem JE, Miller LT (1983) Comparative vitamin B-6 bioavailability from tuna, whole wheat bread, and peanut butter in humans. J Nutr 113:2412–2420

35. Kabir H, Leklem JE, Miller LT (1983) Relationship of the glycosylated vitamin B-6 content of foods of vitamin B-6 bioavailability in humans. Nutr Rep Int 28:709–716

36. Bills ND, Leklem JE, Miller LT (1987) Vitamin B-6 bioavailability in plant foods is inversely correlated with % glycosylated vitamin B-6 (abstract). Fed Proc 46:1487

37. Gregory JF, Trumbo PR, Bailey LB, et al (1991) Bioavailability of pyridoxine-5-β-D-glucoside determined in humans by stable isotopic methods. J Nutr 121:177–186

38. Coburn SP, Mahuren JD (1983) A versatile cation-exchange procedure for measuring the seven major forms of vitamin B-6 in biological samples. Anal Biochem 129:310–317

39. Hollins B, Henderson JM (1986) Analysis of B-6 vitamers in plasma by reversed-phase column liquid chromatography. J Chromatogr 380:67–75

40. Ink SL, Henderson LM (1984) Vitamin B-6 metabolism. Annu Rev Nutr 4:445–470

41. Lumeng L, Ki T-K, Lui A (1985) The interorgan transport and metabolism of vitamin B-6. In Reynolds RD, Leklem JE (eds), Vitamin B-6: its role in health and disease. Liss, New York, pp 35–54

42. Merrill AH, Henderson JM, Wang E, et al (1984) Metabolism of vitamin B-6 by human liver. J Nutr 114:1664–1674

43. Wada H, Snell EE (1961) The enzymatic oxidation of pyridoxine and pyridoxamine phosphates. J Biol Chem 236:2089–2095

44. Lumeng L, Li T-K (1980) Mammalian vitamin B-6 metabolism: regulatory role of protein-binding and the hydrolysis of pyridoxal 5'-phosphate in storage and transport. InTryfiates GP (ed), Vitamin B-6 metabolism and role in growth. Food and Nutrition Press, Westport, CT, pp 27–51

45. Pogell BM (1958) Enzymatic oxidation of pyridoxamine phosphate to pyridoxal phosphate in rabbit liver. J Biol Chem 232:761–766

46. Wozenski JR, Leklem JE, Miller LT (1980) The metabolism of small doses of vitamin B-6 in men. J Nutr 110:275–285

47. Coburn SP, Whyte MP (1988) Role of phosphatases in the regulation of vitamin B-6 metabolism in hypophosphatasia and other disorders. In Leklem JE, Reynolds RD (eds), Clinical and physiological applications of vitamin B-6. Liss, New York, pp 65–93

48. Whyte MP, Mahuren JD, Fedde KN, et al (1988) Perinatal hypophosphatasia: tissue levels of vitamin B-6 are unremarkable despite markedly increased circulating concentrations of pyridoxal 5'-phosphate (evidence for an ectoenzyme role for tissue nonspecific alkaline phosphatase). J Clin Invest 81:1234–1239

49. Coburn SP, Lewis DL, Fink WJ, et al (1988) Estimation of human vitamin B-6 pools through muscle biopsies. Am J Clin Nutr 48:291–294

50. Coburn SP (1990) Location and turnover of vitamin B-6 pools and vitamin B-6 requirements of humans. Ann NY Acad Sci 585:76–85

51. Krebs EG, Fischer EH (1964) Phosphorylase and related enzymes of glycogen metabolism. In Harris RS, Wol IG, Lovaine JA (eds), Vitamin and hormones, vol 22. Academic Press, New York, pp 399–410

52. Merrill AH Jr, Henderson JM (1987) Diseases associated with defects in vitamin B-6 metabolism or utilization. Annu Rev Nutr 7:137–156

53. Leklem JE (1988) Vitamin B-6 metabolism and function in humans. In Leklem JE, Reynolds RE (eds), Clinical and physiological applications of vitamin B-6. Liss, New York, pp 1–26

54. Shultz TD, Leklem JE (1981) Urinary 4-pyridoxic acid, urinary vitamin B-6 and plasma pyridoxal phosphate as measures of vitamin B-6 status and dietary intake of adults. In Leklem JE, Reynolds RD (eds), Methods in vitamin B-6 nutrition. Plenum Press, New York, pp 297–320

55. Sauberlich HE (1968) Section IX Biochemical systems and biochemical detection of deficiency. In Sebrell WH, Harris RS (eds), The vitamins: chemistry, physiology, pathology, assay, 2nd ed, vol 2. Academic Press, New York, pp 44–80

56. Rose DP, Leklem JE, Brown RR, Linkswiler HM (1975) Effect of oral contraceptives and vitamin B-6 deficiency on carbohydrate metabolism. Am J Clin Nutr 28:872–878

57. Black AL, Guirard BM, Snell EE (1978) The behavior of muscle phosphorylase as a reservoir for vitamin B-6 in the rat. J Nutr 108:670–677

58. Angel JF, Mellor RM (1974) Glycogenesis and gluconeogenesis in meal-fed pyridoxine-deprived rats. Nutr Rep Int 9:97–107

59. Leklem LE (1985) Physical activity and vitamin B-6 metabolism in men and women: interrelationship with fuel needs. In Reynolds RD, Leklem JE (eds), Vitamin B-6: its role in health and disease. Liss, New York, pp 221–241

60. Leklem JE, Shultz TD (1983) Increased plasma pyridoxal 5'-phosphate and vitamin B-6 in male adolescents after a 4500-meter run. Am J Clin Nutr 38:541–548

61. Manore M, Leklem JE, Walter MC (1987) Vitamin B-6 metabolism as affected by exercise in trained and untrained women fed diets differing in carbohydrate and vitamin B-6 content. Am J Clin Nutr 46:995–1004

62. Leklem JE, Brown RR, Rose DP, et al (1975) Metabolism of tryptophan and niacin in oral contraceptive users receiving controlled intakes of vitamin B-6. Am J Clin Nutr 28:146–156

63. McHenry EW, Gauvin G (1938) The B vitamins and fat metabolism. I. Effects of thiamine, riboflavin and rice polish concentrate upon body fat. J Biol Chem 125:653–660

64. Audet A, Lupien PJ (1974) Triglyceride metabolism in pyridoxine-deficient rats. J Nutr 104:91–100

65. Abe M, Kishino Y (1982) Pathogenesis of fatty liver in rats fed a high protein diet without pyridoxine. J Nutr 112:205–210

66. Witten PW, Holman RT (1952) Polyethenoid fatty acid metabolism. VI. Effect of pyridoxine on essential fatty acid conversions. Arch Biochem Biophys 41:266–273

67. Cunnane SC, Manku MS, Horrobin DF (1984) Accumulation of linoleic and γ-linolenic acids in tissue lipids of pyridoxine-deficient rats. J Nutr 114:1754–1761

68. Loo G, Smith JT (1986) Effect of pyridoxine deficiency on phospholipid methylation in rat liver microsomes. Lipids 21:409–412

69. Cho YO, Leklem JE (1990) In vivo evidence of vitamin B-6 requirement in carnitine synthesis. J Nutr 120:258–265

70. Chi MS (1984) Vitamin B-6 in cholesterol metabolism. Nutr Res 4:359–362

71. Baysal A, Johnson BA, Linkswiler H (1966) Vitamin B-6 depletion in man: blood vitamin B-6, plasma pyridoxalphosphate, serum cholesterol, serum transaminases and urinary vitamin B-6 and 4-pyridoxic acid. J Nutr 89:19–23

72. Dakshinamurti K (1982) Neurobiology of pyridoxine. In DraperHH (ed), Advances in nutritional research, vol 4. Plenum Press, New York, pp 143–179

73. Bender DA (1984) B vitamins in the nervous system. Neurochem Int 6:297–321

74. Coursin DB (1969) Vitamin B-6 and brain function in animals and man. Ann NY Acad Sci 166:7–15

75. Coursin DB (1954) Convulsive seizures in infants with pyridoxine-deficient diet. JAMA 154:406–408

76. Canham JE, Baker EM, Harding RS, et al (1969) Dietary protein: its relationship to vitamin B-6 requirements and function. Ann NY Acad Sci 166:16–29

77. Grabow JD, Linswiler H (1969) Electroencephalographic and nerve-conduction studies in experimental vitamin B-6 deficiency in adults. Am J Clin Nutr 22:1429–1434

78. Kretsch MJ, Sauberlich HE, Newburn E (1991) Electroencephalographic changes and periodontal status during short-term vitamin B-6 depletion of young, nonpregnant women. Am J Clin Nutr 53:1266–1274

79. Kirksey A, Morre DM, Wasyncquk AZ (1990) Neuronal development in vitamin B-6 deficiency. Ann NY Acad Sci 585: 202–218

80. Wasynczuk A, Kirksey A, Morre DM (1983) Effects of vitamin B-6 deficiency on specific regions of developing rat brain: the extrapyramidal motor system. J Nutr 113:746–754

81. Morre DM, Kirksey A, Das GD (1978) Effects of vitamin B-6 deficiency on the developing central nervous sytem of the rat: gross measurements and cytoarchitectural alterations. J Nutr 108:1250–1259

82. Chang S-J, Kirksey A, Moore DM (1981) Effects of vitamin B-6 deficiency on morphological changes in dendritic trees of purkinje cells in developing cerebellum of rats. J Nutr 111:848–857

83. Chandra RK, Puri S (1985) Vitamin B-6 modulation of immune responses and infection. In Reynolds RD, Leklem JE (eds), Vitamin B-6: its role in health and disease. Liss, New York, pp 163–175

84. Robson LC, Schwarz LC (1975) Vitamin B-6 deficiency and lymphoid system. I. Effect of cellular immunity and in vitro incorporation of ^{3}H-uridine by small lymphocytes. Cell Immunol 16:135–144

85. Cheslock K, McCully MT (1960) Response of human beings to a low-vitamin B-6 diet. J Nutr 70:507–513

86. Rall LC, Meydani SN (1993) Vitamin B-6 and immune competence. Nutr Rev 51:217–225

87. Meydani SN, Ribaya-Mercado JD, Russell RM, et al (1991) Vitamin B-6 deficiency impairs interleukin 2 production and lymphocyte proliferation in elderly adults. Am J Clin Nutr 53:1275–1280

88. Sergeev AV, Bykovskaja SN, Luchanskaja M, Rauschenbach MO (1978) Pyridoxine deficiency and cytotoxicity of T lymphocytes in vitro. Cell Immunol 38:187–192

89. Gridley DS, Stickney DR, Nutter RL, et al (1987) Suppression of tumor growth and enhancement of immune status with high levels of dietary vitamin B-6 in BALB/c mice. J Natl Cancer Inst 78:951–959

90. Ha C, Miller LT, Kerkvliet NI (1984) The effect of vitamin B-6 deficiency on host susceptibility to Maloney sarcoma virus-induced tumor growth in mice. J Nutr 114:938–945

91. Talbott MC, Miller LT, Kerkvliet NI (1987) Pyridoxine supplementation: effect on lymphocyte responses in elderly persons. Am J Clin Nutr 46:659–664

92. Baum MK, Mantero-Atienza E, Shor-Posner G, et al (1991) Association of vitamin B-6 status with parameters of immune function in early HIV-1 infection. J Acquir Immun Defic Syndr 4:1122–1132

93. Salhany JM, Schopfer LM (1993) Pyridoxal 5'-phosphate binds specifically to soluble CD4 protein, the HIV-1 receptor. J Biol Chem 268:7643–7645

94. Schirch LVG, Mason M (1963) Serine transhydroxymethylase. J Biol Chem 238:1032–1037

95. Chen SC, Daron HH, Aull JL (1989) Inhibition of thymidylate synthase by pyridoxal phosphate. Int J Biochem 21:1217–1221

96. Compton MM, Cidlowski JA (1986) Vitamin B-6 and glucocorticoid action. Endocr Rev 7:140–148

97. Allgood V, Cidlowski JA (1991) Novel role for vitamin B-6 in steroid hormone action: a link between nutrition and the endocrine system. J Nutr Biochem 2:523–534

98. Oka T, Komori N, Kkuwahata M, et al (1995) Pyridoxal 5'-phosphate modulates expression of cytosolic aspartate aminotransferase gene by inactivation of glucocorticord receptor. J Nutr Sci Vitaminol 41:363–375

99. Leklem J (1990) Vitamin B-6: a status report. J Nutr 120: 1503–1507

100. Reynolds RD (1995) Biochemical methods for status assessment. In Raiten DJ (ed), Vitamin B-6 metabolism in pregnancy, lactation and infancy. CRC Press, Boca Raton, FL, pp 41–59

101. Miller LT, Leklem JE, Shultz TD (1985) The effect of dietary protein on the metabolism of vitamin B-6 in humans. J Nutr 115:1663–1672

102. Lumeng L, Ryan MP, Li T-K (1978) Validation of the diagnostic value of plasma pyridoxal 5'-phosphate measurements in vitamin B-6 nutrition of the rat. J Nutr 108:545–553

103. Lee CM, Leklem JE (1985) Differences in vitamin B-6 status indicator responses between young and middle-aged women fed constant diets with two levels of vitamin B-6. Am J Clin Nutr 42:226–234

104. Brown RR (1985) The tryptophan load test as an index of vitamin B-6 nutrition. In Leklem JE, Reynolds RD (eds), Methods in vitamin B-6 nutrition. Plenum Press, New York, pp 321–340

105. Linkswiler HM (1981) Methionine metabolite excretion as affected by a vitamin B-6 deficiency. In Leklem JE, Reynolds

JE (eds), Methods in vitamin B-6 nutrition. Plenum Press, New York, pp 373–381

106. Sauberlich JE, Canham JE, Baker EM, et al (1972) Biochemical assessment of the nutritional status of vitamin B-6 in the human. Am J Clin Nutr 25:629–642

107. Dlaery K, Lussier-Cacan S, Selhub J, et al (1995) Homocysteine and coronary artery disease in French Canadian subjects: relation with vitamin B-12, B-6, pyridoxal phosphate, and folate. Am J Cardiol 75:1107–1111

108. Ubbink JB, Vermaak WJH, van der Merwe A, Becker PJ (1993) Vitamin B-12, vitamin B-6 and folate nutritional status in men with hyperhomocysteinemia. Am J Clin Nutr 57:47–53

109. McCormick DB (1989) Two interconnected B vitamins: riboflavin and pyridoxine. Physiol Rev 69:1170–1198

110. Bhagavan HN (1985) Interaction between vitamin B-6 and drugs. In Reynolds RD, Leklem JE (eds), Vitamin B-6: its role in health and disease. Liss, New York, pp 401–415

111. Bassler KH (1988) Megavitamin therapy with pyridoxine. Int J Vitam Nutr Res 58:105–118

112. Stone WJ, Warnock LG, Wagner C (1975) Vitamin B-6 deficiency in uremia. Am J Clin Nutr 28:950–957

113. Lumeng L, Li T-K (1974) Vitamin B-6 metabolism and chronic alcohol abuse: pyridoxal phosophate levels in plasma and the effects of acetaldehyde on pyridoxal phosphate synthesis and degration in human erythrocytes. J Clin Invest 53:693–704

114. Serfontein WJ, Ubbink JB, DeVilliers LS, et al (1985) Plasma pyridoxal-5′-phosphate level as risk index for coronary artery disease. Atherosclerosis 55:357–361

115. Potera C, Rose DP, Brown RR (1977) Vitamin B-6 deficiency in cancer patients. Am J Clin Nutr 30:1677–1679

116. Devita VT, Chabner BA, Livingston DM, Oliverio VT (1971) Anergy and tryptophan metabolism in Hodgkin's disease. Am J Clin Nutr 24:835:840

117. Hollenbeck CB, Leklem JE, Riddle MC, Connor WE (1983) The composition and nutritional adequacy of subject-selected high carbohydrate, low fat diets in insulin-dependent diabetes mellitus. Am J Clin Nutr 38:41–51

118. Dakshinamurti K (1990) Vitamin B-6. Ann NY Acad Sci, vol 585

119. Schaumburg H, Kaplan J, Windebank A, et al (1983) Sensory neuropathy from pyridoxine abuse: a new megavitamin syndrome. New Engl J Med 309:445–448

120. Bernstein AL, Lobitz CS (1988) A clinical and electro-physiologic study of the treatment of painful diabetic neuropathies with pyridoxine. In Leklem JE, Reynolds RE (eds), Clinical and physiological applications and vitamin B-6. Liss, New York, pp 415–423

121. National Research Council (1989) Recommended Dietary Allowances, 10th ed. National Academy Press, Washington, DC

122. Raiten DJ, ed (1995) Vitamin B-6 metabolism in pregnancy, lactation, and infancy. CRC Press, Boca Raton, FL

123. Leklem J, Hansen C, Miller L (1991) Effect of three levels of protein on vitamin B-6 status of adult women [abstract]. FASEB J 5:A557

124. Rose CS, Gyorgy P, Butler M, et al (1976) Age differences in vitamin B-6 status of 617 men. Am J Clin Nutr 29:847–853

125. Ribaya-Mercado JD, Russell RM, Sahyoun N, et al (1991) Vitamin B-6 requirements of elderly men and women. J Nutr 121:1062–1074

126. Driskell JA (1994) Vitamin B-6 requirements of humans. Nutr Res 14:293–324

127. Coburn SP (1994) A critical review of minimal vitamin B-6 requirements for growth in various species with a proposed method of calculation. Vitam Horm 48:259–300

128. Merrill A, Burnham F (1990) Vitamin B-6. In Brown M (ed), Present knowledge in nutrition, 6th ed. International Life Sciences Foundation, Washington, DC, pp 155–162

Chapter 19

Niacin

Robert A. Jacob and Marian E. Swendseid

The term niacin is the generic descriptor for nicotinic acid (pyridine-3-carboxylic acid) and derivatives exhibiting qualitatively the biological activity of nicotinamide (nicotinic acid amide). Nicotinic acid was isolated as a pure chemical substance in 1867, but not until 1937 was it demonstrated to be the anti-black-tongue factor in dogs and the antipellagra vitamin for humans.[1] Before 1937 it had been suggested that pellagra was due to a deficiency of tryptophan in corn, but the biosynthetic pathway for the formation of a niacin derivative from tryptophan was not established until after both nicotinamide and nicotinic acid were shown separately to be antipellagragenic.

Chemistry and Analytical Methods

The structures of nicotinic acid and nicotinamide are shown in Figure 1. Both compounds are stable, white crystalline solids. Nicotinamide is more soluble in water, alcohol, and ether than is nicotinic acid. The acid or amide form can be determined by a chemical reaction with cyanogen bromide and organic bases, by liquid chromatography, or by microbiological methods using a variety of bacteria requiring niacin for growth.[2,3] The active coenzyme forms of niacin, nicotinamide adenine dinucleotide (NAD) and NAD phosphate (NADP), can be determined by enzyme-cycling colorimetric or high-performance liquid chromatography (HPLC) methods.[4,5] A spectrophotometric method for measuring oxidized and reduced pyridine nucleotides in erythrocytes was recently reported, with the caution that traditional methods for quantitating the nucleotides in erythrocytes may be inaccurate because of factors such as protein binding.[6]

Nicotinamide, nicotinic acid, and their metabolites can be measured in blood plasma and urine by newer HPLC techniques as well as traditional chemical methods.[2,7–12] The urinary metabolites of niacin, including the methylated derivatives N^1-methylnicotinamide (NMN) and N^1-methyl-2-pyridone-5-carboxamide (2-pyridone), can be determined by fluorescence or HPLC techniques. Ketones react with NMN in alkaline solution to form a fluorescent product,[12] whereas chemical methods for determining 2-pyridone are more tedious than for NMN. The

biological activity of niacin-containing foods can be determined by the dog pellagra test (black tongue disease) or growth tests in chicks and rats.

Metabolism and Biochemistry

Absorption and transport. Nicotinic acid and nicotinamide are rapidly absorbed from the stomach and the intestine.[13] At low concentrations absorption occurs as Na^+-dependent facilitated diffusion, but at higher concentrations passive diffusion predominates. Three to 4 g of niacin given orally can be almost completely absorbed. Nicotinamide is the major form in the bloodstream and arises from enzymatic hydrolysis of NAD in the intestinal mucosa and liver.[14] NAD and NADP, the main dietary forms of niacin, are hydrolyzed by enzymes in the intestinal mucosa to yield nicotinamide. The intestinal mucosa is rich in niacin conversion enzymes such as NAD glycohydrolase. Nicotinamide is released from NAD in liver and intestines by glycohydrolases and transported to tissues that synthesize their own NAD as needed. Tissues apparently take up both forms of the vitamin by simple diffusion; however, evidence indicates a facilitated transport of niacin into erythrocytes.[15]

Excretion. Excess niacin is methylated in liver to NMN, which is excreted in the urine along with the 2- and 4-pyridone oxidation products of NMN (Figure 2). The two major excretion products are NMN and 2-pyridone; minor amounts of niacin or niacin oxide and hydroxyl forms are also excreted.[16] The pattern of niacin products excreted after niacin ingestion depends somewhat on the amount and form of niacin ingested and the niacin status of the individual.

Biosynthetic pathways and their regulation. Niacin is biosynthesized from quinolinate in all organisms studied. In mammals, quinolinic acid arising from dietary tryptophan through the kynurenine pathway is converted to nicotinic acid ribonucleotide (Figure 2).[17] This conversion is regulated by the enzyme quinolinate phosphoribosyltransferase. In humans the biosynthesis of niacin from tryptophan is an important route for meeting the body's niacin requirement. The efficiency of conversion

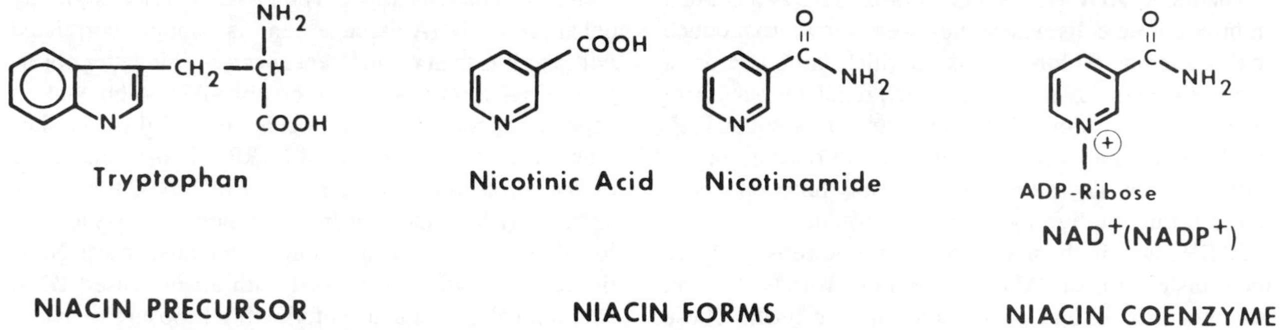

Figure 1. Niacin-related structures.

of dietary tryptophan to niacin is affected by a variety of nutritional and hormonal factors. Deficiencies of vitamin B-6, riboflavin, or iron slow the conversion because these micronutrients are essential cofactors for enzymes involved in the pathway. Conversion efficiency increases with restricted protein, tryptophan, energy, or niacin intakes, because of changes in activities of pathway enzymes including tryptophan oxygenase, quinolinate phosphoribosyltransferase, and picolinate carboxylase.[17] Irrespective of dietary factors, large individual differences in the conversion efficiency of tryptophan to niacin were reported.[18] To estimate nutritional intake or niacin equivalents (NEs) from tryptophan, an average conversion ratio of 60 mg tryptophan to 1 mg niacin was recommended by the Food and Nutrition Board of the National Research Council.[19] This conversion value is based primarily on studies in humans that measured the conversion of tryptophan to niacin metabolites;[20] an exception to the ratio is caused by a threefold increase in conversion efficiency in pregnant women during the third trimester.[21] This increase presumably is due to the stimulation by estrogen of tryptophan oxygenase, the presumably rate-limiting enzyme in the pathway.[22]

An amino acid imbalance, particularly excessive dietary leucine, was reported to antagonize the tryptophan-to-niacin conversion, possibly by altering kynureninase activity.[23] Other studies showed that the addition of 5% leucine to the diet increased the activity of hepatic NADP glycohydrolase and, thereby, decreased NAD concentration. In isolated rat liver cells, 2-oxoisocaproate (the 2-oxo analog of leucine) decreases NAD biosynthesis from both tryptophan and nicotinic acid.[24] Whether excess dietary leucine compromises niacin status, however, remains open to question because some studies in rats and humans showed no effects of excess leucine on niacin metabolism or status.[18,25–27]

The niacin coenzymes NAD and NADP are synthesized in all tissues of the body from nicotinic acid, nicotinamide, or both (Figure 2). Evidence for mitochondrial synthesis of these pyridine nucleotides from nicotinamide was reported.[28] Tissue concentrations of NAD appear to

be regulated by the concentration of extracellular nicotinamide, which in turn is under hepatic control and is hormonally influenced. In liver, excess plasma nicotinamide is converted to storage NAD (i.e., NAD not bound to enzymes) and to metabolites of niacin that are excreted. Tryptophan and nicotinic acid also contribute to storage NAD, and studies suggest that, at least in rats, liver synthesizes NADP predominantly from tryptophan rather than from preformed niacin.[29] The nicotinamide formed in the degradation of NAD can be reconverted to NAD via nicotinamide ribonucleotide. Human tissue cells contain little nicotinamide deamidase, but nicotinamide can be deamidated in the intestinal tract by intestinal microflora.[30] Hydrolysis of hepatic NAD allows release of nicotinamide for transport to tissues that lack the ability to synthesize the NADP coenzymes from tryptophan.

Biochemical functions. Niacin is essential in the form of the coenzymes NAD and NADP in which the nicotinamide moiety acts as electron acceptor or hydrogen donor in many biological redox reactions. Thus, NAD functions as an electron carrier for intracellular respiration as well as a co-dehydrogenase with enzymes involved in the oxidation of fuel molecules, such as glyceraldehyde 3-phosphate, lactate, alcohol, 3-hydroxybutyrate, pyruvate, and α-ketoglutarate dehydrogenases. NADP functions as a hydrogen donor in reductive biosyntheses, such as in fatty acid and steroid syntheses, and like NAD as a codehydrogenase, such as in the oxidation of glucose 6-phosphate to ribose 5-phosphate in the pentose phosphate pathway.

The niacin cofactor NAD is also required for important nonredox reactions. It is the substrate for three classes of enzymes that cleave the β-N-glycosylic bond of NAD to free nicotinamide and catalyze the transfer of ADP-ribose.[31] Two classes catalyze ADP-ribose transfer to proteins: mono-ADP-ribosyltransferases and poly-ADP-ribose polymerase (PARP). A third class of enzymes promotes the formation of cyclic ADP-ribose, which mobilizes calcium from intracellular stores in many types of cells.[32]

The mono-ADP-ribosyltransferases were first studied in prokaryotic cells where they were shown to produce toxins such as diphtheria toxin, which inhibits protein synthesis, and cholera toxin, which regulates adenylate cyclase activity. Mono-ADP-ribosyltransferases and their products have also been identified and purified in eukaryotic cells. These enzymes probably function in signal transduction by modulating G-protein activity.

PARP found in the nuclei of eukaryotic cells catalyzes the transfer of many ADP-ribose units from NAD to an acceptor protein and also to the enzyme itself. These nuclear PARPS seem to function in DNA replication and repair and cell differentiation, but the molecular mecha-

nisms are not yet known. The PARP activity is greatly enhanced by DNA damage[33] and is strongly correlated with the life span of different species. This latter observation suggests that a higher poly-ADP-ribosylation capacity might contribute to genomic stability and thus longer life. Because the K_m of PARP is in the same range as the intracellular concentration of NAD, the niacin status may be important in the response of tissue cells to DNA damage. In niacin-deficient rats, lower NAD tissue levels were correlated with an increased DNA strand break accumulation following exposure to oxidative stress.[34] Cells that are NAD deficient are more sensitive to the toxic effects of carcinogenic alkylating

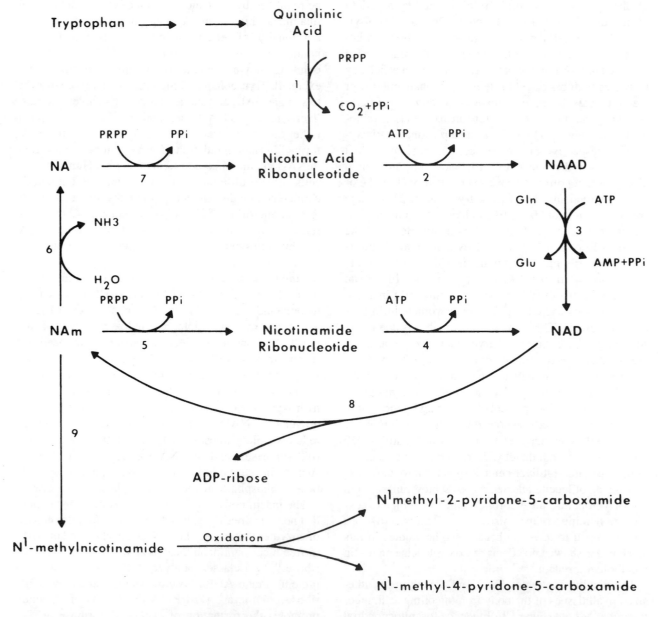

Figure 2. Pathways of niacin metabolism. NA, nicotinic acid; NAm, nicotinamide; NAAD, nicotinic acid adenine dinucleotide; PPPP, phosphoribosyl pyrophosphate. Enzymes: 1, quinolinate phosphoribosyltransferase; 2 & 4, adenyltransferases; 3, NAD synthetase; 5, nicotinamide phosphoribosyltransferase; 6 nicotinamide deamidase; 7, nicotinate phosphoribosyltransferase; 8, poly (ADP-ribose) synthetase or NAD glycohydrolase; 9, N[1]-methyltransferase.

agents. Oxidant or DNA strand-break stressors cause rapid depletion of the cellular NAD pool in lymphocytes and murine macrophages because of excessive poly-ADP-ribose synthesis. The generation of ATP may also be impaired. There are many reports of elevated PARP activity in tumor cells accompanied by low levels of NAD. If a tissue has only a limited capacity to resynthesize NAD from the nicotinamide liberated by the polymerase, an increased PARP activity may result in tissue-specific niacin deficiencies.

Nicotinic acid was found to be part of the glucose tolerance factor, an organochromium complex isolated from yeast that potentiates the insulin response.[35] The role of the niacin moiety in the glucose tolerance factor is unknown.

Biochemical assessment of niacin status. Measurement of the urinary excretion of the two major methylated metabolites, NMN and 2-pyridone, has been used to determine niacin status. The Interdepartmental Committee on Nutrition for National Defense published criteria for interpreting urinary NMN excretion amounts in adults and pregnant women and suggested 24-hour excretions for adults of <5.8 mmol/d as representing deficient niacin status and 5.8–17.5 mmol/d as representing low status.[36] The use of creatinine corrections to allow for use of random fasting urine samples rather than 24-hour collections is fraught with difficulty in interpretation because of differences in creatinine excretion with age.[36] The ratio of 2-pyridone to NMN was suggested as a niacin deficiency marker independent of age and creatinine excretion.[36] Shibata and Matsuo,[37] however, found that the urinary pyridone-NMN ratio in rats and humans was strongly dependent on the level of protein intake and that the ratio was a measure of protein adequacy rather than niacin status. An experimental study of niacin deficiency in adult males found the ratio to be insensitive to a marginal niacin intake of 10 NE/day and not totally reliable for evaluating an intake of 6 NE/day.[26] In contrast, study of a recent outbreak of pellagra in Mozambican women showed that the ratio of 6-pyridone to NMN correlated well with the clinical symptoms, principally dermatitis.[38]

Concentrations of niacin and niacin metabolites in plasma are normally quite low and generally have not been shown to be useful markers of niacin status. Results from an experimental study, however, indicated that 2-pyridone but not NMN in plasma could be a reliable marker of niacin deficiency because 2-pyridone dropped below detection limits after a short period on a low niacin intake.[26] With an oral niacin load (20 mg nicotinamide/70 kg body weight), postdose changes in the 2-pyridone metabolite were more reflective of niacin status than were those of the NMN metabolite. These changes occurred in plasma as well as in urine.[26]

Although Vivian et al.[39] reported a nearly 40% decrease in blood pyridine nucleotides in human subjects fed a niacin-deficient experimental diet, subsequent studies reported mixed results regarding the effects of pellagra or experimental niacin deficiency on concentrations of blood pyridine nucleotides. In the experimental study of niacin deficiency cited above,[26] erythrocyte NAD levels decreased by ≈70% whereas NADP levels remained unchanged when adult male subjects were fed low-niacin diets of either 6 or 10 NE/day.[27] The results suggest that the erythrocyte NAD concentration may serve as a sensitive indicator of niacin depletion and that a ratio of erythrocyte NAD to NADP of <1.0 may identify subjects at risk of developing niacin deficiency.[27] This is consistent with earlier findings of a similar decrease in NAD relative to NADP in fibroblasts grown in niacin-restricted culture.[40]

Requirement for Niacin

The recommended dietary allowance (RDA) expressed as NEs ranges from 13 to 19 NE/d for adults or 1.6 NE/1 MJ (6.6 NE/1000 kcal; 1 NE = 1 mg of niacin).[19] This amount provides for differences in various diets consumed in terms of the bioavailability of niacin and the contribution of tryptophan. Recognizing that variations occur in the amount of tryptophan converted to niacin, the Food and Nutrition Board recommended that an average value of 60 mg tryptophan be considered to be equivalent to 1 mg niacin. The evidence on which these allowances are based were studies in adult men and women conducted during the 1950s, and the allowances were confirmed in later studies. There is no information on niacin requirements of children from infancy through adolescence. In infants, milk from well-nourished mothers appears adequate to meet niacin needs, and on the basis of the niacin content of human milk, the allowance for infants up to age 6 months is 1.9 NE/1 MJ (8 NE/1000 kcal). There is also no direct evidence of niacin requirements during pregnancy and lactation. The RDA provides an increase of 2 NE/day for pregnant women on the basis of an increased energy requirement of 1.26 MJ/day (300 kcal/day). An estimated 1.0–1.3 mg of preformed niacin is secreted daily during lactation. Added to this is an increase of energy expenditure to support lactation, resulting in a recommended additional allowance of 5 NE/day for lactating women.

Food Sources

Niacin is widely distributed in plant and animal foods. Good sources are yeast, meats (including liver), cereals, legumes, and seeds. Milk, green leafy vegetables, and fish as well as coffee and tea also contain appreciable amounts. Niacin is present in uncooked foods mainly as the pyridine nucleotides NAD and NADP, but some hydrolysis of these nucleotides to free forms may occur during food preparation. In plants niacin may be bound to macromolecules and be unavailable to mammals. In wheat there are several forms of bound niacin containing various peptides, hexoses, and pentoses (sometimes referred to as niacinogen or niacytin). In corn the bioavailability of bound niacin is increased by pretreatment with lime water, a procedure used in Central America and Mexico for preparing tortillas. Roasting green coffee beans removes the methyl group from trigonellin (1-methylnicotinic acid), resulting in an increase in nicotinic acid. Some newer varieties of corn contain more tryptophan and niacin than do traditional varieties. Niacin is unique among the vitamins in that an amino acid, tryptophan, is a precursor that can contribute substantially to niacin nutriture by its conversion to a niacin derivative in mammalian liver tissue. Because most proteins contain ≈1% tryptophan, it is theoretically possible to maintain adequate niacin status on a diet devoid of niacin but containing >100 g protein.

Deficiency States

The classic dietary deficiency disease, pellagra, was observed in the mid-18th century in Spain and described more fully a few years later by physicians in northern Italy who used the term pellagra (raw skin) for the first time. The disease is associated with poorer social classes whose chief dietary staple often consists of some type of cereal such as maize (corn) or sorghum. The connection between pellagra and eating maize was shown by Goldberger, who in 1920 conducted epidemiologic studies that indicated that pellagra was a deficiency disease caused by lack of a dietary factor in maize.[1] In 1937 nicotinic acid was established as this factor by its demonstrated effectiveness in curing pellagra.[1] In experimental studies with humans, clinical signs of pellagra develop in 50–60 days after the initiation of a corn diet. The most common signs of a niacin deficiency are changes in the skin; mucosa of the mouth, tongue, stomach, and intestinal tract; and nervous system. The symptoms associated with the skin are most characteristic. A pigmented rash develops symmetrically in areas exposed to sunlight and is similar to a sunburn, although in chronic cases a darker color may develop. Changes in the digestive tract are associated with vomiting, constipation, or diarrhea, and the tongue becomes bright red. Neurological symptoms include depression, apathy, headache, fatigue, and loss of memory. Pellagra was common in the United States and parts of Europe in the early 20th century, but it has now virtually disappeared from industrialized countries except for its occurrence in some alcoholics. It still appears in India and parts of China and Africa, recently reported in Mozambican refugees in Malawi.[41] An analysis of diets described in historical studies of human pellagra indicated that many had NE in excess of the RDA, but a low intake of riboflavin was common. These results suggest that the etiology of the

U.S. pellagra epidemic of the early 1900s has not been completely explained.[42] Deficiencies of other micronutrients required in the tryptophan-to-niacin conversion pathways (e.g., riboflavin, pyridoxine, and iron) may also be involved in the appearance of pellagra.

Pellagra-like syndromes also were described in situations where the absence of dietary niacin deficiency was documented.[43] In each case the pellagra resulted from a reduction in the conversion of tryptophan to niacin. Pellagra sometimes occurs with the carcinoid syndrome where tryptophan is preferentially hydrolyzed to 5-OH-tryptophan and serotonin. Prolonged treatment with the drug Isoniazid also may lead to niacin deficiency by competition of the drug with pyridoxal phosphate, a cofactor required in the tryptophan-to-niacin pathway. Patients with Hartnup's disease, an autosomal recessive disorder, develop pellagra because of a defect in the absorption process for tryptophan and other monocarboxylic amino acids in the intestine and kidney. Nicotinamide treatment (40–250 mg/day) results in marked improvement in skin and neurologic abnormalities.[44]

Niacin deficiency has been produced in dogs, pigs, monkeys, chickens, trout, and rats.[45] Pigs are particularly sensitive and exhibit a scaly dermatitis. There is generally poor growth and lack of appetite as well as inflammation of mouth and tongue mucosa (black tongue disease in dogs). Skin lesions do not always occur, as, for example, in young monkeys. Niacin deficiency states have also been produced in animals by administration of synthetic niacin antagonists, including acetylpyridine, 6-aminonicotinamide, and 2-amino,1,3,4 thiazole. These compounds have teratogenic effects when administered to pregnant animals and some of them have antitumor effects.[46]

Pharmacological Effects and Toxicity

That large doses of nicotinic acid can reduce serum cholesterol concentrations in human subjects was first reported in 1955.[47] Subsequent studies revealed that triacylglycerol concentrations were also decreased and that these effects were not observed when nicotinamide was given. The administration of nicotinic acid in the Coronary Drug Project was associated with a reduction in recurrent myocardial infarctions and in long-term total mortality.[48] Nicotinic acid given as a drug in doses of 1.5–3 g/day decreases total and LDL cholesterol concentrations and increases HDL cholesterol concentrations. There are side effects including flushing of the skin, hyperuricemia, hepatic and ocular abnormalities, and occasional hyperglycemia. These effects are reversed if the drug is reduced in amount or discontinued. The lipid-decreasing effect of nicotinic acid has been extensively investigated, but the mechanism of action is not known. It does not appear related to any vitamin coenzyme function because nicotinamide does not have a similar effect.

Nicotinamide in a dosage of ≈ 25 mg·kg^{-1}·day^{-1} is currently under trial for helping prevent and control diabetes.[49] Nicotinamide has also been shown to act as a tumor-specific radiosensitizer, possibly resulting from its effect on vasorelaxation and increased tumor oxygenation.[50] The pharmacokinetics of nicotinamide in four healthy adults has been reported.[51] Plasma concentrations and clearance rates are dose dependent, with half-life ranging from 1.5 to 9 hours for oral doses of 1–6 g. Peak concentrations ranged from 0.7 to 1.1 mmol/mL after a 6-g dose. The time to peak concentrations was dose independent, with a broad range of 0.7 to 3 hours.

Experiments with rats showed that injections of nicotinamide (1 g/kg) caused phosphaturia that results from an increased NAD concentration in the renal cortex.[52] NAD is an inhibitor or modulator of the Na$^+$-dependent transport of phosphate through the membranes of the proximal kidney tubules. In adult rats large doses of nicotinamide induced activities of drug-metabolizing enzymes, including components of the hepatic microsomal mixed-function oxidase system.[52] Chronic administration of large doses of nicotinamide to rats also produces increased lipid and decreased choline concentrations in liver.[53] The LD$_{50}$ (oral) for the rat is 3.5 g/kg for nicotinamide and 4.5–5.2 g/kg for nicotinic acid. Nicotinamide fed at concentrations of 1–2% of the diet inhibits growth.[54]

References

1. Spies TD, Cooper C, Blankenhorn MA (1938) The use of nicotinic acid in the treatment of pellagra. JAMA 110:622–627

2. Henderson LM (1983) Niacin. Annu Rev Nutr 3:289–307

3. Baker H, Frank O (eds) (1968) Clinical vitaminology, methods, and interpretation. Interscience Publishers, New York

4. Nisselbaum JS, Green S (1969) A simple ultramicromethod for determination of pyridine nucleotides in tissues. Anal Biochem 27:212–217

5. Stocchi V, Cucchiarini L, Canestrari F, et al (1987) A very fast ion-pair reversed-phase HPLC method for the separation of the most significant nucleotides and their degradation products in human red blood cells. Anal Biochem 167:181–190

6. Wagner TC, Scott MD (1994) Single extraction method for the spectrophotometric quantification of oxidized and reduced pyridine nucleotides in erythrocytes. Anal Biochem 222:417–426

7. McKee RW, Kang-Lee YA, Panaqua M, Swendseid ME (1982) Determination of nicotinamide and metabolic products in urine by high performance liquid chromatography. J Chromatogr 230:309–318

8. Shibata K, Kawada T, Iwai K (1987) High performance liquid chromatographic determination of nicotinamide in rat tissue samples and blood after extraction with diethyl ether. J Chromatogr 422:257–262

9. Shibata K, Kawada T, Iwai K (1988) Simultaneous microdetermination of nicotinamide and its major metabolites, N^l-methyl-2-pyridone-5-carboxamide and N^1-methyl-4-pyridone-3-carboxamide, by high performance liquid chromatography. J Chromatogr 424:23–28

10. Stratford MRL, Dennis MF (1992) High-performance liquid chromatographic determination of nicotinamide and its metabolites in human and murine plasma and urine. J Chromatogr 582:145–151

11. Miyauchi Y, Sano N, Nakamura T (1993) Simultaneous determination of nicotinic acid and its 2 metabolites in human plasma using solid-phase extraction in combination with high performance liquid chromatography. Int J Vitam Nutr Res 63:145–149

12. Pelletier O, Brassard R (1977) Automated and manual determination of N^l-methylnicotinamide in urine. Am J Clin Nutr 30:2108–2116

13. Bechgaard H, Jespersen S (1977) GI absorption of niacin in humans. J Pharm Sci 66:871–872

14. Henderson LM, Gross CJ (1979) Metabolism of niacin and niacinamide in perfused rat intestine. J Nutr 109:654–662

15. Lan SJ, Henderson LM (1968) Uptake of nicotinic acid and nicotinamide by rat erythrocytes. J Biol Chem 243:3388–3394

16. Mrocheck JE, Jolley RL, Young DS, Turner WJ (1976) Metabolic response of humans to ingestion of nicotinic acid and nicotinamide. Clin Chem 22:1821–1827

17. Van Eys J (1991) Niacin. In Machlin LH (ed), Handbook of vitamins, 2nd ed. Marcel Dekker, New York, pp 311–340

18. Patterson JI, Brown RR, Linkswiler H, Harper AE (1980) Excretion of tryptophan-niacin metabolites by young men: effects of tryptophan, leucine, and vitamin B$_6$ intakes. Am J Clin Nutr 33:2157–2167

19. National Research Council (1989) Recommended dietary allowances, 10th ed. National Academy Press, Washington, DC

20. Horwitt MK, Harper AE, Henderson LM (1981) Niacin-tryptophan relationships for evaluating niacin equivalents. Am J Clin Nutr 34:423–427

21. Wertz AW, Lojkin ME, Bouchard BS, Derby MB (1958) Tryptophan-niacin relationships in pregnancy. J Nutr 64:339–353

22. Rose DP, Braidman IP (1971) Excretion of tryptophan metabolites as affected by pregnancy, contraceptive steroids, and steroid hormones. Am J Clin Nutr 24:673–683

23. Anonymous (1986) Pellagragenic effect of excess leucine. Nutr Rev 44:26–27

24. Bender DA (1989) Effects of a dietary excess of leucine and of the addition of leucine and 2-oxo-isocaproate on the metabolism of tryptophan and niacin in isolated rat liver cell. Br J Nutr 61:629–640

25. Cook NE, Carpenter KJ (1987) Leucine excess and niacin status in rats. J Nutr 117:519–526

26. Jacob RA, Swendseid ME, McKee RW, et al (1989) Biochemical markers for assessment of niacin status in young men: urinary and blood levels of niacin metabolites. J Nutr 119:591–598

27. Fu CS, Swendseid ME, Jacob RA, McKee RW (1989) Biochemical markers for assessment of niacin status in young men: levels of erythrocyte niacin coenzymes and plasma tryptophan. J Nutr 119:1949–1955

28. Lange RA, Jacobson MK (1977) Synthesis of pyridine nucleotides by the mitochondrial fractions of yeast. Biochem Biophys Res Commun 76:424–428

29. Bender DA, Olufunwa R (1988) Utilization of tryptophan, nicotinamide and nicotinic acid as precursors for nicotinamide nucleotide synthesis in isolated rat liver cells. Br J Nutr 59:279–287

30. Bernofsky C (1980) Physiologic aspects of pyridine nucleotide regulation in mammals. Mol Cell Biochem 33:135–143

31. Lautier D, Lagueux J, Thibodeau J, et al (1993) Molecular and biochemical features of poly(ADP-ribose) metabolism. Mol Cell Biochem 122:171–193

32. Kim H, Jacobson EL, Jacobson MK (1994) NAD glycohydrolases: a possible function in calcium homeostasis. Mol Cell Biochem 138:237–243

33. Stierum RH, Vanherwijnen MHM, Hageman GJ, Kleinjans JCS (1994) Increased poly (ADP-ribose) polymerase activity during repair of (+/−) -anti-benzo[a]pyrene diolepoxide-induced DNA damage in human peripheral blood lymphocytes in vitro. Carcinogenesis 15:745–751

34. Zhang JZ, Henning SM, Swendseid ME (1993) Poly(ADP-ribose) polymerase activity and DNA strand breaks are affected in tissues of niacin-deficient rats. J Nutr 123:1349–1355

35. Mertz W (1975) Effects and metabolism of glucose tolerance factor. Nutr Rev 33:129–135

36. Sauberlich HE, Dowdy RP, Skala JH (1974) Laboratory tests for the assessment of nutritional status. CRC Press, Boca Raton, FL, pp 284–288

37. Shibata K, Matsuo H (1989) Effect of supplementing low protein diets with the limiting amino acids on the excretion of N^l-methylnicotinamide and its pyridones in the rat. J Nutr 119:896–901

38. Dillon JC, Malfait P, Demaux G, Foldihope C (1992) Urinary metabolites of nicotinamide during pellagra. Ann Nutr Metab 36:181–185

39. Vivian VM, Chaloupka MM, Reynolds MS (1958) Some aspects of tryptophan metabolism in human subjects. 1. Nitrogen balances, blood pyridine nucleotides, and urinary excretion of N-methylnicotinamide and N-methyl-2-pyridone-5-carboxamide on a low niacin diet. J Nutr 56:587–598

40. Jacobson EL, Lange RA, Jacobson MK (1979) Pyridine nucleotide synthesis in 3T3 cells. J Cell Physiol 99:417–426

41. Malfait P, Moren A, Dillon JC, et al (1993) An outbreak of pellagra related to changes in dietary niacin among Mozambican refugees in Malawi. Int J Epidemiol 22:504–511

42. Carpenter KJ, Lewin WJ (1985) A reexamination of the composition of diets associated with pellagra. J Nutr 115:543–552

43. McCormick DB (1988) Niacin. In Shils ME, Young VR (eds), Modern nutrition in health and disease, 7th ed. Lea and Febiger, Philadelphia, pp 370–375

44. Halversen K, Halversen S (1963) Hartnup disease. Pediatrics 31:29–38

45. Sauberlich HE (1987) Nutritional aspects of pyridine nucleotides. In Dolphun D, Poulson R, Aramovic O (eds), Pyridine nucleotide coenzymes, vol 2B. John Wiley & Sons, New York, pp 608–609

46. Weiner M, Van Eys J (1983) Nicotinic acid antagonists. In Weiner M (ed), Nicotinic acid: nutrient-cofactor-drug. Marcel Dekker, New York, pp 109–131

47. Altschul Z, Hoffer A, Stephen JD (1955) Influence of nicotinic acid on serum cholesterol in man. Arch Biochem Biophys 54:558–559

48. Canner PL, Berge KG, Wenger NK, et al. (1986) Fifteen-year mortality in Coronary Drug Project patients: long-term benefit with niacin. J Am Coll Cardiol 8:1245–1255

49. Mandruppoulsen T, Reimers JI, Andersen HU (1993) Nicotinamide treatment in the prevention of insulin-dependent diabetes-mellitus. Diabetes Metab Rev 9:295–309

50. Kelleher DK, Vaupel PW (1994) Possible mechanisms involved in tumor radiosensitization following nicotinamide administration. Radiother Oncol 32:47–53

51. Stratford MRL, Rojas A, Hall DW, et al (1992) Pharmacokinetics of nicotinamide and its effect on blood pressure, pulse and body temperature in normal human volunteers. Radiother Oncol 25:37–42

52. Nomura K, Shui M, Sano K, et al (1983) Effect of nicotinamide administration to rats on the liver microsomal drug metabolizing enzymes. Int J Vitam Nutr Res 53:35–43

53. Kang-Lee YA, McKee RW, Wright SM, et al (1982) Metabolic effects of nicotinamide administration to rats. J Nutr 113:215–221

54. Friedrich W (1988) Vitamins. W de Gruyter, New York

Chapter 20

Vitamin B-12

Victor Herbert

A fatal anemia due to "some disorder of the digestive and assimilative organs" was first described by Combe[1] in the 1820s and subsequently in greater detail by Addison in the 1850s.[2] For a century, because this anemia was invariably fatal, it was called pernicious anemia. The Nobel Prize–winning discovery by Minot and Murphy[3] in 1926 proved that the disease could be cured by feeding large quantities of liver. Castle and Townsend[4] showed that the causative mechanism was "an inability to carry out some essential step in the process of gastric digestion." Castle's work was seminal in developing the concept that all deficiencies of vitamin B-12 (or of any vitamin) could arise in one of six fundamental ways: three inadequacies (ingestion, absorption, or utilization) or three increases (requirement, excretion, or destruction).[5] Ironically, Castle did not share the Nobel Prize with Minot and Murphy, who shared it with Whipple, who, with Robscheit-Robbins,[6] showed that beef liver enhanced hemoglobin formation in chronically bled dogs. In 1936, 2 years after the Nobel Prize was awarded for liver therapy of pernicious anemia, it became clear that the dogs responded to liver because of its iron content and not its vitamin content.[7]

The search for the active principle in liver culminated with the isolation of vitamin B-12 in 1948 by a team of Merck scientists in the United States, who beat a Glaxo team in England by 3 weeks.[8,9] Another Nobel Prize (chemistry, 1964) went to Hodgkin for elucidating the chemical structure of vitamin B-12 by x-ray crystallography.

In the past 6 years, there has been increased understanding of vitamin B-12 status and its staging, the role of genetics in determining individual predisposition to deficiency, and increased recognition of selective vitamin deficiency in one cell line rather than another (such as early neural damage resulting from vitamin B-12 deficiency producing cognitive dysfunction before hematological damage produces anemia).[10–15]

Vitamin B-12 is unstable in its coenzymatically active forms.[16] The American and British teams who successfully isolated vitamin B-12 in 1948 were lucky because in the process of isolation they passed their concentrates through a charcoal column. The cyanide in the charcoal replaced the unstable metabolically active adducts attached to the cobalt, resulting in the stable (but vitamin-inactive) molecule cyanocobalamin, which,

because of its stability, has been the primary pharmaceutical form of the vitamin.

Nomenclature

Figure 1 indicates the nomenclature for vitamin B-12.[16–20] The four reduced pyrrole rings linked together become a macrocyclic ring designated corrin because it is the core of the vitamin B-12 molecule. All the compounds containing this ring are designated corrinoids. Corrin resembles the heme of hemoglobin, but has one less α-methene bridge and has cobalt (Co) instead of iron at the center. As the figure indicates, the cobalamins contain the entire structure in the figure, and the permissive (semisystematic or trivial) term "cobalamin" (or "vitamin B-12") is used to describe the vitamin B-12 molecule without the cyanide group. Cobalamin is prefixed by the designation of the anionic R group attached to the cobalt. The permissive names are more widely used than the more cumbersome systematic names. For example, the systematic name for vitamin B-12 is α-(5,6-dimethylbenzimidazolyl)-cobamide cyanide. Cyanocobalamin is the permissive name for vitamin B-12. The term "vitamin B-12" has two meanings. To the chemist, it means only cyanocobalamin. In the nutrition and pharmacology literature, it is a generic term for all the cobamides active in humans. So far, all the cobamides found to play a role in human metabolism have been cobalamins. The two cobalamins currently known to be coenzymatically active in humans are methylcobalamin and 5'-deoxyadenoxyl cobalamin (also known as coenzyme B-12).

About one-third of the "vitamin B-12" in serum is in fact not cobalamins, but other corrinoids, which are metabolically dead for humans but vitamin-active for bacteria. Thus, many microbiological assays find normal vitamin B-12 levels in vitamin B-12–deficient people because the assay is reading as vitamin B-12 what is in fact noncobalamin corrinoids. To avoid this problem, most laboratories use competitive inhibition radioassays that measure only cobalamins and no other corrinoids.[10,21–26]

Sources in Food

All vitamin B-12 found in nature is made by microorganisms. The vitamin is absent in plants except when

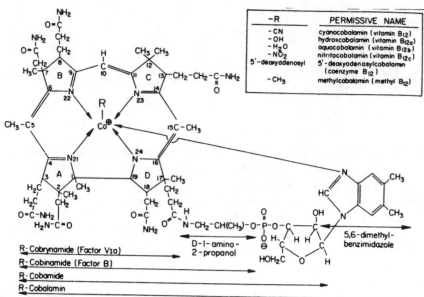

−R	PERMISSIVE NAME
− CN	cyanocobalamin (vitamin B_{12})
− OH	hydroxocobalamin (vitamin B_{12a})
− H_2O	aquocobalamin (vitamin B_{12b})
− NO_2	nitritocobalamin (vitamin B_{12c})
5′-deoxyadenosyl	5′-deoxyadenosylcobalamin (coenzyme B_{12})
− CH_3	methylcobalamin (methyl B_{12})

Figure 1. Structural formula of vitamin B-12. The numbering system for the corrin nucleus is made to correspond to that of the porphin nucleus by omitting the number 20. The corrin nucleus is in the plane of the page. The R group is above it; the rest of the molecule is below it.

they are contaminated by microorganisms.[10,17] Root nodules of certain legumes contain small quantities of vitamin B-12 made by entrapped microorganisms; fermented foods contain minute amounts.[10,17] Fruits, vegetables, grains, and grain products are devoid of vitamin B-12 except when contaminated with fecal matter used as fertilizer. Feces contain a large amount of vitamin B-12 that microorganisms in the colon synthesize. The vitamin is not absorbed from the colon. Some seaweed containing vitamin B-12 from microbial synthesis can help vegetarians ward off vitamin B-12 deficiency,[10,17] but spirulina does not because its "B-12" is not active for humans (except for some true vitamin B-12 from fecal contamination).[17,27]

Strict vegetarians (vegans) develop vitamin B-12 deficiency slowly over a period of many years because of efficient enterohepatic circulation, i.e., they continue to reabsorb the vitamin B-12 we all excrete daily in bile (Figure 2).[11,12,14] Delay in development of vitamin B-12 deficiency in some third-world vegetarian children and adults may also relate in part to cleanliness. The less thoroughly they wash their hands after defecating and the more frequently they suck their fingers, the more they protect themselves against developing vitamin B-12 deficiency. Normal people excrete ≈3.7 nmol vitamin B-12/day in their feces, although a substantial portion of fecal "B-12" may be analogues and not B-12 that is active for humans.[27,28]

The usual dietary sources of vitamin B-12 are meat and meat products (including shellfish, fish, poultry, and eggs) and to a lesser extent milk and milk products. The source of vitamin B-12 in animal products is via the animal's ingestion of animal products and microorganisms containing vitamin B-12, aided by the relatively trivial vitamin B-12–producing activity of microorganisms in the animal's small bowel.[11,12]

Rich sources of vitamin B-12 (>10 μg/100 g wet weight) include organ meats, such as lamb or beef liver, kidney, and heart, and bivalves, such as clams and oysters, which siphon large quantities of vitamin B-12–synthesizing microorganisms from the sea. Moderately large amounts (3–10 μg/100 g wet weight) occur in nonfat dry milk, some seafood (crabs, rockfish, salmon, and sardines), and egg yolk. Moderate amounts (1–3 μg/100 g wet weight) occur in muscle meats, some seafood (lobster, scallops, flounder, haddock, swordfish, and tuna), and fermenting cheeses such as Camembert and Limburger. Fermenting butter and fish sauces of Southeast Asia are also good sources. Fluid milk products, cheddar cheese, and cottage cheese contain <1 μg vitamin B-12/100 g wet weight.

When milk is pasteurized for 2–3 seconds, it loses 7% of its available vitamin B-12; boiling for 2–5 minutes destroys 30%; sterilization in a bottle for 13 minutes at 119–120°C causes a loss of 77%; and rapid sterilization (3–4 seconds) with superheated steam at 143 °C destroys ≈10% of the vitamin.[29] Overprocessed milk as a sole source of vitamin B-12 may be inadequate.[30]

Effects of Megadoses of Vitamin C on Vitamin B-12

Megadoses (500 mg) of vitamin C may adversely affect availability of vitamin B-12 from food, and persons taking even greater megadoses of vitamin C (≥1 g) may develop vitamin B-12 deficiency disease.[31-35] Persons taking megadoses of vitamin C should have their blood checked regularly for evidence of vitamin B-12 deficiency or, preferably, stop taking megadoses of vitamin C, because even taking additional vitamin B-12 might not protect against vitamin B-12 deficiency when megadoses of vitamin C are taken.[32] Herbert et al[21,35] found that 10–30% of vitamin B-12 in multivitamin preparations was converted to analogues worthless to humans, some with anti–B-12 action, by the redox action of vitamin C, iron, and other antioxidant nutrients in those preparations. Vitamin C drives massive free radical generation from iron.[36] Kondo et al[37] found that two of the analogues in a multivitamin preparation blocked vitamin B-12 metabolism in mammalian cells, and suggested that

copper, thiamin, and vitamin C added to animal feeds converted substantial animal feed cobalamin to analogues, some of which had anti–B-12 action and could thus worsen vitamin B-12 deficiency. At pharmacological doses, in the presence of iron, vitamin C is one of the most potent oxidants known, driving iron-catalyzed generation of billions of free radicals, which can not only damage vitamin B-12 but destroy intrinsic factor (IF).[36,38]

Nutritional Requirements

The minimum daily absorbed requirement to sustain normality for vitamin B-12 is only 0.1 μg,[39] so the recommended dietary allowance (RDA) of 2 μg is overgenerous, i.e., it allows a substantial excess for storage.[40,41] Vitamin B-12 requirements have been estimated

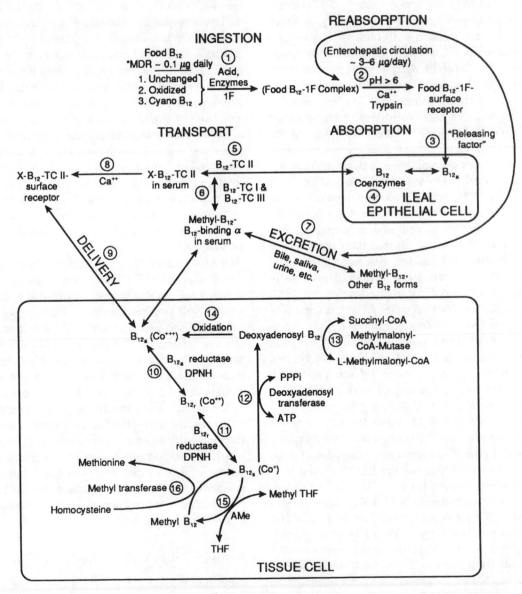

Figure 2. Flow chart of vitamin B-12 metabolism in man. MDR, adult minimum daily requirement from exogenous sources to sustain normality.

from three different types of studies.[10,39,42–44] One type showed that the minimal quantity of daily injected vitamin B-12 that can produce and maintain hematological response in uncomplicated vitamin B-12 deficiency was ≈0.1 µg/d, with 0.5–1 µg producing maximal hematological responses. Another type correlated concentrations of vitamin B-12 in serum and liver in deficient and healthy subjects; moderately deficient individuals had an average liver vitamin B-12 concentration of 0.12 nmol/g wet weight liver that was associated with serum vitamin B-12 concentrations of 59–96 pmol/L and an average total body vitamin B-12 concentration of ≈185 nmol. Individuals with lesser deficiency, with no developed morphological cell damage, had an average liver vitamin B-12 concentration of ≈0.21 nmol/g wet weight that was associated with serum levels between 96 and 148 pmol/L and an average total body vitamin B-12 concentration of ≈390 nmol. The third type of study, in which body stores were correlated with turnover rates of radioactive vitamin B-12, indicated radioactivity turnover of between 0.1% and 0.2% daily regardless of whether body vitamin B-12 stores were normal or reduced.

On the basis of such findings, the joint Food and Agriculture Organization and World Health Organization (FAO/WHO) expert group[42] recommends a daily intake of 1 µg vitamin B-12 for normal adults, allowing a substantial margin above normal physiological requirements. The Food and Nutrition Board of the National Research Council,[40] copying Herbert's[39] recommended dietary intakes (RDIs), suggests 2 µg as the RDA for adults, allowing an even greater margin above normal requirements. Vitamin B-12 is so abundant in the average nonvegetarian diet (3–9 µg/day) that body stores tend to progressively rise throughout life, until genetically predisposed gastric atrophy starts to develop.[12,14,45]

During the latter half of pregnancy, the fetus removes ≈0.2 µg vitamin B-12/day from maternal stores. To compensate, the FAO/WHO group,[42] of which Herbert was a member, recommends the total daily intake of vitamin B-12 be increased in pregnancy to 1.4 µg. The RDA[40] again copied Herbert[39] by adding an extra margin above need to recommend 2.2 µg/day during pregnancy.

About 0.3 µg vitamin B-12 is lost daily in the breast milk of nursing mothers.[42] To compensate for this loss, the FAO/WHO group[42] recommends a total daily intake during lactation of 1.3 µg, and the RDA[40] copied Herbert[39] by recommending 2.6 µg.

Because nutritional vitamin B-12 deficiency in infants is corrected by 0.1 µg vitamin B-12/day, the FAO/WHO group[42] recommends 0.1 µg as the daily intake for infants being fed artificially. Herbert[39] recommended 0.3 µg for infants from birth to 2.9 months, 0.4 µg for infants from 3 to 5.9 months, and 0.5 µg for infants from 6 to 11.9 months. The RDA[40] essentially copies Herbert[39] in recommending 0.3 µg in months 0–5.9 and 0.5 µg in months 6–12. Milk from marginally vitamin B-12–deficient mothers whose serum contains vitamin B-12 concentrations above the lower limit of normal (that is, 148 pmol/L) is usually adequate.

Some argue that the vitamin B-12 RDA for the elderly should be 3 µg to include those with malabsorption due to atrophic gastritis, on the shaky ground that those with this pathology but not yet total gastric atrophy might be able to split adequate vitamin B-12 from 3 µg in their food, even if they no longer can from 2 µg in their food.[39,40,43,46] This argument is obviously specious because the average American's daily vitamin B-12 intake in food is 3–7 µg.[17] An atrophic stomach splits no vitamin B-12 from food. Such an argument betrays ignorance that RDAs are for healthy persons, not those with gastric (or other) pathology. RDAs are defined as follows: "Recommended dietary allowances (RDAs) are the levels of intake of essential nutrients that, on the basis of scientific knowledge, are judged by the Food and Nutrition Board to be adequate to meet the known nutrient needs of practically all healthy persons."[40]

Fenton and Rosenblatt observed some rare infants born with a genetic defect in the enzyme that removes cyanide from cyanocobalamin to render it vitamin-active.[2] In such infants, supplying cyanocobalamin is harmful because it attaches to cobalamin apoenzymes producing a metabolically dead holoenzyme. Humans have no circulating cyanocobalamin unless they are smokers (getting cyanide in tobacco smoke), eat cyanide-containing foods (like bitter cassava or bitter apricot kernels), or take cyanocobalamin parenterally, including via the nasal mucosa.[47]

Genetic factors affect the ability to digest, absorb, and utilize vitamin B-12.[10,14] Genes determine at what age the stomach will stop producing gastric acid and, as we age, when it will stop producing IF. Thus, genes determine when predisposition to vitamin B-12 deficiency will be expressed. Genetics also play a role in elevated levels of homocysteine due to various genetically determined enzyme defects and to the relationship of high homocysteine to vitamin B-12, folate, and vitamin B-6 status.[10,48]

Hematology and endocrinology are connected in part by genetically predisposed autoimmunity, most strikingly seen in multiple endocrine adenopathy syndrome, in which circulating antibodies to hormones and IF are present.[2,49] Just as the presence of circulating antibody to adrenal and thyroid predicts adrenal and thyroid disease, so does the presence of circulating antibody to IF predict pernicious anemia.[2,49]

Assessment of Vitamin B-12 Nutriture

Because progressive gastric atrophy develops in a genetically determined, age-dependent fashion sometime between the age of 50 and 90 years in most people (re-

SEQUENTIAL STAGES OF VITAMIN B₁₂ STATUS
Biochemical and hematological sequence of events as negative vitamin B₁₂ balance progresses.
© 1990, 1995 Victor Herbert (modified 1995 to include homocysteine)

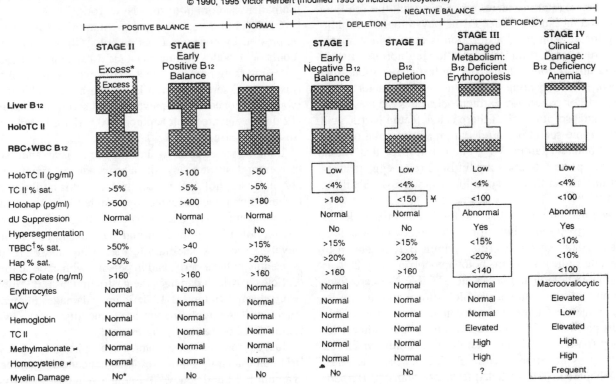

| | POSITIVE BALANCE | | NORMAL | DEPLETION | | DEFICIENCY | |
| | STAGE II | STAGE I Early Positive B₁₂ Balance | Normal | STAGE I Early Negative B₁₂ Balance | STAGE II B₁₂ Depletion | STAGE III Damaged Metabolism: B₁₂ Deficient Erythropoiesis | STAGE IV Clinical Damage: B₁₂ Deficiency Anemia |
	Excess*						
HoloTC II (pg/ml)	>100	>100	>50	Low <4%	Low <4%	Low <4%	Low <4%
TC II % sat.	>5%	>5%	>5%				
Holohap (pg/ml)	>500	>400	>180	>180	<150 ¥	<100	<100
dU Suppression	Normal	Normal	Normal	Normal	Normal	Abnormal	Abnormal
Hypersegmentation	No	No	No	No	No	Yes	Yes
TBBC† % sat.	>50%	>40	>15%	>15%	>15%	<15%	<10%
Hap % sat.	>50%	>40	>20%	>20%	>20%	<20%	<10%
RBC Folate (ng/ml)	>160	>160	>160	>160	>160	<140	<100
Erythrocytes	Normal	Normal	Normal	Normal	Normal	Normal	Macroovalocytic
MCV	Normal	Normal	Normal	Normal	Normal	Normal	Elevated
Hemoglobin	Normal	Normal	Normal	Normal	Normal	Normal	Low
TC II	Normal	Normal	Normal	Normal	Normal	Elevated	Elevated
Methylmalonate ⨯	Normal	Normal	Normal	Normal	Normal	High	High
Homocysteine ⨯	Normal	Normal	Normal	Normal	Normal	High	High
Myelin Damage	No*	No	No	No	No	?	Frequent

* Cyanocobalamin excesses (injected or intranasal) produce transient rise in B₁₂ analogues on B₁₂ delivery protein (TC II); the significance of such rises is unknown (Herbert et al, 1987). Cyanocobalamin acts as an anti-B₁₂ in a rare congenital defect in B₁₂ metabolism.

⨯ In serum and urine.

† TBBC= Total B₁₂ binding capacity.

¥ Low holohaptocorrin correlates with liver cell B₁₂ depletion. There may be hematopoietic cell and glial cell B₁₂ depletion prior to liver cell depletion, and those cells may be in STAGE III or IV negative B₁₂ balance while liver cells are still in STAGE II.

Figure 3. Staging vitamin B-12 status from normal through depletion to deficiency by appropriate laboratory tests. Depletion means low stores (low reserves) but normal biochemical function. Deficiency means not enough nutrient to sustain normal biochemical function (updated to 1995).

ducing the ability to absorb food vitamin B-12), at the age of 50 years and every 5 years thereafter, serum holotranscobalamin II (holoTCII) should be measured.[12,15,50–61] Serum holoTCII is the circulating protein that delivers vitamin B-12 to all DNA-synthesizing cells (Figure 2); if concentrations of this protein are low, daily 25-µg to 1-mg vitamin B-12 tablets (to allow 1% absorption by diffusion) or monthly 250-µg to 1-mg injections of vitamin B-12 should be taken for life.[12]

Negative balance is the descriptor for the situation in which the amount of vitamin B-12 absorbed daily decreases below the amount lost each day (Figure 3). Negative balance rapidly produces depletion, which, if untreated, progresses to deficiency. Low serum holoTCII, the earliest indicator of negative vitamin B-12 balance, is a surrogate Schilling test and a measure of inadequate vitamin B-12 delivery to DNA-synthesizing cells.[60] Reduced absorption of B-12 reduces packaging of B-12

on holoTCII and therefore reduces delivery of B-12 to hematopoietic, brain glial, and other cells that depend solely on surface holoTCII receptors to acquire needed B-12.[12,61,62] Healthy glial cells are important in protecting brain from damage.[61] Because of small B-12 stores, blood and glial cells become deficient while liver cells are still normal.[10,12]

Serum holoTCII is low before total serum vitamin B-12 is low or deficiency occurs (Figure 3), so finding low holoTCII allows giving a monthly vitamin B-12 injection to prevent early negative balance progressing to clinical harm, thereby saving billions of health care dollars.[10,55] The Schilling test measures vitamin B-12 absorption (not stores) through the feeding of radioactive vitamin B-12 to a patient to delineate whether there is malabsorption of vitamin B-12.[34,54,64–67] It is not a measure of vitamin B-12 stores, but a measure of the absorbability of vitamin B-12 at the time the test is done.

If one misperceives the Schilling test as a test for vitamin B-12 deficiency, one often draws wrong conclusions.

When crystalline vitamin B-12 is used, the Schilling test is a measure of whether the physiological machinery for vitamin B-12 absorption is normal in stomach, pancreas, and ileum, thereby allowing normal vitamin B-12 absorption. If the Schilling test shows subnormal absorption, repeating it with the missing factor added (e.g., IF or pancreatic extract) delineates the reason for the malabsorption.[34,54] If there is a defect in gastric acid or enzyme secretion, producing malabsorption of only food-bound vitamin B-12, one can test for that via an animal-protein-bound vitamin B-12 (e.g., egg, meat, or serum), rather than a crystalline vitamin B-12 Schilling test.[34,54,67]

The measurement of serum total vitamin B-12 levels is a relatively late indicator of deficiency because normally ≈80% of total serum vitamin B-12 is bound to the late indicator serum holohaptocorrin; only 20% is on the early indicator serum holoTCII.[12,61] As cell stores slowly fall, the amount of holohaptocorrin (vitamin B-12 on the circulating storage protein haptocorrin) slowly falls pari passu. Holohaptocorrin is in equilibrium with body (particularly liver) vitamin B-12 stores, which fall slowly as negative vitamin B-12 balance progresses; holohaptocorrin has a half-life of 240 hours (V Herbert, unpublished, 1995).[12,60,61] The only receptors for haptocorrin are on vitamin B-12 storage cells (liver cells and reticuloendothelial cells), whereas every DNA-synthesizing cell (including liver and reticuloendothelial cells) has cell surface receptors for TCII, the ubiquitous vitamin B-12–delivery protein.[10,12,60] HoloTCII, made in the ileal enterocytes from intracellularly synthesized TCII and absorbed vitamin B-12, is secreted into the serum with a subsequent half-life of only 6 minutes, and therefore falls below normal within 1 week after vitamin B-12 absorption stops, whereas total serum B-12 (mainly holohaptocorrin) stays "normal" for another 2–4 months.[12,51,58,59,61,66]

By measuring holoTCII, Marcus et al.[68] found that vitamin B-12 depletion was common in the elderly. Subsequently, Pennypacker et al.,[69] looking only for actual deficiency (elevated serum methylmalonic acid and homocysteine), found it in only 14.5% of 152 Veterans Affairs patients aged 65–99 years. On the basis of the earlier work by Marcus et al.,[68] at least another 14.5% of the Pennypacker et al. cases were probably in stage I to stage II negative vitamin B-12 balance (i.e., depletion) (Figure 3), and would have been found if Pennypacker et al.[69] had modernized to assay the same 152 sera for holoTCII.

We found negative vitamin B-12 balance (stages I–IV) in 35% of 150 outpatients of a Bronx Veterans Affairs Medical Center (aged 65–85 years) by screening for low holoTCII. When negative B-12 balance was defined as a serum vitamin B-12 concentration <221 pmol/L (<300 pg/mL), negative balances were found in 37 of 100 outpatient seniors in upstate New York.[70]

Guzik et al.[71] found negative vitamin B-12 balance expressed by concentrations of holoTCII <60 pg/mL) common in both well-nourished (15%) and malnourished (36%) nursing home residents. However, if one looked just at total serum vitamin B-12, the negative balance was often concealed by elevated total serum vitamin B-12 due to elevated holohaptocorrin, perhaps secondary to liver disease.

Looking for circulating antibody to IF is an ancillary screening test for gastric damage–produced vitamin B-12 malabsorption.[49] We recently found this antibody in acquired immune deficiency syndrome (AIDS) patients with vitamin B-12 malabsorption, diagnosed by low serum holoTCII despite normal serum total cobalamin levels.[72] It can be ancillary to measuring holoTCII for screening in the elderly, and in persons with chronic iron deficiency, which damages the gastric mucosa.[12,49] However, chronic vitamin B-12 deficiency damages immune function,[73] so circulating antibody may disappear as vitamin B-12 deficiency progresses.[49]

Just as iron deficiency damages esophageal and gastric mucosa and promotes esophageal cancer,[72] so does vitamin B-12 deficiency.[74,75] Being a vegetarian gave no protection against vitamin B-12 deficiency–related, folic acid deficiency–related, vitamin E deficiency–related, or vitamin A and β-carotene deficiency–related esophageal cancer in vegetarian Chinese.[74–76]

In Padua, Italy, and London (May 20–27, 1993), at an international symposium on Addisonian pernicious anemia, Schilling provided an elegant review of cobalamin absorption tests.[2] The etiology of cobalamin deficiency and staging of vitamin B-12 status were also reviewed.[2] Both Goh et al.[55] and Amin et al.[77] confirmed our staging chart delineation (Figure 3) that low holoTCII precedes high homocysteine or methylmalonic acid as negative vitamin B-12 balance progresses. Also at the symposium, Green, Metz, Allen, and Lindenbaum updated their work on the nerve damage of B-12 deficiency.[2]

Linnell and Bhatt[78] discussed abnormalities in cobalamin metabolism in a subgroup of patients with multiple sclerosis.[2] Our laboratory has been studying two such families, each with two members with multiple sclerosis, with neurologist colleagues at New York Hospital–Cornell Medical Center.[2] In these cases, the evidence so far suggests a common genetic defect producing both disorders, with the vitamin B-12 deficiency leading to expression of an autoimmune multiple sclerosis and vitamin B-12 therapy suppressing further expression.[2]

According to Bottazzo, people of Finnish or Sardinian stock are genetically predisposed to pernicious anemia.[2] Sullivan and Herbert[44] showed that the frequency of pernicious anemia in persons living in Boston's Little Italy was as frequent as that among Boston Irish. When one looks for this disease, one finds it. Pernicious anemia was allegedly rare in China, but our colleague Ran looked for it, and found it was not rare.[79] Black females in their child-bearing years have a genetic predisposition to get pernicious anemia much more frequently than do age-matched white females, as shown by Metz, Hift, and Johnson and Carmel.[2]

As discussed above, there are six ways that one can get vitamin B-12 deficiency. In alcoholism, cobalamin deficiency occurs from a combination of four etiologies: inadequate ingestion and absorption plus increased utilization and excretion.[80] A tabular lexicon of the various disorders that can produce each of the six ways one can get vitamin B-12 deficiency appears elsewhere.[10,81]

Barring instant vitamin B-12 deficiency produced by a vitamin B-12 antagonist or by nitrous oxide anesthesia, the negative balance sequence from normality to deficiency (Figure 3) with respect to vitamin B-12 (or any nutrient) passes through two stages of depletion, followed by two stages of deficiency:[5,10,56,81,82] stage I, low serum vitamin B-12 (serum depletion); stage II, low cell stores of vitamin B-12 (cell depletion); stage III, biochemical deficiency (inadequate biochemical function); and stage IV, clinically manifest deficiency (clinical dysfunction). Stage I negative balance does not necessarily have to go on to Stage II. It may stabilize as Stage I and then go back to normal, as, for example, when diminished vitamin B-12 absorption is transient rather than permanent (Figure 3). Additionally, one may have a deficiency of vitamin B-12 in one cell line before it occurs in another because stores of vitamin B-12 are smaller, utilization is more rapid, or resupply is slower.[15] Such deficiency may be early-mild, or subtle.

Vitamin B-12 may regulate the synthesis of proteins involved in cobalamin absorption, transport, and delivery (IF, haptocorrin, and transcobalamin, and their cell surface receptor proteins),[83] just as Klausner of the National Institutes of Health showed that iron regulates the proteins involved in their synthesis.[84] In *Advances in Thomas Addison's Diseases*, the proceedings of the international symposium held in Padua and London, Jacobsen discusses the up-regulation and down-regulation of these cell surface receptors (Figure 3).[2]

Much of the vitamin B-12 in reticulocytes got there via reticulocyte cell surface cobalamin-TCII receptors that are not on mature red blood cells (RBCs).[83,85] Total RBC vitamin B-12 is largely that in the youngest RBCs. Like serum holoTCII, the measurement of RBC vitamin B-12 may prove to be more useful than that of total serum vitamin B-12 in delineating early vitamin B-12 depletion (Figure 3).[58,86] When subnormal absorption is thought to be due to loss of gastric IF secretion, one can directly assay for IF to prove it.[87]

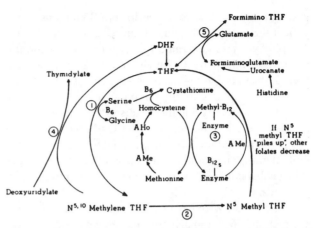

Figure 4. Interrelations in man between vitamin B-12 and folate (and vitamin B-6). Numbers represent enzymes: 1, serine hydroxymethyl-transferase; 2, methylene tetrahydrofolate (THF) reductase; 3, homocysteine transmethylase (methyltransferase); 4, thymidylate synthetase; 5, formininotransferase. AMe, S-adenosylmethionine; DHF, dihydrofolate; B-12, reduced vitamin B-12.

As a general rule, a serum vitamin B-12 concentration <1.11 pmol/L is diagnostic for stage II to III negative vitamin B-12 balance (Figure 3).[5] Vitamin B-12 deficiency in alcoholism is often masked by a holohaptocorrin level that is normal to elevated (but not a normal holoTCII) as the result of excess abnormal haptocorrin released from damaged liver.[80] During pregnancy, when folate deficiency frequently appears,[88] there is a gradual fall in serum vitamin B-12 concentration[17,89] that rises to normal when the patient is treated with folate.

Methylmalonic acid and homocysteine accumulate in serum and are excreted in the urine in increased quantities in stage III negative vitamin B-12 balance (Figures 3 and 4) because vitamin B-12 is required for their normal metabolism (Figures 2 and 4). Most patients with vitamin B-12 deficiency (i.e., those in stage III negative balance) have methylmalonic acidemia but some do not, even after oral loading doses of valine or isoleucine.[62,90–93] Many elderly have harmful hyperhomocysteinemia.[10,12,62,69,78,90–94]

The diagnostic deoxyuridine suppression test (DxdUST) is a useful biochemical assessment of vitamin B-12 (and folic acid) nutriture.[95–102] In this test, bone marrow cells, peripheral blood lymphocytes, or whole-blood samples from an individual are preincubated in test tubes with nonradioactive deoxyuridine and then with a radioactive precursor of DNA.[96–100,103] By the amount of radioactivity incorporated into the DNA of the cells in the absence versus the presence of vitamin B-12 (or folic acid) added to the test tube, not only vitamin B-12 (or folic acid) deficiency but also whether it will be corrected by supplying vitamin B-12 (or folic acid) can be determined. The lymphocyte (and whole-blood) test detects past vitamin B-12 (or folic acid) deficiency even after the start of treatment because resting lymphocytes are impervious to B vitamins and so reflect the nutritional status of the patient at the time the lymphocyte was generated (an average of 1–2 months earlier).[100] If the patient with vitamin B-12 deficiency has a viral illness triggering many newly generated DNA-synthesizing lymphocytes, the lymphocytes will take up injected B-12 therapy and the results of the subsequent diagnostic test will be normal. The DxdUST recognizes lymphocyte vitamin deficiency even when serum and red cell vitamin concentrations are normal,[101] as, for example, when cobalamin metabolism is damaged by nitrous oxide anesthesia.[104,105]

In the book *Advances in Thomas Addison's Diseases*, Carmel and Wickramasinghe discuss how valuable the DxdUST has been to their research; Carmel confirms our staging of vitamin B-12 deficiency (Figure 3), in which results of the DxdUST become abnormal before either methylmalonic acid or homocysteine rise in early vitamin B-12 deficiency.[2,92,106] In discussing negative vitamin B-12 balance, Carmel uses the word "subtle" as a synonym for the words "early" and "mild";[107–109] Carmel[107] also fails to diagnose about half the cases with early negative balance because he has not modernized to measure serum holoTCII.[51,61,108]

Metz reviewed our laboratory effort to create the DxdUST and confirmed the methylfolate trap hypothesis by showing that methylfolate is unable to function as folate in the diagnostic test, i.e., it is trapped in a "metabolically dead" status in vitamin B-12 deficiency.[2,96] The DxdUST is sometimes erroneously referred to as the Killman experiment. Killman had shown that, in vitro, deoxyuridine suppressed incorporation of thymidine into DNA differently in normal and megaloblastic bone marrow cells; however, Killman never determined if this could be corrected in vitro. We converted this biochemical finding into a diagnostic test by adding the missing vitamin or vitamins to bone marrow in additional test tubes, and showed that what was corrected in the additional test tubes (vitamin B-12 or folate or both) was corrected in the patient.[96]

The vitamin B-12 in liver cells is mainly not on haptocorrin but on excess (i.e., well above need) intracellular quantities of vitamin B-12 apoenzymes.[2] The normal liver cell is programmed to make vitamin B-12 apoenzymes in amounts ten times the quantity it needs.[10] Liver-store depletion is measured by low serum holohaptocorrin (B-12 haptocorrin). Liver Kuppfer cell and reticuloendothelial cell surface receptors for holohaptocorrin (and their relative absence on kidney, heart, or spleen cells) were first reported in 1959.[110] Serum holohaptocorrin is in equilibrium with liver B-12 stores.[12,80,83,111] Serum B-12 may be not only normal but actually elevated in liver disease and myeloproliferative disorders because of the release into the serum of abnormal B-12 binders (from the liver in the former and from granulocytes and mononuclear cells in the latter).[5,80,111] These abnormal binders do not deliver B-12 to blood, brain glial, and other DNA-synthesizing cells that have receptors only for B-12 on TCII.[12,62]

Early stage III negative balance is recognized by slowed DNA synthesis, demonstrable biochemically by the DxdUST, and morphologically by an elevated granulocytic leukocyte nuclear lobe average seen on a peripheral blood smear.[5,95–102] These findings precede a rise in serum and urine homocysteine and methylmalonic acid (Figure 3).[10,12,50,51,53,55,62,92]

Selective nutrient deficiency in one cell line but not another is confirmed by therapeutic trials. Within 1–2 weeks after a 1-mg B-12 injection, the degree of granulocyte segmentation in the hematopoietic system falls sharply, and anorexia, malaise, cognitive dysfunction, and paranoia in the neuropsychiatric system all improve. These findings were observed in patients who had normal total serum B-12 concentrations but low serum holoTCII and abnormal peripheral blood DxdUSTs that were corrected in the test tube by B-12.[10,12,50,53]

The enterohepatic circulation of vitamin B-12 is important in cobalamin economy and homeostasis.[12,112,113] Nonvegetarians normally eat ≈3–7 µg vitamin B-12 daily and excrete from their liver into the intestine via their bile 5–10 µg vitamin B-12 each day. If they have no gastric, pancreatic, or small bowel dysfunction interfering with reabsorption, they reabsorb ≈3–5 µg vitamin B-12 from the bile each day. Because of this, an efficient enterohepatic circulation keeps the adult vegan, who eats very little vitamin B-12, from developing vitamin B-12 deficiency disease for 20–30 years.[112] Even as body stores fall and daily vitamin B-12 output in bile falls with body stores to as low as 1 µg, the percentage of vitamin B-12 reabsorbed from bile rises to close to 100% so that the whole 1 µg is reabsorbed.[12]

On the other hand, infants of macrobiotic mothers, who have almost no enterohepatic vitamin B-12 circulation because almost no vitamin B-12 stores were received from their mothers, and therefore have little vitamin B-12 to put in their bile, rapidly develop vitamin B-12 deficiency (see also Ueland[2]).[10,12,17] Unlike the vegetarian whose absorption machinery is normal, a person whose absorption machinery is damaged by a defect in gastric secretion, in pancreatic secretion, or in the gut that results in intestinal malabsorption will develop vitamin B-12 deficiency in 1–3 years because these absorption defects block not only absorption of food vitamin B-12 but also reabsorption of vitamin B-12 excreted into the intestinal tract via the bile.[10,12,54,56,113,114]

Sourial reported vegetarians who had relatively low total serum vitamin B-12, but no biochemical or clinical problems because their holoTCII was adequate.[2] In our laboratory, we found such people have borderline low holoTCII (in the range between 40 and 60 pg/mL) rather than levels below 40.[2,12] These are people who became vegetarians as teenagers or young adults, so they already had significant liver stores of vitamin B-12 that could protect them against vitamin B-12 deficiency for years because of their enterohepatic circulation of vitamin B-12.

Although circulating antibody to human IF is diagnostic for incipient, latent, or full-blown autoimmune pernicious anemia, it does not always mean that pernicious anemia is present.[49] To predict future vitamin B-12 deficiency of any dietary or malabsorptive cause, autoimmune or not, measuring serum holoTCII is almost infallible.[51,58,59–62,72,81]

Our previous studies showed that when radioactive vitamin B-12 is fed to reticulocytes deficient in vitamin B-12, they take up less vitamin B-12 than do vitamin B-12–normal reticulocytes, suggesting that TCII receptors are down-regulated by higher levels of apoTCII.[83,85] Such higher levels of apoTCII occur when there is not enough vitamin B-12 to create holoTCII.

Clinical disease resulting from vitamin B-12 deficiency usually manifests most prominently in blood or neurologic damage, as Lindenbaum and Allen discuss.[2] There may be only mild (subtle) blood damage, manifested by granulocyte hypersegmentation, which, as we first showed, is always accompanied by an abnormal DxdUST.[5,107–109] We suspect the neurologic damage may prove to be associated with increased homocysteine or cobalamin analogues in the brain, although HCY may not yet be clearly elevated in the spinal fluid or circulating blood.[2,12,115,116]

In the northern tier of the United States, major myelin synthesis damage due to vitamin B-12 deficiency with only minor (i.e., abnormal DxdUST and granulocyte hypersegmentation) hematopoietic damage reflects better folate nutriture.[92,116] Persons with a higher economic status can purchase fresh, uncooked high-folate fruits and fruit juices in the colder months (September to April).

Metabolism

A flow chart of vitamin B-12 metabolism in humans is presented in Figure 2 and the interrelations of vitamin B-12 and folate in Figure 4.[5,10,117,118] As indicated in Figure 2, a vitamin B-12–containing enzyme removes the methyl group from methylfolate, thereby regenerating THF from which is made the 5,10-methylene THF required for thymidylate synthesis. Because methylfolate is the predominant form of the vitamin in human serum and liver and because methylfolate only returns to the body's folate pool via the vitamin B-12–dependent step, vitamin B-12 deficiency results in folate being trapped as methylfolate and thus becoming metabolically useless.[118] The folate-trap hypothesis explains the fact that hematological damage of vitamin B-12 deficiency is indistinguishable from that of folate deficiency. In both instances the defective synthesis of DNA results from the same defect in the final common pathway, namely, an inadequate quantity of 5,10-methylene THF to participate adequately in DNA synthesis.[117–121]

Two important facets of the folate-trap hypothesis are that vitamin B-12 is required for folate uptake by cells and that the role of vitamin B-12 in folate polyglutamate synthesis is not in getting from monoglutamate (THF) to polyglutamate but rather in getting from methyl THF to THF, which is the preferred precursor for folate polyglutamates.[117–120] The blockade in getting from methyl THF to THF causes methyl THF to leak from vitamin B-12–deficient red cells. The folate trap may also control folate metabolism by regulating the supply of formate.[10,102,121,122] Metz et al.[96] first reported that formylfolate best corrected the abnormal result of a diagnostic deoxyuridine suppression test in vitamin B-12 deficiency. Some investigators asserted they were unable to demonstrate methylfolate trapping, but in the same study showed such trapping by both a rise in liver methyl THF polyglutamate in the "first 24 hours after nitrous oxide exposure due to cessation of methyl transfer to homocysteine" and a "rise in plasma methylfolate which persists for the duration of the nitrous oxide exposure."[17]

As indicated in Figure 2, for normal vitamin B-12 absorption from food, one needs a normal stomach: gastric acid and enzymes free vitamin B-12 from its peptide bonds in food by proteolysis; the vitamin B-12 then attaches to swallowed salivary protein, and gastric parietal cells secrete IF, the glycoprotein essential for vitamin B-12 absorption from the ileum.[123] Normal absorption also requires a normal pancreas—trypsin and bicarbonate (which raise the pH to above 8) digest the salivary protein, freeing the vitamin B-12 to bind to IF—and a normal ileum, whose cell surface receptors take up the vitamin B-12 complex with IF in the presence of free ionic calcium.[64,113] Patients with pancreatic disease, which reduces available free calcium, cannot absorb vitamin B-12. Their vitamin B-12 absorption is improved by giving them calcium, bicarbonate, or pancreatic extract, each of which increases available free calcium.[64,113] The importance of free calcium for vitamin B-12 absorption was sharply etched in our studies showing that the oral antidiabetic agent, metformin, produced vitamin B-12 malabsorption by tying up free calcium; this was correctable by milk or calcium carbonate tablets.[2,12,65]

Determination of which of these three organs is involved in a specific case of subnormal absorption of vitamin B-12 is made by feeding a small radioactive (for Schilling testing) or nonradioactive dose (for surrogate Schilling testing by measuring holoTCII) of vitamin B-12 with an appropriate addition (gastric acid, enzymes, trypsin, IF, or bicarbonate).[2,12,34,54,65] Bile also may play a role in the normal absorption of vitamin B-12.[80,112] Enterohepatic circulation of vitamin B-12 is of great importance.[10,12,28,112,113]

Methylcobalamin is the form of the vitamin involved in adding a methyl unit to homocysteine to convert it to methionine.[2,118] Coenzyme B-12 (deoxyadenosyl B-12) is involved in the methylmalonic acid-succinate isomerization.[2,12,17,117] The forms of vitamin B-12 involved in other metabolic functions are currently unclear.[2,12]

Nervous System Deprivation of Vitamin B-12

Vitamin B-12 deficiency results in neuropathy.[2,12,78,124–128] Deficiency produces patchy, diffuse, and progressive demyelination; an insidious neuropathy often begins in the peripheral nerves and progresses centrally to the posterior and lateral columns of spinal cord (producing subacute combined degeneration, also called combined system disease and posterolateral sclerosis or funicular degeneration) and to brain (megaloblastic madness).[2,10,50,91,92,127] Frenkel[128] described defects in the fatty acids of myelin in patients with vitamin B-12 deficiency. The role these defects play in demyelination is unclear. Scott et al.[129] reported that nitrous oxide–induced, subacute, combined degeneration in monkeys could be prevented by dietary supplementation with methionine. Their data strongly suggest that the neurological damage of vitamin B-12 deficiency may be due to methyl group deficiency owing to an inability to synthesize methionine and S-adenosyl methionine, or to homocysteine pileup being toxic to the brain. As they noted, cycloleucine, which inhibits activation of methionine to S-adenosyl methionine, causes neurological damage in rodents that is identical to subacute combined degeneration.[129]

Vitamin B-12 (or folate) deficiency, but not depletion, produces elevated serum homocysteine levels. Brattstrom and Ueland indicated independently that accumulated HCY, in deficiency of either vitamin B-12 or folate (or other causes), is both neurotoxic and vasculotoxic, promoting heart attacks, thrombotic strokes, and peripheral vascular occlusions.[2] This phenomenon may be much more widespread than previously appreciated.[130–134] High serum HCY may be reduced toward normal by RDA amounts of folic acid, vitamin B-12, or vitamin B-6, if the high HCY level is related to a deficiency of one of those three vitamins.[2,10,12] If the elevated level is not due to such a deficiency, it still may often be reduced toward normal by pharmacological (well above RDA) doses of folic acid.[2,10,12]

Vitamin B-12 Therapy and Megatherapy

The only established therapeutic use of vitamin B-12 is in treating deficiency of the vitamin.[10,81] When the deficiency is due to inadequate ingestion, as may occur in strict vegetarians, an oral dose of 1 μg/d of the vitamin supplied as food fortification (for example, in cereals and soy products) is adequate treatment.[12]

When the vitamin B-12 deficiency is due to inadequate absorption, 1 μg/d of the vitamin given by injection is adequate therapy.[39,44] A single injection of ≥100 μg will produce complete remission in a patient whose vitamin B-12 deficiency is not complicated by unrelated systemic disease or other factors. The remission is sustained for life by monthly injections of a minimum of 100 μg vitamin B-12.[10]

The only legitimate need for megatherapy with vitamin B-12 is in the very rare patient with a congenital defect in vitamin B-12 metabolism, such as vitamin B-12–responsive methylmalonic acidemia.[135] In fact, prenatal therapy of methylmalonic acidemia is possible with large amounts of vitamin B-12 administered to the mother, although whether such prenatal therapy accomplishes anything is debatable.[136,137] Large injections of hydrocobalamin, by instantly soaking up cyanide, are an effective antidote to acute cyanide poisoning.[138]

Aside from the above indications, the use of vitamin B-12 in various neurological disorders (with the exception of hydrocobalamin for cyanide-induced tobacco amblyopia[139] and to prevent an attack of wine-sulfite–induced asthma) has no known value. The red color of the vitamin along with its almost total lack of known toxicity makes it an almost ideal placebo, and it is so used by many physicians.[10] Unfortunately, it is also used by hustlers who profit from selling it as oral or sublingual tablets, intranasal gels, or injections containing megaquantities of the vitamin at exorbitant prices by indicating that it has a wide range of salutary effects it does not have.[13,140]

A legitimate use of daily oral tablets containing from 25 μg to 1 mg vitamin B-12 is in prevention of vitamin B-12 deficiency in elderly persons with gastric atrophy.[10,12] One percent of free vitamin B-12 is absorbed by mass action in the absence of gastric IF,[10,12] provided it is eaten 1 hour away from any food, because gastric emptying half-time is 30 minutes. (Food protein binds free vitamin B-12, and if there is no gastric acid or enzymes to free vitamin B-12 from food protein, the vitamin can be lost with food waste in the stool).

Summary

Vitamin B-12 is synthesized by bacteria. It is present in all animal, but rarely in plant, foods. It is required by all DNA-synthesizing cells, including those of the hematopoietic and nervous system, to facilitate the cyclic metabolism of folic acid, which is essential for thymidine, and thus DNA, synthesis. It transfers a methyl group from methylfolate, converting vasculotoxic excess homocysteine to methionine, a major one-carbon donor. The average adult requirement for vitamin B-12 is ≈1 μg/d. The RDA for adults is 2 μg/d.[39–41]

The circulating vitamin B-12–delivery protein, TCII, is of prime importance in vitamin B-12 metabolism.[10,12,115] Low serum holoTCII is not only a surrogate Schilling test, but also diagnoses inadequate absorption of vitamin B-12 of any cause months before serum homocysteine and methylmalonic acid are elevated.[10,12,124] Gastric IF is necessary for normal absorption of physiological quantities of vitamin B-12. One percent of pharmacological quantities, eaten apart from food, are absorbed by mass action diffusion. Cobalamin analogues, produced by supplements of vitamin C, may cause more rapid development of vitamin B-12 deficiency.[10,12,21–23,31–33]

When one stops eating vitamin B-12, one passes through four stages of negative cobalamin balance: serum depletion (low holoTCII, i.e., low vitamin B-12 on TCII), cell depletion (falling holohaptocorrin and low red cell vitamin B-12), biochemical deficiency (slowed DNA synthesis, elevated serum homocysteine and methylmalonic acid), and, finally, clinical deficiency (anemia). Serum vitamin B-12 is on two proteins: the circulating vitamin B-12–delivery protein TCII (normally containing 20% of the serum vitamin B-12) and the circulating vitamin B-12–storage protein haptocorrin (normally containing 80% of the serum vitamin B-12). Because TCII is depleted of vitamin B-12 within days after absorption stops, the best screening test for early negative vitamin B-12 balance is measurement of vitamin B-12 on TCII (holoTCII). HoloTCII falls below the bottom of its normal range long before total serum vitamin B-12 (which is mainly vitamin B-12 on haptocorrin) does.

Lack of delivery of vitamin B-12 to the glial cells of brain quickly wipes out their small vitamin B-12 stores; the cells then become vitamin B-12 deficient with build-up of homocysteine.[10,48,63,92,141] Homocysteine, a normal sulfur-containing amino acid at usual levels, is a neurotoxin and vasculotoxin when elevated.[2,10,12,48,55,62,93,94,124–126,131,133]

About one-half of AIDS patients have decreased levels of holoTCII.[60] Herbert et al.[60] and others reported that some cognitive and hematopoietic dysfunction of such AIDS patients is reversed by vitamin B-12 therapy.[142]

Workers who do not measure holoTCII find only the cases of negative B-12 balance in the elderly that have progressed to deficiency;[67,69,107,126] however, they would find the half with predeficiency depletion and be able to treat them and thus prevent deficiency from ever developing if they simply followed the advice to add

holoTCII measurements to their diagnostic armamentarium.[12,50,51,108,124,143] By repeatedly measuring holoTCII, Allen et al.[144] were able to identify intermittent malabsorption of vitamin B-12 due to waxing and waning parasitic infestation as a major factor in the vitamin B-12 deficiency prevalent in rural Mexican communities. Carmel's[67,107] many cases of "mysterious B-12 deficiency of the elderly not due to malabsorption" are almost certainly deficiency due to intermittent B-12 malabsorption that precedes irreversible malabsorption as pernicious anemia gradually progresses.[2,108,145] He fails to diagnose it because he does not measure holoTCII as we and others teach to do.[12,108,143–145]

References

1. Combe JS (1824) History of a case of anaemia. Trans Med Chirurg Soc Edinburgh 1:194–204
2. Bhatt HR, James HVT, Besser GM, et al, eds (1994) Advances in Thomas Addison's diseases, 2 vols. Journal of Endocrinology Ltd, Bristol, United Kingdom
3. Minot GR, Murphy WP (1926) Treatment of pernicious anemia by special diet. JAMA 87:470–476
4. Castle WB, Townsend WC (1929) Observations on the etiologic relationship of achylia gastrica to pernicious anemia. II. The effect of the administration to patients with pernicious anemia of beef muscle after incubation with normal human gastric juice. Am J Med Sci 178:764–777
5. Herbert V (1987) The 1986 Herman Award Lecture: nutrition science as a continually unfolding story: the folate and vitamin B-12 paradigm. Am J Clin Nutr 46:387–402
6. Whipple GH, Robscheit-Robbins FS (1925) Blood regeneration in severe anemia: favorable influence of liver, heart and skeletal muscle in diet. Am J Physiol 72:408–418
7. Whipple GH, Robscheit-Robbins FS (1936) Iron and its utilization in experimental anemia. Am J Med Sci 191:1124–1143
8. Rickes EL, Brink NG, Koniuszy FR, et al (1948) Crystalline vitamin B-12. Science 107:396–397
9. Smith EL, Parker LFJ (1948) Purification of anti-pernicious anaemia factor. Biochem J 43:vii–ix
10. Herbert V, Das KC (1994) Folic acid and vitamin B-12. In Shils ME, Olson JA, Shike M (eds), Modern nutrition in health and disease, 8th ed. Lea & Febiger, Philadelphia, pp 402–425
11. Rauma A-L, Torronen R, Hennine O, et al (1995) Vitamin B-12 status of long-term adherents of a strict uncooked vegan diet ("living food diet") is compromised. J Nutr 125:2511–2515
12. Herbert V (1994) Staging vitamin B-12 status in vegetarians. Am J Clin Nutr 59(suppl):1213S–1222S
13. Herbert V, Subak-Sharpe GJ, eds (1995) Total nutrition: the only guide you'll ever need: from the Mount Sinai School of Medicine. St. Martin's Press, New York
14. Simopoulos A, Herbert V, Jacobson B, eds (1993) Genetic nutrition: designing a diet based on your family medical history. Macmillan, New York (republished as a 1995 softcover book titled The Healing Diet)
15. Herbert V, Cohen L, Kasdan TS, et al (1990) Rediscovering selective nutrient deficiency in one cell line but not another: low serum holotranscobalamin II (holo-TCII) may identify negative vitamin B-12 balance only in cells (ex: hematopoietic) with surface receptors solely for TCII, and not in cells (ex: liver) with receptors also for haptocorrin: in AIDS,

there may be stage IV negative B-12 balance in hematopoietic and neuropsychiatric cells with liver cells only in
stage I-II [abstract]. Clin Res 38:23A

16. Zagalak B, Friedrich W, eds (1979) Vitamin B-12. Proceedings of the Third European Symposium on Vitamin B-12 and
Intrinsic Factor. Walter de Gruyter, New York

17. Herbert V (1988) Vitamin B-12: plant sources, requirements,
and assay. Am J Clin Nutr 48:852–858

18. Babior BM, ed (1975) Cobalamin biochemistry and pathophysiology. John Wiley & Sons, New York

19. IUPAC-IUB Commission on Biochemical Nomenclature
(1974) The nomenclature of corrinoids (1973 recommendations). Biochemistry 13:1550–1560

20. Pratt JM (1972) Inorganic chemistry of vitamin B-12. Academic Press, New York

21. Herbert V, Drivas G, Foscaldi R, et al (1982) Multivita-
min/mineral food supplements containing vitamin B-12
may also contain analogues of vitamin B-12. N Engl J
Med 307:255–256

22. Kolhouse JF, Kondo H, Allen NC, et al (1978) Cobalamin
analogues are present in human plasma and can mask
cobalamin deficiency because current radioisotope dilution assays are not specific for true cobalamin. N Engl J
Med 299:785–792

23. Gottlieb CW, Retief FP, Herbert V (1967) Blockade of vitamin B-12-binding sites in gastric juice, serum and saliva by
analogues and derivatives of vitamin B-12 and by antibody
to intrinsic factor. Biochim Biophys Acta 141:560–572

24. England JM, Linnell JC (1980) Problems of the serum vitamin B-12 assay. Lancet 2:1072–1074

25. Mollin DL, Hoffbrand AV, Ward PG, et al (1980) Interlaboratory comparison of serum vitamin B-12 assay. J Clin
Pathol 33:243–248

26. International Commission for Standardization in Haematology (1986) Proposed serum standard for human serum
vitamin B-12 assay. Br J Haematol 64:809–811

27. Herbert V, Drivas G (1982) Spirulina and vitamin B-12. JAMA
248:3096–3097

28. Kanazawa S, Herbert V, Herzlich B, et al (1983) Removal
of cobalamin analogue in bile by enterohepatic circulation.
Lancet 1:707–708

29. Herbert V (1981) Vitamin B-12. Am J Clin Nutr 34:971-972

30. Herbert V, Manusselis C, Drivas G, et al (1983) Low vitamin B-12 content of heavily processed milks may explain
vitamin B-12 deficiency in young adults in Mexico [abstract].
Clin Res 31:241A

31. Herbert V, Jacob E, Wong K-TJ, et al (1978) Low serum vitamin B-12 levels in patients receiving ascorbic acid in
megadoses: studies concerning the effect of ascorbate on
radioisotope vitamin B-12 assay. Am J Clin Nutr 31:253–258

32. Hines JD (1975) Ascorbic acid and vitamin B-12 deficiency
[letter]. JAMA 234:24

33. Herbert V (1995) Vitamin C supplements and disease: counterpoint [editorial]. J Am Coll Nutr 14:112–113

34. Herbert V (1983) Folic acid and vitamin B-12. In Rothfeld
B (ed), Nuclear medicine in vitro. JB Lippincott, Philadelphia, pp 337–354

35. Herbert V, Landau L, Bash R, et al (1979) Ability of megadoses
of vitamin C to destroy vitamin B-12 and cobinamide and
to reduce absorption of vitamin B-12 (with a note on B-12
radioassays). In Zagalak B, Friedrich W (eds), Vitamin B-
12. Proceedings of the Third European Symposium on Vitamin B-12 and Intrinsic Factor. Walter de Gruyter, New York,
pp 1069–1077

36. Herbert V, Shaw S, Jayatilleke E, Kasdan TS (1994) Most free-
radical injury is iron-related: it is promoted by iron, hemin,

holoferritin and vitamin C, and inhibited by desferoxamine
and apoferritin. Stem Cells 12:289–303

37. Kondo H, Binder MJ, Kolhouse JF, et al (1982) Presence and
formation of cobalamin analogues in multivitamin-mineral
pills. J Clin Invest 70:889–898

38. Shaw S, Herbert V, Colman N, et al (1990) Effect of etha-
nol-generated free radicals on gastric intrinsic factor and
glutathione. Alcohol 7:153–157

39. Herbert V (1987) Recommended dietary intakes (RDI) of
vitamin B-12. Am J Clin Nutr 45:671–678

40. National Research Council (1989) Recommended dietary
allowances, 10th ed. National Academy Press, Washington,
DC

41. Herbert V (1990) The RDA is mainly the work of the 1980–85
(10th) RDA Committee, but with 9th RDA numbers for vitamins A and C [abstract]. FASEB J 4:A374

42. Joint FAO/WHO Expert Group (1988) Requirements of vitamin A, iron, folate, and vitamin B-12. FAO Food and Nutrition Series No. 23. Food and Agriculture Organization, Rome

43. Herbert V (1994) Vitamin B-12 and elderly people. Am J
Clin Nutr 59:1093–1094

44. Sullivan LW, Herbert V (1965) Studies on the minimum
daily requirements for vitamin B-12: hematopoietic responses to 0.1 microgram of cyanocobalamin or coenzyme
B-12 and comparison of their relative potency. N Engl J
Med 272:340–346

45. McLaren DS (1981) The luxus vitamins—A and B-12. Am J
Clin Nutr 34:1611–1616.

46. Russell RM (1994) Reply to V Herbert [letter]. Am J Clin
Nutr 59:1094

47. Herbert V, Kasdan TS, Huebscher T (1987) Nasal vitamin
B-12 gel may not be a reliable alternative to injectable
vitamin B-12; both bind preferentially to TCII and produce analogue increment just on TCII [abstract]. Blood
70(suppl):45A

48. Herbert V (1992) Folate and neural tube defects. Nutr Today 27(6):30–33

49. Herbert V (1967) Immunologic factors in pernicious anemia. Postgrad Med 42:298–303

50. Shaw S, Jayatilleke E, Bauman W, Herbert V (1994) The
mechanism of B-12 malabsorption and depletion due to
Metformin and its reversal with dietary calcium [abstract].
J Am Diabetes Assoc 43(Suppl 1):167A

51. Herbert V (1995) Low serum B-12 on TCII, or low serum
and red cell folate, predict later high serum homocysteine
and even later megaloblastic anemia. Proceedings of the
XIIIth Meeting of the International Society of Haematology
(European and African Division). Turk J Haematol, Vol 14
(Suppl 1), Abstract 204

52. Rothenberg SP, Quadros EV (1995) Transcobalamin II and
the membrane receptor for the transcobalamin II-cobalamin
complex. Ballieres Clin Haematol 8:499–514

53. Herbert V, Fong W, Stopler T, et al (1989) Low serum
holotranscobalamin II (B-12-TCII) diagnoses both negative
B-12 balance (B-12 malabsorption) and reduced B-12 delivery to marrow in AIDS prior to high serum homocysteine
(HCY) [abstract]. Blood 74(suppl 1):6A

54. Herbert V (1975) Detection of malabsorption of vitamin B-
12 due to gastric or intestinal dysfunction. Semin Nucl Med
2:220–234

55. Goh YT, Jacobsen DW, Green R (1991) Diagnosis of functional cobalamin deficiency: utility of transcobalamin II-
bound vitamin B-12 determination in conjunction with total serum homocysteine and methylmalonic acid [abstract].
Blood 78(suppl I):100A

56. Herbert V, Rudick A (1993) Billions will be saved by as-

sessing iron status in all Americans, folate status in all fertile females, and vitamin B-12 status in all after age 55 [abstract]. FASEB J 7:A412

57. Matthews JH (1995) Cobalamin and folate deficiency in the elderly. Ballieres Clin Haematol 8:679–697

58. Das KC, Manusselis C, Herbert V (1991) Determination of vitamin B-12 (cobalamin) in serum and erythrocytes by radioassay, and holotranscobalamin II (holo-TCII) and holo-haptocorrin (holo-TC I and III) in serum by adsorbing holo-TCII on microfine silica. J Nutr Biochem 2:455–464

59. Wickramasinghe SN, Fida S (1993) Correlations between holo-transcobalamin II, holo-haptocorrin, and total B-12 in serum samples from healthy subjects and patients. J Clin Pathol 46:537–539

60. Herbert V, Fong W, Gulle V, Kasdan TS (1990) Low holo-transcobalamin II is the earliest serum marker for subnormal vitamin B-12 (cobalamin) absorption in patients with AIDS. Am J Hematol 34:132–139

61. Herzlich B, Herbert V (1988) Depletion of serum holo-transcobalamin II: an early sign of negative vitamin B-12 balance. Lab Invest 58:332–337

62. Green R (1995) Metabolite assays in cobalamin and folate deficiency. Ballieres Clin Haematol 8:533–566

63. Streit WJ, Kincaid-Colton CA (1995) The brain's immune system. Sci Am 273(5):54–61

64. Carmel R, Rosenberg AH, Lau KS, et al (1969) Vitamin B-12 uptake by human small bowel homogenate and its enhancement by intrinsic factor. Gastroenterology 56:548–555

65. Shaw S, Jayatilleke E, Bauman W, et al (1993) Mechanism of B-12 malabsorption and depletion due to metformin discovered by using serial serum holo-transcobalamin II (holoTCII) (B-12 on TCII) as a surrogate for serial Schilling tests [abstract]. Blood 82(suppl 1):432A

66. Allen RH (1982) Cobalamin (vitamin B-12) absorption and malabsorption. Viewpoints Digestive Dis 14:17–20

67. Carmel R (1995) Malabsorption of food cobalamin. Ballieres Clin Haemat 8:639–655

68. Marcus DL, Shaddick D, Crampz J, et al (1987) Transcobalamin II levels in a hematologically normal elderly population. J Am Geriatr Soc 35:635–638

69. Pennypacker LC, Allen RH, Kelly JP, et al (1992) High prevalence of cobalamin deficiency in elderly outpatients. J Am Geriatr Soc 40:1197–1204

70. Yao Y (1992) Low serum vitamin B-12 in seniors. J Fam Pract 35:524–529

71. Guzik HJ, Tommasulo BC, Mandel FD, et al (1993) Prevalence of negative vitamin B-12 balance in well and malnourished frail elderly [abstract]. J Am Geriatr Soc 41:SA27

72. Herbert V, Shaw S, Jayatilleke E, et al (1990) Evidence in serum for food vitamin B-12 (cobalamin) malabsorption in AIDS: high gastrin, low cobalamin on transcobalamin II, and circulating antibody to intrinsic factor despite normal serum total cobalamin levels [abstract]. Clin Res 38:361A

73. Ran JY, Li XF, Rau HL, et al (1990) Reduced immunologic function in folate and/or B-12 deficiency megaloblastic anemia (MA) and in vegetarians in China [abstract]. Blood 76(suppl 1):217A

74. Herbert V (1993) Nutrient deficiency and esophageal cancer in China. CNI Nutr Week 23(40):6

75. Ran JY, Dou P, Wang LY, et al (1993) Correlation of low serum folate and total B-12 with high incidence of esophageal carcinoma (EC) in Shanxi, China [abstract]. Blood 82(suppl I):532A

76. Herbert V (1992) Diet and cancer prevention. National Council Against Health Fraud Newsletter 15(3):3

77. Amin J, Vu T, Bateman R, et al (1992) Measurement of red cell B-12 and holoTCII levels: the key to the evaluation of true B-12 deficiency? [abstract]. Blood 80:381A

78. Linnell JC, Bhatt HR (1995) Inherited errors of cobalamin metabolism and their management. Ballieres Clin Haematol 8:567–601

79. Herbert V (1982) Megaloblastic anemia in China. Ann Intern Med 97:139-140

80. Kanazawa S, Herbert V (1985) Total corrinoid, cobalamin (vitamin B-12), and cobalamin analogue levels may be normal in serum despite cobalamin depletion in liver in patients with alcoholism. Lab Invest 53:108-110

81. Herbert V, Das KC (1992) Anemias due to nuclear maturation defects (megaloblastic anemias). In Hurst JW (ed), Medicine for the practicing physician, 3rd ed. Butterworth-Heinemann, Boston, pp 851–857

82. Herbert V (1989) Staging nutrient status from too little to too much by appropriate laboratory tests. In Livingston GE (ed), Nutritional status assessment of the individual. Food and Nutrition Press, Trumbull, CT, pp 147–167

83. Shevchuk O, Huebscher T, Herbert V (1988) Evidence that vitamin B-12 regulates synthesis of proteins involved in corrinoid metabolism [abstract]. FASEB J 2:A1086

84. Herbert V (1992) Everyone should be tested for iron disorders. J Am Diet Assoc 92:1502–1509

85. Retief FP, Gottlieb CW, Herbert V (1967) Delivery of Co[57]B-12 to erythrocytes from alpha and beta globulin of normal, B-12-deficient, and chronic myeloid leukemia serum. Blood 29:837–851

86. Tisman G, Vu T, Amin J, et al (1993) Measurement of red blood cell vitamin B-12: a study of the correlation between intracellular B-12 content and concentrations of plasma holotranscobalamin II. Am J Hematol 43:226–229

87. Sullivan LW, Herbert V, Castle WB (1963) In vitro assay for human intrinsic factor. J Clin Invest 42:1443–1458

88. Herbert V (1977) Anemias. In Winick M (ed), Nutritional disorders of American women. John Wiley & Sons, New York, pp 79–90

89. Tisman G, Herbert V, Richards N, et al (1994) Use of simple and reproducible assay for measurement of serum vitamin B-12 bound to its active transport protein transcobalamin II, holotranscobalamin II (HoloTCII) in 104 pregnant patients; evidence that 29% have marked and 38% have moderate reductions of holotranscobalamin II levels due to fetal shunting [abstract]. Mount Sinai School of Medicine, New York, 1994, p H12

90. Kahn SB, Williams WJ, Barness LW, et al (1965) Methylmalonic acid excretion, a sensitive indicator for vitamin B-12 deficiency in man. J Lab Clin Med 66:75–83

91. Lindenbaum J, Healton EB, Savage DB, et al (1988) Neuropsychiatric disorders caused by cobalamin deficiency in the absence of anemia or macrocytosis. N Engl J Med 318:1720–1728

92. Herbert V, Norman EJ, Alston TA, et al (1988) Cobalamin deficiency and neuropsychiatric disorders. N Engl J Med 319:1733–1735

93. Lindenbaum J, Rosenberg IH, Wilson PW, et al (1994) Prevalence of cobalamin deficiency in the Framingham elderly population. Am J Clin Nutr 60:2–11

94. Selhub J, Jacques PF, Wilson PWF, et al (1993) Vitamin status and intake as primary determinants of homocysteinemia in an elderly population. JAMA 270:2693–2698

95. Das KC, Herbert V (1989) In vitro DNA synthesis by megaloblastic bone marrow: effect of folates and cobalamins on thymidine incorporation and de novo thymidine synthesis. Am J Hematol 31:11–20

96. Metz J, Kelly A, Swett VC, et al (1968) Deranged DNA synthesis by bone marrow from vitamin B-12-deficient humans. Br J Haematol 14:575–592

97. Herbert V, Tisman G, Go LT, et al (1973) The dU suppression test using ^{125}IUdR to define biochemical megaloblastosis. Br J Haematol 24:713–723

98. Das KC, Hoffbrand AV (1970) Lymphocyte transformation in megaloblastic anaemia: morphology and DNA synthesis. Br J Haematol 19:459–468

99. Das KC, Manusselis C, Herbert V (1980) Simplifying lymphocyte culture and the deoxyuridine suppression test by using whole blood (0.1 ml) instead of separated lymphocytes. Clin Chem 26:72–77

100. Das KC, Herbert V (1978) The lymphocyte as a marker of past nutritional status: persistence of abnormal lymphocyte deoxyuridine (dU) suppression test and chromosomes in patients with past deficiency of folate and vitamin B-12. Br J Haematol 38:219–233

101. Das KC, Herbert V, Colman N, et al (1978) Unmasking covert folate deficiency in iron-deficient subjects with neutrophil hypersegmentation: dU suppression tests on lymphocytes and bone marrow. Br J Haematol 39:357–375

102. Wickramasinghe SN (1995) Morphology, biology and biochemistry of cobalamin- and folate-deficient bone marrow cells. Ballieres Clin Haematol 8:441–459

103. Das KC, Asiz MA, Colman N, et al (1991) Eliminating false positive and false negative results in lymphocyte diagnostic dU suppression test (DxdUST) for folate deficiency by recognizing different "normal" individuals have different folate stores [abstract]. Blood 78(suppl 10):99A

104. Kondo H, Osborne JL, Kolhouse JF, et al (1981) Nitrous oxide has multiple deleterious effects on cobalamin metabolism. J Clin Invest 67:1270–1283

105. van der Westhuyzen J, Fernandes-Costa F, Metz J, et al (1982) Cobalamin (vitamin B-12) analogues are absent in plasma of fruit bats exposed to nitrous oxide. Proc Soc Exp Biol Med 171:88–91

106. Herbert V (1984) Megaloblastic anemias. Lab Invest 52:3–19

107. Carmel R (1992) Reversal by cobalamin therapy of minimal defects in the deoxyuridine suppression test in patients without anemia: further evidence for a subtle metabolic cobalamin deficiency. J Lab Clin Med 119:240–244

108. Herbert V (1988) Don't ignore low serum cobalamin (vitamin B-12) levels. Arch Intern Med 148:1705–1707

109. Herbert V, Memoli D, McAleer E, et al (1986) What is normal? variation from the individual's norm for granulocyte "lobe average" and holo-transcobalamin II (Holo-TC II) diagnoses vitamin B-12 deficiency before variation from the laboratory norm [abstract]. Clin Res 34:718A

110. Herbert V (1959) Studies on the role of intrinsic factor in vitamin B-12 absorption, transport, and storage. Am J Clin Nutr 7:433–443

111. Jacob E, Baker EJ, Herbert V (1980) Vitamin B-12-binding proteins. Physiol Rev 60:918–959

112. Kanazawa S, Herbert V (1983) Mechanism of enterohepatic circulation of vitamin B-12: movement of vitamin B-12 from bile R-binder to intrinsic factor due to the action of pancreatic trypsin. Trans Assoc Am Physicians 96:336-344

113. Herzlich B, Herbert V (1984) The role of the pancreas in cobalamin (vitamin B-12) absorption. Am J Gastroenterol 79:489–493

114. Herbert V, Scrimshaw N, Solomons N (1995) Nutritional disorders and the alimentary tract. In Haubrich WS, Schaffer F, Berk JE (eds), Gastroenterology, 5th ed, vol 4. WB Saunders, Philadelphia, pp 3240–3254

115. Herbert V, Memoli D, March R, et al (1986) Vitamin B-12 analogue levels tend to rise as cobalamin deficiency develops with cessation of therapy in pernicious anemia [abstract]. Blood 68:46A

116. Herbert V (1990) Nutritional anemias in the elderly. In Prinsley DM, Sandstead HH (eds), Nutrition and aging. Alan R Liss, New York, pp 203–227

117. Herbert V (1971) Recent developments in cobalamin metabolism. In Armstein HRV, Wrighton RJ (eds), The cobalamins. Churchill Livingstone, Edinburgh, pp 2–16

118. Herbert V, Zalusky R (1962) Interrelations of vitamin B-12 and folic acid metabolism: folic acid clearance studies. J Clin Invest 41:1263–1276

119. Noronha JM, Silverman M (1962) On folic acid, vitamin B-12, methionine and formimmunoglutamic acid metabolism. In vitamin B-12 and intrinsic factor, Second European Symposium. Enke, Stuttgart, Germany, pp 728–736

120. Shin YL, Buhring KU, Stokstad ELR (1975) The relationships between vitamin B-12 and folic acid and the effect of methionine on folate metabolism. Mol Cell Biochem 9:97–108

121. Chanarin I (1990) The megaloblastic anemias, 3rd ed. Blackwell, Oxford, United Kingdom

122. Scott JM, Dinn JJ, Wilson P, et al (1981) The methyl-folate trap and the supply of S-adenosylmethionine. Lancet 2:755

123. Herzlich B, Herbert V (1986) Rapid collection of human intrinsic factor uncontaminated with cobalophilin (R binder). Am J Gastroenterol 81:678-680

124. Green R, Kinsella LJ (1995) Current concepts in the diagnosis of cobalamin deficiency. Neurology 45:1435–1440

125. Weir DG, Scott JM (1995) The biochemical basis of the neuropathy in cobalamin deficiency. Ballieres Clin Haematol 8:479–497

126. Savage DG, Lindenbaum J (1995) Neurological complications of acquired cobalamin deficiency: clinical aspects. Ballieres Clin Haematol 8:657–678

127. Jacob E, Herbert V (1980) Vitamin B-12 and the nervous system. In Kumar S (ed), Biochemistry of brain. Pergamon Press, New York, pp 127–142

128. Frenkel EP (1973) Abnormal fatty acid metabolism in peripheral nerves of patients with pernicious anemia. J Clin Invest 52:1237–1245

129. Scott JM, Dinn JJ, Wilson P, et al (1981) Pathogenesis of subacute combined degeneration: a result of methyl group deficiency. Lancet 2:337–340

130. Herbert V, Kasdan TS (1993) Can genetic nutrition be used to predict and prevent heart attacks? the Mount Sinai heart attack prediction and prevention profile [abstract]. Clin Res 41:397A

131. Nygard O, Vollset SE, Refsum H, et al (1995) Total plasma homocysteine and cardiovascular risk profile. JAMA 274:1526–1533

132. Jacobsen DW, Green R, Herbert V, et al (1990) Decreased serum glutathione with normal cysteine and homocysteine levels in patients with AIDS [abstract]. Clin Res 38:556A

133. Green R, Jacobsen DW (1995) Clinical implications of hyperhomocysteinemia. In Bailey LB (ed), Folate in health and disease. Marcel Dekker, New York, pp 75–122

134. Stabler SP, Allen RW, Savage DW, et al (1990) Clinical spectrum and diagnosis of cobalamin deficiency. Blood 76:871–881

135. Fenton WA, Rosenberg LE (1989) Inherited disorders of cobalamin transport and metabolism. In Scriver R, Beaudet AL, Sly WS, Valle D (eds), The metabolic basis of inherited disease. McGraw-Hill, New York, pp 2065–2082

136. Ampola MG, Mahoney MJ, Nakamura E, et al (1975) Prenatal therapy of a patient with vitamin B-12-responsive methylmalonic acidemia. N Engl J Med 293:313–317

137. Nyhan WL (1975) Prenatal treatment of methylmalonic acidemia. N Engl J Med 293:353–354

138. Cottrell JE, Casthely P, Brodie JD, et al (1978) Prevention of nitroprusside-induced cyanide toxicity with hydrocobalamin. N Engl J Med 298:809

139. Wilson J, Linnel JC, Matthews DM (1971) Plasma-cobalamins in neuro-ophthalmological diseases. Lancet 1:259–261

140. Barrett S, Herbert V (1994) The vitamins pushers: how the "health food" industry is selling Americans a bill of goods. Prometheus Press, Amherst, NY

141. Herbert V (1988) B-12 deficiency in AIDS [letter]. JAMA 260:2837

142. Herbert V (1993) Vitamin B-12 deficiency neuropsychiatric damage in acquired immunodeficiency syndrome [letter]. Arch Neurol 50:569

143. Allen LH, Casterline J (1994) Vitamin B-12 deficiency in elderly individuals: diagnosis and requirements. Am J Clin Nutr 60:12–14

144. Allen LH, Rosado JL, Casterline JE, et al (1995) Vitamin B-12 deficiency and malabsorption are highly prevalent in rural Mexican communities. Am J Clin Nutr 62:1013–1019

145. Herbert V (1969) Transient (reversible) malabsorption of vitamin B-12. Br J Haematol 17:213–219

Chapter 21

Folic Acid

Jacob Selhub and Irwin H. Rosenberg

Folic acid is the term most commonly used to refer to a family of vitamers with related biological activity. Other terms, folate, folates, and folacin, are generally interchangeable. Folic acid was isolated in 1943 by a team at Lederle Laboratories that included E. L. Robert Stokstad, and this isolation was followed by the identification and synthesis of pteroylglutamic acid in 1945.[1] Fifteen years earlier Lucy Wills of the Royal Free Hospital in London had described a "new haemopoietic factor" in yeast that cured tropical macrocytic anemia in India. This unknown substance was referred to as "Wills factor" by Watson and Castle when they confirmed that the new hemopoietic principle was found in a different fraction of liver extract from that which was curative for pernicious anemia. Concurrently, factors identified by other methods were assigned candidate vitamin names during that period of the 1930s when it was still possible to aspire to the identification of a new vitamin. Some of those names included "vitamin M" and "vitamin Bc" relating to assay animals, monkey and chick. The relationship of these factors to other factors such as the growth factor for *Lactobacillus casei* was not appreciated.[2] The term "folic acid" was used by Mitchell et al. in 1941[3] to refer to a growth factor in spinach leaves, thus the term folic acid or folate. Other designations for this yet to be determined growth principle were vitamin B-10 and vitamin B-11, and when folic acid was identified as pteroylglutamic acid, those numerical designations dropped out and thus the next and last vitamin to be identified became vitamin B-12.

The metabolic interactions of vitamin B-12 and folic acid and their common association with megaloblastic anemia were an important part of the history of both vitamins. Only in retrospect was it possible to note that "vitamin Bc" was folic acid, "vitamin Bc conjugate" was folylpolyglutamate, and there was yet an additional "extrinsic factor" or anti-pernicious-anemia factor that would eventually become vitamin B-12. If the first half of this century was the era of the identification of all of the known vitamins, including folic acid, and the elaboration of the use of synthetic forms of the vitamin for the treatment of deficiency disease and anemia, then the second half of the century might be appreciated as the period when new research on the absorption, metabolism, and assay characteristics of this vitamin has led to an appreciation of its importance in the diet and its potential for adding to the nutritional defenses against cancer, heart disease, stroke, and birth defects.

Folate Metabolism

Structure and function of folate coenzymes in one-carbon transfer reactions. Folates are a family of compounds that have pteroylglutamic (PteGlu) as a common structure (Figure 1). They differ from each other in the pyrazine ring, which can assume different forms of substitutions, and by the p-aminobenzoylglutamate (PABAGlu) moiety, which can contain additional glutamate residues in gamma peptide linkage. The pyrazine ring may be partially reduced at the 7,8 position ($H_2PteGlu_n$) or fully reduced ($H_4PteGlu_n$). Reduction is catalyzed by dihydrofolate reductase (reaction 2, Figure 2), a target enzyme for cancer chemotherapy. Fully reduced folates ($H_4PteGlu_n$) may be present as such or substituted with a carbon unit of various oxidation levels. At the formate oxidation level the substitution may occupy the 5 position (5-formyl-$H_4PteGlu_n$), the 10 position (10-formyl-$H_4PteGlu_n$), or both positions (5,10-methenyl-$H_4PteGlu_n$). Both the 10-formyl and 5,10-methenyl derivatives serve as respective substrates for the synthesis of C-2 and C-8 of purines (reactions 16 and 17, Figure 2).

At the oxidation level of formaldehyde, the substitution occupies both the 5 and 10 positions (5,10-methylene-$H_4PteGlu_n$). Unlike other substitutions, 5,10-methylene-$H_4PteGlu_n$ is unstable and readily dissociates to formaldehyde and $H_4PteGlu_n$. In spite of this instability, 5,10-methylene-$H_4PteGlu_n$ participates in a number of key reactions. In the de novo synthesis of thymidylate (reaction 14, Figure 2) the methylene group together with two electrons from the pyrazine ring are transferred to form a methyl group that substitutes a hydrogen in the 5 position of the deoxyuridine monophosphate (dUMP). This transfer results in $H_2PteGlu_n$ as a product. Reduction to $H_4PteGlu_n$ is a necessary step to start a new cycle of thymidylate or other folate-dependent syntheses. This

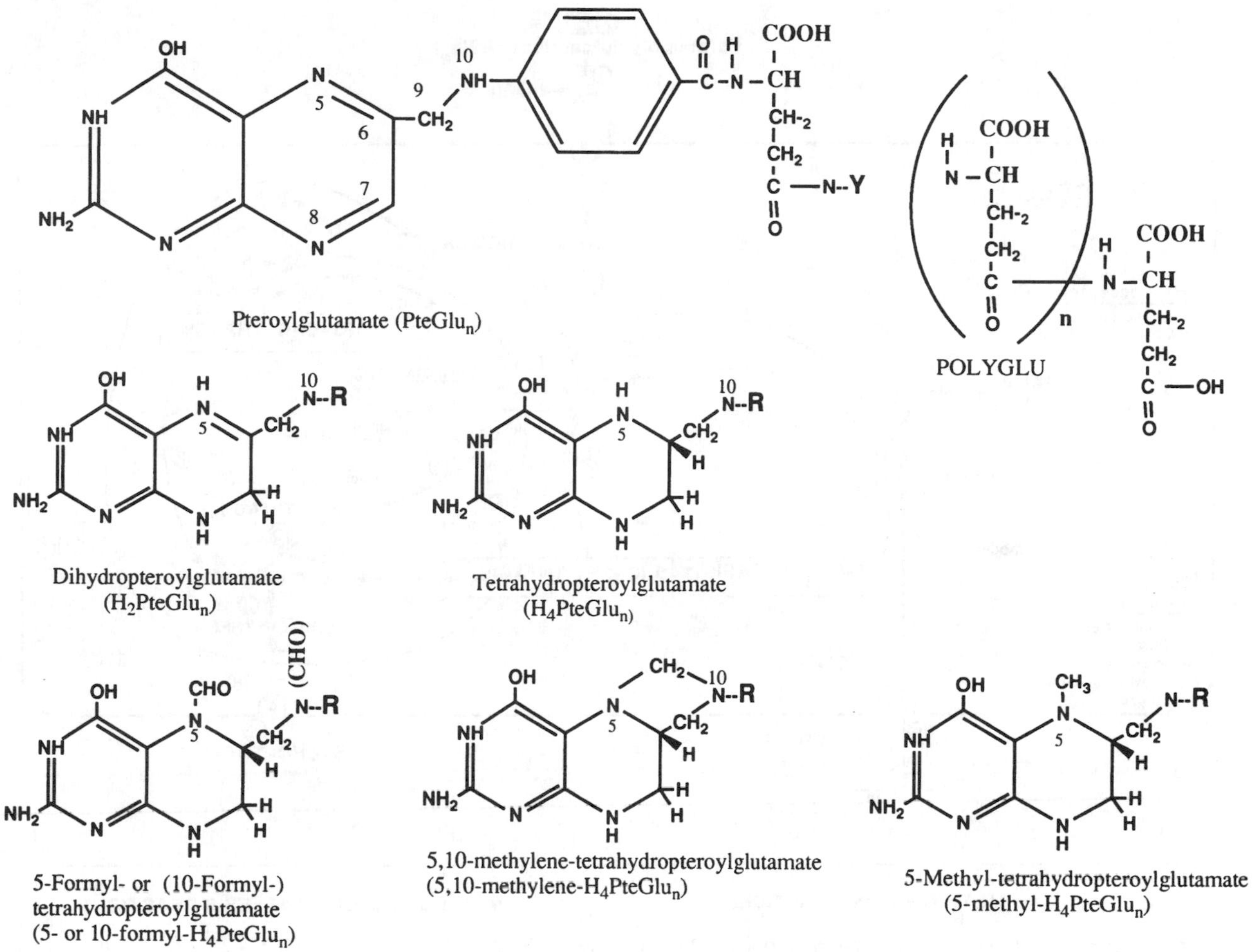

Figure 1. Chemical formulas for pteroylglutamic acid and its derivatives.

necessity provided the basis for choosing dihydrofolate as a target enzyme for cancer chemotherapy. Compounds in the family of antifolate agents, in which the hydroxyl group in the 4 position is replaced by an amino group (aminopterin, methotrexate), are potent inhibitors of dihydrofolate reductase with affinities for the enzyme that are three orders of magnitude higher than the affinity for $H_2PteGlu_n$.

Another reaction for which 5,10-methylene-$H_4PteGlu_n$ serves as substrate is the reversible synthesis of serine from glycine (reaction 4, Figure 2)). The importance of this reaction lies primarily in the opposite direction, where a new carbon unit from serine is acquired by folate coenzymes for use in numerous syntheses. Because serine is formed from glucose, such folate-dependent syntheses are de novo syntheses, as opposed to salvage pathways where proteins and nucleic acids, either from the diet or from within the cell, are degraded to release the respective compounds (purines, pyrimidines, methionine etc.).

At the oxidation level of methanol, substitution occurs at the 5 position (5-methyl-$H_4PteGlu_n$). This methyltetrahydrofolate serves as the methyl donor for homocysteine methylation to methionine (reaction 7, Figure 2) in a reaction that is catalyzed by a methyltransferase which, in animals, contains methyl-B-12 as the prosthetic group and requires catalytic amounts of S-adenosylmethionine (SAM).

Circulating folates are monoglutamyl derivatives mostly in the form of 5-methyl-$H_4PteGlu$. Within the cell, acquisition of additional glutamates (polyglutamylation, reaction 3, Figure 2) renders these folates incapable of cellular exit unless they are converted back to monoglutamyl derivatives.[4-11] $H_4PteGlu$ is the preferred substrate for polyglutamylation while 5-methyl-$H_4PteGlu$ exhibits poor substrate activity.[5-9] The assimilation of circulating folate, i.e., 5-methyl-$H_4PteGlu$, by the cell necessitates demethylation. Such a demethylation can occur only through homocysteine methylation catalyzed by the B-12–dependent methyltrans-

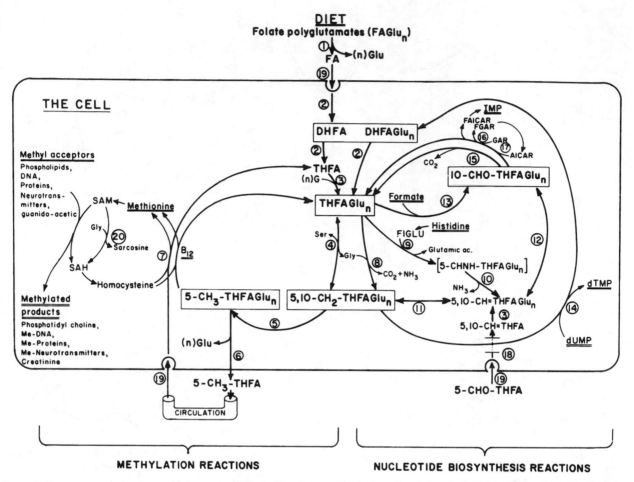

Figure 2. Enzymes and reactions of folate metabolism: 1) γ-glutamyl hydrolase (brush border?) (EC 3.4.22.12), 2) dihydrofolate reductase (EC 1.5.1.3), 3) folylpoly-glutamate synthase (EC 6.3.2.17), 4) serine hydroxymethyl transferase (EC 2.1.2.1), 5) methylenetetrahydrofolate reductase (EC 1.7.99.5), 6) -glutamyl hydrolase (lysosomal?) (EC 3.4.22.12), 7) cobalamin-dependent methionine synthase (EC 2.1.1.13), 8) glycine cleavage enzyme system (EC 1.4.4.2;2.1.2.10), 9) glutamate formimino-transferase (LEC 2.1.2.5), 10) formiminotetrahydrofolate cyclodeaminase (EC 4.3.1.4), 11) methylenetetrahydrofolate dehydrogenase (EC 1.5.1.5), 12) methenyltetrahydrofolate cyclohydrolase (EC 3.5.4.9), 13) formyltetrahydrofolate synthetase (EC 6.3.4.3), 14) thymidylate synthase (EC 2.1.1.45), 15) formyltetrahydrofolate dehydrogenase (EC 1.5.1.6), 16) phosphoribosyl glycinamide (GAR) formyl transferase (EC 2.1.2.2), 17) phosphoribosyl aminoimidazole carboxamide (AICAR) formyl transferase (EC 2.1.2.3), 18) 5-formyltetrahydrofolate cycloligase (EC 6.3.3.2), 19) folate/MTX transport mechanism, and 20) glycine methyl transferase (EC 2.1.1.20).

ferase. Cellular folate depletion is one consequence of vitamin B-12 deficiency.

Polyglutamylation is also associated with greater affinity of enzymes toward their respective substrates, and if a particular substrate acts as an inhibitor of a particular reaction, inhibition potency is increased with increase in the number of glutamate residues.[5–12]

The mechanism of polyglutamylation is consistent with findings showing that the majority of cellular folates contain a total of five or six glutamate residues. However, conditions (folate deficiency, alcoholism, methotrexate therapy, and others) have been described that were found to be associated with elongation of the glutamate chains. The mechanistic basis for these extensions of the glutamate chain remains uncertain.

The involvement of folate in the synthesis of purines, thymidylate, methionine, and serine-glycine interconversion lies in the propensity of $H_4PteGlu_n$ to serve both as a one-carbon acceptor and a one-carbon donor, and also in the capacity of the cell of folate coenzyme interconversions.

The acquisition of a carbon unit by $H_4PteGlu_n$ occurs primarily through the transfer of serine 3-carbon and formation of 5,10-methylene-$H_4PteGlu_n$ (reaction 4, Figure 2). Aside from serving as the source of the methyl group for thymidylate synthesis, the methylene group of 5,10-methylene-$H_4PteGlu_n$ may undergo oxidation to formate or reduction to methanol levels of oxidation.

Oxidation is a reversible reaction that results in the formation of 5,10-methenyl-$H_4PteGlu_n$ (reaction 11,

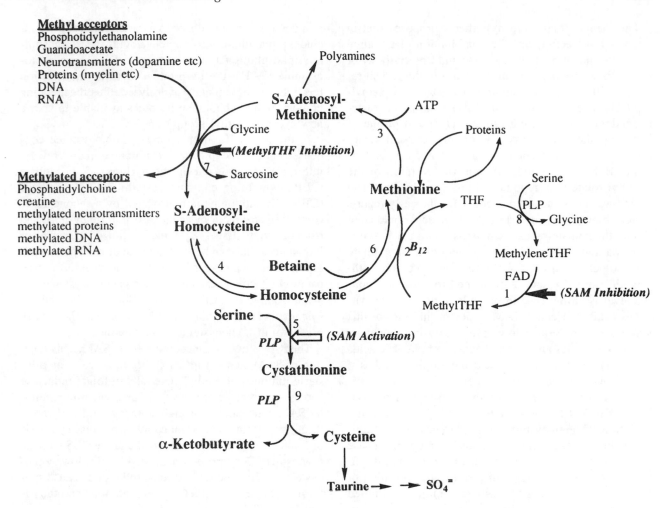

Methyl acceptors
Phosphotidylethanolamine
Guanidoacetate
Neurotransmitters (dopamine etc)
Proteins (myelin etc)
DNA
RNA

Methylated acceptors
Phosphatidylcholine
creatine
methylated neurotransmitters
methylated proteins
methylated DNA
methylated RNA

Figure 3. Homocysteine metabolism in animals. Enzyme reactions that are regulated by SAM and 5-methyltetrahydrofolate (Methyl-THF) are indicated by large arrows. Open arrows indicate activation, closed arrows indicate inhibition. Enzymes: 1) 5,10-methylenetetrahydrofolate reductase; 2) N-5- methyltetrahydrofolate:homocysteine methyltransferase; 3) S-adenosylmethionine synthase; 4) S-adenosylhomocysteine hydrolase; 5) cystathionine β-synthase; 6) betaine:homocysteine methyltransferase; 7) glycine N-methyltransferase; 8) serine hydroxymethylase; 9) γ-cystathionase.

Figure 2). This reaction is catalyzed by a trifunctional enzyme (C_1-THF synthase) that, in addition to the methylenetetrahydrofolate dehydrogenase that is responsible for oxidation, contains methenyltetrahydrofolate cyclohydrolase (reaction 12, Figure 2) and formyltetrahydrofolate synthase (reaction 13, Figure 2). Reactions 11 and 12 provide the substrates for purine synthesis.

The reduction of 5,10-methylene-$H_4PteGlu_n$ to 5-methyl-$H_4PteGlu_n$ (reaction 5, Figure 2) is a physiologically irreversible reaction. Irreversibility renders the regeneration of $H_4PteGlu_n$ dependent on the methylation of homocysteine to methionine by the B-12–dependent methyltransferase.

Regulatory mechanisms. The realization that folates are involved in a number of diverse reactions has prompted efforts to investigate regulatory mechanisms of folate metabolism. According to Krumdieck,[13] folate

metabolism can be regarded as two crucial groups of reactions that compete in the cell for available folates: reactions that lead to the de novo synthesis of methionine and those that lead to the synthesis of nucleic acids (purines and thymidylate). According to this hypothesis, the synthesis of methionine is the more crucial of the two. In addition to its function as a building block for proteins and as source of polyamines, methionine is the precursor of SAM, the universal methyl donor for >100 reactions. Many of these reactions, e.g., phospholipid synthesis and creatine-phosphate synthesis, are vital to the survival of the cell and the organism. This "tug of war" theory proposes that when folate is in short supply, folate coenzymes are directed toward methionine synthesis at the expense of nucleic acid synthesis. The above hypothesis assumes the existence of a coordination between nucleic acid synthesis and methionine synthesis. Such existence is yet to be proven.

The methyl folate trap hypothesis proposes that in vitamin B-12 deficiency, the combination of impaired B-12–dependent methyltransferase and irreversibility of the methylenetetrahydrofolate reductase–dependent reaction will lead to the trapping of folates as 5-methyl-$H_4PteGlu_n$, resulting in the impairment of other folate-dependent syntheses, e.g., thymidylate and purines.[14] This hypothesis explains the common clinical symptoms (i.e., megaloblastic anemia) seen in folate and vitamin B-12 deficiencies. A modified version of the "methyl folate trap hypothesis" proposed by Scott and Weir[15] was constructed to account for the early reports which showed that large doses of folic acid could ameliorate the hematological symptoms seen in B-12–deficient patients but may mask or may even precipitate neurological manifestations. According to this hypothesis, the normal response of the cell to a low methionine level is an increase in methyltetrahydrofolate synthesis. This is because SAM, a potent inhibitor of this synthesis, is also at a low level. As a consequence, folate coenzymes are diverted away from nucleic acids synthesis and toward increased methionine synthesis.

The cell responds to vitamin B-12 deficiency in the same manner as when methionine is limited. However, because in B-12 deficiency the (B-12–dependent) methylation of homocysteine is impaired, the 5-methyl-$H_4PteGlu_n$ formed will accumulate (be trapped) because other folate coenzymes are needed for nucleic acid synthesis, and their absence will result in the cessation of cell proliferation (megaloblastic anemia). The limited methionine that is available is now directed for methylation reactions, which include brain myelin. Intake of large doses of folic acid will provide the necessary coenzymes for nucleic acid synthesis and cell proliferation. Since methionine synthesis is still limited, the increase in cell proliferation will divert the limited supply of methionine away from methylation reactions and toward protein building blocks for newly formed cells. Brain myelin may become increasingly unmethylated under these conditions.

In recent years interest in plasma homocysteine has been growing because epidemiologic data link moderate elevations of plasma homocysteine (hyperhomocysteinemia) to higher prevalence of occlusive vascular disease and stroke.[16–20] Homocysteine is a sulfur amino acid whose metabolism is at the intersection of two metabolic pathways, remethylation and transsulfuration (Figure 3). In remethylation, homocysteine acquires a methyl group from 5-methyl-$H_4PteGlu_n$ or from betaine to form methionine. The reaction with 5-methyl-$H_4PteGlu_n$ occurs in all tissues and is vitamin B-12–dependent, while the reaction with betaine is confined mainly to the liver and is independent of vitamin B-12. A considerable proportion of methionine is then activated by ATP to form SAM. SAM serves primarily as a universal methyl donor to a variety of acceptors including guanidinoacetate, nucleic acids, neurotransmitters, phospholipids, and hormones. S-adenosylhomocysteine (SAH), the by-product of these methylation reactions, is subsequently hydrolyzed, thus regenerating homocysteine, which then becomes available to start a new cycle of methyl-group transfer.

In the transsulfuration pathway, homocysteine condenses with serine to form cystathionine in an irreversible reaction catalyzed by the pyridoxal-5'-phosphate (PLP)–containing enzyme, cystathionine β-synthase (CBS). Cystathionine is hydrolyzed by a second PLP-containing enzyme, γ-cystathionase, to form cysteine and α-ketobutyrate. Excess cysteine is oxidized to taurine or inorganic sulfates and excreted in the urine. Thus, in addition to the synthesis of cysteine, this transsulfuration pathway effectively catabolizes excess homocysteine that is not required for methyl transfer. Note that since homocysteine is not a normal dietary constituent, the dietary precursor of homocysteine is methionine.

The two pathways are coordinated by SAM. This function of SAM stems from its ability to serve as an allosteric inhibitor of methylenetetrahydrofolate reductase and as an activator of CBS.[19–24] Thus, when intracellular SAM concentration is high, homocysteine is diverted through the transsulfuration pathway because synthesis of 5-methyl-$H_4PteGlu_n$ is inhibited and the CBS enzyme is activated. Conversely, when SAM level is low, homocysteine is diverted toward remethylation because synthesis of 5-methyl-$H_4PteGlu_n$ is uninhibited and the activity of CBS is diminished.

A second tier of coordination lies in the propensity of 5-methyl-$H_4PteGlu_n$ to serve as an inhibitor of glycine N-methyltransferase.[25,26] This enzyme serves to regulate the level of cellular SAM. A high intracellular level of SAM will result in an inhibited synthesis of 5-methyl-$H_4PteGlu_n$, and that will release glycine N-methyltransferase from inhibition and allow it to rid the cell of excess SAM. When the concentration of 5-methyl-$H_4PteGlu_n$ is high because of low intracellular SAM level, glycine methylation is inhibited.

Folate compartmentation. Another important method of folate regulation is through compartmentation based on 1) asymmetric distribution of folate coenzymes between cytosol and mitochondria and 2) differential distribution of specific folate coenzymes because of binding proteins.

In liver cells the major pool of folate coenzymes are polyglutamyl derivatives, which are distributed in both the cytosol and mitochondria (Figure 3).[27] In cytosol 45% of total folates are methyl-$H_4PteGlu_n$, 30% are formyl-$H_4PteGlu_n$, and 25% are unsubstituted $H_4PteGlu_n$. In mitochondria only 7% of total folates are methyl-$H_4PteGlu_n$; the remainder are distributed between formyl-$H_4PteGlu_n$ (44%) and unsubstituted $H_4PteGlu_n$ (48%).[28]

CYTOPLASM   **MITOCHONDRIA**

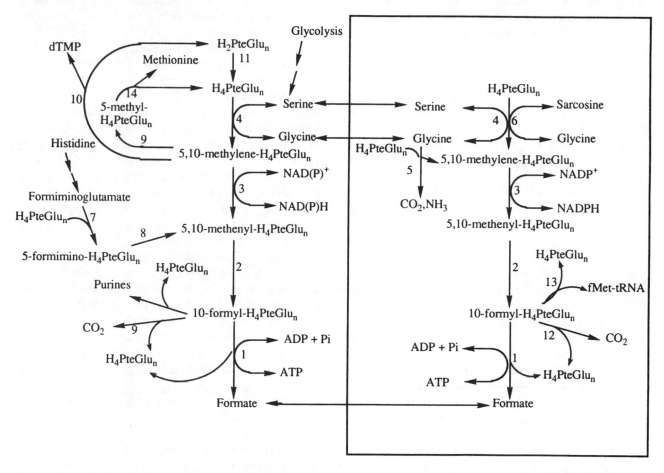

Figure 4. Organization of folate-mediated one-carbon metabolism in eukaryotes. Reactions 1,2, and 3: 10-formyltetrahydrofolate synthase, 5,10-methenyltetrahydrofolate cyclohydrolase, and 5,10-methylenetetrahydrofolate dehydrogenase, respectively, are catalyzed by C1-THF-synthase. The other reactions are catalyzed by: 4) serine hydroxymethylase; 5) glycine cleavage enzyme; 6) sarcosine dehydrogenase; 7) formimino-L-glutamate-tetrahydrofolate 5-formiminotransferase; 8) 5-formiminotetrahydrofolate cyclodeaminase; 9) 5,10-methylenetetrahydrofolate reductase; 10) thymidylate synthase; 11) dihydrofolate reductase; 12) 10- formyltetrahydrofolate dehydrogenase; 13) methionyl-tRNA formyltransferase; 14) N-5-methyltetrahydrofolate:homocysteine methyltransferase.

Folate-dependent enzymes are also distributed in these two compartments. The trifunctional enzyme C1-THF synthase (catalyzes reactions 3, 2, and 1 in Figure 4) is present in both compartments. Folylpolyglutamate synthase is also present in both compartments.[29] On the other hand, dihydrofolate reductase appears to be present in the cytosolic compartment only, whereas the glycine cleavage enzyme, sarcosine dehydrogenase, and dimethylglycine dehydrogenase are all mitochondrial.[29-31]

These distributions of folate coenzymes and folate-dependent enzymes are consistent with the known folate-mediated metabolic activities in each compartment. In the cytosol, folate coenzymes are involved in purine, thymidylate, and methionine syntheses. Serine-glycine interconversion occurs in both compartments, whereas glycine cleavage as well as oxidation of dimethylglycine and sarcosine occur in mitochondria.[32-34] Also in mitochondria, folate coenzymes are involved in the formyl-

ation of initiator transfer RNA for organelle protein synthesis (Figure 4).[35]

Folate-binding proteins (FBP) are either membrane-bound or intracellular.[36-38] The membrane-bound proteins are thought to be involved in folate transport. The high-affinity FBP is located in the brush-border membranes of the proximal tubular cells of kidney and was shown to mediate transport of folate through an endocytic pathway.[39-41] This protein is also found in the choroid plexus and outer placental membranes, where it is thought to function in a similar manner to that in the kidney.[42,43] These high-affinity FBPs appear to transport 5-methyl tetrahydrofolate selectively; hence they are in a way responsible for folate compartmentation. Other folate transport proteins with lower affinity have been described. The recently isolated reduced folate transporter is responsible for the cellular sequestration of reduced folates and methotrexate but not oxidized folates.[37,38]

Intracellular FBPs are distributed in both mitochondria and cytosolic compartments.[44] Two of the three FBPs in the cytosol have been identified as the enzymes 10-formyltetrahydrofolate dehydrogenase and glycine N-methyltransferase.[45,46] The mitochondrial FBPs were shown to correspond to dimethylglycine dehydrogenase and sarcosine dehydrogenase.[47]

Glycine N-methyltransferase, which catalyzes the methylation of glycine by SAM, contains bound 5-methyl-$H_4PteGlu_5$, which also acts as an inhibitor of this reaction.[25,46,48] It has been postulated that this inhibition of the glycine N-methyltransferase enzyme serves to regulate the level of SAM. Both of the mitochondrial FBPs catalyze the oxidative demethylation of their respective substrates to yield free formaldehyde. In the presence of their ligand ($H_4PteGlu_5$) formaldehyde is trapped as 5,10-methylene-$H_4PteGlu_5$ for use in C1-dependent metabolism.

In liver 60% of cytosolic folates and 20% of mitochondrial folates were found to be bound to intracellular FBPs.[49] It is suggested, however, that much cellular folate is bound to the enzymes of folate metabolism, and this binding is important to the sequestration of folate coenzymes for more efficient syntheses, particularly under conditions of limited folate supply.[50–52]

In substrate channeling, the intermediate products of a set of reactions are sequestered into the active site of the next enzyme without a dissociation step.[27] This phenomenon is caused by either a multifunctional enzyme or multienzyme complexes. Among the advantages predicted for such channeling is the high conversion rate that can be attained because the reactions are independent of bulk substrate concentrations and because the reaction intermediates are protected so they are not used for competing reactions. Channeling is susceptible to regulation through changes in the nature and extent of enzyme associations. C1-THF synthase is a trifunctional enzyme with two independent functional domains. One domain contains an overlapping active site shared by methylene-tetrahydrofolate dehydrogenase (reaction 3, Figure 4) and methenyl-tetrahydrofolate cyclohydrolase (reaction 2, Figure 4) on the NH_2 terminal. The other domain contains 10-formyl-tetrahydrofolate synthase activity in the COOH terminal (reaction 1, Figure 4). Channeling occurs between reactions 2 and 3 in the first domain (but not between the two domains), so that when 5,10-methylene-$H_4PteGlu_n$ is used as substrate, no lag period is observed before the final product, 10-formyl-$H_4PteGlu_n$, appears. Intermediates in these series of reactions (e.g., methenyl-$H_4PteGlu_n$) do not compete.

Tissue and Food Folate Analysis

Naturally occurring folates are present in a variety of forms that differ by the state of oxidation and carbon substitution of the pteridine ring and the number of glutamate residues in a γ-peptide linkage with the p-aminobenzoylglutamate moiety. Considerable effort has been directed to devising methods for the analysis of tissue and food folate distribution on the premise that information on folate distribution could provide the basis for understanding folate-dependent metabolism in tissues and folate bioavailability in food products. Initial information on the diversity of tissue and food folate distribution was derived from the use of the differential microbial assay.[53] The assay is based on the differing capacity of bacterial species to utilize different forms of folates. However, because bacteria cannot utilize polyglutamyl folates, extracts require prior treatment with pteroylpolyglutamate hydrolyses (e.g., conjugase) before assay. The information provided by the differential microbial assay is thus limited.

The use of thymidylate synthase to determine 5,10-methylenetetrahydrofolates. An electrophoretic assay method developed by Priest et al. is based on the incorporation of 5,10-methylene-$H_4PteGlu_n$ derivatives into a ternary complex with thymidylate synthase and 5-fluoro-2-deoxy[³H]uridylate.[54,55] Folate with different pteridine ring structures (folic acid , dihydro- and tetrahydrofolate, formyl, and methyltetrahydrofolates) can be identified following their conversion to 5,10-methylene-$H_4PteGlu_n$ using selective combinations of chemical and enzymatic reactions.

An important extension of this procedure is the ability to analyze folate polyglutamates. At pH 8.2 the same ternary complex is negatively charged to an extent that is determined by the number of glutamate residues of the attached folate. The higher the number of residues the more negatively charged the complex, which allows separation by gel electrophoresis. Separated folates are quantified by densitometry after autoradiography.[54,55] This method is suitable for the analysis of folate in small tissue samples, as in cell culture, and it is the only method capable of determining 5,10-methylene-tetrahydrofolate derivatives. However the need to convert all folates quantitatively to 5,10-methylene-tetrahydrofolates renders this method quite tedious. Recently this method was used with some modifications for the analysis of rat liver folates.[56]

Analysis of the glutamic acid chain length distribution. Analysis of the glutamic acid chain length distribution requires cleavage of the folate molecule at the C9-N10 bond and detection of the resulting p-aminobenzoylglutamate moieties as naphthylethylenediamine azo dye derivatives. Krumdieck et al.[57] have taken advantage of the different susceptibility of reduced folates (with and without one-carbon substitution) for oxidative cleavage to develop a differential cleavage approach which divides folates into three pools: pool 1 includes 5,10-methylene-THF, THF, and DHF derivatives; pool

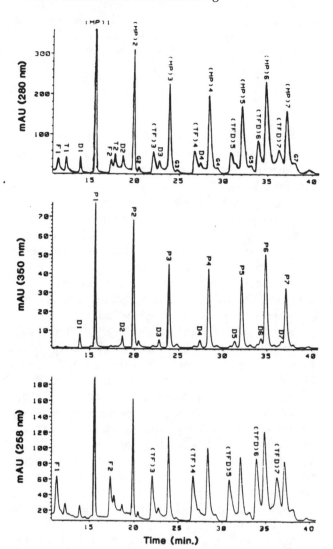

Figure 5. Chromatography of a mixture that contained PteGlu$_{1-7}$ and its various reduced forms, a total of 35 derivatives. Activities shown in the top panel represent absorption values at 282 nm, those in the middle panel 350 nm, and those in the bottom panel 258 nm. Symbols are as follow: F, 10-formyl-H$_4$PteGlu$_{1-7}$; T, H$_4$PteGlu$_{1-7}$; M, 5-methyl-H$_4$PteGlu$_{1-7}$; and P, PteGlu$_{1-7}$. Numbers following symbols refer to numbers of glutamate residues. Reprinted with permission from reference 59.

milk folate-binding protein attached to a Sepharose-4B as the affinity matrix. The HPLC system employs a reverse-phase C$_{18}$ column and a mobile phase that is composed of an acetonitrile gradient and tetrabutyl amino phosphate as an ion-pairing reagent. Figure 5 is the chromatographic pattern of a mixture of 35 forms of folate (with and without a carbon substitution) with glutamate chains ranging from one to seven. The chromatographic pattern is composed of seven clusters representing groups of folates with increasing numbers of glutamate residues. In clusters containing mono- and diglutamyl folates there was a separation between the 10-formyl- (F), the tetrahydro- (T), and the dihydro- (D) derivatives. In clusters containing higher numbers of residues these three folates tended to elute in the same fraction. In each cluster PteGlu$_n$ (P) and corresponding 5-methyl-H$_4$PteGlu$_n$ (M) eluted in the same peak, which was separate from the above three folates. The position of the eluting folate within the cluster provides a first screening for determining the pteridine ring structure. Spectral characteristics from the diode array detector provide the additional detail for final identification. Quantification of the activity peaks is based on individual peak area determined at 280, 258, and 350 nm (Figure 5), and corresponding "peak area extinction coefficients" are determined for each folate at these wavelengths.[59]

This new method of folate analysis has been applied to analysis of mammalian tissues and food products having diverse folate distribution.[60-64] The compositions determined by this method correspond closely with those published using other methods of analysis. Furthermore, the total folate contents estimated by summation of the concentration of the individual components closely correlate ($r=0.954$) with those obtained from the microbial assay using *Lactobacillus casei* after conjugase treatment.[63] This method is technically simple and quite rapid. A total of 24–30 analyses can be accomplished within a week by one person.

Functional Assessment of Folate Status

Folate deficiency can arise in a variety of settings, including alcoholism, low dietary intake, or malabsorption. It is seen under conditions of increased cellular turnover such as pregnancy, cancer, and hemolytic anemia. Several drugs, including sulfasalazine and diphenylhydantoin, interfere with folate absorption or use.

Advanced folate deficiency characteristically causes macrocytic or megaloblastic anemia, with abnormalities on peripheral blood smear and bone marrow examinations. Clinical manifestations of folate deficiency often resemble the hematologic features of vitamin B-12 deficiency. Status of both folate and B-12 should be evaluated in suspected cases.

2 consists of only 5-methyl-THF derivatives; and pool 3 consists of the various isomers of formyl-THF and 5-formimino-THF derivatives.

Combined-affinity chromatography and reverse-phase liquid chromatography (affinity/HPLC) for the analysis of tissue folate distribution. The affinity/HPLC method for folate analysis is based on the use of affinity chromatography for folate purification and a combination of HPLC separation and spectral analyses with a UV diode array detector.[58,59] Affinity chromatography uses a small column containing purified

Table 1. Laboratory assessment of folate nutriture

Measurement	Deficient levels	Low levels	Acceptable levels
Serum folate (nmol/L)	<6.7	6.7–13.2	>13.5
Red cell folate (nmol/L)	<315	315–358	>360

Laboratory tests. Measurement of serum folate is the most widely used method to assess folate status. For most clinical situations it is adequate because low body stores are reflected in low folate levels. A low serum folate level is not always a reflection of depleted body stores, however, because serum folate is sensitive to changes in intakes or temporary changes in folate metabolism.

Since red blood cell folate content is at least ten times the concentration of serum folate, another method of assessing folate status is the measurement of whole-blood folate. This method obviates the need to separate the two blood constituents. The serum acts as a source of conjugase to hydrolyze red cell folylpolyglutamates before microbial assay.[65] A standard method to determine folate levels is by microbial assay with *Lactobacillus casei*. Serum folate levels are determined directly while red cell levels are determined after treatment with conjugase. The method is sufficiently simple for routine use, but it is inadequate for blood samples containing antibiotics or methotrexate, compounds that interfere with bacterial growth.

In recent years, a widely applied technique is to use the high-affinity binding protein derived from milk to determine folate by competitive binding assay.[66] This method is not sensitive to antibiotics or methotrexate. It requires the use of a high pH in the incubation mixture because at physiologic pH the affinity for 5-methyltetrahydrofolate, the main constituent of serum folate, is much lower than for folic acid, which is used as the radioactive standard.[67] Before analysis serum samples must be boiled to destroy endogenous folate-binding protein.

Functional and synthetic product assays. Folate deficiency is associated with alteration of a number of biochemical reactions. The metabolism of histidine to glutamic acid is impaired in folate deficiency, which causes an increase in urinary excretion of formiminoglutamic acid (FIGLU) and urocanic acid. This occurs particularly after a loading dose (2–15 mg) of L-histidine.[68]

Folate deficiency also impairs the de novo synthesis of adenine compounds, and in consequence, there is an increased urinary excretion of adenine precursors such as aminoimidazolecarboxamide.[68]

The deoxyuridine suppression test is based on the capacity of a cell system to synthesize thymidylate de novo from added deoxyuridine (dUMP), a folate-dependent pathway, thereby diminishing (or competing for) incorporation of radioactive thymidine into cellular DNA. In folate deficiency, suppression by deoxyuridine of [³H]thymidine incorporation is diminished. The method uses aspirates of bone marrow or peripheral lymphocytes.[69,70]

Another functional test of folate status uses lymphocytes from patients to determine incorporation of [¹⁴C]formate into serine or methionine in the presence of excess glycine or homocysteine.[71] The method depends upon the presence of tetrahydrofolate coenzymes; hence in deficiency states a decrease in the incorporation of the radioactive formate is observed. The laboratory tests of folate status are summarized in Table 1.

The recognition of plasma homocysteine levels as a functional indicator of folate status stemmed principally from the recognition that moderate elevations of plasma homocysteine levels are associated with increased risk of occlusive vascular disease and stroke.[16–19] Vitamin status and plasma homocysteine concentrations are inversely correlated in nonlinear fashion.[72,73] There is a plasma folate level (≈6 ng/mL) beyond which homocysteine concentrations remain unchanged and below which concentrations increase. Similar though weaker correlations have been observed between (nonfasting) plasma homocysteine and vitamin B-12 and PLP plasma concentrations.[72,74]

Plasma homocysteine also may serve to assess the adequacy of folate intake. Data from the Framingham Study demonstrated a strong inverse correlation between folate intake (estimated by food frequency questionnaire) and plasma homocysteine levels. The pattern is similar to that of plasma folate.[72] An estimated intake of ≈400 μg/day appears to be adequate for maintaining low homocysteine plasma levels.

Folate Absorption and Food Folate Bioavailability

Much of our present knowledge of intestinal absorption of folates is derived from studies that used crystalline folate compounds.[75–78] These studies can be summarized as follows: 1) Intestinal folate absorption occurs at the monoglutamate level; hence hydrolysis of folylpolyglutamates to monoglutamyl derivatives is a necessary step for this process. 2) In man and pig the brush-border membrane of the small intestine contains a pteroylpolyglutamate hydrolase (PPH) that is distinct from that found within the enterocyte, by its pH requirement, size, and sensitivity to inhibitors.[79] It is suggested that in man and pig this brush-border enzyme is, at least in part, responsible for the hydrolysis of dietary folate polyglutamates.[79,80] 3) The intestinal transport of monoglutamyl folates occurs by a carrier-mediated process that is equally shared by reduced and oxidized monoglutamyl derivatives as well as by the antifolate methotrexate. This transport is highly pH dependent, with an optimum pH of 5.0–6.0, and declines sharply with increase in pH. A second transport mechanism is simple diffusion. This transport predominates at higher luminal pH or at pharmacological folate concentrations.

In spite of this information our knowledge of the bioavailability of food folates is fragmentary. The paucity of information stems principally from the complexity of dietary folates, their low level in various foods, the presence of dietary factors such as inhibitors of PPH that could affect folate bioavailability, and the inability to distinguish between newly absorbed folate and endogenous folates. The use of deuterated folate for studying intestinal folate absorption in man is a step in the right direction.[81] The use of these folates in their crystalline form has provided valuable new information about the characteristics of intestinal folate absorption in man.[82,83] Deuterated folates were used for a long-term study to determine body pool and body turnover of folates.[84] The possibility of applying this approach to the study of a variety of parameters, including assessment of folate status and folate requirement, is quite exciting. However, exactly how these deuterated folates can be used to study the absorption of food folates remains to be determined.

Folic Acid and Disease

Beginning with the association of folic acid with macrocytic anemia and even its mistaken role as the anti–pernicious anemia principle in the 1930s, the primary clinical relationship of folic acid has been its hemopoietic effect in the prevention and treatment of macrocytic or megaloblastic anemia. Given the additional nutritional stress of pregnancy, folic acid deficiency and megaloblastic anemia of pregnancy continue to be of worldwide importance. The effects of excessive alcohol and alcoholism on the intake, absorption, metabolism, and utilization of folate have made that pathogenic relationship important. These relationships of folic acid to macrocytic anemia have been well described in previous issues of *Present Knowledge in Nutrition* and in numerous reviews. In the spirit of presenting present and newly emerging knowledge about folic acid nutrition in the clinical arena, we will address some emerging information on inherited abnormalities of folate metabolism and the connection of folic acid with neural tube defects, cancer, and heart disease.

Folate interaction with a common mutation. Like many other congenital disorders, those that are caused by abnormalities in folate metabolism are rare and are in the domain of specialists in genetic and metabolic disorders.[85] In 1988 Kang et al.[86] reported a variant of methylenetetrahydrofolate reductase (MTHFR) that was distinguishable from the normal enzyme by its lower specific activity and its heat sensitivity (thermolability). In subsequent studies the authors suggested that this thermolabile variant was an inherited autosomal recessive trait present in ≈5% of the general population and in 17% of patients with coronary artery disease.[87] A group headed by Rozen[88] isolated the cDNA for human MTHFR and demonstrated that the thermolability is caused by a missense mutation of alanine (ala) to valine (val). Using PCR techniques, a number of laboratories have shown that the frequency in the normal population of homozygous mutant genotype is higher than that predicted by the enzymatic studies of Kang et al.[86] and stands at 12%.

It is too early to predict the importance of this mutation in the prevalence of disease. MTHFR thermolability may be associated with moderate hyperhomocysteinemia.[89] Early evidence implies a higher prevalence of homozygotes for alanine to valine mutations among mothers who have given birth to a child with neural tube defect and also among people with cardiovascular disease.

Folate and cancer. Early clinical studies of folic acid suggested a relationship between megaloblastic morphologic changes in tissues of individuals with folate deficiency and the appearance of precancerous cells. In 1954 Massey and Rubin[90] postulated that cytologically abnormal cells in the stomach might represent a transitional cell type between those cells that characterize the atrophic gastric epithelium in folate deficiency or pernicious anemia, and gastric cancer cells. Two decades later, prospective controlled clinical intervention trials by investigators at the University of Alabama found regression of dysplasia of epithelial cells in the uterine cervix and reversion of metaplasia in tracheobronchus epithelial cells.[91,92] Studies such as these are potentially confounded by the cytological similarities of megaloblastic and dysplastic cells. Since the Alabama studies several more epidemiologic studies have related folate nutrition to precancerous dysplastic changes in cervical epithelium and the colorectal epithelium.[93–105] Animal studies have demonstrated that carcinogen-induced colon cancer is induced more quickly and with greater severity in folate-deficient animals.[104] The relationship of folate to DNA methylation, DNA repair, and oncogene expression have provided the basis for hypotheses relating folate nutriture to cancer risk and prevention. Several trials now underway are exploring the possibility that increased folate intake or supplementation may lessen the risk of developing cancer in stomach and colon or the risk of pre-cancerous colonic polyps progressing to colon cancer.

The most convincing epidemiologic evidence of an association between folate status and colorectal neoplasia was published after a study of >25,000 people showed that increased folate intake was inversely associated with the incidence of adenomatous polyps in the distal half of the colorectum.[105] Thus, a growing body of clinical studies suggest that folate status can modulate the process of carcinogenesis. The evidence is strongest with respect to colorectal cancer, where the effects occur with relatively modest alterations in folate status and may be present when vitamin status is altered within the range of what is presently considered to be normal.

Folate and neural tube defects. One of the most compelling studies relating vitamins and disease was the randomized controlled clinical trial which showed that a nutritional supplement containing folic acid successfully and markedly reduced the occurrence of neural tube defects (spina bifida or anencephaly) in babies when the intervention was administered before conception.[106] This was the culmination of a quarter century of research dominated by observational studies showing that folate supplements protected against some neural tube defects. Another randomized controlled clinical trial had shown that large doses of folic acid (4 mg) administered before pregnancy could successfully prevent the recurrence of a neural tube defect in children born to mothers who had previously had a child with such a defect.[107] Such studies have given rise to recommendations in several countries, including the United States, that women capable of becoming pregnant should consume 400 μg of folate daily. In several countries fortification of flour is under consideration as one approach, along with improved diet, to ensure adequate folate intake. The mechanism by which increased folate intake might affect neural tube defect continues to be uncertain. It is almost certain that neural tube defect occurs as a result of complex genetic and nutritional interactions. Some genetic alterations that have been proposed as participants in the pathogenesis are abnormalities of the methionine synthase gene and polymorphisms of methylene tetrahydrofolate reductase (MTHFR) gene. Preliminary studies suggest that the heat-labile variant of MTHFR is associated with risk of neural tube defect (Blom et al., personal communication). The possibility that elevated homocysteine levels secondary to nutritional or genetic abnormalities might have toxic effects on the fetus at the critical time of neural tube closure is currently under investigation.

Folate, homocysteine, and cardiovascular disease and stroke. The association between plasma homocysteine concentration and thrombo-occlusive heart disease has recently become the subject of many clinical studies that link moderate elevations of plasma homocysteine to symptomatic peripheral vascular, cerebrovascular, and coronary heart disease.[16-18] Pooled results from retrospective studies indicate that fasting plasma homocysteine concentrations in patients with vascular disease are on average 31% higher than in normal subjects. Abnormal plasma homocysteine concentration after an oral methionine challenge is 12 times more prevalent in patients with cardiovascular disease than in normal subjects. Prospective studies of middle-aged male physicians in the United States indicated that plasma homocysteine concentrations of only 17 μmol/L, or 12% above the upper limit of normal, were associated with a 3.4-fold increase in the risk of acute myocardial infarction.[18] In the Framingham Heart Study, the longest observed cohort study on vascular disease, it has been demonstrated that folic acid, vitamin B-12, and vitamin B-6 are determinants of plasma homocysteine levels, with folic acid showing the strongest association (in this and several other studies).[108,109] In that same population, ultrasound demonstrated that homocysteine plasma levels were strong predictors of carotid artery narrowing. Such narrowing is predictive of the risk of both stroke and coronary disease. The pathogenetic mechanisms by which plasma homocysteine may be associated with increased thrombo-occlusive vascular disease have not been clearly established. Possible mechanisms include direct toxic effects of the sulfur amino acid on vascular endothelium, prothrombotic or antithrombolytic effects on platelets or clotting control mechanisms, and the induction of changes in vascular reactivity.

Numerous studies have demonstrated that homocysteine levels are responsive to intervention, the most effective vitamin intervention being folic acid, with or without vitamins B-12 and vitamin B-6. Intervention trials to examine the impact of reduced homocysteine levels on the morbidity and mortality from heart disease and stroke are under development.

Acknowledgment

We are honored to dedicate this chapter to E. L. Robert Stokstad (1933–1995), who contributed so much throughout his life to our present knowledge in nutrition.

References

1. Stokstad ELR (1992) Historical perspective on key advances in the biochemistry and physiology of folates. In Picciano MF, Stokstad LR, Gregory JF III (eds), Folic acid metabolism in health and disease. Wiley-Liss, New York, pp 1–21
2. Rosenberg IH, Goodwin HA (1973) The digestion and absorption of dietary folate. Gastroenterology 60:455–463
3. Mitchell HK, Snell EE, Williams RJ (1941) The concentration of "folic acid." Am Chem Soc 63:2284
4. Horne DW, Patterson D, Cook R (1991) Effect of nitrous oxide inactivation of vitamin B12-dependent methionine synthetase on the subcellular distribution of folate coenzymes in rat liver. Arch Biochem Biophys 272:749–753

5. Osborne CB, Lowe KE, Shane B (1993). Regulation of folate and one-carbon metabolism in mammalian cells. I. Folate metabolism in Chinese hamster ovary cells expressing *Escherichia coli* or human folylpoly-gamma-glutamate synthetase activity. J Biol Chem 269:21657–21664

6. Lowe KE, Osborne CB, Lin BF, et al (1994) Regulation of folate and one-carbon metabolism in mammalian cells. II. Effect of folylpoly-gamma-glutamate synthetase substrate specificity and level on folate metabolism and folylpoly-gamma-glutamate specificity of metabolic cycles of one-carbon metabolism. J Biol Chem 269:21665–21685

7. Lin BF, Huang RF, Shane B (1993) Regulation of folate and one-carbon metabolism in mammalian cells. III. Role of mitochondrial folylpoly-gamma-glutamate synthetase. J Biol Chem 269:21684–21691

8. Kim JS, Lowe KM, Shane B (1993) Regulation of folate and one-carbon metabolism in mammalian cells. IV. Role of folylpoly-gamma-glutamate synthetase in methotrexate metabolism and cytotoxicity. J Biol Chem 269:21692–21697

9. Lin BF, Shane B (1994) Expression of *Escherichia coli* folylpolyglutamate synthetase in the Chinese hamster ovary cell mitochondrion. J Biol Chem 270:9725–9733

10. Taylor RT, Hanna ML (1979) Folate-dependent enzymes in cultured Chinese hamster cells: folylpolyglutamate synthetase and its absence in mutants auxotrophic for glycine + adenosine + thymidine. Arch Biochem Biophys 181: 331–344

11. Bertino JR, Coward JK, Cashmore A, et al (1978) Polyglutamate forms of folate: natural occurrence and role as substrates in mammalian cells. Biochem Soc Trans 4: 875–878

12. Matthews RG, Baugh CM (1982) Interactions of pig liver methylenetetrahydrofolate reductase with methylene-tetrahydro-pteroylpolyglutamate substrates and with dihydropteroylpolyglutamate inhibitors. Biochemistry 19: 2040–2045

13. Krumdieck CL (1985) Role of folate deficiency in carcinogenesis. In Butterworth CE, Hutchinson ML (eds), Nutritional factors in the induction and maintenance of malignancy. Academic Press, New York, pp 225–245

14. Herbert V, Zalusky R (1962) Interrelations of vitamin B12 and folic acid metabolism: folic acid clearance studies. J Clin Invest 41:1263–1278

15. Scott JM, Weir DG (1981) The methyl folate trap: a physiological response in man to prevent methyl group deficiency in kwashiorkor (methionine deficiency) and an explanation for folic-acid induced exacerbation of subacute combined degeneration in pernicious anemia. Lancet 2(8442):337–340

16. Ueland PM, Refsum H, Brattstrom L (1992) Plasma homocysteine and cardiovascular disease. In Francis RBJ (ed), Atherosclerotic cardiovascular disease, hemostasis, and endothelial function. Marcel Dekker, New York, pp 185–236

17. Ueland PM, Refsum H (1991) Plasma homocysteine, a risk factor for vascular disease: plasma levels in health, disease, and drug therapy. J Lab Clin Med 114(5):475–501

18. Stampfer MJ, Malinow MR, Willett WC, et al (1992) A prospective study of plasma homocyst(e)ine and risk of myocardial infarction in US physicians. JAMA 269:897–901

19. Selhub J, Miller JW (1993) The pathogenesis of homocysteinemia: interruption of the coordinate regulation by S-adenosylmethionine of the remethylation and transsulfuration of homocysteine. Am J Clin Nutr 55:131–138

20. Jencks DA, Matthews RG (1989) Allosteric inhibition of methylenetetrahydrofolate reductase by adenosylmethionine. J Biol Chem 1262(6):2487–2493

21. Kutzbach C, Stokstad ELR (1973) Mammalian methylene-tetrahydrofolate reductase: partial purification, properties, and inhibition by S-adenosylmethionine. Biochim Biophys Acta 250:459–479

22. Kutzbach C, Stokstad ELR (1968) Feedback inhibition of methylene-tetrahydrofolate reductase in rat liver by S-adenosylmethionine. Biochim Biophys Acta 139:217–220

23. Finkelstein JD, Kyle WE, Martin JJ, Pick AM (1975) Activation of cystathionine synthase by adenosylmethionine and adenosylethionine. Biochem Biophys Res Commun 66(1):81–89

24. Koracevic D, Djordjevic V (1979) Effect of trypsin, S-adenosylmethionine and ethionine on L-serine sulfhydrase activity. Experientia 33:1010–1011

25. Cook J, Wagner C (1984) Glycine N-methyltransferase is a folate binding protein of rat liver cytosol. Proc Natl Acad Sci USA 81:3631–3634

26. Wagner C, Briggs WT, Cook RJ (1987) Inhibition of glycine N-methyltransferase activity by folate derivatives: implications for regulation of methyl group metabolism. Biochem Biophys Res Commun 127(3):746–752

27. Appling RD (1993) Compartmentation of folate-mediated one-carbon metabolism in eukaryotes. FASEB J 5:2645–2651

28. Horne DW, Patterson D, Cook R (1991) Effect of nitrous oxide inactivation of vitamin B12-dependent methionine synthetase on the subcellular distribution of folate coenzymes in rat liver. Arch Biochem Biophys 272:749–753

29. Wang FK, Kock J, Stokstad ELR (1968) Folate coenzyme pattern, folate linked enzymes and methionine biosynthesis in rat liver mitochondria. J Biochem 346:458–466

30. Motokawa Y, Kikuchi G (1973) Glycine metabolism in rat liver mitochondria. V. Intramitochondrial localization of the reversible glycine cleavage system and serine hydroxymethyltransferase. Arch Biochem Biophys 146:461–466

31. Frisell WR, Patwardhan MV, Mackenzie CG (1965) Quantitative studies on the soluble compartments of light and heavy mitochondria from rat liver. J Biol Chem 240:1849–1855

32. Schirch L (1984). Folates in serine and glycine metabolism. In Blakely RL, Benkovic SJ (eds), Folates and pterins, vol 1. Wiley, New York, pp 399–431

33. Kikuchi G (1975) The glycine cleavage system: composition, reaction mechanism, and physiologic significance. Mol Cell Biochem 1:170–189

34. Lewis KF, Randolph VM, Nemeth E, Frisell WR (1980) Oxidation of one-carbon compounds to formate and carbon dioxide in rat liver mitochondria. Arch Biochem Biophys 187:443–449

35. Staben C, Rabinowitz JC (1984) Formation of formyl-methionyl-tRNA and initiation of protein synthesis. In Blakley RL, Benkovic SJ (eds), Folates and Pterins, vol 1. Wiley, New York, pp 457–495

36. Henderson GB (1992) Folate binding proteins. Annu Rev Nutr 10:319–335

37. Antony AC (1992) The biological chemistry of folate receptors. Blood 79:2827–2840

38. Ratnman M, Freisheim JH (1992) Proteins involved in the transport of folates and antifolates by normal and neoplastic cells. In Picciano MF, Sokstad ELR, Gregory JF III (eds), Folic acid metabolism in health and disease. Wiley-Liss, New York, pp 93–120

39. Selhub J, Emmanuel D, Stavropoulos T, Arnold R (1989) Renal folate absorption and the kidney folate binding protein (FBP). I. Urinary clearance studies. Am J Physiol 252:F750–F756

40. Selhub J, Nakamura S, Carone FA (1989) Renal folate absorption and the kidney folate binding protein. II. Microinfusion studies. Am J Physiol 252:F757–F780

41. Birn H, Selhub J, Christensen EI (1993) Internalization and

intracellular transport of folate-binding protein in rat kidney proximal tubule. Am J Physiol 264(33):C302–C310

42. Spector R (1979) Identification of folate binding protein in choroid plexus. J Biol Chem 252:3364–3372

43. Green T, Ford HC (1984) Human placental microvilli contain high affinity binding sites for folate. J Biol Chem 218:75–82

44. Zamierowski MM, Wagner C (1974) High molecular weight complexes of folic acid in mammalian tissues. Biochem Biophys Res Commun 60:81–89

45. Min H, Shane B, Stokstad ELR (1990) Identification of 10-formyltetrahydrofolate dehydrogenase-hydrolase as a major folate binding protein in liver cytosol. Biochim Biophys Acta 968:348–353

46. Cook RJ, Wagner C (1984) Glycine N-methyltransferase is a folate binding protein of rat liver cytosol. Proc Natl Acad Sci USA 81:3631–3634

47. Wittwer AJ, Wagner C (1981) Identification of the folate-binding proteins of rat liver mitochondria as dimethylglycine dehydrogenase and sarcosine dehydrogenase: purification and folate-binding characteristics. J Biol Chem 256:4102–4108

48. Wagner C, Briggs WT, Cook RJ (1987) Inhibition of glycine N-methyl transferase activity by folate derivatives: implications for regulation of methyl group metabolism. Biochem Biophys Res Commun 127:746–752

49. Zamierowski MM, Wagner C (1979) Effect of folacin deficiency on folacin-binding proteins in the rat. J Nutr 107:1937–1945

50. Matherly LH, Czaijowski A, Muench SP, Psiakis JT (1992) Role for cytosolic folate-binding proteins in the compartmentation of endogenous tetrahydrofolates and the 5-formyl tetrahydrofolate-mediated enhancement of 5-fluoro-2-deoxyuridine antitumor activity in vitro. Cancer Res 50:3262–3270

51. Matherly LH, Muench SP (1992) Evidence for a localized conversion of endogenous tetrahydrofolate cofactors to dihydrofolate as an important element in antifolate action in murine leukemia cells. Biochem Pharmacol 39:2005–2014

52. Strong WB, Schirch V (1991) In vitro conversion of formate to serine: effect of tetrahydropteroylpolyglutamates and serine hydroxymethyltransferase on the rate of 10-formyltetrahydrofolate synthetase. Biochemistry 28:9430–9439

53. Bird OD, McGlohon M, Vaitkus JW (1965) Naturally occurring folates in the blood and liver of the rat. Anal Biochem 12:18–35

54. Priest DG, Happel KK, Doig MT (1980) Electrophoretic identification of poly-g-glutamate chain-lengths of 5,10-methylenetetrahydrofolate using thymidylate synthetase complexes. J Biochem Biophys Methods 3:201–206

55. Priest DG, Happel KK, Magnum M, et al (1981) Tissue folylpolyglutamate chain-length characterization by electrophoresis as thymidylate synthetase-fluorodeoxyuridylate ternary complexes. Anal Biochem 115:163–170

56. Carl GF, Smith JL (1995) Simultaneous measurement of one-carbon and polyglutamate derivatives of folic acid in rat liver using enzymatic interconversions of folates followed by ternary complex formation with thymidylate synthetase and 5-fluorodeoxyuridylic acid: standardization of the method. J Nutr 125(5):1245–1257

57. Krumdieck CL, Tamura T, Eto S (1985) Synthesis and analysis of the pteroylpolyglutamates. Vitam Horm 40:45–94

58. Selhub J, Darcy-Vrillon B, Fell D (1990) Affinity chromatography of naturally occurring folate derivatives. Anal Biochem 169:247–251

59. Selhub J (1991) Determination of tissue folate composition by affinity chromatography followed by high pressure ion pair liquid chromatography. Anal Biochem 184:84–93

60. Selhub J, Seyoum E, Pomfret EA, Zeisel S (1993) Effects of choline deficiency and methotrexate treatment upon liver folate content and distribution. Cancer Res 51:16–21

61. Varela-Moreiras G, Selhub J (1992) Long-term folate deficiency alters folate content and distribution differentially in rat tissues. J Nutr 122:986–993

62. Varela-Moreiras G, Selhub J, Dacosta KA, Zeisel SH (1993) Effect of chronic choline deficiency in rats on liver folate content and distribution. J Nutr Biochem 3:519–522

63. Seyoum E, Selhub J (1993) Combined affinity and ion pair column chromatographies for the analysis of food folate. J Nutr Biochem 4:490–494

64. Hidiroglou N, Camilo ME, Beckehauer HC, et al (1994) Effect of chronic alcohol ingestion on hepatic folate distribution in the rat. Biochem Pharm 47(9):1561–1566

65. McGuire JJ, Coward JK (1984) Pteroylglutamates: biosynthesis, degradation, and function. In Blakley RL, Benkovic SJ (eds), Folates and pterins, vol 1. Wiley, New York, pp 136–180

66. Rothenberg SP, daCosta M (1978) Folate-binding proteins and radioassay for folate. Clin Haematol 5:570–589

67. Givas JK, Gutcho S (1975) pH dependence of the binding of folates to milk binder in radioassay of folates. Clin Chem 21:427–428

68. Sauberlich HE, Dowdy RP, Skala JH (1974) Laboratory tests for the assessment of nutritional status. CRC Press, Boca Raton, FL

69. Das KC, Herbert V (1980) The lymphocyte as a marker of past nutritional status: persistence of abnormal deoxyuridine (dU) suppression test and chromosomes in patients with past deficiency of folate and vitamin B12. Br J Haematol 38:219–233

70. Das KC, Herbert V, Coleman N (1980) Unmasking covert folate deficiency in iron-deficient subjects with neutrophil hypersegmentation: dU suppression tests on lymphocytes and bone marrow. Br J Haematol 39:357–375

71. Ellegaard J, Esmann V (1972) A sensitive test for folic-acid deficiency. Lancet 1:308

72. Selhub J, Jacques PF, Wilson PWF, et al (1993) Vitamin status and intake as primary determinants of homocysteinemia in an elderly population. JAMA 272:2703–2708

73. Kang S, Wong PWK, Norusis M (1989) Homocysteinemia due to folate deficiency. Metabolism 136:458–462

74. Stabler SP, Marcell PD, Podell ER, et al (1990) Elevation of total homocysteine in the serum of patients with cobalamin or folate deficiency detected by capillary gas chromatography-mass spectrometry. J Clin Invest 81:466–474

75. Rosenberg IH, Zimmerman J, Selhub J (1987) Folate transport. Chimioterapia 4:354–358

76. Rosenberg IH, Selhub J (1986) Intestinal absorption of folates In Blakley RL (ed), Folates and pterins, vol 3. Wiley, New York, pp 148–178

77. Halsted CH (1992) Intestinal absorption of dietary folates. In Picciano MF, Sokstad ELR, Gregory JS III (eds), Folic acid metabolism in health and disease. Wiley-Liss Inc. , New York, pp 23–45

78. Mason JB (1992) Intestinal transport of monoglutamyl folates in mammalian systems. In Picciano MF, Sokstad ELR, Gregory JF III (eds), Folic acid metabolism in health and disease. Wiley-Liss Inc., New York, pp 47–63

79. Reisenauer AM, Krumdieck CL, Halsted CH (1979) Folate conjugase: two separate activities in human jejunum. Science 198:196–197

80. Gregory JF, Ink SL, Cerda JJ (1989) Comparison of ptero-

ylpolyglutamate hydrolase (folate conjugase) from porcine and human intestinal brush border membrane. Comp Biochem Physiol 90B:1135–1141

81. Gregory JF III, Toth JP (1992) Stable-isotopic methods for in vivo investigation of folate absorption and metabolism. In Picciano MF, Sokstad ELR, Gregory JF III (eds), Folic acid metabolism in health and disease. Wiley-Liss, New York, pp 151–170

82. Gregory JF III, Bhandari SD, Bailey LB, et al (1992) Relative bioavailability of deuterium-labeled monoglutamyl tetra-hydrofolates and folic acid in human subjects. Am J Clin Nutr 55(6):1147–1153

83. Gregory JF III, Bhandari SD, Bailey LB, et al (1991) Relative bioavailability of deuterium-labeled monoglutamyl and hexaglutamyl folates in human subjects. Am J Clin Nutr 54:736–740

84. van der Porten AE, Gregory JF III, Toth JP, et al (1992) In vivo folate kinetics during chronic supplementation of human subjects with deuterium-labeled folic acid. J Nutr 122(6):1293–1299

85. Rosenblatt DS (1991) Inherited disorders of folate transport and metabolism. In Scriver CR, Beaudet AL, Sly WS, Valle D (eds), The metabolic basis for inherited disease. McGraw-Hill, New York, pp 2049–2064

86. Kang SS, Zhou J, Wong PWK, et al (1990) Intermediate homocysteinemia: a thermolabile variant of methylene-tetrahydrofolate reductase. Am J Hum Genet 43:414–421

87. Kang SS, Wong PWK, Susmano A, et al (1993) Thermolabile methylenetetrahydrofolate reductase: an inherited risk factor for coronary heart disease. Am J Hum Genet 48:536–545

88. Goyette P, Sumner JS, Milos R, et al (1994) Human meth-ylenetetrahydrofolate reductase: isolation of cDNA, mapping and mutation identification. Nature Genetics 7:195–200

89. Frosst P, Blom HJ, Mikos R, et al (1995) A candidate genetic risk factor for vascular disease: a common mutation in methylenetetrahydrofolate reductase. Nature Genetics 10:111–113

90. Massey B, Rubin C (1954) The stomach in pernicious anemia: a cytologic study. Am J Med Sci 227:481–492

91. Butterworth C Jr, Hatch K, Gore H, et al (1984) Improvement in cervical dysplasia associated with folic acid therapy in users of oral contraceptives. Am J Clin Nutr 35:75–84

92. Heimburger D, Alexander C, Birch R, et al (1990) Improvement in bronchial squamous metaplasia in smokers treated with folate and vitamin B12. JAMA 259:1525–1530

93. Butterworth C Jr, Hatch K, Soong SJ, et al (1992) Folate deficiency and cervical dysplasia. JAMA 268:528–533

94. Brock K, Berry G, Mock P, et al (1990) Nutrients in diet and plasma and risk of in situ cervical cancer. J Natl Cancer Inst 82:582–587

95. Verreault R, Chu J, Mandelson M, Shy K (1991) A case-control study of diet and invasive cervical cancer. Int J Cancer 43:1050–1054

96. Ziegler R, Brinton L, Mammon R, et al (1992) Diet and risk of invasive cervical cancer among white women in the United States. Am J Epidemiol 132:432–445

97. Ziegler R, Jones C, Brinton CL, et al (1993) Diet and risk of in situ cervical cancer among white women in the United States. Cancer Causes Control 2:17–29

98. Potischman N, Brinton L, Laiming V, et al (1993) A case control study of serum folate levels and invasive cervical cancer. Cancer Res 51:4807–4811

99. Lashner B, Heidenreich P, Su G, et al (1991) The effect of folate supplementation on the incidence of dysplasia and cancer in chronic ulcerative colitis. Gastroenterology 97:255–259

100. Lashner B (1993) Red blood cell folate is associated with the development of dysplasia and cancer in ulcerative colitis. J Cancer Res Clin Biol 119:549–554

101. Freudenheim J, Graham S, Marshall J, et al (1993) Folate intake and carcinogenesis of the colon and rectum. Int J Epidemiol 20:369–374

102. Benito E, Stiggelbout A, Bosch F, et al (1993) Nutritional factors in colorectal cancer risk: a case-control study in Majorca. Int J Cancer 49:161–168

103. Meyer F, White E (1993) Alcohol and nutrients in relation to colon cancer in middle-aged adults. Am J Epidemiol 138:225–236

104. Cravo M, Mason J, Dayal Y, et al (1992) Folate deficiency enhances the development of colonic neoplasia in dimeth-ylhydrazine-treated rats. Cancer Res 52:5002–5006

105. Giovannucci E, Stampfer M, Colditz G, et al (1993) Folate, methionine, and alcohol intake and risk of colorectal adenoma. J Natl Cancer Inst 87:895–904

106. Czeizel AE (1995) Folic acid in the prevention of neural tube defects. J Pediatr Gastroenterol Nutr 2:4–16

107. Medical Research Council Vitamin Study Research Group (1991) Prevention of neural tube defects: results of the Medical Research Council Vitamin Study. Lancet 338: 131–137

108. Selhub J, Jacques PF, Wilson PWF, et al (1993) Vitamin status and intake as primary determinants of homocysteinemia in an elderly population. JAMA 270:2693–2698

109. Selhub J, Jacques PF, Bostom AG, et al (1995) Association between plasma homocysteine and extracranial carotid artery stenosis. N Engl J Med 332:286–291

Chapter 22

Biotin

Donald M. Mock

This chapter provides a summary of current knowledge of biotin nutrition, references to a few classic observations, and a detailed bibliography of publications since 1989. The reader is referred to the sixth edition of *Present Knowledge in Nutrition* and other recent reviews for additional readings in biotin nutrition.[1-5]

History of Discovery

Although a growth requirement for the "bios" fraction had been demonstrated in yeast, Boas was the first to demonstrate the requirement for biotin in a mammal.[4] In rats fed protein derived from egg white, Boas observed a syndrome of severe dermatitis, hair loss, and neuromuscular dysfunction known as "egg-white injury." A factor present in liver cured the egg-white injury and was named "protective factor X." It is now recognized that the critical event in this "egg-white injury" of both the human and the rat is the highly specific and very tight binding ($K_d = 10^{-15}M$) of biotin by avidin, a glycoprotein found in egg white. Native avidin is resistant to intestinal proteolysis in both the free and biotin-combined form. Thus, dietary avidin (e.g., in diets containing uncooked egg white) is thought to bind and prevent the absorption of both dietary biotin and any biotin synthesized by intestinal bacteria.

Structure, Chemistry, and Biochemistry of Biotin

Structure. The structure of biotin (Figure 1) was independently elucidated by Kogl and by du Vigneaud in the early 1940s.[2,4] Because biotin has three asymmetric carbons in its structure, eight stereoisomers exist; of these only one, designated d-(+)-biotin, is found in nature and is enzymatically active. This compound is generally referred to simply as biotin or D-biotin. Biocytin (ε-N-biotinyl-L-lysine) is about as active as biotin on a mole basis in mammalian growth studies.

Biotin is a bicyclic compound. One of the rings contains a ureido group (-N-CO-N-), and the other contains sulfur and is termed a tetrahydrothiophene ring. The two rings have a boat configuration with respect to each other. The tetrahydrothiophene ring has a valeric acid side chain. On the basis of binding of biotin analogs by avidin and x-ray crystallography of the biotin-avidin complex,[1] the ureido ring of the molecule is the most important region regarding the extraordinarily tight binding of biotin to avidin and to streptavidin, a protein similar to avidin that is excreted by *Streptomyces avidinii*. Other studies suggest that the length of the side chain or the apolar nature of the -CH$_2$- moieties in the side chain also play a role in the binding of biotin to the hydrophobic site on avidin.[1]

Chemical synthesis of biotin. The structure of biotin was confirmed by de novo chemical synthesis by Harrison and co-workers in the 1940s.[4] As reviewed recently, all the early synthetic methods suffered from the disadvantage that either the yield of the proper stereospecific isomer was low or that special intermediates were required to obtain stereospecificity.[4,6] These shortcomings are avoided by the stereospecific synthesis developed by Goldberg and Sternbach in 1949 in the laboratories of Hoffmann-La Roche.[4,6,7] The Goldberg/Sternbach synthesis or modifications thereof are the methods by which biotin is synthesized commercially.[4] Additional stereospecific methods of synthesis have been published recently.[8,9]

Biochemistry of biotin. In mammals, biotin serves as an essential cofactor for four carboxylases, each of which catalyzes a critical step in intermediary metabolism.[10] All four of the mammalian carboxylases catalyze the incorporation of bicarbonate into a substrate as a carboxyl group. Four similar carboxylases, two other carboxylases, two decarboxylases, and a transcarboxylase are found in nonmammalian organisms. All of these biotin-dependent enzymes appear to work by a similar mechanism in all animals.

Attachment of the biotin to the apocarboxylase (Figure 1) is a condensation reaction catalyzed by holocarboxylase synthetase. An amide bond is formed between the carboxyl group of the valeric acid side chain of biotin and the ε-amino group of a specific lysyl residue in the apocarboxylase; these apocarboxylase regions contain sequences of amino acids that tend to be highly conserved within and between species for the individual carboxylases.

Holocarboxylase synthetase (EC 6.3.4.10) is present in both the cytosol and the mitochondria. Studies of human mutant holocarboxylase synthetase indicate that both the mitochondrial and cytoplasmic forms are encoded by one gene.[11] However, in rats Shriver and co-workers[12] have concluded that two different holocarboxylase

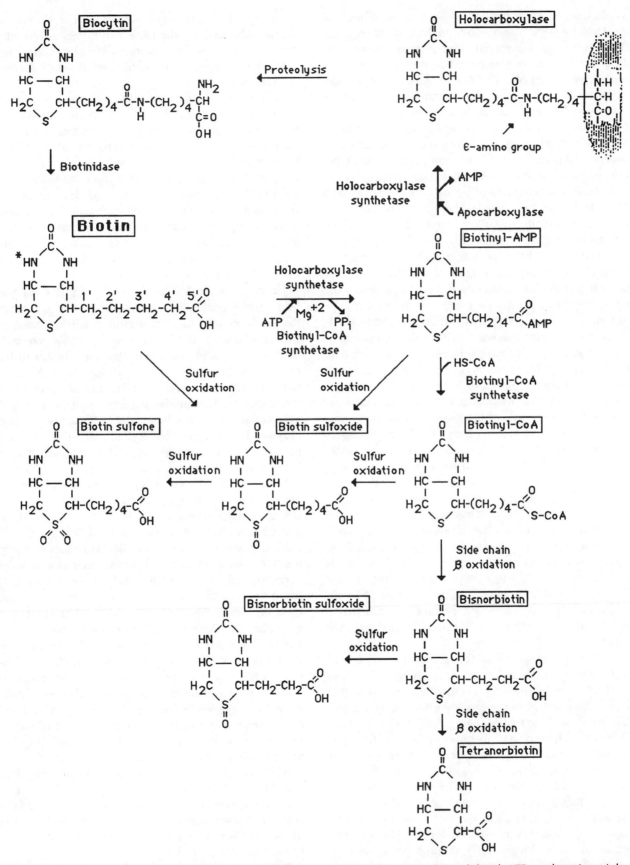

Figure 1. Biotin metabolism. The specific systems leading to the sulfoxides have not been defined. ATP = adenosine triphosphate; AMP = adenosine monophosphate; CoA = coenzyme A; PP$_i$ = pyrophosphate; * = site of attachment of carboxyl moiety.

synthetases catalyze the biotinylation of the mitochondrial and cytosolic carboxylases on the basis of sequence differences and site-specific mutagenesis studies. The holocarboxylase synthetase reaction is driven thermodynamically by hydrolysis of ATP to inorganic phosphate.

Regulation of intracellular mammalian carboxylase activity by biotin remains to be elucidated. However, the interaction of biotin synthesis and production of holo-acetyl-CoA carboxylase in *E. coli* has been extensively studied and reviewed.[13,14] The biotin-protein ligase (specifically, a holoacetyl-CoA carboxylase synthetase in *E. coli*) catalyzes formation of the covalent bond between biotin and a specific lysine residue in the biotin carboxylase carrier protein (BCCP) of acetyl-CoA carboxylase. The biotin-binding domain of BCCP of *E. coli* acetyl-CoA carboxylase has been sequenced.[15] As with the four mammalian carboxylases (Figure 1), the biotinylation of the apocarboxylase proceeds in two steps. First, the holocarboxylase synthetase reacts with biotin and ATP to form a complex between the synthetase and biotinyl-AMP, releasing pyrophosphate. If a suitable amount of the BCCP portion of acetyl-CoA carboxylase is present, the holocarboxylase is formed, and AMP is released. If insufficient apocarboxylase is present, the holocarboxylase synthetase:biotinyl-AMP complex acts to repress further synthesis of biotin by binding to the promoter regions of the biotin operon (bio). These promoters control a cluster of genes that encode enzymes that catalyze biotin synthesis; these enzymes include biotin synthetase, the enzyme complex that converts dethiobiotin to biotin. In its role as a repressor of the bio operon, the holocarboxylase synthetase has been named BirA; this name arose from initial observations on *biotin* intracellular *retention* properties and was found to be allelic to repression of biotin synthesis by biotin (bioR). Biotinyl-AMP acts as a co-repressor through its role in the BirA:biotinyl-AMP complex. Thus, the rate of biotin synthesis is responsive to both the supply of apo-BCCP and the supply of biotin as reflected in the biotinyl-AMP concentration.

Additional research has focused on conversion of dethiobiotin (or an earlier precursor, pimelic acid) to biotin.[16] This is an unusual enzymatic reaction that closes the tetrahydrothiophene ring by inserting a sulfur. These studies used *E. coli* or *Bacillus sphaericus* bioB transformants that overproduce biotin; Ifuku and co-workers[17] have sequenced several point mutations leading to bioB transformants in *E. coli*. Such studies have provided evidence that biotin synthetase is a two-iron two-sulfur enzyme that requires NADPH, S-adenosyl methionine, and Fe^{3+} or Fe^{2+}.[18–20] Flavodoxin is also required, probably as an electron donor.[21] The source of the sulfur in the thiophene ring is probably cysteine or a derivative. Additional studies in cell-free systems have established the cofactor and metal ion requirements.[22–25]

Alanine and acetate serve as carbon sources; carbon dioxide liberated via the tricarboxylic acid cycle may serve as well.[26] The first eukaryotic biotin synthetase has now been cloned and sequenced from the yeast *Saccharomyces cerevisiae*.[27]

In the carboxylase reaction, the carboxyl moiety from bicarbonate dissolved in cell water is first attached to biotin at the ureido nitrogen opposite the side chain; then the carboxyl group is transferred to the substrate. The reaction is driven by the hydrolysis of ATP to ADP and inorganic phosphate. Subsequent reactions in the pathways of the four mammalian carboxylases release CO_2 from the product of the carboxylase reaction. Thus, these reaction sequences rearrange the substrates into more useful intermediates but do not violate the classic observation that mammalian metabolism does not result in the *net* fixation of carbon dioxide.

The common mechanism for the carboxylase reaction begins with tautomerization of the ureido ring to enhance the nucleophilicity of its two nitrogens.[10,28] Because of steric hindrance at the 3'-N (same side of the molecule as the valeric acid side chain that joins biotin to the protein backbone of the carboxylase), the 1'-N reacts uniquely with a carbonyl phosphate that previously was formed by the reaction between bicarbonate and ATP. The product of this reaction is the 1'-N-carboxybiotinyl enzyme. This reactive carboxylate group then is incorporated into the substrate, typically at a carbon with incipient carbanion character.

Three of the four biotin-dependent carboxylases are mitochondrial; the fourth (acetyl-CoA carboxylase, ACC) is found in both the mitochondria and the cytosol. Allred and co-workers[12,29–32] have observed that ACC (EC 6.4.1.2) exists in an active cytosolic form and two largely inactive mitochondrial forms with molecular weights of ≈264,000 and 234,000, respectively. The mitochondrial forms are hypothesized to serve as storage forms that leave the mitochondria and are transformed into the active cytosolic ACC during periods of restricted biotin availability. The decrease of the mitochondrial form with maintenance of the activity of cytosolic ACC is consistent with a storage role.[12] However, maintenance of normal amounts of the three mitochondrial enzymes after 4 weeks of egg-white feeding observed by Allred and co-workers[12] is not consistent with the onset of abnormal organic aciduria after as little as 2 weeks of egg-white feeding in rats and humans.[33,34]

ACC catalyzes the incorporation of bicarbonate into acetyl-CoA to form malonyl-CoA (Figure 2). This three-carbon compound then serves as a substrate for the fatty acid synthetase complex; the net result is the elongation of the fatty acid substrate by two carbons and the loss of the third carbon as CO_2.

Pyruvate carboxylase (PC, EC 6.4.1.1) catalyzes the incorporation of bicarbonate into pyruvate to form ox-

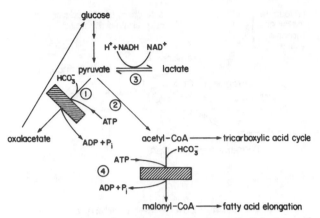

Figure 2. Lactate and pyruvate metabolism. Deficiencies of PC and ACC (▨) can affect the metabolic fate of intermediates related to lactic acid. NAD+ and NADH = oxidized and reduced nicotinamide adenine dinucleotide; ADP = adenosine diphosphate; P_i = inorganic phosphate. Enzymes catalyzing numbered reactions: 1) pyruvate carboxylase (PC), 2) pyruvate dehydrogenase, 3) lactate dehydrogenase, 4) acetyl-CoA carboxylase (ACC). Reprinted by permission of Lippincott-Raven Publishers.[35]

aloacetate, an intermediate in the Kreb's tricarboxylic acid cycle (Figure 2). Thus, PC catalyzes an anapleurotic reaction. In gluconeogenic tissues (i.e., liver and kidney), the oxaloacetate can be converted to glucose. Deficiency of PC has been proposed as the cause of the lactic acidemia, central nervous system lactic acidosis, and abnormalities in glucose regulation observed in biotin deficiency and biotinidase deficiency as discussed below.

Methylcrotonyl-CoA carboxylase (MCC, EC 6.4.1.4) catalyzes an essential step in the degradation of the branch-chained amino acid leucine (Figure 3). Deficient activity of this enzyme (whether due to genetic deficiency of only this carboxylase, multiple carboxylase deficiency, or biotin deficiency) leads to metabolism of its substrate 3-methylcrotonyl-CoA by an alternate pathway to 3-hydroxyisovaleric acid, 3-methylcrotonylglycine, or both.[1,35] Thus, increased urinary excretion of these abnormal metabolites in the urine reflects deficient activity of MCC and can reflect biotin depletion at the tissue level in genetically normal individuals.

Propionyl-CoA carboxylase (PCC, EC 6.4.1.3) catalyzes the incorporation of bicarbonate into propionyl-CoA to form methylmalonyl-CoA, which undergoes isomerization to succinyl-CoA and enters the tricarboxylic acid cycle (Figure 4). The three carbon propionic acid moiety originates from several sources: the catabolism of the branch-chained amino acids isoleucine, valine, methionine, and threonine; the side chain of cholesterol; the oxidation of odd chain length saturated fatty acids; and the metabolism of dietary carbohydrate by intestinal flora. In a fashion analogous to

MCC deficiency, deficiency of PCC leads to increased urinary excretion of 3-hydroxypropionic acid and 2-methylcitric acid.[1,36]

In the normal turnover of cellular proteins, holocarboxylases are degraded to biotin linked to lysine (biocytin) or biotin linked to an oligopeptide containing at most a few amino acid residues (Figure 1). Because the amide bond between biotin and lysine is not hydrolyzed by cellular proteases, the specific hydrolase biotinidase (biotin-amide hydrolase, EC 3.5.1.12) is required to release biotin for recycling.

Genetic deficiencies of holocarboxylase synthetase and biotinidase cause the two distinct types of multiple carboxylase deficiency which were previously designated the neonatal and juvenile forms. Biotinidase deficiency is particularly relevant to understanding biotin deficiency because the clinical manifestations result largely from a secondary biotin deficiency. The biotinidase gene is a single copy gene of 1629 bases encoding a 543 amino acid protein.[37] Its mRNA is present in many tissues including heart, brain, placenta, liver, lung, skeletal muscle, kidney, and pancreas.[37] Highest biotinidase activities are found in serum, liver, kidney, and adrenal gland. The observation that serum concentrations of biotinidase are decreased in patients with impaired liver function suggests that liver is the source of serum biotinidase.[38]

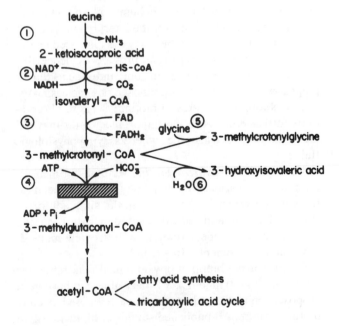

Figure 3. Leucine degradation. A deficiency (▨) of MCC causes increased urinary excretion of 3-methylcrotonylglycine and 3-hydroxyisovaleric acid. FAD and $FADH_2$ = oxidized and reduced flavin adenine dinucleotide. Enzymes catalyzing numbered reactions: 1) leucine-isoleucine transaminase, 2) branched-chain 2-keto acid dehydrogenase, 3) isovaleryl-CoA dehydrogenase, 4) methylcrotonyl-CoA carboxylase (MCC), 5) glycine N-acylase, 6) enoyl hydratase (crotonase). Reprinted by permission of Lippincott-Raven Publishers.[35]

Instead of being incorporated into carboxylases after entering the pools of biotin and its intermediary metabolites, dietary biotin or biotin released by carboxylase turnover may be catabolized. For example, biotinyl-AMP can be converted to biotinyl-CoA by biotinyl-CoA synthetase. This synthetase also catalyzes the formation of biotinyl-AMP from biotin and ATP, thus producing the substrate for formation of biotinyl-CoA. The relation between biotinyl-CoA synthetase and holocarboxylase synthetase as well as the existence and location of intracellular pools of biotinyl-AMP remains unclear. Biotinyl-CoA is oxidized to bisnorbiotin and tetranorbiotin (metabolites with two and four fewer carbons, respectively, in the valeric acid side chain; Figure 1).

Contrary to the tacit assumption of many early biotin balance studies, it now appears that about half of biotin undergoes metabolism before excretion, and thus a significant proportion of the total avidin-binding substances in human urine and plasma and rat urine is attributable to biotin metabolites rather than to biotin per se.[1] The findings of a pioneering study of biotin metabolites in human urine based on paper chromatography and bioassays have been confirmed by recent studies that take advantage of the greater precision and reliability of HPLC/avidin-binding assays.[1,39–41] Biotin, bisnorbiotin, and biotin sulfoxide are present in mole ratios of ≈3:2:1 in human urine and plasma. The presence of substantial amounts of biotin metabolites in human plasma and urine has important implications for the interpretation of both avidin-binding assays and bioassays as discussed below. Moreover, recent observations provide evidence that biotin catabolism is induced in some individuals during pregnancy and by anticonvulsants, thereby increasing the ratio of biotin catabolites to biotin.[42,43] These observations further emphasize the importance of distinguishing biotin from its catabolites when assaying physiologic fluids.

Methods for measuring biotin. Methods for measuring biotin at pharmacologic and physiologic concentrations were extensively reviewed in the sixth edition of PKN.[1] Here methods are discussed with a focus on methods used in recent studies and to review methodological advancements since 1989.

For measuring biotin at physiological concentrations (100 pmol/L–100 nmol/L), a variety of assays have been proposed, and a limited number have been used to study biotin nutriture. All published studies of biotin nutriture have used one of three basic types of biotin assays: bioassays (most studies), avidin-binding assays (several recent studies), or fluorescent derivative assays (two published studies).

Bioassays generally have adequate sensitivity to measure biotin in blood and urine. Precision is limited for the turbidity methods, but a recent modification of the *L. plantarum* assay uses agar plates previously injected

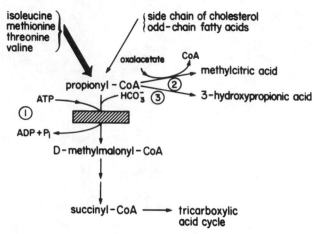

Figure 4. Propionate metabolism. Propionate is derived primarily from amino acid degradation and to a lesser extent from cholesterol and odd-chain fatty acids; a deficiency (▨) of PCC causes increased urinary excretion of methylcitric and 3-hydroxypropionic acids. Enzymes catalyzing numbered reactions: 1) propionyl-CoA carboxylase (PCC), 2) citrate synthetase, 3) β-oxidation or direct ω–hydroxylation. Reprinted by permission of Lippincott-Raven Publishers.[35]

with *L. plantarum* to obtain better precision.[44] Radiometric bioassays offer both sensitivity and precision. However, the bacterial bioassays (and perhaps the eukaryotic bioassays as well) suffer from interference by unrelated substances and from variability of the growth response to biotin analogs; these bioassays can give conflicting results if biotin is bound to protein.[1] For some bioassay organisms, prior acid or enzymatic hydrolysis (or both) is required to release the biotin from protein and thus make the biotin available to the assay organism. In other organisms (e.g., *Klockera brevis*), the detectable biotin decreases with enzymatic hydrolysis consistent with destruction of biotin by some acid hydrolysis regimens.[45]

Avidin-binding assays generally measure the ability of biotin to compete with (^{3}H)biotin, (^{125}I)biotin, or (^{14}C)biotin for binding to avidin (isotope dilution assays); bind to (^{125}I)avidin and thus prevent (^{125}I)avidin or enzyme-coupled avidin from binding to a biotinylated protein adsorbed to plastic (sequential, solid-phase assay); or prevent the binding of a biotinylated enzyme to avidin and thereby prevent the consequent inhibition of an enzyme activity. Other methods detect the postcolumn enhancement of fluorescence activity caused either by the mixing of the column eluate with fluorescent-labeled avidin or by derivatization of biotin and metabolites by a fluorescent agent before separation by HPLC.[46,47] Avidin-binding assays using novel detection systems such as electrochemical detection, bioluminescence linked through glucose-6-phosphate dehydrogenase, or a double antibody technique have been published recently and may offer some advantages in terms of sensitivity.[48–50] Avidin-binding assays have been criticized for being cumbersome, requiring highly specialized equipment or reagents, or performing poorly when applied to biological fluids. Avidin-binding assays detect all avidin-binding substances, although the relative detectability of biotin and analogs varies between analogs and between assays depending on how the assay is conducted (e.g., competitive versus sequential). In a manner analogous to the pioneering work of Wright et al.,[39] assays that couple chromatographic separation of biotin analogs with subsequent avidin-binding assay of the chromatographic fractions are both sensitive and chemically specific. These assays have been used in several recent studies that provide new insights into biotin nutrition.

A problem in the area of biotin analytical technology that remains unaddressed is the disagreement among the various bioassays and avidin-binding assays concerning the true concentration of biotin in human plasma. Reported mean values range from ≈500 pmol/L to >10,000 pmol/L.

Absorption and Transport

Digestion of protein-bound biotin. Neither the mechanism of the intestinal hydrolysis of protein-bound biotin nor the relationship of digestion of protein-bound biotin to its bioavailability has been clearly defined. The content of free biotin and protein-bound biotin in foods is variable, but the majority of biotin in meats and cereals appears to be protein-bound. Wolf et al.[51] have postulated that biotinidase plays a critical role in the release of biotin from covalent binding to protein. Biotinidase in pancreatic juice might be responsible for release of biotin during the luminal phase of proteolysis. Mucosal biotinidase might release biotin from biotinyl oligopeptides, the presumed products of intestinal proteolysis. The role of mucosal biotinidase is not certain because the activity is not enriched in intestinal brush-border membranes.[51]

In view of the observations suggesting that a free carboxyl group is necessary for binding to the intestinal biotin transporter, significant uptake of biotinyl-oligopeptides by the biotin transporter seems unlikely,[52] but this conclusion remains controversial.[53] Alternatively, biotinyl-oligopeptides might be absorbed directly by a nonspecific pathway for peptide absorption.

In patients with biotinidase deficiency, doses of free biotin that do not greatly exceed the estimated dietary intake (50–150 µg/day) appear adequate to prevent the symptoms of biotinidase deficiency, presumably by preventing biotin deficiency.[54] Biotinidase deficiency may contribute to biotin deficiency through impaired intestinal digestion of protein-bound biotin, impaired cellular recycling of biotin, impaired renal salvage, or a combination of these mechanisms.

Intestinal absorption. Early studies using low specific activity radiolabeled biotin and intact tissues such as everted gut sacs indicated that intestinal and renal transport of biotin occurred by simple diffusion.[1] However, given the small amounts of biotin in foodstuffs and animal tissues and the efficient conservation of biotin by the body under most circumstances, simple diffusion is teleologically unattractive.[55] Within the last decade, studies using higher specific activity radiolabeled biotin, brush-border membrane vesicles, and cell culture systems have greatly expanded current knowledge of intestinal and renal transport of biotin.[1,55-60] A biotin transporter is present in the intestinal brush-border membrane. The carrier is highly structurally specific, requiring both a free carboxyl group on the valeric acid side chain and an intact ureido ring, according to most studies; however, not all structure-activity studies have confirmed the need for a free carboxyl group.[61] Studies using normal human tissue, human intestinal cell lines, and intestinal tissue from rabbit and rat reveal that transport of biotin is temperature dependent and occurs against a concentration gradient. Biotin transport is electroneutral because of the 1:1 coupling of biotin (COO^-) with Na^+. Biotin transport also occurs by simple diffusion; diffusion predominates at higher (pharmacological) concentrations. These recent studies of the biotin transporter cast into doubt the conclusion from some earlier studies that biotinidase is the principal biotin-binding protein in the intestinal brush-border membrane.[1]

In rats, biotin transport is up-regulated with maturation from the suckling stage to adulthood, and the site of maximal transport by the biotin transporter shifts from ileum to jejunum. Although carrier-mediated transport of biotin was most active in the proximal small bowel of the rat, Bowman and Rosenberg[62] concluded that absorption of biotin from the proximal colon was still significant, supporting the potential nutritional significance of biotin synthesized by enteric flora. Clinical studies also provide some evidence that biotin can be absorbed from the human colon.[63,64]

In intact rats and CaCo-2 cells, up-regulation of biotin transport occurs in response to biotin deficiency; the mechanism for most of the change appears to be an increased V_{max} (presumably mediated by an increased number of carriers) rather than a change in the carrier affinity. Studies of rabbit intestinal brush-border membrane transport indicate that histidine residues and sulfhydryl groups are important in the normal function of the transporter. The histidine residues are probably located at or near the biotin-binding site.[65]

In contrast to most other investigators, Leon-Del-Rio and co-workers[53] observed only passive diffusion of biotin in the rat, but saturable transport of biocytin. In hamsters they observed saturable transport of biotin but passive diffusion of biocytin. These investigators propose that protein-bound biotin is absorbed mainly in its free form in the hamster but at least partially as biocytin in the rat.

The exit of biotin from the enterocyte (i.e., transport across the basolateral membrane) is also carrier-mediated but is independent of Na[+], is electrogenic, and does not accumulate biotin against a concentration gradient.[66] Said and co-workers[67] investigated the mechanism leading to reduced plasma biotin concentration in a substantial portion of alcoholics. In evacuated gut sacks from rats, they observed that acute ethanol exposure inhibited biotin transport. Chronic ethanol feeding reduced intestinal transport of biotin and decreased plasma concentrations of biotin. These authors speculated that the effects of ethanol on intestinal transport of biotin may contribute to the impaired biotin status associated with chronic alcoholism.

Transport of biotin from intestine to peripheral tissue. Little has been definitively established concerning the transport of biotin to the liver and peripheral tissues from the site of absorption in the intestine. Several articles report biotin plasma levels, pharmacokinetics, and bioavailability after acute or chronic oral, intramuscular, or intravenous administration of biotin in cattle, swine, and human subjects.[68–73]

Investigation of biotin binding to proteins in plasma and serum has proceeded along two distinct lines: investigation of the biotin-binding properties of biotinidase and empirical assessment of covalent and reversible binding of biotin to whole plasma and fractionated plasma proteins. Wolf et al.[74] originally hypothesized that biotinidase might serve as a biotin-binding protein in plasma or perhaps even as a carrier protein for the transport of biotin into the cell. Chuahan and Dakshinamurti[75] provided evidence to support that hypothesis. Biotin binding to purified biotinidase, albumin, α- and β-globulins, and fractionated human serum was assessed by (^{3}H)biotin binding to protein using ammonium sulfate precipitation and by (^{3}H)biotin equilibrium dialysis. These investigators concluded that biotinidase is the only protein in human serum that specifically binds biotin. Others have disagreed.[1] Using (^{3}H)biotin, centrifugal ultrafiltration, and dialysis to assess reversible binding in plasma from the rabbit, pig, and human, Mock and Lankford[76] found that <10% of the total pool of free plus reversibly bound biotin is reversibly bound to plasma macromolecules (presumably protein). A similar biotin-binding system was detected by Mock and Lankford[76] in experiments with physiologic concentrations of human serum albumin. Additional studies determined the proportion of biotin covalently bound to plasma protein.[77] Using acid hydrolysis and (^{3}H)biotinyl-albumin as an index of the completeness of biotin release, the investigators found additional biotin was released by hydrolysis. Overall, the percentages of free, reversibly bound, and covalently bound biotin in human serum are ≈81%, 7%, and 12%, respectively.[77]

The results of the two approaches discussed above apparently conflict. The differences may arise from differences in the experimental approach, the definition of binding, or both. The importance of either type of biotin binding to the transport of biotin from the intestine to the peripheral tissues is not yet clear. The binding detected by Mock and co-workers may represent a structurally nonspecific interaction between hydrophobic portions of the biotin molecule and one or more of the hydrophobic binding sites on a serum protein such as albumin. This binding may be analogous to the binding of apolar optical and fluorescent dyes to the hydrophobic binding sites on albumin and avidin.[78–83]

Uptake of biotin by liver. The uptake of biotin by mammalian liver and peripheral tissues has been the subject of several investigations. Studies of 3T3-L1 fibroblasts, rat hepatocytes isolated by collagenase perfusion, basolateral membrane vesicles from human liver, and Hep G$_2$ human hepatoma cells indicate that uptake of free biotin is mediated both by diffusion and by a specialized carrier system that is dependent upon a Na[+] gradient, temperature, and energy.[60,84–88] Transport is electroneutral (Na[+] to biotin 1:1) and specific for a free carboxyl group, but transport is not strongly specific for the structure in the region of the thiophene ring.[88] In contrast, isolated cultured hepatocytes did not exhibit a carrier-mediated transport system.[89]

Additional studies by Weiner and Wolf[90] in cultured rat hepatocytes demonstrated trapping of biotin, presumably in holocarboxylase enzymes as covalently bound biotin. These studies confirm earlier studies by McCormick and Zhang and emphasize the importance of metabolic trapping of water-soluble vitamins as a mechanism for an intracellular accumulation.[60] After entering the hepatocyte, biotin diffuses into the mitochondria via a pH-dependent process.[91] Said and co-workers[91] have postulated that biotin enters the mitochondria in the neutral protonated form and dissociates into the anionic form in the alkaline mitochondrial environment becoming trapped by the charge.

Transport of biotin into the central nervous system. Using an in situ rat brain perfusion technique and (^{3}H)biotin, Spector and Mock[92] demonstrated that biotin is transported across the blood-brain barrier by a saturable system; the apparent K$_m$ was ≈100 μmol/L (a value several orders of magnitude greater than the concentration of free biotin in plasma). Inhibition of transport by structural analogs suggested that the free carboxylate group in biotin was important to transport. Transfer of biotin directly into the cerebrospinal fluid (CSF) via the choroid plexus did not appear to be an important mechanism of biotin entry into the central nervous system. Other studies using either intravenous or intraventricular injection of (^{3}H)biotin into adult rabbits demonstrated that (^{3}H)biotin was cleared from CSF more rapidly than mannitol, suggesting specific transport systems for biotin uptake into the neurons after biotin crosses the blood-brain barrier.[93] Two hours after intraventricular injection, only minimal metabolism of biotin and covalent binding to brain proteins was observed. However, after 18 hours about one-third of the biotin had been incorporated into brain protein. These findings suggest that biotin enters the brain by a saturable transport system that does not depend upon the subsequent metabolism of biotin or its trapping by incorporation into brain proteins.

In human studies Mock and co-workers have measured the concentrations of free "biotin" (i.e., total avidin-binding substances) in CSF and ultrafiltrates of plasma and found a ratio of 0.85 ± 0.5 for 11 subjects.[1] This result is similar to the CSF:plasma ratios determined for biotin by Spector and Mock[92] in the rabbit, a species that has a specific system for biotin transport across the blood-brain barrier.

Renal handling of biotin. Specific systems for the reabsorption of water-soluble vitamins from the glomerular filtrate may contribute to conservation of water-soluble vitamins.[55] A biotin transport system has been identified by Podevin and Barbarat[94] in both brush-border and basolateral membrane vesicles from rabbit kidney cortex. Uptake by brush-border membrane vesicles was saturable, occurred against a biotin concentration gradient, and was dependent on an inwardly directed Na^+ gradient. The K_m was 28 μM, and transport exhibited structural specificity. In contrast, the uptake of biotin by basolateral membrane vesicles was not sensitive to a Na^+ gradient. In the rat kidney, Spencer and Roth[95] demonstrated a similar system with a K_m of 0.2 μmol/L that was inhibited by equimolar concentrations of biocytin.

In vitro studies of biotin transport by human renal tissue preparations have not been published. Baumgartner and co-workers[96-98] have measured the renal clearance of biotin in vivo and have calculated biotin:creatinine clearance ratios.[95-97] In normal adults and children who are not receiving biotin supplementation, the clearance ratio is ≈ 0.4. In patients with biotinidase deficiency, renal wasting of biotin and biocytin occurs; biotin:creatinine clearance ratios are typically ≥ 1, and half-lives for biotin are $\approx$half of the normal value. The mechanism for the increased renal excretion of biotin in biotinidase deficiency has not been defined, but biotinidase may have a role in the renal handling of biotin. For example, abnormal plasma biotinidase might bind biotin less tightly, increasing the glomerular sieving coefficient, serve less effectively as a reclamation transporter in the renal tubule, or alter cellular salvage of biotin during turnover of renal holocarboxylases.

Placental transport of biotin. Specific systems for transport of biotin from the mother to the fetus have recently been reported.[99-101] Studies using microvillus membrane vesicles and cultured trophoblasts detected a saturable transport system for biotin that was dependent upon Na^+ and actively accumulated biotin within the placenta with slower release into the fetal compartment. However, in the isolated perfused single cotyledon, transport of biotin across the placenta was slow relative to placental accumulation.[99,100] Little evidence of accumulation on the fetal side was detected, suggesting that the overall placental transfer of biotin is most consistent with a passive process. Membrane vesicle transport was sensitive to short-term exposure to ethanol, but overall transfer was not.[100] Further studies using fetal facing (basolateral) membrane vesicles detected a saturable, Na^+ dependent, electroneutral, carrier-mediated uptake process that was not as active as the biotin uptake system in the maternal facing (apical) membrane vesicles.[101]

Transport of biotin into human milk. Using an avidin-binding assay, Mock and co-workers[45] have concluded that >95% of the biotin (i.e., total avidin-binding substances) is present in the skim fraction of human milk rather than in the cell pellet or fat fraction. Less than 3% of total biotin was reversibly bound to macromolecules and <5% was covalently bound to macromolecules. Thus, almost all the biotin in human milk is free in the aqueous compartment of the skim fraction. The concentration of biotin in human milk remains fairly constant between the fore, mid, and hind milk in the same feeding but varies substantially over 24 hours in some women.[102] In a study of eight women, milk from four showed a steady increase in biotin concentration during the first 18 days postpartum.[102] Thereafter biotin concentrations varied substantially for unknown reasons. Measured by the same assay, the concentration of biotin in the aqueous phase of human milk exceeds the concentration in serum by one to two orders of magnitude. It seems likely that there is a transport system that conveys biotin from plasma to milk against a concentration gradient. Studies of the biotin and metabolite profile using an HPLC/avidin-binding assay indicate that bisnorbiotin accounts for $\approx$50% and biotin sulfoxide $\approx$10% of the total biotin plus metabolites in early and transitional human milk. With duration of lactation, the biotin concentration increases, but the bisnorbiotin and biotin sulfoxide concentrations still account for 25% and 8% at 5 weeks postpartum.[103] Current studies provide no evidence for a predominant trapping mechanism or for a soluble biotin-binding protein.

Other Effects of Biotin

Effects of biotin on cell growth, glucose homeostasis, DNA synthesis, and expression of the asialoglycoprotein receptor have been reported and reviewed. No direct relationship to biotin's role as a cofactor for the four carboxylases has been defined.[1,104-106] Whether one or more of the effects will ultimately prove to be the indirect result of carboxylase deficiency remains unclear.

Biotin Deficiency

Circumstances leading to deficiency. The fact that the normal human has a requirement for biotin has been clearly documented in two situations: prolonged consumption of raw egg white and parenteral nutrition without biotin supplementation in patients with short-gut syndrome and other causes of malabsorption.[1] Biotin deficiency also has been clearly demonstrated in biotinidase deficiency.[1] The mechanism by which biotinidase deficiency leads to biotin deficiency probably involves several processes: gastrointestinal absorption of biotin may be decreased because deficiency of biotinidase in pancreatic secretions leads to inadequate release of protein-bound biotin, salvage of biotin at the cellular level may be impaired during normal turnover of proteins to which biotin is linked covalently, and renal loss of biocytin and biotin is abnormally increased.

The clinical findings and biochemical abnormalities caused by biotinidase deficiency are quite similar to those of biotin deficiency, including periorificial dermatitis, conjunctivitis, alopecia, ataxia, and developmental delay.[1] These clinical similarities support the hypothesis that the pathogenesis of biotinidase deficiency involves a secondary biotin deficiency. However, the reported signs and symptoms of biotin deficiency and biotinidase deficiency are not identical. Seizures, irreversible neurosensory hearing loss, and optic atrophy have been observed in biotinidase deficiency but have not been reported in biotin deficiency. However, cerebral atrophy and apparent stretching of the optic nerve were reported in one patient with biotin deficiency. Moreover, Heard et al.[107] have reported that biotin deficiency causes impaired auditory brainstem function in young rats.

As judged by lymphocyte carboxylase activities and plasma biotin levels, Velazquez and co-workers[108,109] detected biotin deficiency in children with severe protein-energy malnutrition. They speculate that biotin deficiency may be responsible for part of the clinical syndrome of protein-energy malnutrition.

Accumulating data provide evidence that long-term anticonvulsant therapy in adults can lead to biotin depletion and that the depletion can be severe enough to interfere with amino acid metabolism. In early reports, Krause and co-workers[110,111] reported decreased plasma concentrations of biotin (assayed by the *Lactobacillus plantarum* bioassay). A later demonstration of increased urinary excretion of 3-hydroxyisovaleric acid in adults receiving long-term anticonvulsant therapy[112] has been confirmed by Mock and Dyken[42] and provides evidence that biotin is depleted at the tissue level.

The mechanism of biotin depletion during anticonvulsant therapy is not known. The anticonvulsants implicated include phenobarbital, phenytoin, carbamazepine, and primidone. These drugs each have a carbamide (-NH-CO-) moiety in their structures, as does biotin; in some cases they incorporate a full ureido group (-NH-CO-NH-). Said and co-workers[59,113] have demonstrated that therapeutic concentrations of primidone and carbamazepine specifically and directly inhibit biotin uptake by brush-border membrane vesicles from human intestine, and they suggest that impaired intestinal absorption is one mechanism leading to biotin deficiency. Mock and co-workers[43] have recently reported substantial increases in the urinary excretion of biotin catabolites, especially bisnorbiotin. The increases are large enough to constitute an important drain on total body pools of biotin and suggest that accelerated catabolism of biotin induced by anticonvulsants may also contribute to reduced biotin status in these individuals. Chuahan and Dakshinamurti[75] have demonstrated that phenobarbital, phenytoin, and carbamazepine displace biotin from biotinidase, conceivably affecting plasma transport, renal handling, or cellular uptake of biotin.

Biotin deficiency has also been reported or inferred in several other circumstances: Leiner's disease is a severe form of seborrheic dermatitis that occurs in infancy. Although a number of studies have reported prompt resolution of the rash with biotin therapy, biotin was ineffective in the only double-blind therapeutic trial.[1,114]

Johnson et al.[115] and Heard et al.[116] have proposed that biotin deficiency may cause sudden infant death syndrome (SIDS) by a pathogenic mechanism analagous to that in chicks. (Biotin deficiency in the chick produces a fatal hypoglycemic disease dubbed "fatty liver-kidney syndrome" because deficient activity of pyruvate carboxylase impairs gluconeogenesis.) They support their hypothesis by demonstrating that hepatic biotin is significantly lower at autopsy of SIDS infants than in infants dying from other causes. Additional studies (activity of hepatic pyruvate carboxylase, excretion of urinary organic acids, and blood glucose) are needed to confirm or refute this hypothesis.

Concerns about the teratogenic effects of biotin deficiency have led to studies of biotin status during human gestation. Some of these studies have detected low plasma concentrations of biotin, others have not.[1] Recent studies by Mock et al.[42] have detected increased 3-hydroxyisovaleric acid in more than half of normal women by the third trimester of pregnancy, and urinary excretion of biotin was abnormally decreased in ≈50% of the women studied.

Patients undergoing chronic hemodialysis have been reported to have low plasma concentrations of biotin.[117] Yatzidis et al.[118] have reported that nine patients on chronic hemodialysis developed either encephalopathy (four patients) or peripheral neuropathy (five patients); all responded to biotin therapy. Blood concentrations of biotin and lactic acid and urinary excretion rates of the characteristic organic acids were not reported. Other investigators have reported that plasma and red cell concentrations of biotin are significantly increased rather than decreased in patients receiving chronic hemodialysis.[119] The etiological role of biotin in uremic neurological disorders and the general applicability of these results remain to be determined.

Reduced blood or liver concentrations of biotin or urinary excretion of biotin have been reported in alcoholics, patients with gastric disease, or inflammatory bowel disease.[4,120,121]

Colombo and co-workers[122] treated women with brittle fingernails using oral doses of biotin (2.5 mg/day). Electron microscopy revealed a 25% increase in nail thickness and improved morphology. The biotin status of the subjects was not assessed.

Clinical findings of frank deficiency.
Whether caused by egg-white feeding or omission of biotin from total parenteral nutrition, the clinical findings of frank biotin deficiency in adults and older children have been similar to those reported by Sydenstricker and co-workers[123] in a pioneering study of egg-white feeding. Typically, the deficiency began to appear gradually after weeks to several years of egg-white feeding.[1] Six months to 3 years typically elapsed between the initiation of total intravenous feeding without biotin and the onset of the findings of biotin deficiency.[1,35] Thinning hair, often with loss of color, was reported in most patients. A skin rash described as scaly (seborrheic) and red (eczematous) was present in most; and in several, the rash was distributed around the eyes, nose, and mouth. Depression, lethargy, hallucinations, and paresthesias of the extremities were prominent neurologic symptoms in the majority of adults.

In the infants who developed biotin deficiency, the signs and symptoms of biotin deficiency began to appear within 3 to 6 months after initiation of total parenteral nutrition; this earlier onset may reflect an increased biotin requirement because of growth. The rash typically appeared first around the eyes, nose, and mouth; ultimately, the ears and perineal orifices were involved (periorificial). The appearance of the rash was similar to that of cutaneous candidiasis (i.e., an erythematous base and crusting exudates); typically, Candida could be cultured from the lesions. The rash of biotin deficiency is quite similar to the rash of zinc deficiency. In infants, hair loss was noted after 6 to 9 months of parenteral nutrition; within 3 to 6 months of the onset of hair loss, two infants lost all hair including eyebrows and lashes. These cutaneous manifestations, in conjunction with an unusual distribution of facial fat, are called biotin deficiency facies. The most striking neurological findings in biotin-deficient infants were hypotonia, lethargy, and developmental delay. A peculiar withdrawn behavior was noted and may reflect the same central nervous system dysfunction diagnosed as depression in the adult patients.

Laboratory findings of biotin deficiency.
Although commonly used to assess biotin status in a variety of clinical populations, the putative indices of biotin status had not been previously studied during progressive biotin deficiency. To address this issue, Mock and co-workers[34] induced progressive biotin deficiency by feeding egg white and measured the urinary excretion of biotin, bisnorbiotin, and 3-hydroxyisovaleric acid. The urinary excretion of biotin declined dramatically with time on the egg-white diet, reaching frankly abnormal values in nine of the eleven subjects by day 20. Bisnorbiotin excretion declined in parallel, providing evidence against an unregulated obligate catabolism of the free biotin pool. By day 14 of egg-white feeding, 3-hydroxyisovaleric acid excretion was abnormally increased in all 11 subjects, providing evidence that biotin depletion reduces the activity of the biotin-dependent enzyme methylcrotonyl-CoA carboxylase and alters intermediary metabolism of leucine earlier in the course of experimental biotin deficiency than previously appreciated. The time course for development of metabolic abnormalities was similar to that observed in the egg-white-fed rat.[33,124] Plasma concentrations of free biotin as measured by HPLC/avidin-binding assay decreased to abnormal values in less than half of the subjects. These studies provide objective confirmation of the impression that blood biotin concentration is not an early or sensitive indicator of impaired biotin status.[125]

Plasma concentrations of biotin (i.e., total avidin-binding substances) are higher in term infants than older children and, for reasons that are not simply related to dietary intake, decline after 3 weeks of breast feeding or feeding of formula containing 11 µg/L of biotin.[126] Infant formulas supplemented with 300 µg biotin/L produce plasma concentrations ≈20-fold greater than normal. Consequences of these higher levels, if any, are unknown.

Odd-chain fatty acid accumulation is a marker of biotin deficiency, according to Kramer et al., Suchy et al., and Mock et al.[127–129] These groups independently demonstrated increases in the percentage composition of odd-chain fatty acids (e.g., 15:0, 17:0, etc.) in hepatic, cardiac, or serum phospholipids in the biotin-deficient rat. Similar accumulation has been reported in the liver of the biotin-deficient chick.[130] Further, Mock and co-workers[131] reported the accumulation of these odd-chain fatty acids in the plasma of patients who developed biotin deficiency during parenteral nutrition. The accumulation of odd-chain fatty acids is thought to result from propionyl-CoA carboxylase deficiency, because genetic deficiency of propionyl-CoA carboxylase results in the accumulation of odd-chain fatty acids in plasma, red blood cells, and liver. Apparently, the accumulation of propionyl-CoA leads to the substitution of a propionyl-CoA moiety for acetyl-CoA (a 3-carbon for a 2-carbon moiety) in the fatty acid elongation reaction and, hence, to the formation of an odd-chain fatty acid.

Biochemical pathogenesis. The mechanisms by which biotin deficiency produces specific signs and symptoms remain to be completely delineated. However, several recent studies have given new insights into the biochemical pathogenesis of biotin deficiency. The tacit assumption of most of these studies is that the clinical findings of biotin deficiency result directly or indirectly from deficient activities of the four biotin-dependent carboxylases.

Sander and co-workers initially suggested that the CNS effects of biotinidase deficiency (and, by implication, biotin deficiency) might be mediated through deficiency of pyruvate carboxylase and the attendant CNS lactic acidosis.[132] Because pyruvate carboxylase activity declined more slowly in brain than in liver during progressive biotin deficiency in the rat, the investigators discounted this mechanism. However, subsequent studies suggest their original hypothesis is correct. Diamantopoulos et al.[54] expanded the hypothesis by proposing that deficiency of brain biotinidase (which Suchy et al.[133] reported was already quite low in normal brain) combined with biotin deficiency leads to a deficiency of brain pyruvate carboxylase and, in turn, to CNS accumulation of lactic acid. This CNS lactic acidosis is postulated to be the primary mediator of the hypotonia, seizures, ataxia, and delayed development seen in biotinidase deficiency. Additional support for the CNS lactic acidosis hypothesis has come from direct measurements of CSF lactic acid in children with either biotinidase deficiency or isolated pyruvate carboxylase deficiency and from the rapid resolution of lactic acidemia and CNS abnormalities in patients who have developed biotin deficiency during parenteral nutrition.[1] The work of Suchy, Rizzo, and Wolf has provided evidence against an etiologic role for disturbances in brain fatty acid composition in the CNS dysfunction.[128]

Several studies have demonstrated abnormalities in metabolism of fatty acids in biotin deficiency and have suggested that these abnormalities are important in the pathogenesis of skin rash and hair loss. Initially, the similarity between cutaneous manifestations of biotin deficiency and essential fatty acid deficiency plus the established role of biotin in lipid synthesis led to dietary intervention with polyunsaturated fatty acid. For example, Munnich et al.[134] have described a 12-year-old boy with multiple carboxylase deficiency in whom the enzymatic defect was almost certainly biotinidase deficiency based on subsequent elucidation of the pathogenesis of multiple carboxylase deficiency by Wolf and co-workers.[135] The child presented with alopecia and periorificial scaly dermatitis. Oral administration of "unsaturated fatty acids composed of 11% C18:1, 71% C18:2, 8% C18:3, and 0.3% C20:4" at a rate of "2–400 mg/day" plus twice daily

topical administration of the same mixture of fatty acids "resulted in dramatic improvement of the dermatologic condition" and hair growth. Lactic acidosis and organic aciduria remained the same. These investigators speculated the deficiency of acetyl-CoA carboxylase led to impaired synthesis or metabolism of long-chain polyunsaturated fatty acids (PUFAs), which was treated by the topical and oral administration of PUFA.

Three studies in the rat support the possibility of abnormal PUFA metabolism as a result of biotin deficiency and as a cause of the cutaneous manifestations. Kramer et al.[127] and Mock et al.[129] have reported significant abnormalities in the phospholipid n-6 fatty acids of blood, liver, and heart. Watkins and Kratzer[130] also found abnormalities of phospholipid n-6 fatty acids in liver and heart of biotin-deficient chicks. It has been speculated that these abnormalities in PUFA composition might result in abnormal composition or metabolism of prostaglandins and related substances derived from these PUFAs.[129,136,137] The question of an etiological role was addressed directly by Mock.[138] Supplementation with n-6 PUFAs as Intralipid prevented the development of the cutaneous manifestations of biotin deficiency in a group of rats who were as biotin deficient (on the basis of biochemical measurements) as the biotin-deficient control group that did not receive the supplemental n-6 fatty acids and did develop the classic rash and hair loss. Mock concluded that an abnormality in n-6 PUFA metabolism plays a pathogenic role in the cutaneous manifestations of biotin deficiency and that the effect of the n-6 PUFA cannot be attributed to biotin sparing.

Other effects of deficiency. Subclinical maternal biotin deficiency has been shown to be teratogenic in several species including chicken, turkey, mouse, rat, and hamster.[1] Fetuses of mouse dams with degrees of biotin deficiency too mild to produce the characteristic cutaneous or CNS findings developed micrognathia, cleft palate, and micromelia.[139–141] The incidence of malformation increased with the degree of biotin deficiency to a maximum incidence of ≈90%. Differences in teratogenic susceptibility among rodent species have been reported, and a corresponding difference in biotin transport from the mother to the fetus has been proposed as the cause.[142] Bain et al.[143] have hypothesized that biotin deficiency affects bone growth via effects on the synthesis of prostaglandins derived from n-6 fatty acid. This effect on bone growth might be the mechanism for the teratogenic effects of biotin deficiency.

Studies of cultured lymphocytes and of in vivo immune responses in rats and mice indicate that biotin is required for normal function of a variety of immunological cells. These functions include production of antibodies, immunological reactivity, protection against sepsis, macrophage function, differentiation of T and B lymphocytes, afferent immune response, and cytotoxic

Table 1. Recommended intake of biotin

Age	Safe and adequate daily oral intakes[a]	Daily parenteral intakes[b]
	(µg)	(µg)
Preterm infants[c]	5	5–8 µg·kg^{-1}
Infants up to 6 month	10	20
Infants up to 1 year	15	20
Children 1–3 year	20	20
Children 4–6 year	25	20
Older children, 7–10 year	30	20
Older children (>11 years) and adults	30–100	60

[a]National Research Council.[145]
[b]Greene et al.[146]
[c]Greene and Smidt.[147]

T-cell response.[1] In humans, Okabe et al.[120] report that patients with Crohn's disease have depressed natural killer cell activity that was responsive to biotin supplementation. In patients with biotinidase deficiency, Cowan et al.[144] have demonstrated defects in both T-cell and B-cell immunity.

Diagnosis of biotin deficiency. The diagnosis of biotin deficiency has been established by demonstrating reduced urinary excretion of biotin, increased urinary excretion of the characteristic organic acids discussed earlier, and resolution of the signs and symptoms of deficiency in response to biotin supplementation. Plasma and serum levels of biotin, whether measured by bioassay or avidin-binding assay, have not uniformly reflected biotin deficiency.[125]

Clinical response to administration of biotin has been dramatic in all well-documented cases of biotin deficiency. The rash healed within a few weeks, and healthy hair generally grew by 1–2 months. Hypotonia, lethargy, and depression generally resolved within 1–2 weeks, followed by accelerated mental and motor development in infants.

Treatment of biotin deficiency. Pharmacological doses of biotin (1–10 mg) have been used to treat most patients. For two patients parenteral administration of 100 µg /day of biotin was adequate to cause resolution of the signs and symptoms of biotin deficiency and to prevent their recurrence.[1] However, abnormal organic aciduria persisted for at least 10 weeks in one patient receiving 100 mg/day, suggesting that this dose may not have been adequate to restore tissue biotin levels to normal over that time. Could this degree of tissue biotin deficiency be sufficient to cause significant, if subtle, morbidity? If so, should a loading dose of 1 or 10 mg for 1 or 2 weeks be given as initial therapy for acquired biotin deficiency? There are currently no data on which to base answers to these questions.

Requirements and Allowances

Data providing an accurate estimate of the biotin requirements for infants, children, and adults are lacking, and as a result, recommendations often conflict.[1,145] Data for an accurate estimate of the requirement for biotin administered parenterally are also lacking. For parenteral administration, uncertainty about the true metabolic requirement for biotin is compounded by lack of information concerning the effects of infusing biotin continuously as opposed to intermittent postprandial absorption into the intestinal portal blood. Despite these limitations, recommendations have been formulated for oral biotin intakes by all ages from infant through adult, for oral and parenteral intake of biotin by preterm infants, and for parenteral intake by all ages from infant through adult.[145-147] These recommendations are given in Table 1. One published study of parenterally supplemented infants found normal plasma levels of biotin in term infants supplemented at 20 µg/day and increased plasma levels of biotin in preterm infants supplemented at 13 µg/day.[148] (Note that the units for plasma biotin should be pg/mL in Moore et al.[148])

An important factor in the current uncertainty concerning biotin requirements is the possibility that biotin synthesized by intestinal bacteria (referred to hereafter as bacterial biotin) may contribute significantly to absorbed biotin. If so, the required intake would be reduced and might be dependent on factors that influence the density and species distribution of intestinal flora. For example, it is conceivable that interruption of absorption of bacterial biotin is a critical event in both biotin deficiency from egg-white ingestion and biotin deficiency during parenteral nutrition. In the former, bacterial biotin may be bound by avidin; in the latter, reduced intestinal surface for absorption, rapid transit time, and antibiotic suppression of gut bacteria may lead to reduced absorption of bacterial biotin. Unfortunately, few data are available for assessing the actual magnitude of absorbed bacterial biotin.

Dietary Sources of Biotin

There is no published evidence that biotin can be synthesized by mammals; thus, higher animals must derive biotin from exogenous sources. The ultimate source of biotin appears to be de novo synthesis by bacteria, primitive eukaryotic organisms such as yeast, molds, and algae, and some plant species.

Most measurements of biotin content of foods used bioassays. Despite the limitations of interfering substances, protein binding, and lack of chemical specificity, there is reasonably good agreement among the published reports, and some worthwhile generalizations can be made.[149-153] Biotin is widely distributed in natural foodstuffs, but the absolute content of even the richest sources is low when compared to the content of most other water-soluble vitamins. Foods relatively rich in biotin include egg yolk, liver, and some vegetables. According to Hardinge and Crooks,[149] the average dietary biotin intake of the Swiss population is ≈70 μg/day. This figure is in reasonable agreement with the estimated dietary intake of biotin in a composite Canadian diet (62 μg/day) and the actual analysis of the diet (60 μg/day).[154] Calculated intake of biotin for the British population was 35 μg/day.[155,156]

Toxicity

Toxicity has not been reported in individuals who have received daily doses of as much as 200 mg orally and 20 mg intravenously to treat biotin-responsive inborn errors of metabolism and acquired biotin deficiency.

Acknowledgments

Many thanks to Nell Mock for the art work in the figures.

References

1. Mock DM (1989) Biotin. In Brown M (ed), Present knowledge in nutrition, 6th ed. International Life Sciences Institute, Washington, DC, pp 189–207
2. Bhatia D, Borenstein B, Gaby S, et al (1992) Vitamins, part XIII: Biotin. In Hui YU (ed), Encyclopedia of food science and technology, vol 4. John Wiley & Sons, New York, pp 2764–2770
3. Combs GF Jr (1992) The vitamins. Fundamental Aspects in Nutrition and Health, vol 1. Academic Press Limited, Ithaca, NY
4. Bonjour J-P (1991) Biotin. In Machlin LJ (ed), Handbook of vitamins, 2nd ed. Marcel Dekker, New York, pp 393–427
5. Mock DM (1992) Biotin in human milk: when, where, and in what form? In Picciano MF, Lonnerdal B (eds), Mechanisms regulating lactation and infant nutrient utilization. John Wiley & Sons, New York, pp 213–219
6. Marquet A (1977) New aspects of the chemistry of biotin and some analogs. Pure Appl Chem 49:183–196
7. Sternbach LH (1963) Biotin. In Florkin M, Stotz EG (eds), Comprehensive biochemistry, vol 2. Elsevier, New York, pp 66–81
8. Miljkovic D, Velimirovic S, Csanadi J, Popsavin V (1989) Studies directed towards stereospecific synthesis of oxybiotin, biotin, and their analogs: preparation of some new 2,5, anhydro-xylitol derivatives. J Carbohydrate Chem 8:457–467
9. Deroose FD, DeClercq PJ (1995) Novel enantioselective syntheses of (+)-biotin. J Org Chem 60:321–330
10. McCormick D (1996) Bio-organic mechanisms important to coenzyme functions. In Handbook of vitamins, 3rd ed. Marcel Dekker, New York (in press)
11. Sweetman L, Nyhan WL (1986) Inheritable biotin-treatable disorders and associated phenomena. Annu Rev Nutr 6:317–343
12. Shriver BJ, Roman-Shriver C, Allred JB (1993) Depletion and repletion of biotinyl enzymes in liver of biotin-deficient rats: evidence of a biotin storage system. J Nutr 123:1140–1149
13. Brandsch R (1994) Regulation of gene expression by cofactors derived from B vitamins. J Nutr Sci Vitaminol 40:371–399
14. Cronan JE Jr (1989) The E. coli bio operon: transcriptional repression by an essential protein modification enzyme. Cell 58:427–429
15. Chapman-Smith A, Turner DL, Cronan JE, et al (1994) Expression, biotinylation and purification of a biotin-domain peptide from the biotin carboxy carrier protein of Escherichia coli acetyl-CoA carboxylase. Biochem J 302:881–887
16. Ohsawa I, Kisou T, Kodama K, et al (1992) Bioconversion of pimelic acid into biotin by Bacillus sphaericus bioB transformants. J Ferment Bioengineering 73:121–124
17. Ifuku O, Haze S, Kishimoto J, et al (1993) Sequencing analysis of mutation points in the biotin operon of biotin-overproducing Escherichia coli mutants. Biosci Biotech Biochem 57:760–765
18. Sanyal I, Cohen D, Flint G (1993) Biotin synthase: purification, characterization as a (2FE-2S) cluster protein, and in vitro activity of the Escherichia coli bioB gene product. Biochemistry 33:3625–3631
19. Bower S, Perkins J, Yocum RR, et al (1995) Cloning and characterization of the Bacillus subtilis birA gene encoding a repressor of the biotin operon. J Bacteriol 177:2572–2575
20. Ohshiro T, Yamamoto M, Tse Sum Bui B, et al (1995) Stimulatory factors for enzymatic biotin synthesis from dethiobiotin in cell-free extracts of Escherichia coli. Biosci Biotech Biochem 59:943–944
21. Ifuku O, Koga N, Haze S, et al (1994) Flavodoxin is required for conversion of dethiobiotin to biotin in Escherichia coli. Eur J Biochem 224:173–178
22. Fujisawa A, Abe T, Ohsawa I, et al (1993) Bioconversion of dethiobiotin into biotin by resting cells and protoplasts of Bacillus sphaericus bioB transformant. Biosci Biotech Biochem 57:740–744
23. Ohshiro T, Yamamoto M, Izumi Y, et al (1994) Enzymatic conversion of dethiobiotin to biotin in cell-free extracts of a Bacillus sphaericus bioB transformant. Biosci Biotech Biochem 58:1738–1741
24. Florentin D, Tse Sum Bui B, Marquet A, et al (1994) On the mechanism of biotin synthase of Bacillus sphaericus. C R Acad Sci III 317:485–488
25. Fujisawa A, Abe T, Ohsawa I, et al (1993) Bioconversion of dethiobiotin to biotin by a cell-free system of a bioYB transformant of Bacillus sphaericus. FEMS Microbiol Lett 110:1–4
26. Ifuku O, Miyaoka H, Koga N, et al (1994) Origin of carbon atoms of biotin ${}^{13}C$-NMR studies on biotin biosynthesis in Escherichia coli. Eur J Biochem 220:585–591
27. Zhang S, Sanyal I, Bulboaca GH, et al (1994) The gene for biotin synthase from Saccharomyces cerevisiae: cloning, sequencing, and complementation of Escherichia coli strains lacking biotin synthase. Arch Biochem Biophys 309:29–35
28. Knowles JR (1989) The mechanism of biotin-dependent enzymes. Annu Rev Biochem 58:195
29. Allred J, Roman-Lopez CR (1988) Enzymatically inactive forms of acetyl-CoA carboxylase in rat liver mitochondria. Biochem J 251:881–885
30. Allred J, Roman-Lopez C, Jurin R, McCune S (1989) Mitochondrial storage forms of acetyl-CoA carboxylase: mobilization/activation accounts for increased activity of the enzyme in liver of genetically obese Zucker rats. J Nutr 119:478–483
31. Allred JB, Roman-Lopez CR, Pope TS, Goodson J (1985) Dietary dependent distribution of acetyl-CoA carboxylase between cytoplasm and mitochondria of rat liver. Biochem Biophys Res Commun 129:453–460

32. Roman-Lopez, Shriver B, Joseph C, Allred J (1989) Mitochondrial acetyl-CoA carboxylase: time course of mobilization/activation in liver of refed rats. Biochem J 260:927–930

33. Mock NI, Mock DM (1992) Biotin deficiency in rats: disturbances of leucine metabolism is detectable early. J Nutr 122:1493–1499

34. Mock NI, Mock DM, Malik M, Bishop MW (1995) Urinary excretion of biotin and 3-hydroxyisovaleric acid (3-HIA) are early indicators of biotin deficiency [abstract]. FASEB J 9:A985

35. Mock DM (1986) Water-soluble vitamin supplementation and the importance of biotin. In Lebenthal E (ed), Textbook on total parenteral nutrition in children: indications, complications, and pathophysiological considerations. Raven Press, New York, pp 89–108

36. Liu Y, Shigematsu Y, Nakai A, et al (1993) The effects of biotin deficiency on organic acid metabolism: increase in propionyl coenzyme A-related organic acids in biotin-deficient rats. Metab Clin Exp 42:1392–1397

37. Cole H, Reynolds TR, Lockyer JM, et al (1994) Human serum biotinidase cDNA cloning, sequence, and characterization. J Biochem 269:6566–6570

38. Grier RE, Heard GS, Watkins P, Wolf B (1989) Low biotinidase activities in the sera of patients with impaired liver function: evidence that the liver is the source of serum biotinidase. Clin Chim Acta 186:397–400

39. Wright LD, Cresson EL, Driscoll CA (1956) Biotin derivatives in human urine. Proc Soc Exp Biol Med 91:248–252

40. Mock DM, Lankford G, Cazin J Jr (1993) Biotin and biotin analogs in human urine: biotin accounts for only half of the total. J Nutr 123:1844–1851

41. Mock D, Lankford GL, Mock NI (1995) Biotin accounts for only half of the total avidin-binding substances in human serum. J Nutr 125:941–946

42. Mock D, Mock N, Stratton S, Stadler D (1995) Urinary excretion of biotin decreases during pregnancy, providing evidence of decreased biotin status [abstract]. FASEB J 9:A155

43. Mock D, Dyken M (1995) Biotin deficiency results from long-term therapy with anticonvulsants. Gastroenterology 108:A740

44. Fukui T, Iinuma K, Oizumi J, Izumi Y (1994) Agar plate method using *Lactobacillus plantarum* for biotin determination in serum and urine. J Nutr Sci Vitaminol 40:491–498

45. Mock DM, Mock NI, Langbehn SE (1992) Biotin in human milk: methods, location, and chemical form. J Nutr 122:535–545

46. Przyjazny A, Hentz NG, Bachass LG (1993) Sensitive and selective liquid chromatographic postcolumn reaction detection system for biotin and biocytin using a homogeneous fluorophore-linked assay. J Chromatogr 654:79–86

47. Stein J, Hahn A, Lembcke B, Rehner G (1992) High-performance liquid chromatographic determination of biotin in biological materials after crown ether-catalyzed fluorescence derivatization with panacyl bromide. Anal Biochem 200:89–94

48. Sugawara K, Tanaka S, Nakamura H (1994) Electrochemical determination of avidin-biotin binding using an electroactive biotin derivative as a marker. Bioelectrochemistry Bioenergetics 33:205–207

49. Terouanne B, Bencheich M, Balaguer P, et al (1989) Bioluminescent assays using glucose-6-phosphate dehydrogenase: application to biotin and streptavidin detection. Anal Biochem 180:43–49

50. Thuy LP, Sweetman L, Nyhan WL (1991) A new immunochemical assay for biotin. Clin Chim Acta 202:191–198

51. Wolf B, Heard G, McVoy JRS, Raetz HM (1984) Biotinidase deficiency: the possible role of biotinidase in the processing of dietary protein-bound biotin. J Inherit Metab Dis 7:121–122

52. Said HM, Thuy LP, Sweetman L, Schatzman B (1993) Transport of the biotin dietary derivative biocytin (N-biotinyl-L-lysine) in rat small intestine. Gastroenterology 104:75–80

53. Leon-Del-Rio A, Vizcaino G, Robles-Diaz G, Gonzalez-Noriega A (1990) Association of pancreatic biotinidase activity and intestinal uptake of biotin and biocytin in hamster and rat. Ann Nutr Metab 34:266–272

54. Diamantopoulos N, Painter MJ, Wolf B, et al (1986) Biotinidase deficiency: accumulation of lactate in the brain and response to physiologic doses of biotin. Neurology 36:1107–1109

55. Bowman BB, McCormick DB, Rosenberg IH (1989) Epithelial transport of water-soluble vitamins. Annu Rev Nutr 9:187–199

56. Ma TY, Dyer DL, Said HM (1994) Human intestinal cell line CaCo-2: a useful model for studying cellular and molecular regulation of biotin uptake. Biochim Biophys Acta 1189:81–88

57. Said HM, Derweesh I (1991) Carrier-mediated mechanism for biotin transport in rabbit intestine—studies with brush-border membrane vesicles. Am J Physiol 261:R94–R97

58. Said HM, Horne DW, Mock DM (1989) Effect of aging on intestinal biotin transport in the rat. Exp Gerontol 25:67–73

59. Said HM, Mock DM, Collins JC (1989) Regulation of biotin intestinal transport in the rat: effect of biotin deficiency and supplementation. Am J Physiol. 25:G306–G311

60. McCormick D, Zhang Z (1993) Cellular assimilation of water-soluble vitamins in the mammal: riboflavin, B6, biotin, and C. Proc Soc Exp Biol Med 202:265–270

61. Ng K-Y, Borchardt RT (1993) Biotin transport in a human intestinal epithelial cell line (CaCo-2). Life Sci 53:1121–1127

62. Bowman BB, Rosenberg I (1987) Biotin absorption by distal rat intestine. J Nutr 117:2121–2126

63. Sorrell MF, Frank O, Thomson AD, et al (1971) Absorption of vitamins from the large intestine in vivo. Nutr Rep Int 3:143–148

64. Oppel TW (1948) Studies of biotin metabolism in man. IV. Studies of the mechanism of absorption of biotin and the effect of biotin administration on a few cases of seborrhea and other conditions. Am J Med Sci 215:76–83

65. Said HM, Mohammadkhani R (1992) Involvement of histidine residues and sulfhydryl groups in the function of the biotin transport carrier of rabbit intestinal brush-border membrane. Biochim Biophys Acta 1107:238–244

66. Said HM, Redha R, Nylander W (1988) Biotin transport in basolateral membrane vesicles of human intestine. Gastroenterology 94:1157–1163

67. Said HM, Sharifian A, Bagherzadeh A, Mock D (1990) Effect of chronic ethanol feeding and acute ethanol exposure in vitro on intestinal transport of biotin. Am J Clin Nutr 52:1083–1086

68. Frigg M, Straub C, Hartmann D (1993) The bioavailability of supplemental biotin in cattle. Int J Vitam Nutr Res 63:122–128

69. Bryant KL, Kornegay ET, Knight JW, Notter DR (1989) Uptake and clearance rates of biotin in pig plasma following biotin injections. Int J Vitam Nutr Res 60:52–57

70. Misir R, Blair R (1988) Biotin bioavailability from protein supplements and cereal grains for weanling pigs. Can J Anim Sci 68:523–532

71. Bitsch R, Sal I, Hotzel D (1988) Studies on bioavailability of oral biotin doses for humans. Int J Vitam Nutr Res 59:65–71

72. Clevidence B, Marshall M (1988) Biotin levels in plasma and urine of healthy adults consuming physiological levels of biotin. Nutr Res 8:1109–1118

73. Mock D, Mock N (1994) Serum concentrations of biotin and biotin analogs increase during acute and chronic biotin supplementation [abstract]. FASEB J 8:A921

74. Wolf B, Grier RE, McVoy JRS, Heard GS (1985) Biotinidase deficiency: a novel vitamin recycling defect. J Inherit Metab Dis 8:53–58

75. Chuahan J, Dakshinamurti K (1988) Role of human serum biotinidase as biotin-binding protein. Biochem J 256:265–270

76. Mock DM, Lankford G (1990) Studies of the reversible binding of biotin to human plasma. J Nutr 120:375–381

77. Mock DM, Malik MI (1992) Distribution of biotin in human plasma: most of the biotin is not bound to protein. Am J Clin Nutr 56:427–432

78. Green NM (1975) Avidin. Adv Protein Chem 29:85–133

79. Green NM (1970) Spectrophotometric determination of avidin and biotin. In McCormick DB, Wright LD (eds), Methods in enzymology, vol 18, part A. Academic Press, New York, pp 418–424

80. Green NM (1965) A spectrophotometric assay for avidin and biotin based on binding of dyes by avidin. Biochem J 94:23c–24c

81. Mock DM, Horowitz P (1990) A fluorometric assay for avidin-biotin interaction. In Wilchek M, Bayer EA (eds), Methods in enzymology, vol 184. Academic Press, San Diego, pp 234–240

82. Mock DM, Lankford GL, Horowitz P (1988) A study of the interaction of avidin with 2-anilinonaphthalene-6-sulfonic acid as a probe of the biotin binding site. Biochim Biophys Acta 956:23–29

83. Mock DM, Lankford G, DuBois D, Horowitz P (1985) A fluorometric assay for the biotin-avidin interaction based on displacement of the fluorescent probe 2-anilinonaphthalene-6-sulfonic acid. Anal Biochem 151:178–181

84. Cohen ND, Thomas M (1982) Biotin transport into fully differentiated 3T3-L1 cells. Biochem Biophys Res Commun 108:1508–1516

85. Bowers-Komro DM, McCormick DB (1985) Biotin uptake by isolated rat liver hepatocytes. Ann NY Acad 447:350–358

86. Said HM, Hoefs J, Mohammadkhani R, Horne D (1992) Biotin transport in human liver basolateral membrane vesicles: a carrier-mediated, Na+ gradient-dependent process. Gastroenterology 102:2120–2125

87. Said HJ, Korchid S, Horne DW (1990) Transport of biotin in basolateral membrane vesicles of rat liver. Am J Physiol 259:G865–G872

88. Said HM, Ma TY, Kamanna VS (1994) Uptake of biotin by human hepatoma cell line, Hep G(2): a carrier-mediated process similar to that of normal liver. J Cell Physiol 161:483–489

89. Weiner D, Wolf B (1990) Biotin uptake in cultured hepatocytes from normal and biotin-deficient rats. Biochem Med Metab Biol 44:271–281

90. Weiner D, Wolf B (1991) Biotin uptake, utilization, and efflux in normal and biotin-deficient rat hepatocytes. Biochem Med Metab Biol 46:344–363

91. Said HM, McAlister-Henn L, Mohammadkhani R, Horne DW (1992) Uptake of biotin by isolated rat liver mitochondria. Am J Physiol 263:G81–G86

92. Spector R, Mock DM (1987) Biotin transport through the blood-brain barrier. J Neurochem 48:400–404

93. Spector R, Mock DM (1988) Biotin transport and metabolism in the central nervous system. Neurochem Res 13:213–219

94. Podevin R-A, Barbarat B (1986) Biotin uptake mechanisms in brush-border and basolateral membrane vesicles isolated from rabbit kidney cortex. Biochim Biophys Acta 856:471–481

95. Spencer PD, Roth KS (1988) On the uptake of biotin by the rat renal tubule. Biochem Med Metab Biol 40:95–100

96. Baumgartner ER, Sourmala T, Wick H (1985) Biotin-responsive multiple carboxylase deficiency (MCD): deficient biotinidase activity associated with renal loss of biotin. J Inherit Metab Dis 8:59–64

97. Baumgartner ER, Sourmala T, Wick H (1985) Biotinidase deficiency: factors responsible for the increased biotin requirement. J Inherit Metab Dis 8:59–64

98. Baumgartner ER, Sourmala T, Wick H (1985) Biotinidase deficiency associated with renal loss of biocytin and biotin. J Inherit Metab Dis 7:123–125

99. Karl P, Fisher SE (1992) Biotin transport in microvillous membrane vesicles, cultured trophoblasts and the isolated perfused cotyledon of the human placenta. Am J Physiol 262:C302–C308

100. Schenker S, Hu Z, Johnson RF, et al (1993) Human placental biotin transport: normal characteristics and effect of ethanol. Alcohol Clin Exp Res 17:566–575

101. Hu Z-Q, Henderson GI, Schenker S, Mock DM (1994) Biotin uptake by basolateral membrane of human placenta: normal characteristics and role of ethanol. Proc Soc Exp Biol Med 206:404–408

102. Mock DM, Mock NI, Dankle JA (1992) Secretory patterns of biotin in human milk. J Nutr 122:546–552

103. Stratton S, Mock N, Mock D (1996) Biotin and biotin metabolites in human milk: the metabolites are not negligible. J Invest Med 44:58A

104. Maebashi M, Makino Y, Furukawa Y, et al (1993) Therapeutic evaluation of the effect of biotin on hyperglycemia in patients with non-insulin dependent diabetes mellitus. J Clin Biochem Nutr 14:211–218

105. Reddi A, DeAngelis B, Frank O, et al (1988) Biotin supplementation improves glucose and insulin tolerances in genetically diabetic KK mice. Life Sci 42:1323–1330

106. Collins JC, Paietta E, Green R, et al (1988) Biotin-dependent expression of the asialoglycoprotein receptor in HepG2. J Biol Chem 263:11280–11283

107. Heard GS, Lenhardt ML, Bowie RM, et al (1989) Increased central conduction time (CTT) but no hearing loss (HL) in young biotin deficient rats [abstract]. FASEB J 3:A1242

108. Velazquez A, Martin-del-Campo C, Baez A, et al (1988) Biotin deficiency in protein-energy malnutrition. Eur J Clin Nutr 43:169–173

109. Velazquez A, Teran M, Baez A, et al (1995) Biotin supplementation affects lymphocyte carboxylases and plasma biotin in severe protein-energy malnutrition. Am J Clin Nutr 61:385–391

110. Krause K-H, Berlit P, Bonjour J-P (1982) Impaired biotin status in anticonvulsant therapy. Ann Neurol 12:485–486

111. Krause K-H, Berlit P, Bonjour J-P (1982) Vitamin status in patients on chronic anticonvulsant therapy. Int J Vitam Nutr Res 52:375–385

112. Krause K-H, Kochen W, Berli PT, Bonjour J-P (1984) Excretion of organic acids associated with biotin deficiency in chronic anticonvulsant therapy. Int J Vitam Nutr Res 54:217–222

113. Said HM, Reyadh R, Nylander W (1989) Biotin transport and anticonvulsant drugs. Am J Clin Nutr 49:127–131

114. Erlichman M, Goldstein R, Levi E, et al (1981) Infantile flexural seborrhoeic dermatitis: neither biotin nor essential fatty acid deficiency. Arch Dis Child 567:560–562

115. Johnson AR, Hood RL, Emery JL (1980) Biotin and the sudden infant death syndrome. Nature 285:159–160

116. Heard GS, Hood RL, Johnson AR (1983) Hepatic biotin and the sudden infant death syndrome. Med J Aust 2:305–306

117. Livaniou E, Evangelatos GP, Ithakissios DS, et al (1987) Serum biotin levels in patients undergoing chronic hemodialysis. Nephron 46:331–332

118. Yatzidis H, Koutisicos D, Agroyannis B, et al (1984) Biotin in the management of uremic neurologic disorders. Nephron 36:183–186

119. DeBari V, Frank O, Baker H, Needle M (1984) Water soluble vitamins in granulocytes, erythrocytes, and plasma obtained from chronic hemodialysis patients. Am J Clin Nutr 39:410–415

120. Bonjour J-P (1981) Biotin-dependent enzymes in inborn errors of metabolism in human. World Rev Nutr Diet 38:1–88

121. Okabe N, Urabe K, Fujita K, et al (1988) Biotin effects in Crohn's disease. Dig Dis Sci 33:1495–1496

122. Colombo VE, Gerber F, Bronhofer M, Floersheim GL (1990) Treatment of brittle fingernails and onychoschizia with biotin: scanning electron microscopy. J Am Acad Dermatol 23:1127–1132

123. Sydenstricker VP, Singal SA, Briggs AP, et al (1942) Observations on the "egg white injury" in man. JAMA 118:1199–1200

124. Mock DM, Jackson H, Lankford GL, et al (1989) Quantitation of urinary 3-hydroxyisovaleric acid using deuterated 3-hydroxyisovaleric acid as internal standard. Biomed Environ Mass Spectrom 18:652–656

125. Bonjour J-P (1985) Biotin in human nutrition. Ann NY Acad Sci 447: 97–104

126. Livaniou E, Mantagos S, Kakabakos S, et al (1991) Plasma biotin levels in neonates. Biol Neonat 59:209–212

127. Kramer TR, Briske-Anderson M, Johnson SB, Holman RT (1984) Effects of biotin deficiency on polyunsaturated fatty acid metabolism in rats. J Nutr 114:2047–2052

128. Suchy SF, Rizzo WB, Wolf B (1986) Effect of biotin deficiency and supplementation on lipid metabolism in rats: saturated fatty acids. Am J Clin Nutr 44:475–480

129. Mock DM, Mock NI, Johnson SB, Holman RT (1988) Effects of biotin deficiency on plasma and tissue fatty acid composition: evidence for abnormalities in rats. Pediatr Res 24:396–403

130. Watkins BA, Kratzer FH (1987) Tissue lipid fatty acid composition of biotin-adequate and biotin-deficient chicks. Poult Sci 66:306–313

131. Mock DM, Johnson SB, Holman RT (1988) Effects of biotin deficiency on serum fatty acid composition: evidence for abnormalities in humans. J Nutr 118:342–348

132. Sanders JE, Pachman S, Townsend JJ (1982) Brain pyruvate carboxylase activity and the pathophysiology of biotin-dependent diseases. Neurology 32:878–880

133. Suchy SF, McVoy JRS, Wolf B (1985) Neurologic symptoms of biotinidase deficiency: possible explanation. Neurology 35:1510–1511

134. Munnich A, Saudubray JM, Coude FK, et al (1980) Fatty-acid-responsive alopecia in multiple carboxylase deficiency. Lancet 1:1080–1081

135. Wolf B, Grier RE, Allen RJ, et al (1983) Biotinidase deficiency: the enzymatic defect in late-onset multiple carboxylase deficiency. Clin Chim Acta 131:273–281

136. Marshall MW (1987) The nutritional importance of biotin—an update. Nutr Today 22:26–30

137. Watkins BA, Kratzer FH (1987) Dietary biotin effects on polyunsaturated fatty acids in chick tissue lipids and prostaglandin E$_2$ levels in freeze-clamped hearts. Poult. Sci 66:1818–1828

138. Mock DM (1988) Evidence for a pathogenetic role of fatty acid (FA) abnormalities in the cutaneous manifestations of biotin deficiency (abstract). FASEB J 2:A1204

139. Watanabe T, Endo A (1990) Teratogenic effects of maternal biotin deficiency in mouse embryos examined at midgestation. Teratology 42:295–300

140. Watanabe T (1993) Dietary biotin deficiency affects reproductive function and prenatal development in hamsters. J Nutr 123:2101–2108

141. Watanabe T, Dakshinamurti K, Persaud TVN (1995) Biotin influences palatal development of mouse embryos in organ culture. J Nutr 125:2114–2121

142. Watanabe T, Endo A (1989) Species and strain differences in teratogenic effects of biotin deficiency in rodents. Am Inst Nutr 119:255–261

143. Bain SD, Newbrey JW, Watkins BA (1988) Biotin deficiency may alter tibiotarsal bone growth and modeling in broiler chicks. Poult Sci 67:590–595

144. Cowan MJ, Wara DW, Packman S, et al (1979) Multiple biotin-dependent carboxylase deficiencies associated with defects in T-cell and B-cell immunity. Lancet July 21:115–118

145. National Research Council (1989) Recommended Dietary Allowances, 10th ed. National Academy Press, Washington, DC, pp 165–169

146. Greene HL, Hambridge KM, Schanler R, Tsang RC (1988) Guidelines for the use of vitamins, trace elements, calcium, magnesium, and phosphorus in infants and children receiving total parenteral nutrition: report of the Subcommittee on Pediatric Parenteral Nutrient Requirements for the Committee on Clinical Practice Issues of the American Society for Clinical Nutrition. Am J Clin Nutr 48:1324–1342

147. Greene H, Smidt L (1993) Nutritional needs of the preterm infant: water soluble vitamins: C, B1, B2, B6, niacin, pantothenic acid, and biotin. In Tsang RC, Lucas A, Uauy R, Zlotkin S (eds) Nutritional needs of the preterm infant. Williams and Wilkins, Baltimore, MD, pp 121–133

148. Moore MC, Greene HL, Phillips B (1986) Evaluation of a pediatrics multiple vitamin preparation for total parenteral nutrition in infants and children: I. Blood levels of water-soluble vitamins. Pediatrics 77:530–538

149. Hardinge MG, Crooks H (1961) Lesser known vitamins in food. J Am Diet Assoc 38:240–245

150. Wilson J, Lorenz K (1979) Biotin and choline in foods—nutritional importance and methods of analysis: a review. Food Chem 4:115–129

151. Hoppner K, Lampi B (1983) The biotin content of breakfast cereals. Nutr Rep Int 284:793–798

152. Pennington JAT, ed (1989) Bowes and Church's food values of portions commonly used, 15th ed. J J P Lippincott Co., Philadelphia

153. Guilarte TR (1985) Analysis of biotin levels in selected foods using a radiometric-microbiological method. Nutr Rep Int 324:837–845

154. Hoppner K, Lampi B, Smith DC (1978) An appraisal of the daily intakes of vitamin B12, pantothenic acid and biotin from a composite Canadian diet. Can Inst Food Sci Technol J 11:71–74

155. Bull NL, Buss DH (1982) Biotin, panthothenic acid and vitamin E in the British household food supply. Hum Nutr Appl Nutr 36A:125–129

156. Lewis J, Buss DH (1988) Trace nutrients: minerals and vitamins in the British household food supply. Br J Nutr 60:413–424

Chapter 23

Pantothenic Acid

Nora Plesofsky-Vig

In 1933 pantothenic acid was shown to be an essential factor for the growth of yeast;[1] shortly thereafter it was identified as the nutrient that cured chickens of vitamin-deficiency-induced dermatitis.[2] Although the synthesis of pantothenic acid was accomplished by Williams and Major in 1940,[3] it was not until 1947 that coenzyme A (CoA) was demonstrated by Lipmann and colleagues[4] to be the biologically functional form of pantothenic acid. They showed that CoA was an essential cofactor for the acetylation of sulfonamide in liver and for the production of acetylcholine in brain. The central roles of CoA in the respiratory tricarboxylic acid cycle, fatty acid synthesis and degradation, and other metabolic and regulatory processes have since been elucidated.

Pantothenic acid is formed in microorganisms by the amide linkage of pantoic acid to β-alanine (Figure 1).[5] The main biological route of CoA synthesis is through phosphorylation of the free acid to form pantothenic acid 4′-phosphate, which, upon condensation with cysteine and decarboxylation, yields 4′-phosphopantetheine, whose metabolite pantetheine is an essential growth factor for the yogurt-producing *Lactobacillus bulgaricus*. Coenzyme A is produced by anhydride attachment of adenosine 5′-monophosphate to 4′-phosphopantetheine, followed by phosphorylation at the ribose 3′-hydroxyl (Figure 1). The active sulfhydryl group of CoA, derived from cysteine, is frequently esterified to acetate or other acyl groups. In certain cases, instead of being linked to diphospho-adenosine in CoA, the 4′-phosphopantetheine is covalently linked to a protein.[6] These include proteins that are active in fatty acid metabolism, such as the acyl carrier protein of bacteria and mitochondria and the fatty acid synthetase of eukaryotes, where serine forms a phosphodiester linkage to 4′-phosphopantetheine. Also modified by phosphopantetheine are the citrate lyase of anaerobic bacteria and enzymes involved in the nonribosomal synthesis of peptide antibiotics, such as tyrocidine and gramicidin S.

CoA and other pantothenate-containing molecules participate in two types of reactions, acyl group transfer and condensation.[7] Acyl group transfer occurs by nucleophilic addition to the carbonyl group that is thioesterified to CoA, followed by new ester bond formation and displacement of CoA. In condensation reactions, the α-carbon of the esterified acyl group is acidified by the thioester with CoA and it attaches to an electrophilic center, leading to carbon-carbon bond formation or cleavage. During respiratory metabolism, the first step of the tricarboxylic acid cycle is the condensation of acetyl-CoA with oxaloacetic acid to yield citric acid. Fatty acid synthesis involves acetate and malonate transfer from CoA, as well as condensation of these groups into the growing fatty acid chain.[8]

Absorption, Transport, Storage, and Turnover

CoA from dietary sources is hydrolyzed in the intestinal lumen to pantothenic acid, which is absorbed into the bloodstream by a sodium-dependent transport mechanism.[9] After pantothenic acid is circulated in the plasma, it is taken up into most cells by cotransport with sodium ions, and the placental absorption of pantothenate from maternal circulation also occurs by sodium cotransport.[10] The enzyme pantothenate kinase, which catalyzes the first step in the conversion of pantothenate to CoA, is the primary site of control of CoA synthesis in bacteria and rat hearts.[11] Tissue CoA levels appear to be independent of pantothenate availability.[12] Mitochondria may be the final site of CoA synthesis, since 95% of CoA is located in mitochondria and CoA itself does not cross the mitochondrial membrane; nevertheless, all required synthetic enzymes have been found in the cytosol.[11] Pantothenate is released from CoA by multiple steps of hydrolysis, the final, unique step being the hydrolysis of pantetheine to pantothenate and cysteamine.[13] Free pantothenic acid is excreted in urine.

Biochemical Functions

Macromolecular syntheses. Pantothenic acid plays a central role in many metabolic processes.[7] It is essential to the synthesis of fatty acids and membrane phospholipids, including sphingolipids, as well as to the oxidative degradation of fatty acids and amino acids. The synthesis of amino acids such as leucine, arginine, and methionine includes a pantothenate-dependent step. Pantothenic acid, in CoA, is also required for synthesis of isoprenoid-derived compounds, such as cholesterol, steroid hormones, dolichol, vitamin A, vitamin D, and heme A. Further, CoA is essential to the synthesis of δ-amino-levulinic acid, a precursor of the corrin ring in vitamin B_{12} and the porphyrin rings in hemoglobin and cytochromes.

It contributes an essential acetyl group to the neurotransmitter acetylcholine and to the sugars N-acetylglucosamine, N-acetylgalactosamine, and N-acetylneuraminic acid, components of glycoproteins and glycolipids.

Protein acetylation. Through its recently described role as a donor of acetate and fatty acyl groups to proteins,[6]

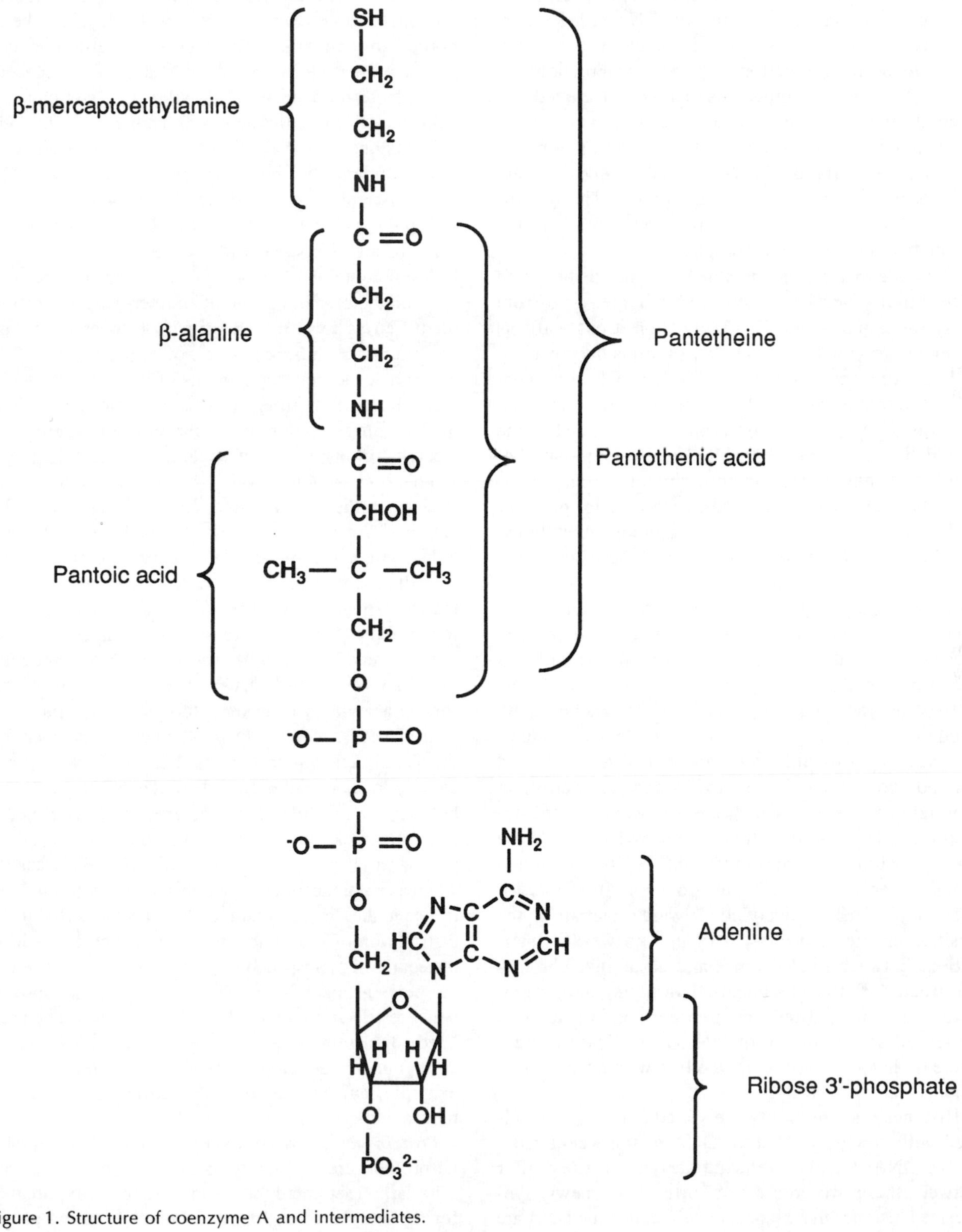

Figure 1. Structure of coenzyme A and intermediates.

CoA affects a wide range of cellular processes, including steps in signal transduction. The addition of acetate to the N-terminal amino acid of proteins is a common modification, occurring in 50–90% of eukaryotic proteins.[14] It was earlier suggested, on the basis of in vitro experiments, that this modification protects proteins from proteolytic degradation, but more recent experiments have yielded contradictory results.[15] Nevertheless, N-terminal acetylation was shown in *Saccharomyces cerevisiae* to be important for cell cycle progression and sexual development, processes that were disrupted in a strain defective in N-terminal acetyltransferase activity.[16] Acetylation influences the structure of certain proteins, for example, increasing the N-terminal α-helical content of calpactin I, a calcium-binding protein.[17] This modification was required for calpactin I assembly with the regulatory subunit of the complex.

There are mammalian peptide hormones that become N-terminally acetylated during their cleavage from polyprotein precursors. This acetylation strongly affects hormone activity. Pro-opiomelanocortin is the precursor of both adrenocorticotropin (ACTH) and β-lipotropin. ACTH in turn is processed to α-melanocyte-stimulating hormone (MSH), and β-lipotropin is processed to the opioid β-endorphin.[18] Both MSH and β-endorphin become N-terminally acetylated in the intermediate pituitary, but neither is acetylated in the anterior pituitary and only MSH is acetylated in the brain.[6] Acetylation has different effects on the activities of these hormones, stimulating α-MSH activity but inhibiting β-endorphin, which becomes unable to bind to opioid receptors.[19] In this case, acetylation appears to be a tissue-specific mechanism for differentially regulating the activities of two products of a single precursor.

Two important classes of proteins are reversibly acetylated on the ε-amino group of internal lysine residues: histones and α-tubulin. A tetramer of histones H3 and H4 and two histone dimers of H2A and H2B constitute a protein core around which DNA is wound in the nucleosome. These four histones are acetylated on lysine residues within their amino terminal regions, with histones H3 and H4 each having four possible sites for acetylation. Histone acetylation, which neutralizes the positive charge of lysines, is thought to weaken interactions between nucleosomes and destabilize chromatin structure.[20] It results in partial unfolding of the chromatin, as indicated by increased chromatin solubility, increased susceptibility of DNA to nucleases, and a decrease in the negative supercoiling within the nucleosome.[21,22]

Histones that are highly acetylated tend to be associated with newly synthesized DNA or transcriptionally active DNA, but the preferred acetylation sites differ between these two processes.[6] Furthermore, newly synthesized histones that associate with replicating DNA are only transiently acetylated, whereas histones in transcriptionally active DNA are dynamically acetylated. Use of an antibody that is reactive against the ε-acetyl lysine of histones demonstrated that the acetylated chromatin fraction from chick embryo erythrocytes was strongly enriched in the transcriptionally active α-D-globin gene sequences.[23] The acetylation of histone H4, particularly on Lys16, was shown by mutational analysis to be important for activating transcription of certain genes in *S. cerevisiae*.[24] During DNA replication, H4 is diacetylated before its deposition, possibly in a complex with H3, onto chromatin, where it assembles with the other core histones.[25] Acetylation of the deposited histones inhibits binding of the internucleosomal histone H1 to newly assembled chromatin.[26] Other chromatin-associated proteins, such as the high-mobility-group proteins I and II, are also subject to acetylation.

A subset of α-tubulin has also been shown to be acetylated on the ε-amino group of an internal lysine residue, identified as Lys40.[27] The dimer of α- and β-tubulin constitutes the building block of microtubules. These essential structural components of the cytoskeleton affect cell shape, motility, and organelle movement; in the nucleus microtubules guide chromosome segregation. Acetylation of α-tubulin apparently occurs in the assembled microtubule, which proved to be a better substrate than the tubulin dimer for the isolated acetylase activity.[28] Acetylation appears to stabilize the microtubules, which become resistant to agents such as colchicine that depolymerize unmodified microtubules. Furthermore, treatment with drugs such as taxol that stabilize microtubules leads to increased α-tubulin acetylation.[29]

Acetylated microtubules show a distinct intracellular distribution,[6] which is detected by an antibody specific for the acetylated form of α-tubulin. In migrating human 3T3 cells, acetylated microtubules are excluded from the leading-edge microtubules. They are located preferentially in axons rather than dendrites of rat cerebellum, but they are excluded from the growth cones of neurite tips.[30] In chick muscle fibers, they underlie motor endplates, participating in vesicle and organelle transport, whereas the unacetylated cytoplasmic microtubules contribute to the flexible alteration of cell shape. The nuclear distribution of acetylated microtubules changes during the course of meiosis and mitosis,[31] tending to move from the poles at metaphase to the spindle at anaphase and being restricted to the midbody by telophase. The acetylated population of microtubules also becomes polarized as asymmetry develops during cell differentiation, for example, during the preimplantation development of mouse embryo cells.[32]

Protein acylation with myristic acid. Several cellular proteins are covalently modified with myristic acid, a 14-carbon saturated fatty acid.[6] Sequence requirements for myristoylation at free N-terminal α-amino groups, the most common site for modification, are much more stringent than for the analogous acetylation. It absolutely requires an N-terminal glycine, originally in the second position; a small uncharged subterminal residue and a serine in the sixth position are important. The isolated myristoyl transferase shows a specific preference for myristoyl-CoA over other possible acyl-CoA donors.[33] Myristate modifies proteins that are located in the cytoplasm, as well as proteins associated with the plasma membrane, the endoplasmic reticulum, and the nuclear membrane. N-terminal myristoylation, which occurs cotranslationally and is irreversible, may be required for a protein to bind to membranes, but it is rarely sufficient for membrane association, which requires additional protein modifications or cofactors. Modification with a second hydrophobic moiety, in addition to myristate, has been observed to direct certain proteins to particular membrane locations.[34] It was demonstrated in S. cerevisiae that N-terminal myristoylation is essential for cell viability because disruption of the gene for N-myristoyl transferase was recessively lethal.[35]

There are many cellular proteins whose N-terminal myristoylation has been described and characterized.[6] These include enzymes, such as NADH-cytochrome b_5 reductase and the endothelial nitric oxide synthase,[36] as well as proteins that participate in signal transduction, such as cAMP-dependent protein kinase and the B subunit of calcineurin, a calmodulin-dependent protein phosphatase. An N-myristoylated protein that is an alanine-rich protein kinase C substrate (MARCKS) has been identified as an actin filament cross-linking protein that may be involved in the cytoskeletal rearrangements of stimulated cells. Myristoylation of MARCKS is required for its initial binding to the plasma membrane, but cell activation causes MARCKS to become phosphorylated and to dissociate from membranes, relocalizing to the cytosol.[37]

The pp60[src] protein is a viral oncogenic tyrosine kinase that is N-myristoylated.[6] A mutagenized, nonmyristoylated pp60[src] retained enzymatic activity but did not associate with the plasma membrane and was unable to transform cells. As a result of the pp60[src] mutation, a small group of membrane-associated proteins had decreased tyrosine phosphorylation.[38] A myristic acid analogue with reduced hydrophobicity also prevented pp60[src] from associating with membranes, suggesting its possible use as an antitumor agent.[39] When the cellular Src protein was mutagenized at its N-terminal glycine, and hence nonmyristoylated, its kinase activity in mitosis was blocked, presumably because a membrane-bound phosphatase regulates activity of the cellular Src protein.[40] Although pp60[src] itself is not additionally modified with palmitic acid, many members of this tyrosine kinase family are palmitoylated within the six N-terminal residues as well as N-terminally myristoylated.[34] N-termi-

nal myristoylation of viral structural proteins is required for formation of mature mammalian retroviruses, papovaviruses, and picornaviruses.[6]

N-terminal myristoylation occurs on a subset of the α subunits of G proteins, the heterotrimeric GTP-binding proteins that mediate transmembrane signaling from a wide range of hormone and neurotransmitter agonists.[41] This modification occurs on members of the G_i and G_o subfamilies, and it was found to affect α subunit interaction with the βγ subunits and to be required for signal transduction by $α_{12}$.[42] Like the Src-related tyrosine kinases, certain myristoylated α subunits are also modified with palmitate near the N-terminal myristate.[43]

ADP-ribosylation factors (ARFs) are N-myristoylated monomeric GTP-binding proteins that regulate intracellular vesicular transport and activate phospholipase D. Although they are predominantly cytosolic, ARFs also localize to the Golgi, where they copurify with non-clathrin-coated transport vesicles. Both myristoylation and GTP are required for the binding of ARFs to membranes,[44] and myristoylation has been proposed to stabilize the N-terminus in an amphipathic α-helix that contributes to the interaction between ARFs and membranes. GTP hydrolysis and guanine nucleotide exchange likely regulate the cycling of myristoylated ARF between soluble and membrane-associated forms as a part of regulated vesicle transport.

For a small number of cellular proteins, myristoylation occurs on the ε-amino groups of internal lysine residues. These include the insulin receptor, the interleukin-1 α and β precursors, tumor necrosis factor α precursor, and the μ immunoglobulin heavy chain, which becomes acylated during transport through the Golgi complex.[45–48] The core subunit I of cytochrome c oxidase becomes internally myristoylated in Neurospora crassa, suggesting that mitochondria contain the enzymatic components required to myristoylate this mitochondrially encoded protein.[49]

Protein acylation with palmitic acid. Palmitate is an abundant, 16-carbon saturated fatty acid that is added to viral and cellular proteins posttranslationally and reversibly, typically by an ester bond to a serine or cysteine residue.[6] Being more hydrophobic than myristate, palmitate causes modified proteins to associate with membranes, most often the plasma membrane. The addition and removal of palmitate provides a mechanism for cellular regulation of a protein's location and consequent activity. Enzymes with palmitoyl transferase activity show little apparent substrate specificity in terms of the fatty acyl group that is transferred from CoA or the sequence requirements for the addition. Certain proteins that are N-myristoylated are also modified with palmitate, including the Src-related tyrosine kinases (but not Src itself), a subset of the G protein α subunits, and endothelial nitric oxide synthase.[34,43,50] By increasing a protein's membrane affinity, prior myristoylation appears to facilitate transfer of palmitate to dually acylated proteins.[51] It has been proposed that dual acylation of Src-related kinases directs their association with glycosyl phosphatidylinositol–anchored outer membrane proteins, an association that may help to transduce extracellular signals in immune system cells.[52]

Many G protein α subunits are esterified to palmitate at the third-position cysteine. Mutation of this cysteine in $G_o1\alpha$ caused relocalization of the subunit from an exclusively membrane location to a distribution between the cytosol and the membrane, despite the retention of N-terminal myristoylation.[53] $G_{s\alpha}$, the G protein α subunit that mediates hormonal stimulation of cAMP synthesis, required palmitate both for membrane localization of the subunit and for its stimulation of adenylyl cyclase.[54] Modification with palmitate appears to be a mechanism for regulating $G_{s\alpha}$ activity in vivo, with α_s becoming rapidly depalmitoylated after binding GTP in response to hormonal activation. The depalmitoylated α subunit is released from the membrane and translocates to the cytosol.[54]

Esterification to palmitate is also characteristic of most viral and cellular Ras proteins, which are monomeric GTP-binding proteins. The mammalian Ras protein is an essential part of a signal transduction pathway, required for activation of the mitogen-activated protein kinase cascade.[55] Palmitoylation occurs close to the carboxyl end of the proteins, near C-terminal isoprenyl and methyl modifications. Palmitate addition is required for oncogenic Ras proteins to associate strongly with membranes and to transform cells.[6] Palmitoylation of the Ras2 protein of S. cerevisiae was shown to be required for its efficient membrane localization.[56]

Many transmembrane receptors are esterified to palmitate in their cytoplasmic domains. These include the iron-transferrin receptor, the insulin receptor, and the nicotinic acetylcholine receptor, as well as several membrane glycoproteins of immune system cells. Several G protein-coupled receptors have a conserved cysteine in their cytoplasmic tail that is modified by palmitic acid. The structure of these receptors is characterized by seven transmembrane α-helices that are linked by three intracellular and three extracellular loops. Palmitoylation, which is thought to lead to the formation of a fourth intracellular loop, occurs in the photoreceptor rhodopsin, dopamine (D_1 and D_2) receptors, the β_2-adrenergic receptor, the α_{2A}-adrenergic receptor, thyrotropin-releasing hormone receptor, and the choriogonadotropin receptor. The biological effects of palmitoylation appear to vary for these receptors. For both the dopamine receptor[57] and the β_2-adrenergic receptor,[58] palmitate is added shortly after the receptor is exposed to agonist, and this modification contributes to agonist-dependent desensitization of the receptor. For the α_{2A}-adrenergic

receptor, palmitoylation contributes to down-regulation of receptor number,[59] whereas for thyrotropin-releasing hormone and choriogonadotropin receptors, palmitoylation slows internalization of the receptors after prolonged agonist exposure.[60]

Several proteins that link plasma membrane components to intracellular or extracellular proteins are modified with palmitate. These include gap-junction proteins of heart and eye lens and cytoskeleton-attachment proteins such as ankyrin and vinculin.[6,61] Spectrin, which is a major component of the erythrocyte cytoskeleton, is itself palmitoylated in its β subunit, and this acylated subpopulation is more tightly associated with the cell membrane than is unmodified spectrin.[62] Palmitoylation of the transmembrane glycoprotein GP85 is required for its high-affinity binding to ankyrin,[63] suggesting that palmitoylation may be important for protein, as well as membrane, interactions.

Analyses of vesicular transport of proteins destined for the cell surface have shown that palmitoyl-CoA is required for reconstituting transport through the Golgi stacks in vitro.[64] Both the budding of vesicles from donor Golgi, which involves cisternal membrane fusion, and fusion of these vesicles with acceptor Golgi cisternae depended on the addition of fatty acyl-CoA. Vesicle budding was inhibited by addition of either a nonhydrolyzable analogue of palmitoyl-CoA or an inhibitor of acyl-CoA synthetase. Molecules that accept the required acyl group have not been identified.

Several differentiated cells have characteristic proteins that are palmitoylated. In epidermal keratinocytes, a transglutaminase cross-links peptides into an envelope that contributes to cell cohesiveness, and reduced transglutaminase activity in individuals is associated with severe skin disorders.[65] The transglutaminase requires modification with palmitate for its anchorage in the keratinocyte membrane.[66] Pulmonary surfactant has a major peptide component, SP-C, that contains two esterified palmitate groups.[67] The glycoprotein of gastric mucus, which is also fatty acylated, includes a protease-resistant fraction that is highly acylated with 20 mol fatty acid/mol glycoprotein.[68] In cystic fibrosis patients this protease-resistance fraction is more highly acylated with 66 mol fatty acid/mol glycoprotein, probably contributing to the insoluble mucous secretions of these patients.

In developing brains, GAP-43 is a major component of the growth cone membranes of elongating axons, and SNAP-25 is a synaptic protein involved in later stages of axon growth. The reversible acylation of both of these proteins has been proposed to be important for growth cone motility and process outgrowth.[69] The unacylated form of GAP-43 stimulates the heterotrimeric GTP-binding protein G_o, whereas the addition of palmitate to GAP-43 blocks this activity.[70] Nitric oxide, which inhibits the growth of cultured neurites and causes growth cone collapse, also inhibits the acylation of GAP-43 and SNAP-25, along with that of other neuronal proteins. The effect of nitric oxide on neurite growth, which may contribute to the regulation of process outgrowth and remodeling in vivo, was proposed to be due, at least in part, to its inhibition of neuronal protein acylation.[69]

Isoprenylation of proteins. Farnesyl and geranyl-geranyl are isoprenoid compounds whose synthesis requires CoA. These two isoprenoids become covalently attached to certain proteins at their mature carboxyl termini. This modification is accompanied either by the addition of palmitate or by a series of basic amino acids nearby. Although Ras-related proteins and most cellular proteins are modified by the 20-carbon geranyl-geranyl, Ras itself is modified by the 15-carbon farnesyl.[71] Prenylation, which increases membrane-affinity, is necessary for oncogenic Ras proteins to transform cells. The cellular Ras protein, a critical component of the mitogen-activated protein kinase cascade, acts by directing the protein kinase Raf to the plasma membrane. Ras was dispensable, however, when a farnesylation signal was added to Raf, which localized by itself to the correct membrane site.[55] Nuclear lamins A and B are isoprenylated, as are several γ subunits of heterotrimeric G proteins, including retinal transducin.[71]

Mammalian Rab proteins are monomeric GTP-binding proteins, related to Ras, that associate with specific organellar membranes and are proposed to regulate specific stages of vesicular transport to the cell surface.[72] The cycling of Rab proteins between cytosolic and membrane-bound forms is related to vesicular movement between organelles via membrane budding and fusion. C-terminal modification of Rab proteins with geranyl-geranyl was found to be necessary for membrane binding as well as for interaction of a Rab protein with a specific GDP dissociation inhibitor that releases the Rab protein from membranes.[73] Retinal degradation or choroideremia in human cells is associated with a defect in a protein that has sequence homology to GDP dissociation inhibitors.[71]

Deficiency

The effects of a pantothenate-deficient diet have been studied in several animal species.[74] Rats deficient in pantothenate develop hypertrophy of the adrenal cortex, followed by hemorrhage and necrosis; they also show increased resistance to certain viral infections. Deficiency in dogs produces hypoglycemia, gastrointestinal symptoms, rapid respiration and heart beat, and convulsions. There is depressed heme synthesis in monkeys, leading to anemia. When pantothenic acid–deficient mice were exercised, they displayed lower stamina and had lower liver and muscle glycogen levels.[12] Pantothenate-deficient chickens show dermatitis, poor feathering, and axon and

myelin degeneration within the spinal cord. Deficiency-induced dermatitis and graying in mice was reversed by administration of pantothenic acid, but the once-popular idea that pantothenate might restore hair color in humans proved fruitless.

Because of the widespread availability of pantothenic acid, humans rarely are deficient in it. However, deficiency has been detected under conditions of severe malnutrition. World War II prisoners of war in the Philippines, Japan, and Burma suffered from a disease in which their toes became numb and they experienced painful burning sensations in their feet. Pantothenic acid was specifically required to relieve these symptoms of nutritional melalgia.[75] When pantothenic acid deficiency was induced in humans by combined administration of the antagonist ω-methylpantothenate and a pantothenate-deficient diet, the most common symptoms were headache, fatigue, insomnia, intestinal disturbances, and paresthesia of hands and feet. Also reported were a decrease in the eosinopenic response to ACTH, a loss of antibody production, and increased sensitivity to insulin.[76]

Requirement

Although formal recommended dietary allowances (RDA) have not been established for pantothenic acid, the recommended daily intake is 18–32 μmol (4–7 mg) pantothenic acid for adults. The recommended amount is lower for younger age groups, being 9 μmol (2 mg) daily for infants and 18–23 μmol (4–5 mg) daily for children 7–10 years of age.[77] These recommendations are consistent with the actual pantothenate content of the average American diet, estimated in one analysis at 5.8 mg/day.[12,78] However, a study of adolescents showed that despite a pantothenate intake of < 4 mg/day by some subjects, blood concentrations of the vitamin were in the normal range (0.91–2.74 μmol/L), and urinary excretion was highly correlated with dietary intake.[79]

Food and Other Sources

Pantothenic acid is widely distributed in nature, being essential for all forms of life. Dietary sources that are particularly rich in pantothenate, having at least 50 μg/g dry weight, are liver, kidney, yeast, egg yolk, and broccoli. Royal bee jelly (511 μg/g) and ovaries of tuna and cod (2.32 mg/g) have extremely high levels of pantothenic acid.[74] Human milk is rich in pantothenate, which increases five-fold within 4 days after parturition, from 2.2 to 11.2 μmol/L (48 to 245 μg/dL); cow's milk has a similar pantothenate content.[74] Pantothenic acid is relatively stable at neutral pH. Nevertheless, cooking is reported to destroy 15–50% of the vitamin in meat, and the processing of vegetables was associated with pantothenate losses of 37–78%.[12] Panthenol, the alcohol derivative of pantothenic acid, is widely used as a supplement in multivitamin preparations because it is more stable than pantothenate, to which it is converted by humans after intake.[80] The calcium and sodium salts of D-pantothenate are also available as supplements.

Excess, Toxicity

High oral doses of calcium pantothenate were not toxic to rats, dogs, rabbits, or humans. However, the lethal dose for mice (LD_{50}), leading to respiratory failure, was determined to be 42 mmol (10 g)/kg.[74]

Summary

Pantothenic acid is a ubiquitous vitamin in which humans are rarely deficient. It is converted in the body to CoA, the form in which it accomplishes most of its biological functions. The essential roles pantothenic acid plays in the synthesis and acetylation of small molecules and in respiratory metabolism have long been recognized. Pantothenate is also required for the modification of numerous proteins with acetyl and fatty acyl groups, modifications that affect protein localization and activity. Many proteins involved in signal transduction are acylated, as are several proteins of erythrocytes, the immune system, the nervous system, and hormonally responsive cells.

References

1. Williams RJ, Lyman CM, Goodyear GH, et al (1933) "Pantothenic acid," a growth determinant of universal biological occurrence. J Am Chem Soc 55:2912–2927
2. Wagner AF, Folders K (1964) Vitamins and coenzymes. Interscience/John Wiley & Sons, New York
3. Williams RJ, Major RT (1940) The structure of pantothenic acid. Science 91:246
4. Lipmann F, Kaplan NO, Novelli GD, et al (1947) Coenzyme for acetylation, a pantothenic acid derivative. J Biol Chem 167:869–870
5. Brown G (1959) The metabolism of pantothenic acid. J Biol Chem 234:370–378
6. Plesofsky-Vig N, Brambl R (1988) Pantothenic acid and coenzyme A in cellular modification of proteins. Annu Rev Nutr 8:461–482
7. Metzler DE (1977) Biochemistry. Academic Press, New York
8. Wakil SJ, Stoops JK, Joshi VC (1983) Fatty acid synthesis and its regulation. Annu Rev Biochem 52:537–579
9. Fenstermacher DK, Rose RC (1986) Absorption of pantothenic acid in rat and chick intestine. Am J Physiol 250:G155–G160
10. Grassl SM (1992) Human placental brush-border membrane Na⁺-pantothenate cotransport. J Biol Chem 267:22902–22906
11. Robishaw JD, Berkich D, Neely JR (1982) Rate-limiting step and control of coenzyme A synthesis in cardiac muscle. J Biol Chem 257:10967–10972
12. Tahiliani AG, Beinlich CJ (1991) Pantothenic acid in health and disease. Vitam Horm 46:165–228
13. Wittwer CT, Burkhard D, Ririe K, et al (1983) Purification and properties of a pantetheine hydrolysing enzyme from pig kidney. J Biol Chem 258:9733–9738
14. Driessen HPC, de Jong WW, Tesser GI, Bloemendal H (1985) The mechanism of N-terminal acetylation of proteins. CRC Crit Rev Biochem 18:281–306
15. Gonen H, Smith CE, Siegel NR, et al (1994) Protein synthesis elongation factor EF-1α is essential for ubiquitin-dependent degradation of certain Nα-acetylated proteins and may be substituted for by the bacterial elongation factor EF-Tu. Proc Natl Acad Sci USA 91:7648–7652
16. Mullen JR, Kayne PS, Moerschell RP, et al (1989) Identification and characterization of genes and mutants for an N-terminal acetyltransferase from yeast. EMBO J 8:2067–2075
17. Johnsson N, Marriott G, Weber K (1988) p36, the major cytoplasmic substrate of src tyrosine protein kinase, binds to its p11 regulatory subunit via a short amino-terminal amphiphatic helix. EMBO J 7:2435–2442
18. Herbert E, Uhler M (1982) Biosynthesis of polyprotein precursors to regulatory peptides. Cell 30:1–2
19. O'Donohue TL, Handelmann GE, Miller RL, Jacobowitz DM (1982) N-acetylation regulates the behavioral activity of α-melanotropin in a multineurotransmitter neuron. Science 215:1125–1127
20. Csordas A (1990) On the biological role of histone acetylation. Biochem J 265:23–38
21. Ridsdale JA, Hendzel MJ, Delcuve GP, Davie JR (1990) Histone acetylation alters the capacity of the H1 histones to condense transcriptionally active/competent chromatin. J Biol Chem 265:5150–5156
22. Norton VG, Imai BS, Yau P, Bradbury EM (1989) Histone acetylation reduces nucleosome core particle linking number change. Cell 57:449–457
23. Hebbes TR, Thorne AW, Crane-Robinson C (1988) A direct link between core histone acetylation and transcriptionally active chromatin. EMBO J 7:1395–1402
24. Durrin LK, Mann RK, Kayne PS, Grunstein M (1991) Yeast histone H4 N-terminal sequence is required for promoter activation in vivo. Cell 65:1023–1031
25. Perry CA, Dadd CA, Allis CD, Annunziato AT (1993) Analysis of nucleosome assembly and histone exchange using antibodies specific for acetylated H4. Biochemistry 32:13605–13614
26. Perry CA, Annunziato AT (1991) Histone acetylation reduces H1-mediated nucleosome interactions during chromatin assembly. Exp Cell Res 196:337–345
27. Edde B, Rossier J, Le Caer JP, et al (1991) A combination of posttranslational modifications is responsible for the production of neuronal alpha-tubulin heterogeneity. J Cell Biochem 46:134–142
28. Maruta H, Greer K, Rosenbaum JL (1986) The acetylation of alpha-tubulin and its relationship to the assembly and disassembly of microtubules. J Cell Biol 103:571–579
29. Piperno G, LeDizet M, Chang X-J (1987) Microtubules containing acetylated α-tubulin in mammalian cells in culture. J Cell Biol 104:289–302
30. Robson SJ, Burgoyne RD (1989) Differential localisation of tyrosinated, detyrosinated, and acetylated alpha-tubulins in neurites and growth cones of dorsal root ganglion neurons. Cell Motil Cytoskeleton 12:273–282
31. Schatten G, Simerly C, Asai DJ, et al (1988) Acetylated α-tubulin in microtubules during mouse fertilization and early development. Dev Biol 130:74–86
32. Houliston E, Maro B (1989) Posttranslational modification of distinct microtubule subpopulations during cell polarization and differentiation in the mouse preimplantation embryo. J Cell Biol 108:543–551

33. Towler DA, Adams SP, Eubanks SR, et al (1987) Purification and characterization of yeast myristoylCoA:protein N-myristoyltransferase. Proc Natl Acad Sci USA 84:2708–2712

34. Resh MD (1994) Myristylation and palmitylation of Src family members: the fats of the matter. Cell 76:411–413

35. Duronio RJ, Towler DA, Heuckeroth RO, Gordon JI (1989) Disruption of the yeast N-myristoyl transferase gene causes recessive lethality. Science 243:796–800

36. Liu J, Sessa WC (1994) Identification of covalently bound amino-terminal myristic acid in endothelial nitric oxide synthase. J Biol Chem 269:11691–11694

37. Taniguchi H, Manenti S (1993) Interaction of myristoylated alanine-rich protein kinase C substrate (MARCKS) with membrane phospholipids. J Biol Chem 268:9960–9963

38. Linder ME, Burr JG (1988) Nonmyristoylated p60^{v-src} fails to phosphorylate proteins of 115–120kDa in chicken embryo fibroblasts. Proc Natl Acad Sci USA 85:2608–2612

39. Heuckeroth RO, Gordon JI (1989) Altered membrane association of p60^{v-src} and a murine 63-kDa N-myristoyl protein after incorporation of an oxygen-substituted analog of myristic acid. Proc Natl Acad Sci USA 86:5262–5266

40. Bagrodia S, Taylor SJ, Shalloway D (1993) Myristylation is required for Tyr-527 dephosphorylation and activation of pp60^{c-src} in mitosis. Mol Cell Biol 13:1464–1470

41. Mumby SM, Linder ME (1994) Myristoylation of G-protein α subunits. Methods Enzymol 237:254–268

42. Gallego C, Gupta SK, Winitz S, et al (1992) Myristoylation of the G$α_{i2}$ polypeptide, a G protein α subunit, is required for its signaling and transformation functions. Proc Natl Acad Sci USA 89:9695–9699

43. Mumby SM, Kleuss C, Gilman AG (1994) Receptor regulation of G-protein palmitoylation. Proc Natl Acad Sci USA 91:2800–2804

44. Haun RS, Tsai S-C, Adamik R, et al (1993) Effect of myristoylation on GTP-dependent binding of ADP-ribosylation factor to Golgi. J Biol Chem 268:7064–7068

45. Hedo JA, Collier E, Watkinson A (1987) Myristyl and palmityl acylation of the insulin receptor. J Biol Chem 262:954–957

46. Stevenson FT, Bursten SL, Fanton C, et al (1993) The 31-kDa precursor of interleukin 1α is myristoylated on specific lysines within the 16-kDa N-terminal propiece. Proc Natl Acad Sci USA 90:7245–7249

47. Stevenson FT, Bursten SL, Locksley RM, Lovett DH (1992) Myristyl acylation of the tumor necrosis factor α precursor on specific lysine residues. J Exp Med 176:1053–1062

48. Pillai S, Baltimore D (1987) Myristoylation and the posttranslational acquisition of hydrophobicity by the membrane immunoglobulin heavy-chain polypeptide in B lymphocytes. Proc Natl Acad Sci USA 84:7654–7658

49. Vassilev AO, Plesofsky-Vig N, Brambl R (1995) Cytochrome c oxidase in Neurospora crassa contains myristic acid covalently linked to subunit 1. Proc Natl Acad Sci USA 92:8680–8684

50. Robinson, LJ, Busconi L, Michel T (1995) Agonist-modulated palmitoylation of endothelial nitric oxide synthase. J Biol Chem 270:995–998

51. Degtyarev MY, Spiegel AM, Jones TLZ (1994) Palmitoylation of a G protein α$_i$ subunit requires membrane localization not myristoylation. J Biol Chem 269:30898–30903

52. Shenoy-Scaria AM, Gauen LKT, Kwong J, et al (1993) Palmitylation of an amino-terminal cysteine motif of protein tyrosine kinases p56^{lck} and p59^{fyn} mediates interaction with glycosyl-phosphatidylinositol-anchored proteins. Mol Cell Biol 13:6385–6392

53. Grassie MA, McCallum JF, Guzzi F, et al (1994) The palmitoylation status of the G-protein G$_o$1α regulates its avidity of interaction with the plasma membrane. Biochem J 302:913–920

54. Wedegaertner PB, Bourne HR (1994) Activation and depalmitoylation of G$_{sα}$. Cell 77:1063–1070

55. Stokoe D, Macdonald SG, Cadwallader K, et al (1994) Activation of Raf as a result of recruitment to the plasma membrane. Science 264:1463–1467

56. Kuroda Y, Suzuki N, Kataoka T (1993) The effect of posttranslational modifications on the interaction of Ras2 with adenylyl cyclase. Science 259:683–686

57. Ng GYK, Mouillac B, George SR, et al (1994) Desensitization, phosphorylation and palmitoylation of the human dopamine D$_1$ receptor. Eur J Pharmacol 267:7–19

58. Mouillac B, Caron M, Bonin H, et al (1992) Agonist-modulated palmitoylation of β$_2$-adrenergic receptor in Sf9 cells. J Biol Chem 267:21733–21737

59. Eason MG, Jacinto MT, Theiss CT, Liggett SB (1994) The palmitoylated cysteine of the cytoplasmic tail of α$_{2A}$-adrenergic receptors confers subtype-specific agonist-promoted downregulation. Proc Natl Acad Sci USA 91:11178–11182

60. Kawate N, Menon KMJ (1994) Palmitoylation of luteinizing hormone/human choriogonadotropin receptors in transfected cells. J Biol Chem 269:30651–30658

61. Manenti S, Dunia I, Benedetti EL (1990) Fatty acid acylation of lens fiber plasma membrane proteins. MP26 and α-crystallin are palmitoylated. FEBS Lett 262:356–358

62. Mariani M, Maretzki D, Lutz HU (1993) A tightly membrane-associated subpopulation of spectrin is ^{3}H-palmitoylated. J Biol Chem 268:12996–13001

63. Bourguignon LYW, Kalomiris EL, Lokeshwar VB (1991) Acylation of the lymphoma transmembrane glycoprotein, GP85, may be required for GP85-ankyrin interaction. J Biol Chem 266:11761–11765

64. Pfanner N, Orci L, Glick BS, et al (1989) Fatty acyl-coenzyme A is required for budding of transport vesicles from Golgi cisternae. Cell 59:95–102

65. Huber M, Rettler I, Bernasconi K, et al (1995) Mutations of keratinocyte transglutaminase in lamellar ichthyosis. Science 267:525–528

66. Chakravarty R, Rice RH (1989) Acylation of keratinocyte transglutaminase by palmitic and myristic acids in the membrane anchorage region. J Biol Chem 264:625–629

67. Curstedt T, Johansson J, Persson P, et al (1990) Hydrophobic surfactant-associated polypeptides: SP-C is a lipopeptide with two palmitoylated cysteine residues, whereas SP-B lacks covalently linked fatty acyl groups. Proc Natl Acad Sci USA 87:2985–2989

68. Slomiany A, Jozwiak Z, Takagi A, Slomiany BL (1984) The role of covalently bound fatty acids in the degradation of human gastric mucus glycoprotein. Arch Biochem Biophys 229:560–567

69. Hess DT, Patterson SI, Smith DS, Skene JHP (1993) Neuronal growth cone collapse and inhibition of protein fatty acylation by nitric oxide. Nature 366:562–565

70. Sudo Y, Valenzuela D, Beck-Sickinger AG, et al (1992) Palmitoylation alters protein activity: blockade of G$_o$ stimulation by GAP-43. EMBO J 11:2095–2102

71. Marshall CJ (1993) Protein prenylation: a mediator of protein-protein interactions. Science 259:1865–1866

72. Farnsworth CC, Seabra MC, Ericsson LH (1994) Rab geranylgeranyl transferase catalyzes the geranylgeranylation of adjacent cysteines in the small GTPases Rab1A, Rab3A, and Rab5A. Proc Natl Acad Sci USA 91:11963–11967

73. Araki S, Kaibuchi K, Sasaki T, et al (1991) Role of the C-terminal region of smg p25A in its interaction with mem-

branes and the GDP/GTP exchange protein. Mol Cell Biol 11:1438–1447

74. Robinson FA (1966) The vitamin co-factors of enzyme systems. Pergamon Press, Oxford

75. Glusman M (1947) The syndrome of "burning feet" (nutritional melalgia) as manifestion of nutritional deficiency. Am J Med 3:211–223

76. Hodges RE, Ohlson MA, Bean WB (1958) Pantothenic acid deficiency in man. J Clin Invest 37:1642–1657

77. Food and Nutrition Board, National Research Council (1989) Recommended dietary allowances, 10th ed. National Academy Press, Washington, DC

78. Tarr JB, Tamura T, Stokstad ELR (1981) Availability of vitamin B_6 and pantothenate in an average American diet in man. Am J Clin Nutr 34:1328–1337

79. Eissenstat BR, Wyse BW, Hansen RG (1986) Pantothenic acid status of adolescents. Am J Clin Nutr 44:931–937

80. Bird OD, Thompson RQ (1967) Pantothenic acid. In Gyorgy P, Pearson WN (eds), The vitamins, Vol 7, 2nd ed. Academic Press, New York, pp 209–241

Chapter 24

Calcium
and Phosphorus

Claude D. Arnaud and Sarah D. Sanchez

Calcium

Calcium is responsible for structural functions involving the skeleton and soft tissues and regulatory functions such as neuromuscular transmission of chemical and electrical stimuli, cellular secretion, and blood clotting. More than 99% of body calcium is in the skeleton.

Calcium is the most abundant divalent cation in the human body, making up 1.5–2.0% of its total weight. All living things possess powerful mechanisms to conserve calcium and to maintain constant cellular and extracellular fluid (ECF) calcium concentrations.[1-3] The physiological functions of calcium are so vital to survival that in the face of severe dietary deficiency or abnormal losses, the same mechanisms can demineralize bone to prevent even minor hypocalcemia. Bone provides a vital and readily available source of calcium for the maintenance of normal ECF calcium concentrations, ≈50% of which is ionized (Ca^{2+}) and physiologically active.

The endocrine system that helps maintain calcium homeostasis in vertebrates is integrated and complex.[4,5] It involves the interaction of two polypeptide hormones, parathyroid hormone (PTH) and calcitonin (CT), and a sterol hormone, 1,25-dihydroxycholecalciferol (calcitriol).[6-8] Biosynthesis and secretion of the polypeptide hormones are regulated by a negative feedback mechanism involving ECF Ca^{2+}. The biosynthesis of calcitriol from the major circulating metabolite of vitamin D, 25-hydroxycholecalciferol (calcidiol), takes place in the kidney and is regulated by PTH and CT as well as by concentrations of calcium and phosphate in the ECF. Other hormones, such as insulin, cortisol, growth hormone, thyroxine, epinephrine, estrogen, and testosterone, together with several growth factors (e.g., the insulin-like growth factors IGF1 and 2) and some compounds not yet identified, as well as certain physical phenomena, have roles in modifying and regulating organ responses to PTH, CT, and calcitriol.[9]

The relationships among the major components that maintain calcium homeostasis are illustrated in Figure 1.[2] Each of the three overlapping feedback loops involves one of the target organs of the calciotropic hormones and the four controlling elements, plasma calcium, PTH, CT, and calcitriol. The left limbs of the loops depict physiological events that increase plasma calcium and the right limbs depict events that decrease plasma calcium. Under physiological conditions there are small fluctuations in plasma calcium. Decreases in plasma calcium increase PTH secretion and decrease CT secretion. These changes in hormone secretion lead to increased bone resorption, decreased renal excretion of calcium, and increased intestinal calcium absorption via PTH stimulation of calcitriol production (left side of figure). As a consequence, plasma calcium increases slightly above its physiological concentrations, inhibiting PTH secretion and stimulating CT secretion. These changes in plasma hormone concentrations decrease bone resorption, increase renal calcium excretion, and decrease intestinal absorption of calcium (right side of figure), causing plasma calcium to fall slightly below the physiologic concentration. This sequence of events occurs within microseconds and is constantly repeated so that plasma calcium is maintained at physiologic concentrations with minimal oscillation. The "butterfly" scheme in the figure not only demonstrates the relationships among elements that control mineral homeostasis under physiological conditions but also illustrates adaptive responses to various specific perturbations.

Phosphorus

A major element in hydroxyapatite, phosphorus is a key inorganic constituent of bone. In cells, it is an important part of many life-sustaining compounds, such as phospholipids, phosphoproteins, and nucleic acids; the hormonal second messengers cyclic adenosine monophosphate, cyclic guanine monophosphate, and inositol polyphosphates; and 2,3-diphosphoglycerate, which is the regulator of oxygen release by hemoglobin. Phosphorus is also the repository of metabolic energy in the

245

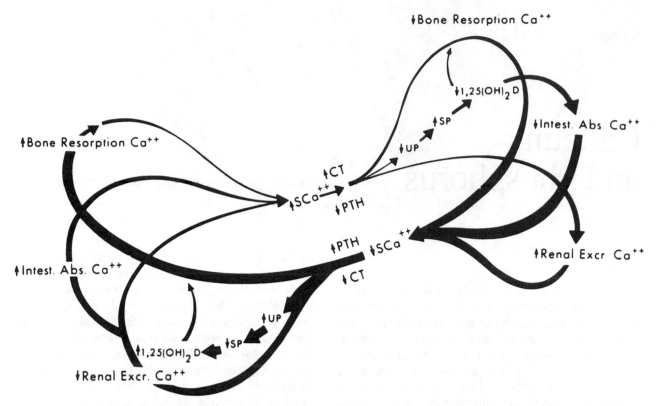

Figure 1. Regulation of calcium homeostasis. Three overlapping control loops interlock and relate to one another through the level of blood concentrations of ionic calcium, parathyroid hormone (PTH), and calcitonin (CT). Each loop involves a calciotropic hormone target organ (bone, intestine, or kidney). The limbs on the left depict physiological events that increase blood concentrations of serum calcium (SCa^{2+}), and the limbs on the right, events that decrease this concentration. UP, urine phosphorus: SP, serum phosphorus. From reference 2. (Used with permission.)

form of the high-energy phosphate bond, an allosteric regulator of many enzymes, and an active participant in many physiological buffer systems. Serum concentrations of phosphate serve as one of the regulators of the rate of renal production of calcitriol.

Dietary Phosphorus

Spencer et al.[10] showed that an increase in phosphorus intake from 800 mg/day [the recommended dietary allowance (RDA)[11]] to 2000 mg/day in adult males failed to affect calcium balance regardless of the calcium intake, which ranged from 200 to 2000 mg/day. Similarly, Heaney and Recker[12] reported that varying phosphorus intake had no effect on overall calcium balance in perimenopausal women. Both groups observed that urinary calcium excretion varied inversely with dietary phosphorus, implying that fecal calcium excretion must have varied directly with dietary phosphorus because there was no change in calcium balance. It thus appears that changes in phosphorus intake by normal adult humans have important effects on calcium metabolism (decreased intestinal calcium absorption and decreased renal excretion of calcium) but that these effects prob-

ably cancel one another so that calcium balance is not affected.

The mechanism by which increased dietary phosphorus might decrease intestinal absorption of calcium has been investigated. Portale et al.[13] showed that increasing dietary phosphorus from a low intake of <500 mg/day to 3000 mg/day decreased the production rate of calcitriol so that its serum concentration fell from a level 80% greater than normal to the low-normal range. This observation suggests that the ability to adapt to decreases or increases in dietary phosphorus depends on the ability of the kidney to respond by increasing or decreasing its production of calcitriol, respectively.

The question arises, therefore, whether increases in dietary phosphorus might adversely influence calcium economy in those whose kidneys have a limited capacity to produce calcitriol or who need to be in positive calcium balance. There is considerable evidence in animals that diets containing more phosphorus than calcium cause hyperparathyroidism and bone loss.[14-19] Almost all these reports concern young (growing) or aged animals, whereas in humans investigations of the influence of high-phosphate diets on calcium metabolism were performed in young or middle-aged adults.[20-23] In this regard,

Portale et al[24] reported that normal phosphorus intake was sufficient to suppress plasma concentrations of calcitriol in children with moderate renal insufficiency. No studies of the influence of dietary phosphorus on calcium and bone metabolism have been reported in other populations that may be unduly sensitive to increments in dietary phosphorus above the RDA (e.g., the young who are building bone or the elderly who have a decreased ability to absorb or conserve calcium even though concern was expressed previously that high phosphorus intakes may contribute to age-related bone loss in humans).[20,25]

Plasma Calcium and Phosphate

Plasma calcium is distributed in three major fractions: ionized, protein-bound, and complexed.[26] The ionized form (Ca^{2+}), the only biologically active species, constitutes 46–50% of total calcium. The protein-bound fraction, roughly equivalent to the ionized fraction in amount, is biologically inert. The calcium bound to plasma proteins [albumin (80%) and globulin (20%)], however, is important as a readily available reservoir of this important cation. Because the binding of calcium to these proteins obeys the mass-law equation, calcium can dissociate from its binding sites as a first-line defense against hypocalcemia. Moreover, hyperproteinemia (e.g., hyperglobulinemia in myelomatosis) can increase, and hypoproteinemia (e.g., hypoalbuminemia in cirrhosis of the liver and nephrosis) can decrease total plasma calcium. The only means of accurately determining the plasma concentration of Ca^{2+} in hypoproteinemic or hyperproteinemic states is to measure it directly by an ion-sensitive electrode procedure. The fraction of calcium that is complexed to organic (e.g., citrate) and inorganic (e.g., phosphate or sulfate) acids is small ($\approx 8\%$) and, like the ionized fraction, is ultrafilterable (diffusible). Complexed calcium probably has little importance as a reservoir for ionized calcium, but in states of hyperphosphatemia such as may exist in chronic renal failure, excessive complexing of calcium with phosphate may contribute to the decrease in plasma ionized calcium observed in this condition.

The normal range for total serum calcium is narrow (2.2–2.5 mmol/L) and the same is true for the ionized fraction. Thus, values for total calcium <2.2 mmol/L, assuming that plasma protein concentrations are normal, reflect clinically significant hypocalcemia, and values >2.5 mmol/L reflect hypercalcemia. Hypocalcemia produces a myriad of symptoms and, when severe, can result in tetany and possibly convulsions.[27] Hypercalcemia can produce functional changes in most organ systems, which may lead to a confusing variety of symptoms and objective findings.[28]

The serum calcium concentration varies little despite large changes in dietary calcium because of the adaptive alterations by which the endocrine system regulates this mineral (Figure 1). Minor diurnal changes (decreases in the afternoon) have been recorded. In addition, serum calcium concentration decreases with age in men but not in women, probably because of a decrease in serum albumin concentration in men. Total (but not ionized) serum calcium concentration also decreases in pregnancy, and this change may be due to the decrease in serum albumin concentration caused by plasma volume expansion.

In contrast to plasma calcium, only 15% of plasma phosphate is bound to proteins. The rest is ultrafilterable and consists mainly of free HPO_4^{2-} and $NaHPO_4^{1-}$ (85%), with free $H_2PO_4^{1-}$ making up the remainder (15%). By convention, plasma phosphate is expressed as the amount of elemental phosphorus measured. Compared with calcium, serum phosphate concentration has a wider range of normal values (0.8–1.6 mmol/L). Moreover, increases or decreases in dietary phosphorus are promptly reflected in changes in the same direction in serum phosphorus and urinary phosphorus excretion. There are also marked diurnal variations in serum and urinary phosphorus excretion (both may as much as double in the afternoon and evening) even during a fast. These variations are caused in part by diurnal changes in plasma cortisol. Serum phosphorus concentrations in young children are almost double those in adults and increase slightly with age in women, a poorly understood finding that may relate to the increased bone turnover in these groups.

Severe hypophosphatemia (<0.5 mmol/L) can cause both skeletal myopathy and cardiomyopathy.[26] These conditions may lead to rhabdomyolysis. The levels of 2,3-diphosphoglyceric acid and adenosine triphosphate (ATP) in erythrocytes may also decrease; the decrease in 2,3-diphosphoglyceric acid in turn may decrease oxygen delivery to tissues, and the decrease in ATP may cause hemolytic anemia. Chronic moderate hypophosphatemia frequently results in osteomalacia or rickets. Generally, restoration of serum phosphate concentration to normal corrects abnormal organ function in hypophosphatemic conditions.

Acute, severe hyperphosphatemia such as might be induced by intravenous phosphate infusion can cause hypocalcemia severe enough to cause tetany and even death.[26] The less severe hyperphosphatemia induced by phosphate ingestion rarely causes symptoms; if patients have associated disorders with a tendency toward hypocalcemia (e.g., mild hypoparathyroidism or chronic renal failure), however, frank hypocalcemia can be precipitated.

Interrelation of Plasma Calcium and Phosphorus

The physiological importance of the relationship between circulating Ca^{2+} and free phosphate is poorly understood, especially regarding the formation and dissolution of amorphous calcium phosphate [$Ca_3(PO_4)_2$] and hydroxyapatite [$Ca_{10}(PO_4)_6(OH)_6$] in bone. Available evidence, however, indicates that the ion product of normal plasma concentrations of calcium and phosphate (the Ca × P ion product) is considerably higher than is necessary to form these two compounds. Thus, compared with bone, plasma is supersaturated with calcium and phosphate, and this is probably an important driving force in bone mineralization. The positive effect of vitamin D on bone mineralization is probably indirect and resides in its ability to maintain the Ca × P ion product within the normal range by increasing calcium and phosphate absorption from the gut and resorption from bone (Figure 1).

The biological significance of the Ca × P ion product has been questioned in recent years, but it is important to recognize that concentration products <0.7 mmol/L usually reflect a mineralization defect in bone and those >2.2 mmol/L reflect a propensity toward soft tissue calcification. There are exceptions to these numerical guidelines, but short of directly measuring changes in bone formation in biopsy specimens or changes in calcium content in soft tissues, determining the Ca × P ion product may provide the best indirect indication of these pathological changes.

Calcium and Phosphate Economy

The amounts of dietary calcium and phosphate required to maintain metabolic balance (dietary intake equal to urinary and fecal excretion) vary with physiological need, intestinal absorption, and kidney retention.[26] Dietary deprivation of calcium or phosphorus induces adaptive changes in the production and secretion of the calciotropic hormones that minimize the development of negative balance of these two ions (Figure 1). In the case of calcium, only 30–50% of ingested calcium is normally absorbed (fractional absorption). With decreased intake, serum calcium decreases slightly, and the sequence of events depicted in the left limbs of the feedback loops in the figure is activated. In severe chronic dietary deficiency of calcium in normal subjects, increased PTH secretion stimulates increased plasma calcitriol production, which increases fractional intestinal calcium absorption. It also reduces renal calcium excretion, but this response is less important because of the relatively small percentage of filtered calcium that is excreted. Such changes reduce the consequences of this perturbation on overall body calcium economy. The tradeoff for this adaptive response is chronic hyperparathyroidism, a condition that can induce progressive demineralization of bones. Thus, as is the case for most adaptive mechanisms, they are beneficial when applied over a relatively short period of time, but when applied chronically, can have destructive effects of considerable consequence.

Whereas the intestine plays the major adaptive role in dietary calcium deficiency, the kidney plays the major adaptive role in dietary phosphate deficiency. This is because 70–80% of dietary phosphorus is normally absorbed, and practically all (>80%) absorbed phosphorus is excreted by the kidney. Thus, any increase in fractional intestinal absorption of phosphorus in response to dietary deprivation would have little influence in preventing negative balance, but reducing renal excretion by only 50%, for example, would have an effect comparable to that of almost tripling the dietary intake. Reductions of renal excretion of this magnitude and greater occur rapidly and are sustained for long periods of time in response to dietary deprivation of phosphorus. The mechanism involved in this response is not entirely understood. The hypophosphatemia that occurs in phosphate deficiency is associated with increased production of calcitriol, increased intestinal absorption of calcium, mild hypercalcemia, and a decrease in PTH secretion (Figure 1, left, middle limb), increased renal tubular reabsorption of phosphate, and hypophosphaturia. It is well established, however, that efficient renal phosphate conservation in response to dietary phosphate deprivation occurs in parathyroidectomized animals, a finding that casts doubt on whether the calciotropic hormone response to phosphorus deprivation is singularly responsible for the observed hypophosphaturia in this condition.

Bone

Bone is unique as a living tissue in that it is not only rigid and resistant to forces that would ordinarily break brittle materials, but also light enough to be moved by coordinated muscle contractions.[29] These characteristics are a function of the strategic location of two major types of bone. Cortical bone, composed of densely packed mineralized collagen laid down in layers, provides rigidity and is the major component of tubular bones. Trabecular (cancellous) bone is spongy in appearance, provides strength and elasticity, and constitutes the major portion of the axial skeleton. Defective or scanty cortical bone leads to long-bone fractures whereas defective or scanty trabecular bone leads to vertebral fractures. Fractures of long bones also may occur when normal trabecular bone reinforcement is lacking.

Two-thirds of the weight of bone is due to minerals and the remainder to water and collagen. Minor organic components, such as proteoglycans, lipids, noncollagenous proteins, and acidic proteins containing γ-carboxyglutamic acid, are probably very important, but their functions are poorly understood.

The mineral of bone exists in two forms. The major form consists of hydroxyapatite in crystals of variable maturity. The remainder is amorphous calcium phosphate, which lacks a coherent x-ray diffraction pattern, has a lower ratio of calcium to phosphate than does pure hydroxyapatite, occurs in regions of active bone formation, and is present in larger quantities in young bone.

Bone is resorbed and formed continuously throughout life, and these important processes depend on three major types of bone cells, each with different functions. Osteoblasts form new bone on surfaces of bone previously resorbed by osteoclasts. The osteoblasts are thought to be derived from a population of dividing cells on bone surfaces that arise from mesenchymal cells in bone connective tissue. Osteoblasts are actively involved in the synthesis of matrix components of bone (primarily collagen) and probably facilitate the movement of mineral ions between ECF and bone surfaces. The physiological importance of such ion transport by osteoblasts, if it occurs at all, is controversial, but there is widespread agreement that osteoblast-mediated transport of calcium and phosphate is involved in the mineralization of collagen, which in turn is crucial to bone formation. During bone formation osteoblasts gradually become encased in the bone matrix that they have produced.

Once encased, osteoblast function and morphology change, and osteoblasts become osteocytes. Protein synthesis decreases markedly, and the cells develop multiple processes that reach out through lacunae in bone tissue to "communicate" with other osteocyte processes within a bone unit (osteon) and also with the cell processes of surface osteoblasts. The physiological importance of osteocytes is controversial, but they are believed to act as a cellular syncytium that permits translocation of mineral in and out of regions of bone removed from surfaces.

The osteoclast is a multinucleated giant cell that is responsible for bone resorption. It is probably derived from circulating mononucleated macrophages, which differentiate into mature osteoclasts by fusion in the bone environment. These cells contain all of the enzymatic components that, when secreted, solubilize matrix and release calcium and phosphate. Once released, mineral is transported through the osteoclast into the ECF and ultimately into blood. Opinion has varied over the years concerning the relative importance to extracellular mineral homeostasis of the resorption of bone osteoclasts and of the translocation of mineral from the surface of bone into the extracellular space by surface osteoblasts.

Two types of bone structure, woven and lamellar, may be observed microscopically in cortical or trabecular bone. Woven bone is a normal constituent of embryonic bone and usually reflects disease in adult bone. Lamellar bone is stronger and more slowly formed. It replaces woven bone progressively after birth. Woven bone is characterized by nonparallelism of collagen fibers, many osteocytes per unit area of matrix, and mineral that is poorly incorporated into collagen fibrils. Lamellar bone has a parallel arrangement of collagen fibers, few osteocytes per unit area of matrix, and a mineral phase that is within the collagen fibrils. Cortical lamellar bone is present in concentric layers surrounding vascular channels that comprise the haversian systems of cortical bone (osteons). By contrast, the lamellar bone of trabeculae is layered in long sheaves and sheets.

The term "modeling" denotes processes involved in formation of the macroscopic skeleton. Thus, modeling ceases at maturity (18–20 years). The term "remodeling" denotes processes occurring at bone surfaces before and after adult development that maintain the structural integrity of bone. Remodeling abnormalities responsible for metabolic bone diseases involve alterations in the balance between bone formation and bone resorption and lead to diminished structural integrity of bone, ultimately compromising its functions.

Normally, despite continuous bone remodeling, there is little net gain or loss of skeletal mass after longitudinal growth has ceased. This finding led to the view that bone resorption and formation are closely coupled and that coupling is the result of the coordinated activity of packets of interacting osteoblasts and osteoclasts. These packets have been called basic multicellular units. The temporal activity of a unit is characterized by osteoclastic resorption of a defined quantity of bone (on the surface in trabecular bone and by actual excavation in cortical bone) followed by osteoblast repair of the defect. Such repair consists of the laying down and subsequent mineralization of collagen (osteoid).

Thus, the driving force for changing net bone mass is intrinsic to the cellular processes that govern bone resorption and formation, and functional uncoupling of these cellular processes is required to either increase or decrease bone mass. By contrast, the major mineral ions of bone (calcium, phosphorus, and magnesium) play a more passive role in any mass changes that occur in bone. They must be present at physiological concentrations in ECF for bone mineralization (formation) to occur normally. Dietary minerals contribute to this physiological state by helping to replace minerals that have been lost either by obligatory processes (in urine, stool, and sweat) or by normal distribution to bone and soft tissues. Hence, calcium balance generally reflects the degree of coupling of bone formation and resorption. Negative balances are recorded when bone resorption exceeds formation, and positive balances are recorded when bone formation exceeds bone resorption.

Calcium Bioavailability

The 1989 RDAs for calcium are listed in Table 1.[11] It is important to recognize, however, that dietary calcium can appear in ECF and be deposited in bone only if it is absorbed by the intestine. It was a long-held belief

Table 1. Recommended dietary allowances for calcium

Category and age	RDA (mg/day)
Infants	
0–0.5 year	400
0.5–1.0 year	600
Children, 1–10 years	800
Adolescents and adults	
11–24 years	1200
25 to ≥50 years	800

From reference 11.

that the absorbability of calcium from food and preparations used for supplements could be predicted by their solubility in vitro.[30] Heaney et al.,[31] however, recently measured the absorption of calcium in women from biosynthetically [45]Ca-labeled food and various supplements. They found that calcium solubility in vitro had little relationship to calcium absorbability in vivo in the range (0.1–10.0 mmol/L) within which the commonly used calcium sources lie. This is of considerable interest because it suggests that the influence of stomach and intestinal pH may be irrelevant to the absorbability of calcium from commonly used sources. This was suggested by the earlier finding that calcium as the carbonate is absorbed normally in pentagastrin-resistant or pharmacologically induced achlorhydria, so long as that salt was ingested with food. It also raises the possibility that there may be a mechanism whereby the intestine can absorb calcium as chelated complexes because such complexes can exist in large amounts at the pH of intestinal juice. Finally, the studies of Heaney et al.[31] showed conclusively that calcium in spinach is much less well absorbed than the calcium in kale. This might have been expected because spinach, but not kale, contains large quantities of oxalate. Heaney et al.,[32,33] however, make the important point in two other papers that spinach calcium is even more poorly absorbed than oxalate calcium, suggesting that unknown factors that do not relate to anionic determinants may exert large previously underappreciated effects on calcium absorption.

Interactions of Calcium with Other Nutrients

Although studies over the past half century established that high amounts of dietary protein taken as an isolated nutrient increase renal calcium excretion,[34,35] epidemiologic studies showed no adverse effect of high amounts of dietary protein on either the rate of hip fracture or metacarpal cortical bone mass.[36,37]

Dietary fiber chelates calcium and other minerals in the gastrointestinal tract, and this observation led to concern that high-fiber diets may increase risk of bone loss and osteoporotic fracture.[38–40] Although there is evidence in some[41–43] but not all[44] studies that consumption of high amounts of dietary fiber (in particular wheat bran) may interfere with the absorption of calcium, there is little evidence that high-fiber diets alone induce calcium deficiency in individuals who otherwise consume a balanced diet.

Genetically Programmed Bone Mass

The level of bone mass achieved at skeletal maturity (peak or maximal bone mass) is a major factor modifying the risk of osteoporosis. The more bone mass available before age-related bone loss occurs, the less likely it will decrease to a level at which fracture will occur.[45–47] Normally, longitudinal bone growth is completed some time during the second decade of life. It is axiomatic that positive calcium balance is needed for this to occur, and it is easy to calculate that the required average daily body retention of calcium during this 20-year period is approximately 110 mg/day for females and 140 mg/day for males. During the adolescent growth spurt, the required calcium retention is two to three times higher than those average values.[48,49] To achieve such retention, the RDA for calcium has been set at 1200 mg/day for people 11–24 years of age.[11] If obligatory losses of calcium in urine, feces, and sweat are not greater than average, the RDAs for calcium are adequate provided that 50% of the ingested calcium is absorbed. A lower percentage of absorption or calcium intakes <1200 mg/day without compensatory increases in the absorption rate would not provide adequate calcium for peak bone growth. Unfortunately, the studies of Miller et al.[50] showing that the absorption fraction for calcium in children and adolescents averaged only 35% were not available to the National Research Council at the time it last established new RDAs for calcium. If the Food and Nutrition Board had known that calcium absorption in those groups was one-third lower than they had assumed, they might have recommended a higher RDA for calcium.

Johnston et al.[51] recently addressed the key question of whether calcium supplements could influence bone mass in children. In a double-blind, placebo-controlled study using identical twins, bone mineral density was significantly greater in the group that received calcium supplements of 700 mg/day than in the group that did not receive supplements (whose mean calcium intake was ≈850 mg/day). In a similar study with adolescent girls, Lloyd et al.[52] showed that bone density was greater in the group that received a calcium supplement of 350 mg/day than in the group that received no supplement (whose mean calcium intake was 880 mg/day). It thus appears that an increase in calcium intake well above that which has been considered reasonable can increase bone mass in children and adolescents. What is not known is whether such increases in bone density persist and ultimately become an intrinsic part of the peak bone mass.

Opinion varies as to the age at which bone mass peaks. Until recently, the only data concerning this issue were collected in cross-sectional studies. Those studies suggest that metacarpal cortical area,[48] phalangeal density,[53] combined cortical thickness,[36] and bone mineral content of the spine[54] increased until sometime during the middle of the third or the early part of the fourth decade of life. The only longitudinal data that deal with this issue come from a 4-year study of women aged 19-30 years performed by Recker et al.[55] The data showed progressive increases in forearm and spine bone density and total body calcium in this age range when subjects had average calcium intakes of ≈700 mg/day. Calcium intake and physical exercise correlated positively and protein intake and age correlated negatively with gain in bone density. No gain was observed at the age of ≈29 years. All the foregoing data imply that peak bone mass may not be achieved until 5–10 years after longitudinal bone growth has ceased. During this period, cortical porosity, which increases during the adolescent growth spurt, is probably filled in and bone cortices become thicker.

In contrast, Bonjour et al[56] showed in cross-sectional studies that the gain in bone mineral content in Swiss children slowed by the age of 18 years. This suggested to the authors that skeletal accumulation of calcium did not occur after longitudinal bone growth ceased. Clearly, further studies of Swiss subjects older than 18 years (preferably longitudinal) need to be done before such a conclusion can be drawn.

Calcium Intake and Bone Mass

Several published reports showed either no relationship or only a modestly positive one between dietary calcium and cortical bone mass. Garn et al.[57] found the same rate of loss of metacarpal cortical mass in ≈5800 subjects from seven countries despite wide variations in calcium intake among groups. In fact, low calcium intakes in some ethnic groups were associated with bone mass values higher than those in groups with high lifelong calcium intakes. On the other hand, in the Ten-State Nutrition Survey, Garn et al.[57] found a statistically significant increase in metacarpal cortical area in persons in the highest compared with the lowest percentile of calcium intake. In a similar analysis using data available from the NHANES I study, [58,59] Stanton (Stanton MF, unpublished observation, 1980) found a significant positive correlation between calcium intake and metacarpal cortical width for all subjects ($n = 2250$). When white women ($n = 960$) were excluded, the significance of the correlation disappeared.

Matkovic et al.[36] investigated metacarpal bone mass and the incidence of hip fracture in two regions of Yugoslavia whose inhabitants ingested greatly different quantities of calcium (500 compared with 1100 mg/day,

contained largely in dairy products). The inhabitants of the high-calcium district ingested more energy, fat, and protein and less carbohydrate than did the inhabitants of the low-calcium district. The regions were similar, however, in their agrarian economy and, except for a significantly longer lower limb length in the high-calcium district, the inhabitants' age, weight, and other anthropometric indexes were identical. The inhabitants of the high-calcium district had a 50% lower incidence of hip fractures and a significant increase in metacarpal cortical bone volume compared with the inhabitants of the low-calcium district. This difference could have been due to the prevention of bone loss, but because the differences in bone mass as a function of age were constant, it is more likely that the high lifelong intake of calcium in this population increased peak cortical bone mass. In contrast to the decreased incidence in hip fractures observed in the high-calcium district, the incidence of fractures of the distal forearm (distal 3 cm of the radius or ulna) was the same in the two regions. This finding is of interest because the sites of fracture at the hip generally are considered to be composed mainly of cortical bone whereas those at the wrist are mainly of trabecular bone. The results of a study reported by Anderson and Tylavsky[60] are highly relevant in this regard. These investigators related current and lifelong calcium intake to bone mineral content measured by single-photon absorptiometry at the distal radius (mixture of cortical and trabecular bone) and at the midshaft of the radius (largely cortical bone) in residents of four North Carolina communities. They found a positive correlation of bone mineral content with calcium intake at the midshaft site but no correlation at the distal site.

Several clinical studies examined the relationship of calcium intake to bone mass. Using radiogrammetry, Smith and Frame,[61] Smith and Rizak,[62] and Garn[48] found no relation between current calcium intake and current bone mass. Similarly, Laval-Jeanet et al.[63] and Pacifici et al.[64] showed no correlation of calcium intake to vertebral density as measured by quantitative computed tomography. Most recently, Riggs et al.[65] found no relationship between calcium intakes (range, 260–2003 mg/day; mean, 922 mg/day) of 106 normal women, aged 23–84 years, and the rates of change in bone mineral density at the midradius (determined by single-photon absorptiometry) and the lumbar spine (determined by dual-photon absorptiometry) over a mean period of 4.1 years.

In contrast to the negative observations made by Laval-Jeanet et al.[63] and Pacifici et al.[64] using quantitative computed tomography of the spine, Kanders et al.,[65] using dual-photon absorptiometry, found a greater bone mineral content of L2–L4 vertebrae in young women with a high calcium intake than in those with a low intake. In addition, in a longitudinal study of 76 healthy postmenopausal women, Dawson-Hughes et al.[67] found that women with dietary intakes of <405 mg/day lost spinal bone density at a significantly greater rate than did those with intakes >777 mg/day ($p < 0.026$).

Calcium and Hypertension

Within the past decade, considerable new evidence from human studies has suggested a role for dietary calcium in blood pressure regulation. Views and theories are still in conflict, however, partly because of the wide range of findings. For example, in an analysis of data from NHANES I, McCarron et al.[68] concluded that reduced calcium intake was the best predictor of increased blood pressure among all variables analyzed. Similar conclusions were reached in studies conducted in California, Puerto Rico, and the Netherlands.[69–71]

Other investigators reached different conclusions. Feinleib et al.[72] reanalyzed the NHANES I data studied by McCarron et al.,[68] controlling for age and weight of subjects, and found no significant association between calcium intake and blood pressure. Harlan et al.[73] found systolic blood pressure and calcium intake to be negatively correlated in women but positively correlated in men. Gruchaw et al.[74] concluded that dietary calcium was not a significant predictor of blood pressure. In a large prospective study of omnivorous Japanese men in Hawaii, Reed et al.[75] found inverse associations between intakes of calcium, potassium, protein, and milk (determined from 24-hour dietary recalls) and both systolic and diastolic blood pressure, although it was not possible to determine whether any of these dietary components had an independent effect on blood pressure.

The inconsistency among epidemiologic findings may be, in part, a result of the high degree of colinearity among other dietary factors associated with blood pressure (e.g., potassium and protein) and the limitations in the methods of assessing calcium intake in noninstitutionalized populations.[76,77]

Acute elevations of serum calcium by intravenous infusion of calcium sharply raises blood pressure.[78] Chronic hypercalcemia due to primary hyperparathyroidism is frequently accompanied by hypertension, which is often reversible after the hyperparathyroidism is cured by removing abnormal parathyroid tissue.[79,80] Serum calcium within the normal range has also been shown to correlate with high blood pressure.[81,82]

Hypertensive patients have been shown to have mild hypercalciuria and lower levels of serum ionized and ultrafilterable calcium than do normotensive patients, even in the absence of differences in total serum calcium.[83,84,85] Postnov and Orlov[86] reported that the cells of hypertensive patients bind calcium less avidly than do those of normotensives, and Erne et al.[87] found increased calcium levels in platelets from hypertensive patients. Resnick et al.,[88] working with hypertensive patients, reported alterations in the serum concentrations of the calcium-regulating hormones (PTH, CT, and calcitriol) associated with differences in the renin-aldosterone system. Although all these reported changes indicate that calcium metabolism is probably perturbed in primary hypertension, it is not clear whether the changes are the cause or the result of the hypertension. Taken together, these results do not support any single coherent theory of disordered blood pressure regulation.

Many intervention studies of calcium supplementation demonstrate a mild, short-term reduction in blood pressure in certain normotensive and hypertensive subjects.[89–93] Several carefully performed investigations using randomized, double-blind, placebo-controlled designs, however, suggest that oral calcium supplementation for as long as 6 months has little or no effect on blood pressure.[94–96] Furthermore, there is evidence that in some patients with hypertension and high levels of plasma renin, blood pressure may actually rise in response to calcium supplementation.[97] Finally, two recent studies evaluated the effect of calcium supplementation or dietary calcium intake on pregnancy-induced hypertension and the development of preeclampsia.[98,99] Sanchez-Ramos et al.[98] gave 2 g oral elemental calcium daily ($n = 29$) or placebo ($n = 34$) to 63 nulliparous angiotensin-sensitive pregnant women in a randomized, double-blind clinical trial. Significantly more patients in the placebo group developed hypertension, preeclampsia, or both than in the calcium-treated group. The authors concluded that calcium supplementation given in pregnancy to high-risk nulliparous women reduces the incidence of pregnancy-induced hypertension. The other study, performed by Marcoux et al.,[99] found no relationship between dietary calcium intake and preeclampsia. The odds ratio for the risk of developing gestational hypertension, however, progressively decreased from 1.00 in the lowest quartile of dietary calcium intake to 0.81, 0.66, and 0.60 in the highest.

Acknowledgment. Supported in part by a grant from the USPHS, 5 RO1 AG10925, entitled Building Bone in Osteoporosis with PTH and Estrogen.

References

1. Exton JH (1986) Mechanisms involved in calcium-mobilizing responses. In Greengard P, Robison GA (eds), Advances in cyclic nucleotide and protein phosphorylation research. Raven Press, New York, pp 211–262
2. Arnaud CD (1978) Calcium homeostasis: regulatory elements and their integration. Fed Proc 37:2557–2560
3. Arnaud CD (1988) Mineral and bone homeostasis. In Wyngaarden JB, Smith LH, Plum F (eds), Cecil textbook of medicine, 18th ed. WB Saunders, Philadelphia, pp 1469–1479
4. Aurbach GD, Marx SJ, Spiegel AM (1985) Parathyroid hormone, calcitonin and the calciferols. In Wilson JD, Foster

DW (eds), Williams textbook of endocrinology, 7th ed. WB Saunders, Philadelphia, pp 1137–1217

5. Neer RM (1989) Calcium and inorganic phosphate homeostasis. In DeGroot LJ, Besser GM, Cahill GF, et al (eds), Endocrinology, vol 2, 2nd ed. WB Saunders, Philadelphia, pp 927–953

6. Rosenblatt M, Kronenberg HM, Potts JT Jr (1989) Parathyroid hormone: physiology, chemistry, biosynthesis, secretion, metabolism, and mode of action. In DeGroot LJ, Besser GM, Cahill GF, et al (eds), Endocrinology, vol 2, 2nd ed. WB Saunders, Philadelphia, pp 848–891

7. MacIntyre I (1989) Calcitonin: physiology, biosynthesis, secretion, metabolism and mode of action. In DeGroot LJ, Besser GM, Cahill GF, et al (eds), Endocrinology, vol 2, 2nd ed. WB Saunders, Philadelphia, pp 892–901

8. Holick MF (1989) Vitamin D: biosynthesis, metabolism, and mode of action. In DeGroot LJ, Besser GM, Cahill GF, et al (eds), Endocrinology, vol 2, 2nd ed. WB Saunders, Philadelphia, pp 902–926

9. Centrala M, Canalis E (1985) Local regulators of skeletal growth: a perspective. Endocrinol Rev 6:544–551

10. Spencer H, Kramer L, Osis D, Norris C (1978) Effect of phosphorus on the absorption of calcium and on the calcium balance in man. J Nutr 108:447–457

11. National Research Council (1989) Recommended dietary allowances, 10th ed. National Academy Press, Washington, DC

12. Heaney RP, Recker RR (1982) Effects of nitrogen, phosphorus and caffeine on calcium balance in women. J Lab Clin Med 99:46–55

13. Portale AA, Halloran BP, Murphy MM, Morris RC (1986) Oral intake of phosphorus can determine the serum concentration of 1,25-dihydroxyvitamin D by determining its production rate in humans. J Clin Invest 77:7–12

14. Draper HH, Bell RR (1979) Nutrition and osteoporosis. In Draper HH (ed), Advances in nutritional research, vol 2. Plenum Press, New York, pp 79–106

15. Draper HH, Sie TL, Bergan JG (1972) Osteoporosis in aging rats induced by high phosphorus diets. J Nutr 102:1133–1142

16. Krishnarao GV, Draper HH (1972) Influence of dietary phosphate on bone resorption in senescent mice. J Nutr 102:1143–1145

17. Krook L (1968) Dietary calcium-phosphorus and lameness in the horse. Cornell Vet 58(suppl 1):59–73

18. Miller RM (1969) Nutritional secondary hyperparathyroidism. A review of etiology, symptomatology and treatment in companion animals. Vet Med Small Anim Clin 64:400–408

19. Saville PD, Krook L (1969) Gravimetric and isotopic studies in nutritional hyperparathyroidism in beagles. Clin Orthop 62:15–24

20. Bell RR, Draper HH, Tszeng DYM, et al (1977) Physiological responses of human adults to foods containing phosphate additives. J Nutr 107:42–50

21. Leichsenring JM, Norris LM, Lamison SA, et al (1951) The effect of level of intake on calcium and phosphorus metabolism in college women. J Nutr 45:407–418

22. Malm OJ (1953) On phosphates and phosphoric acid as dietary factors in the calcium balance of man. Scand Clin Lab Invest 5:75–84

23. Zemel MB, Linkswiler HM (1981) Calcium metabolism in the young adult male as affected by levels and form of phosphorus intake and level of calcium intake. J Nutr 111:315–324

24. Portale AA, Booth BE, Halloran BP, Morris RC Jr (1984) Effect of dietary phosphorus on circulating concentrations of 1,25-dihydroxyvitamin D and immunoreactive parathyroid hormone in children with moderate renal insufficiency. J Clin Invest 73:1580–1589

25. Lutwak L (1975) Metabolic and diagnostic considerations of bone. Ann Lab Clin Sci 5:185–194

26. Bringhurst FR (1989) Calcium and phosphate distribution, turnover and metabolic actions. In DeGroot LJ, Besser GM, Cahill GF, et al (eds), Endocrinology, vol 2, 2nd ed. WB Saunders, Philadelphia, pp 805–843

27. Parfitt AM (1989) Surgical, idiopathic, and other varieties of parathyroid hormone-deficient hypoparathyroidism. In DeGroot LJ, Besser GM, Cahill GF, et al (eds), Endocrinology, vol 2, 2nd ed. WB Saunders, Philadelphia, pp 1049–1064

28. Habener JF, Potts JT Jr (1989) Primary hyperparathyroidism clinical features. In DeGroot LJ, Besser GM, Cahill GF, et al (eds), Endocrinology, vol 2, 2nd ed. WB Saunders, Philadelphia, pp 954–966

29. Krane SM, Schiller AL (1989) Metabolic bone disease: introduction and classification. In DeGroot LJ, Besser GM, Cahill GF, et al (eds), Endocrinology, vol 2, 2nd ed. WB Saunders, Philadelphia, pp 1151–1164

30. Pak CYC, Avioli LV (1988) Factors affecting absorbability of calcium from calcium salts and food. Calcif Tissue Int 43:55–66

31. Heaney RP, Recker RR, Weaver CM (1990) Absorbability of calcium sources: the limited role of solubility. Calcif Tissue Int 46:300–304

32. Heaney RP, Weaver CM (1989) Oxalate: effect on calcium absorption. Am J Clin Nutr 50:830–832

33. Heaney RP, Weaver CM, Recker RR (1988) Calcium absorbability from spinach. Am J Clin Nutr 47:707–709

34. Allen LH, Oddoye EA, Margen S (1979) Protein-induced hypercalciuria: a longer term study. Am J Clin Nutr 32:741–749

35. Anand JJB, Linkswiler HM (1974) Effect of protein intake on calcium balance of young men given 500 mg calcium daily. J Nutr 104:695–700

36. Matkovic V, Kostial K, Simonovic I, et al (1979) Bone status and fracture rates in two regions of Yugoslavia. Am J Clin Nutr 32:540–549

37. Garn SM, Solomon MA, Friedl J (1981) Calcium intake and bone quality in the elderly. Ecol Food Nutr 10:131–133

38. Dobbs RJ, Baird IM (1977) The effect of whole meal and white bread on iron absorption in normal people. Br Med J 1:1641–1642

39. Ismail-Beigi F, Reinhold JG, Faraji B, Abadi P (1977) Effects of cellulose added to diets of low and high fiber content upon the metabolism of calcium, magnesium, zinc and phosphorus in man. J Nutr 107:510–518

40. McCance RA, Widdowson EM (1942) Mineral metabolism of healthy adults on white and brown bread dietaries. J Physiol 101:44–85

41. JH Cummings, Hill MJ, Jivraj T, et al (1979) The effect of meat protein and dietary fiber on colonic function and metabolism. I. Changes in bowel habit, bile acid excretion and calcium absorption. Am J Clin Nutr 32:2086–2093

42. Reinhold JG, Faradji B, Abadi P, Ismail-Beigi F (1976) Decreased absorption of calcium, magnesium, zinc and phosphorus by humans due to fiber and phosphorus consumption as wheat bread. J Nutr 106:493–503

43. Sandstead HH, Klevay LM, Jacob RA, et al (1979) Effect of dietary fiber and protein level on mineral element metabolism. In Inglett GE, Falkehaged SI (eds), Dietary fibers, chemistry and nutrition. Academic Press, New York, pp 147–156

44. Stasse-Wolthuis M, Albers HF, van Jeveren JG, et al (1980) Influence of dietary fiber from vegetables and fruits, bran or citrus pectin on serum lipids, fecal lipids, and colonic function. Am J Clin Nutr 33:1745–1756

45. Heaney RP (1986) Calcium, bone health and osteoporosis. In Peck WA (ed), Bone and mineral research, annual 4: a yearly survey of developments in the field of bone and mineral metabolism. Elsevier, New York, pp 255–301

46. Heaney RP (1992) Nutritional factors in osteoporosis. Annu Rev Nutr 13:287–316

47. Matkovic V (1992) Calcium intake and peak bone mass. N Engl J Med 327:119–120

48. Garn SM (1970) The earlier gain and later loss of cortical bone. Charles C Thomas, Springfield, IL

49. Nordin BEC, Horsman A, Marshall DH, et al (1979) Calcium requirement and calcium therapy. Clin Orthop 140:216–239

50. Miller JZ, Smith DL, Flora L (1989) Calcium absorption in children estimated from single and double stable calcium isotope techniques. Clin Chim Acta 183:107–113

51. Johnston CC Jr, Miller JZ, Slemenda CW, et al (1992) Calcium supplementation and increases in bone mineral density in children. N Eng J Med 327:82–87

52. Lloyd T, Andon MB, Rollings N, et al (1993) Calcium supplementation and bone mineral density in adolescent girls. JAMA 270:841–844

53. Albanese AA, Edelson AH, Lorenze EJ, et al (1975) Problems of bone health in the elderly. NY State J Med 75:326–336

54. Krolner B, Pors Nielsen S (1982) Bone mineral content of the lumbar spine in normal and osteoporotic women: cross-sectional and longitudinal studies. Clin Sci 62:329–336

55. Recker RR, Davies KM, Hinders SM, et al (1992) Bone gain in young adult women. JAMA 268:2403–2408

56. Bonjour J-P, Theintz G, Buchs B (1991) Critical years and stages of puberty for spinal and femoral bone mass accumulation during adolescence. J Clin Endocrinol Metab 73:555–563

57. Garn SM, Rohmann CG, Wagner B, et al (1969) Population similarities in the onset and rate of adult endosteal bone loss. Clin Orthop 65:51–60

58. Abraham S, Carroll MD, Dresser CN, Johnson CL (1977) Dietary intake findings, United States 1971–1974. National Center for Health Statistics, Hyattsville, MD [HEW publication no. (HRA) 77-1647]

59. National Center for Health Statistics (1978) Dietary intake source data, United States, 1971–1974. National Center for Health Statistics, Hyattsville, MD [HEW publication no. (PHS) 79-1221]

60. Anderson JJB, Tylvasky FA (1984) Diet and osteopenia in elderly Caucasian women. In Christiansen C, Arnaud CD, Nordin BEC, et al (eds), Proceedings of the Copenhagen International Symposium on Osteoporosis. Department of Clinical Chemistry, Glostrup Hospital, Copenhagen, Denmark, pp 299–304

61. Smith RW Jr, Frame B (1965) Concurrent axial and appendicular osteoporosis: its relation to calcium consumption. N Engl J Med 273:72–78

62. Smith RW Jr, Rizak J (1966) Epidemiologic studies of osteoporosis in women of Puerto Rico and Southwest Michigan with special reference to age, race, nationality and to other associated findings. Clin Orthop 45:31–48

63. Laval-Jeanet AM, Paul G, Bergot C, et al (1984) Correlation between vertebral bone density measurement and nutritional status. In Christiansen C, Arnaud CD, Nordin BEC, et al (eds), Proceedings of the Copenhagen International Symposium

on Osteoporosis. Department of Clinical Chemistry, Glostrup Hospital, Copenhagen, Denmark, pp 305–309

64. Pacifici R, Droke D, Smith S, et al (1985) Quantitative computer tomographic (QCT) analysis of vertebral bone mineral (VBM) in a female population [abstract]. Clin Res 33:615A

65. Riggs BL, Wahner HW, Melton LJ III, et al (1987) Dietary calcium intake and rates of bone loss in women. J Clin Invest 80:979–982

66. Kanders B, Lindsay R, Dempster D, et al (1984) Determinants of bone mass in young healthy women. In Christiansen C, Arnaud CD, Nordin BEC, et al (eds), Proceedings of the Copenhagen international symposium on osteoporosis. Department of Clinical Chemistry, Glostrup Hospital, Copenhagen, Denmark, pp 337–340

67. Dawson-Hughes B, Jacques P, Shipp C (1987) Dietary calcium intake and bone loss from the spine in healthy postmenopausal women. Am J Clin Nutr 46:685–687

68. McCarron DA, Morris CD, Henry HJ, Stanton JL (1984) Blood pressure and nutrient intake in the United States. Science 224:1392–1398

69. Ackley S, Barrett-Connor D, Suarez L (1983) Dairy products, calcium, and blood pressure. Am J Clin Nutr 38:457–461

70. Garcia-Palmieri MR, Costas R Jr, Cruz-Vidal M, et al (1984) Milk consumption, calcium intake, and decreased hypertension in Puerto Rico. Puerto Rico heart health program study. Hypertension 6:322–328

71. Kok FJ, Vandenbroucke JP, Van der Heide-Wessel C, Van der Heide RM (1986) Dietary sodium, calcium, and potassium, and blood pressure. Am J Epidemiol 123:1043–1048

72. Feinleib M, Lenfant C, Miller SA (1984) Hypertension and calcium. Science 226:384–389

73. Harlan WR, Hull AL, Schmouder RL, et al (1984) Blood pressure and nutrition in adults. The National health and nutrition examination survey. Am J Epidemiol 120:17–28

74. Gruchaw HW, Sobocinski KA, Barboriak JJ (1985) Alcohol, nutrient intake, and hypertension in US adults. JAMA 253:1567–1570

75. Reed D, McGee D, Yano K, Hankin J (1985) Diet, blood pressure, and multicolinearity. Hypertension 7:405–410

76. Kaplan NM, Meese RB (1986) The calcium deficiency hypothesis of hypertension: a critique. Ann Intern Med 105:947–955

77. Lau K, Eby B (1985) The role of calcium in genetic hypertension. Hypertension 7:657–667

78. Weidmann P, Massry SG, Coburn JW, et al (1972) Blood pressure effects of acute hypercalcemia: studies in patients with chronic renal failure. Ann Intern Med 76:741–745

79. Rosenthal FD, Roy S (1972) Hypertension and hyperparathyroidism. Br Med J 4:396–397

80. Blum M, Kirsten M, Worth MH Jr (1977) Reversible hypertension, caused by the hypercalcemia of hyperparathyroidism, vitamin D toxicity, and calcium infusion. JAMA 237:262–263

81. Bianchetti MG, Beretta-Piccoli C, Weidamn P, et al (1983) Calcium and blood pressure regulation in normal hypertensive subjects. Hypertension 5:1157–1165

82. Kesteloot H (1984) Epidemiological studies on the relationship between sodium, potassium, calcium, and magnesium and arterial blood pressure. J Clin Cardiovasc Pharmacol 6:S192–S196

83. Morris CD, Henry HJ, McCarron DA (1984) Discordance of hypertensives' dietary Ca^{2+} intake and urinary Ca^{2+} excretion. Clin Res 32:57a

84. Strazzullo P, Siani A, Guglielmi S, et al (1986) Controlled trial of long-term oral calcium supplementation in essential hypertension. Hypertension 8:1084–1088

85. Folsom AR, Smith CL, Prineas RJ, Grimm RH Jr (1986) Serum calcium fractions in essential hypertensive and matched normotensive subjects. Hypertension 8:11–15

86. Postnov YV, Orlov SA (1985) Ion transport across plasma membrane in primary hypertension. Physiol Rev 65:904–945

87. P Erne, Bolli P, Burgisser E, Buhler FR (1984) Correlation of platelet calcium with blood pressure: effect of antihypertensive therapy. N Engl J Med 310:1084–1088

88. Resnick LM, Muller FB, Laragh JH (1986) Calcium-regulating hormones in essential hypertension: relation to plasma renin activity and sodium metabolism. Ann Intern Med 105:649–654

89. Belizan JM, Villar J, Pineda O, et al (1983) Reduction of blood pressure with calcium supplementation in young adults. JAMA 249:1161–1165

90. Grobbee DE, Hofman A (1986) Effect of calcium supplementation on diastolic blood pressure in young people with mild hypertension. Lancet 2:703–707

91. McCarron DA, Morris CD (1985) Blood pressure response to oral calcium in persons with mild to moderate hypertension: a randomized, double-blind, placebo-controlled, crossover trial. Ann Intern Med 103:825–831

92. Resnick LM, Gupta RK, Laragh JH (1984) Intracellular free magnesium in erythrocytes of essential hypertension: relation to blood pressure and serum divalent cations. Proc Natl Acad Sci USA 81:6511–6515

93. Singer DRJ, Markandu ND, Cappuccio FP, et al (1985) Does oral calcium lower blood pressure: a double-blind study. J Hypertens 3:661

94. Tanji JL, Lew EY, Wong GY (1991) Dietary calcium supplementation as a treatment for mild hypertension. J Am Board Fam Prac 4:145–150

95. Galloe AM, Graudal N, Moller J, et al (1993) Effect of oral calcium supplementation on blood pressure in patients with previously untreated hypertension: a randomized, double-blind, placebo-controlled, crossover study. J Hum Hypertens 7:43–45

96. Yamamoto ME, Applegate WB, Klag MJ, et al (1995) Lack of blood pressure effect with calcium and magnesium supplementation in adults with high-normal blood pressure: results from Phase I of the trials of hypertension prevention (TOHP). Ann Epidemiol 5:96–107

97. Resnick LM, Nicholson JP, Laragh JH (1984) Outpatient therapy of essential hypertension with dietary calcium supplementation. J Am Coll Cardiol 3:616

98. Sanchez-Ramos L, Briones DK, Kaunitz AM, et al (1994) Prevention of pregnancy-induced hypertension by calcium supplementation in angiotensin II-sensitive patients. Obstet Gynecol 84:349–353

99. Marcoux S, Brisson J, Fabia J (1991) Calcium intake from dairy products and supplements and the risks of preeclampsia and gestational hypertension. Am J Epidemiol 133:1266–1272

Chapter 25

Magnesium

Maurice E. Shils

Magnesium is essential for a wide range of fundamental cellular reactions. Hence, it is not surprising that magnesium deficiency in an organism may lead to serious biochemical and symptomatic changes. McCollum and associates made the first systematic observations of magnesium deficiency in rats and dogs in the early 1930s.[1] The first description of clinical depletion in humans was published in 1934 in a small number of patients with various underlying diseases.[1] Flink and associates in the early 1950s documented magnesium depletion in alcoholic patients and in patients receiving magnesium-free intravenous solutions.[1] Magnesium deficiency does not appear to be a problem in healthy people; however, an increasing number of clinical disorders associated with magnesium depletion have been recognized. Experimental and clinical observations revealed fascinating interrelations of this ion with other electrolytes, second messengers, hormone receptors, parathyroid hormone secretion and action, vitamin D metabolism, and bone function.

Body Compartments[1]

Adult humans weighing 70 kg contain ≈834–1200 mmol (≈20–28 g) of magnesium. Approximately 60–65% of the total is present in bone, ≈27% is in muscle, another 6–7% is in other cells, and only ≈1% is in extracellular fluid. Muscle, liver, heart, and other soft tissues contain about the same amount, e.g., 7–10 mmol (14–20 mEq)/kg wet weight. Erythrocyte content varies from 1.7 to 2.7 mmol/L, depending on the age of the cells and the analytic measurement used. As the erythrocytes age, the magnesium content slowly decreases. Mononuclear blood cells contain about 3.0 fmol/cell. Normal serum concentrations vary somewhat depending on analytic methods. With atomic absorption spectrophotometry, the usual range for neonates, older children, and adults is 0.7–0.9 mmol (1.4–1.8 mEq)/L. It exists free (≈55%); in complexes with citrate, phosphate, and other ions (≈13%); and protein bound (≈32%). Spinal fluid has 1.4–1.8 times the concentration of magnesium in serum.

Most intracellular magnesium is associated with organic compounds, particularly with ATP. Hence, relatively small changes in the amount of associated magnesium will result in major changes in the amount of free intracellular magnesium ($[Mg^{2+}]_i$) . Total intracellular magnesium concentration varies from ≈6 to 10 mmol/kg wet weight depending on the tissue, except for erythrocytes, which have less. The range often given for $[Mg^{2+}]_i$ in many cells is 0.3–0.6 mmol.

Biochemical and Physiological Functions[1]

Magnesium is involved in at least 300 enzymatic steps in intermediary metabolism. A brief listing of some of the magnesium-dependent metabolic reactions is sufficient to demonstrate the essential nature of this ion. In the glycolytic cycle converting glucose to pyruvate, there are seven key enzymes that require Mg^{2+} alone or associated with ATP or AMP. Thiamin pyrophosphate (TPP), which is formed by an Mg^{2+}-dependent enzyme, plays a role in oxidative decarboxylation of alpha ketoacids in the transketolase reaction and in enzymatic steps of pyruvate dehydrogenase complex converting pyruvate to acetyl CoA. The enzyme converting succinyl CoA to succinate in the citric acid cycle requires GMP and Mg^{2+}.

In the beta oxidation of fatty acids, the first step involving acylCoA synthetase requires ATP and Mg^{2+}. In fatty acid synthesis the commitment step is the carboxylation of acetyl CoA to malonyl CoA by the carboxylase that requires ATP, Mg^{2+}, and bicarbonate. Protein synthesis, which is dependent on energy derived from ATP or GTP, requires Mg^{2+}. This ion is also involved in ribosome particle aggregation and in the interaction of ribosomes, messenger RNA, and the amino acid acyl-transfer RNA molecule. More than 100 protein kinases catalyze the transfer of the gamma phosphate of Mg ATP to a protein substrate. Mg^{2+} is required for the formation of a second messenger, cyclic adenosine monophosphate (cyclic AMP), by adenylate cyclase.

The increased information about concentrations of $[Mg^{2+}]_i$ has led to the concept that regulated changes in its concentration are compatible with its function as a physiologic modulator affecting, e.g., cardiac physiology with coupling of neurotransmitters and enzymes to receptors, with activation of proteins and with modulation of various types of ion channels.[2]

Analytic Procedures

Atomic absorption spectrophotometry, which until recently was the procedure usually used in clinical chemistry laboratories, has been replaced by automated colorimetric methods. However, atomic absorption spectrophotometry still remains the analytic standard.[3]

Ionized serum magnesium may be determined by various techniques noted below in the section on nutriture assessment. $[Mg^{2+}]_i$ may be determined by nuclear magnetic resonance methods, fluorescence indicators, or ion selective microelectrodes.[1] Radioactive ^{28}Mg and stable ^{25}Mg or ^{26}Mg isotopes were used in absorption studies[4,5] and in tracer studies in infants.[6]

Homeostatic Mechanisms

The homeostasis of the individual with respect to mineral balance depends on the amount ingested, intestinal and renal absorption and excretion, and all factors affecting them.

Dietary intake. The amount of magnesium ingested is critical for maintaining homeostasis. Magnesium is widely distributed in plant and animal sources but in greatly differing concentrations.[1] Issues concerning the reliability of intake data of various population groups in the United States, the recommended dietary allowances (RDAs), and the adequacy of the American diet are discussed below.

Gastrointestinal absorption: laboratory animals. Studies in rats that used segment perfusion or everted intestinal sacs have mostly shown that magnesium is better absorbed in the ileum and colon than in the jejunum.[7] In stripped rat mucosa, magnesium was secreted across the duodenum but absorbed in the ileum and in the colon, where both passive and nonpassive cellular transport processes exist.[8]

Gastrointestinal absorption: human studies. The percentage of ingested magnesium absorbed by healthy individuals is influenced by the concentration of magnesium in the diet and, to a variable extent, by the presence of inhibiting or promoting dietary components. As the amounts of ingested magnesium (as ^{28}Mg or magnesium acetate) were increased from very small to large amounts in the same healthy subjects, fractional absorption fell progressively from approximately 65–77% with intakes of 0.3–1.5 mmol (7–36 mg) to 11–14% with intakes of 40 mmol (960–1000 mg).[5,9] A plot of absorption as a function of intake had a curved portion that was compatible with a saturable process (facilitated diffusion or active absorption) and a linear function compatible with passive diffusion,[9] as was suggested by Milla et al.[10] to occur in children. Through the use of intestinal perfusion techniques in human subjects, magnesium was noted to be absorbed in both the jejunum and ileum; it was fully saturable in the ileum but not in the jejunum.[11] Hence, in humans as in rats, colonic absorption of Mg^{2+} is significant.

With a daily magnesium intake of 7.9–14.3 mmol (189–342 mg), healthy adult males in long-term balance studies excreted 35–68% in stool with a fixed daily calcium intake of 5 mmol (200 mg).[12] When free-living adults eating self-selected diets were evaluated periodically over the course of 1 year, absorption of magnesium by men averaged 21% and by women 27%; their average daily intakes were 13.4 mmol (323 mg) and 9.75 mmol (234 mg), respectively.[13]

The influence of dietary calcium and phosphate on magnesium absorption has been reviewed.[1,7,9,14,15] The data appear increasingly to favor the concept that, unlike the situation for calcium and phosphate, magnesium absorption in eumagnesemic individuals is not calcitriol dependent when relatively physiological doses are administered.[16–18]

Renal regulation.[1,19] Approximately 70% of serum magnesium is ultrafiltrable. Consequently, the kidney plays a critical role in magnesium homeostasis. One-third of the filtered ion is absorbed in the proximal convoluted tubule. The thick ascending limb of the loop of Henle appears to be the major site of magnesium reabsorption in the kidney and the major site of control of excretion: 50–60% of filtered magnesium is reabsorbed between the thin descending limb and the early distal tubule. Changes in concentration of magnesium in the tubular lumen and in the plasma affect renal absorption in this segment. The healthy kidney reabsorbs ≈95% of filtered magnesium. Tubular secretion, if it occurs, must be a minor factor.

When magnesium intake is suddenly and severely restricted (e.g., from 4–8 to <0.5 mmol/day) in humans with normal kidney function, magnesium output becomes very small (e.g., <0.3 mmol) within 5–7 days.[20] Supplementing usual dietary intake increases urinary excretion without significantly altering serum concentrations provided that renal function is normal and the amounts given do not exceed maximum filtration and excretion capacities. The intestinal and renal absorptive and excretory mechanisms in normal individuals permit homeostasis to occur over a wide range of intakes.

Despite a significant degree of renal disease with its progressive loss of functioning nephrons, serum magnesium with usual daily intakes is well maintained as the result of increased excretion of a larger than normal filtered load per nephron until creatinine or inulin clearance declines below ≈10 mL/minute.[21]

Dietary Needs for Health

Numerous factors affect the estimated requirements for healthy individuals, including biologic need, bioavailability of magnesium as consumed, and accuracy in estimating intake and retention. Metabolic balance studies are an important source of quantitative data on requirements. Because of methodological problems, including those of collection periods and analytic techniques, skepticism is advised concerning older data.[1,22] Data from more recent balance studies also vary considerably.[1,22]

The 1989 RDA for adults of both sexes is accepted to be 4.5 mg (0.19 mmol)/kg, which is the upper value for magnesium equilibrium in the accepted balance studies.[22] The specific 1989 RDA values for males and females 19 years and older are 350 and 280 mg, respectively; values are 320 mg for pregnant women and 355 mg and 340 mg for the first 6 months and second 6 months of lactation, respectively. Females aged 11–14 and 15–18 years have RDAs of 280 and 300 mg; for males in these age groups the values are 270 and 400 mg, respectively. The RDA for infants of 40–60 mg increases progressively to 170 mg for the age group 7–10 years.[22]

Most infants and children aged 1–5 years in the United States consistently ingest magnesium at amounts at or above the RDAs; for example, children at the 50th percentile have intakes at the RDA or higher.[23,24]

As of 1989 it was considered that "there is less than 75% analytical data for important sources of this food component."[23] The analyzed values for magnesium (from the U.S. Department of Agriculture database) for the 234 foods representing the core foods of the U.S. food supply were 115–124% above the calculated values.[24,25]

Per capita availability (based on disappearance data) of magnesium in the U.S. food supply has been essentially stable at ≈350 mg/day (14.6 mmol/day) since the 1950s, with perhaps a small increase in the early 1980s.[23] This value differs markedly from actual intake data. The mean daily analyzed intakes in the Total Diet Study for females aged 14–16, 25–30, and 60–65 years were (in decreasing amounts for older people) 194–187 mg; those for males were 297–250 mg.[24]

Serum magnesium concentrations were determined by atomic absorption spectrophotometry on a U.S. population sample of 15,820 persons between 1971 and 1974 in the first National Health and Nutrition Examination Survey.[26] Ninety-five percent of adults aged 18–74 had serum concentrations in the range 0.75–0.96 mmol/L (1.50–1.92 mEq/L) . The levels of the lowest fifth percentile were at or above the lower normal values generally used in clinical laboratories (i.e., 0.70–0.73 mmol/L).

Magnesium Deficiency

Hypomagnesemia is the hallmark of experimental depletion in all species studied.

Laboratory species. Although most studied, rats are not representative of other species for certain deficiency signs, e.g., hyperemia, repetitive (and usually acutely fatal) tonic-clonic convulsions, the associated normal-to-high concentrations of serum calcium, and the associated decreased concentrations of parathyroid hormone (PTH).[1] Mice on the same diet developed no hyperemia, became hypocalcemic in association with hypomagnesemia, and died with a single abrupt and massive convulsion.[1] Deficient dogs and monkeys also on the same diet developed spasticity, tremors, and occasionally nonfatal convulsions with hypocalcemia; increasing calcium intake did not increase serum calcium nor prevent the neuromuscular changes. Unlike humans, deficient rats become hyperparathyroid.[27] With the usual proportionally high calcium content of magnesium-deficient diets, calcification of soft tissues was noted in several species.[28]

Human magnesium deficiency. Symptomatic human deficiency usually develops in a setting of predisposing and complicating disease states (Table 1). These disease states often cause intakes of magnesium to be impaired, reduce intestinal or renal absorption, or both, leading to increased losses.

Experimental human studies. Various groups attempted to induce symptomatic magnesium deficiency in human volunteers.[1] In the one study in which symptomatic depletion occurred after a control period, the experimental diet provided ≈0.4 mmol (10 mg) magnesium/day.[20] Plasma magnesium decreased progressively to concentrations that were 10–30% of control values. Erythrocyte magnesium decreased more slowly and to a lesser degree. Urine and fecal magnesium decreased to extremely low concentrations within 7 days. Hypomagnesemia, hypocalcemia, and hypokalemia were present in all of the consistently symptomatic patients. Good intestinal absorption of calcium and low urinary calcium output resulted in positive calcium balance. Most subjects developed hypokalemia and negative potassium balance that resulted from increased urinary losses. Serum sodium remained normal, with the subjects being in positive sodium balance. Abnormal neuromuscular function occurred in five of the seven subjects after deficiency periods ranging from 25 to 110 days.

All symptoms and signs (including personality changes and gastrointestinal symptoms) reverted to normal with reinstitution of magnesium. Serum magnesium returned to normal rapidly; however, there was a delayed return to normal of serum calcium and potassium. Potassium balances became strongly positive as sodium balances became negative.

Table 1. Clinical conditions contributing to magnesium depletion[a]

Malabsorption syndromes
  Inflammatory bowel disease[29,30]
  Gluten enteropathy; sprue[29,30]
  Intestinal fistulas, bypass, or resection[29,30]
  Bile insufficiency states[29,30]
  Immune diseases with villous atrophy[29,30]
  Radiation enteritis[29,30]
  Lymphangiectasia; other fat absorptive defects[29,30]
  Primary idiopathic hypomagnesemia[10,31]
  Gastrointestinal infections[29,30]

Renal dysfunction with excessive losses
  Tubular diseases[19,32]
  Metabolic disorders[19]
  Hormonal effects[19]
  Nephrotoxic drugs and diuretics[19]

Endocrine disorders[33–37]
  Diabetes mellitus[33–37]
  Hyperaldosteronism[33–37]
  Hyperparathyroidism with hypercalcemia[33–37]
  Postparathyroidectomy ("hungry bone" syndrome)[38]
  Hyperthyroidism[33–37]

Pediatric genetic and familial disorders
  Primary idiopathic hypomagnesemia[10,31,39]
  Renal wasting syndrome[32]
  Bartter's syndrome[1]
  Infants of diabetic or hyperparathyroid mothers[1]
  Transient neonatal hypomagnesemic hypocalcemia[1]

Inadequate intake, provision, and retention of magnesium
  Alcoholism[40]
  Protein-calorie malnutrition (usually with infection)[41,42]

[a]Reproduced with modification from reference 1 with permission.

The signs and symptoms noted above in experimental deficiency were described individually or in various combinations in clinical cases of hypomagnesemia. Neuromuscular, gastrointestinal, and personality changes occurred. They include positive Trousseau and Chvostek signs, muscle fasciculations, tremor, muscle spasm, personality changes, anorexia, nausea, and vomiting. Frank tetany, myoclonic jerks, convulsions, and coma have been reported. Convulsions with or without coma occur more frequently in acutely deficient infants than in adults.

In humans the closest related condition to experimental magnesium deficiency is an uncommon congenital primary hypomagnesemia related to a specific defect in intestinal absorption of this ion.[10,39] Hypomagnesemia, hypomagnesuria, hypocalcemia, hypokalemia, and tetany, often with convulsions, occur and are corrected with magnesium supplements. Vitamin D is ineffective in maintaining normocalcemia.

Comparison of human experimental and clinical depletion states. In contrast to the hypomagnesemia occurring in experimental depletion, there are many reports of normal serum or plasma magnesium concentrations in patients who are deemed to be magnesium deficient. These patients' illnesses are varied and usually without associated significant intestinal malabsorption. Such patients may have depressed muscle or cell magnesium or decreased excretion of a load of injected magnesium.[1] However, symptomatic patients with difficulties absorbing magnesium by either the intestinal tract or kidney usually have hypomagnesemia. Because of this reported variability, it has been claimed that serum magnesium is not a good indicator of systemic magnesium depletion in clinical states and that other indicators (e.g., magnesium concentration in mononuclear cells[43,44] or in tissues) are better guides to magnesium nutriture in clinical situations.

The rather bewildering combinations of contradictory variations in the clinical literature on magnesium deficiency reporting on magnesium concentrations in various body fluids and cells emphasize the difficulty in ascribing cause and effect to a specific nutrient deficiency in uncontrolled clinical situations. Deficiency of one or more critical nutrients or a metabolic abnormality may affect use or retention of other nutrients. For example, magnesium deficiency per se depletes serum and cellular potassium, whereas potassium depletion reduces cellular magnesium content;[1] protein catabolism and chronic acidosis cause loss of cellular constituents and decreases in bone and muscle magnesium.[45]

Reports of clinical cases believed to involve magnesium deficiency should include clinical and biochemical data sufficient to permit evaluation of whether the observed changes (or lack of changes) in magnesium concentrations in tissues and serum reflect primary, secondary, or tertiary causes of magnesium depletion.

Sequence of changes in magnesium deficiency and repletion in humans. The factor that initiates hypocalcemia appears to be failure of the normal heterionic exchange of bone calcium for magnesium at the labile bone-mineral surface.[46] Impairment of responsiveness to PTH of the osteoclast receptor then occurs with reduction of active bone resorption.[47] Hypocalcemia progresses despite increased concentration of circulating PTH and with refractoriness to parathyroid extract. As depletion progresses, secretion of PTH diminishes to low levels despite adequate intraparathyroid gland hormonal reserves.[48,49] The biochemical and clinical signs and symptoms of severe magnesium depletion are present at this stage. With administration of adequate magnesium, serum magnesium increases rapidly, permitting heterionic calcium exchange to begin with little or no immediate detectable change in circulating calcium.[22,48,49] The rise in serum PTH may be very rapid with bolus injections of magnesium;[49] PTH receptors on osteoclasts eventually regain responsiveness, serum calcium increases, and then plasma PTH concentrations decrease appropriately. Electrolyte abnormalities recede and clinical signs and symptoms disappear at varied rates.

Vitamin D concentrations and resistance in magnesium deficiency. The calcemic effect of vitamin D, even at high doses, was blunted in the presence of magnesium depletion in rickets, malabsorption syndromes, and idiopathic or surgically induced hypoparathyroidism.[1] Despite low concentrations of calcitriol in most reported cases of magnesium depletion, serum calcium increased after magnesium repletion.[1,50]

Citrate concentrations. Patients depleted of magnesium either chronically or acutely had a markedly decreased content of citrate in their urine, secondary to increased renal tubular citrate reabsorption.[51] Hypocitraturia is a risk factor for oxalate stones in people with hyperoxaluria.

Magnesium depletion in various disease states. The multiple causes of magnesium depletion emphasize that this condition is not a rare occurrence in acutely or chronically ill patients (Table 1).

Management of depletion. The amount, route, and duration of magnesium administration will depend on the severity of depletion and its etiology. Symptomatic deficiency (paresthesias, latent or active tetany) is best treated by intravenous or intramuscular magnesium administration in conjunction with appropriate therapy for the underlying condition and with correction of other electrolyte and acid-base abnormalities. Various dosage schedules have been advocated;[1,52,53] these must always significantly exceed the measured daily losses. Intravenous calcium administration in the treatment of hypocalcemia secondary to magnesium deficiency is usually unnecessary unless incipient or overt tetany is apparent; in this case, a slow calcium infusion begun with magnesium therapy is usually necessary only for 1 or 2 days. The return to the normal range of serum magnesium with magnesium therapy is relatively rapid, but the repletion of magnesium lost from bone and other tissues requires longer magnesium administration. For the chronically depleted asymptomatic patient, frequent oral doses may be sufficient for repletion.

Prolonged magnesium therapy that cannot be met adequately by increased oral intake may be administered in three ways: 1) by intramuscular injection of magnesium salts, which is painful and may lead to sterile abscesses and fibroses; 2) by the old-fashioned but useful hypodermic clysis with dilute magnesium in isotonic solutions, which are infused slowly and periodically through a very small bore needle inserted just under the abdominal skin; and 3) by the intravenous route, which may be peripheral, percutaneous, or via a tunneled central venous catheter.

In the treatment of symptomatic magnesium depletion in infants, a relatively small amount of intravenous or intramuscular magnesium is rapidly effective in controlling neuromuscular signs and restoring serum concentrations.[1] In cases of chronic malabsorption (e.g., primary hypomagnesemia), 0.5–0.75 mmol/kg (1.0–1.5 mEq/kg) in multiple divided oral doses should be tested; this dosage schedule raises serum values to near normal without inducing diarrhea.[31]

Magnesium and Cardiovascular Disease: A Possible Role for Magnesium Depletion?

An inverse relation has been postulated between magnesium intake and nutriture and the development of coronary artery disease (CAD) and its sequelae.[54] Earlier reports noted decreased prevalence of deaths from CAD in areas where the water is hard (i.e., high in calcium, magnesium, and fluoride). However, because of conflicting data, there is no consensus regarding the role of hard water as a factor in the prevalence of CAD.[1]

Serum and heart magnesium concentrations in acute myocardial infarction. Older reports noted decreased serum or plasma values soon after or on admission to hospital of patients with acute myocardial infarction. More recent data contradict these claims with evidence that the time of drawing blood is critical in detecting changes;[55] that such patients often have preexisting congestive heart failure, arrythmias, or both[56,57] and use diuretics or digitalis drugs that may influence serum magnesium concentrations;[56,58] and that serum levels are influenced by the degree of postinfarction lipolysis[59] and pain.[60] Positive correlations between plasma and erythrocyte magnesium and creatine kinase isoenzyme MB (an indicator of infarct size) suggested that magnesium exited the myocardial cells at the time of the infarction and entered the extracellular compartment in proportion to cardiac enzyme activities.[61] A larger decrease in myocardial magnesium was noted in men with a history of angina who died suddenly of heart disease as compared with men without prior angina.[62]

In summary, the causes and significance of the decreased magnesium content in ischemic hearts are not clear because of the many complicating factors that are difficult to control.

Myocardial infarction, arrhythmias, mortality, and magnesium infusion. Meta-analyses of many recent reports suggested that intravenous magnesium given early after suspected acute myocardial infarction reduces the frequency of serious arrhythmias and mortality.[63,64] The report of a major randomized, double-blinded, placebo-controlled study with >2000 patients (LIMIT-2) also indicated some benefit.[65] In this study, mortality from all causes was 7.8% in the magnesium group and 10.3% in the placebo group (p=0.04). Left ventricular failure was reduced by an average of 25% (p=0.009) in the magnesium group followed in the coronary care unit.

Several hypotheses were tested because of claims made in prior studies; it was concluded that there was "no effect" modification by magnesium related to diuretic therapy, magnesium was acting pharmacologically rather than by correcting a deficit, magnesium did not affect the progression to acute myocardial infarction in patients with unstable CAD, and magnesium did not have anti-arrhythmic actions.

The Fourth International Study of Infarct Survival was a much larger randomized trial with 58,050 patients with suspected acute myocardial infarction; the study was designed to assess the benefits and risks of three treatments versus placebo or open control.[66] One treatment was intravenous magnesium sulfate given over 24 hours versus open control; the magnesium infusion was 8 mmol (192 mg) in 15 minutes followed by 72 mmol infused over 24 hours. There was no significant reduction in 5-week mortality either overall (2216 magnesium allocated deaths [7.64%] versus 2103 [7.24%] control deaths) or in any subgroup examined (i.e., treated early or late, in the presence or absence of fibrinolytic or antiplatelet therapies, or at high risk of death). There was a significant excess of mortality with magnesium in heart failure patients or those in cardiogenic shock. The conclusion was that intravenous magnesium was ineffective.

Hypertension. There are such contradictory reports differentiating serum magnesium levels in hypertensive subjects from those in nonhypertensive subjects that no conclusions can be drawn on this point.[1] Of more relevance are the results of a series of intervention studies. Several studies reported that hypertensive patients receiving thiazide diuretics who were also given magnesium supplements had a subsequent drop in blood pressure.[67,68] Others reported no effect of magnesium compared with a placebo in patients with various degrees of hypertension, all of whom initially had normal serum magnesium.[69,70] An 8-month controlled study in subjects with mild hypertension who were not receiving diuretics compared the effects of placebo, potassium alone, and potassium combined with magnesium; potassium alone or with magnesium caused a significant drop in blood pressure, but the addition of magnesium had no effect over that of potassium alone.[71] These and other data suggest that there is no antihypertensive effect of magnesium given in physiological amounts. Magnesium supplements may lower pressures in hypertensive subjects who have become magnesium depleted with chronic diuretic use.[70]

Assessment of Magnesium Nutriture

The desirability of having a reliable marker or markers for diagnosing magnesium depletion and its severity is obvious both for clinical usefulness and for providing more precise data on magnesium requirements in healthy individuals.

Total versus ionized magnesium in serum and plasma. Protein-bound magnesium is subject to variations associated with changes in albumin and acid-base conditions (acidosis decreases and alkalosis increases the bonding); hence, the level of ionized or ultrafilterable magnesium may be a somewhat more relevant determinant of deficiency in certain situations than is total serum magnesium.[72,73] Ultrafilterable magnesium in serum or plasma obtained by micropartition after centrifugation with measurement by atomic absorption spectrophotometry correlated closely (r=0.94) with magnesium analyzed by an ion-selective electrode.

Free intracellular Mg^{2+}. The measurement of the free intracellular phase of magnesium partition is likely to prove valuable to our understanding of the roles of Mg^{2+}. Such studies are beginning. For example, when P nuclear magnetic resonance spectroscopy was applied to erythrocytes obtained from 24 normal subjects before and after 3 weeks of a magnesium-restricted diet, the $[Mg^{2+}]_i$ fell from 209±9.8 to 162±9.3 μmol/L (p<0.001).[74]

Blood mononuclear cells. Variations in the proportion of isolated lymphocytes and monocytes in the analytic sample can influence the magnesium results.[75] The concentration of magnesium in human mononuclear cells has been claimed to be a better guide to magnesium nutriture than is the serum concentration.[43,76] However, in patients with mild to severe congestive heart failure, magnesium concentrations in serum, circulating mononuclear cells, and skeletal muscle were of little predictive value in assessing the magnesium status of myocardial muscle.[77]

Concentration of magnesium in urine. A fairly rapid entry of magnesium into one or more body pools is indicated by its increased retention when given as an intravenous infusion to magnesium-depleted patients. This retention may be assessed by a semiquantitative load test involving measurement of urinary magnesium after an infusion of a given amount of magnesium salt.[78,79]

Hypermagnesemia and Magnesium Toxicity

Induced hypermagnesemia with normal renal function. Pharmacological effects of increased levels of magnesium were noted in in vitro and in vivo studies.[1] Mg^{2+} is interdependent and often competitive with Ca^{2+}.[80] Peripheral and coronary artery vasodilation may occur by competition with Ca^{2+} in vascular smooth muscle.[81] Acute doubling of serum magnesium concentrations causes hypotension and increased renal blood flow in patients in association with prostacyclin release from endothelium.[82] Increased prostacyclin can inhibit platelet adhesion and aggregation.[83] Woods and Fletcher[84] attribute a short-term and a long-term benefit of magnesium given to patients with acute myocardial infarction to its early effect in being present (as an inhibitor of

[Ca²⁺]ᵢ) in the critical first 1–2 minutes of reperfusion, thus protecting myocardial function.

High-dose parenteral magnesium sulfate is the drug of choice in North America for preventing eclamptic convulsions that may occur with severe hypertension in late pregnancy or during labor.[85] It has been given also in an effort to prevent premature labor; a loading dose is followed by maintenance doses to maintain high serum concentrations (e.g., 2.0–3.0 mmol (4–6 mEq)/L) or slightly greater.[86] The high doses used clinically rarely cause toxicity because the magnesium is excreted rapidly and the patients are closely monitored. With the rise in serum magnesium, a fall in PTH may occur with an associated hypocalcemia.[86–88]

Magnesium toxicity. In contrast to the planned experimental or therapeutic hypermagnesemia noted above, elevated serum levels can occur when magnesium-containing drugs, usually antacids or cathartics, are ingested chronically by individuals with serious renal insufficiency; this occurs because ≥20% of Mg²⁺ from various salts may be absorbed. In acute renal failure with oliguria with metabolic acidosis and trauma, tissue release in association with magnesium ingestion or parenteral administration may result in toxicity.

The toxic effects of magnesium excess progress to lethal in their severity with increasing serum concentration.[89] Nausea, vomiting, and hypotension may occur at 1.5–4.5 mmol/L (3–9 mEq/L); bradycardia and urinary retention also may occur in this range. Electrocardiographic changes, hyporeflexia, and secondary central nervous system depression may appear at 2.5–5 mmol/L (5–10 mEq/L) followed at higher concentrations by life-threatening respiratory depression, coma, and asystolic cardiac arrest.[89]

Calcium infusion can counteract magnesium toxicity. Avoidance of magnesium-containing medications in patients with significant renal disease is recommended unless there is good reason and close monitoring. Hypermagnesemia should be suspected in instances of low anion gap in stable patients and a normal anion gap in severely ill acidotic patients.

References

1. Shils ME (1994) Magnesium. In Shils ME, Olson JA, Shike M (eds), Modern nutrition in health and disease, 8th ed. Lea and Febiger, Philadelphia, pp 164–184
2. White RE, Hartzell HC (1989) Magnesium ions in cardiac function: regulation of ion channels and second messengers. Biochem Pharmacol 38:859–867
3. Elin RJ (1991–1992) Determination of serum magnesium concentrations by clinical laboratories. Magnes Trace Elem 10:60–66
4. Schwartz R (1982) ²⁶Mg as a probe in research in the role of magnesium in nutrition and metabolism. Fed Proc 41:2709–2713
5. Roth P, Werner E (1979) Intestinal absorption of magnesium in man. Int J Appl Radiat Isot 30:523–526
6. Schuttez SA, Ziegler EE, Nelson SE, et al (1990) Feasiblilty of using the stable isotope ²⁵Mg to study Mg metabolism in infants. Pediatr Res 27:36–40
7. Hardwich LL, Jones, MR, Brautbar N, et al (1991) Magnesium absorption: mechanisms and the influence of vitamin D, calcium and phosphate. J Nutr 121:13–23
8. Karbach U (1989) Cellular mediated and diffusive magnesium transport across the colon descendens of the rat. Gastroenterology 96:1282–1299
9. Fine KD, Santa Ana CA, Porter JL, et al (1991) Intestinal absorption of magnesium from food and supplements. J Clin Invest 88:396–402
10. Milla PJ, Agget PJ, Wolff OH, et al (1991) Studies in primary hypomagnesemia: evidence for defective carrier-mediated intestinal transport of magnesium. Gut 20:1028–1033
11. Brannan PG, Vergne-Marini P, Pak CYC, et al (1976) Magnesium absorption in the human small intestine: results in normal subjects, patients with chronic renal disease, and in patients with absorptive hypercalcemia. J Clin Invest 57:1412–1418
12. Spencer H, Lesniak M, Gatza LA, et al (1980) Magnesium absorption and metabolism in patients with chronic renal failure and in patients with normal renal function. Gastroenterology 79:26–34
13. Lakshmann FL, Rao RB, Kim WW (1984) Magnesium intakes, balances and blood levels of adults consuming self-selected diets. Am J Clin Nutr 40(suppl 6):1380–1389
14. Spencer H, Osis D (1988) Studies of magnesium metabolism in man: original data and review. Magnesium 7:271–280
15. Lewis NM, Marcus MSK, Behling AR, et al (1989) Calcium supplements and milk: effects on acid-base balances and on retention of calcium, magnesium, and phosphorus. Am J Clin Nutr 49:527–533
16. Hodgkinson A, Marshall DH, Nordin BEE (1979) Vitamin D and magnesium absorption in man. Clin Sci 57:121–123
17. Wilz DR, Gray RW, Dominquez JH, et al (1979) Plasma 1,25 (OH)₂ vitamin D concentrations and net intestinal calcium, phosphate and magnesium absorption in humans. Am J Clin Nutr 32:2052–2060
18. Norman DA, Fordtran JS, Brinkley LJ, et al (1981) Jejunal and ileal adaptation to alterations in dietary calcium: changes in calcium and magnesium absorption and pathogenic role of parathyroid hormones and 1,25 dihydroxy vitamin D. J Clin Invest 67:1599–1603
19. Quamme GA, Dirks JH (1992) The physiology of renal magnesium handling. In Wyndhagen EE (ed), Handbook of physiology, section 8, Renal physiology, vol 2. Oxford University Press, New York, pp 1917–1935
20. Shils ME (1969) Experimental human magnesium deficiency. Medicine (Baltimore) 48:61–85
21. Steele TH, Wen S–F, Evenson MA, et al (1968) The contribution of the chronically diseased kidney to magnesium homeostasis in man. J Lab Clin Med 71:455–463
22. National Research Council (1989) Recommended dietary allowances, 10th ed. National Academy Press, Washington, DC
23. U.S. Department of Health and Human Services, U.S. Department of Agriculture (1989) Nutrition monitoring in the US: an update report on nutrition monitoring [DHHS publication no. 89-1255]. U.S. Government Printing Office, Hyattsville, MD
24. Pennington JAT, Wilson DB (1990) Daily intakes of nine nutritional elements: analyzed vs calculated values. J Am Diet Assoc 90:375–381
25. Pennington JAT, Young B (1991) Total diet study nutritional elements, 1982–1989. J Am Diet Assoc 91:179–183

26. Lowenstein FW, Stanton MF (1986) Serum magnesium levels in the United States: 1971–74. J Am Coll Nutr 5:399–414

27. Anast CS, Forte LF (1983) Parathyroid function and magnesium depletion in the rat. Endocrinology 113:184–189

28. Shils ME (1995) Magnesium. In O'Dell BL, Sunde R (eds), Handbook of nutritionally essential mineral elements. Marcel Dekker, New York, in press

29. Motil KJ, Altschuler SI, Grand R (1985) Mineral balance during nutritional supplementation in adolescents with Crohn's disease and growth failure. J Pediatr 107:473–479

30. Booth CC, Barbouris N, Hanna S, et al (1963) Incidence of hypomagnesemia in intestinal malabsorption. Br Med J 2:141–144

31. Stromme JH, Steen-Johnson J, Harnaes K, et al (1981) Familial hypomagnesemia—a follow–up examination of three patients after 9 to 12 years of treatment. Pediatr Res 15:1134–1139

32. Evans RA, Carter JN, George CRP, et al (1981) The congenital magnesium losing kidney. Q J Med 197:39–52

33. Butler AM (1950) Diabetic coma. N Engl J Med 234:648–656

34. Mimouni F, Miodovnik M, Tsang RC, et al (1987) Polycythemia, hypomagnesemia and hypocalcemia in infants of diabetic mothers. Obstet Gynecol 70:85–88

35. Fort P, Lifshitz F (1986) Magnesium status in children with insulin dependent diabetes mellitus. J Am Coll Nutr 5:69–78

36. Sjögren A, Floren CH, Nilsson A (1988) Magnesium, potassium and zinc deficiency in IDDM related to levels of glycosylated hemoglobin. Diabetes 35:459–463

37. Sjögren AJ, Floren CH, Nilsson A (1988) Magnesium, potassium and zinc deficiency in subjects with type II diabetes mellitus. Acta Med Scand 224:461–465

38. Jones CT, Sellwood RA, Evanson JM (1973) Symptomatic hypomagnesemia after parathyroidectomy. Br Med J 3:391–392

39. Yamamoto T, Kabata H, Yagi H, et al (1985) Primary hypomagnesemia with secondary hypocalcemia: report of a case and review of the world literature. Magnesium 4:153–164

40. Flink EB (1986) Magnesium deficiency in alcoholism. Alcoholism 10:590–594

41. Rosen EU, Campbell PO, Moosa GM (1970) Hypomagnesemia and magnesium therapy in protein–calorie malnutrition. J Pediatr 77:709–714

42. Nichols BL, Alvarado J, Hazelwood CF, et al (1978) Magnesium supplementation in protein-calorie malnutrition. Am J Clin Nutr 31:176–188

43. Reinhart RA (1988) Magnesium metabolism: a review with special reference to relationship between intracellular content and serum levels. Arch Intern Med 148:2415–2420

44. Ryan MF, Ryan MR (1979) Lymphocyte electrolyte alterations during magnesium deficiency in the rat. Isr J Med Sci 148:108–109

45. Drenick EJ, Hunt IF, Swendseid ME (1969) Magnesium depletion during prolonged fasting of obese males. J Clin Endocrinol Metab 29:1341–1348

46. Johannesson AJ, Raisz LG (1983) Effects of low medium magnesium concentration on bone resorption in response to parathyroid hormone and 1,25-dihydroxyvitamin D in organ culture. Endocrinology 113:2294–2298

47. Freitag JJ, Martin KJ, Conrades ME, et al (1979) Evidence for skeletal resistance to parathyroid hormone in magnesium deficiency: studies in isolated perfused bone. J Clin Invest 64:1238–1244

48. Anast CS, Winnacker JL, Forte LR, et al (1976) Impaired release of parathyroid hormone in magnesium deificiency. J Clin Endocrinol Metab 42:707–717

49. Rude RK, Oldham SB, Sharp CF Jr, et al (1978) Parathyroid hormone secretion in magnesium deficiency. J Clin Endocrinol Metab 47:800–806

50. Fuss M, Cogan E, Gillet C, et al (1985) Magnesium administration reverses the hypocalcemia secondary to hypomagnesemia despite low circulating levels of 25-hydroxyvitamin D and 1,25-dihydroxyvitamin D. Clin Endocrinol Metab 22:807–815

51. Rudman D, Dedonis JL, Fountain MT, et al (1980) Hypocitraturia in patients with gastrointestinal malabsorption. N Engl J Med 303:657–661

52. Flink EB (1969) Therapy of magnesium deficiency. NY Acad Sci 162:901–905

53. Olinger ML (1989) Disorders of calcium and magnesium metabolism. Emerg Med Clin North Am 7:795–822

54. Altura BM, Altura BT (1965) New perspectives on the role of magnesium in the pathophysiology of the cardiovascular system. I. Clinical aspects. Magnesium 4:226–244

55. Speich M (1987) Magnesium and creatinine kinase in myocardial failure: new data. Clin Chem 33:739–740

56. Rector WG, DeWood MA, Williams RV, et al (1981) Serum magnesium and copper levels in myocardial infarction. Am J Med Sci 281:25–29

57. Dyckner T (1960) Serum magnesium in acute myocardial infarction: relations to arrhythmias. Acta Med Scand 207:59–66

58. Manthey J, Stoeppler M, Morgenstern W, et al (1981) Magnesium and trace metals: risk factors for coronary heart disease? Association between blood levels and angiographic findings. Circulation 64:722–729

59. Flink EB, Brick JE, Shane SR (1981) Alterations of long-chain free fatty acids and magnesium concentrations in acute myocardial infarction. Arch Intern Med 141:441–443

60. Abraham AS, Shaoul R, Shimonovitz E, et al (1980) Serum magnesium levels in acute medical and surgical conditions. Biochem Med 24:21–26

61. Johnson CJ, Peterson DR, Surith EK (1979) Myocardial tissue concentrations of magnesium and potassium in men dying suddenly from ischemic heart disease. Am J Clin Nutr 32:967–970

62. Speich M, Bousquet B, Nicholas G (1980) Concentrations of magnesium, calcium, potassium and sodium in human heart muscle after acute myocardial infarction. Clin Chem 26:1662–1665

63. Teo KK, Yusuf S, Collins R, et al (1991) Effects of intravenous magnesium in suspected acute myocardial infarction: overview of randomized trial. Br Med J 303:1499–1503

64. Lau J, Antman EM, Jimenez-Silva J, et al (1992) Cumulative meta-analysis of therapeutic trials for myocardial infarction. N Engl J Med 327:248–254

65. Woods KL, Fletcher S, Roffe C, et al (1992) Intravenous magnesium sulphate in suspected acute myocardial infarction: results of the second Leicester Intravenous Magnesium Intervention Trial (LIMIT-2). Lancet 339:1553–1558

66. Collins R, Peto R, Flather M, et al, for ISIS-4 (Fourth International Study of Infarct Survival Collaborative Group) (1995) ISIS-4: a randomised factorial trial assessing early oral captopril, oral mononitrate, and intravenous magnesium sulphate in 58,050 patients with suspected acute myocardial infarction. Lancet 345:669–685

67. Dyckner T, Wester PO (1983) Effect of magnesium on blood pressure. Br J Med 286:1847–1849

68. Reyes AJ, Leary WP, Acosta-Barrios TW, et al (1984) Magnesium supplementation in hypertension treated with hydrochlorothiazide. Curr Ther Res 36:332–340

69. Cappuccio FP, Markandur ND, Beynon GW, et al (1985) Lack

of effect of oral magnesium on high blood pressure: a double-blind study. Br Med J 291:235–238

70. Zemel PC, Zemel MB, Urberg M, et al (1990) Metabolic and hemodynamic effects of magnesium supplementation in patients with essential hypertension. Am J Clin Nutr 52:665–669

71. Patki PS, Singh J, Gokhale SV, et al (1990) Effects of potassium and magnesium in essential hypertension: a double-blind, placebo-controlled crossover study. Br Med J 301:521–523

72. Zaloga GP, Wilkens R, Tourville J, et al (1987) A simple method for determining physiologically active calcium and magnesium concentrations in critically ill patients. Crit Care Med 15:813–816

73. Altura BT, Altura BM (1991–1992) Measurement of ionized magnesium in whole blood, plasma and serum with a new ion-selective electrode in healthy and diseased human subjects. Magnes Trace Elem 10:90–98

74. Rude RK, Stephen A, Nadler J (1991–1992) Determination of red blood cell intracellular free magnesium depletion. Magnes Trace Elem 10:117–121

75. Yang XY, Hosseini JM, Ruddel ME, et al (1989) Comparison of magnesium in human lymphocytes and mononuclear blood cells. Magnesium 8:100–105

76. Ryzen E (1989) Magnesium homeostasis in critically ill patients. Magnesium 8:201–212

77. Ralston MA, Murnane MR, Kelley RE, et al (1989) Magnesium content of serum, circulating mononuclear cells, skeletal muscle, and myocardium in congestive heart failure. Ciruclation 80:573–580

78. Ryzen E, Elbaum N, Singer FR, et al (1985) Parenteral magnesium tolerance testing in the evaluation of magnesium deficiency. Magnesium 4:137–147

79. Rasmussen HS, McNair P, Goransson L, et al (1988) Magnesium deficiency in patients with ischemic heart disease with and without acute myocardial infarction uncovered by an intravenous loading test. Arch Intern Med 148:329–332

80. Levine BS, Coburn JW (1984) Magnesium, the mimic/antagonist of calcium [editorial]. N Engl J Med 310:1253–1254

81. Altura BM, Altura BT (1981) Magnesium ions and contraction of vascular smooth muscles: relationship to some vascular diseases. Fed Proc 40:2672–2679

82. Rude R, Manoogian C, Ehrlich P, et al (1989) Mechanisms of blood pressure regulation by magnesium in man. Magnesium 8:266–273

83. Watson KV, Moldow CF, Ogburn PL, et al (1986) Magnesium sulfate: rationale for its use in pre-eclampsia. Proc Natl Acad Sci USA 83:1075–1078

84. Woods KL, Fletcher S (1994) Long-term outcome after intravenous magnesium sulphate in suspected acute myocardial infarction: the second Leicester Intravenous Magnesium Intervention Trial (LIMIT-2). Lancet 343:816–819

85. Cunningham FG, Lindheimer MD (1992) Hypertension in pregnancy. N Engl J Med 326:927–932

86. Cholst IN, Steinberg SF, Tropper PJ, et al (1984) The influence of hypermagnesemia on serum calcium and parathyroid hormone levels in human subjects. N Engl J Med 310:1221–1225

87. Cruikshank DP, Pitkin RM, Reynolds WA, et al (1979) Effects of magnesium sulfate treatment on perinatal calcium metabolism. I. Maternal and fetal responses. Am J Obstet Gynecol 134:243–249

88. Eisenbud E, LoBue CL (1976) Hypocalcemia after therapeutic use of magnesium sulfate. Arch Intern Med 136:688–691

90. Mordes JP, Wacker EC (1979) Excess magnesium. Pharmacol Rev 29:274–300

Chapter 26

Salt, Water, and Extracellular Volume Regulation

Friedrich C. Luft

Claude Bernard[1] was the first to appreciate and draw attention to the body's compartments in terms of an internal environment (*milieu interieur*). He suggested that the extracellular fluid provided an internal environment, a medium in which all cells are bathed. The internal environment constitutes the extracellular compartment. Its solutes and their concentrations are tightly regulated to permit cell growth, function, and survival. Indeed, the volume of the cells themselves (intracellular compartment), their cytosolic solute concentrations, and their water content are dictated by the constituents of the extracellular compartment and their respective concentrations. Bernard was aware that the extracellular compartment consisted of a solution of ≈0.9% sodium chloride and that the predominant cation in intracellular fluid was potassium.

Homer Smith[2] noted the crucial role of the kidneys in the regulation of the constituents and the volume of both the extracellular and intracellular compartments. He presented a convincing teleological argument that the extracellular compartment contains constituents and concentrations similar to the Precambrian seas, which presumably bathed the earliest primordial unicellular organisms. Further, he suggested that eons earlier the prototype molecules and organelles of cells may have developed in solutions more akin to today's intracellular compartment, that is, a solution that was relatively high in potassium and phosphate and low in sodium and chloride. Smith argued that the maintenance of the extracellular compartment dictated the evolutionary changes observed in both kidney structure and function. Kidneys of diverse organisms, existing in aquatic environments, fresh water, or sea water, as well as kidneys of animals living in various terrestrial environments have in common the task of guarding and regulating the external and the internal compartment. They perform this function by regulating the sodium, chloride, and potassium content and concentration in the body. Further, they regulate the concentration of solutes in both compartments within extremely narrow limits. This function permits the body's cells to thrive and perform their various functions,

a process and a concept termed homeostasis by Claude Bernard.[1]

Body Compartments

The total body water (TBW) in the ideal, prototypic, 70-kg human is ≈0.6 of the body's weight or 40 L (3). Two-thirds of this water resides inside cells (intracellular fluid compartment, or ICF) and one-third exists outside cells (extracellular fluid compartment, or ECF). A minor portion of the TBW exists in the intestines, the anterior chamber of the eyes, and the subarachnoid space and is termed the transcellular compartment. This compartment makes up <1 L of the TBW. By far the most important solutes of the ECF are the electrolytes sodium (135–145 mmol/L) and chloride (98–108 mmol/L). The concentration of potassium in the ECF is much less (3.5–4.5 mmol/L). In the ICF, potassium is the predominant cation, whereas the concentrations of sodium and chloride are negligible. The water content of cells varies with cell type. Muscle cells have a much higher water content than do fat cells. Therefore, the ICF and TBW are closely related to lean body mass.[3]

Sodium, chloride, and potassium are important constituents of the diet. They are virtually completely absorbed in the upper small intestine and they are eliminated in the urine. If sweating is not excessive and if diarrhea is not present, >98% of the ingested sodium and chloride appear in the urine.[3] More than 85% of ingested potassium appears in the urine as well.[3] In Figure 1, TBW, ICF, and ECF are represented as a box. The mouth provides an entrance and the kidneys provide an exit. Immediately apparent is the concept of homeostasis in terms of "what goes in must come out." Violation of this principle results in either expansion (more in than out) or contraction (more out than in) of the boxes shown in Figures 2 and 3. Renal disease may decrease the capacity of the body to eliminate sodium, chloride, and water (Figure 2). Figure 3 illustrates the result of sodium, chloride, and water losses as may occur in Addison's disease, a condition in which mineralocorticoid hormones

BODY WATER DISTRIBUTION

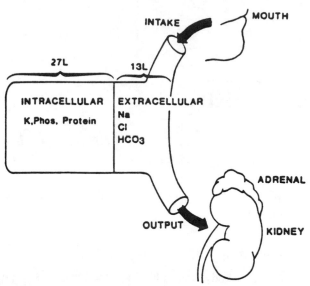

Figure 1. The total body water (40 L) is distributed as intracellular (ICF, 27 L) and extracellular (ECF, 13 L) fluid. Fluids and electrolytes enter via the mouth and are excreted via the kidneys.

are not produced because of failure of the adrenal cortex. Although mineralocorticoids influence <2% of sodium and chloride reabsorption, gradual decreases in the ECF occur in Addison's disease. The consequences of volume contraction are hypotension, shock, and death.

The methods of analysis for sodium, potassium, and chloride are well established and include flame photometry and, for sodium and potassium, ion-specific electrodes.[4] Chloride is measured by silver nitrate titration or more commonly by automated methods.[4]

The absorption of these electrolytes, their transport across cell membranes, and their transport across the renal epithelium occur via active and passive transport involving energy-dependent mechanisms and physical forces.[4] Rather than concentrating on details of transcellular transport and biochemical function, this discussion will be concerned with volume-regulating functions of sodium and chloride.

Sodium, Chloride, and Volume-regulating Systems

The predominant cation and anion in the ECF are sodium and chloride. Normally they cannot be replaced to a great extent by other cations or anions. Therefore, regulation of both sodium and chloride, in terms of both total amount and concentration, is responsible for the regulation of the ECF. Restriction of dietary chloride without restriction of sodium prevents expansion of the ECF. Similarly, concomitant administration of sodium

with an anion other than chloride fails to expand the ECF. The interdependence of sodium and chloride in the process of regulating the ECF is outlined in detail elsewhere.[5] However, because this discussion will concern itself with compartment regulation and its effect on volume and blood pressure, the ions sodium and chloride will be discussed together.

The atomic weight of sodium is 23 whereas that of chloride is 35.5. Thus, 1 g of sodium contains 44 mmol and 1 g chloride contains 28 mmol. One gram of salt, on the other hand, contains 17 mmol Na and 17 mmol Cl. Because food products may be labeled in terms of either grams or milligrams of sodium or salt, the content of these ions in foods is often misleading and confusing.

The intake of sodium and chloride is mainly from salt and varies greatly among countries. For example, the mean daily intake per person is >240 mmol/day in certain parts of northern China, 200 mmol/day in Finland, 150 mmol/day in the United States and western Europe, and <30 mmol/day in the Amazon jungle, the New Guinea highlands, and the Kalahari Desert.[6] The range in sodium and chloride intake is vast; the Yanamamo Indians of Brazil ingest <1 mmol/day of sodium and chloride. In experimental settings, intakes >1500 mmol/day have been tolerated by normal humans for short periods without apparent ill effects.[7] Thus, the kidneys are able to cope with widely differing intakes of sodium and chloride as well as with sudden changes in intake.

The overall control systems for sodium and chloride are imperfectly defined. Adaptation to different levels

VOLUME EXPANSION

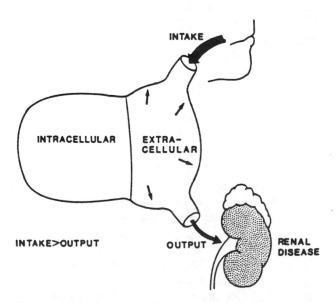

Figure 2. If intake cannot be eliminated, as is the case in certain forms of renal disease, the volume of the compartments must necessarily increase. If sodium, chloride, and water are retained, edema, hypertension, and eventual pulmonary edema develop.

of sodium chloride intake is physiologically quite complicated, with well-documented changes in plasma renin activity, plasma angiotensin II concentration, aldosterone production, atrial natriuretic peptide concentration, sympathetic nervous system tone, substances of gut origin, and perhaps concentration of the elusive natriuretic hormone sodium-potassium-dependent ATPase (Na^+K^+-ATPase), which is thought to be produced in the hypothalamus. These and probably other adaptations help to minimize, but not completely eliminate, the effect of changes in sodium intake on ECF and total body sodium. Thus, the greater the sodium chloride intake, the greater the ECF, the plasma volume, the blood volume, and the cardiac output. However, the principles of Figures 2 and 3 still apply: whatever goes in must come out.

Strauss et al.[8] observed that when sodium chloride intake is suddenly reduced to very low levels, urinary sodium and chloride excretion decrease exponentially over 4 or 5 days to virtually zero (to match the intake). They showed that if even a small amount of salt is ingested, sodium and chloride are immediately excreted. However, if extra sodium and chloride are forced from the body, either through sweating or administered diuretics, any ingested sodium and chloride is retained in the body until the deficit is restored. Hollenberg[9] refined this observation and coined the term *homeostasis set point*, a state between surfeit and deficit or a level of sodium and chloride in the body that is defended. Simpson[10] termed this point the basal level of body sodium and chloride. He proposed the following model for body sodium and chloride based on the principles first described by Strauss:

> When intake is very low, the basal level of sodium and chloride is maintained just sufficient to cover obligatory losses from the skin and bowel. Urinary excretion rates at this state are also very low but must approximate intake.

If the body sodium and chloride decrease below the basal level for any reason, the body will exist in a state of true sodium chloride deficit. Any ingested salt will be retained in the body until the deficit of sodium chloride is made up.

When body sodium lies above the basal level (which it does in most of the world's peoples), the body is in a state of surfeit and the extra sodium and chloride (amount in the body above basal levels) is excreted. The rate of excretion of sodium and chloride is exponentially related to the amount of extra sodium and chloride in the body. As emphasized by Hollenberg,[9] the body sodium and chloride is continuously running downhill toward the basal level and is constantly being increased by further intake of sodium and chloride.

The Yanamamo Indians of Brazil are able to maintain homeostasis with a salt intake barely sufficient to maintain the basal level of body sodium and chloride

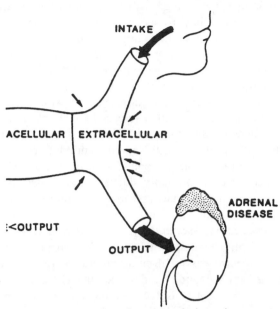

VOLUME CONTRACTION

Figure 3. If the excretion of water and electrolytes exceeds intake, as may occur if sweating is excessive, diarrhea is present, or the kidneys are unable to retain sodium and chloride (e.g., Addison's disease), volume contraction will occur. Blood pressure will fall until shock results.

(<1 mmol/day).[6] However, this ability is a function of the development of homeostatic mechanisms and normal kidney function. Healthy Americans can maintain homeostasis at intakes of sodium and chloride of <10 mmol/day. Whether or not such a low intake is either healthy or desirable for acculturated man[11] is a matter of debate.

Mechanisms of Volume Control

Control of the ECF is essential to maintenance of the internal environment in terms of both ECF constituents and blood pressure. The basic paradigm of redundancy in biological control systems has resulted in several control systems that may be distinguished in a hierarchical fashion as follows:

Behavioral central mechanisms. Behavioral mechanisms exist that control solute and water intake. Particularly relevant to this discussion are salt appetite and thirst.[12,13] Salt appetite is an overriding driving force for sodium and chloride intake in omnivores and particularly in herbivores. Much evidence indicates that the brain renin-angiotensin system is important in this regard.[14] Intracerebroventricular injection of angiotensin II stimulates salt appetite whereas the central administration of captopril, a drug that inhibits the formation of angiotensin II, diminishes salt appetite.

The thirst center influences not only TBW, but also the concentration of the solutes of the body. This concentration is maintained within incredibly narrow limits. An increase in plasma osmolality >288 mmol/L (increase in sodium >140 mmol/L) stimulates the thirst center. Drinking behavior or the search for water ensues. A decrease in plasma osmolality below this level causes a cessation of drinking behavior. In response to these changes in osmolality, arginine vasopressin, the antidiuretic hormone, is either released (>288 mOsmol/L) or inhibited (<288 mOsmol/L). This hormone acts on the renal collecting system.[15] Hemodynamic influences either raise or lower the set point of the osmoreceptor mechanisms, which is normally situated at 288 mOsmol/L. Robertson showed that resetting the osmoreceptor requires the participation of opioid-secreting neurons.[16]

Hormonal systems that influence salt and water balance. Examples include the renin-angiotensin-aldosterone axis, vasopressin, atrial natriuretic peptide, intestinal vasoactive peptides, and the putative Na^+K^+-ATPase, which all control or influence renal sodium and chloride excretion and in addition have other homeostatically relevant extrarenal sites of action.[17]

The circulating renin-angiotensin-aldosterone axis plays a critical role in regulating the basal body sodium and chloride levels. Its suppression enables sodium and chloride to be eliminated from the body. Renin cleaves angiotensinogen, a peptide of hepatic origin, to produce angiotensin I. Angiotensin I is in turn cleaved to angiotensin II, the active material, by the angiotensin-converting enzyme, also termed kininase II.

Angiotensin II, a potent vasoconstrictor, operates on the nephron directly to promote sodium and chloride retention but also stimulates the adrenal cortex to release aldosterone into the circulation. Aldosterone has its main action on the collecting duct and the most distal part of the distal tubule. The maintenance of basal body sodium and chloride is dependent on sodium and chloride reabsorption by these structures.

Adrenalectomized people or those with Addison's disease are unable to tolerate a very low sodium chloride intake. Their basal body sodium chloride content may fall too low to sustain life. On the other end of the scale is primary hyperaldosteronism, the inappropriate release of aldosterone by an adrenal adenoma. Patients with this disorder have arterial hypertension and a total body sodium and chloride content ≈16% above normal values.[10] Any increased intake of sodium or chloride by such individuals is characterized by very rapid excretion, termed *exaggerated natriuresis*. Aldosterone (the renin-angiotensin-aldosterone axis) plays a dominant role in the maintenance of the basal body sodium and chloride content. A potential role for atrial natriuretic peptide and other natriuretic factors, either identified or putative, is not as well defined.

Neural mechanisms of salt and water control. The sympathetic nervous system is a major regulatory mechanism controlling the excretion of sodium and chloride by the kidneys.[18] The sympathetic nervous system may cause sodium and chloride retention by at least three mechanisms: alterations in renal blood flow; initiation of release of renin by the juxtaglomerular apparatus, an innervated structure; and direct effects on the renal tubule via either α or β receptors or both. The role of the sympathetic nervous system in sodium and chloride homeostasis was reviewed by DiBona.[18] The sympathetic nervous system is activated during sodium depletion and suppressed during sodium excess.[19] Disturbances in sympathetic nervous system tone may lead to hypertension by influencing the basal sodium and chloride content of the body.

Intrarenal mechanisms of salt and water control. Intrarenal mechanisms of sodium and chloride handling are also important in the control of basal sodium and chloride content of the body. These mechanisms include locally released autocoid tissue hormones, including renal tissue angiotensin, prostaglandins, kinins, endothelial relaxing factor, endothelin, and less well defined factors.[17] Physical factors, including the oncotic pressure of plasma proteins in the blood bathing the renal tubules, are also important. A high filtration fraction results in a higher oncotic pressure of the plasma exiting the glomerulus and therefore an increase in sodium and chloride reabsorption (glomerular tubular balance).

Salt Intake, Salt Excretion, and Blood Pressure

Our discussion has emphasized that the kidney is solely responsible for salt excretion and volume regulation. Selkurt et al.[20] were the first to recognize a predictable relationship between renal salt excretion and blood pressure. They studied an isolated perfused kidney and realized that higher renal perfusion pressures facilitated salt excretion (pressure natriuresis). A relationship between salt intake–salt excretion and blood pressure (renal function curve) has also been shown for humans.[21] With all regulatory systems intact, this relationship is extremely steep, and sodium (chloride) intakes >600 mmol/day are necessary to cause an increased blood pressure in normal individuals.[7] In primary and secondary hypertension, these relationships are altered.[22] In most primary hypertension, the relationship generally remains extremely steep, namely, a state of salt resistance. In some forms of secondary hypertension, such as primary aldosteronism, the relationship becomes flatter (salt sensitive). Some patients with primary hypertension, low-renin hypertension, type II diabetes, and hypertension; elderly people; and obese people are also relatively salt sensitive. In other forms of secondary hypertension, such as renal vascular hypertension, the relationship remains steep.

Requirements and Allowances for Sodium and Chloride

It is impossible to determine a minimum daily requirement for sodium and chloride. Although the Yanamamo Indians are able to regulate their internal environment with an extremely low sodium chloride intake, it is by no means established that such an intake is advisable for acculturated peoples. As the above discussion indicates, the regulation of basal body sodium and chloride requires normal kidneys as well as intact central, humoral, and intrarenal mechanisms. The regulatory systems also are influenced by age. The Intersalt study indicates that salt intake of the world's population (except for four unacculturated centers) ranges from 100 to 240 mmol sodium and chloride per day.[6]

Some authorities have recommended that dietary sodium and chloride intake should be curtailed to <100 mmol/day in the hope that the development of hypertension, increase in blood pressure with age, and cardiovascular disease morbidity and mortality may thus be alleviated. The wisdom of such an approach in terms of a public health strategy for nonhypertensive normal individuals is currently under debate and is not yet thoroughly established.[11] Clinical abnormalities, signs, and symptoms of electrolyte disorders are reviewed elsewhere.[23]

Salt and Blood Pressure

Dietary salt intake has been associated with blood pressure regulation and with hypertension. The evidence is based on epidemiologic observations and animal, cell culture, and therapeutic studies. A comprehensive review of this material is beyond the scope of this chapter; however, pertinent highlights will be presented.

Population studies. The most comprehensive epidemiologic study of salt intake and blood pressure was the Intersalt study. This study was specifically performed to test three hypotheses: 1) dietary salt intake is related to blood pressure across populations, 2) dietary salt intake is related to the prevalence of hypertension within populations, and 3) dietary potassium intake is inversely related to both. Secondary hypotheses concerned the effects of body mass index and alcohol intake on blood pressure.

In the Intersalt study, 200 people from each of 52 centers worldwide had blood pressure and 24-hour urine measurements after following a strict, uniform protocol. Among the entire 10,079 men and women aged 20–59 years, sodium excretion in individual subjects within separate centers was significantly related to systolic blood

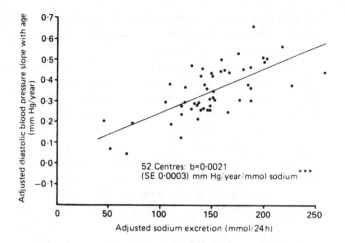

Figure 4. Cross-center plot of diastolic blood pressure slope with age on median sodium excretion and fitted regression line for 52 centers, also adjusted for body mass index and alcohol intake.[6] The plot was constructed with a common initial intercept for all centers (see text). (Reprinted with permission.)

pressure but not to diastolic blood pressure, mean blood pressure, or the prevalence of hypertension. In four remote, rural, unacculturated populations, sodium excretion was <50 mmol/day and blood pressure values were low. In the other 48 centers with sodium excretion >100 mmol/day, sodium excretion was significantly related to the slope of blood pressure increases with increasing age (Figure 4).

In Western societies, blood pressure increases with age, ≈40–50 mm Hg over the lifetime of an individual. According to the Intersalt data, ≈20% of this increase could be attributed to dietary salt intake. If indeed the increase in blood pressure with increasing age could be attenuated by 20%, such a maneuver could have important public health implications. However, the Intersalt figure was constructed with a common intercept for all populations. This assumption implies that all the centers began at a common starting point of blood pressure, and indeed this was not the case. Furthermore, epidemiologic data pose hypotheses; they do not test them. Prospective clinical trials are necessary for that purpose.

In short, hypothesis 1 was answered with a definite "maybe." Systolic blood pressure was related to salt intake across populations, but to a degree that a 2 mm Hg increase in blood pressure could be attributed to a 100 mmol increase in sodium intake. Hypothesis 2 was not clearly supported. Hypothesis 3 was supported; however, body mass index and alcohol consumption had strong, independent effects on blood pressure.

To test the notion that reduced salt intake would decrease the increase in blood pressure with advancing age would require prospective studies that are impractical and cost-ineffective for various reasons. Nevertheless, some experts believe the data at hand are convincing and that health care policy should be implemented to reduce salt intake without such evidence.

Intervention studies. In the Trials of Hypertension Prevention, a moderate reduction of dietary sodium intake reduced the blood pressure of people with high-normal blood pressure (80–89 mm Hg diastolic).[24] In this 18-month study, 327 subjects reduced their 24-hour sodium excretion by an average of 55 mmol/day, whereas 417 randomized control subjects continued on their usual intake (although their average 24-hour sodium excretion was 11 mmol lower after 18 months than at baseline). The lower sodium intake of the active group was associated with a statistically significant reduction in blood pressure of 1.7/0.9 mmHg and a decrease in the incidence of borderline hypertension from 11% in the control group to 9% in the active group. Although the <2 mm Hg fall in blood pressure may not seem like much in an individual patient, a population-wide reduction of even such a small degree could have a major impact in reducing the incidence of hypertension and, possibly, cardiovascular complications.

Numerous controlled studies were performed on hypertensive subjects to determine whether or not sodium restriction will reduce established high blood pressure. These data were analyzed by Cutler et al.,[25] who excluded trials that had confounded designs, compared intake levels beyond the usual range in the population, and did not publish blood pressure and sodium excretion values. Nevertheless, they were able to include 23 trials involving 1536 subjects. Hypertensive individuals decreased their blood pressure by 4.9/2.6 mm Hg; normotensive individuals decreased theirs by about half that amount. This degree of decrease would have been predicted from the Intersalt study.

Risks of rigid dietary sodium and chloride restriction. If dietary sodium is restricted to very low levels in individuals who cannot retain the ions adequately, a variety of complications may ensue. These include less cardiovascular reserve with salt depletion, particularly in hot weather; inability to reconstitute losses, particularly from the gastrointestinal tract; dangers to patients with salt-wasting nephritis or Addison's disease; undesirable activation of the renin-angiotensin-system; and decreased intake of other nutrients when salt intake is curtailed.[23] Figure 3 reviews the pathophysiology of these possible complications. Generally, a decrease in sodium and chloride intake to <50 mmol/day would have to occur before such complications would ensue.

Enthusiasts never tire of describing how easy this intervention is to achieve.[26] Nevertheless, perusal of the studies performed indicates that compliance was generally disappointing. Further, food manufacturers report that low-salt products frequently remain on the shelves and are not accepted by the public. Whether or not this be-havior is related to public ignorance, a failure of salt labeling laws to have been legislated, or poor cooperation because of a recalcitrant industry or because of other as yet undefined reasons is uncertain. Possibly, the mechanisms of the dietary set point in acculturated societies (an issue of salt appetite) is not yet sufficiently defined. Additional research into these issues appears warranted.

References

1. Bernard C (1865) An introduction to the study of experimental medicine (translated by HC Green, 1957). Dover Publications, Inc, New York
2. Smith HW (1959) From fish to philosopher: the story of our internal environment. CIBA Pharmaceutical Products, Inc, Summit, NY
3. Pitts RF (1974) Physiology of the kidney and body fluids. Year Book Medical Publishers Inc, Chicago, IL
4. Maxwell MH, Kleeman CR, Narins RG (1987) Clinical disorders of fluid and electrolyte metabolism. McGraw-Hill Book Company, New York
5. Blaustein MP (1985) Sodium, chloride, extracellular fluid volume, and hypertension. Hypertension 7:834–835
6. The Intersalt Cooperative Research Group (1988) Intersalt: an international study of electrolyte excretion and blood pressure: results for 24 hour urinary sodium and potassium excretion. Br Med J 297:319–328
7. Luft FC, Rankin LI, Bloch R, et al (1979) Cardiovascular and humoral responses to extremes of sodium intake in normal white and black men. Circulation 60:697–706
8. Strauss MB, Lamdin E, Smith WP, Bleifer DJ (1958) Surfeit and deficit of sodium: a kinetic concept of sodium excretion. Arch Intern Med 102:527–536
9. Hollenberg NK (1980) Set point for sodium homeostasis: surfeit, deficit, and their implications. Kidney Int 17:423–429
10. Simpson FO (1988) Sodium intake, body sodium, and sodium excretion. Lancet 2:25–28
11. Swales JD (1988) Salt has only small importance in hypertension. Br Med J 297:307–308
12. Epstein AN (1986) Hormonal synergy as the cause of salt appetite. In De Caro G, Epstein AN, Massi M (eds), The physiology of thirst and sodium appetite, Series A: Life sciences, vol 105. Plenum, New York
13. Fitzsimmons JT (1986) Endogenous angiotensin and sodium appetite. In De Caro G, Epstein AN, Massi M (eds), The physiology of thirst and sodium appetite, Series A: Life sciences, vol 105. Plenum, New York
14. Robertson JLS (1984) The Franz Gross memorial lecture: the renin-aldosterone connection: past, present, and future. J Hypertens 2(suppl 3):1–14
15. Robertson JLS (1987) Salt, volume, and hypertension: causation or correlation? Kidney Int 32:590–602
16. Robertson GL (1987) Physiology of ADH secretion. Kidney Int 32(suppl 31) S20–S26
17. Ritz E, Mann J, Schmid M (1988) Salt and volume regulating systems. In Rettig R, Ganten D, Luft FC (eds), Salt and hypertension. Springer Verlag, Berlin, pp 12–17
18. DiBona GF (1982) The renal nerves in renal adaptation to dietary Na restriction. Am J Physiol 245:F322–F328
19. Luft FC, Rankin LI, Henry DP, et al (1979) Plasma and urinary norepinephrine values at extremes of sodium intake in normal man. Hypertension 1:261–266

20. Selkurt EE, Hall PW, Spencer MP (1949) Influence of graded arterial pressure decrement on renal clearance of creatinine, p-aminohippurate, and sodium. Am J Physiol 159:369–376

21. Guyton AC (1987) Renal function curve: a key to understanding the pathogenesis of hypertension. Hypertension 10:1–15

22. Kimura G (1987) Renal function curve in patients with secondary forms of hypertension. Hypertension 10:11–15

23. Weiner M, Epstein FH (1970) Signs and symptoms of electrolyte disorders. Yale J Biol Med 43:76–109

24. Trials of Hypertension Prevention Collaborative Research Group (1992) The effects of nonpharmacologic interventions on blood pressure of persons with high normal levels: results of the Trials of Hypertension Prevention, Phase I. JAMA 267:1213–1220

25. Cutler JA, Follmann D, Elliott P, Suh I (1991) An overview of randomized trials of sodium reduction and blood pressure. Hypertension 17(suppl I):I-27–I-33

26. Kaplan N (1994) Salt and blood pressure. In Izzo JL, Black HR (eds), Hypertension primer. American Heart Association, Dallas, TX, pp 167–169

Chapter 27

Potassium and Its Regulation   *Friedrich C. Luft*

Potassium is the major intracellular cation in the body. Although intracellular potassium concentration approximates 140 mmol/L, that in the extracellular compartment is narrowly maintained at only 3.5–5.5 mmol/L.[1] The total amount of potassium in the body approaches 3000–4000 mmol. Potassium has an atomic weight of 39. Thus, 1 g potassium contains 25 mmol. Because skeletal muscle has the highest potassium concentrations, the total amount of potassium is closely correlated with the lean body mass. On the basis of these values it can be calculated that ≈2% of total body potassium is outside cells (extracellular) whereas 98% resides inside cells.

Potassium serves a variety of crucial functions in energy metabolism, membrane transport, and maintenance of the potential difference across cell membranes.[2] The latter function is particularly important to all neuromuscular and endocrine cells, whose function is determined by their ability to depolarize and to repolarize. The transfer of signals down nervous pathways, the resultant contraction of muscle groups, the release of an exocrine glandular product or an endocrine hormone, and the propagation of a depolarization wave in smooth muscle or the myocardium all depend upon electrical excitability.

The potential difference across cell membranes is defined by the relationship between the intracellular and extracellular potassium concentrations. The relationship was first described by Nernst, and may be simplified as follows:

$$E = -61.5 \log K_i/K_e,$$

where E is the potential difference in millivolts and K_i is the intracellular concentration and K_e the extracellular potassium concentration. The resting membrane potential and the threshold potential of a cardiac cell are shown in Figure 1. An increase in the extracellular potassium concentration (hyperkalemia) decreases the resting potential (making it less negative) and moves it toward the threshold potential. Such a shift results in the cell being closer to the threshold potential. Should the threshold potential be reached by a further increase in the extracellular potassium concentration, such a cell would depolarize spontaneously and might not be able

to repolarize again (repolarization block). Such a cell is rendered nonfunctional. However, should the extracellular potassium concentration decrease (hypokalemia), the resting membrane potential would become more negative (greater) and the stimulus required to bring the cell to the threshold potential would also have to become greater. Conceivably, no stimulus may be sufficient to depolarize such a cell (depolarization block).

In either event (hyperkalemia or hypokalemia) the cell may become nonfunctional. It will come as no surprise that the signs and symptoms of hyperkalemia and hypokalemia are similar: weakness, lethargy, gastric

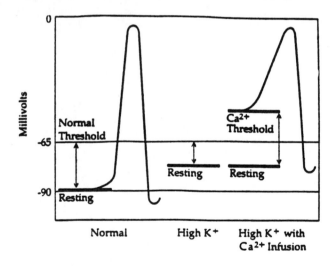

Figure 1. Symptoms that occur in hyperkalemic patients usually result from alterations in electrical excitability of nerve and muscle cell membranes. In the normal action potential curve (left), the difference between the resting membrane potential and the threshold for excitability (arrow) is roughly 25 mV. An increase in plasma K^+ (center) decreases the resting potential (less negative) and decreases the difference between the resting membrane potential and the threshold potential (arrow). This in turn alters the nature of membrane depolarization. Calcium administration raises the threshold potential (right), minimizing the adverse membrane effects of hyperkalemia by returning the difference between the resting and threshold potentials to normal. Hypokalemia would in turn increase the resting membrane potential (more negative), thereby increasing the distance between resting and threshold potential. Both hyperkalemia and hypokalemia thus interfere with the cell's ability to depolarize normally.

HYPERKALEMIA

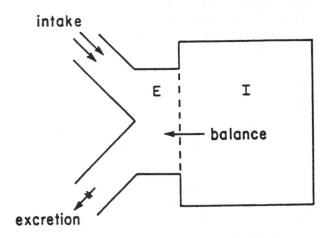

Figure 2. Potassium is almost all (98%) intracellular. The relationship between intracellular and extracellular potassium determines the potential difference across cell membranes. Hyperkalemia can develop if intake exceeds excretion, if excretion is impaired, or if potassium moves from the inside to the outside of cells.

hypomotility, cardiac arrhythmias, and conduction disturbances. Both hyperkalemia and hypokalemia can be lethal. Cardiac arrhythmias and conduction disturbances can be deadly because of failure of the heart to perfuse blood through the vascular bed. The relationship between K_i and K_e is important. The intracellular potassium concentration clearly also influences the membrane potential. Thus, a chronic increase in K_i protects against hyperkalemia, whereas hypokalemia is better tolerated when the intracellular potassium concentration is also reduced. These states of affairs come to be when the changes are chronic rather than acute.

Extracellular potassium concentration is a function of two variables: the total body potassium content and the relative distribution of potassium between the extracellular fluid compartment (ECF) and the intracellular fluid compartment (ICF). The total body potassium content is determined by the difference between potassium intake and excretion. The second variable is a function of internal potassium balance. Figures 2 and 3, respectively, show how hyperkalemia and hypokalemia may arise.

Absorption, Transport, Storage, and Turnover

Potassium enters the body through the diet and is eliminated almost exclusively by the kidneys under normal circumstances. An increase in the ECF potassium concentration may occur because of either increased potassium intake, decreased renal excretion of potassium, or a shift in potassium balance across cell membranes from the inside to the outside of cells. Similarly, a decrease in the ECF potassium concentration can result only from

a decrease in potassium intake, an increase in potassium excretion, or a shift of potassium from outside to inside cells. Clearly, combinations of these disorders may exist simultaneously.

Because only 2% of the total body potassium is outside cells, measurement of the ECF potassium concentration is a relatively crude estimate of the total body potassium, and serious errors in interpretation may result if total body potassium is estimated from the extracellular value. Unfortunately, measurement of the total body potassium content is difficult and cumbersome. Sterns et al.[1] plotted the results of several studies and found that despite considerable variability, a crude estimate of total body potassium deficit can be made if hypokalemia is present. According to their estimate, a chronic decrease in the serum concentration of 0.27 mmol/L represents a decrease in total body potassium by ≈100 mmol.

Potassium intake depends on diet composition.[1,2] For example, the American diet provides ≈50–80 mmol potassium/day.[2] Urinary excretion approaches intake, albeit in a somewhat less accurate fashion than for sodium and chloride. Nevertheless, if there are no concomitant gastrointestinal losses and if renal failure is not present, urinary potassium excretion is an acceptable estimate of daily potassium intake. Potassium is freely filtered at the glomerulus, reabsorbed in the proximal tubule, and secreted in the distal tubule, a process facilitated by the hormone aldosterone. Details on this process are outlined elsewhere.[2]

Factors Altering Internal Potassium Balance

Changes in cell mass. Changes in the size of the ICF may alter the internal potassium balance.[1,3] During

HYPOKALEMIA

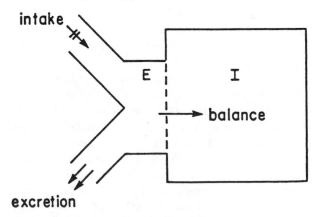

Figure 3. Hypokalemia can develop if the intake of potassium is less than the losses, if potassium losses (e.g., renal losses and diarrhea) exceed intake, or if potassium moves from the outside to the inside of cells.

chronic starvation, cell mass decreases as a result of cellular protein and potassium losses from the body. Similarly, if cell mass increases as a result of growth or refeeding, potassium is retained by the body in proportion to the retention of nitrogen. Many chronically starved individuals are hypokalemic, suggesting that potassium losses in these patients are out of proportion to nitrogen losses, so that true potassium depletion, as well as decreased cell mass, may result. Refeeding of protein with resultant anabolism and cell growth and recovery may increase potassium requirements and aggravate hypokalemia if the requirements are not met. The same may occur if a chronic vitamin deficiency is treated in patients who are depleted in total body potassium. Examples include the treatment of vitamin B-12 or folic acid deficiency. Acute changes in cell mass from cell destruction, such as may occur from rhabdomyolysis or from hemolysis, may result in large endogenous potassium infusion, which may overwhelm the renal excretory capacity. Hyperkalemia, which may be life-threatening, may result.

Changes in tonicity. When hypertonic solutions are infused intravenously, the resulting increase in osmolality of the ECF results in a shift of fluid from the ICF to the ECF. The resulting cellular dehydration results in a shift of potassium from inside cells to outside cells, thereby increasing the concentration of potassium in the ECF.[3] This effect may be clinically important. Hypertonic solutions both of glucose and of sodium bicarbonate are frequently given to treat hyperkalemia. If these solutions are infused quickly, the resulting cellular dehydration may cause potassium to move to the extracelluar space and thus obviate the desired clinical response.

Acid-base disturbances. Under most circumstances, when extracellular pH decreases, potassium exits from cells and the plasma potassium concentration increases. The converse occurs when extracellular pH increases. However, metabolic and respiratory acidosis differ in regard to their effect on ECF potassium.[4] Chronic respiratory acidosis does not influence internal potassium balance, whereas acute respiratory acidosis may, depending on the duration of the disturbance.[4] Furthermore, the effect of metabolic acidosis on internal potassium balance depends on the type of metabolic acidosis. For example, the effects of mineral acids, such as hydrochloric acid, are greater than the effects of organic acids, such as lactic acid. Metabolic alkalosis is almost invariably associated with a negative internal potassium balance. Hyperkalemia may be treated by precipitating metabolic alkalosis via the administration of sodium bicarbonate.

The effects of acid-base disturbances on internal potassium balance are complex and variable. The following generalizations are of clinical significance:

- Patients with metabolic alkalosis are usually hypokalemic; however, the primary cause is total body potassium depletion rather than a redistribution of potassium within the body.
- If renal function is adequate, metabolic acidosis also results in total body potassium depletion. Internal shifts of potassium from inside to outside the cells are accompanied by increases in urinary potassium excretion.
- Respiratory acid-base disturbances generally do not cause much change in internal potassium balance.
- In hyperkalemic patients, the administration of glucose and insulin should cause a prompt movement of potassium from outside to inside cells regardless of the plasma pH.

The administration of alkali (sodium bicarbonate) will cause a prompt movement of potassium from the outside to the inside of cells, if metabolic acidosis is present. Otherwise, bicarbonate is less effective in shifting potassium to the inside of cells than are glucose and insulin. Beta-adrenergic agonists also move potassium from the outside to the inside of cells.[5,6] Calcium gluconate infusion, which directly counteracts the cardiac toxicity of hyperkalemia, alters the threshold potential (Figure 1) but does not change the potassium concentration per se. Potassium may also be removed from the body with the administration of cationic exchange resins or dialysis.

Hormones. Insulin directly stimulates net potassium uptake by skeletal muscle and hepatic cells.[7] Aldosterone promotes renal potassium excretion.[1,2] Catecholamines directly affect internal potassium balance. Beta-agonists promote hypokalemia by enhancing the uptake of potassium by muscle. Alpha-agonists promote hyperkalemia by promoting the release of potassium from liver.[5,6] Epinephrine has primarily beta but also some alpha effects. Thus, its effects may be biphasic, that is, hypokalemia followed by hyperkalemia at very high doses. Norepinephrine, which is primarily an alpha-agonist, tends to cause hyperkalemia by promoting the release of potassium from liver.

Drugs. Cardiac glycosides inhibit Na^+K^+-ATPase. These drugs inhibit the net uptake of potassium. Succinylcholine induces a prolonged, dose-related increase in the ionic permeability of muscle cells and consequently a prolonged efflux of potassium.[8] Beta-blockers interfere with the deposition of potassium into muscle cells by pure beta-agonists or by epinephrine.[5,6]

Exercise. Exercise causes release of potassium from skeletal muscle. As a result, the systemic plasma potassium concentration increases to a degree determined by the extent of the exercise.

Requirements and Allowances for Potassium

The kidneys are responsible for potassium elimination and retention. However, the range in which the kidneys operate to maintain homeostasis of this cation is not as great as for sodium. Potassium ingestion throughout the world ranges from 50 to 200 mmol/day. An intake <50 mmol/day markedly impairs the palatability of food. An intake >200 mmol/day may cause hyperkalemia, although with adaptation potassium elimination by the kidneys and the gastrointestinal tract (the latter particularly if renal function is diminished) is enhanced.[1,2]

Authorities have argued that a diet high in potassium and low in sodium (low urinary sodium-potassium ratio) favors lower blood pressure. A dietary intake of 1 mmol/kg body weight is deemed an appropriate minimum. Such a level would indicate an average intake of 75 mmol/day. If the Americans who participated in the Intersalt study are representative,[9] then many (if not most) Americans ingest less potassium than they should. A high intake of processed ("fast") foods and avoidance of fresh fruits and vegetables may contribute to this low potassium intake. In some segments of society, the relatively high costs of fresh fruits and vegetables may contribute to a relatively low potassium intake.

Potassium and Blood Pressure

Various mechanisms have been proposed to explain a blood pressure–lowering effect of potassium. These include a direct natriuretic effect, suppression of the renin-angiotensin system and the sympathetic nervous system, an effect on kallikreins and eicosanoids, improvement of baroreceptor function, antagonism of the effects of natriuretic hormone, and a direct effect on peripheral vascular resistance. Many studies have demonstrated a short-term natriuretic effect; however, it has not been proven that such effects result in long-term reductions in ECF and circulating fluid volume.

Cross-sectional epidemiologic studies from the United States, Japan, England, Scotland, Sweden, Belgium, Kenya, Zaire, and China all identified an inverse relationship between blood pressure and potassium in the diet, urine, total body (estimates), or serum. In the Intersalt study, an inverse association between 24-hour potassium excretion and systolic blood pressure was observed in 39 of 52 centers.[9] A similar pattern for diastolic blood pressure was observed in 35 of the 52 centers. The four unacculturated societies that participated in Intersalt all had a high potassium consumption, so that the urinary sodium-potassium ratio ranged from 0.01 to 1.78.

Numerous intervention trials have been performed to test the notion that a high potassium intake lowers blood pressure. The rice and fruit diet of the Kempner diet was characterized by a relatively high content of potassium and a low sodium-potassium ratio. The diet was also extremely low in protein and calories. Fifty years ago, the Kempner diet was the extent of therapeutic options for patients with severe hypertension.[10] Numerous other studies have been performed since. A meta-analysis conducted by Cappuccio and MacGregor[11] included 19 prospective randomized and nonrandomized trials. A reduction in supine systolic and diastolic blood pressures of 5.9/3.4 mm Hg was reported. Whelton et al.[12] identified 36 trials involving 2585 participants. A pooled analysis gave results not too different from those reported by Cappuccio and MacGregor.[11] Systolic and diastolic blood pressures decreased by 5.1/3.0 mm Hg.

In addition to its hypotensive effects, potassium supplementation may have independent vasculoprotective properties. In a series of animal models, including both spontaneously hypertensive and Dahl salt-sensitive rats, Tobian[13] reported that addition of either potassium chloride or potassium citrate markedly reduced the probability of death from stroke. An analysis of the Rancho-Bernardo cohort noted that a 40% reduction in 12-year mortality was inversely related to intake of fruits and vegetables. This result is consistent with a protective effect of potassium.[14]

Potassium supplementation tends to lower blood pressure in both hypertensive and normotensive individuals,[11,12,14] and potassium may play a role in the treatment and prevention of hypertension. However, in hypertensive individuals, potassium supplementation is likely to be less important than such nonpharmacological measures as weight reduction, alcohol moderation, increased exercise, and reduced salt intake. Potassium supplementation may play an especially important role in lowering blood pressure in certain groups, such as elderly people and African Americans.

Potassium Supplements

Fruits and vegetables are the best sources of potassium.[15] However, in potassium-depleted individuals, fruits and vegetables may not be sufficient to replace the deficit. An important strategy is to decrease or minimize the body's potassium losses. Under certain circumstances, this may be impossible. Thus, it is important to determine the nature of the potassium loss.

An acid-base disturbance invariably accompanies chronic hypokalemia. For instance, in potassium losses induced by chronic diarrhea or by classic renal tubular acidosis, bicarbonate is concomitantly lost or not appropriately replaced. In such instances, potassium should be replaced as potassium bicarbonate or potassium citrate. The citrate is then promptly metabolized to bicarbonate.

Potassium losses engendered by thiazide diuretics result in chronic metabolic alkalosis and hypochloremia. In such patients, potassium should be supplemented in the form of potassium chloride. A reduced dietary salt intake also minimizes potassium losses in patients receiving thiazide diuretics.

References

1. Sterns RH, Malcolm C, Feif PU, Singer I (1981) Internal potassium balance and the control of the plasma potassium concentration. Medicine 60:339–354
2. Black RM (1993) Acid-base and potassium balance. In Rubenstein E, Federman DD (eds), Scientific American medicine. Scientific American Inc, New York, p 23
3. Moreno M, Murphy C, Goldsmith C (1969) Increase in serum potassium resulting from the administration of hypertonic mannitol and other solutions. J Lab Clin Med 73:291–298
4. Schwartz WB, Brackett NC, Cohen JJ (1965) The response of extracellular hydrogen ion concentration to graded degrees of chronic hypercapnia: the physiologic limits of the defense of pH. J Clin Invest 36:373–382
5. Todd EP, Vick RL (1971) Kaleotropic effect of epinephrine: analysis with adrenergic agonists and antagonists. Am J Physiol 220:1963–1969
6. Castro-Tavares J (1976) A comparison between the influence of pindolol and propranolol on the response of plasma potassium to catecholamines. Arzneimittelforschung Drug Res 26:238–241
7. DeFronzo R, Felig P, Ferrannini E, Wahren J (1980) Effects of graded doses of insulin on splanchnic and peripheral potassium metabolism in man. Am J Physiol 238:E421–E427
8. Gronert GA, Tehye RA (1975) Pathophysiology of hyperkalemia induced by succinylcholine. Anesthesiology 43:89–99
9. Intersalt Cooperative Research Group (1988) Intersalt: an international study of electrolyte excretion and blood pressure: results for 24 hour urinary sodium and potassium excretion. Br Med J 297:319–328
10. Kempner W (1944) Treatment of a kidney disease and hypertensive vascular disease with rice diet. NC Med J 5:125–133, 273–274
11. Cappuccio FP, MacGregor GA (1991) Does potassium supplementation lower blood pressure? A metaanalysis of published trials. J Hypertens 9:465–473
12. Whelton PK, Appel LA, Seidler AJ, et al (1992) Potassium supplementation in the treatment and prevention of hypertension [abstract]. J Hypertens 10(suppl 4):S108
13. Tobian L (1986) High potassium diets markedly protect against stroke deaths from kidney disease in hypertensive rats, a possible legacy from prehistoric times. Can J Physiol Pharmacol 64:840–848
14. Whelton PK (1993) Potassium and blood pressure. In Izzo JL Jr, Black HR (eds), Hypertension primer. American Heart Association Press, Dallas, TX, pp 170–172
15. Working Group on Primary Prevention of Hypertension (1993) Report of the National High Blood Pressure Education Program Working Group on Primary Prevention of Hypertension. Arch Intern Med 153:186–208

Chapter 28

Iron

Ray Yip and Peter R. Dallman

Iron is one of the most investigated and best understood of nutrients. Research on iron nutrition has been facilitated by the relative ease of sampling blood and red cells, which represent the major functional pool of iron in the body. To a large extent, iron metabolism and factors leading to iron deficiency are well defined. Iron deficiency is the most common nutritional deficit worldwide and yet it can be successfully prevented on a population basis.[1-5] In recent years, concern about iron overload in developed countries has spurred research in this area.

Total body iron averages ≈3.8 g in men and ≈2.3 g in women. The iron-containing compounds in the body are grouped into two categories, functional (known to serve a metabolic or enzymatic function) and storage (used for storage and transport of iron). Approximately two-thirds of total body iron is functional iron, and most of this is in the form of hemoglobin within circulating erythrocytes. Other iron-containing enzymes and myoglobin make up about 15% of functional iron. About one-third of total body iron in men is in the form of iron stores, whereas in women storage iron accounts for only about one-eighth. Nutritional iron deficiency is commonly regarded as an insufficient iron supply to meet the need for functional iron after storage iron has been depleted. At the cellular level, iron deficiency can also result from insufficient release of storage iron despite ample iron intake and stores—e.g., anemia of chronic disease. Under circumstances of iron overload, iron stores become disproportionately large, and in severe cases can be more than 10× the functional iron component.

Historical background. The scientific method was first applied to the study of iron nutrition when early in the eighteenth century it was shown that iron was a major constituent of blood.[6,7] Menghini drew attention to the iron content of blood by lifting particles of dried, powdered blood with a magnet. The widespread therapeutic use of iron tablets began in 1832 with a report by Blaud on the efficacy of treating young women in whom "coloring matter was lacking in the blood." Convincing proof that inorganic iron could be used for hemoglobin synthesis came in 1932 from Castle and coworkers,[8] who found that the amount of iron given parenterally to patients with hypochromic anemia cor-

responded closely to the amount of iron gained in circulating hemoglobin. In the past few decades, absorption studies using radioactive isotopes of iron led to the realization that dietary inorganic iron had to be in soluble form to be well absorbed.

Bunge in 1892 described the special vulnerability of infants to iron deficiency. The author found that milk was an unusually poor source of iron, and predicted that excessive feeding of milk could lead to iron deficiency after neonatal iron reserves were depleted. In 1928, Mackay was among the first to demonstrate that iron deficiency was the reason for anemia prevalent among infants in East London, and she showed that anemia could be alleviated by providing iron-fortified powdered milk.[9] Nevertheless, the practice of adding iron to infants' diets did not become widespread in the United States until the 1960s, and is still not common in a number of developed countries.

Chemistry

Chemical properties of iron. Iron is element 26 of the periodic table and has an atomic weight of 55.85. Iron is the fourth most common element on earth after oxygen, silicon, and aluminum. In solid form, iron exists as a metal or in iron-containing compounds. In aqueous solution, iron exists in two oxidation states, Fe^{2+}, the ferrous form, and Fe^{3+}, the ferric form. A special property of iron is how easily it changes between these two forms, which enables iron to serve as a catalyst in redox reactions by donating or accepting electrons. Some of the key biological activities of iron-containing compounds relating to oxygen and energy metabolism depend on the reactive property or high redox potential of iron.

Within living organisms, the potentially harmful reactivity and oxidative potential of iron are carefully modulated by the binding of iron to carrier protein or by the presence of other molecules with antioxidant properties. When not properly controlled, redox reactions can cause significant damage to cellular components like fatty acids, proteins, and nucleic acids. Iron catalyzes the Fenton reaction, one of the best known processes for

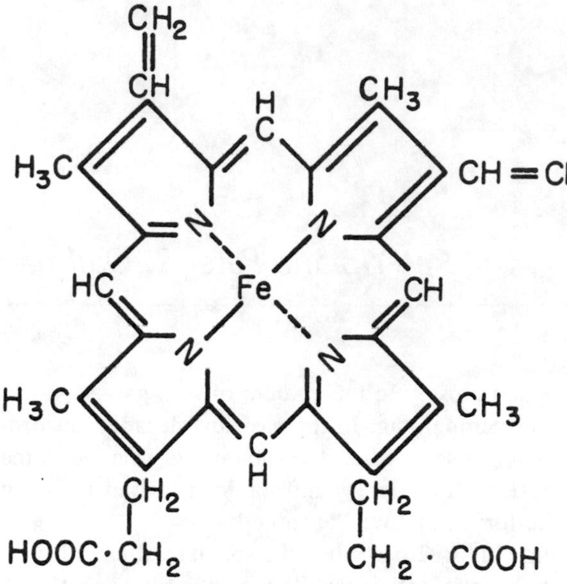

Figure 1. The chemical structure of heme- or ferroprotoporphyrin 9. The same structure without the iron in the center is protoporphyrin 9. The combining of iron with protoporphyrin 9 to form heme requires facilitation by ferrochelatase or heme synthetase.

converting superoxide and hydrogen peroxide to very reactive free radicals.[10]

Free radicals such as hydroxyl radicals cause peroxidation or cross-linking of membrane lipids and intracellular compounds, leading to cell aging and death. Although this is part of the normal aging process of cells,[11] the presence of increased oxidative stress is thought to lead to premature cell aging.

Iron-containing compounds.[12,13] Most functional iron is in the form of heme proteins, i.e., proteins with an iron-porphyrin prosthetic group. The basic structure of heme consists of a protoporphyrin-9 molecule with one iron atom (Figure 1). The unique chemical property of heme is its easy loading and unloading of oxygen. The best-known heme-containing molecule is hemoglobin, which has a molecular weight of 68,000 and is made up of four heme subunits, each with a polypeptide chain of globin attached. Myoglobin, the heme compound in muscle, has a structure similar to hemoglobin except it consists of only one heme and one globin chain. A number of enzymes also contain iron, but these account for less than 3% of the total body iron.

Stored iron exists in two principal forms, ferritin and hemosiderin.[12] Apoferritin, the protein portion of ferritin, consists of 24 polypeptide subunits that form a raspberry-like spherical cluster around hydrated ferric phosphate within the hollow center. There are two subunits of ferritin: heart isoferritin with a molecular weight of 21,000, and liver isoferritin with a molecular weight of 19,000.

On average, ferritin contains ≈25% iron by weight, although ferritin molecules vary in iron content and may contain up to 4000 atoms of iron. Roughly the other half of storage iron in liver is made up of hemosiderin, a heterogeneous group of large iron-salt-protein aggregates. Hemosiderin will react with antibodies to ferritin, and is therefore believed to represent ferritin in various stages of degradation.

Iron Metabolism[13,14]

Three main factors affect iron balance and metabolism: intake, stores, and loss. With respect to iron intake, the two determinants are the quantity and bioavailability of iron in the diet and the capacity to absorb iron. The dietary sources of iron are reviewed below. Iron metabolism is unusual in that iron absorption from the gastrointestinal tract is the primary regulatory mechanism of iron balance. The amount of iron absorbed from food can vary from <1 to >50%.[15,16] The percentage absorbed depends on the type of food eaten and the interaction between the food and regulatory mechanisms in the intestinal mucosa that reflect the body's physiological need for iron.

Iron absorption.[16] Iron absorption is influenced by dietary iron content, bioavailability of dietary iron, amount of storage iron, and rate of erythrocyte production. With respect to diet, nonheme and heme iron are absorbed by different mechanisms.[17] Nonheme iron consists primarily of iron salts, is found mainly in plant and dairy products, and accounts for most of the iron in the diet, usually >85%. Absorption of nonheme iron is strongly influenced by its solubility in the upper part of the small intestine, which in turn depends on how the meal as a whole affects iron solubility. In general, nonheme iron absorption is influenced by solubility enhancers and inhibitors consumed during the same meal.

Heme iron comes primarily from hemoglobin and myoglobin in meat, poultry, and fish. Although heme iron accounts for a smaller proportion of iron in the diet than nonheme iron, it is absorbed ≈2–3× more readily than nonheme iron and is less affected by other dietary constituents. Men absorb an average of ≈6% of total dietary iron compared with ≈13% for women of childbearing age.[18] The higher absorption of iron by women relates to their lower body iron stores and helps to compensate for iron losses through menstruation.

A number of factors are known to enhance or inhibit nonheme iron absorption. The best known enhancer is vitamin C (ascorbic acid).[16] Factors present in meat also enhance nonheme iron absorption,[19] while iron absorption from meals consisting of whole-grain cereals and legumes tends to be poor. The addition of even relatively small amounts of meat or vitamin C to food increases iron absorption from the entire meal. Nonheme iron absorption from a meal containing meat, fish, or chicken is ≈4× greater than from equivalent portions of milk, cheese, or eggs.[20]

Dietary inhibitors of nonheme iron absorption include calcium phosphate, bran, phytic acid (present in unprocessed whole-grain products), and polyphenols (in tea and some vegetables).[18] Coffee may also inhibit iron absorption, but the responsible constituent has not been identified.[21]

Iron entry into the body is regulated by mucosal cells of the small intestine, but the mechanism by which iron absorption is regulated remains uncertain.[22] There appear to be different pathways for the uptake of heme iron and nonheme iron. Body iron stores as well as hematologic status as reflected by hemoglobin level are strong determinants of intestinal uptake of nonheme iron. Individuals who have either low iron stores or iron deficiency and those who are anemic absorb greater fractions of nonheme iron from the diet than nonanemic individuals with ample iron stores.[16] The percentage of nonheme iron that is absorbed can be as high as 50% in subjects with severe iron deficiency anemia. Absorption is enhanced for both heme and nonheme iron, but is more pronounced for nonheme iron. Compared with men, women and children have lower iron stores, and consequently absorb a greater percentage of iron from the diet. This is most striking during pregnancy: as iron stores decline throughout gestation, iron absorption steadily becomes more efficient. Conversely, the high iron stores typical of men and postmenopausal women reduce the percentage of iron absorbed, thereby offering some protection against iron overload.

Iron transport. Transport of iron from the breakdown of hemoglobin or from the intestine to the tissues is accomplished by the plasma transport protein, transferrin. Transferrin delivers iron to the tissues by means of cell membrane receptors specific for transferrin.[24] The receptors bind the transferrin-iron complex at the cell surface and carry it into the cell, where iron is released. Less than 1% of the total body iron is in the transport pool, in transit from intestinal mucosa or reticuloendothelial cells to tissues with high iron requirements, such as the bone marrow, where erythrocytes are produced. The iron supply is reflected by the iron saturation of transferrin: a low saturation indicates undersupply or deficiency and a high saturation indicates oversupply.

The affinity of transferrin receptors for transferrin appears to be constant in various tissues. Tissues such as erythroid precursors, placenta, and liver that have a high iron uptake contain large numbers of transferrin receptors. The genes for both transferrin and transferrin receptor are located on chromosome 3. The number of receptors is highly regulated.[25,26] When cells are in an iron-rich environment, the number of receptors decreases. Conversely, when iron supply to the cells is inadequate because of iron deficiency or increased iron demand related to high cell turnover, the number of transferrin receptors increases. Since the concentration of transferrin receptors in serum is in proportion to that on the cell surface, serum transferrin receptors are another biochemical indicator that can be used to assess iron status.[27]

Iron storage. The foremost iron storage compounds are ferritin and hemosiderin, which are present primarily in the liver, reticuloendothelial cells, and bone marrow.[28,29] The total amount of storage iron varies widely without apparent impairment of body function. Storage iron may be almost entirely depleted before iron-deficiency anemia develops, and a >20-fold increase over normal average iron stores may occur before there is evidence of tissue damage. Iron is stored in the liver mainly in parenchymal cells or hepatocytes, with a smaller portion in reticuloendothelial cells or Kupffer cells. In bone marrow and spleen, stored iron is mainly within reticuloendothelial cells. Stored iron serves as a reservoir to supply cellular iron needs, mainly for hemoglobin production. The iron bound to ferritin is more readily mobilized than iron bound to hemosiderin. With long-term negative iron balance, iron stores are depleted before the onset of tissue iron deficiency. With positive iron balance, iron stores can gradually increase even when the percentage of dietary iron that is absorbed is relatively low—e.g., in postmenopausal women and with increasing age in men. When storage iron is pathologically increased, as in hemochromatosis, the only effective means of reducing iron stores in order to avoid tissue damage is by phlebotomy.

Infants are born with a substantial endowment of stored iron roughly proportional to birth weight. On average, iron stores of a full-term infant can meet the infant's iron needs until ≈6 months of age.[30] Because preterm and low-birth-weight infants are born with much less storage iron and because they experience a higher rate of growth during infancy than full-term babies, their iron stores become depleted much sooner, often by 2–3 months of age; hence low-birth-weight and preterm infants are more vulnerable to iron deficiency. After iron stores are exhausted, at ≈6 months of age up to 24 months of age, substantial iron stores are difficult to accumulate even when iron intake is adequate because of the high iron requirement related to rapid growth. After 2 years of age, as growth rate slows, iron stores start to build and the risk of iron deficiency declines.[31] Throughout adulthood iron stores gradually increase in men. In women stores are low until menopause, after which they increase.

Iron turnover and loss. Erythrocyte destruction and production is responsible for most iron turnover. Erythrocytes contain ≈2/3 of total body iron and have a normal life-span of 120 days. To replace 1/120 of erythrocytes, the daily iron turnover for an adult is ≈20 mg, but most of the iron of degraded erythrocytes is recaptured for the synthesis of hemoglobin. In contrast to hemoglobin, tissue iron compounds vary widely in their life spans and are subject to random degradation at rates similar to the rates of turnover of the subcellular structures with which they are associated; e.g., cytochrome c of rat skeletal muscle has a half-life of 6 days.[32]

Iron losses occur primarily (0.6 mg/day) in the feces from bile, desquamated mucosal cells, and the loss of minute amounts of blood.[33] Smaller amounts of iron are lost in desquamated skin cells and in sweat (0.2–0.3 mg/day). Urinary losses are minor (<0.1 mg/day). In men, total losses average 1.0 mg/day (range 0.5–2.0 mg/day). Premenopausal women must also replace the iron lost in menstrual blood—average blood loss 30–40 mL/cycle or 0.4–0.5 mg/day—which combined with other losses makes a total average loss of 1.3 mg/day. Some women whose blood loss is greater than 80 mL/cycle are unable to maintain a positive iron balance.[34]

The most common reason for abnormal blood loss in certain infants and young children is sensitivity to protein in cow's milk, which manifests as increased occult blood loss from the gastrointestinal tract.[35] In many tropical countries, hookworm infection is a major cause of gastrointestinal blood loss contributing to iron deficiency in older children and adults. In developed countries, intestinal iron losses in adults are usually associated with the chronic use of drugs such as aspirin or with bleeding ulcers or tumors.[36]

Iron needs for growth are greatest in infants and adolescents. During childhood, ≈40 mg iron is required to produce essential iron compounds (hemoglobin, myoglobin, and enzyme iron) for each kilogram of weight gain. Allowing for iron stores of 300 mg, an extra 5 mg iron/kg weight gain is required, for a total 45 mg/kg.

Accurate measurements of iron losses are not available for children, but given that most losses are from intestinal mucosa and skin, one can extrapolate from the 1.0 mg/day in men on the basis of body surface area. By this approach, infants average 0.2 mg/day iron losses and children aged 6–11 years average 0.5 mg/day. For a 6-month-old infant, the combined iron requirement for loss and growth is ≈0.8 mg/day, which is only slightly lower than for adult men. This relatively high requirement makes older infants and younger children vulnerable to iron deficiency.

Physiology

Among iron compounds serving major biological functions, the best known are heme-containing: hemoglobin for oxygen transport, myoglobin for muscle storage of oxygen, and cytochromes for oxidative production of cellular energy in the form of ATP.

Hemoglobin.[37] Hemoglobin plays a critical role in transferring oxygen from lung to tissues. Its structure of four hemes and four globin chains provides an efficient mechanism to combine with oxygen without being oxidized. A remarkable feature of hemoglobin is its ability to become almost fully oxygenated during the short erythrocyte transit time in pulmonary circulation, and then to become largely deoxygenated as erythrocytes traverse tissue capillaries. A number of factors affect the oxygen affinity of hemoglobin as measured by the oxygen dissociation curve: partial pressure of oxygen, pH, temperature, and organic phosphate content. With moderate anemia, biochemical changes to improve oxygen unloading to tissues compensate for the reduced oxygen carrying capacity of blood. With severe anemia, however, the markedly reduced hemoglobin content decreases oxygen delivery and can lead to chronic tissue hypoxia. Even though a lack of iron is the most common reason for anemia, many other pathological conditions can affect hemoglobin or erythrocyte production, leading to anemia and a reduced oxygen carrying capacity of blood.

Myoglobin. Myoglobin consists of a single heme with a single globin chain. Myoglobin is present only in muscles, where it accounts for ≈5 mg/g of tissue. The primary function of myoglobin is to transport and store oxygen within muscle and to release it to meet increased metabolic needs during muscle contraction. Myoglobin makes up ≈10% of total body iron. In rats, skeletal muscle myoglobin decreases with iron deficiency.

Cytochromes.[39] Cytochromes are heme-containing compounds critical to respiration and energy metabolism through their role in mitochondrial electron transport. Cytochromes a, b, and c are essential to the production of cellular energy by oxidative phosphorylation: they serve as electron carriers in transforming adenosine diphosphate (ADP) to adenosine triphosphate (ATP), the primary energy-storage compound. Animals with significant iron deficiency show depleted levels of cytochromes b and c and limited rates of oxidation by the electron transport chain.

Cytochrome c is a pink protein and is the most easily isolated and best characterized of the cytochromes. Like myoglobin, cytochrome c is made up of one globin chain and one heme group containing one iron atom. The cytochrome c concentration in man ranges from 5 to 100 μg/g of tissue, and is highest in tissues such as heart muscle that have a high rate of oxygen utilization.

Cytochrome P450 is located in microsomal membranes of liver cells and intestinal mucosal cells.[39] The primary function of this cytochrome is the breakdown of various endogenous compounds and chemicals or toxins from external sources by oxidative degradation.

Other iron-containing enzymes. Nonheme iron-containing enzymes such as the iron-sulfur complexes of NADH dehydrogenase and succinate dehydrogenase are also involved in energy metabolism.[13] These enzymes are required for the first reaction in the electron transport chain, and account for more iron in mitochondria than do cytochromes. In iron-deficient rats, these dehydrogenases are severely depleted.

Another group of iron-containing enzymes known as hydrogen peroxidases act on reactive molecules that are by-products of oxygen metabolism. Hydrogen peroxidases protect against accumulation of hydrogen peroxide (H_2O_2), a molecule with a high reactive potential, especially in its ionic form (HO_2^-). The high reactive potential of hydrogen peroxide makes it potentially damaging to biologically active molecules.[10] Catalase and peroxidase are heme-containing enzymes that use hydrogen peroxide as a substrate and convert it to water and oxygen. Studies of rat and human erythrocytes have shown increased lipid peroxidative damage with increasing iron deficiency.[40,41] Lecithin cholesterol acyl transferase (LCAT), an enzyme known to protect against lipid peroxidation, also shows reduced activitiy in iron-deficient rats.[42]

Other enzymes that require iron for their function include aconitase, an enzyme of the tricarboxylic acid cycle; phosphoenolpyruvate carboxykinase, a rate-limiting enzyme in the gluconeogenic pathway; and ribonucleotide reductase, an enzyme required for DNA synthesis.

Iron Deficiency

Iron deficiency is the most common nutritional deficiency in the United States and worldwide, affecting mainly older infants, young children, and women of childbearing age.[1,2] In developing countries it is estimated that 30–40% of young children and premenopausal women are affected by iron deficiency.[3] Young children are most susceptible to iron deficiency because they require relatively high amounts of iron for rapid growth during the first 2 years of life, and their usual diet is low in iron unless added as a nutritional supplement.[30] According to the U.S. third National Health and Nutrition Examination Survey (1991), ≈5% of children aged 1–2 years had evidence of iron deficiency on biochemical tests, and half of these are also anemic. Among older children, few show evidence of significant iron deficiency until the rapid growth period that occurs during puberty. Adolescent females are at high risk of iron deficiency because of a combination of rapid growth and menstrual blood loss.

Stages of iron deficiency. A number of hematological and biochemical tests reflecting different aspects of iron metabolism are used to characterize the iron nutritional status. Serum ferritin is the test of choice for assessing iron stores. Stainable iron of a bone marrow aspirate can be used for the same purpose but involves a more elaborate and somewhat painful procedure. Serum iron concentration (Fe), total iron binding capacity (TIBC), and transferrin saturation (Fe/TIBC) reflect iron supply to tissues. Protoporphyrin, the precursor of heme, is elevated in erythrocytes when the supply of iron for heme synthesis is insufficient.[43] Similarly, transferrin receptors respond to an insufficient iron supply to cells and become elevated on cell surfaces and in plasma.[27] Erythrocyte size—measured as mean corpuscular volume (MCV)—and hemoglobin concentration are reduced as a consequence of significant iron deficiency. Another measure reflects the variability of erythrocyte size and is called red cell distribution width (RDW). This value is elevated in iron deficiency, when red cell size becomes increasingly variable.[44]

One should distinguish between anemia and iron-deficiency anemia. Anemia occurs when hemoglobin production is sufficiently depressed to result in a hemoglobin concentration or hematocrit below the central 90% or 95% of range for healthy persons of the same age and sex.[45] A corollary of this definition is that 2.5% or 5.0% of healthy individuals will be considered anemic. There are many causes of anemia other than iron deficiency, notably infection and even mild inflammatory disease.[46,47] A diagnosis of iron-deficiency anemia is made when anemia is accompanied by laboratory evidence of iron deficiency, such as low serum ferritin, or when there is a rise in hemoglobin in response to iron treatment. Table 1 lists the age- and sex-specific hemoglobin and hematocrit values for a normal U.S. population.[48,49] Values for gestational stage are based on four European studies in which all women received iron supplementation.[49] In the United States, hemoglobin values are significantly lower among blacks than whites—8 g/L for adults, 4 g/L for children <5 years[50]—and the difference cannot be attributed to iron nutritional status.[51] Race-specific values should be considered to better compare test results and help detect iron deficiency among different racial and ethnic groups.[50-52]

Iron status is assessed by measuring iron-related laboratory parameters singly or in combination. For example, transferrin saturation and serum ferritin become elevated with excessive iron stores, hence are useful indicators of iron overload. Iron status is expressed as one of five stages ranging from iron overload to severe iron deficiency. Figure 2 is a diagrammatic representation of these five stages in relation to key tests.

In theory, iron depletion can be categorized into three stages ranging from mild to severe.[53] The first stage involves only decreased iron stores as measured by decreased serum ferritin. This stage is not associated with adverse physiological consequences, but does represent increased vulnerability from long-term marginal iron balance that might progress to a more severe deficiency with functional consequences. With low iron stores, there is a compensatory increase in iron absorption that often helps prevent progression to more severe stages. The

Table 1. Estimated normal mean values and lower limits of normal (5th percentile) for hemoglobin and hematocrit[a]

Age (years)	Hemoglobin (g/L)		Hematocrit	
	Mean	Lower limit	Mean	Lower limit
Male and females				
0.5–1.9	123	110	0.359	0.330
2.0–4.9	125	112	0.363	0.340
5.0–7.9	128	114	0.372	0.345
8.0–11.9	132	116	0.384	0.350
Males				
12.0–14.9	140	123	0.405	0.370
15.0–17.9	148	126	0.430	0.380
18+	153	135	0.445	0.400
Females				
12.0–14.9	134	118	0.390	0.355
15.0–17.9	135	120	0.390	0.380
18+ (not pregnant)	135	120	0.390	0.380
Pregnancy				
1st trimester	122	110	0.365	0.330
2nd trimester	116	105	0.350	0.320
3rd trimester	121	110	0.360	0.330

[a]All data are based on venous blood. Persons who had laboratory evidence of iron deficiency or inflammatory disease were excluded. Adapted from Yip et al.[48,49]

second stage of iron depletion is characterized by biochemical changes that reflect a lack of sufficient iron for normal production of hemoglobin and other essential iron compounds, but as yet there is no frank anemia. Typically there is decreased transferrin saturation or increased erythrocyte protoporphyrin, serum transferrin receptor, or RDW. Because the hemoglobin concentration does not yet fall below levels considered indicative of anemia, this stage is often described as iron deficiency without anemia. The third stage of iron depletion is frank iron-deficiency anemia, which varies in severity according to how low the hemoglobin concentration is. In the United States, most cases of iron-deficiency anemia among children and women are mild, characterized by a hemoglobin within 10 g/L of the lower limit of nor-

mal for that group.[2] Iron deficiency, however, can result in severe anemia, defined as hemoglobin <70 g/L by the World Health Organization.[3] In certain developing countries, severe iron deficiency anemia is common.[54]

Assessing iron deficiency in populations. One strategy for determining iron status in a population is to perform multiple tests such as the ferritin model used by the U.S. second National Health and Nutrition Examination Survey (NHANES II), which consisted of serum ferritin, transferrin saturation, and erythrocyte protoporphyrin.[55] A subject was considered iron deficient if two or more tests were abnormal. Another three-test combination measures mean corpuscular volume, transferrin saturation, and erythrocyte protoporphyrin, and is called the MCV model.[55] The advantage of a multiple-test approach is that while singly the individual tests are not very specific for iron deficiency, in combination their specificity is much higher. Their main drawback is relatively high cost and difficulty in maintaining good quality control over several tests.

An alternative population-based approach that is more feasible for developing countries is to use anemia as an indicator, recognizing that anemia is not specific for iron deficiency. Because of their vulnerability to iron deficiency, young children and menstruating women are often the target of anemia assessments, yet studies of men within the same population can yield valuable clues to the relationship between anemia and iron deficiency.[54,56] In developed countries and many developing areas where poor dietary iron intake is the principal reason for anemia of children and women, few men ever develop iron deficiency anemia because their iron requirements are relatively low. This indicates that iron deficiency is the

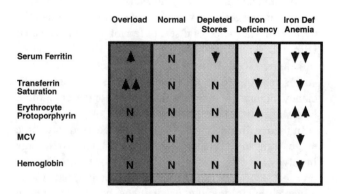

Figure 2. Stages of iron status as reflected by the behavior of different hematologic and iron biochemistry tests. Iron overload is characterized by elevated serum ferritin and transferrin saturation. Iron deficiency can be further divided into three stages: iron depletion, iron deficiency without anemia, and iron deficiency anemia.

main cause of anemia. If men are found to have a significant level of anemia, reasons other than poor dietary iron intake are likely to exist.[54] Malaria, hookworm infection, and nutritional deficiencies besides iron may cause anemia that shows no predilection for women and children.

Causes of iron deficiency by age. Infants older than 6 months and young children are very vulnerable to iron deficiency because of depletion of iron stores from rapid growth, low iron content of most infant diets, and early feeding of cow's milk, which may promote increased gastrointestinal blood loss.[35,57] The combination of rapid growth, depleted stores, and low iron content of the diet results in a peak period of iron deficiency between 9 and 18 months of age.

Because a milk-based diet provides most of the energy consumed during the first year of life, the iron content of various milk products and the bioavailability of iron are strong predictors of iron nutritional status.[58] Infants consuming mainly iron-fortified formula are at low risk of iron deficiency, but those fed nonfortified formulas or whole cow's milk have a 30–40% risk of iron deficiency by 9 month of age, and this risk is likely to be greater by 12 months. Breast-fed infants without adequate iron from other food sources are also at risk of iron deficiency by 9 to 12 months.[58] Iron-deficiency anemia may develop as early as 3 months after birth in premature infants and twins whose neonatal iron stores are smaller and whose weight gain is proportionately greater than for full-term single infants.[53]

The risk of iron deficiency among preadolescent children in developed countries is low because of a slower growth rate and consumption of a mixed diet with ample iron. In many developing countries, however, the combination of poor dietary iron bioavailability and gastrointestinal blood loss due to hookworm infection can result in a high prevalence of iron-deficiency anemia among school-age children.

Iron requirements climb at puberty. Boys gain an average of 10 kg in weight during the peak year of their growth spurt, and their hemoglobin concentration simultaneously rises toward values characteristic of adult men.[48,59] This double burden of providing iron for a larger body size and larger erythrocyte mass is ≅25% increase in total body iron during the year of peak growth. The iron need of adolescent girls is also large. Their average weight gain of 9 kg during the peak year of the growth spurt—sometime between 10 and 12 years of age—is almost as great as that of boys, and the onset of menstruation imposes additional iron needs.

Two factors predispose to iron-deficiency anemia in women: menorrhagia (excessive blood loss during menstruation) and pregnancy. Heavy blood loss (>80 mL/month) occurs in ≈10% of women, and frequently leads to iron-deficiency anemia.[5] Intrauterine devices for contraception increase menorrhagia to 30–50%.[60] Oral contraceptives, on the other hand, decrease menstrual blood loss by about half, and are rarely associated with menorrhagia.[61] Women with menorrhagia are characteristically unaware of their greater-than-normal menstrual blood loss,[34] and for this reason anemia screening at the time of routine health examination is worthwhile.

Iron-deficiency anemia may develop during pregnancy because of the increased iron requirements to supply the expanding blood volume of the mother and the rapidly growing fetus and placenta (Figure 3).[5,62–66] The amount of iron required during the last half of pregnancy cannot be easily met by diet, and therefore the risk of iron deficiency is high, especially toward the end of pregnancy.[65] Healthy women who are not pregnant average ≈2.3 g of total body iron; only ≈0.3 g of this amount is storage iron. The total iron required during pregnancy averages 1 g, and thus greatly exceeds the amount of storage iron available to most women.[62] As pregnancy progresses, reduced iron stores trigger an increase in the efficiency of dietary iron absorption; nevertheless, some women will deplete their iron stores and become anemic. Lower-income U.S. women have consistently shown a 30% prevalence of anemia during the third trimester of pregnancy.[68] Routine iron supplementation is necessary to prevent iron deficiency anemia during pregnancy.

Iron stores increase throughout adult life in men and postmenopausal women,[31] who rarely exhibit nutritional iron deficiency. In elderly people anemia is more commonly associated with chronic inflammatory conditions (e.g., arthritis) than with iron deficiency.[47] The few cases of iron-deficiency anemia among the elderly are usually caused by gastrointestinal blood loss from chronic use of drugs such as aspirin or from lesions or tumors, and not by inadequate iron intake.[36]

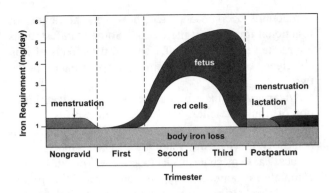

Figure 3. Iron requirement of women before and during pregnancy. Reprinted with permission from Bothwell et al.[66]

Consequences of Iron Deficiency

Unless the anemia is severe, the clinical manifestations of iron deficiency tend to be subtle. As the essential iron compounds become depleted, however, the degree of functional impairment increases.[69] Some manifestations are related to anemia itself, some to the effects of iron deficiency on tissues, and some to a combination of the two.

Anemia. Anemia is by far the best known manifestation of iron deficiency. Mild anemia in itself is of little health consequence in sedentary individuals, since compensatory mechanisms maintain oxygen supply to the tissues. These mechanisms include the following: 1) more complete extraction of oxygen from hemoglobin by tissues; 2) redistribution of blood flow to vital organs, primarily the myocardium and brain, at the expense of other tissues; and 3) increased cardiac output.[70] When anemia becomes severe (hemoglobin <70 g/L), these adaptive mechanisms cannot compensate for the decreased oxygen-carrying capacity of the blood, and acidosis develops. Very severe anemia (hemoglobin <40 g/L), which can result from iron deficiency in combination with other diseases, is associated with increased childhood and maternal mortality,[71,72] particularly at times of increased physiological stress—e.g., during an acute febrile illness or peripartum, when acute blood loss may overwhelm an already stressed capacity for oxygen delivery and cardiovascular function.[73]

Work performance. Anemia causes a substantial reduction in work capacity. This effect is particularly evident when hemoglobin concentration falls below 100 g/L, which is 20–40 g/L below the lower limit of normal for adults. Studies in humans indicate that even a mild degree of anemia can decrease performance during brief but intense exercise.[74] Among men working on a rubber plantation in Indonesia and women working on a tea plantation in Sri Lanka, the productivity of iron-deficient individuals was significantly less than that of workers with normal hemoglobin concentrations.[75,76] After supplementation with iron, the iron-deficient subjects showed improved performance, and the greatest improvement was seen in those who had the lowest hemoglobin concentrations initially.

Impaired work performance in humans certainly can be related to anemia per se, but tissue abnormalities may also be responsible to an undetermined degree. Experiments with rats show that dietary iron deficiency causes marked impairment in oxidative energy production in skeletal muscle.[77,78] This manifests as decreased capacity for prolonged exercise, less efficient glucose oxidation, and increased use of the gluconeogenic pathway by which lactate from the muscle is converted to glucose in the liver.[79]

Behavior and intellectual performance. Mounting evidence points to impaired psychomotor development and intellectual performance as well as changes in behavior resulting from iron deficiency.[80] Studies of infants between 6 months and 2 years of age show a statistically significant decrease in responsiveness and activity, with increased body tension, fearfulness, and tendency to fatigue in association with iron deficiency anemia.[81] The long-term significance of these changes has not been determined. Of particular interest is the observation that abnormalities are most profound in older infants (19–24 months) whose iron deficiency is presumed to have existed for the longest time.[82] Even infants with mild iron-deficiency anemia do not score as well as infants with no laboratory evidence of iron deficiency or evidence merely of depleted iron stores.[81,83,84] The possibility of behavioral abnormalities assumes importance because the rapid rate of growth and differentiation of brain cells during infancy might be expected to make the brain particularly vulnerable to deficiencies in the supply of nutrients. Even though there is good evidence that the developmental deficits can be corrected with iron treatment,[83–85] other studies suggest that abnormalities are not fully corrected.[80]

Body temperature regulation. Also characteristic of iron-deficiency anemia is an impaired capacity to maintain body temperature in a cold environment. This abnormality appears to be related to decreased secretion of thyroid-stimulating hormone and thyroid hormone.[86] Impaired heat production appears to result from the anemia itself, since a blood transfusion corrects the abnormality. Furthermore, rats fed iron-adequate diets show impaired heat production when they are made anemic by bleeding.

Immunity and resistance to infections. Laboratory evidence of decreased resistance to infection is characteristic of iron deficiency both in humans and experimental animals.[87] Despite numerous studies showing impaired resistance to infection under laboratory conditions, and even though iron-deficient children show abnormal lymphocyte and neutrophil function, an increased rate of infections from iron deficiency per se has not been documented. Iron-deficiency anemia and infections are common among poor populations, but a cause-and-effect relationship, although plausible, has not been established.[87]

Lead poisoning. Animal and human studies demonstrate increased absorption of lead associated with iron deficiency.[88,89] In the United States, young children who have iron deficiency have a 3–4× higher prevalence of lead poisoning than children who are not iron-deficient.[90,91] The increased efficiency of iron absorption among iron-deficient subjects is well established; unfortunately, this increased absorptive capacity is not specific to iron, and other divalent metals, including toxic heavy metals such as lead and cadmium, are also absorbed at a faster rate.[92]

Adverse pregnancy outcomes. Anemia of early pregnancy has been associated with preterm delivery, low birth weight, and fetal death in a number of epidemiological studies.[93,94] One study indicates that the increased risk of preterm births is associated specifically with iron-deficiency anemia, rather than anemia itself.[97] An association of late-pregnancy anemia with these consequences is more difficult to interpret, given that hemoglobin is normally lower in the second trimester than in the third.[95,96] These studies were conducted in developed countries, where severe iron-deficiency anemia during pregnancy is rare, and therefore a stronger relationship is possible in developing countries, where severe anemia during pregnancy is more common.[54]

Prevention of Iron Deficiency

Iron deficiency can be prevented by increasing the content and bioavailability of iron in the diet. Iron absorption is improved by including meat, fish, poultry, and ascorbic acid–rich foods in meals, and by decreasing consumption of tea and milk with meals. Iron-fortified cereal products augment the iron content of the diet; those with added ascorbic acid also enhance iron absorption. Parental awareness of what constitutes an appropriate diet is especially important for infants, whose diet is relatively simple. Iron nutrition can be improved by breast feeding or giving iron-fortified formula during the first year to infants who are not breast-fed. When solid foods become part of the infant's diet, iron-fortified infant cereals are a source of iron. These infant-feeding practices have been widely adopted over the past 10–15 years, and have contributed to the striking decline in anemia among older infants and young children in the United States.[98,99] The improved iron nutritional status observed among young children can also be partly attributed to increased use of bioavailable iron compounds to fortify cereal products.

There has probably been a substantial decline in anemia among premenopausal women too. The best evidence comes from Sweden, where 30% of women of fertile age were anemic in 1965, compared with 7% in 1975.[4] The difference was attributed to several factors, including increased use of iron supplements, increased iron fortification of foods, increased use of birth-control pills which decrease menstrual blood loss, and increased intake of ascorbic acid. Most of these factors also apply to women in the United States.

Iron fortification.[100] Ferrous sulfate is commonly used to fortify infant formula and other products sold in cans and jars, as well as bread and other bakery products that have a short shelf-life. Because ferrous sulfate is highly soluble, it is as well absorbed as the intrinsic iron in these foods. Unfortunately, many foods that are marketed and stored for long periods in air-permeable packages are not suitable for fortification with ferrous sulfate because most highly soluble forms of iron promote fat oxidation and rancidity. For this reason, elemental iron powders are commonly used to fortify such foods in North America,

while the relatively nonreactive and insoluble ferric orthophosphate and ferric pyrophosphate are widely used in Europe. The effectiveness of this type of iron fortification in preventing iron-deficiency anemia is not as well documented, but there is some evidence that these compounds also help prevent iron-deficiency anemia.[101]

Iron supplementation. The absorption of iron from tablets or liquid supplements is influenced by dose, iron stores of the recipient, whether it is taken with or between meals, and whether it is taken alone or as part of a vitamin-mineral supplement.[52] In general, iron absorption from supplements is greatest in iron-deficient individuals, because absorption is inversely proportional to iron stores. Iron is absorbed twice as well when given between meals rather than with meals, and absorption is enhanced when the iron supplement is taken with water or juice rather than with tea, coffee, or milk.

Slow-release iron supplements decrease side effects when large doses are given, but are more expensive than the standard ferrous sulfate, ferrous gluconate, and ferrous fumarate. A slow-release preparation may be better absorbed than ferrous sulfate when given with a meal, but it is less well absorbed under fasting conditions.

Among women of childbearing years, iron is commonly taken as part of a vitamin-mineral tablet, yet calcium carbonate and magnesium oxide in these preparations appear to inhibit iron absorption.[102,103] Since less iron is absorbed from certain multivitamin-mineral supplements than from an equivalent amount of iron given alone, it seems advisable to select products that contain ≈60 mg of iron, rather than the recommended dose of 30 mg, to allow for the anticipated lower absorption. It would also be best to select a formulation that contains no more than 250 mg calcium. The single most effective technique for improving compliance with iron supplements is to simplify the treatment regimen,[104] i.e., once/day rather than 3×/day.[105]

Screening and Diagnosis of Iron Deficiency

The manifestations of iron deficiency are usually too subtle to prompt consultation with a physician. Typically, iron deficiency is suspected on the basis of dietary history and low hemoglobin concentration or hematocrit (Table 1) obtained on routine health maintenance visits. A low MCV is strong supportive evidence of iron deficiency. If the history and blood count seem in accord with iron deficiency, a therapeutic trial with iron may be indicated without further confirmatory tests, especially if the anemia is mild, i.e., hemoglobin within 10 g/L of lower limit of normal. Hemoglobin and hematocrit determinations on blood from skin punctures have a substantial sampling error, however. If the results are borderline or only slightly below the normal range, a repeat hemoglobin analysis on venous blood will often be normal. A finding of anemia on venous blood is a sounder basis for a decision regarding a therapeutic trial or the necessity for additional laboratory tests.

The most common tests are erythrocyte protoporphyrin, serum ferritin, and transferrin saturation. The choice of tests depends on local circumstances, convenience, and availability. In recent years, a simplified outpatient laboratory measure of erythrocyte protoporphyrin, the hematofluorometer method, has been used in screening for childhood lead poisoning. This simplified test can also be used to screen for iron deficiency, since most children who have elevated erythrocyte protoporphyrin are iron deficient,[106] but only a small minority actually have elevated lead levels. The screening cutoff for erythrocyte protoporphyrin is 0.35 mg/L of whole blood or 3.0 µg/g of hemoglobin. Current lead-screening programs for children do not use erythrocyte protoporphyrin as the primary measure of lead poisoning, but the test is still useful in screening for iron deficiency.

Treatment for Iron Deficiency

Gastrointestinal side effects are the most common problem encountered in the treatment of iron deficiency. The risk of side effects is directly proportional to the iron dose,[107] and symptoms usually result from larger-than-necessary doses of iron compounds amounting to >120 mg/day of elemental iron. Ferrous sulfate is the least expensive and most widely used form of oral iron. A total dose equivalent to 60 mg of elemental iron (300 mg ferrous sulfate) per day is ample for an adult if given between meals, first thing in the morning, or at bedtime. For infants ≈1 year of age, 30 mg/day (2–3 mg/kg) of elemental iron first thing in the morning rarely causes side effects; this dose is also appropriate and adequate for older children and adolescents. Fortunately, the smaller the dose and the more severe the anemia, the greater the percentage of iron absorbed. A response to treatment should be evident after 1 month, when the deficit in hemoglobin is partially corrected, usually with a rise >10 g/L. Even after a significant hemoglobin response, iron treatment should be continued for another 2–3 months. If there is no correction of anemia after 1 month of iron treatment, further laboratory evaluation (e.g., with serum ferritin) is indicated to either confirm the presence of iron deficiency or determine other causes of anemia.

Iron Requirement and Recommended Daily Allowances

Estimates of average requirements for absorbed iron in adults are based on careful experimental measurements of iron losses. The amount of additional iron that is needed by growing infants and children is calculated from average weight gain and estimates of iron necessary to supply that gain, with iron as hemoglobin, myoglobin, and iron enzymes. Once it is estimated how much absorbed iron is needed for growth and replacement of losses, an assumption must be made about the percentage of iron that is absorbed from the diet. This will depend largely on the nature of the diet. A figure of 5% has been used for diets in which cereals and legumes predominate and that are low in animal tissue protein and ascorbic acid;[108] such diets are typical of many developing countries. A value of 15% is proposed for more varied diets that are rich in meat and ascorbic acid; 10% is used as an intermediate figure,[108] and for the United States, a working figure of 12.5% seems reasonable. Thus, iron need for growth plus replacement of losses is multiplied by eight to arrive at mean dietary iron requirement.

Recommended daily allowances (RDA) for dietary iron provide for individuals whose needs are greater than average. A factor of 1.25 (based on a coefficient of variation of 15%) is used for the calculation, and the resulting quantity represents sufficient iron to meet the needs of most of the population.[109] This figure, however, does not take into account the ≈10% of women whose menstrual blood loss is >80 mL/month, who might develop iron deficiency despite good diets and and who might require supplemental iron.[34]

The current RDA for iron is based on average iron stores of 300 mg and average daily iron losses of 1 mg for men and 1.5 mg for women.[110] With a factor of variation of 1.25, the estimated requirement for absorbed iron is 1.3 mg/day for men and 1.8 mg/day for women. Assuming 10–15% absorption of dietary iron in the United States, the estimated RDA is 10 mg/day for men and 15 mg/day for women.[110] Pregnant women face increased iron demand for fetal and maternal tissue growth, and their RDA is 30 mg/day. This level of iron intake usually cannot be met by dietary sources, and routine iron supplementation is recommended. For nursing mothers, the iron needed to produce breast milk is approximately 0.15–0.3 mg/day, which is equivalent to the iron saved by cessation of menstrual blood loss during lactation,[111] and therefore their iron requirement is the baseline 15 mg/day. For infants and children 6 months–3 years of age, the iron RDA of 10 mg/day is calculated on the need for 1 mg absorbed iron/kg/day. For preterm or low-birth-weight infants, the requirement is 2 mg/kg/day because of lower iron stores at birth and greater rate of growth than term or normal-weight infants.[30]

Dietary Sources of Iron

The dietary source of iron strongly influences the efficiency of iron absorption, which ranges from <1% to >20%. Nonheme iron in foods of vegetable origin is at the lower end of the range, dairy products are in the middle, and meat is at the upper end. About 10% of the small amount of iron in unfortified formulas or whole milk is absorbed. The iron content of breast milk is similar to that of cow's milk, but about 50% of iron in breast milk is absorbed, hence breast milk is a better source of iron than nonfortified formula or cow's milk.[30] Its better absorption efficiency does not entirely make up for its low iron content, however, and after age 6 months breast-fed infants require an additional source of dietary iron to meet their iron requirement.[58]

Meat is a good source of iron because much of it is in the form of heme iron, which is absorbed 2–3× more completely than nonheme iron. In addition, factors in meat promote nonheme iron absorption from the entire meal. NHANES II surveyed the diet of adult women and estimated 31% of iron was from meat sources and 25% was from iron added to food (mainly cereal and wheat flour–based products).[112] Nonheme iron absorption can be enhanced by ascorbic acid ingested with the meal, and ascorbic acid intake is relatively high in the United States—ranging from 76 to 112 mg/day, well above the current RDA of 60 mg/day.[110,113]

Iron Excess and Toxicity

The toxic potential of iron derives from its principal biological property, the ability to exist in two oxidation states: Fe^{2+} (ferrous form) and Fe^{3+} (ferric form). Iron serves as a catalyst in redox reactions by donating or accepting electrons. Some redox reactions, when not properly modulated by antioxidants or iron-binding proteins, can damage cellular components such as fatty acids, proteins, and nucleic acids. A number of health disorders are related to short- or long-term exposure to iron in amounts exceeding the physiological capacity to protect against its reactivity. These pathological conditions range from acute iron poisoning to organ damage due to chronic iron overload.[114] In recent years there has also been concern that "iron overnutrition" among otherwise healthy individuals may lead to increased risk of chronic diseases.

Acute iron toxicity or poisoning. Iron poisoning is a well-defined short-term disorder that occurs following the ingestion of inappropriately large doses of therapeutic iron.[115] Iron toxicity is the most dramatic form of iron excess, and can lead to severe organ damage and death within hours or days. The problem occurs mainly among young children who swallow iron tablets intended for women in the household.[116] The lethal dose of iron is relatively large, ≈200–250 mg/kg, compared with a therapeutic dose of 2–5 mg/kg/day. Iron toxicity becomes significant when the amount of ingested and absorbed iron exceeds that which can be bound to transferrin in the plasma, or when transferrin saturation approaches 100%. The most pronounced local effect of iron poisoning is hemorrhagic necrosis of the gastrointestinal tract, manifested by vomiting and bloody diarrhea, that results from strong acids produced by interaction of iron with hydrochloric acid in the stomach. Systemic effects include coagulation defects, metabolic acidosis, and shock. The metabolic acidosis is attributed to conversion of ferrous iron to ferric iron, releasing hydrogen ions and accumulating lactic acid and citric acid from iron-induced mitochondrial injury.[117]

Hemolytic anemia of preterm infants. The best documented subacute form of iron-induced tissue damage is nonimmune hemolytic anemia occurring among preterm infants deficient in vitamin E who receive iron-fortified formula or oral iron supplements.[118,119] Because the plasma of preterm infants lacks antioxidant capacity, peroxidative damage from increased iron intake can be significant. In contrast, infants supplemented with alpha-tocopherol or who are not deficient in vitamin E show little effect on erythrocyte survival from additional iron intake. Since hemolysis was identified as a consequence of oxidative damage and was found to be preventable by alpha-tocopherol, it has become common practice to give supplemental vitamin E to all preterm infants. Another contributor to hemolytic anemia of premature infants was the high polyunsaturated fat content of infant formula, whose fatty acids rendered erythrocyte cell membranes more susceptible to oxidative damage.[119] This form of hemolytic anemia is now a thing of the past, since current infant formulas contain high proportions of vitamin E and are low in polyunsaturated fatty acids.

Chronic iron toxicity and iron overload. Over the long term, excessive accumulation of body iron not only can result in excessive iron stores, but also can damage various organs when iron cannot be adequately contained in stores. Hemosiderosis refers to increased iron stores in the form of hemosiderin; hemochromatosis refers to excessive storage iron that causes organ damage, often as fibrosis. Iron overload is a nonspecific term for increased total body iron content with or without organ damage. The main routes of excessive iron uptake are oral ingestion and transfusion. The oral route can result in iron overload through either increased absorption or excessive intake.

Hereditary hemochromatosis.[120] The best known and perhaps the most common form of chronic iron overload is hereditary hemochromatosis, a genetic defect in the regulation of iron absorption. Individuals who have homozygous hereditary hemochromatosis absorb more iron than normal. There is evidence that heterozygous individuals also have increased iron absorption but to a lesser extent, so that no iron overload or tissue damage ensues. The frequency of homozygosity is approximately 3–4:1000 in populations of European extraction, while heterozygosity is estimated to be ≈1:10.[121] Age at onset and clinical presentation vary widely; rare cases manifest in late childhood, while others never show evidence of tissue damage. Clinical signs of organ damage from iron overload usually become evident during the third to fifth decade of life in men and after menopause in women. Clinical manifestations appear when total body iron accumulation reaches 20–40 g or about 10× normal. Most affected are liver, pancreas, heart, joints, and pituitary gland. Iron accumulates in parenchymal cells, resulting in cirrhosis, diabetes, heart failure, arthritis, and sexual dysfunction. Transferrin saturation is the most helpful test for screening and diagnosis of hereditary hemochromatosis: a >60% level is 80% sensitive in detecting affected individuals, even without clinical signs of iron overload.[122] The primary treatment is phlebotomy to reduce the body iron load. Phlebotomy that is started before clinical signs appear can avert significant organ damage; after clinical signs, phlebotomy will prevent progression of organ damage but will not reverse existing damage. For this reason, prophylactic screening of asymptomatic cases is recommended.[122]

Iron overload from excessive oral intake. A less common form of iron overload is related to excessive oral iron intake without a defect in iron absorption. The best known example is Bantu-type hemochromatosis, a syndrome seen among Bantu tribesmen in southern Africa who consume large quantities of maize beer high in iron (40–80 mg/L). The high iron content comes from using iron containers for brewing the acid beer, which increases iron solubility.[123] Recent evidence suggests that genetic factors may also contribute to iron overload among Africans who have very high iron intakes.[124]

Iron overload from repeated transfusions for severe anemia. The second major route of iron overload is blood transfusions, and typically occurs among persons who have severe and refractory anemia and depend on repeated transfusion—e.g., beta thalassemia major, a hereditary defect in hemoglobin production. Sideroblastic anemias are due to inherited or acquired disorders of hemoglobin synthesis resulting in ineffective erythropoiesis.[125] Other transfusion-dependent conditions include anemia from bone marrow failure and various types of severe chronic hemolytic anemia. In hemolytic disorders the severe anemia also increases gastrointestinal iron absorption, which can contribute significantly to the iron burden beyond what comes from transfusions.

One unit of transfused blood (500 mL) contains ≈200–250 mg of iron in hemoglobin form, equivalent to the amount of dietary iron absorbed over 150–200 days. Transfusion of 6–12 units of blood/year may lead to clinically evident iron overload. Since phlebotomy is not an option in persons with severe anemia, iron chelation therapy is commonly used to mobilize the excess iron.

Relationship Between Iron Status and Risk of Disease

In recent years there has been speculation that the public may be adversely affected by high levels of iron in food or by high iron stores. This concern arose from observations of a possible association between high levels of transferrin saturation or serum ferritin and cancer or coronary heart disease.[126,127] The hypothesis is that, through unknown mechanisms, the risk of certain chronic diseases may increase with iron stores at the high end of normal range. At present, the validity of these associations is obscure and elucidation will require consistent findings by multiple observers.

Iron status and risk of cancer. Experimental studies show that high iron levels promote carcinogenesis or faster rates of tumor growth.[128] Among the epidemiological studies, the best known is by Steves et al.,[126] who followed a cohort of Americans for 10 years. The authors reported that men who had higher levels of transferrin saturation had a greater incidence of cancer mortality. This relationship was not observed among women, nor could the finding be substantiated when the follow-up period was extended to 17 years or the data reanalyzed by others.[129,130] An earlier study found increased incidence of hepatic carcinoma among Taiwanese men whose serum ferritin levels were elevated.[131] This finding can be explained by chronic hepatitis, a well known cause of liver cancer; hepatitis itself can cause an elevation in serum ferritin.[132] The only strong evidence linking iron overload with cancer is the increased risk of hepatic carcinoma among individuals with hemochromatosis. This association is attributed to chronic injury to hepatic tissues from extremely high levels of iron in liver.

Iron status and risk of coronary heart disease. The most significant epidemiologic study indicating an association between high iron stores and increased risk of coronary heart disease is by Salonen et al.[127] The researchers found that Finnish men whose serum ferritin levels were high (>200 μg/L) at the beginning of the study had a 2.2-fold increased incidence of acute myocardial infarction during the 3-year follow-up. The authors hypothesized that free radicals induced by free iron cause increased peroxidation of low-density lipoprotein and thereby contribute to atherogenesis. An alternative explanation is the mounting evidence for an inflammatory component associated with coronary heart disease, given that serum ferritin functions as an acute reactant and becomes elevated with inflammatory processes.[133]

Since the Finnish report, other studies in the United States and Finland have examined the possible relationship of coronary heart disease with high iron status and have found no association.[130,134,135] A recent review of coronary heart disease among persons with severe iron overload from hereditary hemochromatosis showed an incidence of heart disease no higher than expected for the general population.[120] The results of the Finnish study could be explained by preexisting, subclinical coronary heart disease.

Summary

The field of iron nutrition has undergone considerable changes in recent years. Increasing attention is being paid to the effects of iron deficiency beyond the familiar anemia. In the pediatric population, for instance, there is strong evidence that significant iron deficiency contributes to developmental and behavioral disturbances, underscoring the importance of iron balance as a child health issue. It is also reassuring to note that much that has been learned about iron nutrition in infancy and childhood has been translated into action, primarily as improved infant diets responsible for a decrease in iron-deficiency anemia in the United States.

Regarding women of childbearing age, the other major risk group for iron deficiency, there is enhanced awareness that a negative iron balance cannot always be overcome by improvements in diet. The question remains whether iron-deficiency anemia affects the outcome of pregnancy. If so, the effort to prevent iron deficiency among women of childbearing age must be given high priority.

The most important shift in the field of iron nutrition over the past decade is the increasing concern about iron overnutrition. To a large extent this concern was fueled by epidemiologic observations of associations between elevated levels of serum ferritin or transferrin saturation and cancer or coronary heart disease. These associations are not strong and may possibly relate to the nature of observational studies. However, heart disease and cancer account for most deaths in developed countries, and any hint of increased risk from iron cannot be ignored. The potential impact of high iron stores on health outcomes should be better investigated. At present there is evidence to support active prevention and control of well-defined iron overload disorders, especially hereditary hemochromatosis. A screening program for hereditary hemochromatosis that uses biochemical tests such as transferrin saturation and serum ferritin will also identify persons with iron deficiency who may benefit from further evaluation and intervention. Eventually, the implementation of effective screening and treatment procedures will likely reduce morbidity related to iron overload.

References

1. Pilch SM, Senti FR (1984) Assessment of the iron nutritional status of the U.S. population based on the data collected in the second National Health and Nutrition Examination Survey, 1976–1980. Federation of American Societies for Experimental Biology, Bethesda, MD, p 65

2. Dallman PR, Yip R, Johnson C (1984) Prevalence and causes of anemia in the United States, 1976–1980. Am J Clin Nutr 39:437–445

3. DeMaeyer E, Adiels-Tegman M, Rayston E (1985) The prevalence of anemia in the world. World Health Stat Q 38:302–316

4. Hallberg L, Bengtsson C, Garby L, et al (1979) An analysis of factors leading to a reduction in iron deficiency in Swedish women. Bull World Health Organ 57:947–954

5. Bothwell TH, Charlton RW, Cook JD, Finch CA (1979) Iron metabolism in man. Blackwell Scientific, Oxford

6. McCay CM (1973) Notes on the history of nutrition research. Bern, Huber, pp 138–144, 156–171

7. McCollum EV (1957) A history of nutrition. Houghton Mifflin, Boston, pp 334–358

8. Heath CW, Strauss MB, Castle WB (1932) Quantitative aspects of iron deficiency in hypochromic anemia. J Clin Invest 11:91–110

9. Mackay HM (1928) Anaemia in infancy: prevalence and prevention. Arch Dis Child 3:117–146

10. Halliwell B, Gutteridge JMC (1990) Role of free radicals and catalytic metal ions in human disease: an overview. Methods Enzymol 186:1–85

11. Stocks J, Offerman EL, Modell CB, Dormandy TL (1972) The susceptibility to autooxidation of human red cell lipids in health and disease. Br J Haematol 23:713–736

12. Halliday JW, Ramm GA, Powell LW (1994) The cellular iron processing and storage. In Brock JH, Halliday JW, Pippard MJ, Powell LW (eds), Iron metabolism in health and disease. WB Saunders, London, pp 97–121

13. Dallman PR (1986) Biochemical basis for the manifestations of iron deficiency. Annu Rev Nutr 6:13–40

14. Yip R, Mehra M (1995) Individual functional roles of metal ions in vivo: iron. In Berthon G (ed), Handbook on metal ligands interactions of biological fluid. Marcel Dekker, New York, pp 207–217

15. Hallberg L (1981) Bioavailability of iron in man. Annu Rev Nutr 1:123–147

16. Skikne B, Baynes RD (1994) Iron absorption. In Brock JH, Halliday JW, Pippard MJ, Powell LW (eds), Iron metabolism in health and disease. WB Saunders, London, pp 151–187

17. Björn-Rasmussen E , Hallberg L, Isaksson B, Arvidsson B (1974) Food iron absorption in man: application of the two-pool extrinsic tag method to measure heme and non-heme iron absorption from the whole diet. J Clin Invest 52:247–255

18. Charlton RW, Bothwell TH (1983) Iron absorption. Annu Rev Med 34:55–68

19. Cook JD, Monsen ER (1976) Food iron absorption in human subjects. III. Comparison of the effect of animal proteins on nonheme iron absorption. Am J Clin Nutr 29:859–867

20. Rossander L, Hallberg L, Björn-Rasmussen E (1979) Absorption of iron from breakfast meals. Am J Clin Nutr 32:2484–2489

21. Morck TA, Lynch SR, Cook JD (1983) Inhibition of food iron absorption by coffee. Am J Clin Nutr 37:416–420

22. Peters TJ, Raja KB, Simpson RJ, Snape S (1988) Mechanisms and regulation of iron absorption. Ann NY Acad Sci 526:141–147

23. Davidson LA, Lönnerdal B (1988) Specific binding of lactoferrin to brush-border membrane: ontogeny and effect of glycan chain. Am J Physiol 25J:G580–G585

24. Huebers HA, Finch CA (1987) The physiology of transferrin and transferrin receptors. Physiol Rev 67:520–581

25. Casey JL, Hentze MW, Koeller DM, et al. (1988) Iron-responsive elements: regulatory RNA sequences that control in RNA levels and translation. Science 240:924–928

26. Casey JL, DiJeso B, Rao K, et al (1988) The promoter region of the human transferrin receptor gene. Ann NY Acad Sci 526:54–64

27. Skikne BS, Flowers CH, Cook JD (1990) Serum transferrin receptor: a quantitative measure of tissue iron deficiency. Blood 75:1870–1876

28. Hershko C (1977) Storage iron regulation. Prog Hematol 10:105–148

29. Deiss A (1983) Iron metabolism in reticuloendothelial cells. Semin Hematol 20:81–90

30. Dallman PR, Siimes MA, Stekel A (1980) Iron deficiency in infancy and childhood. Am J Clin Nutr 33:86–118

31. Yip R (1994) Age related changes in iron metabolism. In Brock JH, Halliday JW, Pippard MJ, Powell LW (eds), Iron metabolism in health and disease. WB Saunders, London, pp 427–448

32. Booth FW, Holloszy JO (1977) Cytochrome c turnover in rat skeletal muscles. J Biol Chem 252:416–419

33. Green R, Charlton RW, Seffel H, et al (1968) Body iron excretion in man: a collaborative study. Am J Med 45:336–353

34. Hallberg L, Högdahl A, Nilsson L, Rybo G (1966) Menstrual blood loss—a population study. Acta Obstet Gynecol Scand 45:320–351

35. Ziegler EE, Fomon SJ, Nelson SE, et al (1990) Cow milk feeding in infancy: further observations on blood loss from the gastrointestinal tract. J Pediatr 116:11–18

36. Rockey DC, Cello JP (1993) Evaluation of the gastrointestinal tract in patients with iron-deficiency anemia. N Engl J Med 329:1691–1695

37. Finch CA, Lenfant C (1972) Oxygen transport in men. N Engl J Med 286:407–410

38. Hargreaves RM, Street M, Hoy T, et al (1981) Myoglobin depletion in childhood iron deficiency. Br J Haematol 47:399–401

39. Dallman PR (1974) Tissue effects of iron deficiency. In Jacobs A, Worwood M (eds), Iron in biochemistry and medicine. Academic Press, London

40. Yip R, Mohandas N, Jain SK, et al (1982) Red cell deformability in iron deficiency. In Saltman P, Hegenauer J (eds), The biochemistry and physiology of iron. Elsevier, Amsterdam, pp 617–619

41. Jain SK, Yip R, Joesch RM, et al (1983) Evidence of peroxidative damage to the erythrocyte membrane in iron deficiency. Am J Clin Nutr 37:26–30

42. Jain SK, Yip R, Dallman PR, Shohet SB (1982) Reduced lecithin cholesterol acetyltransferase in iron deficient rats. J Nutr 112:1230–1232

43. Labbe RF, Rettmer RL (1988) Zinc protoporphyrin: a product of iron-deficient erythropoesis. Semin Hematol 26:40–46

44. Novak RW (1987) Red blood cell distribution width in pediatric microcytic anemias. Pediatrics 80:251–254

45. Yip R (1989) Iron status defined. In Filer LJ Jr (ed), Dietary iron: birth to two years. Raven Press, New York, pp 19–36

46. Reeves JD, Yip R, Kiley VA, Dallman PR (1984) Iron deficiency in infants: the influence of mild antecedent infection. J Pediatr 105:874–879

47. Yip R, Dallman PR (1988) The role of inflammation and iron deficiency as causes of anemia. Am J Clin Nutr 48:1295–1300

48. Yip R, Johnson C, Dallman PR (1984) Age-related changes in laboratory values used in the diagnosis of anemia and iron deficiency. Am J Clin Nutr 39:427–436

49. Centers for Disease Control (1989) CDC criteria for anemia in children and childbearing age women. MMWR 38:400–404

50. Johnson-Spear M, Yip R (1994) Hemoglobin difference between black and white women with comparable iron status: justification for race-specific anemia criteria. Am J Clin Nutr 60:117–121

51. Perry GS, Byers T, Yip R, Margen S (1992) Iron nutrition does not account for the hemoglobin differences between blacks and whites. J Nutr 122:1417–1424

52. Earl R, Woeteki C, eds (1993) Iron deficiency anemia: recommended guidelines for prevention, detection and management among US children and women of childbearing age. National Academy Press, Washington, DC

53. Dallman PR, Yip R, Oski FA (1992) Iron deficiency and related nutritional anemias. In Nathan DG, Oski FA (eds), Hematology of infancy and childhood. WB Saunders, Philadelphia, pp 413–450

54. Yip R (1994) Iron deficiency: contemporary scientific issues and international programmatic approaches. J Nutr 124:1479S–1490S

55. Expert Scientific Working Group (1985) Summary of a report on assessment of iron nutritional status of the United States population. Am J Clin Nutr 42:1318–1330

56. Yip R, Gove S, Farah BH, Mursal HM (1990) Rapid assessment of hematological status of refugees in Somalia: the potential value of hemoglobin distribution curves in assessing iron nutrition status. In Hercberg S, Galan P, Dupin H, Colloque (eds), Recent knowledge on iron and folate deficiencies in the world. Volume 197. INSERM, Paris, pp 193–196

57. Fomon SJ, Ziegler EE, Nelson SE, Edwards BB (1981) Cow milk feeding in infancy: gastrointestinal blood loss and iron nutritional status. J Pediatr 98:540–545

58. Pizarro F, Yip R, Dallman PR, et al (1991) Iron status with different infant feeding regimens: relevance to screening and prevention of iron deficiency. J Pediatr 118:687–692

59. Dallman PR (1992) Changing iron needs from birth through adolescence. In Fomon SJ, Zlotkin S (eds), Nutritional anemias. Raven Press, New York, pp 29–38

60. Israel R, Shaw ST, Martin MA (1974) Comparative quantitation of menstrual blood loss with the Lippes loop, Dalkon shield, and Copper T intrauterine devices. Contraception 10:63–71

61. Hefnawi F, Askalani H, Zaki K (1974) Menstrual blood loss with copper intrauterine devices. Contraception 9:133–139

62. Hallberg L (1988) Iron balance in pregnancy. In Beyer H (ed), Vitamins and minerals in pregnancy and lactation. Volume 16, Nestle Nutrition Workshop Series. Raven Press, New York, pp 115–126

63. Svanberg B, Arvidsson B, Norrby A, et al (1975) Absorption of supplemental iron during pregnancy. Acta Obstet Gynecol Scand Suppl 48:87–108

64. Puolakka J (1980) Serum ferritin as a measure of iron stores during pregnancy. Acta Obstet Gynecol Scand Suppl 95:1–63

65. Taylor DJ, Mallen C, McDougall N, Lind T (1982) Effect of iron supplementation on serum ferritin levels during and after pregnancy. Br J Obstet Gynaecol 89:1011–1017

66. Bothwell TH, Charlton RW, Cook JD, Finch CA (1979) Iron metabolism in man. Blackwell, Oxford

67. Cook JD, Finch CA (1979) Assessing iron status of a population. Am J Clin Nutr 32:2115–2119

68. Perry G, Yip R, Zykowski C (1995) Nutritional risk factors among low-income US women. Semin Perinatol 19:211–221

69. Dallman PR (1982) Manifestations of iron deficiency. Semin Hematol 19:19–30

70. Varat MA, Adolph RJ, Fowler NO (1972) Cardiovascular effects of anemia. Am Heart J 83:416–426

71. Van den Broeck J, Eeckels R, Vuylsteke J (1993) Influence of nutritional status on child mortality in rural Zaire. Lancet 341:1491–1495

72. World Health Organization (1992) The prevalence of anemia in women: a tabulation of available information. World Health Organization, Geneva

73. Lackritz EM, Campbell CC, Ruebush TK, et al (1992) Effect of blood transfusion on survival among children in a Kenyan hospital. Lancet 340:524–528

74. Viteri FE, Torun B (1974) Anemia and physical work capacity. Clin Hematol 3:609–626

75. Basta SS, Soekiman MS, Karyadi D, Scrimshaw NS (1979) Iron deficiency anemia and the productivity of adult males in Indonesia. Am J Clin Nutr 32:916–925

76. Edgerton VR, Gardner GW, Ohira Y, et al (1979) Iron-deficiency anemia and its effect on worker productivity and activity patterns. Br Med J 2:1546–1549

77. Finch CA, Miller LR, Inamdar AR, et al (1976) Iron deficiency in the rat: physiological and biochemical studies of muscle dysfunction. J Clin Invest 59:447–453

78. McLane JA, Fell RD, McKay RH, et al (1981) Physiological and biochemical effects of iron deficiency on rat skeletal muscle function. Am J Physiol 241:C47–C54

79. Davies KJA, Donovan CM, Refino CA, et al (1984) Distinguishing effects of anemia and muscle iron deficiency on exercise bioenergetics in the rat. Am J Physiol 246:E535–E543

80. Lozoff B (1988) Behavioral alterations in iron deficiency. Adv Pediatr 35:331–359

81. Lozoff B, Brittenham GM, Viteri FE, et al (1982) The effects of short-term oral iron therapy on developmental deficient anemic infants. J Pediatr 100:351–357

82. Lozoff B, Brittenham GM, Viteri FE, et al (1982) Developmental deficient infants: effects of age and severity of iron lack. J Pediatr 101:948–952

83. Oski FA, Honig AS, Helu B, Howanitz P (1983) Effect of iron therapy on behavior performance in nonanemic, iron-deficient infants. Pediatrics 71:877–880

84. Walter T, Kovalskys J, Stekel A (1983) Effect of mild iron deficiency on infant mental development scores. J Pediatr 104:710–713

85. Idjradinata P, Pollitt E (1993) Reversal of developmental delays in iron-deficient anemic infants treated with iron. Lancet 341:1–4

86. Beard J, Green W, Miller L, Finch CA (1984) Effect of iron-deficiency anemia on hormone levels and thermoregulation during cold exposure. Am J Physiol 247:R114–R119

87. Dallman PR (1987) Iron deficiency and the immune response. Am J Clin Nutr 46:329–334

88. Watson WS, Morrison J, Bethel MIF, et al (1986) Food iron and lead absorption in humans. Am J Clin Nutr 44:248–256

89. Watson WS, Hume RM, Moore MR (1980) Oral absorption of lead and iron. Lancet 2:236–237

90. Yip R, Norris TN, Anderson AS (1981) Iron status of children with elevated blood lead concentrations. J Pediatr 98:922–925

91. Yip R (1990) Multiple interactions between childhood iron deficiency and lead poisoning: evidence that childhood lead poisoning is an adverse consequence of iron deficiency. In Hercberg S, Galan P, Dupin H, Colloque (eds), Recent knowledge on iron and folate deficiencies in the world. Volume 197. INSERM, Paris, pp 523–532

92. Mahaffey KR (1981) Nutritional factors in lead poisoning. Nutr Rev 31:353–362

93. Garn SM, Ridella SA, Petzold AS, Falkner F (1981) Maternal hematologic levels and pregnancy outcomes. Semin Perinatol 5:155–162

94. Murphy JF, O'Riordan J, Newcombe RG, et al (1986) Relation of haemoglobin levels in first and second trimesters to outcome of pregnancy. Lancet 1:992–994

95. Lieberman E, Ryan KJ, Monson RR, Schoenbaum SC (1987) Risk factors accounting for racial difference in the rate of premature birth. N Engl J Med 317:743–748

96. Klebanoff MA, Shiono PH, Berendes HW, Rhoads GG (1990) Facts and artifacts about anemia and preterm delivery. JAMA 262:511–515

97. Scholl TO, Hediger ML, Fischer RL, Shearer JW (1992) Anemia vs iron deficiency, increased risk of preterm delivery in a prospective study. Am J Clin Nutr 55:985–988

98. Yip R, Blinkin NJ, Fleshood L, Trowbridge FL (1987) Declining prevalence of anemia among low-income children in the United States. JAMA 258:1619–1623

99. Yip R, Walsh KM, Goldfarb MG, Binkin NV (1987) Declining prevalence of anemia in childhood in a middle class setting: a pediatric success story? Pediatrics 80:330–334

100. Bothwell TH, Macphail P (1992) Prevention of iron deficiency by food fortification. In Fomon SJ, Zlotkin S (eds), Nutritional anemias. Volume 30. Nestle Nutrition Workshop Series. Raven Press, New York, pp 183–192

101. Walter T, Dallman PR, Pizarro F, et al (1993) Effectiveness of iron fortified infant cereal in prevention of iron deficiency anemia. Pediatrics 91:976–982

102. Babior BM, Peters WA, Briden PM, Cetrulo CL (1985) Pregnant women's absorption of iron from prenatal supplements. J Reprod Med 30:355–357

103. Seligman PA, Caskey JH, Frazier JL, et al (1983) Measurements of iron absorption from prenatal multivitamin-mineral supplements. Obstet Gynecol 61:356–362

104. Bonnar J, Goldberg A, Smith JA (1969) Do pregnant women take their iron? Lancet 1:547–548

105. Porter AMW (1969) Drug defaulting in a general practice. Br Med J 1:218–222

106. Yip R, Schwartz S, Deinard A (1983) Screening for iron deficiency with erythrocyte protoporphyrin test. Pediatrics 72:214–219

107. Solvell L (1970) Oral iron therapy—side effects. In Hallberg L (ed), Iron deficiency: pathogenesis, clinical aspects, therapy. Academic Press, London, pp 573–583

108. Monsen ER, Hallberg L, Layrisse M, et al. (1978) Estimation of available dietary iron. Am J Clin Nutr 31:134–141

109. FAO/WHO (1989) Requirements of vitamin A, iron, folate and vitamin B-2. Report of a joint FAO/WHO Expert Group. World Health Organization, Geneva

110. National Research Council (1989) Recommended dietary allowances, 10th ed. National Academy Press, Washington, DC

111. Lönnerdal B, Keen CL, Hurley LS (1981) Iron, copper, zinc, and manganese in milk. Annu Rev Nutr 1:149–174

112. Murphy SP, Calloway DH (1986) Nutrients intake of women in NHANES II emphasizing trace minerals, fiber, and phytate. J Am Diet Assoc 86:1366–1372

113. Raper ND, Rothenal JC, Woteki CE (1984) Estimates of available iron in diets of individuals 1 year old and older in the Nationwide Food Consumption Survey. J Am Diet Assoc 84:783–787

114. Yip R (1995) Toxicity of essential and beneficial metal irons—iron. In Berthon G (ed), Handbook on metal ligands interactions of biological fluid. Marcel Dekker, New York

115. Banner W Jr, Tong TG (1986) Iron poisoning. Pediatr Clin North Am 33:393–409

116. Centers for Disease Control (1993) Toddler deaths resulting from ingestion of iron supplements—Los Angeles, 1992–1993. MMWR 42:111–113

117. Witzlben CL, Buck BE (1971) Iron overload hepatotoxicity: a postulated pathogenesis. Clin Toxicol 4:579–583

118. Melhorn DK, Gross S (1971) Vitamin E dependent anemia in preterm infants. I. Effect of large dose of medicinal iron. J Pediatr 79:569–580

119. Williams ME, Shott RJ, Oski FA (1975) Role of dietary iron and fat on vitamin E deficiency anemia. N Engl J Med 292:887–890

120. Powell LW, Jazwinska E, Halliday JW (1994) Primary iron overload. In Brock JH, Halliday JW, Pippard MJ, Powell LW (eds), Iron metabolism in health and disease. WB Saunders, London, pp 227–270

121. Edwards CQ, Griffen LM, Goldgar D, et al (1988) The prevalence of hemochromatosis among 11,065 presumably healthy blood donors. N Engl J Med 318:1355–1362

122. Haddow JE, Ledue TB (1994) Preventing manifestation of hereditary haemochromatosis through population based screening. J Med Screening 1:16–21

123. Bothwell TH, Seftel H, Jacobs P, et al (1964) Iron overload in Bantu subjects: study on availability of iron in Bantu beer. Am J Clin Nutr 14:47–51

124. Gordeuk V, Mukiibi J, Hasstedt SJ, et al (1992) Iron overload in Africa: interaction between a gene and dietary iron content. N Engl J Med 326:95–100

125. Bottomley S (1982) Sideroblastic anemia. Clin Haematol 11:389–409

126. Steves RG, Jones DY, Micozzi MS, Taylor PR (1988) Body iron stores and the risk of cancer. N Engl J Med 319:1047–1052

127. Salonen JY, Nyyssonen K, Korpela H, et al (1992) High stored iron levels are associated with excess risk of myocardial infarction in Western Finnish men. Circulation 86:803–811

128. Beard J (1993) Iron-dependent pathologies. In Earl R, Woteki C (eds), Iron deficiency anemia: recommended guidelines for prevention, detection and management among US children and women of childbearing age. National Academy Press, Washington, DC, pp 99–111

129. Yip R, Williamson DF, Byer T (1991) Is there an association between iron nutrition status and the risk of cancer? Am J Clin Nutr 53:30

130. Sempos CT, Looker AC, Gillum RF, Makuc DM (1994) Body iron stores and the risk of coronary heart disease. N Engl J Med 330:1119–1124

131. Steves RG, Beasley RP, Blumburg BS (1986) Iron-binding proteins and risk of cancer in Taiwan. J Natl Cancer Inst 76:605–610

132. Lipschitz DA, Cook JD, Finch CA (1974) A clinical evaluation of serum ferritin as an index of iron stores. N Engl J Med 290:1213–1216

133. Alexander RW (1994) Inflammation and coronary heart disease. N Engl J Med 331:468–469

134. Stampfer MJ, Grodstein F, Rosenberg I, et al (1993) A prospective study of plasma ferritin and risk of myocardial infarction in US physicians. Circulation 87:11

135. Giles WH, Anda RF, Williamson DF, et al (1994) Body iron stores and the risk of coronary heart disease. N Engl J Med 331:1159–1160

Chapter 29

Zinc

Robert J. Cousins

There are many centers of activity providing new information about the nutritional significance of zinc. These include molecular and isotopic approaches to zinc status assessment; molecular characterization of cellular zinc transport systems; understanding the role of zinc in cognition and central nervous system activity; zinc as a determinant of immune system development and maintenance of host defense, including hydroxyl radical protection; zinc and apoptotic cell death; and the molecular biology of zinc including transcriptional control of specific genes and zinc finger proteins associated with cellular proliferation and differentiation and intracellular signaling.

Chemistry

Zinc is a small ion (0.065 nm) and has a concentrated 2+ charge (Zn^{2+}). It is a strong Lewis acid (electron acceptor). Cu^{2+} and Fe^{3+} are stronger and weaker Lewis acids, respectively. Zn^{2+} does not exhibit redox chemistry, which may explain in part why it has biological functions where free radical generation would be deleterious. Because zinc is a Lewis acid, it binds strongly to thiolate and amine electron donors. Zinc also exhibits fast ligand exchange, which is important in its catalytic role in metalloenzymes. Ability to provide a highly localized charge center makes Zn^{2+} a very good attacking group, particularly where sites are constrained and where substrate binding is weak.[1,2]

Zinc has important structural roles as a result of its unique chemistry. Concentrations of free Zn^{2+} in cells are very low, perhaps ≤ 1 nmol/L. Intracellular binding of Zn^{2+} is believed to follow the Irving-Williams order of divalent cations (Cu > Zn ≥ Ni > Co > Fe > Mn > Mg > Ca). This is interpreted to mean that intracellular copper concentrations must be kept low to allow zinc to exercise its weaker binding potential. Greater than 95% of the body zinc content is intracellular. The high zinc content of specific organs or compartments is developed through intracellular sites of high zinc binding affinity and through regulated influx-efflux transport systems.[2] Intracellular zinc chemistry involves primarily thiolate and imidazole ligands. Binding of Zn^{2+} to thiolate ligands is believed to constitute an important mechanism to regulate intracellular levels of this micronutrient.

Understanding of the biological role of zinc has been greatly aided through the use of zinc radionuclides (predominantly ⁶⁵Zn), stable isotopes, and analytical instrumentation, principally atomic absorption spectrophotometry (AAS) and inductively coupled plasma emission (ICP). Zinc radioisotopes and their half-lives are ⁶⁵Zn, 245 days; ⁶⁵ᵐZn, 14 hours; and ⁶³Zn, 39 minutes. Methods of radioisotope assay include gamma ray spectrometry, liquid scintillation spectrometry, and autoradiography. Stable isotopes of zinc and their natural abundances are ⁶⁴Zn, 49%; ⁶⁶Zn, 29%; ⁶⁷Zn, 4%; ⁶⁸Zn, 19%; and ⁷⁰Zn, 1%.[3] Current methods of stable isotope analysis include thermal ionization mass spectrometry, fast atom bombardment mass spectrometry, and inductively coupled plasma mass spectrometry.[4] AAS is the technique most widely used to measure zinc in biological samples. AAS at 213.8 nm, the most commonly used wavelength of spectral absorption, provides sensitivity to <1.5 μmol/L (0.1 mg/L). ICP allows for comparable sensitivity and fewer matrix effects than does AAS combined with simultaneous analysis for many other elements of interest but does so with slightly less precision. Zinc has a high volatility temperature; consequently dry ashing methods to digest tissues and foods for subsequent zinc analysis by AAS or ICP are usually performed at 550 °C.[5] Wet ashing with nitric and other acids is also a widely used preparative method for these zinc assays.[5] Cell suspensions can be hydrolyzed in NaOH with detergent (e.g., sodium dodecyl sulfate) for zinc quantitation.[6] Reference standards for zinc analyses by AAS and ICP are available as solid materials and solutions from the National Institute of Standards and Technology.[7] Energy dispersive x-ray microanalysis of biological samples during electron microscopy provides information on the subcellular localization of zinc.[8] Fluorescent probes [e.g., Zinquin, ethyl (2-methyl-8-*p*-toluenesulphonamido-6-quinolyloxy) acetate] to measure free zinc concentrations within cells during altered physiologic conditions hold promise of defining important changes in cellular zinc created by dietary or physiologic changes.[9]

Absorption and Metabolism

The zinc content of the human body (1.5–2.5 g) approaches that of iron.[10,11] This level is maintained with absorption of about 5 mg/day. Zinc is absorbed from the small intestine, primarily the duodenum and jejunum but also the ileum.[12,13] Lumen perfusion studies in humans suggest that the jejunum exhibits the highest zinc absorption rate.[14] Absorption of zinc also occurs from rat colon.[15] However, when animal studies and those with humans are merged, there is no consensus as to the anatomical region that is quantitatively most important for zinc absorption. Under controlled conditions, apparent absorption of zinc is 33%.[16] Extent of digestion, transit time, and binding to specific factors (e.g., phytic acid), influence the quantitative significance of each intestinal region on the absorption process.

Homeostatic control of zinc metabolism involves a balance between absorption of dietary zinc and endogenous secretions through adaptive regulation programmed by the dietary zinc supply.[17] The intestine is the key organ in maintaining that balance. When isolated from systemic influences and pancreatic secretions, the intestine retains evidence of adaptation to absorption programmed by previous dietary intake.[18–20] This suggests that adaptation of absorption to dietary zinc intake is controlled in intestine. When true absorption is measured, which eliminates endogenous zinc as a factor in calculations, low zinc intake increases the efficiency of absorption. This suggests that up-regulation of zinc uptake upon dietary zinc restriction occurs in humans as in experimental animals.[21,22] Decreased secretion of endogenous zinc during zinc depletion in humans has been a consistent finding.[17,21–23] This is in the range of 20–70 μmol/day. The origin of endogenous zinc is not known but most likely is a mixture of secretions from pancreatic and intestinal cells.

Experimental approaches to elucidate the mechanism of zinc absorption have been directed at brush-border uptake, intracellular diffusion, basolateral transport, and plasma (corporeal) phases. Zinc absorption has been repeatedly shown to involve a mediated (saturable) component and a nonmediated (nonsaturable) component. These appear to be a function of the luminal zinc concentration.[13] Kinetic estimates of absorption are usually obtained through combined measurements of brush-border uptake and total transepithelial zinc movement; therefore the site responsible for generating saturable kinetics is not certain. In rats, the luminal zinc concentration after a meal is ≈80 μmol/L. Thus, intestinal uptake with a K_m of 30–100 μmol/L (average ≈75 μmol/L), as measured by many different approaches, is realistic.[19,24-29] Zinc absorption increases when a zinc-deficient diet is fed. Kinetic evidence from rats suggests this occurs through an increase in transfer rate

(from 60 to 180 nmol Zn·g tissue^{-1}·30 minutes^{-1}) rather than a change in K_m (affinity).[24,25] Carrier-mediated zinc absorption increases during the neonatal period in rats.[30] In humans, the rate of zinc absorption from perfused jejunum is proportional to the luminal zinc concentration over the range 0.1–1.8 mmol/L and is saturable >1.8 mmol/L.[14] The maximal absorption rate is 582 nmol·minutes^{-1}·40 cm^{-1}. A luminal zinc concentration after a meal is estimated at 100 μmol/L for humans.[31] This is similar to that calculated for rats and suggests that under normal dietary conditions zinc is absorbed by the mediated mechanism.

A major portion of zinc is absorbed by a carrier-mediated process that is most active at low luminal zinc concentrations.[19,20,26] However, zinc transport across the apical membrane of enterocytes is difficult to approach experimentally. Brush-border transport has a nonmediated (diffusion) component at high zinc concentrations.[25,28] However, the brush-border transport process does not appear to require energy. Alternatively, nonmediated (nonsaturable) intestinal zinc uptake may partly reflect paracellular transport rather than transcellular movement. Factors influencing observed transport rates include presence of complex-forming substances (e.g., histidine) and artifactual phenomena (e.g., membrane binding without actual transport).[32] Zinc uptake could be mediated by a zinc receptor (transporter), chelated zinc, endocytotic vesicle formation, or zinc channel in the membrane or through cotransport with an anion.[27] Experimental evidence is against anion cotransport, but active transport as a peptide zinc complex (Gly-Gly-His) using a peptide carrier system is possible.[29] Consequently, with these mechanistic options unresolved, the absorbable form of food zinc is unclear.

The intracellular phase of zinc absorption (transcellular movement) has been extensively studied. Zinc newly acquired from the intestinal lumen is bound to many different molecular species. Two have been identified: metallothionein (MT) and cysteine-rich intestinal protein (CRIP).[33,34] Although the association of zinc with CRIP is correlated to absorption, it is not likely to act in transcellular zinc movement. Tissue-specific expression, developmental increases just before weaning, and abundance in Paneth cells suggest a role for this double-zinc finger protein in proliferation-differentiation or host defense.[35] In contrast, MT gene expression in intestine is directly correlated to dietary zinc intake.[36] Zinc absorption declines as MT synthesis is elevated in response to dietary zinc.[20,37] Binding of newly acquired intestinal zinc to MT follows synthesis, and the regulation of absorption does not occur if synthesis is inhibited.[38] Zinc flux in the mucosal-to-serosal direction is inversely related to cellular MT whereas zinc transfer in the serosal-to-mucosal direction is directly related.[20] MT is envisioned as an expandable zinc pool within enterocytes that is able to impede zinc movement out of these cells by acting as a transient intracellular buffer of Zn^{2+} movement.[13] MT may also be secreted at the apical and serosal surfaces of enterocytes. With long-term feeding of zinc-rich diets to rats, intestinal MT may adapt to a low level of abundance.[39] As an alternative for transcellular zinc movement, a vesicular transfer mechanism has been proposed that is similar to one proposed for calcium. This model is based on decreased zinc transport by Caco 2 cells in culture when treated with quinacrine, a lysosome-disrupting agent.[40]

Extrusion of zinc from enterocytes appears as a linear function of the luminal zinc concentration.[28,41] If the enterocytes contain ≈ 20 µg/g and 1% is free zinc, the intracellular concentration is, at best, 3 µmol/L whereas that of the plasma is 15 µmol/L. This suggests that a pump is needed to counter the uphill zinc gradient. An ATPase may provide the energy to drive zinc efflux from enterocytes.[26,41] Basolateral membrane vesicles (BLMVs) show very appreciable zinc transport with saturable and nonsaturable kinetics evident.[41] The K_m and V_{max} of BLMV transport were not altered by dietary zinc intake. A zinc transporter similar to that in kidney cells may regulate zinc cellular efflux in enterocytes.[42] Zinc transport in the serosal-to-mucosal direction has been reported.[20,24,43,44] This may contribute to endogenous zinc secretion, fecal zinc loss, and homeostatic control.

The nonmediated (nonsaturable) component of zinc absorption is observed at higher luminal zinc concentrations.[18,24] Although this mode of luminal-to-vascular zinc transport could represent a linear phase of transcellular movement, it more likely represents primarily paracellular diffusion. Zinc at large luminal concentrations may be absorbed by this route (e.g., during consumption of supplements). Some zinc chelates may be absorbed by this route as well.

As components of the diet are degraded, zinc is presented to enterocytes as smaller zinc-binding ligands, primarily peptides, amino acids, and nucleotides, and perhaps to a limited extent as free zinc.[12,13] Solubility may be an important factor, determining zinc uptake by enterocytes in these situations.[45,46] Many factors have been reported to promote or antagonize zinc absorption.[47,48] Gastric acid secretion inhibition may lower zinc absorption in humans.[49] Histidine and cysteine, which have high zinc binding constants, inhibit zinc absorption in some systems and not others.[32,50] EDTA improves zinc utilization in some species during specific feeding situations.[10–13] In rats, Zn-EDTA and Zn-methionine complexes reduce uptake and absorption.[51] Although widely discussed, citric acid and picolinic acid do not appear to consistently stimulate zinc absorption.[47,48,52,53] Picolinic acid may promote urinary zinc excretion and lead to negative zinc balance.[53] Phytate has been shown to reduce zinc absorption by a variety of experimental techniques and in actual feeding situations, probably by reducing the solubility of zinc in forms needed for brush-border uptake.[10,12,46,48] Phytate was a contributing factor in human zinc deficiency reported in the Middle East in the 1960s.[54] It also accounts for the lower zinc absorption in soy-based infant formulas.[47] A folic acid-zinc interaction has been widely studied but appears not to have quantitative significance.[55,56]

Some minerals in the diet may alter zinc absorption. Inorganic iron in pharmacological doses may decrease zinc uptake.[12,47] Other studies suggest heme iron has the same effect, but the capacity to absorb iron does not influence zinc uptake.[57] Zinc may bind to an integrin isoform as has been postulated as a component of the Fe^{2+} uptake mechanism. Copper appears to have little direct effect on zinc absorption.[12,48] Evidence suggests that calcium and zinc are transported by distinctly different mechanisms.[27] This may explain why calcium appears to have little effect on zinc absorption in rats and why neither vitamin D nor 1,25-dihydroxychole-calciferol affects zinc absorption[58,59] except in tissue culture.[40] Calcium supplements, however, may lower zinc absorption through an effect within the intestinal lumen that increases zinc loss.[60] High levels of calcium cause parakeratosis in pigs, a skin disorder produced through concomitant zinc restriction.[10,12] A variety of physiological factors including fasting; pregnancy; and disease processes, including infection, surgery, pancreatic insufficiency, and alcoholism may sometimes alter zinc absorption.[10,12,44,48]

Albumin appears to be the major portal carrier for newly absorbed zinc.[18,61] Changes in the systemic level of albumin may alter zinc absorption.[61] Absorption of zinc also occurs via the skin, but its quantitative significance in zinc acquisition is unknown.[62] Placental zinc transport appears to reflect maternal zinc status and physiological conditions, including alcohol intake.[63]

Plasma zinc comprises only 0.1% of the body zinc.[10,12] Although its concentration is normally maintained within strict limits, it comprises a compartment that can fluctuate markedly in response to specific physiological stimuli and dietary intake.[48,63] Normally in animals and humans, plasma zinc concentrations are maintained at ≈ 1 µg/mL.[48,63] Up to 12 plasma proteins bind zinc in vitro, but albumin and α_2-macroglobulin contain most of the plasma zinc (70% and 20–40%, respectively).[64] There is a large molar excess of albumin compared with zinc. Albumin and zinc have an association constant of 10^6 mol/L. It is believed that this relatively low binding affinity for zinc, commonly referred to as loosely bound zinc, is important for the mechanism of plasma zinc exchange with cells.[48,63] Other plasma proteins binding some zinc are transferrin, histidine-rich glycoprotein, and perhaps metallothionein. Endocytotic intake of transferrin may contribute to zinc uptake by some cell types.[63] Less than 1% of the plasma zinc is bound to low-molecular-weight complexes (primarily with cysteine and histidine). These complexes may have roles in zinc uptake by cells.[48,63] Free Zn^{2+} in plasma is estimated to be 2×10^{-10} mol/L (0.01% of plasma zinc).[65] More than 80% of blood zinc is found in cells, mostly in erythrocytes; carbonic anhydrases account for most of the zinc (>85%), with ≈5% accounted for by Cu/Zn superoxide dismutase.[63] Reticulocytes contain metallothionein in amounts that reflect zinc intake.[66-68] In human blood, erythrocytes contain ≈1 mg zinc/10^6 cells whereas mononuclear and polynuclear cells contain ≤6 mg zinc/10^6 cells.[69]

The plasma zinc level responds markedly to external stimuli, including fluctuations in zinc intake, fasting, and various acute stresses, such as infection.[48,63,70-72] A reproducible reduction in the level (15%) occurs postprandially, perhaps related to meal-induced changes in insulin and glucose.[73] Most reductions in plasma zinc levels are believed to reflect increased hepatic zinc uptake, perhaps resulting from hormonal control. The increase in plasma zinc on fasting results from hormonally regulated catabolic changes wherein a portion of the large reserve of zinc in muscle (57% of body zinc) is mobilized.[71] This response to fasting is observed in zinc-depleted rats also.[70] In experimental zinc depletion, plasma zinc levels are reduced with severe restriction but not with moderate restriction.[56,63,74] Hypozincemia associated with infection could be a host defense mechanism where zinc clearance from plasma would decrease zinc availability. Perhaps related to homeostatic control of plasma zinc levels is the in vitro evidence that has shown that superantigens can bind zinc, influencing their biological activity.[75]

Kinetic modeling experiments with human subjects and animals have provided valuable data on how zinc metabolic compartments are used. Through the use of ^{65}Zn as a tracer, two phases of turnover (rapid ≅12.5 days and slow ≅300 days) were detected in humans.[76,77] Very reactive tissues are liver, followed by pancreas, kidney, and spleen; slow turnover is found in central nervous system and bone. A similar model was developed in rats, and high metabolic activity of zinc in bone marrow was documented.[78] These kinetic models respond to metabolic changes regulated by hormones.[78,79] Specifically, glucocorticoid hormone produces a decrease in plasma zinc and concomitant increase in hepatic uptake.[79] Kinetic data suggest an exchangeable zinc pool whose size depends on zinc intake.[80] Size of this pool was estimated at 2.4–2.8 mmol (157–183 mg) Zn and decreased by 26–32% in severe zinc restriction for 1 week. Individual cell types may have very high rates of zinc turnover; for example, turnover was estimated to be 30 hours in rat hepatocytes.[81] There appears to be little zinc available as a stored reserve. Consequently, when adaptation to intake fails, deficiency occurs rapidly.[82]

Considerable evidence from tracer studies and isolated cells suggests that the zinc-binding-protein MT is a factor in regulating zinc metabolism. Included in this concept is that MT is inducible by dietary zinc via the metal response element (MRE) and MTF-1 mechanism of transcriptional regulation (described later).[36,83] Dietary regulation of MT expression appears to constitute an autoregulation system wherein increased MT synthesis is linked to increased zinc binding within cells. MT may act as a Zn^{2+} buffer, controlling the free Zn^{2+} level or helping to coordinate an intracellular pool that is responsive to both hormones and diet. Probes capable of fluorescence upon forming complexes with Zn^{2+} within cells may reveal the nature of the labile intracellular zinc pool.[9] One such fluoroprobe (Zinquin) has shown that free intracellular zinc concentrations in hepatocytes are stimulated by glucocorticoids and interleukin 6 and are related to MT.[9] The MT promoter contains response elements required for regulation by a variety of hormones and cytokines.[84] Reduction in plasma zinc has been shown by kinetic modeling to coincide with MT synthesis and zinc binding by the MT kinetic compartment.[78] Transgenic mice have been developed where the MT gene has been inactivated (knock out; null mutation) by homologous recombination techniques.[85] These animals develop normally but are sensitive to cadmium toxicity. This suggests that MT is not necessary for development but may be important for homeostatic responses to stresses, processing of a fluctuating dietary zinc supply, or both. Zinc transporters that regulate influx or efflux may allow cells to adapt further to differences in zinc intake independent of MT. Concentration of excess zinc within intracellular vesicles is possible and has been predicted on the basis of zinc chemistry.[1,2]

Cytokines, primarily interleukins 1 and 6, influence zinc metabolism. It is believed that a stress, such as acute infection where endotoxins are produced, leads to secretion of cytokines that have multiple effects, including activation of immune cells. Tracer studies show that interleukin 1 increases ^{65}Zn uptake into liver, bone marrow, and thymus, with less going to bone, skin, and intestine. This differential zinc turnover is believed to be a defensive host response.[86] Interleukin 6, a major regulator of the acute-phase response, directly increases zinc uptake by hepatocytes.[87] These changes occur concurrently with changes in MT expression and cellular defense. Maternally administered, interleukin 1 produces zinc-related changes in fetal MT expression, which may have implications for fetal development.[68]

Homeostatic control of zinc metabolism is maintained primarily by fecal excretion of endogenous zinc.[88] At zinc intakes of 7, 15, and 30 mg/day, human subjects have fecal zinc losses of 6.8, 14.4, and 30.1 mg/day, respectively.[17] Reduction in fecal zinc as a function of duration of depletion is observed within days.[88] Severe zinc restriction (0.3 mg zinc/day) in humans reduces fecal zinc loss from >10 mg/day to <1 mg/day.[16] Endogenous losses are a mix of pancreatic and intestinal secretions. Meals stimulate endogenous zinc secretion, and over half of zinc in the intestinal lumen can be so derived.[89] Renal zinc loss is low and not significantly influenced by zinc intake.[17] Urinary zinc responds to changes in muscle catabolism.[90] Glucagon may regulate zinc reabsorption by the distal renal tubule.[91]

Physiological (Biochemical) Function

The biochemical functions of zinc that determine physiological effects have received extensive study. However, the signs of altered zinc status are diverse and have not been assigned to a defect in a specific function.[10,11] The ubiquitous distribution of zinc among cells, coupled with zinc being the most abundant intracellular trace element, points to very basic functions.[1,2] Three different functions—catalytic, structural, and regulatory—define the role of zinc in biology.

Catalytic roles are found in enzymes from all six classes of enzymes.[92] Examples are the RNA nucleotide transferases (RNA polymerases I, II, and III), alkaline phosphatase, and the carbonic anhydrases. Although well over 200 zinc metalloenzymes have been characterized, when the same enzyme from different sources (plant, microbial, and animal) is counted only once, >50 enzymes are found to contain zinc. An enzyme is generally considered a zinc metalloenzyme if removal of zinc causes reduction in activity without affecting the enzyme protein irreversibly and reconstitution with zinc restores activity. How zinc is donated to apometalloenzyme proteins is not known but may involve post-translational modification (metal donation), perhaps coordinated by the endoplasmic reticulum or vesicular zinc compartments.

The literature is filled with examples of zinc metalloenzymes that are influenced by the dietary zinc supply.[10] However, unequivocal evidence of a direct link between zinc deficiency and toxicity signs and individual enzymes has not appeared in complex organisms. It is generally believed that a physiological defect would occur only if the zinc-requiring enzyme was acting at a rate-limiting step in a critical biochemical pathway or process. The relationship of zinc nutrition to alcoholic liver disease focused on the zinc metalloenzyme alcohol dehydrogenase (EC 1.1.1.1), which is a historical example of a potential zinc metalloenzyme–disease relationship.[10] The growth response seen in zinc-supplemented children is a more recent example relating to protein synthesis, perhaps through augmented RNA polymerase activity.[93] The most definitive demonstration of a relationship between zinc status and RNA synthesis was with the eukaryotic single cell organism *Euglena*.[94]

The structural function of zinc is a rapidly expanding area of biological investigation. Structural roles for zinc in metalloenzymes exist. The cytosolic enzyme CuZn superoxide dismutase (Cu/Zn SOD) is an example; copper functions at the catalytic site whereas zinc has a role in structure.[10] The zinc finger motif in proteins represents an extremely important structural role. Zinc fingers tend to have the following general structure: -C-X_2-C-X_n-C-X_2-C-, where C designates cysteine and X designates other amino acids. This structural arrangement allows zinc to be bound as a tetrahedral complex with four cysteines. Zinc fingers with some histidines replacing cysteines are also very abundant. Zinc-finger proteins were first identified in 1985 in frog (*Xenopus*) oocyte transcription factor TFIIIA; estimates are that up to 1% of the human genome (300–700 human genes) codes for these proteins.[95] Classic examples of zinc-finger transcription factors are the retinoic acid and calcitriol (1,25-dihydroxycholecalciferol) receptors.[95] Originally considered to be DNA-binding domains of transcription factors in the cell nucleus, zinc-finger proteins were later shown to have a broader cellular distribution and biochemical role. Some zinc-finger proteins are involved in functions requiring protein-protein interactions, most of which appear to affect cellular differentiation or proliferation, but zinc-finger motifs are also found among signal transduction factors and may play a role in cell adhesion.[95,96] Evidence suggests that zinc is redistributed within cellular sites during signal transduction.[97] The zinc-finger regions of protein kinases may be necessary for that intracellular translocation.[95] The ever-expanding list of recognized cell-surface receptors includes many with zinc-finger (zinc-binding) domains.[95] Interest in zinc-finger motifs is intense because they are potential targets for therapeutic intervention with drugs.[98] Zinc may influence turnover of labile mRNA in cells through a structural role.[99]

The influence of zinc nutrition on zinc-finger-containing cellular components needs to be defined. However, three points are clear: 1) considering their abundance, zinc fingers contribute to the overall zinc requirement; 2) they provide a rationale for the tight homeostatic control of zinc metabolism; and 3) they may explain previous suggestions that zinc has roles in membrane receptor action, cellular proliferation and development, and other very basic but critical biochemical roles. Dietary zinc may interact directly with zinc in some zinc-finger and related motifs found in proteins. Removal of zinc from zinc-finger proteins may cause a loss of function, as was demonstrated in vitro for the transcription factor SP1 with the use of apometallothionein.[100]

A third generalized biochemical role for zinc is as a stimulator of transacting factors responsible for regulating gene expression. The only well-studied example of this role is in the expression of MT or MT-like proteins.[101]

The basic components are a metal-binding transcription factor (MTF) and an MRE in the promoter of the regulated gene. The MTF acquires zinc in the cell cytosol or nucleus and then is able to interact with the MRE to stimulate transcription. Dietary zinc is taken up by cell nuclei in proportion to the zinc intake level, suggesting a close relation between nuclear zinc and the dietary zinc supply.[36] Zinc fingers of the MTF may allow it to respond directly to zinc for MRE binding, or a separate metal-binding inhibitor may bind zinc, which then liberates the MTF for MRE binding.[83]

The distribution of MRE regulation mechanisms within the genome has not been established. Zinc transporters may be MRE-MTF-regulated systems and may control intracellular zinc levels by this mechanism.[42] Two genes expressed in liver and associated with the acute phase response—C-reactive protein and α_1-acid glycoprotein—appear to be regulated by metals via MREs.[102] For individual genes, MTF regulation could be positive or negative as a function of zinc occupancy. The use of dietary zinc as a common regulator of gene expression via MREs may occur so that under conditions of a diminished dietary zinc supply some zinc-requiring processes are limited as a nutrient energy conservation or defensive mechanism.

It is difficult to reconcile these biochemical functions with established physiological effects of zinc function. These include effects in lipid peroxidation, apoptosis, proliferation and differentiation, and immunity. Consequently, the literature is filled with anecdotal descriptions of putative zinc-responsive physiological effects. The biochemical basis for these is even more clouded. Two of these are discussed below.

Beneficial effects of zinc in protection against various noxious agents (including organic compounds), χ and γ radiation, and infectious agents (endotoxins, etc.) have been well documented. There is no common mechanism of action specifically related to zinc. For example, zinc's role in prevention of lipid peroxidation could be via Cu/Zn SOD activity, MT, inhibition of the cytochrome P450 system, or through an as yet unrecognized biological function.[10,11,103–105] MT has been shown to scavenge hydroxyl (OH•) radicals in vitro and hence may act as an inducible antioxidant.[83,87,104,106,107] The OH• radical is among the most reactive of the reactive oxygen intermediates associated with oxidative stress. The up-regulation of MT synthesis by mediators of host defense (e.g., interleukins 1 and 6) during the acute response or during postischemic stress associated with surgery, when large amounts of OH• radicals are produced, supports the in vitro findings.[86,87,107] However, data conflict as to the beneficial effects of zinc and how they are mediated.[6,103,108] Frequently, zinc is referred to as cytoprotective, a designation that seems appropriate on the balance of available data.

Zinc may act as a regulator of apoptotic cell death.[109,110] The biochemical role has not been defined. At high zinc levels (>500 μmol/L), in vitro evidence suggests that zinc inhibits apoptosis induced by glucocorticoids.[111] Zinc may act by endonuclease inactivation, poly(ADP-ribose) synthetase inhibition, or stimulation of protein kinase C activity. A chelatable pool of zinc in cells may interact directly with protein kinase C via its zinc-finger-like domain and influence translocation and hence signal transduction.[97] Flow cytometry data have shown that zinc at lower (<200 μmol/L) concentrations may induce apoptosis by a process that requires protein synthesis.[112] The applicability of these in vitro studies to the intact animal remains to be defined. Similarly, the exact mechanism of zinc-related effects or the specificity of this apoptotic process compared with that found in malnutrition has not been defined.

Deficiency

Zinc-deficiency signs are the result of diminution of one or more of the biological functions of zinc. This nutritional deficiency is a type II deficiency, where the first response is a reduction in growth without an apparent reduction in tissue concentrations.[82] A reduction in food intake appears to be a most sensitive response to a reduction in the dietary zinc supply.[113] The anorexia and cyclic food intake of animals (chicks and rats) fed zinc-deficient diets are well documented.[113,114] Poor appetite also tends to be a clinical feature of zinc deficiency in children.[10,54,82] The mechanism of this zinc-related anorexia is complex. Possible mechanisms include release of opiates, cholecystokinin, or neuropeptide Y with sites of action in the brain (possibly hypothalamic) or intestine.[113,115,116] Curiously, force feeding a zinc-deficient diet by stomach tube to rats is fatal.[117] The function of this reduction in intake may be for the purpose of adaptation since, by limiting growth, tissue zinc levels are conserved for critical functions. Cell culture studies suggest that it is difficult to markedly deplete cells of essential zinc unless zinc chelators are added to the medium.[118,119] As a consequence of this avid zinc retention by cells, diagnosis of zinc deficiency through measures of tissue levels is not possible.[82,120]

The reduction in growth with reduced zinc in the diet is coincident with a reduction in endogenous losses.[10,88,120] As tissues conserve zinc, it has been suggested that only a small cellular pool of zinc is exchangeable.[80,82,120] Data obtained with stable zinc isotopes as tracers support the concept of a labile exchangeable zinc pool.[80] Signs of deficiency may occur when that pool is depleted. In rats the plasma zinc concentration drops rapidly when zinc is removed from the diet.[63] This also correlates to a reduction in MT-bound zinc.[38] Cellular zinc is primarily tightly bound to constituents with markedly different rates of turnover. However, a labile pool may function to help control intracellular processes and thus contribute to zinc homeostasis. Clinical manifestations of zinc deficiency result when altered zinc metabolism is such that homeostatic controls cannot supply the various body pools necessary for maintaining biochemical functions.[88,120] Ordinarily, fluctuations in the dietary zinc supply may be met by using the reserves from muscle, where >50% of the body zinc in humans is located. Fasting increases plasma zinc in humans and rats and may reflect this redistribution.[63,71] Increased hepatic MT synthesis during fasting may represent a hormonally regulated conservation mechanism for zinc.[70] In addition, hepatic fatty acid composition and lipid accumulation are observed in zinc-deficient rats.[121]

Overt signs of zinc deficiency have been well documented in animals and humans. In animals they include retarded growth, depressed immune function, skin lesions, depressed appetite, skeletal abnormalities, and impaired reproductive ability.[10,11] Classical studies documented diet-related zinc deficiency in humans where growth reduction (to the point of dwarfism) and sexual immaturity were among the findings;[54] in swine, severe skin lesions (called parakeratosis) were observed.[10] Nevertheless, human zinc deficiency has been a challenge to clearly define.

Congenital zinc deficiency caused by zinc malabsorption was documented as acrodermatitis enteropathica in humans and adema disease in dairy cattle.[122,123] These conditions result in skin lesions and impaired immunity (exhibited as susceptibility to infection) and both are reversible by zinc supplementation. Acrodermatitis enteropathica is associated with *Candida albicans* infections, and adema disease produces thymic atrophy.[10] These inherited disorders demonstrate a link between zinc deficiency and immune function in animals and humans. Originally, the lack of a factor required for absorption was believed to be the defect responsible for these genetic disorders.[12]

The exact biochemical basis for compromised immunity in zinc-deficient subjects has not been established.[124] Reduced zinc intake clearly results in thymic atrophy in pigs and cattle and reduced T-helper cell function in mice.[125] Total parenteral nutrition (TPN) without adequate zinc leads to decreased natural killer cell activity.[126] Recent intervention experiments have suggested that zinc may improve such immune indicators as T-lymphocyte responsiveness in malnourished children.[127] Zinc supplementation in vitro increases antibody production in aged cells.[128] Similarly, zinc increases peripheral blood mononuclear cell synthesis of interferon γ, interleukins 1 and 6, tumor necrosis factor α and interleukin 2 receptor, and proliferation of concanavalin A–stimulated cells.[129,130] Zinc within physiologic concentrations may control the secretion and production of these immune regulators and

could be important in situations requiring monocyte activation.[129] The molecular mechanisms responsible could relate to any of the three basic functions of zinc. Zinc may be needed for structure and activity of thymulin, a nine-amino-acid peptide found in plasma that stimulates T-cell development.[131] Perhaps a related event is that interleukin 1 stimulates MT-associated zinc uptake by thymocytes in vitro before thymulin release.[132] Chelation of zinc in adult thymocyte cultures leads to DNA fragmentation and cell death.[110] In contrast, apoptosis was not induced by zinc chelation in immature thymocytes. It was speculated that intracellular zinc may alter the cell selection process through apoptosis. High zinc concentrations may inhibit apoptosis via modulating protein kinase C activity.[97,110] Flow cytometry data have clearly shown that early B cells in bone marrow are depleted in nutritional zinc deficiency.[133] This could occur through increased apoptosis signaled by zinc deficiency. Other mechanisms could explain altered immune cell growth found in zinc deficiency.

Other features of cell proliferation and differentiation relate to zinc nutrition and deficiency. Bone zinc deposition reflects dietary zinc intake, which may change during bone remodeling produced by changes in osteoblastic and osteoclastic activity as regulated by growth factors, cytokines, and hormones.[10,11] Furthermore, bone zinc appears to provide a mobilizable source or pool of zinc that reflects dietary zinc intake.[134] This is supported with metabolic studies where interleukin 1 depressed [65]Zn incorporation into calcified bone as zinc was diverted to marrow and liver.[86] The high proliferative rate of progenitor and stem cells of the bone marrow and the active, cytokine-responsive zinc metabolism of bone marrow cells suggest that this is a target of zinc deficiency.[86,133] In addition, zinc deficiency in early development influences teratogenic changes in fetuses.[135]

Seizures may occur in children with acute zinc deficiency, and behavioral abnormalities are found in individuals with the acrodermatitis enteropathica genotype.[136] Their etiology is not clear, but specific regions of the brain associated with neuronal activity and memory (e.g., hippocampus) are very rich in zinc.[137] Specifically, zinc is actively taken up by and stored in synaptic vesicles, is released from nerve terminals, and may act in synaptic transmission. Nevertheless, the consequences of zinc deprivation on behavior in humans remain an unexplained area.[11]

Apart from the marked growth reduction and immune dysfunction defining human zinc deficiency, other clinical manifestations of zinc deficiency may be subtle and less pronounced. The clinical literature is abundant with descriptions of a more subjective nature that describe dysfunctions that may have zinc-dependent components or be in some way related to zinc.[136] Reduced plasma zinc concentrations are common in inflammatory bowel disease, which may indicate reduced zinc absorption or increased zinc losses, and may respond to zinc therapy.[15,138] An interaction between zinc and folic acid has been the subject of much study. The intestinal folate conjugase is a zinc metalloenzyme. Although folate metabolism is altered in zinc-deficient rats, no changes are noted in humans with low zinc intake.[55] Folate does not appear to influence zinc status in humans fed normal- or low-zinc diets.[56]

Our current understanding of human zinc deficiency, much of which may be marginal deficiency, is based on responses to zinc supplementation. The attempt to augment immunocompetence in elderly subjects without signs of zinc deficiency is an example.[139] The effect of supplemental zinc was negative. It is reasoned that supplemental zinc may be beneficial only "in subjects with preexisting dietary or laboratory evidence of zinc deficiency."[140] Alcoholism, perhaps accompanied by pancreatic or liver disease, may result in marginal zinc deficiency because of reduced absorption or retention.[136] A similar scenario could be developed to rationalize zinc-responsive disorders affecting other cell types and tissues. For example, in age-related macular degeneration, a photic injury to the zinc-rich retinal pigment epithelium in the macular region may lead to oxidative damage and cause degeneration. Zinc supplementation, under some dietary conditions, may reverse or protect against the injury caused by light.[141] Zinc-related taste and smell dysfunction and skin disorders have been reported.[10,11,136,142] If truly zinc responsive, these may be explained on the same basis of a response to preexisting marginal zinc deficiency.[10] Recent evidence supports a zinc effect on growth and cognitive improvement in malnourished children in developing countries.[93] In growth retardation associated with the failure-to-thrive syndrome, zinc supplements are not uniformly effective.[143] An acrodermatitis enteropathica–like condition in humans may be caused by low zinc levels in breast milk.[144] This may be similar to the congenital condition in mice (lethal milk) where inadequate amounts of zinc are transferred to the maternal milk supply, causing terminal zinc deficiency in nursing pups.[145]

Requirement and Status Assessment

Recent surveys indicate that American males consume 90% and females consume 81% of the recommended dietary allowance (RDA) for zinc.[146,147] Other estimates of intake range from 47% to 67% of the RDA.[12] It is estimated that 70% of zinc consumed by the U.S. population is from animal products.[148] The World Health Organization estimates lactating women need to absorb 5.5 mg Zn/day. Consequently, fractional absorption of zinc from the daily diet is a very important factor in meeting this need.[12]

Physiological factors undoubtedly influence the zinc requirement to some extent. RDAs are determined on the basis of age, sex, pregnancy, and lactation.[88,147] The RDA for zinc is 5 mg/day for infants, 10 mg/day for children under 10 years, 15 mg/day for males over 10 years, 12 mg/day for females over 10 years, 15 mg/day during pregnancy, and 19 and 16 mg/day for lactation during the first and second 6 months, respectively. A fractional absorption of 20% is assumed. There is close agreement on zinc requirements among species.[10] Where data are available, age, growth, pregnancy, and lactation are determinants of the zinc requirements in animals. The term "true (physiological) zinc requirement" refers to the amount of zinc needed to replace all endogenous losses and supply zinc needed for fetal growth, lactation, and increased body mass.[88] RDAs have been estimated by a variety of methods: balance studies, measures of total endogenous zinc losses, and radioactive and stable isotope studies of zinc turnover. Guidelines for zinc intake during TPN are available.[149,150] Zinc as zinc sulfate is preferred for infusion solutions, which usually contain <10 mg Zn/L; for TPN, zinc requirements are 2.5–4 mg/day for adults and 100-300 μg/kg body weight for children.

Assessment of zinc status in humans has proven to be difficult. The development of AAS and its applicability to aqueous solutions has made the measurement of plasma zinc concentrations a standard and routine practice. Normally, plasma zinc is maintained at 12–18 μmol/L (0.8–1.2 μg/mL). As indicated above, physiological changes can influence this concentration. Nevertheless, dietary zinc restriction has been shown to reduce plasma zinc levels by ≤50% under experimental conditions.[63] In extensive experiments with human subjects under controlled and field conditions, plasma zinc has been shown to be a poor index of zinc status.[10,63,120] It is reasoned that plasma zinc is reduced in humans only when the exchangeable zinc pool has been depleted.[80] Leukocyte zinc, erythrocyte zinc, hair zinc, and saliva zinc are among variables also suggested as assessment measures, but they are not viewed as good indices of status.[63] A zinc tolerance test was proposed as a method to detect low zinc status.[151] The basis of this assessment method is the observed increase in plasma zinc concentration within hours after consumption of an oral dose of zinc (25–50 mg). A lower response curve is presumed to indicate better zinc status (low absorption). Although widely used in zinc absorption and clinical studies, the method is not recognized as a method of choice for status assessment.[12,63]

An alternative approach to assessment is to use a functional outcome (i.e., metalloenzyme activity or zinc-induced processes). Plasma alkaline phosphatase (EC 3.1.3.1) has been the most commonly used enzyme for zinc status assessment, particularly in survey conditions.[10,11] The enzyme may be of value in monitoring zinc status during TPN.[152] The angiotensin-converting enzyme (EC 3.4.15.1) has shown some value as an index.[153] Overall zinc metalloenzymes have not proven to be indicative of dietary zinc status.[10,11] Synthesis of MT, which is zinc dependent, reflects zinc intake in both rats and humans. (The mechanistic basis was presented in a previous section.) In rats, zinc deficiency markedly reduced plasma and erythrocyte MT levels measured by radioimmunoassay.[66,154] In human subjects, zinc depletion or supplementation produced the response of erythrocyte MT expected of zinc-dependent events programmed during reticulocyte development in the bone marrow.[67,68] Erythrocyte MT is actually in reticulocytes, because MT in erythroid cells decreases early in the erythrocyte's life span in peripheral blood.[66–68] Erythrocyte MT may be a useful index for differentiating between low and adequate zinc intake and could be used to monitor zinc supplementation programs.[67,155] Plasma MT has potential as an index of zinc status in humans. However, in rats plasma MT is sensitive to physiological stimuli.[156] Assessment using both plasma zinc and plasma MT may be a method for differentiating between the exchangeable zinc pool size and tissue zinc redistribution.[120] Monocyte MT mRNA may provide an alternative method of assessment using reverse-transcription polymerase chain reaction technology.

Food and Other Sources

Foods vary greatly in their inherent zinc content, with red meat and shellfish constituting the best sources of zinc. Foods of vegetable origin tend to be low in zinc except for the embryo portion of grains, such as wheat germ. The presence of phytic acid in plant products is a major factor that limits zinc bioavailability from these sources (as discussed earlier).[12] It has been argued, on this basis, that vegetarians are more likely to have a compromised zinc supply. The zinc–phytic acid complex is insoluble and poorly absorbed from the gastrointestinal tract. Certain food preparation practices, such as leavening of bread through the action of yeast, allows the phytase activity to substantially lower the phytate content of breads and similar products.[12] Phytate in unleavened bread was believed to be a contributing factor to the development of human zinc deficiency, as first described in the Middle East.[54]

Total zinc content of the diet provides only a gross estimate of zinc intake. Bioavailable zinc is the portion that is absorbed and used.[12] Most zinc in foods is bound to proteins and nucleic acids, usually in stable complexes that require substantial digestive activity to render zinc readily available.[12,13] Numerous other components in foods provide ligands for zinc binding; some improve zinc absorption whereas others do not.[47] Because the mechanism of zinc absorption is not known, their mode of action is not clear. Some zinc complexes, when consumed in large amounts, may be absorbed by the paracellular route, which bypasses transcellular absorptive mechanisms. Inhibitory factors in zinc absorption are found in soy protein (high phytate content), wheat and corn flour, coffee, tea, various beans, cheeses, and cow's milk. Inhibitory components include phytate, oxalate, fiber, EDTA, and polyphenols (tannins).[12,47] Calcium supplements may increase fecal zinc loss and thereby influence zinc absorption.[60] Roles of enhancers of zinc absorption have not been well studied.

Methods to assess zinc bioavailability include metabolic studies with foods intrinsically or extrinsically labeled with stable or radioactive isotopes, intestinal lavage, balance studies, zinc tolerance tests, growth measurements, and slope ratio assay.[12] In some cases, the method of expression (e.g., true absorption versus apparent absorption) can produce differing results. As an example, using true absorption as a measure, the absorption of zinc from beef was 55% and from high-fiber cereal it was 15%. Under the same conditions, calculated apparent absorption was 15% and −25%, respectively.[157] Accounting for endogenous zinc losses appears to provide a more realistic estimate of bioavailability.

Zinc bioavailability is greater from human milk than cow's milk or soy protein. There was speculation that a low-molecular-weight component in human milk was responsible. Numerous experiments have failed to definitively support a role for either picolinic acid or citric acid as the factor responsible.[52,53] Proteins in human milk, which bind most of the zinc, are believed to be more easily digestible than casein, the major protein in cow's milk.[12] This may explain the higher zinc bioavailability from human milk.

Zinc supplements, either zinc alone or combined mineral or vitamin-mineral preparations, are widely used. Reasons for using zinc supplements include concern that dietary intake may not provide sufficient zinc (as in a vegetarian diet) or belief that zinc has health-promoting properties.

Excess and Toxicity

The dietary aspects of zinc toxicity have been well reviewed.[158,159] Acute zinc toxicity results in gastric distress, dizziness, and nausea. This can be a complicating factor in zinc supplementation studies, with an emetic effect occurring at >150 mg zinc/day. Death has occurred with large TPN doses of zinc.[160] Gastric problems are observed in chronic toxicity.[158] Among other chronic effects are reductions in immune function (decrease in lymphocyte stimulation to phytohemagglutinin) and high-density lipoprotein (HDL) cholesterol reported with very high supplements (300 mg zinc/day). A depression in

PRESENT KNOWLEDGE IN NUTRITION, 7th Edition

lymphocyte stimulation was not observed at 100 mg zinc/day. In contrast, supplementation at 150 mg zinc/day in females decreased low-density lipoprotein and lowered serum ceruloplasmin ferroxidase activity. No significant changes in HDL were found. In elderly subjects, 100 mg zinc/day did not improve immunocompetence and did not alter total serum cholesterol or HDL cholesterol.[139] High dietary zinc intake in chickens produces a pause in egg production and molting via precipitous decreases in food intake.[161] Feeding zinc to chickens at 100 mg/kg diet produced pancreatic acinar cell exocrine dysfunction.[162] The mechanism is unknown.

Hypocupremia observed when sickle cell anemia patients were treated with 150 mg zinc/day resulted from a zinc-induced copper deficiency.[163] Subsequently, this occurrence was used as a way to decrease copper absorption in Wilson's disease, a copper accumulation disorder. Presumably, zinc-induced intestinal MT binds copper preferentially and leads to copper loss via desquamation of enterocytes.[164] Sideroblastic anemia, with marked cellular changes in marrow aspirates, was observed secondary to copper deficiency induced by high zinc intakes.[165]

A number of emerging issues relate to zinc toxicity via supplementation. The first is that MT can be induced by zinc in bone marrow cells.[68] This response may be part of a protective effect for stem cells. Animal studies suggest that the hematotoxic effects of some chemotherapeutic agents can be circumvented to allow larger doses of drug to be used for treatment by feeding high-zinc diets to induce bone marrow MT.[166] The presence of increased MT expression in cells clearly is cytoprotective against certain chemotherapeutic drugs.[167]

Zinc is found in abundance in the central nervous system, where brain alone accounts for 1.5% of total body zinc.[10] Turnover of brain zinc is slow, and areas of high zinc content occur, such as hippocampus. Homeostatic controls allow these sites to avidly conserve zinc in zinc deficiency.[137,168] Synaptic vesicles of nerve terminals actively take up zinc. Stimulation of nerve fibers, particularly in the hippocampus, causes release of zinc.[137] MT III isoform and cysteine-rich intestinal protein are found in this area and must reflect a zinc-related function.[169,170] High concentrations of zinc at the end of axons (synaptic boutons) have been suggested as a factor contributing to Alzheimer's disease.[171] Specifically, when added to isolated Aβ amyloid protein, zinc caused protein aggregation similar to the amyloid plaque formation found in Alzheimer's patients. The role of Aβ as a primary factor in this disorder is a matter of debate. These findings have important implications for zinc supplementation in elderly people.

On balance, zinc should be considered a relatively nontoxic micronutrient in moderate supplementation levels. The concern is that nutrient imbalances and interactions caused by selective supplementation may produce toxicity not encountered with usual dietary practices.

Summary

Zinc nutrition is a very active area of research. State-of-the-art methods are being applied toward the goal of improving our understanding of absorption mechanisms, cellular transport, and metabolism and toward development of biomarkers for status assessment. The role for zinc in gene regulation has been expanded with identification of zinc-finger domains in proteins. The wide distribution of zinc-finger domains suggests their involvement in many critical cellular functions, particularly for protein-protein interactions that influence proliferation and differentiation. The zinc adequacy of diets composed of highly processed foods continues to be an issue with regard to both humans and animals. Successful zinc intervention therapy in developing countries suggests that zinc deficiency is still of medical interest. Newer biochemical evidence suggests that oversupplementation with zinc could have deleterious consequences.

References

1. da Silva JJR, Williams RJP, eds (1991) The biological chemistry of the elements: the inorganic chemistry of life. Clarendon Press, Oxford
2. Williams RJP (1984) Zinc: what is its role in biology? Endeavour 8:65–70
3. Budavara S, ed (1989) The Merck index, 11th ed. Merck & Co, Inc, Rahway, NJ, pp 1597–1601
4. Turnlund JR (1989) The use of stable isotopes in mineral nutrition research. J Nutr 199:7–14
5. Hendricks DG (1994) Mineral analysis by traditional methods. In Neilsen SS (ed), Introduction to the chemical analysis of foods. Jones and Bartlett Publishers, Boston, MA, pp 123–135
6. Coppen DE, Richardson DE, Cousins RJ (1988) Zinc suppression of free radicals induced in cultures of rat hepatocytes by iron, t-butyl hydroperoxide and 3-methylindole. Proc Soc Exp Biol Med 189:100–109
7. Trahey NM, ed (1992) Standard reference materials catalog 1992–93. National Institute of Standards and Technology, special publication 260. US Government Printing Office, Washington DC
8. Farkas I, Szerdahelyi P, Kása P (1988) An indirect method for quantitation of cellular zinc content of Timm-stained cerebellar samples by energy dispersive X-ray microanalysis. Histochemistry 89:493–497
9. Coyle P, Zalewski PD, Philcox JC, et al (1994) Measurement of zinc in hepatocytes by using a fluorescent probe, Zinquin: relationship to metallothionein and intracellular zinc. Biochem J 303:781–786
10. Hambidge KM, Casey CE, Krebs NF (1986) Zinc. In Mertz W (ed), Trace elements in human and animal nutrition II. Academic Press, Orlando, FL, pp 1–37
11. Mills CF, ed (1989) Zinc in human biology. Springer-Verlag, New York, pp 371–381

12. Solomons NW, Cousins RJ (1984) Zinc. In Solomons NW, Rosenberg IH (eds), Absorption and malabsorption of mineral nutrients. Alan R Liss, New York, pp 125–197

13. Cousins RJ (1989) Theoretical and practical aspects of zinc uptake and absorption. In Laszlo JA, Dintzis FR (eds), Mineral absorption in the monogastric GI tract: chemical, nutritional and physiological aspects. Plenum, New York, pp 3–12

14. Lee HH, Prasad AS, Brewer GJ, Owyang C (1989) Zinc absorption in human small intestine. Am J Physiol 256:G87–G91

15. Naveh Y, Lee-Ambrose LM, Samuelson DA, Cousins RJ (1993) Malabsorption of zinc in rats with acetic acid-induced enteritis and colitis. J Nutr 123:1389–1395

16. Baer MT, King JC (1984) Tissue zinc levels and zinc excretion during experimental zinc depletion in young men. Am J Clin Nutr 39:556–570

17. Jackson MJ, Jones FA, Edwards RHT, et al (1984) Zinc homeostasis in man: studies using a new stable isotope-dilution technique. Br J Nutr 51:199–208

18. Smith KT, Cousins RJ (1980) Quantitative aspects of zinc absorption by isolated, vascularly perfused rat intestine. J Nutr 110:316–323

19. Steel L, Cousins RJ (1985) Kinetics of zinc absorption by luminally and vascularly perfused rat intestine. Am J Physiol 248:G46–G53

20. Hoadley JE, Leinart AS, Cousins RJ (1988) Relationship of ^{65}Zn absorption kinetics to intestinal metallothionein in rats: effects of zinc depletion and fasting. J Nutr 118:497–502

21. Ziegler EE, Serfass RE, Nelson SE, et al (1989) Effect of low zinc intake on absorption and excretion of zinc by infants studied with ^{70}Zn as extrinsic tag. J Nutr 119:1647–1653

22. Lee D-Y, Prasad AS, Hydrick-Adair C, et al (1993) Homeostasis of zinc in marginal human zinc deficiency: role of absorption and endogenous excretion of zinc. J Lab Clin Med 122:549–556

23. Taylor CM, Bacon JR, Aggett PJ, Bremner I (1991) Homeostatic regulation of zinc absorption and endogenous losses in zinc-deprived men. Am J Clin Nutr 53:755–763

24. Hoadley JE, Leinart AS, Cousins RJ (1987) Kinetic analysis of zinc uptake and serosal transfer by vascularly perfused rat intestine. Am J Physiol 252:G825–G831

25. Menard MP, Cousins RJ (1983) Zinc transport by brush border membrane vesicles from rat intestine. J Nutr 113:1434–1442

26. Raffaniello RD, Wapnir RA (1989) Zinc uptake by isolated rat enterocytes: effect of low molecular weight ligands. Proc Soc Exp Biol Med 192:219–224

27. Tacnet F, Watkins DW, Ripoche P (1990) Studies of zinc transport into brush-border membrane vesicles isolated from pig small intestine. Biochim Biophys Acta 1024:323–330

28. Raffaniello RD, Lee S-Y, Teichberg S, Wapnir RA (1992) Distinct mechanisms of zinc uptake at the apical and basolateral membranes of Caco-2 cells. J Cell Physiol 152:356–361

29. Tacnet F, Lauthier F, Ripoche P (1993) Mechanisms of zinc transport into pig small intestine brush-border membrane vesicles. J Physiol 465:57–72

30. Ghishan FK, Sobo G (1983) Intestinal maturation: in vivo zinc transport. Pediatr Res 17:148–151

31. Steinhardt HJ, Adibi SA (1984) Interaction between transport of zinc and other solutes in human intestine. Am J Physiol 247:G176–G182

32. Wapnir RA, Khani DE, Bayne MA, Lifshitz F (1983) Absorption of zinc by the rat ileum: effects of histidine and other low-molecular-weight ligands. J Nutr 113:1346–1354

33. Richards MP, Cousins RJ (1977) Isolation of an intestinal metallothionein induced by parenteral zinc. Biochem Biophys Res Commun 75:286–294

34. Hempe JM, Cousins RJ (1991) Cysteine-rich intestinal protein binds zinc during transmucosal zinc transport. Proc Natl Acad Sci USA 88:9671–9674

35. Levenson CW, Shay NF, Lee-Ambrose LM, Cousins RJ (1993) Regulation of cysteine-rich intestinal protein by dexamethasone in the neonatal rat. Proc Natl Acad Sci USA 90:712–715

36. Cousins RJ, Lee-Ambrose LM (1992) Nuclear zinc uptake and interactions and metallothionein gene expression are influenced by dietary zinc in rats. J Nutr 122:56–64

37. Coppen DE, Davies NT (1987) Studies on the effects of dietary zinc dose on ^{65}Zn absorption in vivo and on the effects of Zn status on ^{65}Zn absorption and body loss in young rats. Br J Nutr 57:35–44

38. Richards MP, Cousins RJ (1975) Mammalian zinc homeostasis: requirement for RNA and metallothionein synthesis. Biochem Biophys Res Commun 64:1215–1223

39. Reeves PG (1995) Adaptation responses in rats to long-term feeding of high-zinc diets: emphasis on intestinal metallothionein. J Nutr Biochem 6:48–54

40. Fleet JC, Turnbull AJ, Bourcier M, Wood RJ (1993) Vitamin D-sensitive and quinacrine-sensitive zinc transport in human intestinal cell line Caco-2. Am J Physiol 264:G1037–G1045

41. Oestreicher P, Cousins RJ (1989) Zinc uptake by basolateral membrane vesicles from rat small intestine. J Nutr 119:639–646

42. Palmiter RD, Findley SD (1995) Cloning and functional characterization of a mammalian zinc transporter that confers resistance to zinc. EMBO J 14:639–649

43. Kowarski S, Blair-Stanek CS, Schachter D (1974) Active transport of zinc and identification of zinc-binding protein in rat jejunal mucosa. Am J Physiol 226:401–407

44. Urban E, Campbell ME (1984) In vivo zinc transport by rat small intestine after extensive small bowel resection. Am J Physiol 247:G88–G94

45. Turnbull AJ, Blakeborough P, Thompson RPH (1990) The effects of dietary ligands on zinc uptake at the porcine intestinal brush-border membrane. Br J Nutr 64:733–741

46. Han O, Failla ML, Hill AD, et al (1994) Inositol phosphates inhibit uptake and transport of iron and zinc by a human intestinal cell line. J Nutr 124:580–587

47. Sandström B, Lönnerdal B (1989) Promoters and antagonists of zinc absorption. In Mills CF (ed), Zinc in human biology. Springer-Verlag, New York, pp 57–78

48. Cousins RJ (1985) Absorption, transport and hepatic metabolism of copper and zinc: special reference to metallothionein and ceruloplasmin. Physiol Rev 65:238–309

49. Sturniolo GC, Montino MC, Rossetto L, et al (1991) Inhibition of gastric acid secretion reduces zinc absorption in man. J Am Coll Nutr 10:372–375

50. Schölmerich J, Freudemann A, Köttgen E, et al (1987) Bioavailability of zinc from zinc-histidine complexes. I. Comparison with zinc sulfate in healthy men. Am J Clin Nutr 45:1480–1486

51. Hempe JM, Cousins RJ (1989) Effect of EDTA and zinc-methionine complex on zinc absorption by rat intestine. J Nutr 119:1179–1187

52. Roth HP, Kirchgessner M (1985) Utilization of zinc from picolinic or citric acid complexes in relation to dietary protein source in rats. J Nutr 115:1641–1645

53. Seal CJ, Heaton FW (1985) Effect of dietary picolinic acid on the metabolism of exogenous and endogenous zinc in the rat. J Nutr 115:986–993

54. Prasad AS (1979) Zinc in human nutrition. CRC Press, Boca Raton, FL, 84 pp

55. Tamura T (1995) Nutrient interaction of folate and zinc. In Bailey LB (ed), Folate in health and disease. Marcel Dekker, New York, pp 287–308

56. Kauwell GPA, Bailey LB, Gregory JF, et al (1995) Zinc status is not adversely affected by folic acid supplementation and zinc intake does not impair folate utilization in human subjects. J Nutr 125:66–72

57. Valberg LS, Flanagan PR, Chamberlain MJ (1984) Effects of iron, tin, and copper on zinc absorption. Am J Clin Nutr 40:536–541

58. Southon S, Wright AJA, Fairweather-Tait SJ (1989) The effect of combined dietary iron, calcium and folic acid supplementation on apparent ^{65}Zn absorption and Zn status in pregnant rats. Br J Nutr 62:415–423

59. Koo SI, Fullmer CS, Wasserman RH (1980) Effect of cholecalciferol and 1,25-dihydroxycholecalciferol on the intestinal absorption of zinc in the chick. J Nutr 110:1813–1818

60. Wood R, Zheng J (1995) Calcium supplementation reduces intestinal zinc absorption and balance in humans [abstract]. FASEB J 9:A283

61. Smith KT, Failla ML, Cousins RJ (1979) Identification of albumin as the plasma carrier for zinc absorption by perfused rat intestine. Biochem J 184:627–633

62. Keen CL, Hurley LS (1977) Zinc absorption through skin: correction of zinc deficiency in the rat. Am J Clin Nutr 30:528–530

63. Cousins RJ (1989) Systemic transport of zinc. In Mills CF (ed), Zinc in human biology. Springer-Verlag, New York, pp 79–93

64. Scott BJ, Bradwell AR (1983) Identification of the serum binding proteins for iron, zinc, cadmium, nickel, and calcium. Clin Chem 29:629–633

65. Magneson GR, Puvathingal JM, Roy WJ (1987) The concentrations of free Mg^{2+} and free Zn^{2+} in equine blood plasma. J Biol Chem 262:11140–11145

66. Robertson A, Morrison JM, Wood AM, Bremner I (1989) Effects of iron deficiency on metallothionein-I concentrations in blood and tissues of rats. J Nutr 119:439–445

67. Grider A, Bailey LB, Cousins RJ (1990) Erythrocyte metallothionein as an index of zinc status in humans. Proc Natl Acad Sci USA 87:1259–1262

68. Huber KL, Cousins RJ (1988) Maternal zinc deprivation and interleukin-1 influence metallothionein gene expression and zinc metabolism of rats. J Nutr 118:1570–1576

69. Milne DB, Ralston NVC, Wallwork JC (1985) Zinc content of cellular components of blood: methods for cell separation and analysis evaluated. Clin Chem 31:65–69

70. Richards MP, Cousins RJ (1976) Metallothionein and its relationship to the metabolism of dietary zinc in rats. J Nutr 106:1591–1599

71. Henry RW, Elmes ME (1975) Plasma zinc in acute starvation. Br Med J 4:625–626

72. Falchuk KH (1977) Effect of acute disease and ACTH on serum zinc proteins. N Engl J Med 296:1129–1134

73. King JC, Hambidge KM, Westcott JL, et al (1994) Daily variation in plasma zinc concentrations in women fed meals at six-hour intervals. J Nutr 124:508–516

74. Gordon PR, Woodruff CW, Anderson HL, O'Dell BL (1982) Effect of acute zinc deprivation on plasma zinc and platelet aggregation in adult males. Am J Clin Nutr 35:113–119

75. Fraser JD, Urban RG, Strominger JL, Robinson H (1992) Zinc regulates the function of two superantigens. Proc Natl Acad Sci USA 89:5507–5511

76. Foster DM, Aamodt RL, Henkin RI, Berman M (1979) Zinc metabolism in humans: a kinetic model. Am J Physiol 237:R340–R349

77. Wastney ME, Aamodt RL, Rumble WF, Henkin RI (1986) Kinetic analysis of zinc metabolism and its regulation in normal humans. Am J Physiol 251:R398–R408

78. Dunn MA, Cousins RJ (1989) Kinetics of zinc metabolism in the rat: effect of dibutyryl cAMP. Am J Physiol 256:E420–E430

79. Henkin RI, Foster DM, Aamodt RL, Berman M (1984) Zinc metabolism in adrenal cortical insufficiency: effects of carbohydrate-active steroids. Metabolism 33:491–501

80. Miller LV, Hambidge KM, Naake VL, et al (1994) Size of the zinc pools that exchange rapidly with plasma zinc in humans: alternative techniques for measuring and relation to dietary zinc intake. J Nutr 124:268–276

81. Pattison SE, Cousins RJ (1986) Kinetics of zinc uptake and exchange by primary cultures of rat hepatocytes. Am J Physiol 250:E677–E685

82. Golden MNH (1989) The diagnosis of zinc deficiency. In Mills CF (ed), Zinc in human biology. Springer-Verlag, New York, pp 323–333

83. Palmiter RD (1994) Regulation of metallothionein genes by heavy metals appears to be mediated by a zinc-sensitive inhibitor that interacts with a constitutively active transcription factor, MTF-1. Proc Natl Acad Sci USA 91:1219–1223

84. Dunn MA, Blalock TL, Cousins RJ (1987) Metallothionein. Proc Soc Exp Biol Med 185:107–119

85. Masters BA, Kelly EJ, Quaife CJ, et al (1994) Targeted disruption of metallothionein I and II genes increases sensitivity to cadmium. Proc Natl Acad Sci USA 91:584–588

86. Cousins RJ, Leinart AS (1988) Tissue-specific regulation of zinc metabolism and metallothionein genes by interleukin 1. FASEB J 2:2884–2890

87. Schroeder JJ, Cousins RJ (1990) Interleukin 6 regulates metallothionein gene expression and zinc metabolism in hepatocyte monolayer cultures. Proc Natl Acad Sci USA 87:3137–3141

88. King JC, Turnlund JR (1989) Human zinc requirements. In Mills CF (ed), Zinc in human biology. Springer-Verlag, New York, pp 335–350

89. Matseshe JW, Phillips SF, Malagelada JR, McCall GT (1980) Recovery of dietary iron and zinc from the proximal intestine of healthy man: studies of different meals and supplements. Am J Clin Nutr 33:1946–1953

90. Fell GS, Fleck A, Cuthbertson DP, et al (1973) Urinary zinc levels as an indication of muscle catabolism. Lancet 2:280–282

91. Victery W, Levenson R, Vander AJ (1981) Effect of glucagon on zinc excretion in anesthetized dogs. Am J Physiol 240:F299–F305

92. Vallee BL, Galdes A (1984) The metallobiochemistry of zinc enzymes. In Meister A (ed), Advances in enzymology. John Wiley, New York, pp 283–429

93. Rivera J, Brown KH, Santizo MC, et al (1995) Effects of zinc supplementation on the growth of young Guatemalan children [abstract]. FASEB J 9:A164

94. Falchuk KH, Fawcett DW, Vallee BL (1975) Role of zinc in cell division of *Euglena gracilis*. J Cell Sci 17:57–78.

95. Klug A, Schwabe JWR (1995) Zinc fingers. FASEB J 9:597–604

96. Dawid IB, Toyama R, Taira M (1995) LIM domain proteins. C R Acad Sci Paris 318:295–306

97. Forbes IJ, Zalewski PD, Giannakis C, et al (1990) Interaction between protein kinase C and regulatory ligand is enhanced by a chelatable pool of cellular zinc. Biochim Biophys Acta 1053:113–117

98. Wu H, Yang W-P, Barbas CF (1995) Building zinc fingers by selection: toward a therapeutic application. Proc Natl Acad Sci USA 92:344–348

99. Taylor GA, Blackshear PJ (1995) Zinc inhibits turnover of labile mRNAs in intact cells. J Cell Physiol 162:378–387

100. Zeng J, Heuchel R, Schaffner W, Kägi JHR (1991) Thionein (apometallothionein) can modulate DNA binding and transcription activation by zinc finger containing factor Sp1. FEBS Lett 279:310–312

101. Cousins RJ (1994) Metal elements and gene expression. In Olson RE (ed), Annual review of nutrition. Annual Reviews Inc, Palo Alto, CA, pp 449–469

102. Yiangou M, Ge X, Carter KC, Papaconstantinou J (1991) Induction of several acute-phase protein genes by heavy metals: a new class of metal-responsive genes. Biochemistry 30:3798–3806

103. Willson RL (1989) Zinc and iron in free radical pathology and cellular control. In Mills CF (ed), Zinc in human biology. Springer-Verlag, New York, pp 147–172

104. Thornalley PJ, Vasak M (1985) Possible role for metallothionein in protection against radiation-induced oxidative stress. Biochim Biophys Acta 827:36–44

105. Barch DH, Fox CC, Rosche WA, et al (1992) Inhibition of rat methylbenzylnitrosamine metabolism by dietary zinc and zinc in vitro. Gastroenterology 103:800–806

106. Schwarz MA (1994) Cytoplasmic metallothionein overexpression protects NIH 3T3 cells from tert-butyl hydroperoxide toxicity. J Biol Chem 269:15238–15243

107. Powell SR, Hall D, Aiuto L, et al (1994) Zinc improves postischemic recovery of isolated rat hearts through inhibition of oxidative stress. Am J Physiol 266:H2497–H2507

108. Xu Z, Squires EJ, Bray TM (1994) Effects of dietary zinc deficiency on the hepatic microsomal cytochrome P450 2B in rats. Can J Physiol Pharmacol 72:211–216

109. Thompson CB (1995) Apoptosis in the pathogenesis and treatment of disease. Science 267:1456–1462

110. McCabe MJ, Jiang SA, Orrenius S (1993) Chelation of intracellular zinc triggers apoptosis in mature thymocytes. Lab Invest 69:101–110

111. Zalewski PD, Forbes IJ, Seamark RF, et al (1994) Flux of intracellular labile zinc during apoptosis (gene-directed cell death) revealed by a specific chemical probe, Zinquin. Chem Biol 1:153–161

112. Telford WG, Fraker PJ (1995) Preferential induction of apoptosis in mouse CD4$^+$CD8$\alpha\beta$TCR^{lo}CD3ϵ^{lo} thymocytes by zinc. J Cell Physiol 164:259–270

113. O'Dell BL, Reeves PG (1989) Zinc status and food intake. In Mills CF (ed), Zinc in human biology. Springer-Verlag, New York, pp 173–181

114. Chesters JK, Quarterman J (1970) Effects of zinc deficiency on food intake and feeding patterns of rats. Br J Nutr 24:1061–1069

115. Blanchard RK, Cousins RJ (1995) Differential display of dietary zinc regulated rat intestinal mRNAs [abstract]. FASEB J 9:A866

116. Shay NF, Beverly JL, Rains TM, et al (1995) Central administration of neuropeptide Y restores intake to normal levels in zinc deficient rats [abstract]. FASEB J 9:A867

117. Flanagan PR (1984) A model to produce pure zinc deficiency in rats and its use to demonstrate that dietary phytate increases the excretion of endogenous zinc. J Nutr 114:493–502

118. Chesters JK (1989) Biochemistry of zinc in cell division and tissue growth. In Mills CF (ed), Zinc in human biology. Springer-Verlag, New York, pp 109–118

119. Schroeder JJ, Cousins RJ (1991) Maintenance of zinc-dependent hepatic functions in rat hepatocytes cultured in medium without added zinc. J Nutr 121:844–853

120. King JC (1990) Assessment of zinc status. J Nutr 120:1474–1479

121. Eder K, Kirchgessner M (1994) Dietary fat influences the effect of zinc deficiency on liver lipids and fatty acids in rats forcefed equal quantities of diet. J Nutr 124:1917–1926

122. Moynahan EJ (1974) Acrodermatitis enteropathica: a lethal inherited human zinc-deficiency disorder. Lancet ii:399–400

123. Flagstad T (1976) Lethal trait A 46 in cattle: intestinal zinc absorption. Nord Vet Med 28:160–169

124. Keen CL, Gershwin ME (1990) Zinc deficiency and immune function. In Olson RE (ed), Annual review of nutrition. Annual Reviews Inc, Palo Alto, CA, pp 415–431

125. Fraker PJ, DePasquale-Jardieu P, Zwickl CM, Luecke RW (1978) Regeneration of T-cell helper function in zinc deficient adult mice. Proc Natl Acad Sci USA 75:5660–5664

126. Allen JI, Perri RT, McClain CJ, Kay NE (1983) Alterations in human natural killer cell activity and monocyte cytotoxicity induced by zinc deficiency. J Lab Clin Med 102:577–589

127. Kramer TR, Udomkesmalee E, Dhanamitta S, et al (1993) Lymphocyte responsiveness of children supplemented with vitamin A and zinc. Am J Clin Nutr 58:566–570

128. Winchurch RA, Togo J, Adler WH (1987) Supplemental zinc (Zn^{2+}) restores antibody formation in cultures of aged spleen cells. II. Effects on mediator production. Eur J Immunol 17:127–132

129. Driessen C, Hirv K, Rink L, Kirchner H (1994) Induction of cytokines by zinc ions in human peripheral blood mononuclear cells and separated monocytes. Lymphokine Cytokine Res 13:15–20

130. Malavé I, Rodriguez J, Araujo Z, Rojas I (1990) Effect of zinc on the proliferative response of human lymphocytes: mechanism of its mitogenic action. Immunopharmacology 20:1–10

131. Dardenne M, Pleau JM, Nabarra B, et al (1982) Contribution of zinc and other metals to the biological activity of the serum thymic factor. Proc Natl Acad Sci USA 79:5370–5373

132. Coto JA, Hadden EM, Sauro M, et al (1992) Interleukin 1 regulates secretion of zinc-thymulin by human thymic epithelial cells and its action on T-lymphocyte proliferation and nuclear protein kinase C. Proc Natl Acad Sci USA 89:7752–7756

133. King LE, Osati-Ashtiani F, Fraker PJ (1995) Depletion of cells of the B lineage in the bone marrow of zinc-deficient mice. Immunology 85:69–73

134. Bobilya DJ, Johanning GL, Veum TL, O'Dell BL (1994) Chronological loss of bone zinc during dietary zinc deprivation in neonatal pigs. Am J Clin Nutr 59:649–653

135. Clegg MS, Keen CL, Hurley LS (1989) Biochemical pathologies of zinc deficiency. In Mills CF (ed), Zinc in human biology. Springer-Verlag, New York, pp 129–145

136. Aggett PJ (1989) Severe zinc deficiency. In Mills CF (ed), Zinc in human biology. Springer-Verlag, New York, pp 259–279

137. Xie X, Smart TG (1991) A physiological role for endogenous zinc in rat hippocampal synaptic neurotransmission. Nature 349:521–524

138. Hendricks KM, Walker WA (1988) Zinc deficiency in inflammatory bowel disease. Nutr Rev 12:401–408

139. Bogden JD, Oleske JM, Lavenhar MA, et al (1988) Zinc and immunocompetence in elderly people: effects of zinc supplementation for 3 months. Am J Clin Nutr 48:655–663

140. Life Sciences Research Office (1991) Zinc and immune function in the elderly. Federation of American Societies for Experimental Biology, Bethesda, MD

141. Newsome DA, Swartz M, Leone NC, et al (1988) Oral zinc in macular degeneration. Arch Ophthalmol 106:192–198

142. Henkin RI, Aamodt RL, Agarwal RP, Foster DM (1982) The role of zinc in taste and smell. In Prasad AS (ed), Clinical, biochemical, and nutritional aspects of trace elements. Alan R Liss, New York, pp 161–188

143. Walravens PA, Hambidge KM, Koepfer DM (1989) Zinc supplementation in infants with a nutritional pattern of failure to thrive: a double-blind, controlled study. Pediatrics 83:532–538

144. Lee MG, Hong KT, Kim JJ (1990) Transient symptomatic zinc deficiency in a full-term breast-fed infant. J Am Acad Dermatol 23:375–379

145. Lee D-Y, Shay NF, Cousins RJ (1992) Altered zinc metabolism occurs in murine lethal milk syndrome. J Nutr 122:2233–2238

146. Moser-Veillon PB (1990) Zinc: consumption patterns and dietary recommendations. J Am Diet Assoc 90:1089–1093

147. National Research Council (1989) Recommended dietary allowances, 10th ed. National Academy Press, Washington, DC

148. Welsh SO, Marston RM (1982) Zinc levels of the US food supply: 1909–1980. Food Technol 36:70–76

149. American Medical Association (1979) Guidelines for essential trace element preparations for parenteral use. JAMA 241:2051–2054

150. Solomons NW (1991) Zinc. In Baumgartner TG (ed), Clinical guide to parenteral micronutrition, 2nd ed. Lyphomed, Chicago, pp 215–233

151. Sullivan JF, Jetton MM, Burch RE (1979) A zinc tolerance test. J Lab Clin Med 93:485–492

152. Kasarskis EJ, Shuna A (1980) Serum alkaline phosphatase after treatment of zinc deficiency in humans. Am J Clin Nutr 33:2609–2612

153. Dahlheim H, White CL, Rothemund J, et al (1989) Effect of zinc depletion on angiotensin I-converting enzyme in arterial walls and plasma of the rat. Miner Electrolyte Metab 15:125–129

154. Sato M, Mehra RK, Bremner I (1984) Measurement of plasma metallothionein-1 in the assessment of the zinc status of zinc-deficient and stressed rats. J Nutr 114:1683–1689

155. Thomas EA, Bailey LB, Kauwell GA, et al (1992) Erythrocyte metallothionein response to dietary zinc in humans. J Nutr 122:2408–2414

156. Bremner I, Morrison JN, Wood AM, Arthur JR (1987) Effects of changes in dietary zinc, copper and selenium supply and of endotoxin administration on metallothionein I concentrations in blood cells and urine in the rat. J Nutr 117:1595–1602

157. Zheng J, Mason JB, Rosenberg IH, Wood RJ (1993) Measurement of zinc bioavailability from beef and a ready-to-eat high-fiber breakfast cereal in humans: application of whole-gut lavage technique. Am J Clin Nutr 58:902–907

158. Fosmire G (1990) Zinc toxicity. Am J Clin Nutr 51:225–227

159. Fox MRS (1989) Zinc excess. In Mills CF (ed), Zinc in human biology. Springer-Verlag, New York, pp 365–370

160. Brocks A, Reid H, Glazer G, et al (1977) Acute intravenous zinc poisoning. Br Med J 1:1390–1391

161. McCormick CC, Cunningham DL (1984) High dietary zinc and fasting as methods of forced resting: a performance comparison. Poultry Sci 63:1201–1206

162. Lü J, Combs GF (1988) Effect of excess dietary zinc on pancreatic exocrine function in the chick. J Nutr 118:681–689

163. Prasad AS, Brewer GJ, Shoomaker EB, Rabbani P (1978) Hypocupremia induced by zinc therapy in adults. JAMA 240:2166–2168

164. Yuzbasiyan-Gurkan V, Grider A, Nostrant T, et al (1992) Treatment of Wilson's disease with zinc: X. Intestinal metallothionein induction. J Lab Clin Med 120:380–386

165. Fiske DN, McCoy HE, Kitchens CS (1994) Zinc-induced sideroblastic anemia: report of a case, review of the literature, and description of the hematologic syndrome. Am J Hematol 46:147–150

166. Doz F, Berens ME, Deschepper CF, et al (1992) Experimental basis for increasing the therapeutic index of cis-diaminedicarboxylatocyclobutaneplatinum(II) in brain tumor therapy by a high-zinc diet. Cancer Chemother Pharmacol 29:219–226

167. Kelley SL, Basu A, Teicher BA, et al (1988) Overexpression of metallothionein confers resistance to anticancer drugs. Science 241:1813–1815

168. Dreosti IE (1989) Neurobiology of zinc. In Mills CF (ed), Zinc in human biology. Springer-Verlag, New York, pp 235–247

169. Masters BA, Quaife CJ, Erickson JC, et al (1994) Metallothionein III is expressed in neurons that sequester zinc in synaptic vesicles. J Neurosci 14:5844–5857

170. Khoo C, Hallquist NA, Cousins RJ (1995) Carbon-tetrachloride-induced inflammation increases cysteine-rich intestinal protein expression in the hippocampus and immune tissues [abstract]. FASEB J 9:A867

171. Bush AI, Pettingell WH, Multhaup G, et al (1994) Rapid induction of Alzheimer Aβ amyloid formation by zinc. Science 265:1464–1467

Chapter 30

Copper

Maria C. Linder

Copper (atomic number 29) is a transition metal widely distributed in nature. Although not among the most abundant on earth, it has been estimated that 6.7 and 5×10^{12} kg, respectively, are present in our tillable soils and water, along with another 2.9×10^{10} and 2.4×10^{5} kg, respectively, in plants and animals.[1] Water of the ocean surface contains ≈1 ppb, but concentrations increase linearly with depth,[2] ≈100-fold per 1000 m. Fresh water concentrations are lower and more variable (from ≈0.1 to 1.0 ng/g). In solution, as well as in living organisms, copper is found almost exclusively in the +2 and +1 valence states, the former predominating. At neutral pH in aqueous media (as in most cells and organisms) copper ions form hydroxides that precipitate out of solution unless chelated by organic molecules.

The redox chemistry of this element makes it particularly suited for releasing and accepting electrons and especially for the direct transfer of electrons to molecular oxygen. Thus many electron transfer and oxidation-reduction reactions involving oxygen are catalyzed by copper-containing enzymes in biological systems. Some of these enzymes are fundamental to life as we know it.

Recognition of copper as an essential element for plants and animals was based on studies pioneered by McHargue (in plants and mollusks)[3,4] and Hart et al.[5] (in animals). The essentiality of copper was considered established upon being reviewed by Hoagland[6] and then others in the 1930s.[7]

Concentrations of copper in living organisms average 1–2 µg/g with some exceptions (Table 1).[7] This is lower than soil concentrations (3–100 µg/g)[8] but much higher than water concentrations. Recent estimates suggest that the average human adult contains a total of ≈110 mg of copper. Kidneys have the highest copper concentrations (Table 1), followed by liver and brain and then heart and whole bone. Blood and muscle concentrations are ≈1 µg/g, whereas the concentration in the gastrointestinal tract is about twice as high. (Finger- and toenails are very rich in copper, and hair concentrations are also significant.) In newborns, concentrations of liver copper are much higher than in adults (≈40 µg/g), reflecting prenatal storage of the element. Most of this copper is used for new tissue in the first 6 months of life.

Because of their weight and volume, muscle and skeleton probably contain ≈25% and 42% of total body copper, respectively. Liver and brain are next (≈9%), and blood has ≈5% (60% of which is in the plasma). Concentrations in animal tissues tend to be similar but slightly lower than those in humans, except in plasma, which tends to be the same.

Absorption, Transport, Storage, and Turnover

Absorption. In humans and animals, absorption of copper occurs primarily in the duodenum, although the rest of the small intestine (and perhaps even the colon) is capable of uptake. Whether absorption occurs in the stomach is unclear.[7] The efficiency of gastrointestinal copper uptake by human adults from normal foodstuffs is quite high, values for apparent absorption ranging from 55% to 75% and not varying appreciably with age and sex

Table 1. Concentrations of copper in living organisms[a]

Organism	Overall concentration µg/g (ppm)
Humans	1.7
Blood (whole)[b]	1.1
Plasma	1.05
Kidney	12
Liver	6.2
Brain	5.2
Heart	4.8
Skeleton	4.1
Skeletal muscle	0.9
Hair	20
Nails	8–20
Animals	1.5–2.5
Fowl	0.5–3
Fish (sea)	2–3
(freshwater)	0.4–3
Shellfish	3–37
Insects	3–31
Arthropods	4–30
Plants	
Flesh	0.5–3
Nuts, seeds	3–37

[a]Modified from Linder.[7]
[b]All human tissue values are for adults.

(except perhaps being greater in young women).[7,9,10] In studies with rats, actual absorption rates of 30–50% (per 24 hours) were reported for intakes within the normal range. Uptake efficiency plummets to <10% when intake is excessive. In both rats and humans there is evidence that uptake at least partly responds to need, and thus, some endogenous regulation of absorption is exercised.

Absorption is a two-step process involving uptake (probably of Cu^{2+}) into mucosal cells by crossing their brush border and transfer across the basolateral membrane for entry into blood and internal tissues. Evidence suggests that brush-border uptake is via nonmediated diffusion and serosal transfer is mainly via an energy-dependent saturable carrier.[7] Uptake into mucosal cells does not guarantee further transfer into the body per se, because variable amounts will be held back by mucosal cell proteins, notably metallothioneins. The concentration of basolateral transporters may vary with physiological condition and perhaps even with copper status, although this remains to be examined. The transporter in the basolateral membrane responsible for pumping copper into blood and interstitial fluid is probably the P-type ATPase recently cloned in connection with Menkes disease.[11–14] (The Menkes gene apparently encodes a defective copper-specific, energy-requiring transporter. An inherited Menkes gene is not immediately lethal to newborns, partly because infants are born with copper stores and probably also because some absorption occurs by other mechanisms.) Basolateral membrane carriers used by other metal ions (notably Zn^{2+} and Cd^{2+}) may be involved,[7,15] as this would explain some of the antagonism between these ions and copper under extreme conditions of intake. A further explanation is that zinc and cadmium ions also induce metallothioneins in the intestinal mucosa, thus providing a trap for Cu^{2+} in these cells. However, in normal mammals, copper absorption is significantly depressed only when Zn^{2+} or Cd^{2+} is given in very great excess. Chronic intake of excess zinc is prescribed for patients with copper overload caused by Wilson disease to minimize copper absorption. The copper retained in metallothionein in the enterocytes is lost when these cells slough off (life span 3–5 days in adult humans).

Reports have been both positive and negative concerning an antagonism for absorption between copper and iron.[15] The most recent report shows an inverse correlation between liver copper concentrations in rats and low, normal, or very high dietary iron intakes (7, 40, and 389 mg Fe/kg diet).[16] Both apparent absorption and biliary excretion of copper were reduced with excessive iron intakes. Plasma copper and ceruloplasmin concentrations (measured by enzyme activity) were depressed 30–40%, but liver copper was only ≈10% lower than normal. So, if there is a consistent effect of iron on copper absorption, it is also relatively mild and seen only under extreme conditions.

Other dietary factors that influence copper absorption include chelating agents (such as amino acids and citrate), which enhance absorption, and intestinal binding agents (such as bile and fiber), which inhibit absorption. Under certain conditions, ascorbic acid may decrease absorption, though this remains controversial. Cu^+ may be less well absorbed than Cu^{2+}, and ascorbate can reduce Cu^{2+} to Cu^+. Such a reduction could thus explain the 37% decrease in uptake (over 3 hours, originally reported by Van Campen and Gross[17] for ligated duodenal segments in rats). However, those studies used very large, unphysiological doses and have not been corroborated by others in rats[7] and in humans under real-life conditions (i.e., retention of ^{65}Cu while on diets differing in ascorbate content from 5 to 605 mg/day).

Transport. After being absorbed by the intestine, copper rapidly enters the blood circulation and quickly is deposited mainly in liver. This pattern is evident from studies in several species, including rats[18,19] and humans.[20,21] In rats, virtually all of the element that enters blood is gone from the circulation after 2 hours[19] and can be found almost exclusively in liver, kidney, and liver-derived products.[7] These products include the bile (thought to be the main excretory route for copper) and ceruloplasmin (a major α_2-glycoprotein that accounts for 60–65% of the copper in human plasma and serum[22,23]). After its initial virtual disappearance from blood, newly absorbed copper thus reappears in the circulation in ceruloplasmin. The copper in ceruloplasmin is not part of the exchangeable plasma copper pool and is not directly transferred to other copper components of the plasma. However, it is available for uptake by cells in most tissues of the body, as demonstrated repeatedly by animal and cell culture studies with ^{67}Cu[7,19,24,25] and from modeling of data from stable isotope studies in humans.[21] Acute inhibition of liver ceruloplasmin synthesis (during which copper is incorporated into the protein) also inhibits uptake of newly absorbed copper by nonhepatic tissues.[26] Nevertheless, there appears to be redundancy, and other copper sources are used when ceruloplasmin is not available. In the first reported case of a human with defective ceruloplasmin gene expression, no changes in copper status were immediately obvious.[27] Also, nonhepatic cells take up copper from transcuprein[19] and even from albumin.[7,19,24]

All of this implies that transport and distribution of copper occurs in two phases, the first involving transfer from intestine to liver and kidney and the second involving transfer from liver to most other parts of the body. During the second phase of distribution, copper is normally carried by ceruloplasmin, which appears as the only plasma component bearing newly absorbed copper after initial liver (and kidney) deposition.

During the first phase of distribution, specific proteins also appear to be involved. It is well established that albumin (by far the most abundant plasma protein) is a site for copper binding. In most species, the N-terminus of albumin contains a high-affinity copper binding site.[7,28,29] However, albumin is not essential for normal transport and distribution of incoming copper, as demonstrated in Nagase analbuminemic rats[30] and consistent with the observation that some animals (notably dogs) have no high-affinity copper binding site on their albumin. In rats,[19] humans,[22,23] and some other mammals,[31] a much larger protein ($\approx$270 kDa) accounts for about the same amount of plasma copper as albumin (10–20% of the total). Based on in vitro labeling with $^{67}Cu^{2+}$, this protein and albumin are the main components of the exchangeable plasma copper pool. They directly bind added Cu^{2+} and exchange the metal ion between them. It seems likely that this protein (transcuprein) is a more specific carrier for newly absorbed copper than is albumin and that it targets the copper mainly to liver. Transcuprein rapidly exchanges copper with albumin, probably by direct protein-protein interactions.[32] When only one protein is present, release rates for copper from either protein are very slow.

Whether low-molecular-weight copper complexes (e.g., copper-dihistidine) play a significant role in copper transport remains unclear. In vitro studies with unphysiologically high concentrations of copper-dihistidine demonstrate uptake by a saturable carrier with an apparent K_m of 10^{-8} mol/L. Copper in low-molecular-weight complexes (including dihistidine) is probably $\approx 0.5 \times 10^{-10}$ mol/L in vivo,[7,33] and not all of that is part of the exchangeable plasma copper pool.[7] Albumin can inhibit cell uptake of copper from the dihistidine complex.[34,35] Thus it seems likely that albumin and transcuprein are the main (or even the only) carriers in blood involved with the transfer of newly absorbed copper to liver and kidney and that transcuprein rather than albumin actually aids uptake by hepatic cells.

Storage. In general, copper cannot be considered a metal that is stored. It usually enters the body from the intestine with ease and is also readily excreted. Although there appears to be some regulation of absorption in relation to need, more being absorbed in deficiency and less in the face of copper adequacy, copper homeostasis is maintained mainly through excretion. Thus, when excess amounts are administered parenterally (as by injection into rats), the excess tends to disappear within a few days, even with large doses.[36] Nevertheless, cells in most or all tissues are equipped to temporarily sequester the excess in the form of copper thionein (copper complexed with the small, high-cysteine protein, metallothionein). As already mentioned in connection with intestinal absorption, metallothionein also binds other divalent metal ions, such as Zn^{2+}, but copper can displace most of them from metallothionein. In liver and kidney cells, influx of excess copper may also induce increased

Table 2. Copper concentration of adult human body fluids and gastrointestinal juices (average values)[a]

	Concentration (µg/g)	Secretion (µg/day)
Body fluid		
Blood plasma	1.05	
Lymph	1.2	
Cerebrospinal fluid	5	
Synovial fluid	0.2–0.5	
Urine	0.02–0.05	30–75
Gastrointestinal juice		
Saliva	0.22	330–450
Gastric juice	0.39	1000
Bile	4.0	2500?
Duodenal juices	0.17	400–2200

[a]Modified from Linder.[7]

expression of the protein.[37] Binding to metallothionein also is a mechanism for detoxifying copper ions that can otherwise catalyze the formation of oxygen radicals.[38]

A few species of mammals tend to accumulate stores of copper thionein, particularly in liver. This is a general tendency in dogs, which have much higher liver concentrations than do other species (80 vs. 5–6 µg/g in humans, rats, and pigs).[7,31,38,39] Deliberate storage of the trace element (again in metallothionein) also occurs in liver of fetuses before birth, probably in all mammals, from where it is thought to provide copper for the rapid growth of the suckling infant. (Milk is not rich in copper.[7,40])

Turnover and excretion. In animals and humans little copper is excreted via the urine, and most leaves the body after being returned to the digestive tract. Clearly the bile is a major (or the major) excretory route. Ligation of the bile duct results in accumulation of copper in liver, and when genetic traits reduce the rate of biliary copper excretion, liver copper concentrations rise and can lead to tissue damage. In the inherited human condition of Wilson disease, copper will accumulate not just in liver but also in other tissues (including brain).[41–43] Unless heavily treated with specific chelating agents that allow enhanced urinary copper losses, this disease results in early death. The defective gene in question probably encodes a copper transporter (also a P-type ATPase) that transfers the metal from hepatocytes into the bile. Whether this involves transfer across membranes of lysosomes (which contribute copper to bile)[44] or across a portion of the plasma membrane (which forms the bile canaliculi) is still to be determined.

The bile is probably not the only significant net excretory route for copper from the body, as ligation of the bile duct reduces whole-body copper turnover only by $\approx$50% (at least in rats).[36] Also, substantial amounts of copper are released into the gastrointestinal tract with saliva as well as with gastric, intestinal, and pancreatic juices (Table 2). Indeed, the total amount of copper secreted daily into the digestive tract ($\approx$5 mg) is more than three times as much as that received on average from the usual diet of human adults ($\approx$0.6–1.6 mg). Most of this copper is reabsorbed, because net fecal excretion (comprising >90% of copper losses) balances net intake. Very little copper is lost daily in the urine (<0.07mg) or from skin, hair, and nails. Most of the copper in bile appears not to be reabsorbable, at least in rats, in apparent contrast to that in gastric fluid and saliva.[7,45,46] This makes bile the most likely source of excretable copper entering the digestive tract. Thus, for net excretion, most copper in tissues must first return to liver.

Although we understand something about the distribution of incoming copper, many questions remain about how it returns to liver and enters the bile. Plasma ceruloplasmin itself returns and enters the bile,[47–49] probably being absorbed into hepatic cells by receptor-mediated endocytosis involving galactose receptors. (Desialylated plasma glycoproteins, as a group, are thought to be removed from the circulation by this mechanism.[50]) Desialylation of ceruloplasmin was reported to occur in liver endothelial cells "guarding" the space of Disse and during its transcytosis into that space.[51] Some or all of this ceruloplasmin (with some copper) enters the bile itself, although the molecular state of biliary ceruloplasmin is still in question. A recent abstract reports the presence of 126-kDa material,[52] which would correspond to partially deglycosylated plasma ceruloplasmin; earlier reports indicate the presence of ceruloplasmin fragments[47] and that most biliary copper is bound to two low-molecular-weight components ($\leq$5 kDa).[7] Some newly absorbed copper that enters hepatocytes as ions also finds its way more directly into the bile, especially when large doses are administered.[53] Most likely, much of the copper in peripheral tissues returns to liver via the same mechanism used by copper newly absorbed from the intestine. Upon release as Cu^{2+} into interstitial fluid, it would join the exchangeable plasma copper pool (binding to albumin and transcuprein) and thus find its way back to liver (and kidney).

Johnson et al.[9] used [67]Cu to study the turnover of whole-body copper in men and women under 59 years of age and obtained half-life values of $\approx$25 and 19 days, respectively. Turnover remained the same in older women but fell to 13–16 days in older men. There was also preliminary evidence of a copper compartment with a much slower rate of turnover. The presence of at least two compartments that turn over at different rates had been shown in rats after injection of [67]Cu.[36] One compartment had a relatively short half-life of 67 hours and the other was much longer (>200 hours). What these fast and slow turnover compartments may be is still unknown. However, the two sets of compartments identified in the two species probably are not the same, because collection of turnover data in humans began several days after administration of the stable isotope whereas that in rats began right after administration. The fast turnover compartment in rats (which may reflect biliary excretion of administered ionic copper) was thus probably missed in the human studies. If so, the slower turnover compartment in the rats ($t_{1/2}$ > 200 hours) may correspond to the 19–20-day half-life compartment in humans, and there would be a third body compartment that turns over even more slowly.

Biochemical and Physiological Functions

The current roster of known copper-containing enzymes is listed in Table 3. Most of these are present in vertebrates. Some are fundamental to the life and survival of living cells, some are unique to vertebrates or mammals, and others are unique to species other than mammals.

As already mentioned, cytochrome c oxidase and its coenzyme cytochrome c are among the most conserved proteins in nature and found in every living cell, where they function in respiration. Respiration reflects the delivery and use of molecular oxygen so that the carbohydrate, fat, and amino acid fuels can be oxidized to generate cell energy. Most cell energy is transiently held in the form of ATP, derived from oxidative phosphorylation involving the electron transport chain of mitochondria (or bacterial cell membranes), the terminal components of which are cytochrome c and its oxidase. Thus, as with most other copper enzymes, cytochrome c oxidase is the site where molecular oxygen is bound and reduced.

At least three copper enzymes appear to have a role in antioxidant defense. These are the widely distributed intracellular and extracellular superoxide dismutases (SODs), extracellular ceruloplasmin, and the mainly intracellular copper thioneins. Intracellular cytosolic SODs most often contain one zinc and one copper atom in each active site (Cu/Zn SOD), but some bacterial and mitochondrial SODs contain manganese or iron ions instead. The extracellular SOD of blood plasma is related only functionally and because it contains copper. All SODs catalyze the conversion of superoxide anions to peroxides. These can then be converted to H_2O by catalase or the selenium-dependent glutathione peroxidase. If the SOD gene is knocked out (as done in yeasts[54]), tolerance of oxygen radicals is markedly diminished. Recent studies with purified copper thioneins indicate that this protein, formerly thought to function merely in storage and detoxification of copper, also has free radical scavenging activity.[55,56] Because most mammalian metallothioneins usually have zinc rather than copper as their constituent metal ion, this activity of copper thionein is not likely to be important except when excess copper has accumulated.

Table 3. Copper-containing enzymes in mammals and other phyla

Enzyme/protein	Distribution and function
Cytochrome c oxidase[a]	Ubiquitous in mitochondria; last component in the electron transport chain of oxidative phosphorylation: reduction of O_2.
Cu/Zn superoxide dismutase	Ubiquitous in cytosol; protection against oxygen radicals: dismutation of superoxide to peroxide and O_2.
Tyrosinase (catecholoxidase /phenolase)[a]	Widely distributed; melanin production in mammals (in melanosomes) and diverse functions in plants and fungi: oxidative polymerization of tyrosines, oxidation of monophenols and o-diphenols to quinones.
Lysyl oxidase[a,b]	Mammals (vertebrates?), extracellular in connective tissue; cross-linking of collagen and elastin: oxidative cross-linking of lysine residues.
Dopamine-4-monooxygenase[a,b]	Mammals (vertebrates?), in central nervous system and adrenal medullary cells; formation of epinephrine and norepinephrine: hydroxylation of dopamine.
α-Amidating enzyme[b]	Mammals (vertebrates?), in granules of neurohypophysis; modification of neuropeptides: oxidative removal of carbons of C-terminal glycine residue, leaving α-amino.
Amine and diamine oxidases[a,b]	Widely distributed (mammals, plants, fungi, etc.); intracellular and extracellular; oxidative inactivation (?) of histamine, tyramine, and polyamines: oxidative deamination.
Ceruloplasmin[a,c]	Vertebrates, in blood plasma and other extracellular fluids; free radical scavenger and role in promoting flux of iron out of storage sites: oxidation of Fe^{2+} to Fe^{3+}.
Ferroxidase II[a]	Vertebrates (?), in blood plasma; function unknown, but like ceruloplasmin can oxidize Fe^{2+} to Fe^{3+}.
Extracellular SOD	Vertebrates, in blood plasma and probably other extracellular fluids; part of antioxidant defense system(?): dismutation of O_2^- to H_2O_2 and H_2O.
Ascorbate oxidase[a]	Plants and fungi, mainly intracellular; function unclear but in plants may play a role in fruit maturation and protection of wounds; oxidizes ascorbate, catechols, flavonoids, and hydroxycinnamic acid; in terms of reactivity, belongs to the family of blue copper oxygenases that include laccase and ceruloplasmin.
Laccase[a]	Plants and fungi, mostly extracellular; oxidative polymerization of phenolic compounds to seal wounds (trees); decomposition of lignin (polyphenolic)? (fungi): oxidation of benzene diols; belongs to the family of blue copper oxygenases.
Phenylalanine-4-monooxygenase[a]	Ubiquitous (?) intracellular enzyme; has either iron or copper as a cofactor (mammalian enzyme is iron dependent); synthesis of tyrosine and degradation of phenylalanine: hydroxylation of phenylalanine.
Metallothionein[c]	Ubiquitous, intracellular, with traces that are extracellular in body fluids; high cysteine-containing divalent metal ion storage protein that has some superoxide dismutase activity when bound to copper.

[a]Reaction requires molecular mono- or di-oxygen.
[b]6-Hydroxy dopa or pyrroloquinoline quinone is a cofactor for the enzyme.
[c]Also plays nonenzymatic roles (see Table 4).

Ceruloplasmin (like the less abundant extracellular SOD) is positioned to deal with oxygen radicals outside cells. Because of a trinuclear cluster of copper atoms plus one or two additional feeder copper atoms, excess electrons are thought to be able to enter and be dissipated. Thus, ceruloplasmin is not an SOD, but rather a scavenger of several types of oxygen radicals.[57,58] Ceruloplasmin is probably bound to cell surface receptors in the plasma membranes of most cells[7,11] and may protect unsaturated fatty acids that are particularly vulnerable to oxidation and destruction by hydroxyl radicals.

Several other copper enzymes are involved in molecular oxygen–requiring reactions that lead to cross-linking or polymerization of amino acids or other substituents. These include the extracellular lysyl oxidase of connective tissue, which is needed for proper maturation of collagen and elastin. As such, it is fundamental to the functioning and formation of connective tissue, including that needed for wound healing and maintaining the integrity of blood vessels (strengthened by elastic fibers). The melanin polymer that protects our skin against excess ultraviolet light and determines the pigmentation of our eyes and hair is formed from tyrosine with the aid of the copper-containing enzyme tyrosinase. (The same enzyme catalyzes reactions with similar but different substrates in plants and other organisms, and its functions there are not well understood.[7]) Ascorbate oxidase and laccase, found in plants and fungi but not in mammals, also may catalyze molecular oxygen-requiring oxidations that lead to polymer formation, as with latex sap (laccase) or wound covering films (ascorbate oxidase).

Table 4. Nonenzymatic functions of copper-binding proteins

Protein	Distribution and function
Albumin	Vertebrates, in blood plasma and extracellular fluids; part of the exchangeable plasma copper pool; carrier of ionic copper in circulation and binder of excess copper; carries a high-affinity N-terminal copper binding site.
Ceruloplasmin	Vertebrates, in blood plasma and extracellular fluids; not part of the exchangeble plasma copper pool; source of copper for cells; scavenger of oxygen radicals; ferroxidase; in terms of reactivity, belongs to the family of blue copper oxygenases that includes laccase and ascorbate oxidase.
Transcuprein	Vertebrates?, in blood plasma; part of the exchangeable plasma copper pool; binds copper with even higher affinity than albumin; exchanges copper with albumin.
Metallothioneins	Ubiquitous, intracellular, with traces that are extracellular in body fluids; high-cysteine divalent metal ion storage protein: affinity for Cu^{2+} is higher than that for most other metal ions.
Factors V and VIII	Mammals, extracellular in blood plasma; nonenzyme proteins necessary for blood clotting; portions homologous to ceruloplasmin.
Cartilage matrix glycoprotein	Mammals, intracellular substituent of chondrocytes and some other cells; considerable homology with ceruloplasmin; like lysyl oxidase, appears to support connective tissue function.
Hemocyanin	Molluscs and arthropods, in the circulatory fluid; substitutes for hemoglobin in carrying oxygen (bound to pairs of copper atoms); belongs to the tyrosinase family of blue copper monooxygenases.
Plastocyanin	Plants, in chloroplasts; part of the electron transport system used in photosynthesis: transfers electrons from cytochrome b_6-f to photosystem I.

The formation and inactivation of hormones appears to be another copper enzyme–catalyzed function. Biosynthesis of the catecholamines epinephrine (released from the adrenal medulla in stress) and norepinephrine (the major neurotransmitter of the sympathetic nervous system) is dependent on hydroxylation of dopamine by dopamine-β-monooxygenase (hence the previous name, dopamine-β-hydroxylase). Maturation of several neuropeptide hormones in the anterior pituitary of mammals requires the partial removal of a C-terminal glycine residue, leaving the glycine amino nitrogen as an amide group attached to the carboxylate of the next-to-last amino acid. This reaction is carried out by an α-amidating enzyme. The inactivation of several bioactive amines, including the monoamines histamine, tyramine, dopamine, and serotonin and the diamines spermidine and putrescine, is thought to be catalyzed by extracellular and intracellular copper-dependent amine and diamine oxidases. Copper may also aid in the action of some small peptide hormones (the enkephalins) by helping them to achieve an optimal conformation for binding to their receptors.[59,60]

There is good evidence that copper enzymes are also important for normal metabolism and functioning of iron in the mammal. Cu/Zn SOD is an important enzyme for erythrocytes (which are particularly exposed to oxygen), but in addition, ceruloplasmin and another copper-dependent enzyme (ferroxidase II) may both play a role in the flow of iron that supports hematopoiesis. The hypothesis is that iron released from storage sites (such as liver ferritin) would be in the Fe^{2+} valence state and that ceruloplasmin (also known as ferroxidase I) and ferroxidase II

oxidize this iron to Fe^{3+} so that it can bind to its transfer protein in the plasma.[61] (Transferrin only binds Fe^{3+}.) A low activity of the ferroxidases would thus result in a diminished flow of iron back to the bone marrow and thus reduce the rate of erythrocyte formation.

Almost without exception, copper-dependent enzymes catalyze reactions that involve molecular oxygen (Table 3), and the exceptions mostly involve oxygen radicals. Several of the enzymes also have (or may have) the recently discovered 6-hydroxy dopa or pyrroloquinoline quinone as a cofactor (Table 3). The enzymes can also be partially grouped according to the state and number of their copper atoms. There are the blue copper proteins, with multiple copper atoms in at least three different liganded states (types 1, 2, and 3), exemplified by ceruloplasmin, laccase, and ascorbate oxidase (as well as plastocyanin). This group appears to contain a three-atom copper cluster that is involved in electron transfer and is the site for binding of the oxygen (except in plastocyanin). One or two additional blue copper atoms are thought to feed in electrons from the periphery of the proteins. Although there is copper ligation and reaction homology, little amino acid sequence homology is noted among these proteins. The other group is that of the hemocyanins and tyrosinases, which have at their active center a pair of type 3 copper atoms.

As partially described, copper proteins also have several nonenzymatic functions (Table 4), including copper distribution (ceruloplasmin, albumin, transcuprein), temporary storage (metallothioneins), and electron transport (plastocyanin, ceruloplasmin?). Additional functions include oxygen transport in molluscs and arthropods (where hemocyanin substitutes for hemoglobin), blood clotting in mammals and humans (via nonenzymatically active factors V and VIII), and a newly discovered glycoprotein of unknown function in cartilage (cartilage matrix glycoprotein).[62,63] Portions of blood clotting factors and especially cartilage matrix glycoprotein have considerable sequence homology with ceruloplasmin. (Cartilage matrix glycoprotein also has p-phenylene diamine oxidase activity.) Blood clotting factors contain one copper atom, are probably secreted by endothelial cells lining blood vessels, and are activated through cleavage by thrombin.[7]

Copper Deficiency

At the cellular level. From discussion of the functions of copper enzymes and copper-binding proteins in the last section, the effects of copper deficiency in mammals can already be surmised. At the cellular level, deficiency would result in a reduction in the capacity to carry out respiration and oxidative phosphorylation and thus in a deficit in energy supply. This would slow down various cell activities, from active transport to transcription, translation, and other biosynthetic processes. Even in moderate copper deficiency, the activity of cytochrome c oxidase is reduced in cells of several organs, notably liver and heart.[7,64] However, it is also clear that (except perhaps in muscle) normal cells carry an excess capacity and rarely exercise their electron transport systems at maximum rates, so moderate reductions of cytochrome c oxidase activity alone are not likely to be life threatening in the short term.

The next most likely enzymatic activity to be reduced in copper deficiency is that of Cu/Zn SOD, which would be expected to enhance the fragility of cell membranes in general because unsaturated lipids in the cell periphery are particularly vulnerable to oxidative damage. Indeed, deficiency results in a shortened life span of erythrocytes[65,66] and leads to enhanced accumulation of lipid oxidation products in these cells.[67] Although in mammals specialized tissues requiring copper are more likely to be spared, a severe deficiency of copper in cells of the central nervous system and adrenal medulla will depress formation of copper-dependent catecholamines. Reduced levels of norepinephrine (and increased dopamine) and reduced urinary excretion of catecholamine metabolites have been shown in brains of copper-depleted mice and rats.[68–70]

Copper deficiency in animals. When the diet is deficient in copper, abundant studies in animals indicate that three copper proteins are the most immediately affected. Plasma ceruloplasmin concentrations and activities plummet within days of placing rats on a low-copper diet and become undetectable within 1–3 weeks;[7,64] cytosolic SOD in liver and erythrocytes decreases 50% in 1–2 weeks (but decreases by <20% in other tissues); and mitochondrial cytochrome c oxidase decreases dramatically in the heart (>30% in the first week and >50% by 3 weeks) and also decreases in other tissues (20–25% by 3 weeks; in liver ATP production is also impaired).[71] Muscle levels of cytochrome c oxidase may also drop by >50% after several weeks.[64] After maturation of the central nervous system of animals, which occurs early in life, the brain shows much more resistance to dietary copper deprivation. Thus, brain function (including its ability to form ATP) is much less likely to be impaired than that of liver and heart, and only a severe deficiency, developing from deprivation of the mother during fetal development and continuing into the suckling period, results in substantial changes in brain copper enzyme activities and function.[69,72]

When ceruloplasmin concentrations fall to low levels, replenishment of copper lost from cells probably is also markedly reduced. The activity of lysyl oxidase (secreted by connective tissue cells) in bone, lung, and other tissues is especially vulnerable to copper deficiency,[73] and repletion is particularly responsive to intravenous ceruloplasmin administration.[74] (Intracellular enzymes may be less vulnerable because they are not lost from cells by secretion and the intracellular copper can be recycled.) Thus, one of the hallmarks of severe copper deficiency in mammals is the loss of integrity of elastic and connective tissue, resulting in increased fragility of the blood vessel wall, abnormal elastin, vascular lesions (especially in the arteries), and a greater likelihood of aneurysms. An additional copper-influenced phenomenon involving blood vessels may be angiogenesis, which is the development of the vascular system of blood vessels and capillaries. In some systems (in vivo and in vitro) angiogenesis has been stimulated by copper complexes, particularly of copper with heparin.[75] Amine oxidase-dependent remodeling may also be involved.[76] In sheep, where pigmentation and structure of the wool depend on sufficient copper, a reduction in its availability results in less tyrosinase activity and alters color. (Hair structure in humans is also changed in the copper deficiency of Menkes disease, resulting in stiffness and kinking.) A reduction in tyrosinase activity and alteration of wool in sheep also appears to be the particular consequence of their grazing on forage high in molybdenum and sulfur. The stable thiomolybdates of copper formed, though absorbed and circulating, do not release copper and prevent its availability for biological functions.[77,78]

A major effect of long-term copper deficiency usually is the development of a hypochromic, microcytic anemia that is reversed by copper administration.[15,66,79,80] A deficiency of white blood cells (leukopenia) and a reduction in the rate of granulopoiesis also occur. Possible reasons for the anemia include a decrease in the availability of copper for formation of erythrocyte Cu/Zn

SOD, an enzyme that accounts for much of the copper in erythrocytes.[7] Whether this results in feedback inhibition of erythropoiesis (as with iron) is unknown. The relative lack of SOD in these cells (along with the great reduction in circulating ceruloplasmin that also occurs) is accompanied by a shortening of the erythrocyte life span,[66] which is thought to result from an enhanced vulnerability of the cell membrane to oxidative damage. The decreased erythropoiesis of copper deficiency is accompanied by a decrease in the content and biosynthesis of heme in reticulocyte mitochondria.[65] (Decreases in heme formation were also documented in liver and brain as a consequence of copper deficiency.[81]) Nevertheless, the effect of copper deprivation is not due to a need for copper on the part of the enzymes of porphyrin and heme biosynthesis, nor is it due to a lack of iron in the mitochondria (as might be expected from decreases in iron flow to bone marrow). It is therefore still unknown just where the defect lies, and a decreased rate of ATP formation (that is due to a lower respiratory capacity) could conceivably be involved.

Two other aspects of iron metabolism may be vulnerable. First, as mentioned in the last section, ceruloplasmin can oxidize Fe^{2+}, which may be required for binding of iron (as Fe^{3+}) to plasma transferrin, because iron may be released as Fe^{2+} from intracellular ferritin upon reduction and chelation. (There is some evidence that mucosal iron crossing the basolateral membrane and entering the portal blood is also mostly Fe^{2+}.[82]) In any event, there is considerable evidence in animal models that copper deficiency results in the accumulation of iron in liver[7] and that this is accompanied by a reduction in transferrin iron saturation, at least in the initial stages.[65,83] There is also evidence for[82,83] and against[15] a reduction in release of diet-derived mucosal iron into blood. Intravascular infusion of ceruloplasmin apparently causes an almost immediate release of liver iron to transferrin in the circulation, as shown in pigs and dogs.[15,84–87] Ceruloplasmin has an effect on intestinal iron release in rats;[82] the effect is so rapid that ceruloplasmin synthesis or entry into cells cannot be involved. Possibly an iron transporter in the plasma membrane requires ceruloplasmin as a cofactor (oxidizing agent) for release of the iron. In yeast, a ceruloplasmin homologue (FET3) positioned on the outside of the cell membrane was found to be necessary for the efflux of iron.[88,89] The recent discovery of a defective ceruloplasmin gene in a patient with hemosiderosis reemphasizes the apparent importance of this protein to mammalian iron flux.[27]

In any event, many unresolved questions and contradictory findings underline our lack of exact knowledge about the mechanisms of this copper deficiency effect. Although as little as 1% of the normal ceruloplasmin concentration is sufficient to maintain the normal outflow of iron from liver,[7] anemia can occur even when there is still some ceruloplasmin.[66] Very low ceruloplasmin concentrations do not necessarily lead to anemia, as shown by Prohaska[90,91] in mice and by Fields et al.[92,93] in rats. Thus, it appears the two phenomena can be dissociated.

A final phenomenon often observed during copper deficiency, which may also be linked to iron, is cardiac hypertrophy, involving hypertrophy of cardiac mitochondria. The mitochondrial swelling may be linked to a dysfunction of electron transport (from reduced cytochrome c oxidase activity).[94] As shown in rats, and also in pigs and humans, the heart can exhibit electrocardiographic changes[95,96] and a decreased production of ventricular norepinephrine.[72,97] The anemia of copper deficiency may in itself be a factor in the development of these symptoms. Studies in mice showed that anemia precedes development of cardiac hypertrophy,[72] and Fields et al.[97] found that transfusion of erythrocytes into copper-deficient rats will reverse it. However, this may be only part of the story, because antioxidants also protect against the hypertrophy,[98] and a reduction in copper enzyme-dependent antioxidant activity resulting in membrane damage may also be occurring.

In addition, alterations in lipid and glucose metabolism have also been observed to occur in copper deficiency, although the exact role of copper (and indeed, whether it has any direct role) is still to be determined. Symptoms observed are hypercholesterolemia and hypertriacylglyceridemia as well as glucose intolerance and enhanced sorbitol production. The inconsistency of observations by different investigators about the development of elevated blood cholesterol and triacylglycerol suggests that other factors are not being controlled and may be more directly involved.[7] Concerning the carbohydrates, although the pancreas tends to be damaged in copper deficiency, perhaps through increased peroxidation, this is true for the exocrine part and not for the cells that secrete and release insulin.[7,99] One area that may help to explain some long-term effects of copper deficiency, such as insulin resistance and diabetes-like effects, concerns formation of sugar alcohols. These are implicated in much of the pathology of long-term diabetes, perhaps through the formation of protein adducts that can induce autoimmune responses.[100] Fields et al.[101] and Lewis et al.[102] reported increases in tissue sorbitol concentrations in copper-deficient rats on high-fructose diets. Nevertheless, the activities of the enzymes responsible for sorbitol production or removal (aldose reductase and sorbitol dehydrogenase) apparently are not dependent on dietary copper status.

Finally, both fertility and immunity may depend in some way upon copper sufficiency. O'Dell et al.[103] first determined that copper-deficient rats produced markedly fewer offspring and that the pups were born with impaired hematopoiesis and abnormally developed bone and vasculature. These symptoms may all be explained by the needs for copper-dependent enzymes and processes already addressed, including effects on heme biosynthesis, maturation of collagen and elastic fibers (as well as angiogenesis) involved in vascular development, and bone formation. In addition, sperm motility is reduced with copper deficiency, which may be due to decreases in cytochrome c oxidase leading to less ATP availability.[7,104] With regard to immunity, an increased susceptibility to infection in copper deficiency was first reported by Prohaska and Lukasewycz[105] in mice and Boyne and Arthur[106] in steers. Since then, many studies have confirmed and extended the observations. There appear to be hyporesponsiveness of lymphoid cells to mitogens;[107] decreased production of antibodies;[108] decreased activity of natural killer cells;[108] decreased thymus weight, levels of thymic hormone, and splenic T cells;[109,110,111,112] and decreased antimicrobial activity of phagocytes.[7] Again, it is unclear whether these effects are specific for immune cells, involving as yet unknown copper-dependent factors, or whether they are mainly a response to decreased energy availability plus increased oxidative damage induced by lack of cytochrome c oxidase and SOD, respectively.

Copper deficiency in humans. Most of the obvious symptoms of copper deficiency already described for animals have also been observed in humans, beginning with the anemia, leukopenia, and especially neutropenia;[66,113–115] decreases in ceruloplasmin and erythrocyte Cu/Zn SOD;[116] hypercholesterolemia;[117,118] increased turnover of erythrocytes;[66] and development of abnormal electrocardiographic patterns.[96] There is no reason to believe that humans differ significantly in their responses from those of other mammals.

Requirement

There is no set requirement for intake of dietary copper (no recommended dietary allowance), although 2.0–3.0 mg is considered to be a safe and adequate intake for human adults, with lower suggested intakes for infants and children (Table 5).[119] In terms of overall dietary concentration, the intake recommended for humans is on the low end of that recommended for animals, including larger animals such as sheep and pigs. This difference may reflect the more rapid growth rates of the animal species indicated and the customary composition of the diets on which they are raised. In any event, the two- to threefold higher concentrations of copper in animal feeds are unlikely to be toxic to humans.

Actual intakes of copper by human adults on self-selected diets have been variously estimated at slightly more than 1 mg/day, on average, but vary considerably (0.6–1.6 mg/day);[7] one study recorded values of 1.2–1.3 mg for men and 0.9–1.2 mg/day for women.[9] Intakes

Table 5. Estimated safe and adequate daily dietary intakes of copper recommended for humans and animals[a]

Species	Age (years)	Recommended intake (μg/g diet)	(mg/day)
Humans	0–0.5		0.5–0.7
	0.5–1		0.7–1.0
	1–3		1.0–1.5
	4–6		1.5–2.0
	7–21		2.0–3.0
	>21	2–3	2.0–3.0
Rabbits		3	
Mice		4.5	
Rats		5	
Pigs, sheep, cats		5	
Dogs		7.3	

[a]From Solomons.[119]

required to achieve zero balance were reported as 1.2–1.3 mg in 1980,[120] but more recent studies with young men and women on diets of 0.8–7.5 mg/day[121] indicated that even at the low intakes copper balance appeared to be maintained for the 42 days of the study. Moreover, there appeared to be an adaptation to levels of intake, so that there was a greater efficiency of absorption at lower intakes, and vice versa. Thus, actual needs may be <1 mg/day for adults, which is very close to values for actual consumption. (Indeed, there is little evidence of copper deficiency within the populations of industrialized nations.) At the same time, there appears to be no harm in having a higher intake, such as the levels estimated to be safe and adequate for humans and animals (Table 5).[119]

Food and Other Sources of Copper

Almost all of the copper entering the digestive tract of humans comes from solid rather than liquid foods or water. Food sources vary ≈100-fold, from values as low as 0.3 μg/g in some vegetables to values as high as 37 μg/g in nuts and shellfish.[7] In general, oysters and other shellfish have the highest concentrations (averaging 12–37 μg/g); then nuts (3–37 μg/g); grains, other seeds, and legumes (3–8 μg/g); fish (2–3 μg/g); poultry (0.5–3 μg/g); vegetables (0.3–3 μg/g); fruits (0.4–1.5 μg/g); and muscle meats (0.9–1 μg/g). In seeds and other grains, the bran and germ have most of the element, and thus the refining of flour removes most of the copper originally present. Despite copper piping, only trace amounts normally leach into the drinking water.[11]

Copper Excess and Toxicity

Copper is relatively nontoxic to most mammals and birds, including rodents, poultry, pigs, and humans.

Excess intakes of copper causing acute or even chronic toxic effects are rare. Nevertheless, there have been instances when children accidentally ingested $CuSO_4$ used as a pesticide on certain crops[122] and when there has been more chronic excess intake, as in the case of "Indian childhood cirrhosis."[23] In the latter instance it was determined that some of the women in India heated milk formula in brass pots that leached a great deal of the metal into the liquid. This resulted in the development of liver cirrhosis, one of the most common symptoms of copper toxicosis. The same pathology is observed when animals are chronically fed excessive amounts of copper (e.g., 2000 $\mu g/g$ in pig feed)[123,124] and when inherited defects in copper excretion result in accumulation of the metal in liver and other tissues (e.g., in Wilson disease in humans,[11] in Long Evans Cinnamon rats,[125] and in many dogs [Bedlington terriers in particular][31]). Sheep are more sensitive than most other mammals.[122] With very high intakes (such as 2000 $\mu g/g$), the digestive tract is also injured[124] and there is damage to additional internal organs, including the kidney (renal tubules) and brain. Hemolysis of erythrocytes can occur and is a major response to acute toxic doses.[126]

Most toxic effects of copper probably result from the production of oxygen radicals by Cu^+ chelates, such as when ascorbate reduces Cu^{2+}.[38,127,128] (The toxic effects of the herbicide paraquat has even been ascribed to such a complex.[38,129]) In liver, the first recipient of most of the incoming dietary copper, damage from oxygen radicals causes scar tissue to form, leading to changes in tissue architecture and a reduction in liver function. Scarring of other tissues and damage to cell membranes (e.g., in kidney tubules and erythrocytes) will lead to cell lysis and connective tissue deposition.

Summary

Copper is an essential nutrient needed for the function of many important enzymes, electron transporters, and other factors. One of these (cytochrome c oxidase) is fundamental to generation of usable ATP energy by almost all living cells; others play major roles in the protection of cells and cell membranes against oxidative damage, the integrity of connective tissue and blood vessels, the formation of skin and hair pigments, the production of neurotransmitters and other hormones, and perhaps also in aspects of iron metabolism involving heme biosynthesis and flux of iron out of critical sites in liver and intestine. The fact that copper has such ubiquitous and basic biochemical roles in metabolism potentially places all cells in jeopardy when a dietary deficiency arises.

In contrast to some other metals, notably iron, copper is relatively easily absorbed and excreted from the body. Foods have a wide range of copper concentrations, but normal dietary intakes appear to be in the range of requirements. Overt deficiencies are very rare. Excess intakes are relatively well tolerated within a 10–100-fold range. Toxic intakes hardly ever occur. No recommended dietary allowance has been established, but doses of 2–3 mg/day are considered safe and adequate.

References

1. Nriagu JO (1980) Zinc in the environment. Health effects (Part 2). Wiley, New York, p 480
2. Owen CA Jr (1982) Biochemical aspects of copper: copper deficiency and toxicity. Physiological aspects of copper. Noyes, Park Ridge, NJ
3. McHargue JS (1927) The proportion and significance of copper, iron, manganese and zinc in some molluscs and crustaceans. Trans Kentucky Acad Sci 2:46–52
4. McHargue JS (1927) Significance of the occurrence of manganese, copper, zinc, nickel, and cobalt in Kentucky blue grass. Indust Eng Chem 19:274–276
5. Hart EB, Steenbock H, Waddell J, Elvehjem CA (1928) Iron in nutrition: copper as a supplement to iron for hemoglobin building in the rat. J Biol Chem 77:797–812
6. Hoagland DR (1932) Mineral nutrition in plants. Annu Rev Biochem 1:618–636
7. Linder M (1991) The biochemistry of copper. Plenum, New York
8. Stevenson EJ (1986) Cycles of soil. Wiley-Interscience, New York
9. Johnson PE, Milne DB, Lykken GI (1992) Effect of age and sex on copper absorption, biological half-life, and status in humans. Am J Clin Nutr 1992;56:917–925
10. Turnlund JR, Keyes WR, Anderson HL, Acord LL (1989) Copper absorption and retention in young men at three levels of dietary copper using the stable isotope, ^{65}Cu. Am J Clin Nutr 49:870–878
11. Linder MC, Hazegh-Azam M (1995) Copper biochemistry and molecular biology. In Oliveras M, Uauy R (eds), WHO report on copper and health, in press
12. Mercer J, Livingston J, Hall B, et al (1993) Isolation of a partial candidate gene for Menkes disease by positional cloning. Nature Genet 3:20–25.
13. Vulpe C, Levinson B, Whitney S, et al (1993) Isolation of a candidate gene for Menkes disease and evidence that it encodes a copper-transporting ATPase. Nature Genet 3:7–13
14. Chelly J, Tumer Z, Tonnesen T, et al (1993) Isolation of a candidate gene for Menkes disease that encodes a potential heavy metal binding protein. Nature Genet 3:14–19
15. Linder MC (1993) Interactions between copper and iron in mammalian metabolism. In Elsenhans B, Forth W, Schumann K (eds), Metal-metal interactions. Bertelsmann Foundation, Gutersloh, Germany, pp 11–41
16. Yu S, West CE, Beynen AC (1994) Increasing intakes of iron reduce status, absorption and biliary excretion of copper in rats. Br J Nutr 71:887–895
17. Van Campen DR, Gross E (1968) Influence of ascorbic acid on the absorption of copper by rats. J Nutr 95:617–622
18. Owen CA Jr (1965) Metabolism of radiocopper (Cu^{64}) in the rat. Am J Physiol 209:900–904
19. Weiss KC, Linder MC, Los Alamos Radiological Medicine Group (1985) Copper transport in rats involving a new plasma protein. Am J Physiol 249:E77–E88
20. Walshe JM (1983) Hudson Memorial Lecture: Wilson's dis-

ease: genetics and biochemistry—their relevance to therapy. J Inher Metab Dis 6:51–58

21. Scott KC, Turnlund JR (1994) Compartment model of copper metabolism in adult men. J Nutr Biochem 5:342–350

22. Wirth PL, Linder MC (1985) Distribution of copper among components of human serum. J Natl Cancer Inst 75:277–284

23. Barrow L, Tanner MS (1988) Copper distribution among serum proteins in paediatric liver disorders and malignancies. Eur J Clin Invest 18:555–560

24. Harris, ED (1991) Copper transport: an overview. Proc Soc Exp Biol Med 37:130–140

25. Percival SS, Harris ED (1990) Copper transport from ceruloplasmin: characterization of the cellular uptake mechanism. Am J Physiol 258:C140–C146

26. Lee SH, Lancey R, Montaser A, et al (1993) Transfer of copper from mother to fetus during the latter part of gestation in the rat. Proc Soc Exp Biol Med 203:428–439

27. Yoshida K, Furihata K, Takeda S, et al (1995) A mutation in the ceruloplasmin gene is associated with systemic hemosiderosis in humans. Nature Genet 9:267–272

28. Breslow E (1964) Comparison of cupric ion-binding sites in myoglobin derivatives and serum albumin. J Biol Chem 239:3252–3259

29. Lau SJ, Sarkar B (1971) Ternary co-ordination complex between human serum albumin, copper(II) and histidine. J Biol Chem 246:5938–5943

30. Vargas EJ, Shoho AR, Linder MC (1994) Copper transport in the Nagase analbuminemic rat. Am J Physiol 267:G259–G269

31. Montaser A, Tetreault C, Linder MC (1992) Comparison of copper binding proteins in dog serum with those in other species. Proc Soc Exp Biol Med 200:321–329

32. Tsai MT, Dinh CT, Linder MC (1992) Interactions of transcuprein and albumin in copper transport [abstract]. FASEB J 6:922

33. May PM, Linder PW, Williams DR (1977) Computer simulation of metal-ion equilibria in biofluids: models for the low-molecular-weight complex distribution of calcium(II), magnesium(II), manganese(II), iron(III), copper(II), zinc(II), and lead(II) ions In human blood plasma. J Chem Soc 588–594

34. Ettinger MJ, Darwish HM, Schmitt RC (1986) Mechanism of copper transport from plasma to hepatocytes. Fed Proc 45:2800–2804

35. McArdle HJ, Guthrie JR, Ackland ML, Danks DM (1987) Albumin has no role in the uptake of copper by human fibroblasts. J Inorg Biochem 31:123–131

36. Linder MC, Roboz M (1986) Turnover and excretion of copper in rats as measured with [67]Cu. Am J Physiol 251:E551–E555

37. Yagle MK, Palmiter RD (1985) Coordinate regulation of mouse metallothionein-I and metallothionein-II genes by heavy metal glucocorticoids. Mol Cell Biol 5:291–294

38. Kadiiska MB, Hanna PM, Mason RP (1993) In vivo ESR spin trapping evidence for hydroxyl radical-mediated toxicity of paraquat and copper in rats. Toxicol Appl Pharmacol 123:187–192

39. Goresky CA, Holmes TH, Sass-Kortsak A (1968) The initial uptake of copper by the liver in the dog. Can J Physiol Pharmacol 46:771–784

40. Linder MC, Munro HN (1973) Iron and copper metabolism in development. Enzyme 15:111–138

41. Yamaguchi Y, Heiny ME, Gitlin JD (1993) Isolation and characterization of a human liver cDNA as a candidate gene for Wilson disease. Biochem Biophys Res Commun 197:271–277

42. Bull PC, Thomas GR, Rommens JM, et al (1993) The Wilson disease gene is a putative copper transporting P-type ATPase similar to the Menkes gene. Nature Genet 5:327–337

43. Tanzi RE, Petrukhin K, Chernov I, et al (1993) The Wilson disease gene is a copper transporting ATPase with homology to the Menkes disease gene. Nature Genet 5:344–348

44. Gross JB, Myers BM, Kost LJ, Kuntz SM, LaRusso NF (1989) Biliary copper excretion by hepatocyte lysosomes in the rat. J Clin Invest 83:30–39

45. Gollan JL (1975) Studies on the nature of complexes formed by copper with human alimentary secretions and their influence on copper absorption in the rat. Clin Sci Mol Med 49:237–245

46. Farrer PA, Mistilis SP (1968) Copper metabolism in the rat: studies of the biliary excretion and intestinal absorption of ^{64}Cu-labeled copper. Birth Defects 4:14–22

47. Kressner MS, Stockert RJ, Morell AG, Sternlieb I (1984) Origins of biliary copper. Hepatology 4:867–870

48. Gregoriadis G, Morell AG, Sternlieb I, Scheinberg IH (1970) Catabolism of desialylated ceruloplasmin in the liver. J Biol Chem 245:5833–5837

49. van den Hamer CJA, Morell AG, Scheinberg IH (1970) Physical and chemical studies on ceruloplasmin. IX. The role of galactosyl residues in the clearance of ceruloplasmin from the circulation. J Biol Chem 245:4397–4402

50. Stockert RK, Haimes HB, Morell AG (1980) Endocytosis of asialoglycoprotein enzyme conjugates by hepatocytes. Lab Invest 43:556–563

51. Omoto E, Tavassoli M (1989) The role of endosomal traffic in the transendothelial transport of ceruloplasmin in the liver. Biochem Biophys Res Commun 162:554–561

52. Chowrimootoo GFE, Seymour CA (1994) The role of caeruloplasmin in copper excretion. Biochem Soc Trans 22:190S

53. Harada M, Sakisaka S, Yoshitake M, et al (1993) Biliary copper excretion in acutely and chronically copper-loaded rats. Hepatology 17:111–117

54. Bermingham-McDonogh O, Gralla EB, Valentine JS (1988) The copper, zinc superoxide dismutase gene of *Saccharomyces cerevisiae*: cloning, sequencing, and biological activity. Proc Natl Acad Sci USA 85:4789–4793

55. Felix K, Lengfelder E, Hartmann HJ, Weser U (1993) A pulse radiolytic study on the reaction of hydroxyl and superoxide radicals with yeast Cu(I)-thionein. Biochim Biophys Acta 1203:104–108

56. Sato M, Bremner I (1993) Oxygen free radicals and metallothionein. Free Radic Biol Med 14:325–337

57. Goldstein IM, Charo IF (1982) Ceruloplasmin: an acute phase reactant and anti-oxidant. Lymphokines 8:373–411

58. Gutteridge JMC (1985) Inhibition of the Fenton reaction by the protein caeruloplasmin and other copper complexes: assessment of ferroxidase and radical scavenging activities. Chem Biol Interact 56:113–120

59. Sadee W, Pfeiffer A, Herz A (1982) Opiate receptor: multiple effects of metal ions. J Neurochem 39:659–667

60. Pettit LD, Formicka-Koslowska G (1982) A suggested role for copper in the biological activity of neuropeptides. Neurol Sci Lett 50:53–56

61. Frieden E (1986) Perspectives on copper biochemistry. Clin Physiol Biochem 4:11–19

62. Fife RS, Kluve-Beckerman B, Houser DS, et al (1993) Evidence that a 550,000 dalton cartilage matrix glycoprotein is a chondrocyte membrane associated protein closely related to ceruloplasmin. J Biol Chem 268:4407–4411

63. Fife RS, Moody S, Houser D, Proctor C (1994) Studies of

copper transport in cultured bovine chondrocytes. Biochim Biophys Acta 1201:19–22

64. Paynter DI, Moir RJ, Underwood EJ (1979) Changes in activity of the Cu-Zn superoxide dismutase enzyme in tissues of the rat with changes in dietary copper. J Nutr 109:1570–1576

65. Williams DM, Loukopoulos D, Lee GR, Cartwright GE (1976) Role of copper in mitochondrial iron metabolism. Blood 48:77–85

66. Hirase N, Abe Y, Sadamura S, et al (1992) Anemia and neutropenia in a case of copper deficiency: role of copper in normal hematopoiesis. Acta Haematol 87:195–197

67. Jain SK, Williams DM (1988) Copper deficiency anemia: altered red blood cell lipids and viscosity in rats. Am J Clin Nutr 48:637–640

68. Prohaska JR, Cox DA (1983) Decreased brain ascorbate levels in copper-deficient mice and in brindled mice. J Nutr 113:2623–2629

69. Prohaska JR, Bailey WR (1994) Regional specificity in alteration of rat brain copper and catecholamines following perinatal copper deficiency. J Neurochem 63:1551–1557

70. Morgan RF, O'Dell BL (1977) Effect of copper deficiency on the concentrations of catecholamines and related enzyme activities in the rat brain. J Neurochem 28:207–213

71. Weisenberg E, Harbreich A, Mager J (1980) Biochemical lesions in copper-deficient rats caused by secondary iron deficiency: derangement of protein synthesis and impairment of energy metabolism. Biochem J 188:633–641

72. Gross AM, Prohaska JR (1990) Copper-deficient mice have higher cardiac norepinephrine turnover. J Nutr 120:88–96

73. Rucker RB, Riggins RS, Laughlin R, et al (1975) Effects of nutritional copper deficiency on the biomechanical properties of bone and arterial elastin in the chick. J Nutr 105:1062–1067

74. Dameron CT, Harris ED (1987) Regulation of aortic CuZn-superoxide dismutase with copper: ceruloplasmin and albumin re-activate and transfer copper to the enzyme in culture. Biochem J 248:669–675

75. Alessandri G, Raju K, Gullino PM (1983) Mobilization of capillary endothelium in vitro induced by effectors of angiogenesis in vivo. Cancer Res 43:1790–1797

76. Ziche M, Jones J, Gullino PM (1987) Role of prostaglandin E1 and copper in angiogenesis. J Natl Cancer Inst 69:475–482

77. Suttle NF (1980) The role of thiomolybdates in the nutritional interactions of copper, molybdenum, and sulphur: fact of fantasy? Ann NY Acad Sci 355:195–205

78. Mason J (1982) The putative role of thiomolybdates in the pathogenesis of Mo-induced hypocupraemia and molybdenosis: some recent developments. Ir Vet J 36:164–166

79. Lahey ME, Gubler CJ, Chase MS, et al (1952) Studies on copper metabolism. II. Hematologic manifestations of copper deficiency in swine. Blood 7:1053–1074

80. Fujita M, Itakura T, Takagi Y, Okada A (1989) Copper deficiency during total parenteral nutrition: clinical analysis of three cases. J Parent Enter Nutr 13:421–425

81. Prohaska JR (1988) Biochemical functions of copper in animals. In Prasad AS (ed), Essential and toxic trace elements in human health and disease. Alan R Liss, New York, pp 105–124

82. Wollenberg P, Mahlberg R, Rummel W (1990) The valency state of absorbed iron appearing in the portal blood and ceruloplasmin substitution. Biol Metals 3:1–7

83. Lee GR, Nacht S, Lukens JN, Cartwright GE (1968) Iron metabolism in copper-deficient swine. J Clin Invest 47:2058–2069

84. Ragan HA, Nacht S, Lee GR, et al (1969) Effect of ceruloplasmin on plasma iron in copper deficient swine. Am J Physiol 217:1320–1323

85. Osaki S, Johnson DA (1969) Mobilization of liver iron by ferroxidase (ceruloplasmin). J Biol Chem 244:5757–5766

86. Osaki S, Johnson DA, Frieden E (1966) The possible significance of the ferrous oxidase activity of ceruloplasmin in normal human serum. J Biol Chem 241:2746–2751

87. Roeser HP, Lee GR, Nacht S, Cartwright GE (1970) The role of ceruloplasmin in iron metabolism. J Clin Invest 49:2408–2417

88. Askwith CE, Eide D, Van Ho A, et al (1994) The FET3 gene of S. cerevisiae encodes a multicopper oxidase required for ferrous iron uptake. Cell 76:403–410

89. Dancis A, Yuan DS, Moehle C, et al (1994) Molecular characterization of a copper transport protein in S. cerevisiae: an unexpected role for copper in iron transport. Cell 76:393–402

90. Prohaska JR (1981) Comparison between dietary and genetic copper deficiency in mice: copper dependent anemia. Nutr Res 1:159–167

91. Prohaska JR (1984) Repletion of copper-deficient mice and brindled mice with copper or iron. J Nutr 114:422–430

92. Fields M, Holbrook J, Scholfield J, et al (1986) Effect of fructose or starch on copper-67 absorption and excretion by the rat. J Nutr 116:625–632

93. Fields M, Holbrook J, Scholfield J, et al (1986) Development of copper deficiency in rats fed fructose or starch: weekly measurements of copper indices in blood. Proc Soc Exp Biol Med 181:120–124

94. Bode AM, Miller LA, Faber J, Saari JT (1992) Mitochondrial respiration in heart, liver, and kidney of copper-deficient rats. J Nutr Biochem 3:668–672

95. Kopp SJ, Klevay LM, Feliksik JM (1983) Physiologic and metabolic characterization of a cardiomyopathy induced by chronic copper deficiency. Am J Physiol 245:H855–H859

96. Klevay LM (1985) Atrial thrombosis, abnormal electrocardigrams and sudden death in mice due to copper deficiency. Atherosclerosis 54:213–224

97. Fields M, Lewis CG, Lure MD (1991) Anemia plays a major role in cardiac hypertrophy of copper deficiency. Metab Clin Exp 40:1–3

98. Johnson WT, Saari JT (1989) Dietary supplementation with t-butylhydroquinone reduces cardiac hypertrophy and anemia associated with copper deficiency in rats. Nutr Res 9:1355–1662

99. Lewis CG, Fields M, Craft N, et al (1987) Changes in pancreatic enzyme specific activities of rats fed a high-fructose, low-copper diet. J Am Coll Nutr 7:27–34

100. Linder MC (1991) Nutritional biochemistry and metabolism. New York, Elsevier

101. Fields M, Lewis CG, Beal T (1989) Accumulation of sorbitol in copper deficiency: dependency on gender and type of dietary carbohydrate. Metab Clin Exp 38:371–375

102. Lewis CG, Fields M, Beal T (1990) Effect of changing the type of dietary carbohydrate or copper level of copper-deficient, fructose-fed rats on tissue sorbitol concentrations. J Nutr Biochem 1:160–166

103. O'Dell BL, Hardwick BC, Reynolds G (1961) Mineral deficiencies of milk and congenital malformations in the rat. J Nutr 73:151–156

104. Morisawa M, Mohri H (1972) Heavy metals and spermatozoan motility. I. Distribution of iron, zinc and copper in sea urchin spermatozoa. Exp Cell Res 70:311–315

105. Prohaska JR, Lukasewycz OA (1981) Copper deficiency supresses the immune response of mice. Science 213:559–561

106. Boyne R, Arthur JR (1981) Effects of selenium and copper deficiency on neutrophil function in cattle. J Comp Pathol 91:271–276

107. Kramer TR, Johnson WT, Briske-Anderson M (1988) Influence of iron and the sex of rats on hematological, biochemical, and immunological changes during copper deficiency. J Nutr 118:214–221

108. Lukasewycz OA, Prohaska JR (1990) The immune response in copper deficiency. Ann NY Acad Sci 587:147–159

109. Koller LM, Mulhern SA, Frankel NC, et al (1987) Immune dysfunction in rats fed a diet deficient in copper. Am J Clin Nutr 45:997–1006

110. Mulhern SA, Koller LM (1988) Severe or marginal copper deficiency results in a graded reduction in immune system status of mice. J Nutr 118:1041–1047

111. Vyas D, Chandra RK (1983) Thymic factor activity, lymphocyte stimulation response and antibody producing cells in copper deficiency. Nutr Res 3:343–349

112. Lukasewycz OA, Prohaska JR, Meyer SG, et al (1985) Alterations in lymphocyte subpopulations in copper-deficient mice. Infect Immun 48:644–647

113. Dunlap WM, James GW III, Hume DM (1974) Anemia and neutropenia caused by copper deficiency. Ann Intern Med 80:470–476

114. Vilter RW, Ozian RC, Hess RC, et al (1974) Manifestations of copper deficiency in a patient with systemic sclerosis on intravenous hyperalimentation. N Engl J Med 291:188–191

115. Zidar BL, Shadduck RK, Ziegler Z, Winkelstein A (1977) Observations on the anemia and neutropenia of human copper deficiency. Am J Hematol 3:177–185

116. Klevay LM, Inman L, Johnson LK, et al (1984) Increased cholesterol in plasma in a young man during experimental copper depletion. Metabolism 33:1112–1118

117. Klevay LM, Canfield WK, Gallagher SK, et al (1986) Decreased glucose tolerance in two men during experimental copper depletion. Nutr Rep Int 33:371–382

118. Reiser S, Powell A, Yang CY, Canary JJ (1987) Effect of copper intake on blood cholesterol and its lipoprotein distribution in men. Nutr Rep Intl 36:641–649

119. Solomons N (1988) Zinc and copper. In Shils ME, Young VR (eds), Modern nutrition in health and disease, 7th ed. Lea & Febiger, Philadelphia, pp 238–262

120. Klevay LM, Ceck SJ, Jacob RA, et al (1980) The human requirement for copper. 1. Healthy men fed conventional American diets. Am J Clin Nutr 33:45–50

121. Turnlund JR (1991) Copper absorption and gastrointestinal excretion in humans: the impact of adaptation to dietary copper intake on copper deficiency and toxicity. In Momcilovic B (ed), Trace elements in man and animal (TEMA-7). Institute for Medical Research and Occupational Health of Zagreb, Zagreb, pp 34/1–34/3

122. Davis GK, Mertz W (1987) Copper. In Mertz W (ed), Trace elements in human and animal nutrition, 5th ed, Vol 1. Academic Press, New York, pp 301–364

123. Evering W, Haywood S, Brenner I, et al (1991) The protective role of metallothionein in copper overload. In Momcilovic B (ed), Trace elements in man and animal (TEMA-7). Institute for Medical Research and Occupational Health of Zagreb, Zagreb, pp 2/8–2/9

124. Chang WF, Wu FM, Shyu JJ, et al (1991) Clinical and pathological studies of swine copper intoxication. Zhonghua Minguo Shouyi Xuehui Zazhi 18:97–108 (CA 118:249416)

125. Yukitoshi Y, Heiny ME, Shimizu N, et al (1994) Expression of the Wilson disease gene is deficient in the Long-Evans Cinnamon rat. Biochem J 301:1–4

126. Linder MC, Houle PA, Isaacs E, et al (1979) Copper regulation of ceruloplasmin in copper deficient rats. Enzyme 24:23–35

127. Lind SE, McDonagh JR, Smith CJ (1993) Oxidative inactivation of plasmin and other serine proteases by copper and ascorbate. Blood 82:1522–1531

128. Shah MA, Bergethon PR, Boak AM, et al (1992) Oxidation of peptidyl lysine by copper complexes of pyrroloquinoline quinone and other quinones: a model for oxidative pathochemistry. Biochim Biophys Acta 1159:311–318

129. Kadiiska MA, Hanna PM, Jordan SJ, Mason RP (1993) Electron spin resonance evidence for free radical generation in copper-treated vitamin E- and selenium-deficient rats: in vivo spin-trapping investigation. Molec Pharmacol 44:222–227

Chapter 31

Selenium

Orville A. Levander and Raymond F. Burk

In 1957 Schwarz and Foltz[1] showed that traces of dietary selenium prevented liver necrosis in rats deficient in vitamin E. Soon thereafter selenium was used widely in agriculture to prevent a variety of selenium- and vitamin E-responsive conditions in livestock and poultry, such as white muscle disease in sheep and cattle, hepatosis dietetica in swine, exudative diathesis in chickens, and gizzard myopathy in turkeys.[2] Supplementation of feeds with selenium resulted in great economic gains for animal producers.

Signs of selenium deficiency have not been observed in free-living animals whose diets are adequate in vitamin E. A "pure" deficiency of selenium uncomplicated by simultaneous vitamin E deficiency has been seen only in laboratory animals under experimental conditions. Rats fed a low-selenium diet adequate in vitamin E through two generations exhibited poor growth, sparse hair coats, cataracts, and reproductive failure.[3] Nutritional pancreatic atrophy (NPA) was produced in chicks fed amino acid-based diets severely deficient in selenium.[4] NPA was originally considered the only well-documented specific organ lesion resulting from uncomplicated selenium deficiency in any species, but the atrophy was found to respond also to high levels of dietary vitamin E and other antioxidants.[5] NPA can be produced in chicks by feeding a practical-type diet composed of ingredients from a selenium-deficient region of China, but the severity of the atrophy is reduced, thereby suggesting that a factor associated with the practical diet may provide partial protection from NPA in the selenium-deficient chick.[6]

Despite the difficulties encountered in producing a pure selenium deficiency in animals, selenium is considered an essential element for humans. It is a constituent of the enzyme glutathione peroxidase isolated from human red blood cells, and in China selenium deficiency has been associated with two diseases of childhood.[7,8]

Body Compartments

Most selenium in animal tissues is present in two compartments or forms (Figure 1). One of these is selenomethionine, which is incorporated in place of methionine in a variety of proteins, and the other is selenocysteine in selenoproteins such as glutathione peroxidase, iodothyronine deiodinase, and selenoprotein

P. Other forms may be present because tissue selenium has not been fully characterized.

Selenomethionine in tissues is derived from the diet because it cannot be synthesized in the body. This form of selenium is not regulated by the selenium status of the animal and can be regarded as an unregulated storage compartment. When dietary selenium supply is interrupted, turnover of the selenomethionine pool provides selenium to the organism. This has been demonstrated in human beings who moved from areas of high selenium intake to areas of low intake. Blood selenium levels declined slowly for a year before reaching levels typical of the low-selenium area.[9] Glutathione peroxidase activity in red blood cells was similar in subjects residing in the two areas, suggesting that the fall in selenium concentration was at the expense of the selenomethionine compartment, with the selenocysteine compartment being maintained.

Selenocysteine is the form of selenium known to account for its biological activities. Most evidence suggests that the selenocysteine compartment is tightly regulated (see Metabolism section). Such regulation is necessary because this reactive compound would likely interfere with biochemical function if it were free in the cell. Selenocysteine is incorporated into proteins by a specific mechanism, and there is no evidence that it substitutes for cysteine in animal systems. Selenium incorporation into tRNA has been demonstrated, indicating

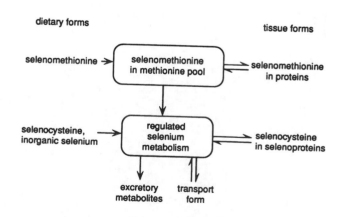

Figure 1. Relationships of dietary forms (left) to tissue forms (right) of selenium. Excretory metabolites and the transport form are also present in tissues but only in relatively small quantities.

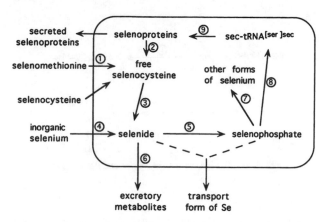

Figure 2. Regulated selenium metabolism. An outline of selenium metabolism is shown based on reactions that are known to take place. The box represents the cell. The circled numbers indicate 1) the transsulfuration pathway, 2) proteolytic breakdown of proteins, 3) selenocysteine β-lyase, 4) reduction by glutathione, 5) selenophosphate synthetase, 6) methylation, 7) replacement of sulfur in tRNA by selenium, 8) replacement of oxygen in serine with selenium to produce selenocysteine, and 9) decoding of UGA in mRNA with insertion of selenocysteine into primary structure of protein. The origin and identity of the transport form of selenium is unknown. It might arise from selenide or selenophosphate as indicated by the broken lines.

that there may be other biologically active forms of the element than selenocysteine.[10]

Methods of Analysis and Assessment of Selenium Status

Selenium concentration can be determined with great accuracy by a variety of methods. Fluorometry, neutron activation analysis, atomic absorption, and mass spectrometry have been used to measure the element in fluids and tissues. Biologically active selenium can be estimated by measuring glutathione peroxidase activity and selenoprotein P concentration.[11,12]

The use of these measurements in the assessment of selenium status requires an understanding of selenium metabolism. As indicated above and illustrated in Figure 1, intake of the element as selenomethionine results in a higher tissue selenium concentration than intake of the same amount of the element in other forms, because some of the selenomethionine will be present in proteins substituting for methionine. Selenium released by catabolism of selenomethionine then will be present as selenocysteine in selenoproteins. Thus, selenium from selenomethionine enters both major tissue selenium compartments.

Intake of the element in inorganic form or in the form of selenocysteine affects only the selenocysteine compartment. This compartment is regulated and measurements of it are useful in detecting selenium deficiency

because selenoprotein concentrations decline in that situation. The selenocysteine compartment is not useful to assess selenium status once the selenium requirement has been met because selenoprotein concentrations are not responsive to excess selenium. Selenoproteins that have been measured to assess the selenocysteine compartment are blood and liver glutathione peroxidase and plasma selenoprotein P.[12]

Additional biochemical changes can be used to judge the severity of selenium deficiency in experimental animals. In the rat, plasma glutathione concentration and liver glutathione S-transferase activity increase in severe selenium deficiency.[11] Concentrations of selenoprotein mRNAs are also affected by selenium deficiency and might be useful in assessing its severity.[13,14]

Metabolism

Seleno amino acids are the principal dietary forms of the element for free-living animals. Selenium is often supplied in inorganic form in experimental diets and in supplements.

Absorption of selenium does not appear to be regulated, and most studies have shown it to be high (>50%). Selenomethionine is absorbed by the same mechanism as methionine, but little is known about selenocysteine absorption. Inorganic selenium absorption is efficient and is not affected by selenium status.[15,16]

Available evidence suggests that selenomethionine follows methionine metabolic pathways. It is not known to have a physiological function separate from that of methionine.

Regulated selenium metabolism is organized to meet several needs. One is to maintain a low free concentration of the highly reactive compound selenocysteine. Selenocysteine is incorporated into proteins by a mechanism over which free selenocysteine has no influence. Another is to achieve selenium homeostasis. The pathway does this by regulating the formation of methylated excretory metabolites.

Figure 2 is an outline of regulated selenium metabolism. Selenium forms entering the pathway are converted to selenide. Selenomethionine derived from the diet or from protein catabolism is converted to selenocysteine by transsulfuration.[17] Selenocysteine derived from selenomethionine, the diet, or selenoprotein catabolism yields selenide via selenocysteine β-lyase.[18] Inorganic selenium (selenite) reacts with glutathione to yield selenide.[19] Thus, selenide appears to be the first common form of selenium in the regulated selenium pathway. It has several potential fates.

One fate of selenide is metabolism to selenophosphate, an anabolic form of the element that appears to be committed to the synthesis of selenoproteins and selenotRNAs. Selenophosphate synthetase carries out this reaction with the consumption of ATP.[20] Selenide is also a substrate for methylation enzymes that produce urinary and breath excretory metabolites of selenium.[21,22] Thus, conversion of selenide to selenophosphate has characteristics of a regulatory reaction. Stimulation of this reaction would increase the proportion of selenide being converted to selenophosphate while decreasing the proportion entering the excretory pathway. This would conserve selenium and is the situation observed in selenium deficiency. Inhibition of the reaction would cause a rise in selenide concentration leading to an increase in selenium excretion. This situation is observed when selenium is available in amounts greater than needed for selenoprotein synthesis. Selenophosphate synthetase cDNA has recently been isolated from a human cDNA library.[20] Study of this enzyme might allow characterization of its regulation.

A small molecule transport form of selenium has been shown to be produced by the intestine and released into the portal blood within minutes of administration of inorganic selenium by gastric tube.[23] The identity of this compound has not been established, but it might arise from selenide or selenophosphate because of its small size and rapid formation. No information is available on production of this transport form of selenium by extraintestinal tissues.

Selenoprotein synthesis has been characterized in prokaryotes, and some of its major features in animals have been established (Figure 3A).[24] tRNA[Ser]Sec, a unique tRNA with the anticodon for UGA, is charged with serine by seryl-tRNA ligase.[27] ser-tRNA[Ser]Sec is converted to sec-tRNA[Ser]Sec by a process requiring selenophosphate (SePO$_3^{3-}$) as substrate. A pyridoxal phosphate enzyme, selenocysteine synthetase, carries out the conversion of serine to selenocysteine in prokaryotes. The same conversion takes place in eukaryotes, but the enzyme catalyzing it has not been identified. The UGA in the open reading frame of the selenoprotein mRNA is decoded with insertion of selenocysteine into the primary structure of the protein. This step requires the SECIS motif in the mRNA (Figure 3B) and one or more protein elongation factors.

Selenoprotein synthesis is regulated transcriptionally by tissue specificity, cell development, and environmental factors.[28-30] Nutritional availability of selenium has important effects on selenoprotein mRNAs through post-transcriptional mechanisms. Liver cellular glutathione peroxidase (GSHPx-1) contains ≈25% of the selenium in the rat.[31] In selenium deficiency the liver GSHPx-1 mRNA concentration decreases more rapidly than does mRNA concentration of other selenoproteins, and for this reason a buffer role for GSHPx-1 has been proposed.[13,14,32] It is postulated that GSHPx-1 is down-regulated so that less abundant, but more essential, selenoproteins can be maintained with the limited selenium available.

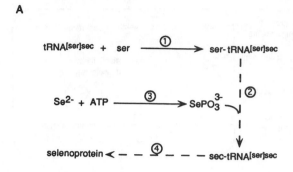

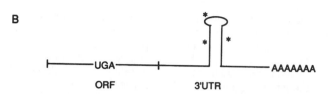

Figure 3. *Panel A.* Outline of selenoprotein synthesis. Solid lines indicate reactions that have been characterized, and broken lines indicate ones that have not yet been characterized. The circled numbers indicate 1) seryl-tRNA ligase, 2) selenocysteine synthetase function (characterized in bacteria but not in animals), 3) selenophosphate synthetase, and 4) elongation factor (characterized in bacteria but not in animals) and SECIS motif in selenoprotein mRNA. *Panel B.* Representation of a selenoprotein mRNA. The open reading frame (ORF) contains a UGA codon that is decoded as selenocysteine. The 3′ untranslated region (3′UTR) contains a stem-loop structure necessary for the decoding of the UGA as selenocysteine. The asterisks on the stem loop indicate the locations of conserved nucleotide sequences. One of these is present on the loop and the other two are present on bulges from the stem. The stem loop with its conserved sequences constitutes the SECIS motif.[25] This figure was adapted from reference 26.

Biochemical Function

The metabolic effects of selenium deficiency include susceptibility to certain types of oxidative injury, alterations in thyroid hormone metabolism, increased susceptibility to injury by mercury, alterations in activities of biotransformation enzymes, and an increase in plasma glutathione concentration.[11,33-36] Selenoproteins are generally thought to account for the effects of the element.

Four selenium-dependent glutathione peroxidases have been characterized and designated GSHPx's 1–4 by Genome Data Bank.[26] They reduce hydroperoxides using GSH as the hydrogen donor. GSHPx-1 is cellular glutathione peroxidase and was shown to be a selenoprotein in 1973.[37] It is the most abundant selenoprotein in the rat and appears to be present in virtually all cells. It reduces H$_2$O$_2$ and free hydroperoxides. GSHPx-2, also known as GSHPx-GI because it is localized to the gastrointestinal tract, is intracellular and has substrate specificity similar to GSHPx-1. It has been postulated to metabolize hydroperoxides that are absorbed from the diet.[38]

GSHPx-3, the extracellular or plasma glutathione peroxidase, is secreted primarily by kidney but is also produced in liver and breast tissue.[39] It can reduce hydroperoxides esterified to phospholipids as well as free hydroperoxides.[40] Extracellular glutathione peroxidase appears to complement the intracellular forms by controlling hydroperoxides outside of cells. GSHPx-4, the enzyme known as phospholipid hydroperoxide glutathione peroxidase, is a monomer while GSHPx's 1–3 are homotetramers.[41] GSHPx-4 is present in many tissues but is most abundant in testis. It is found in membrane fractions and free in the cytosol.[42] This enzyme has been suggested to play a major role in protecting against lipid peroxidation because it is the only intracellular glutathione peroxidase that can reduce fatty acid hydroperoxides present in phospholipids. The glutathione peroxidases are part of the defenses of the organism against oxidative injury.

Iodothyronine deiodinases remove iodine from thyroid hormone molecules. This process activates T_4 and inactivates T_3. Type I iodothyronine deiodinase is a selenoprotein and its physiological role is to provide T_3 to peripheral tissues from T_4 secreted by the thyroid gland.[34,35] It is found in liver, kidney, and thyroid tissue. Selenium deficiency causes the activity of the type I enzyme to decline; but loss of this activity is largely compensated for by a rise in plasma T_4, which prevents hypothyroidism. Type II iodothyronine deiodinase is present in the brain, pituitary, brown fat, and placenta.[34] It regulates intracellular T_3 in these tissues and controls thyroid-stimulating hormone secretion, and it was recently shown to be a selenoprotein.[43] Type III iodothyronine deiodinase, which inactivates T_3 and degrades other thyroid hormones, also was recently shown to be a selenoprotein, although little is known about its function in selenium deficiency.[44]

Animal studies have shown that combined selenium deficiency and iodine deficiency leads to more severe hypothyroidism than does iodine deficiency alone.[35] Some evidence suggests that cretinism in newborns may be a consequence of combined deficiencies of these two elements in mothers.[35]

Selenoprotein P is an abundant extracellular selenoprotein that contains multiple selenocysteine residues in its primary structure.[45] It is synthesized by many tissues and may have an oxidant defense role in the extracellular space.[33] Selenoprotein W is a muscle protein that has been shown to contain selenocysteine.[46] Selenium deficiency causes the concentration of selenoprotein W to decrease, and it may be involved in the pathogenesis of muscular degeneration seen in combined selenium–vitamin E deficiency.[46]

More selenoproteins will be characterized. It has been estimated that 50–100 of them are present in animals.[47] Bacteria contain biologically active forms of selenium other than selenocysteine, and analogous compounds are probably present in animals.[48] Much remains to be learned about the biochemical function of selenium.

Deficiency

Selenium deficiency has been associated with Keshan disease, an endemic cardiomyopathy that primarily affects children and women of childbearing age in some areas of China.[8] Several indices of selenium status are depressed in such patients, and diets from endemic areas are extremely low in the element because of the selenium-poor soils there. Large-scale intervention trials have demonstrated conclusively the efficacy of selenium supplementation in controlling Keshan disease.[49]

However, certain features of the disease cannot be explained solely on the basis of selenium deficiency. For example, seasonal and annual fluctuations in the incidence of the disease were more consistent with an infectious rather than a nutritional etiology. Indeed, Chinese scientists found that selenium-deficient mice were less resistant to heart damage due to coxsackievirus B_4 isolated from a Keshan disease victim than selenium-adequate mice.[50] Beck et al.[51] confirmed these results and showed that a myocarditic strain of coxsackievirus B_3 (CVB3/20) caused greater cardiopathology in selenium-deficient mice than in selenium-supplemented mice. Moreover, inoculation of a benign (amyocarditic) strain of coxsackievirus B_3 (CVB3/0) into selenium-deficient mice resulted in a moderate degree of heart damage whereas no damage was observed in selenium-adequate mice given the CVB3/0.[52] When virus was isolated from selenium-deficient mice inoculated with the CVB3/0, passed through cell culture, and then reinoculated into normal mice, the heart damage persisted. This suggested that the benign virus had undergone a genotypic change that accounted for its increased virulence. When the genome of the virus that was passed through the selenium-deficient host was sequenced, it was found that the RNA had changed at six of the seven sites thought to be associated with virulence.[53] As far as the authors were aware, this was the first reported instance in which host nutritional status had an influence on the genetic makeup of a pathogen. If the results were applicable to other RNA viruses, such as polio, hepatitis, influenza, or HIV, the public health implications could be considerable.

Although the viral changes discussed above are presented only in the context of selenium deficiency, it should be pointed out that similar viral changes were also observed in vitamin E–deficient mice.[54] Since marginal vitamin E status is often seen in populations in which

Keshan disease is endemic, the relative contributions of selenium and/or vitamin E deficiency to the etiology of Keshan disease need to be determined.[55]

Kashin-Beck disease, an endemic osteoarthritis that occurs during the preadolescent or adolescent years, is another disease that has been linked to low-selenium status in China.[8,56] However, the selenium deficiency hypothesis does not seem to be as widely accepted for Kashin-Beck disease as for Keshan disease, and other etiological theories (mycotoxins in grain, mineral imbalance, organic contaminants in drinking water) have been proposed.[57] An animal model in which selenium-deficient mice are given fulvic acid in the drinking water has been suggested as an approach to study the pathogenesis of this condition.[58]

In past years selenium was not generally added to fluids used for total parenteral nutrition (TPN). As a result, several cases of biochemical selenium deficiency (low plasma or blood selenium levels, depressed glutathione peroxidase activity) were reported. Despite these reports of impaired selenium status, no clinical syndrome characteristic of selenium deficiency was seen in such patients.[59] Cardiomyopathy and skeletal muscle weakness have been observed in a few intravenously fed individuals who were not supplemented with selenium.[60–62] Currently, there are no official guidelines for the doses or forms of selenium supplements to be administered to TPN patients.[63]

Several experiments with rodent models indicate a protective effect of selenium against tumorigenesis, although high (i.e., nonnutritional, >0.25 µg/g dry diet) doses of selenium are generally used.[64] Because of the high dietary intakes needed to demonstrate an anticarcinogenic effect, attempts are being made to develop new anticancer selenium compounds with low toxicity.[65] One potential chemopreventive agent with such desirable properties is triphenylselenonium chloride, a lipophilic monocationic compound.[66] Of the materials thus far tested, triphenylselenonium chloride has the largest chemopreventive index (ratio of the maximum tolerable dose to the effective dose inhibiting tumor yield by 50%). Feeding this compound at a level of 30 ppm selenium in the diet reduced the yield of mammary tumors by ≈70% in rats treated with dimethylbenzanthracene whereas the maximum tolerated dose was >200 ppm selenium. The mechanism by which selenium protects against cancer in these rodent models is not known, but the elevated intakes needed for protection suggest that something is involved other than the selenoenzymes and selenoproteins responsive to nutritional quantities of dietary selenium (the glutathione peroxidases, selenoprotein P, the iodothyronine deiodinases, etc.).

Despite the considerable success in obtaining protective effects of elevated dietary intakes of selenium against cancer in laboratory animals, recent attempts to identify similar protective effects of selenium against human cancer at dietary intakes typically found in the United States were unsuccessful. Two large cohort studies (62,641 subjects) failed to find any inverse relationship between the selenium content of toenails (assumed to provide a reasonably stable estimate of selenium intake over a period of years) and cancer risk in women.[67,68] However, these two studies were criticized on the basis of an insufficiently large selenium gradient in the study population and certain methodological difficulties involved in the use of toenail selenium level as a biomarker of selenium status.[69,70] A nutrition intervention trial involving almost 30,000 subjects from a poorly nourished rural population in China showed that a combined supplement of selenium, vitamin E, and β-carotene reduced overall cancer mortality by 13%, but the relevance of these results to better nourished Western populations is not clear.[71–73] Selenium supplements are currently being given in a double-blinded cancer prevention trial in the southeastern United States, and it is hoped that the results of that study will furnish more definitive information regarding the use of selenium compounds as chemopreventive agents.[70]

In order to guard against any possible deleterious effects of poor selenium status on human health, the Ministry of Agriculture and Forestry of Finland started supplementing the fertilizer used in that country with selenium in the fall of 1984.[74] The Finnish diet tended to be quite low in selenium because soils in the region are deficient in the mineral. As the selenium from fertilizer worked its way through the food chain, the selenium intake from the Finnish diet increased from 30–40 µg/day to almost 100 µg/day and plasma selenium concentrations in the general population rose accordingly. Despite this well-documented improvement in the overall selenium status on a national scale, no dramatic change in cancer mortality or incidence attributable to selenium has been seen during the 8-year course (1984–1992) of this intervention program.[74]

Requirements and Allowances

In 1980 the Food and Nutrition Board of the U.S. National Academy of Sciences proposed an estimated safe and adequate daily dietary intake of selenium of 50–200 µg for adults.[75] This range was extrapolated from animal experiments because few data about selenium in human nutrition were available. Most mammals appear to require ~0.1 µg selenium/g dry diet. If humans consumed 500 g of (dry) diet daily, then they would require 50 µg of selenium per day, the lower limit of the safe and adequate range. However, some workers have found that the young of certain animals need >0.1 µg/g diet, so the validity of human requirements extrapolated from animal studies is uncertain.[76]

Balance studies often have been used to estimate human requirements for various minerals, but the pitfalls in the use of balance data for this purpose are well known.[77] A comparison of balance studies from China, New Zealand, and the United States revealed that metabolic balance could be achieved over a wide range of selenium intakes (9–80 µg/day).[78] Balance was maintained in persons with low selenium intakes by a decreased urinary and fecal excretion of selenium. Thus, balance studies do not appear particularly helpful in delineating human requirements for selenium.

On the basis of dietary surveys, scientists in China determined the dietary selenium intake needed to prevent Keshan disease. The disease is absent in areas where the dietary intake averages 19 and 14 µg/day for adult men and women, respectively.[79] This very low intake could be considered a "minimum daily requirement" for selenium.

Chinese scientists also have estimated what they called a "physiological" selenium requirement based on maximization of plasma glutathione peroxidase activity. The diets of men living in a Keshan disease area (average dietary selenium intake of 10 µg/day) were supplemented with graded doses of selenomethionine for several months. Individuals consuming a total of ≥40 µg selenium/day had similar enzyme values, and this intake was considered the physiological requirement under these conditions.[79]

The Food and Nutrition Board used the above experiment as the basis for its 1989 recommended dietary allowance (RDA) for selenium.[80] The Chinese value was adjusted to account for differences in body weight and to incorporate an appropriate safety factor. RDAs for selenium of 70 and 55 µg/day were calculated for adult men and women, respectively.[81] The selenium RDA for younger age groups was extrapolated downward according to metabolic body size. More recently, the Panel on Dietary Reference Values of the British Committee on Medical Aspects of Food Policy adopted 75 and 60 µg/day as their reference nutrient intake (RNI) for adult males and females, respectively.[82] The RNI is defined as an intake two standard deviations above the estimated average requirement and is presumed to satisfy the nutritional needs of 97.5% of the population.

Sources

The selenium content of foods varies widely (µg/g fresh weight): organ meats and seafoods, 0.4–1.5; muscle meats, 0.1–0.4; cereals and grains, <0.1–>0.8; dairy products, <0.1–0.3; and fruits and vegetables, <0.1.[83] The primary factor affecting the selenium content of plant foods is the amount of selenium available in the soil for uptake by plants in a given area. For example, corn, rice, and soybeans collected in an area of China with human selenosis contained an average of 8.1, 4.0, and 11.9 µg/g, respectively, whereas the same foods taken from a Keshan disease area contained only 0.005, 0.007, and 0.010 µg/g.[84] Animal products also show some variation in selenium content. However, the extreme values are moderated somewhat because animals tend to conserve selenium under conditions of deficiency and excrete it under conditions of excessive exposure.

Data from nationwide food surveys analyzed by the U.S. Food and Drug Administration show that the average selenium intake by adults between 1974 and 1982 was 108 µg/day, with annual values of 83–129 µg/day.[85] Thus, the well-balanced North American diet appears to provide ample selenium to satisfy the RDA for this element. The national diets of countries with soils poor in selenium furnish lower quantities of selenium. For example, dietary selenium intakes in New Zealand were reported to be 28–32 µg/day.[83]

High dietary selenium intakes occur in areas with naturally seleniferous soils. In one region of China where endemic human selenosis was seen, intakes as high as 6690 µg/day were reported.[84] The source of selenium in this food chain was a highly seleniferous coal that lost its selenium to the soil because of weathering.

Animal models have shown great variation in the nutritional bioavailability of selenium in different foods. On the basis of increased hepatic glutathione peroxidase activity in selenium-depleted rats, selenium fed as mushrooms, tuna, wheat, beef kidney, and Brazil nuts had 5%, 57%, 83%, 97%, and 124% of the availability of sodium selenite, respectively.[86,87] A bioavailability trial carried out with men of low-selenium status in Finland showed that a number of variables had to be considered in such studies, including short-term increases in glutathione peroxidase activity, long-term tissue retention of selenium, and metabolic conversion of retained forms of selenium to biologically active forms.[88]

Toxicity

Human selenium poisoning from consumption of toxic foods containing high levels of selenium was reported in Enshi County, China, where chronically intoxicated individuals ingested an average of 4.99 mg selenium/day in a vegetable diet.[84] Signs of selenosis included loss of hair and nails, skin lesions, tooth decay, and abnormalities of the nervous system. Concomitant fluorosis may have been a complicating factor in the appearance of the latter two signs.[8] Acutely poisoned persons (loss of hair in 3–4 days) may have consumed as much as 38 mg selenium/day.[89]

Human selenium poisoning was reported in 13 persons in the United States who consumed a "health food" supplement that contained ~182 times more selenium than stated on the label.[90–92] The total amount of selenium thought to be ingested by the victims was 27–2387 mg. The most common symptoms were nausea, vomiting, hair loss, nail changes, irritability, fatigue, and peripheral neuropathy.

The biochemical basis of selenium toxicity is not fully understood, but several possible reaction mechanisms have been suggested, such as interference with sulfur metabolism, catalytic oxidation of sulfhydryl groups, and inhibition of protein synthesis.[93]

Although there are no sensitive and specific biochemical indicators of dietary selenium overexposure,[83] toxicological standards for selenium have been proposed on the basis of clinical signs of selenosis such as loss of hair or nails.[83] For example, a follow-up study carried out in the endemic selenosis zone of China was used by the U.S. Environmental Protection Agency to calculate a reference dose (RfD) for selenium.[94–96] The RfD is defined as "an estimate (with uncertainty spanning perhaps an order of magnitude) of a daily exposure to the human population (including sensitive subgroups) that is likely to be without appreciable risk of deleterious effects during a lifetime."[97] The basis of the RfD was a no-observed-adverse-effect level (NOAEL) of 853 µg/day calculated from a regression equation relating whole-blood selenium concentrations to dietary selenium intake in persons exhibiting no clinical signs of selenosis. A study from the United States corroborated the estimate for the NOAEL, since no signs of selenium poisoning were seen in persons from South Dakota or Wyoming who consumed as much as 724 µg/day.[98] The individuals in the Chinese survey weighed an average of 55 kg, so the NOAEL on a body weight basis was 853/55 or 15 $\mu g \cdot kg^{-1} \cdot day^{-1}$. The RfD calculation included an uncertainty factor of 3 applied to the NOAEL (to account for sensitive individuals) and yielded a value of 5 $\mu g \cdot kg^{-1} \cdot day^{-1}$. Thus, for the standard 70 kg Western male, the RfD would be 350 µg/day. In their report on dietary reference values,[82] the British recommended that the maximum safe selenium intake from all sources should be 450 µg/day for adult males.[82] Until better indices of selenium overexposure are developed, it would seem imprudent (and unnecessary from the nutritional point of view) to consume routinely more than the 200 µg upper limit of the Food and Nutrition Board's 1980 estimated safe and adequate daily dietary intake.[75]

References

1. Schwarz K, Foltz CM (1957) Selenium as an integral part of factor 3 against dietary necrotic liver degeneration. J Am Chem Soc 79:3292–3293
2. Board on Agriculture, Committee on Animal Nutrition, National Research Council (1983) Selenium in nutrition, revised ed. National Academy of Sciences, Washington, DC
3. McCoy KEM, Weswig PH (1969) Some selenium responses in the rat not related to vitamin E. J Nutr 98:383–389
4. Thompson JN, Scott ML (1969) Role of selenium in the nutrition of the chick. J Nutr 97:335–342
5. Whitacre ME, Combs GF Jr, Combs SB, Parker RS (1987) Influence of dietary vitamin E on nutritional pancreatic atrophy in selenium-deficient chicks. J Nutr 117:460–467
6. Combs GF Jr, Liu CH, Lu ZH, Su Q (1984) Uncomplicated selenium deficiency produced in chicks fed corn-soy-based diet. J Nutr 114:964–976
7. Awasthi YC, Beutler E, Srivastava SK (1975) Purification and properties of human erythrocyte glutathione peroxidase. J Biol Chem 250:5144–5149
8. Yang G, Ge K, Chen J, Chen X (1988) Selenium-related endemic diseases and the daily selenium requirement of humans. World Rev Nutr Diet 55:98–152
9. Robinson MF (1976) The moonstone: more about selenium. J Hum Nutr 30:79–91
10. Wittwer AJ, Ching W-M (1989) Selenium-containing tRNA^{Glu} and tRNA^{Lys} from Escherichia coli: purification, codon specificity and translational activity. Biofactors 2:27–34
11. Hill KE, Burk RF, Lane JM (1987) Effect of selenium depletion and repletion on plasma glutathione and glutathione-dependent enzymes in the rat. J Nutr 117:99–104
12. Yang JG, Hill KE, Burk RF (1989) Dietary selenium controls rat plasma selenoprotein P concentration. J Nutr 119:1010–1012
13. Sunde RA, Dyer JA, Moran TV, et al (1993) Phospholipid hydroperoxide glutathione peroxidase: full-length pig blastocyst cDNA sequence and regulation by selenium status. Biochem Biophys Res Commun 193:905–911
14. Hill KE, Lyons PR, Burk RF (1992) Differential regulation of rat liver selenoprotein mRNAs in selenium deficiency. Biochem Biophys Res Commun 185:260–263
15. Whanger PD, Pedersen ND, Hatfield J, Weswig PH (1976) Absorption of selenite and selenomethionine from ligated digestive tract segments in rats. Proc Soc Exp Biol Med 153:295–297
16. Brown DG, Burk RF, Seely RJ, Kiker KW (1972) Effect of dietary selenium on the gastrointestinal absorption of $^{75}SeO_3^{2-}$. Int J Vitam Nutr Res 42:588–591
17. Esaki N, Nakamura T, Tanaka H, et al (1981) Enzymatic synthesis of selenocysteine in rat liver. Biochemistry 20:4492–4500
18. Esaki N, Nakamura T, Tanaka H, Soda K (1982) Selenocysteine lyase, a novel enzyme that specifically acts on selenocysteine: mammalian distribution and purification and properties of pig liver enzyme. J Biol Chem 257:4386–4391
19. Ganther HE (1979) Metabolism of hydrogen selenide and methylated selenides. In Draper HH (ed), Advances in Nutritional Research, vol 2. Plenum, New York, pp 107–128
20. Berry J, Harney JW, Low SC (1995) Cloning and expression of the human selenium donor protein, the homolog of prokaryotic SELD. FASEB J 9:A286
21. Mozier NM, McConnell KP, Hoffman JL (1988) S-adenosyl-L-methionine:thioether S-methyltransferase, a new enzyme in sulfur and selenium metabolism. J Biol Chem 263:4527–4531
22. Bopp BA, Sonders RC, Kesterson JW (1982) Metabolic fate of selected selenium compounds in laboratory animals and man. Drug Metab Rev 13:271–318
23. Kato T, Read R, Rozga J, Burk RF (1992) Evidence for intestinal release of absorbed selenium in a form with high hepatic extraction. Am J Physiol 262:G854–G858
24. Böck A (1994) Incorporation of selenium into bacterial selenoproteins. In Burk RF (ed), Selenium in biology and human health. Springer-Verlag, New York, pp 9–24
25. Berry MJ, Banu L, Chen Y, et al (1991) Recognition of UGA

as a selenocysteine codon in type I deiodinase requires sequences in the 3' untranslated region. Nature 353:273–276

26. Burk RF (1996) Selenium-dependent glutathione peroxidases. In Guengerich FP (ed), Comprehensive toxicology, vol 3, Biotransformation. Pergamon, Oxford, in press

27. Hatfield DL, Choi IS, Ohama T, et al (1994) Selenocysteine tRNA[Ser]Sec isoacceptors as central components in seleno-protein biosynthesis in eukaryotes. In Burk RF (ed), Selenium in biology and human health. Springer-Verlag, New York, pp 25–44

28. O'Prey J, Ramsay S, Chambers I, Harrison PR (1993) Transcriptional up-regulation of the mouse cytosolic glutathione peroxidase gene in erythroid cells is due to a tissue-specific 3' enhancer containing functionally important CACC/GT motifs and binding sites for GATA and Ets transcription factors. Mol Cell Biol 13:6290–6303

29. Shen Q, Chada S, Whitney C, Newburger PE (1994) Regulation of the human cellular glutathione peroxidase gene during in vitro myeloid and monocytic differentiation. Blood 84:3202–3208

30. Cowan DB, Weisel RD, Williams WG, Mickle DAG (1993) Identification of oxygen responsive elements in the 5'-flanking region of the human glutathione peroxidase gene. J Biol Chem 268:26904–26910

31. Hawkes WC, Wilhelmsen EC, Tappel AL (1985) Abundance and tissue distribution of selenocysteine-containing proteins in the rat. J Inorg Biochem 23:77–92

32. Sunde RA (1994) Intracellular glutathione peroxidases—structure, regulation, and function. In Burk RF (ed), Selenium in biology and human health. Springer-Verlag, New York, pp 45–77

33. Burk RF, Hill KE, Awad JA, et al (1995) Pathogenesis of diquat-induced liver necrosis in selenium-deficient rats: assessment of the roles of lipid peroxidation and selenoprotein P. Hepatology 21:561–569

34. Berry MJ, Larsen PR (1992) The role of selenium in thyroid hormone action. Endocr Rev 13:207–219

35. Arthur JR, Beckett GJ (1994) Roles of selenium in type I iodothyronine 5'-deiodinase and in thyroid hormone and iodine metabolism. In Burk RF (ed), Selenium in biology and human health. Springer-Verlag, New York, pp 93–115

36. Reiter R, Wendel A (1983) Selenium and drug metabolism. I. multiple modulations of mouse liver enzymes. Biochem Pharmacol 32:3063–3067

37. Rotruck JT, Pope AL, Ganther HE, et al (1973) Selenium: biochemical role as a component of glutathione peroxidase. Science 179:588–590

38. Chu F-F, Doroshow JH, Esworthy RS (1993) Expression, characterization, and tissue distribution of a new cellular selenium-dependent glutathione peroxidase, GSHPx-GI. J Biol Chem 268:2571–2576

39. Maser RL, Magenheimer BS, Calvet JP (1994) Mouse plasma glutathione peroxidase: cDNA sequence analysis and renal proximal tubular expression and secretion. J Biol Chem 269:27066–27073

40. Yamamoto Y, Takahashi K (1993) Glutathione peroxidase isolated from plasma reduces phospholipid hydroperoxides. Arch Biochem Biophys 305:541–545

41. Brigelius-Flohe R, Aumann K-D, Blöcker H, et al (1994) Phospholipid-hydroperoxide glutathione peroxidase: genomic DNA, cDNA, and deduced amino acid sequence. J Biol Chem 269:7342–7348

42. Roveri A, Maiorino M, Nisii C, Ursini F (1994) Purification and characterization of phospholipid hydroperoxide glutathione peroxidase from rat testis mitochondrial membranes. Biochim Biophys Acta 1208:211–221

43. Davey JC, Becker KB, Schneider MJ, et al (1995) Cloning of a cDNA for the type II iodothyronine deiodinase. J Biol Chem 270:26786–26789

44. Croteau W, Whittemore SL, Schneider MJ, St Germain DL (1995) Cloning and expression of a cDNA for a mammalian type III iodothyronine deiodinase. J Biol Chem 270:16569–16575

45. Burk RF, Hill KE (1994) Selenoprotein P: a selenium-rich extracellular glycoprotein. J Nutr 124:1891–1897

46. Vendeland SC, Beilstein MA, Chen CL, et al (1993) Purification and properties of selenoprotein W from rat muscle. J Biol Chem 268:17103–17107

47. Burk RF, Hill KE (1993) Regulation of selenoproteins. Annu Rev Nutr 13:65–81

48. Gladyshev VN, Khangulov SV, Axley MJ, Stadtman TC (1994) Coordination of selenium to molybdenum in formate dehydrogenase H from Escherichia coli. Proc Natl Acad Sci 91:7708–7711

49. Yang G, Chen J, Wen Z, et al (1984) The role of selenium in Keshan disease. Adv Nutr Res 6:203–231

50. Bai J, Wu S, Ge K, et al (1980) The combined effect of selenium deficiency and viral infection on the myocardium of mice. Acta Acad Med Sin 2:29–31

51. Beck MA, Kolbeck PC, Shi Q, et al (1994) Increased virulence of a human enterovirus (coxsackievirus B3) in selenium-deficient mice. J Infect Dis 170:351–357

52. Beck MA, Kolbeck PC, Rohr LH, et al (1994) Benign human enterovirus becomes virulent in selenium-deficient mice. J Med Virol 43:166–170

53. Beck MA, Shi Q, Morris VC, Levander OA (1995) Rapid genomic evolution of a non-virulent coxsackievirus B3 in selenium-deficient mice results in selection of identical virulent isolates. Nature Med 1:433–436

54. Beck MA, Kolbeck PC, Rohr LH, et al (1994) Vitamin E deficiency intensifies the myocardial injury of coxsackievirus B3 infection of mice. J Nutr 124:345–358

55. Xia Y, Piao J, Hill KE, Burk RF (1994) Keshan disease and selenium status of populations in China. In Burk RF (ed), Selenium in biology and human health. Springer-Verlag, New York, pp 182–196

56. Allander E (1994) Kashin-Beck disease: an analysis of research and public health activities based on a bibliography 1849–1992. Scand J Rheum 23:1–36

57. World Health Organization (1990) Kashin-Beck disease and non-communicable diseases. Chinese Academy of Preventive Medicine, Beijing, China

58. Yang C, Wolf E, Roser K, et al (1993) Selenium deficiency and fulvic acid supplementation induces fibrosis of cartilage and disturbs subchondral ossification in knee joints of mice: an animal model study of Kashin-Beck disease. Virchows Archiv A Pathol Anat 423:483–491

59. Levander OA, Burk RF (1986) Report of the 1986 A.S.P.E.N. Research Workshop on Selenium in Clinical Nutrition. J Parenter Enter Nutr 10:545–549

60. Fleming CR, McCull JT, O'Brien JF, et al (1984) Selenium status in patients receiving home parenteral nutrition. J Parenter Enter Nutr 8:258–262

61. van Rij AM, Thomson CD, Lyons JM, et al (1986) Selenium deficiency in total parenteral nutrition. Am J Clin Nutr 32:2076–2085

62. Brown MR, Cohen HJ, Lyons JM, et al (1986) Proximal muscle weakness and selenium deficiency associated with long-term parenteral nutrition. Am J Clin Nutr 43:549–554

63. AMA Department of Foods and Nutrition (1979) Guidelines for essential trace element preparations for parenteral use. JAMA 241:2051–2054

64. Combs GF Jr, Combs SB (1986) The role of selenium in nutrition. Academic Press, Orlando, FL

65. Ip C, Ganther HE (1994) Novel strategies in selenium cancer chemoprevention research. In Burk RF (ed), Selenium in biology and human health. Springer-Verlag, New York, pp 170–180

66. Ip C, Thompson H, Ganther H (1994) Activity of triphenyl-selenonium chloride in mammary cancer prevention. Carcinogenesis 15:2879–2882

67. Hunter DJ, Morris JS, Stampfer MJ, et al (1990) A prospective study of selenium status and breast cancer risk. JAMA 264:1128–1131

68. Garland M, Morris JS, Stampfer MJ, et al (1995) Prospective study of toenail selenium levels and cancer among women. J Natl Cancer Inst 87:497–505

69. Schrauzer GN (1991) Selenium and breast cancer. JAMA 265:28

70. Clark LC, Alberts DS (1995) Selenium and cancer: risk or protection? J Natl Cancer Inst 87:473–475

71. Blot WJ, Li J-Y, Taylor PR, et al (1993) Nutrition intervention trials in Linxian, China: supplementation with specific vitamin/mineral combinations, cancer incidence, and disease-specific mortality in the general population. J Natl Cancer Inst 85:1483–1492

72. Benner SE, Hong WK (1993) Clinical chemoprevention: developing a cancer prevention strategy. J Natl Cancer Inst 85:1446–1447

73. Smigel K (1993) News: dietary supplements reduce cancer deaths in China. J Natl Cancer Inst 85:1448–1450

74. Varo P, Alfthan G, Huttunen JK, Aro A (1994) Nationwide selenium supplementation in Finland—effects on diet, blood and tissue levels, and health. In Burk RF (ed), Selenium in biology and human health. Springer-Verlag, New York, pp 199–218

75. National Research Council (1980) Recommended dietary allowances, 9th ed. National Academy Press, Washington, DC

76. Meyer RW, Mahan DC, Moxon AL (1981) Value of dietary selenium and vitamin E for weanling swine as measured by performance and tissue selenium and glutathione peroxidase activities. J Anim Sci 52:302–311

77. Mertz W (1987) Use and misuse of balance studies. J Nutr 117:1811–1813

78. Levander OA (1986) Selenium. In Mertz W (ed), Trace elements in human and animal nutrition, 5th ed. Academic Press, Orlando, FL, pp 209–279

79. Yang G, Zhu L, Liu S, et al (1987) Human selenium requirements in China. In Combs GF Jr, Spallholz JE, Levander OA, Oldfield JE (eds), Selenium in biology and medicine, part B. AVI Publishing Co, Westport, CT, pp 589–607

80. National Research Council (1989) Recommended dietary allowances, 10th ed. National Academy Press, Washington, DC

81. Levander OA (1991) Scientific rationale for the 1989 recommended dietary allowance for selenium. J Am Diet Assoc 91:1572–1576

82. Department of Health (1991) Dietary reference values for food energy and nutrients for the United Kingdom (Report on Health and Social Subjects, No. 41). HMSO, London

83. International Programme of Chemical Safety (1987) Selenium, Environmental Health Criteria 58. World Health Organization, Geneva

84. Yang GQ, Wang S, Zhou R, Sun S (1983) Endemic selenium intoxication of humans in China. Am J Clin Nutr 37:872–881

85. Pennington JAT, Wilson DB, Newell RF, et al (1984) Selected minerals in foods surveys, 1974 to 1981/82. J Am Diet Assoc 84:771–780

86. Levander OA (1983) Considerations in the design of selenium bioavailability studies. Fed Proc 42:324–329

87. Chansler MW, Mutanen M, Morris VC, Levander OA (1986) Nutritional bioavailability to rats of selenium in Brazil nuts and mushrooms. Nutr Res 6:1419–1428

88. Levander OA, Alfthan G, Arvilommi H, et al (1983) Bioavailability of selenium to Finnish men as assessed by platelet glutathione peroxidase activity and other blood parameters. Am J Clin Nutr 37:887–897

89. Yang GQ (1985) Keshan disease: an endemic selenium-related deficiency disease. In Chandra RK (ed), Trace elements in nutrition of children. Raven Press, New York, pp 273–290

90. Jensen R, Clossons W, Rothenberg R (1984) Selenium intoxication—New York. MMWR 33:157–158

91. Anonymous (1984) Toxicity with superpotent selenium. FDA Bull 14:19

92. Helzlsouer K, Jacobs R, Morris S (1985) Acute selenium intoxication in the United States. Fed Proc 44:1670

93. Levander OA (1983) Selenium: biochemical actions, interactions, and some human health implications. In Prasad AS (ed), Clinical, biochemical, and nutritional aspects of trace elements. Alan R Liss, New York, pp 345–368

94. Yang G, Zhou R, Yin S, et al (1989) Studies of safe maximal daily dietary selenium intake in a seleniferous area of China. I. Selenium intake and tissue selenium levels of the inhabitants. J Trace Elem Electrolytes Health Dis 3:77–87

95. Yang G, Yin S, Zhou R, et al (1989) Studies of safe maximal daily dietary Se-intake in a seleniferous area in China. II. Relation between Se-intake and the manifestation of clinical signs and certain biochemical alterations in blood and urine. J Trace Elem Electrolytes Health Dis 3:123–130

96. Abernathy CO, Cantilli R, Du JT, Levander OA (1993) Essentiality versus toxicity: some considerations in the risk assessment of essential trace elements. In Saxena J (ed), Hazard assessment of chemicals, vol 8. Taylor and Francis, Washington, DC, pp 81–113

97. Poirier KA (1994) Summary of the derivation of the reference dose for selenium. In Mertz W, Abernathy CO, Olin SS (eds), Risk assessment of essential elements. ILSI Press, Washington, DC, pp 157–166

98. Longnecker MP, Taylor PR, Levander OA, et al (1991) Selenium in diet, blood, and toenails in relation to human health in a seleniferous area. Am J Clin Nutr 53:1288–1294

Chapter 32

Fluoride

Kathy R. Phipps

Fluoride is the only nutrient that has been demonstrated to reduce the prevalence and severity of dental caries in both children and adults. Because of fluoride's positive impact on dental health, the National Research Council's Food and Nutrition Board considers it to be a "beneficial element for humans."[1] At one time fluoride was considered an essential nutrient,[2] but the Food and Nutrition Board has backed away from that position because an essential role for fluoride could not be confirmed. Although fluoride is no longer considered an essential factor for human growth and development, many believe that there is an optimal dose of systemic fluoride for maximal benefit against dental caries. On the basis of empirical evidence, it appears that 0.05–0.07 mg/kg body weight per day is a fair estimate of that optimal dose.[3]

Sources of Ingested Fluoride

Fluoride is ubiquitous, occurring in minute amounts in all foodstuffs and water supplies. The major influence on total fluoride intake, however, is probably the fluoride content of drinking water. In the United States, ≈52% of the population receives water with a fluoride concentration adjusted to between 0.7 and 1.2 mg/L.[4] An additional 4% receives naturally fluoridated water with a concentration of ≥0.7 mg/L. To calculate total fluoride intake, sources other than water, such as milk, infant formulas, beverages, food, and other fluoride products, must also be considered.

The fluoride content of breast milk is <0.01 mg/L.[5,6] The fluoride contents of ready-to-feed milk-based and soy-based infant formulas are 0.05–0.37 mg/L and 0.17–0.38 mg/L, respectively. When powdered and concentrated liquid formulas are reconstituted with deionized water, fluoride levels are similar to those of ready-to-feed products. When reconstituted with fluoridated water, however, infant formulas contain higher amounts of fluoride. Thus, a 6-week-old infant who is exclusively breast-fed will have a mean daily fluoride intake of <0.01 mg/kg body weight compared with a mean daily intake of 0.01–0.07 mg/kg body weight if a ready-to-feed formula is used and 0.10–0.23 mg/kg body weight if formula is used and 0.10–0.23 mg/kg body weight if formula is reconstituted with water containing 1.0 mg fluoride/L.[7]

The fluoride content of processed beverages closely matches the fluoride content of water used in processing. Because of this, there is considerable variation in the fluoride content of processed beverages, ranging from 0.03 to 6.8 mg/L.[7] Another beverage that contains fluoride is tea. Raw tea leaves may contain as much as 400 mg fluoride/kg, and the fluoride content of tea has been found to range from 0.1 to 4.2 mg/L when brewed with deionized water.[8,9]

Chicken, fish, and seafood products may also contain high levels of fluoride, especially if bone and shell are included in the processing. Canned fish may contain up to 40 mg fluoride/kg, whereas dried seafood can contain up to 290 mg/kg.[10] Evaluation of chicken products indicates that they contain between 0.6 and 10.6 mg fluoride/kg.[11,12]

In addition to foods and beverages, children may ingest fluoride from a variety of therapeutic fluoride products such as toothpaste and fluoride supplements. In the United States, the fluoride concentration of toothpaste ranges from 1000 to 1500 mg/kg; the average 2–3-year-old ingests 28–65% of the dentifrice used to brush teeth.[13,14] Fluoride supplements also play an important role in a child's daily fluoride intake. Table 1 presents the revised fluoride dosage schedule adopted in 1994 by the American Dental Association Council on Dental Therapeutics and the American Academy of Pediatric Dentistry.[15,16] Fluoride supplements are not recommended until a child is 6 months old, which coincides with the eruption of the primary teeth.

Because of differences in fluoride content of similar products and wide variations in consumption patterns, estimates of fluoride intake for children and adults are difficult to obtain. For an adult male residing in a fluoridated community, estimates of daily fluoride intake from food and beverages range from 1 to 3 mg/day. This range is reduced to ≤1.0 mg/day in a nonfluoridated area.[17] When all sources of fluoride are taken into account, the daily fluoride intake of 6-month-old infants has been estimated to be 0.01–0.29 mg/kg body weight; that of a 12-month-old infant,

Table 1. Fluoride supplement dosage schedule[15,16]

Age	Fluoride supplement at different concentrations of fluoride in drinking water		
	<0.3 mg/L	0.3–0.6 mg/L	>0.7 mg/L
	mg/d		
0–6 months	0	0	0
6 months–3 years	0.25	0	0
3–6 years	0.50	0.25	0
6–16 years	1.00	0.50	0

0.02–0.25 mg/kg; and that of 2–3-year-old children, 0.02–0.24 mg/kg.[7]

Physiology and Metabolism of Fluoride

Studies in both animals and humans have shown that ≈75–90% of ingested fluoride is absorbed rapidly and readily from the gastrointestinal tract, with the remaining 10–25% being excreted in feces.[18] The half-time for absorption is ≈30 minutes, so peak plasma concentrations usually occur within 30–60 minutes. The mechanism of fluoride absorption has been determined to be diffusion.

Once fluoride is absorbed, it passes into the blood for distribution throughout the body and for partial excretion. From plasma, fluoride complexes with calcified tissues and is distributed to either the extracellular or intracellular spaces of the soft tissues or is excreted. Most of the ionic fluoride retained in the body enters into calcified tissues (bone and developing teeth) either by substituting for the hydroxyl ion or bicarbonate ion in hydroxyapatite in bone or enamel to form fluoroapatite or by ionic exchange within the hydration shell of the crystalline surface.[18] Approximately 50% of the fluoride absorbed each day is deposited in the calcified tissues within 24 hours, resulting in ≈99% of the body burden of fluoride being associated with calcified tissues.[19]

Although fluoride has a high affinity for bone, it is not irreversibly bound in bone but forms a reversible sequestered pool.[20] Fluoride in bone can be remobilized, either rapidly by interstitial ionic exchange or slowly as a result of the ongoing process of bone remodeling. The process of bone remodeling is more active in the young, which is why fluoride deposition in bone is inversely proportional to age.[20]

Renal excretion is the predominant route for removal of inorganic fluoride from the body, with ≈50% of the daily intake being cleared by the kidneys. Fluoride is freely filtered through the glomerular capillaries and undergoes tubular reabsorption in varying degrees. The renal clearance of fluoride is directly related to urinary pH and, under some conditions, to urinary flow rate.[21,22] Because of this, factors that affect urinary pH, such as diet, drugs, metabolic or respiratory disorders, and altitude of residence, can affect how much absorbed fluoride is retained.

Health Benefits of Fluoride

Dental caries. That fluoride has substantial benefits in the prevention of tooth decay is well documented. Numerous studies taken together clearly establish a causal relationship between fluoride and the prevention of dental caries.[18] The mechanism of the effect of fluoride in reducing caries has been a controversial topic, but a consensus has emerged in recent years about the most important mechanisms.[23] Three main mechanisms have been proposed to account for the anticaries effect of fluoride.[24] First, the topical effect of a constant infusion of low-concentration fluoride into the oral cavity is to enhance remineralization during the repeated cycles of demineralization and remineralization in the early stages of the carious process. Second, fluoride in plaque inhibits glycolysis, the process by which sugar is metabolized by bacteria to produce acid. Third, there is evidence that preeruptive fluoride exerts some degree of caries inhibition; it acts via incorporation into the developing enamel hydroxyapatite crystal, thus reducing enamel solubility.

Osteoporosis. The testing of fluoride as a therapeutic agent for the treatment of osteoporosis began in the early 1960s.[25] The initial therapeutic studies indicated that although the fluoride-treated patients had increased bone formation, the new bone was poorly mineralized. By decreasing the fluoride dose and supplementing it with calcium, the new bone appeared to be normally calcified. Since the 1960s numerous clinical studies evaluating the effects of therapeutic doses of fluoride on bone cells, skeletal histology, bone density, and fracture rates have been conducted and several reviews have been published.[26–28] However, fluoride is not currently approved by the Food and Drug Administration for treatment of osteoporosis.

Most investigators agree that fluoride 1) stimulates bone formation by osteoblastic stimulation, 2) increases bone formation earlier and to a larger extent in trabecular bone than in cortical bone, and 3) increases spinal bone density.[29] The efficacy of fluoride as a therapeutic agent, however, is a controversial topic. One controlled trial of sodium fluoride concluded that a fluoride-calcium regimen was not effective in treating postmenopausal osteoporosis.[30] In this study, continuous supplementation with sodium fluoride and calcium carbonate increased the bone mineral density of the lumbar spine but did not reduce the rate of vertebral fractures per person-year of follow-up. Of concern was the fact that the fluoride-calcium group, compared with the placebo-calcium group, had a substantial loss of bone from the shaft of the radius. In addition, the fluoride-calcium group had nonvertebral fractures 3.2 times more often than did the placebo-calcium group. These nonvertebral fractures included Colles' fractures and fractures of the humerus, ribs, pelvis, proximal femur, and tibia. Some of these fractures were incomplete or stress fractures of the lower extremity, a fairly common side effect of fluoride therapy.

Another clinical trial of the effectiveness of fluoride in the treatment of osteoporosis found a statistically significant decrease in the individual rate of new vertebral fracture after ≈2.5 years of a therapy consisting of intermittent slow-release sodium fluoride plus continuous calcium citrate.[31] This study also found that radial-shaft bone density did not change significantly in either the treatment or the placebo group and no participant had micro fractures or hip fractures.

To explain the different outcomes of these two studies, it was postulated that the higher and continuous dosage of a more bioavailable form of fluoride in the Riggs et al. study may have caused a rapid growth of trabecular bone at the expense of cortical bone.[31] This hypothesis has led to the conclusion that the clinical response to fluoride depends on formulation, dose, and mode of delivery.

The hypothesis that fluoride therapy increases trabecular bone mass at the expense of cortical bone mass has reopened the research into the effect of waterborne fluoride on bone mass and hip fracture rates. During the past 10 years, nine ecological studies have addressed the relationship between hip fracture incidence and water fluoridation. These studies have presented conflicting results, with two showing a protective association, four showing no association, and three showing a negative association between fluoridation and hip fracture incidence.[29] Those finding a negative association reported the relative risks for hip fracture in fluoridated communities compared with nonfluoridated communities to be in the range of 1.08–1.27 for women and 1.17–1.41 for men. These are low relative risks, so that any increased risk of hip fracture in fluoridated communities is likely to be very slight.

Each of these epidemiologic studies contained basic design flaws that make the interpretation of results difficult. Lack of control for confounding variables was the most critical flaw present in each study. Although sex and race were generally controlled for, menopausal state and estrogen use were not addressed. Because these studies were epidemiologic in design, actual fluoride exposure is unknown because individual fluoride histories were not obtained. On the basis of the available literature, there is no association between the ingestion of water containing 0.7–1.2 mg/L fluoride and osteoporosis or fractures.

Health Risks of Fluoride

The health effects (both benefits and risks) of fluoride depend on the applied dose, ranging from physi-

ological through pharmacological to toxicological. To fully understand the effects of fluoride, the concept of dose-response is important. A dose-response relationship is defined as a relationship in which a change in amount, intensity, or duration of exposure is associated with a change, either an increase or a decrease, in risk of a specified outcome.[32] In general, the health risks of fluoride exposure can be divided into two categories: acute and chronic.

Acute toxicity. The literature contains a wide range of estimates of the acute toxic dose of fluoride. On the basis of a review of the literature, Hodge and Smith[33] concluded that the "certainly lethal dose" of sodium fluoride for a 70-kg person was 5–10 g when taken orally. This corresponds to a fluoride dose of 32–64 mg fluoride/kg. The "probably toxic dose" (PTD) of fluoride is 5 mg fluoride/kg of body weight.[34] The PTD is defined as "the minimum dose that could cause toxic signs and symptoms, including death, and that should trigger immediate therapeutic intervention and hospitalization."[35] The "safely tolerated dose" (STD) has been estimated to be 3–5 mg fluoride/kg.[36]

The signs and symptoms of acute fluoride toxicity are nausea, vomiting, diarrhea, abdominal pain, excessive salivation and lacrimation, pulmonary disturbances, cardiac insufficiency and weakness, convulsions, sensory disturbances, paralysis, and coma.[37] In severe poisoning, vomiting should be induced immediately with syrup of ipecac or by digital stimulation. The affected individual should be taken to the hospital for further treatment. If it is certain that an amount below the STD has been ingested, the symptoms should be limited to gastrointestinal distress (nausea and vomiting). Calcium given orally, such as in milk or ice cream, will relieve gastrointestinal symptoms. At intakes <5 mg fluoride/kg, induced vomiting is not recommended.[38]

Chronic toxicity. The only known adverse effect associated with the chronic ingestion of relatively low levels of fluoride (1–2 mg/L in the drinking water) is dental fluorosis, which is hypomineralization of enamel resulting from excess fluoride reaching teeth during developmental stages.[39] Dental fluorosis is considered to be a dose-response condition; severity ranges from barely discernible, even to a trained observer, to the most severe manifestation of stained and pitted enamel. Several detailed reviews of the literature concerning fluorosis data over time have concluded that the prevalence of dental fluorosis in optimally fluoridated areas ranges from 8% to 51%, compared with a range of 3–26% in nonfluoridated areas.[40,41] These ranges include all degrees of severity, although ≈90% of dental fluorosis cases recorded in the United States are mild to very mild.[42] Because dental fluorosis is a function of total fluoride intake during critical developmental periods, most dental researchers believe that the best approach to stabilizing its prevalence and severity is to control fluoride ingestion from foods, processed beverages, and dental products rather than reduce the recommended concentrations of fluoride in drinking water.[43,44]

Chronic ingestion of high doses of fluoride can cause skeletal fluorosis, and it has been speculated that crippling skeletal fluorosis might occur in people who ingest 10–25 mg fluoride/day for 7–20 years.[42,45] The asymptomatic preclinical stage of skeletal fluorosis is characterized by slight increases in bone mass that are detectable radiographically and bone-ash fluoride concentrations of 3500–5500 mg/kg. As a reference, the usual fluoride content in bone ash from individuals who have ingested optimally fluoridated water (0.7–1.2 mg/L) is <1500 mg/kg. As the stages of skeletal fluorosis progress, symptoms range from occasional stiffness or pain in the joints to chronic joint pain, osteoporosis of long bones, and, in severe cases, muscle wasting and neurological defects.[46] Skeletal fluorosis in the United States is rare, with only six cases being reported during the past 30 years. The most recent case involved a 54-year-old female with osteosclerosis. Investigation disclosed the cause of her osteosclerosis to be fluorosis secondary to the ingestion of well water containing 8 mg fluoride/L for 7 years.[45]

The National Research Council, Committee on Toxicology, Subcommittee on Health Effects of Ingested Fluoride,[42] recently reviewed the effects of ingested fluoride on the renal system and the gastrointestinal system in addition to the genotoxicity and carcinogenicity of fluoride. On the basis of available data, the subcommittee believes that the ingestion of fluoride at currently recommended concentrations is not likely to produce renal toxicity, is not likely to produce adverse effects in the gastrointestinal system, is not genotoxic at the concentrations found in plasma of most people in the United States, and is not associated with increased cancer risk in humans.[42]

References

1. National Research Council (1989) Recommended dietary allowances, 10th ed. National Academy Press, Washington, DC, pp 235–240
2. National Research Council (1974) Recommended dietary allowances, 8th ed. National Academy Press, Washington, DC, pp 98–99
3. Burt BA (1992) The changing patterns of systemic fluoride intake. J Dent Res 71:1228–1237
4. US Department of Health and Human Services, Centers for Disease Control and Prevention (1993). Fluoridation census, 1992. CDC, Atlanta
5. Ekstrand J, Spak CJ, Falch J, et al (1984) Distribution of fluoride to human breast milk following intake of high doses of fluoride. Caries Res 18:93–95
6. Dirks OB, Jongeling-Eijndhoven JM, Flissebaalje TD, Gedalia I (1974) Total and free ionic fluoride in human and cow's milk as determined by gas-liquid chromatography and the fluoride electrode. Caries Res 8:181–186
7. Levy SM, Kiritsy MC, Warren JJ (1995) Sources of fluoride intake in children. J Public Health Dent 55:39–52
8. Duckworth SC, Duckworth R (1978) The ingestion of fluoride in tea. Br Dent J 145:368–370
9. Hargreaves JA, Stahl MJ (1986) Fluoride content of teas [abstract]. J Dent Res 65(Spec Iss):B176
10. Wei SHY, Hatab FN (1987) Fluoride content of dried sea foods [abstract]. J Dent Res 66(Spec Iss):957
11. Singer L, Ophaug R (1979) Total fluoride intake of infants. Pediatrics 63:460–466
12. Wiatrowski E, Kramer L, Osis D, Spencer H (1975) Dietary fluoride intake of infants. Pediatrics 55:517–522
13. Stookey GK (1990) Critical evaluation of the composition and use of topical fluorides. J Dent Res 69(Spec Iss):805–812
14. Levy SM (1994) Review of fluoride exposures and ingestion. Commun Dent Oral Epidemiol 22:173–180
15. Anonymous (1994) New fluoride guidelines proposed. J Am Dent Assoc 125:366
16. American Academy of Pediatrics (1995) Fluoride supplementation for childres: interim policy recommendations. Pediatrics 95:777
17. Burt BA, Eklund SA (1992) Dentistry, dental practice, and the community, 4th ed. WB Saunders, Philadelphia, p 140
18. Ad-hoc Subcommittee of Fluoride (1991) Review of fluoride benefits and risks. Department of Health and Human Services, Public Health Service, Washington, DC
19. Whitford GM (1983) Fluorides: metabolism, mechanisms of action and safety. Dent Hyg 57:16–18, 20–22, 24–29
20. Whitford GM (1990) The physiological and toxicological characteristics of fluoride. J Dent Res 69(Spec Iss):539–549
21. Whitford GM, Pashley DH, Stringer GE (1976) Fluoride renal clearance: a pH-dependent event. Am J Physiol 230:527–532
22. Chen PS, Smith FA, Gardner DE (1956) Renal clearance of fluoride. Proc Soc Exp Biol Med 92:879–883
23. Murry JJ, Rugg-Gunn AJ, Jenkins GN, eds (1991) Fluorides in caries prevention. Wright, Boston, pp 295–323
24. Koulourides T (1990) Summary of session II: fluoride and the caries process. J Dent Res 69(Spec Iss):558
25. Rich C, Ensinck J (1961) Effect of sodium fluoride on calcium metabolism of human beings. Nature 191:184–185
26. Pak CY (1989) Fluoride and osteoporosis. Proc Soc Exp Biol Med 191:278–286
27. Gruber HE, Baylink DJ (1991) The effects of fluoride on bone. Clin Orthop 267:264–277
28. Kleerekoper M, Mendlovic DB (1993) Sodium fluoride therapy of postmenopausal osteoporosis. Endocr Rev 14:312–323
29. Phipps KP (1995) Fluoride and bone health. J Public Health Dent 55:53–56
30. Riggs BL, Hodgson SF, O'Fallon WM, et al (1990) Effect of fluoride treatment on the fracture rate in postmenopausal women with osteoporosis. New Engl J Med 322:802–809
31. Pak CYC, Sakhaee K, Piziak V, et al (1994) Slow release sodium fluoride in the management of postmenopausal osteoporosis: a randomized controlled trial. Ann Intern Med 120:625–632
32. Last J (1983) A dictionary of epidemiology. Oxford, New York
33. Hodge HC, Smith FA (1965) Biological properties of inorganic fluorides. In Simonds JH (ed), Fluorine chemistry, Vol IV. Academic Press, New York, pp 2–37
34. Whitford GM (1990) The physiological and toxicological characteristics of fluoride. J Dent Res 69(Spec Iss):539–549
35. Whitford GM (1987) Fluoride in dental products: safety considerations. J Dent Res 66:1056–1060
36. Payless JS, Tinanoff N (1985) Diagnosis and treatment of acute fluoride toxicity. J Am Dental Assoc 110:209–211

37. Duxbury AJ, Leach FN, Duxbury JT (1982) Acute fluoride toxicity. Br Dent J 153:64–66

38. Bayless JM, Tinanoff N (1985) Diagnosis and treatment of acute fluoride toxicity. J Am Dent Assoc 110:209–211

39. Fejerskov O, Manji F, Baelum V (1990) The nature and mechanisms of dental fluorosis in man. J Dent Res 69(Spec Iss):692–700

40. Szpunar SM, Burt BA (1987) Trends in the prevalence of dental fluorosis in the United States: a review. J Public Health Dent 47:71–79

41. Pendrys DG, Stamm JW (1990) Relationship of total fluoride intake to beneficial effects and enamel fluorosis. J Public Health Dent 69(Spec Iss):529–538

42. National Research Council (1993) Health effects of ingested fluoride. National Academy Press, Washington, DC

43. Rozier RG (1991) Reaction paper: appropriate uses of fluoride, considerations for the '90s. J Public Health Dent 51:56–59

44. Szpunar SM, Burt BA (1992) Evaluation of appropriate use of dietary fluoride supplements in the US. Commun Dent Oral Epidemiol 20:148–154

45. Felsenfeld AJ, Roberts MA (1991) A report of fluorosis in the United States secondary to drinking well water. JAMA 265:486–488

46. Smith FA, Hodge HC (1979) Airborne fluorides and man. Crit Rev Environ Control 9:1–25

Chapter 33

Manganese

Carl L. Keen and Sheri Zidenberg-Cherr

Manganese is a metal that has been recognized since the Roman Empire; its name, which is derived from a Greek word for magic, is appropriate given its wide range of metabolic functions and the diverse abnormalities that can result from either its deficiency or toxicity. The essentiality of manganese was established in 1931 when it was demonstrated that a deficit of this substance resulted in poor growth and impaired reproduction in rodents.[1,2] Manganese deficiency has long been recognized as a practical problem in the swine and poultry industries, and during the past decade there has been increasing interest in the concept that manganese deficiency may be a factor contributing to the development or progression of some human diseases.[3] Manganese toxicity is also recognized as a significant health hazard for both domestic animals and humans. This chapter briefly summarizes some of the recent literature related to manganese nutrition, metabolism, and metabolic function. Because of space constraints, review articles rather than original sources are cited in many cases; the reader is directed to these reviews for the original citations and for a more comprehensive discussion of the topics.

Chemistry

Manganese is a transition element located in the 7a column on the periodic table. It can exist in 11 oxidation states from –3 to +7, with the most common valences being +2, +4, and +7. The +2 valence is the predominant form in biological systems, the +4 valence occurs in MnO_2, and the +7 valence is found in permanganate.[4] Free Mn^{2+} has a strong isotropic electron paramagnetic resonance signal that can be used to determine its concentration in the low micromolar range.[5]

Manganese[3+] is also critical in biological systems. For example, Mn^{3+} is the oxidative state of manganese in manganese superoxide dismutase (MnSOD), it is the form in which transferrin binds manganese, and it is probably the form of manganese that interacts with Fe^{3+}.[6,7] Given its smaller ionic radius, the chelation of Mn^{3+} in biological systems would be predicted to be stronger than that of Mn^{2+}. Cycling between Mn^{3+} and Mn^{2+} has been suggested to be potentially deleterious to biological systems because it can involve the generation of free radicals; however, some have argued that at low concentrations, manganese is typically associated with free radical clearance, rather than production.[8–11]

The solution chemistry of Mn^{2+} is relatively simple. The aquo ion is resistant to oxidation in acidic or neutral solutions. It does not begin to hydrolyze until pH 10; therefore, free Mn^{2+} can be present in neutral solutions at relatively high concentrations. Divalent manganese is a d^5 ion and typically forms high-spin complexes lacking crystal field stabilization energies. The above properties, along with its large ionic radius and small charge to radius ratio, result in manganese forming weak complexes relative to other first-row divalent ions such as Ni^{2+} and Cu^{2+}.

Absorption, Transport, Storage, and Turnover

At present, our understanding of the mechanisms regulating the uptake and retention of manganese in humans and experimental animals is limited. Conventional chemical balance techniques have serious limitations with regard to manganese, given the low retention of the element from single meals, the rapid reexcretion of absorbed manganese via bile into the feces, and the slow turnover of manganese pools in the body. Manganese has only one stable isotope; thus, stable isotope techniques based on isotope ratios cannot be used to study manganese absorption. Recently, an increasing number of studies on the absorption and excretion of manganese have been performed using [54]Mn, a γ-emitter with a half-life of 312 days. The use of [54]Mn as an extrinsic label to study manganese uptake from a number of food products, including meat, lettuce, wheat, and dairy products, has been validated.[12,13] Typically in these studies, single radiolabeled meals are fed and whole-body retention measurements are done over a 4-week period. After the excretion of the nonabsorbed isotope, the slow body retention measurements are used to calculate initial fractional absorption.[12]

In studies in which [54]Mn-labeled test meals have been used, the efficiency of manganese absorption in adult humans has been reported to range from 1% to 15%; in contrast, values higher than 25% have been reported from balance studies.[12–15] Given the inherent difficulties associated with chemical balance studies, the absorption values obtained using [54]Mn-labeled meals are probably more accurate. Manganese absorption and retention are higher in young rats than in adults, partly as a consequence of immature excretory pathways.[16] In addition, the ontogenic expression of many manganese-dependent processes is most robust during the early postnatal period; thus, a higher retention of manganese during this time period would be predicted. Human infants have also been reported to retain relatively more manganese from a meal than adults.[17] Taken together, these observations have led to the suggestion that neonates may be particularly susceptible to manganese toxicosis.[18] Hambidge and Krebs[19] have suggested that the recommended maximum level for manganese in infant formulas is 0.12 μg/kJ (50 μg/100 kcal), a value that is considerably lower than that currently found in many commercial formulas.

Manganese absorption is thought to occur throughout the length of the small intestine. In contrast to many of the other essential minerals, the level of manganese in a meal does not have a pronounced effect on the percent absorbed, suggesting that manganese homeostasis is primarily achieved by excretion. At present, there are little data concerning the influence of individual dietary constituents on manganese absorption. High levels of fiber, iron, calcium, and phosphorus have been reported to increase dietary manganese requirements in experimental animals, but with the exception of iron, these factors have only minimal effects on manganese absorption in humans.[13,20-22] Phytate has been shown to inhibit manganese absorption in both experimental animals and humans.[14] Presumably, phytate complexes with manganese to form low-solubility manganese complexes in the intestinal tract, resulting in a reduction in the fraction of soluble manganese available for absorption. In contrast to iron, ascorbic acid does not markedly enhance manganese uptake.[14] Ethanol consumption has been reported to be associated with increased liver manganese concentrations in several species including humans. Although it has been suggested that this increase is due in part to an ethanol-induced increase in manganese absorption, it is more likely a consequence of ethanol-induced increases in liver MnSOD content.[23] High levels of dietary aluminum have been reported to result in low tissue manganese concentrations, possibly as a consequence of aluminum-associated reductions in manganese uptake.[24] Manganese absorption has been reported to be higher in adult women than in adult men, while retention has been reported to be longer in men.[25] Although these differences may be related to iron status, they may also reflect hormonal effects on manganese absorption.

There is a dearth of information regarding the mechanisms by which manganese is taken up and transported across the enterocyte. Based on their similar physiochemical properties, it can be predicted that manganese and iron share some common absorptive and transport mechanisms. The absorption of manganese from a meal can be inversely related to the iron content of the meal as well as the iron status of the individual.[18,26,27] Chronic iron supplementation (60 mg/day for 124 days) has been associated with low levels of serum manganese and lymphocyte MnSOD activity.[27]

Although these observations support the concept that manganese and iron share a common transport pathway, metal-specific intestinal transport proteins have yet to be identified for manganese. Based on studies with brush-border membrane vesicles, Bell et al.[28] reported that the mucosal transport of manganese occurs through a nonsaturable, simple diffusion process when manganese is present at concentrations ranging from 1 to 90 mol/L. However, using intestinal perfusion techniques, Garcia-Aranda et al.[29] reported that the intestinal absorption of manganese is a rapidly saturable process that involves a high-affinity, low-capacity, active-transport mechanism. One interpretation of these reports is that the membrane vesicle studies reflect the initial uptake of manganese, while the perfusion studies reflect manganese uptake across the mucosal membrane and its subsequent serosal transfer. A high-affinity, low-capacity intestinal transfer system for manganese would be valuable as it would help to ensure that the uptake of manganese from diets low in the element would be efficient while partially protecting the animal from absorbing excessive amounts of the element. However, as was noted, current evidence suggests that manganese homeostasis is achieved primarily through excretion rather than absorption.

Manganese entering into the portal blood from the gastrointestinal tract may either remain free (≈0.02 μmol/L) or rapidly become associated with α_2-macroglobulin in a 1:1 ratio.[7] From the portal circulation, the bulk of the absorbed manganese is transported to the liver, where it is rapidly taken up.[30] The uptake of Mn^{2+} by isolated hepatocytes has been reported to occur by a unidirectional, saturable process with the properties of passive mediated transport.[31] A small fraction of the absorbed manganese enters the systemic circulation where it becomes oxidized to Mn^{3+} and bound to transferrin (K_a ≈$10^{10}M^{-1}$).[7] There is speculation that this oxidation step may be catalyzed by ceruloplasmin.

On entering the liver, manganese enters at least five metabolic pools. One pool represents manganese taken up by the lysosomes, from which it is thought to be transferred subsequently to the bile canaliculus. The regulation of manganese is thought to be maintained partly through biliary excretion of the element; up to 50% of manganese injected intravenously can be recovered in the feces within 24 hours. A second pool of manganese is associated with the mitochondria. Mitochondria have a large capacity for manganese uptake, and it is thought that mitochondrial uptake and release of manganese and calcium are related. A third pool of manganese is found in the nuclear fraction of the cell; the roles of nuclear manganese have not been delineated. A fourth manganese pool is incorporated into newly synthesized manganese proteins. The fifth identified intracellular pool of manganese is free Mn^{2+}; fluctuations in this pool may be an important regulator of cellular metabolic control in a manner analogous to free Ca^{2+} and Mg^{2+}.[6,31]

The mechanisms by which manganese is transported to, and taken up by, extrahepatic tissues have not been identified. Transferrin is the major manganese-binding protein in plasma, although up to 10–20% of the manganese in plasma can be associated with albumin and α_2-macroglobulin.[7] While the mechanisms by which manganese is taken up by extrahepatic tissue are still poorly understood, transferrin-mediated manganese uptake across the blood-brain barrier is well established, and neuroblastoma cells in culture have been shown to take up manganese-transferrin complexes.[32,33] Manganese uptake by extrahepatic tissue does not appear to be increased under conditions of manganese deficiency, suggesting a lack of inducible manganese-transport proteins.[30]

Currently, there is only limited information concerning the hormonal regulation of manganese metabolism. Fluxes in the concentrations of adrenal, pancreatic, and pituitary-gonadal axis hormones can affect tissue manganese concentrations.[34] However, it is not clear to what extent hormone-induced changes in tissue manganese concentrations are due to alterations in cellular uptake of manganese or to changes in the expression of manganese metalloenzymes or manganese-activated enzymes.

In marked contrast to most other essential mineral elements, there does not appear to be any appreciable "stores" of manganese in the body. This lack of manganese storage proteins may contribute to the considerable toxicity of this element when there are high cellular concentrations of this metal.

Biochemical Functions

An average human has between ≈200 and 400 μmol of manganese, which is fairly uniform in distribution throughout the body.[6] There is relatively little variation among species with regard to tissue manganese concentrations; bone, liver, pancreas, and kidney tend to have high concentrations of manganese (20–50 nmol/g). Brain, heart, lung, and muscle manganese concentrations are typically <20 nmol/g; blood and serum concentrations are 200 and 20 nmol/L, respectively. Manganese tends to be highest in tissues rich in mitochondria, as its concentration is higher in mitochondria than in cytoplasm or other cell organelles. High concentrations of manganese are normally found in pigmented structures, such as retina, dark skin, and melanin granules. Bone can account for up to 25% of total body manganese because

of its mass, but bone manganese is not thought to be a readily mobilizable pool. In contrast to several other essential trace elements, the fetus does not accrue stores of manganese prior to birth, and fetal tissue manganese concentrations are markedly lower than those found in adults.

Manganese functions in part as a constituent of metalloenzymes and as an enzyme activator. Manganese-containing enzymes include arginase, pyruvate carboxylase, and MnSOD. Arginase, the cytosolic enzyme responsible for urea formation, contains 4 mol Mn^{2+}/mol enzyme. The activity of arginase is affected by diet, with concentrations in manganese-deficient rats being <50% of controls. Despite this marked influence of manganese deficiency on arginase activity, the functional significance of this reduction has not been agreed on, although Brock et al.[35] have recently reported that manganese deficiency-induced reductions in arginase activity can result in elevated plasma ammonia concentrations and low urea concentrations. Kuhn et al.[36] have argued that manganese binding by arginase is also critical for the putative pH-sensing function that has been ascribed for this enzyme in the ornithine cycle. With streptozotocin-induced diabetes, liver and kidney manganese concentrations can be elevated; this increase is associated with an increase in arginase activity.[34] Whether this finding implies an increased manganese requirement for diabetics has not been determined, although it should be noted that studies to date have not indicated a heightened sensitivity of manganese-deficient animals to diabetes-associated abnormalities.[37]

Pyruvate carboxylase, the enzyme that catalyzes the first step of carbohydrate synthesis from pyruvate, contains 4 mol Mn^{2+}/mol enzyme. Although the activity of this enzyme can be slightly lower in manganese-deficient animals than in controls, gluconeogenesis is not markedly inhibited in manganese-deficient animals.[38]

Manganese superoxide dismutase catalyzes the disproportionation of $O\cdot_2^-$ to H_2O_2 and O_2. The activity of MnSOD in tissues of manganese-deficient rats can be significantly lower than in controls. That this reduction is functionally significant is suggested by the observation of high levels of hepatic mitochondrial lipid peroxidation in deficient rats compared with controls.[39] The reduction in MnSOD activity that occurs following the induction of manganese deficiency has been reported to be due to a transcriptional block.[40] Tissue MnSOD activity can be increased by several diverse stressors, including alcohol, ozone, interleukin-1, and tumor necrosis factor-α, presumably as a consequence of stressor-associated increases in cellular free radical (or oxidized target) concentrations.[39,41] This increase in MnSOD activity can be attenuated in manganese-deficient animals, potentially increasing their sensitivity to these insults.[39]

For manganese-activated reactions, the metal can act by binding either to the substrate (such as adenosine triphosphate [ATP]) or directly to the protein, resulting in conformational changes. In contrast to the relatively few manganese metalloenzymes, there are a large number of manganese-activated enzymes, including hydrolases, kinases, decarboxylases, and transferases.[6,42] Many of these metal activations are nonspecific in that other metal ions, particularly Mg^{2+}, can replace Mn^{2+}. One exception to the nonspecific manganese activation of enzymes is the manganese-specific activation of glycosyltransferases. Several manganese deficiency–induced abnormalities have been attributed to a low activity of this enzyme class (see the following discussion). A second example of an enzyme that may be specifically activated by manganese is phosphoenolpyruvate carboxykinase; low activities of this enzyme have been reported in manganese-deficient animals.[38]

A third example of a manganese-activated enzyme is glutamine synthetase. The enzyme, which is found in high concentrations in brain, catalyzes the reaction:

$$NH_3 + glutamate + ATP \rightarrow glutamine + ADP + P_i.$$

Surprisingly, brain glutamine synthetase activity can be normal even in severely manganese-deficient animals, suggesting that this enzyme has either a high priority for the element or that magnesium can substitute for it when manganese is lacking.[43] However, it should also be noted that this enzyme can be inactivated by oxygen radicals; thus, a manganese deficiency–induced reduction in MnSOD activity theoretically could act to depress the activity of this enzyme.[44]

Deficiency Signs

Manganese deficiency has been demonstrated in a number of species, including rats, mice, pigs, and cattle.[3] Signs of manganese deficiency include impaired growth, skeletal abnormalities, impaired reproductive performance, ataxia, and defects in lipid and carbohydrate metabolism.

The effects of manganese deficiency on bone development have been studied extensively, partly because the first abnormality to be recognized as resulting from an inadequate intake of this element was perosis in chickens.[3] It is now recognized that in most species, manganese deficiency can result in shortened and thickened limbs, curvature of the spine, and swollen and enlarged joints.[3,45] The basic biochemical defect underlying the development of these bone defects is a reduction in proteoglycan synthesis secondary to a reduction in the activities of glycosyl transferase. These manganese-activated enzymes are needed for the synthesis of chondroitin sulfate side chains of proteoglycan molecules.[45] Strause et al.[46] have reported that manganese deficiency

in adult rats can result in an inhibition of both osteoblast and osteoclast activity. This observation is particularly noteworthy, given the reports that women with osteoporosis tend to have low blood manganese concentrations and that the provision of manganese supplements might be associated with an improvement in bone health in postmenopausal women.[47,48]

A dramatic sign of manganese deficiency can be severe ataxia if the deficiency occurs in utero. This ataxia, which is irreversible, is characterized by incoordination, lack of equilibrium, and retraction of the head. This condition is the result of impaired development of the otoliths, the calcified structures in the inner ear responsible for normal body-righting reflexes. The otoliths are made up of otoconia, small crystalline structures embedded in an amorphous, proteoglycan-rich matrix. In manganese-deficient animals there is a deficit of proteoglycans in the otolith matrix, and in cells and matrix of the otic cartilage. Thus, it is thought that the block in otolith development is secondary to depressed proteoglycan synthesis because of low activity of manganese-requiring glycosyltransferases.[6] To date, otolith defects attributable to manganese deficiency have not been reported for humans.

Defects in carbohydrate metabolism, in addition to those already described, have been shown in manganese-deficient rats and guinea pigs. In the guinea pig, perinatal manganese deficiency results in severe pancreatic abnormalities, with animals exhibiting aplasia or marked hypoplasia of all cellular components. When manganese-deficient guinea pigs are given a glucose challenge, they respond with a diabetic-type glucose tolerance curve. Manganese supplementation completely reverses the abnormalities in pancreas and glucose tolerance observed in these animals.[6]

In addition to its effect on pancreatic tissue integrity, manganese deficiency can directly impair pancreatic insulin synthesis and secretion. In rats, manganese deficiency results in depressed pancreatic insulin synthesis and enhanced intracellular insulin degradation as well as a depression in the insulin secretory process.[38] The mechanisms underlying the effects of manganese on pancreatic insulin metabolism have not been delineated, but they are thought to be multifactorial. For example, the flux of islet cell manganese from the cell surface to an intracellular pool may be a critical signal for insulin release.[49,50] Insulin mRNA concentrations can be markedly decreased in manganese-deficient rats compared with controls, a finding consistent with the observation of depressed insulin synthesis in these animals.[38] Finally, the effect of manganese deficiency on insulin production also may be due to the destruction of pancreatic β-cells. Diabetogenic agents such as streptozotocin are thought to function via the production of high concentrations of superoxide radicals. The activity of MnSOD in pancreatic islet cells is low relative to other tissues; thus a manganese deficiency–induced reduction in MnSOD activity could render the pancreas particularly susceptible to free radical damage.[6]

In addition to reduced insulin production, manganese deficiency may also affect glucose metabolism by a reduction in the number of glucose transporters in adipose tissue.[51] The mechanism behind this effect has not been identified.

In addition to its effect on endocrine function, manganese deficiency can affect pancreatic exocrine function. For example, manganese-deficient rats can be characterized by an increase in pancreatic amylase content. The mechanism underlying this effect of manganese deficiency has not been delineated; however, it is thought to involve a shift in amylase synthesis or degradation because secretagogue-stimulated acinar secretion is comparable in control and manganese-deficient rats.[52–54]

While the influence of manganese deficiency on carbohydrate metabolism has been demonstrated primarily in experimental animals, there is one report of an insulin-resistant diabetic patient who responded to oral doses of manganese chloride (5 mg of Mn as $MnCl_2$) with decreasing blood glucose concentrations.[55] The rationale for testing the use of manganese in this patient was his reported use of an extract of lucerne, an old South African folk medicine, to treat his diabetes. On analysis the extract was found to contain high concentrations of manganese. Although this is an intriguing case report, others have reported a lack of an effect of oral manganese supplements for either insulin-resistant or insulin-sensitive diabetic subjects, and low blood manganese concentrations have not been found to be a characteristic of diabetics.[56,57]

Abnormal lipid metabolism can result from manganese deficiency, and a lipotropic role for this element has been suggested.[6] Severely manganese-deficient animals can be characterized by high liver fat concentrations, hypocholesterolemia, and low high-density lipoprotein concentrations. Deficient animals can also be characterized by a shift to smaller plasma high-density lipoprotein particles, lower high-density lipoprotein apolipoprotein (apo E) concentrations, and higher apo C concentrations.[58,59]

Abnormal lipid metabolism has been suggested as one of the factors contributing to the development of ultrastructural abnormalities in the tissues of manganese-deficient animals. Reported ultrastructural changes include alterations in the integrity of cell membranes, swollen and irregular endoplasmic reticulum, and elongated mitochondria with stacked cristae. The effect of manganese deficiency on cell membrane integrity could be caused by either an effect of the deficiency on membrane lipid composition or an increased rate of membrane lipid peroxidation or both, because the activity of MnSOD is lower in manganese-deficient animals than in controls.[39] If this is so, it is interesting that the genetically obese (ob/ob) mouse is characterized by low tissue manganese concentrations and MnSOD activity compared with those of lean litter mates.[60] It is not known if the low manganese status of the ob/ob mouse contributes to the pathological expression of this genotype.

It is evident that a deficiency of manganese can result in a number of biochemical and structural defects in experimental animals. That manganese deficiency could potentially be a problem in humans was first suggested by Doisy[61] in 1972, who described a male subject who developed manganese deficiency after its accidental omission from a purified diet that was being used to investigate the effects of vitamin K deficiency. The diet, which was fed for 4 months, provided approximately 0.3 mg Mn/day. Signs that were associated with the feeding of this diet that are not normally considered consequences of vitamin K deficiency included weight loss, reddening of the subject's black hair, dermatitis, reduced growth of hair and nails, and hypocholesterolemia.

The effects of chronic manganese deficiency in young men was investigated by Friedman et al.[62] As part of a manganese balance study, seven male subjects were fed manganese-deficient diets (0.11 mg/day) for 39 days. During the depletion period, all of the subjects were in negative manganese balance and five of the subjects developed a fleeting dermatitis (miliaria crystallina) that disappeared with manganese repletion. Serum calcium, phosphorus, and alkaline phosphatase concentrations increased significantly during the depletion period, consistent with the suggestion by Strause et al.[47] that manganese deficiency may affect bone remodeling.

Although the study of Friedman et al.[62] leaves many unanswered questions about the etiology of the metabolic defects observed during the manganese depletion period, it is a critical study as it indicates the rapidity with which biochemical and metabolic disturbances can occur as a result of low manganese intake in humans. While manganese deficiency has not been documented in humans consuming natural diets, several disease states have been linked to possible disturbances in manganese metabolism.[18] For example, some epileptics have been reported to have low blood manganese concentrations, and low tissue manganese concentrations have been reported in children with maple syrup urine disease and phenylketonuria. Manganese deficiency has also been suggested as a potential underlying factor in the development of joint disease, hip abnormalities, osteoporosis, and congenital malformations.[18] Although it is evident from this that the potential role of manganese deficiency in the etiology or promulgation of several human abnormalities is an area of active research, it should be stressed that evidence for widespread manganese deficiency in human populations is lacking.

Genetic Disorders That Interact with Manganese

The importance of manganese during prenatal development is illustrated in several genetic mutants that possess errors of manganese metabolism. Interactions affecting development can be classified into two groups. The first type of interaction involves a single-mutant gene with a phenotypic expression that can be reduced or prevented by prenatal, postnatal, or perinatal nutritional manipulation. The second type involves strain differences that produce differential responses to a dietary deficiency of the element.

An example of the first group of gene-nutrient interactions is the mutant gene *pallid* in mice. This gene is characterized by pale coat color and ataxia caused by missing or absent otoliths. In an early study in the area of gene-nutrient interactions, Erway et al.[63] demonstrated that supplementing the diet of pallid mice with high amounts of manganese (2000 g Mn/g diet versus a control value of 45 g Mn/g diet) during pregnancy will prevent the occurrence of abnormal otolith development and congenital ataxia in their offspring. The mutant gene itself and the effect of the gene on pigmentation are unaltered by manganese supplementation. The biochemical lesion underlying the enhanced requirement of the pallid mouse for manganese has yet to be identified.

A gene analogous to *pallid, screwneck,* has been identified in mink. This mutant is characterized by a pale coat color, abnormal or missing otoliths in the inner ear, and ataxia. The genetic lesion has been shown to be alleviated by dietary manganese supplementation.[6] Similar to the situation for *pallid,* the biochemical lesions caused by *screwneck* have not been identified.

Representative of the second category of gene-nutrient interactions is the observation that when pregnant mice of several different strains are fed diets containing either a normal (45 g Mn/g diet) or a low amount of manganese (3 g Mn/g diet), the effects on otolith development of the fetuses depend on the mother's genetic background. Most strains show normal otolith development when fed the normal amount of manganese; however, with the lower manganese diet, some strains show up to 30% of normal otolith development in their fetuses, whereas others show only 5% of normal otolith development.[6] The biochemical differences underlying these strain variations are not known, but possible sites include differences in manganese absorption by the mother, maternal blood manganese transport, placental manganese transport, and fetal requirements for glycosyltransferase enzymes. A second example of strain variation in response to manganese deficiency is the observation that Wistar rats differ from RICO rats in that manganese deficiency results in a reduction in hepatic fatty acid synthesis in the former but not the latter strain.[64]

A final example of a rat strain that may be characterized by abnormal manganese metabolism is the genetically epilepsy-prone rat. This rat is characterized by low tissue manganese concentrations compared with those of control rats.[65] This observation is intriguing given the observations that manganese-deficient rats are more susceptible to convulsions than are normal rats, and that whole-blood manganese concentrations are lower in subgroups of humans with epilepsy than in control subjects.[66] Although it is premature to suggest that manganese deficiency is a causative factor for epilepsy in either humans or genetically epilepsy-prone rats, this is an area that merits further investigation.

One human autosomal-recessive genetic disorder that has been reported to be characterized by abnormal manganese metabolism is prolidase deficiency. Prolidase is a manganese-activated dipeptidase with absolute specificity for dipeptides with carboxyl terminal amino acids. The clinical findings in prolidase deficiency include skin ulcers and recurrent infections, mild mental retardation, and bone abnormalities. Patients with this disorder have been reported to have elevated erythrocyte manganese concentrations; however, both erythrocyte prolidase and arginase activities are lower than in normal individuals.[67] These observations suggest that there may be a block in the intracellular transfer of manganese in these individuals.

Requirements and Allowances

The 1989 Recommended Dietary Allowances state that the estimated safe and adequate daily dietary intakes for manganese should be 0.3–1.0 mg/day for infants, 1.0–3.0 mg/day for children, and 2.0–5.0 mg/day for adults.[68] The lower range for the estimated safe and adequate daily dietary intakes figure for adults was based on the review of a number of balance studies in which equilibrium or accretion of manganese occurred whenever the intake was ≥ 2.5 mg/day. According to the results from the Food and Drug Administration's Total Diet Study (1982–1986), manganese intakes were within the estimated safe and adequate daily dietary intake range for young children, teenage boys, adult men, and older men.[69] Intakes for infants tended to exceed the estimated safe and adequate daily dietary intakes, whereas teenage, adult, and older women had manganese intakes that were slightly lower than the appropriate estimated safe and adequate daily dietary intake ranges. Results from the Total Diet Study are encouraging; it should be noted that, on the basis of evaluation of several recent balance studies, it has been argued that the lower range of the recommendation for manganese for adults (2 mg/day) is too low, and that it should be increased to 3.5 mg/day.[70] If this recommendation were followed, a significant proportion of the female population would have intakes <50% of this value.

Specific recommendations for pregnancy and lactation have not been made.

Food and Other Sources

Manganese is widely distributed in the biosphere; it constitutes approximately 0.1% of the earth's crust, making it the 12th most abundant element. Manganese is a component of numerous complex materials, including pyrolusite, manganite, rhoclochrosite, rhodanite, braunite, and pyrochroite. The chemical forms of manganese found in natural deposits include oxides, sulfides, carbonates, and silicates. Water concentrations of manganese are typically between 1 and 100 µg/L, with most values being below 10 µg/L. Typical airborne concentrations of manganese in nonindustrial areas range from 0.05 to 0.10 µg/m³; values around manganese-emitting industries can be markedly higher, often in the range of 1–5 mg/m³.[18,71] Anthropogenic sources of manganese are predominantly from the manufacturing of steel, alloys, and iron products. Manganese is also used in dry cell batteries as an oxidizing agent and as a component of fertilizers, fungicides, and numerous other products. Airborne concentrations of manganese can also be increased as a consequence of the use of manganese-containing antiknock compounds in gasoline.[18,71]

Manganese concentrations in typical food products range from 0.2 µg/g (meat, dairy products, poultry, fish) to 20 µg/g (nuts, cereals, dried fruit). Vegetables typically contain intermediate levels (0.5–2 µg/g). Relatively high concentrations of manganese are found in tea and coffee (300–600 µg/mL), and these sources can account for as much as 10% of daily manganese intake for some individuals. Typical commercial dietary manganese supplements provide 2.5–5 mg of the element as a chloride or carbonate complex.

Toxicity

In domestic animals the major reported biochemical lesion associated with dietary manganese toxicosis is an induction of iron deficiency that may result from an inhibitory effect of manganese on iron absorption.[3] Additional signs of manganese toxicity in domestic animals can include depressed growth, depressed appetite, and altered brain function.[3]

In humans, manganese toxicity represents a serious health hazard, resulting in severe abnormalities of the central nervous system.[18] In its more severe forms, manganese toxicity can result in a syndrome characterized by severe psychiatric symptoms, including hyperirritability, violent acts, hallucinations, disturbances of libido, and incoordination. The toxicity results in a permanent crippling of the extrapyramidal system, the morphological lesions of which are similar to Parkinson's disease. Although the majority of reported cases of manganese toxicity have been in individuals exposed to excessive airborne amounts of the element (>5 mg/m³), subtle signs of manganese toxicity, including delayed reaction time, impaired motor coordination, and impaired memory, have been observed in workers exposed to airborne manganese concentrations <1 mg/m³.[72,73] Manganese toxicity has been reported in an individual who consumed high amounts of manganese supplements over a period of years.[74] There have been a number of cases of manganese toxicity in individuals who consume water containing high manganese concentrations.[18,75,76]

There has been concern recently that the risk for manganese toxicity may be increasing in some geographical areas because of the use of methylcyclopentadenyl manganese tricarbonyl in gasoline as an antiknock agent. However, there is little evidence that air, water, or food manganese concentrations have markedly increased in geographical areas in which this fuel additive has been used.[18,71] In addition to extensive neural damage, reproductive and immune system dysfunction, nephritis, testicular damage, pancreatitis, and hepatic damage can occur with manganese toxicity, but the frequency of these disorders is not known.[18] Manganese is known to be mutagenic in nonmammalian systems, but mutagenicity has not been reported in mammalian systems.[18] High levels of dietary manganese have not been reported to be teratogenic in the absence of overt signs of maternal toxicity.[77] High levels of brain manganese have been reported in subjects with amyotrophic lateral sclerosis, and it has been suggested that this increase may contribute to the progression of the disease.[78]

Several recent papers have described the development of manganese toxicity in individuals with compromised liver function or compromised biliary pathways or both.[79-83] Significantly, these individuals may have abnormal magnetic resonance image (MRI) patterns, which can improve following the alleviation of the manganese toxicity. For example, in some cases improvements in brain function have been achieved after liver transplant.[79-81]

The mechanism or mechanisms underlying the cellular toxicity of manganese have not been absolutely identified, although there is evidence that they involve manganese-initiated catechol autoxidation and excessive tissue oxidative damage.[18,84] Abnormal carbohydrate metabolism may also underlie some of the effects of manganese toxicosis, given the observation that insulin production can be impaired in animals subjected to high amounts of the element.[18]

Biomarkers for Manganese Status

At present, reliable biomarkers for the assessment of manganese status have not been identified. Whole-blood manganese concentrations have been reported to be reflective of soft tissue manganese concentrations in rats; however, it is not known if a similar relationship is also true for humans.[85] Plasma manganese concentrations have been shown to be reduced in subjects fed diets low in manganese and slightly higher than normal in subjects given manganese supplements.[27,62] Lymphocyte MnSOD activity has been reported to be sensitive to dietary manganese intake, but as discussed earlier, a number of diverse stressors can influence the synthesis of this enzyme.[27] Urinary manganese excretion has not been found to be sensitive to dietary manganese intake.[27] With respect to the diagnosis of manganese toxicosis, the use of MRI appears to be promising as the images associated with manganese toxicity are relatively specific.[79–83] Although it is relatively expensive, the use of MRI to detect cases of manganese toxicity may be particularly useful as a means of identifying susceptible individuals in, or around, manganese-emitting factories. In addition, the method may be useful in the evaluation of patients with liver failure.

Summary

The absorption of manganese is not well regulated, and there is little evidence of homeostatic mechanisms controlling the rates of uptake and efflux from the gut. Absorbed manganese is transported via α_2-macroglobulin and transferrin; the ligand or ligands responsible for transferring manganese to extrahepatic tissue have not been agreed on. Despite significant amounts of manganese in the environment, tissue concentrations of the element are typically low.

Fluctuations in the intracellular concentration of free Mn^{2+} may provide a critical regulatory role for some metabolic processes. Spontaneous manganese deficiency can occur in domestic animals and avian species. The incidence of spontaneous manganese deficiency in humans is unknown; however, several disease states are characterized by low blood manganese concentrations. At the biochemical level, manganese deficiency is reflected by low tissue arginase, glycosyl transferase, and MnSOD activities. Manganese-deficient animals can be characterized by abnormal pancreatic function as evidenced by low insulin and high amylase production. Consistent with this biochemistry, manganese-deficient animals are characterized by connective tissue defects and abnormalities in lipid and carbohydrate metabolism.

Manganese is essential for normal brain function, partly through its role in the metabolism of biogenic amines. Manganese toxicity is a serious health hazard, resulting in a permanently crippling neurological disorder of the extrapyramidal system. Manganese toxicity occurs primarily in individuals exposed to high levels of manganese in the air in certain work environments; however, isolated cases of manganese toxicosis occurring from dietary exposure have been reported.

The adequacy of manganese nutrition in humans has not been well characterized, partly because of a lack of good biomarkers for manganese status. However, given the findings of abnormal manganese metabolism in several disease states, it is evident that increased attention should be given to delineating the role of this element in human health and disease.

References

1. Kemmerer AR, Elvehjem CA, Hart EB (1931) Studies on the relation of manganese to the nutrition of the mouse. J Biol Chem 92:623–630
2. Orent ER, McCollum EV (1931) Effects of deprivation of manganese in the rat. J Biol Chem 92:651–678
3. Hurley LS, Keen CL (1987) Manganese. In Underwood E, Mertz E (eds), Trace elements in human health and animal nutrition. Academic Press, New York, pp 185–223
4. Reed GH (1986) Manganese: an overview of chemical properties. In Schramm VL, Wedler FC (eds), Manganese in metabolism and enzyme function. Academic Press, Orlando, FL, pp 313–326
5. Ash DE (1986) Methods of Mn (II) determination. In Schramm VL, Wedler FC (eds), Manganese in metabolism and enzyme function. Academic Press, Orlando, FL, pp 327–356
6. Keen CL, Lonnerdal B, Hurley LS (1984) Manganese. In Frieden E (ed), Biochemistry of the essential ultratrace elements. Plenum Publishing Co, New York, pp 89–132
7. Critchfield JW, Keen CL (1992) Manganese^{+2} exhibits dynamic binding to multiple ligands in human plasma. Metabolism 41:1087–1092
8. Segura-Aguilar J, Lind C (1989) On the mechanisms of the Mn^{3+}-induced neurotoxicity of dopamine: prevention of quinone-derived oxygen toxicity by DR diaphorase and superoxide dismutase. Chem Biol Interact 72:309–324
9. Oteiza PI, Fraga CF, Keen CL (1993) Aluminum has both oxidant and antioxidant effects in mouse brain membranes. Arch Biochem Biophys 300:517–521
10. Coassin M, Ursini F, Bindoli A (1992) Antioxidant effect of manganese. Arch Biochem Biophys 299:330–333
11. Singh RK, Kooreman KM, Babbs CF, et al (1992) Potential use of simple manganese salts as antioxidant drugs in horses. Am J Vet Res 53:1822–1829
12. Davidsson L, Cederblad A, Hagebo E, et al (1988) Intrinsic and extrinsic labeling for studies of manganese absorption in humans. J Nutr 118:1517–1521
13. Johnson PE, Lykken GI, Korynta ED (1991) Absorption and biological half-life in humans of intrinsic and extrinsic ^{54}Mn tracers from foods of plant origins. J Nutr 121:711–717
14. Davidsson L, Almgren A, Juillerat MA, Hurrell RF (1995) Manganese absorption in humans: the effect of phytic acid and ascorbic acid in soy formula. Am J Clin Nutr 62:984–987
15. Freeland-Graves JH, Behmardi F, Bales CW, et al. (1988) Metabolic balance of manganese in young men consuming diets containing five levels of dietary manganese. J Nutr 118:764–773
16. Keen CL, Bell JG, Lonnerdal B (1986) The effect of age on manganese uptake and retention from milk and infant formulas in rats. J Nutr 116:395–402
17. Wirth FH Jr, Numerof B, Pleban P, Neylan MJ (1990) Effect of lactose on mineral absorption in preterm infants. J Pediatr 117:283–287

18. Keen CL, Zidenberg-Cherr S, Lonnerdal B (1994) Nutritional and toxicological aspects of manganese intake: an overview. In Mertz W, Abernathy CO, Olin SS (eds), Risk assesment of essential elements. ILSI Press, Washington DC, pp 221–235

19. Hambidge KM, Krebs NF (1989) Upper limits of zinc, copper and manganese in infant formulas. J Nutr 19:1861–1864

20. Lonnerdal B, Keen CL, Bell JG, Sandstrom B (1987) Manganese uptake and retention: experimental animal and human studies. In Kies C (ed), Nutritional bioavailability of manganese. American Chemical Society, Washington, DC, pp 9–20

21. Davidsson L, Cederblad A, Lonnerdal B, Sandstrom B (1991) The effect of individual dietary components on manganese absorption in humans. Am J Clin Nutr 54:1065–1070

22. Johnson PE, Lykken GI (1991) Manganese and calcium absorption and balance in young women fed diets with varying amounts of manganese and calcium. J Trace Elem Exp Med 4:19–35

23. Halsted CH, Keen CL (1990) Alcoholism and micronutrient metabolism and deficiencies. Eur J Gastroenterol Hepatol 2:399–405

24. Golub M, Han B, Keen CL, Gershwin ME (1993) Developmental patterns of aluminum in mouse brain and effects of dietary aluminum excess on manganese deficiency. Toxicology 81:33–47

25. Finley JW, Johnson PE, Johnson LK (1994) Sex affects manganese absorption and retention by humans from a diet adequate in manganese. Am J Clin Nutr 60:949–955

26. Rossander-Hulten L, Brune M, Sanstrom B, et al (1991) Competitive inhibition of iron absorption by manganese and zinc in humans. Am J Clin Nutr 54:152–156

27. Davis CD, Greger JL (1992) Longitudinal changes of manganese-dependent superoxide dismutase and other indexes of manganese and iron status in women. Am J Clin Nutr 55:747–752

28. Bell JB, Keen CL, Lonnerdal B (1989) Higher retention of manganese in suckling than in adult rats is not due to maturational differences in manganese uptake by rat small intestine. J Toxicol Environ Health 26:387–398

29. Garcia-Aranda JA, Wapnir JA, Lifshitz F (1983) In vivo intestinal absorption of manganese in the rat. J Nutr 113:2601–2607

30. Keen CL, Zidenberg-Cherr S, Lonnerdal B (1987) Dietary manganese toxicity and deficiency: effects on cellular manganese metabolism. In Kies C (ed), Nutritional bioavailability of manganese. American Chemical Society, Washington DC, pp 21–34

31. Schramm VL, Brandt M (1986) The manganese (II) economy of rat hepatocytes. Fed Proc 45:2817–2820

32. Aschner M, Gannon M (1994) Manganese (Mn) transport across the rat blood-brain barrier: saturable and transferrin-dependent transport mechanisms. Brain Res Bull 33:345–349

33. Suarez N, Eriksson H (1993) Receptor-mediated endocytosis of a manganese complex of transferrin into neuroblastoma (SHSY5Y) cells in culture. J Neurochem 61:127–131

34. Failla ML (1986) Hormonal regulation of manganese metabolism. In Schramm VL, Wedler FC (eds), Manganese in metabolism and enzyme function. Academic Press, Orlando, FL, pp 93–105

35. Brock AA, Chapman SA, Ulman EA, Wu G (1994) Dietary manganese deficiency decreases rat hepatic arginase activity. J Nutr 124:340–344

36. Kuhn NJ, Ward S, Piponski M, Young TW (1995) Purification of human hepatic arginase and its manganese (II)-dependent and pH-dependent interconversion between active and inactive forms: a possible pH-sensing function of the enzyme on the ornithine cycle. Arch Biochem Biophys 320:24–34

37. Thompson KH, Lee M (1993) Effects of manganese and vitamin E deficiencies on antioxidant enzymes in streptozotocin-diabetic rats. J Nutr Biochem 4:476–481

38. Baly DL, Walter RM Jr, Keen CL (1994) Manganese metabolism and diabetes. In Klimis-Tavantzis DJ (ed), Manganese in health and disease. CRC Press, Boca Raton, FL, pp 101–113

39. Zidenberg-Cherr S, Keen CL (1991) Essential trace elements in antioxidant processes. In Dreosti IE (ed), Trace elements, micronutrients, and free radicals. Humana Press, New Jersey, pp 107–127

40. Borrello S, De Leo ME, Galeotti T (1992) Transcriptional regulation of MnSOD by manganese in the liver of manganese-deficient mice and during rat development. Biochem Int 28:595–601

41. Akashi M, Hachiya M, Paquette RL, et al (1995) Irradiation increases manganese superoxide dismutase mRNA levels in human fibroblasts: possible mechanisms for its accumulation. J Biol Chem 270:15864–15869

42. Wedler FC (1994) Biochemical and nutritional role of manganese: an overview. In Klimis-Tavantzis DJ (ed), Manganese in health and disease. CRC Press, Boca Raton, FL, pp 1–37

43. Critchfield JW, Carl GF, Keen CL (1993) The influence of manganese supplementation on seizure onset and severity, and brain monoamines in the genetically epilepsy prone rat. Epilepsy Res 14:3–10

44. Schor NF (1988) Inactivation of mammalian brain glutamine synthetase by oxygen radicals. Brain Res 456:17–21

45. Liu AC, Heinrichs BS, Leach RM Jr (1994) Influence of manganese deficiency on the characteristics of proteoglycans of avian epiphyseal growth plate cartilage. Poult Sci 73:663–669

46. Strause L, Saltman P, Glowacki J (1987) The effect of deficiencies of manganese and copper on osteoinduction and on resorption of bone particles in rats. Calcif Tissue Int 41:145–150

47. Strause L, Saltman P, Smith KT, et al (1994) Spinal bone loss in postmenopausal women supplemented with calcium and trace minerals. J Nutr 124:1060–1064

48. Freeland-Graves J, Llanes C (1994) Models to study manganese deficiency. In Klimis-Tavantzis DJ (ed), Manganese in health and disease. CRC Press, Boca Raton, FL, pp 39–86

49. Rorsman P, Hellman B (1983) The interaction between manganese and calcium fluxes in pancreatic β-cells. Biochem J 210:307–314

50. Korc M, Schoni MH (1988) Quin 2 and manganese define multiple alterations in cellular calcium homeostasis in diabetic rat pancreas. Diabetes 73:13–20

51. Baly DL, Schneiderman JS, Garcia-Welsh AL (1990) Effect of manganese deficiency on insulin binding, glucose transport and metabolism in rat adipocytes. J Nutr 120:1075–1079

52. Werner L, Korc M, Brannon PM (1987) Effects of manganese deficiency and dietary composition on rat pancreatic enzyme content. J Nutr 117:2079–2085

53. Chang SC, Brannon PM, Korc M (1990) Effects of dietary manganese deficiency on rat pancreatic amylase mRNA levels. J Nutr 120:1228–1234

54. Korc M (1993) Manganese as a modulator of signal transduction pathways. Prog Clin Biol Res 380:235–255

55. Rubenstein AH, Levin NW, Elliott GA (1962) Manganese-induced hypoglycemia. Lancet 2:1348–1351

56. Walter RM Jr, Aoki TT, Keen CL (1991) Acute oral manganese administration does not consistently affect glucose tolerance in non-diabetic and type II diabetic humans. J Trace Elem Exp Med 4:73–79

57. Walter RM, Uriu-Hare JY, Olin KL, et al (1991) Copper, zinc, manganese, and magnesium status and complications of diabetes mellitus. Diabetes Care 14:1050–1056

58. Kawano J, Ney DN, Keen CL, Schneeman BO (1987) Altered high density lipoprotein composition in manganese-deficient Sprague-Dawley and Wistar rats. J Nutr 117:902–906

59. Davis CD, Ney DM, Greger JL (1990) Manganese, iron and lipid interactions in rats. J Nutr 120:507–513

60. Begin-Heick N, Deeks JR (1987) Hypercorticism and manganese metabolism in brown adipose tissue of the obese mouse. J Nutr 117:1708–1714

61. Doisy E Jr (1972) Micronutrient controls of biosynthesis of clotting proteins and cholesterol. In Hemphill D (ed), Trace substances in environmental health, vol VI. University of Missouri, Columbia, pp 193–199

62. Friedman BJ, Freeland-Graves JH, Bales CW, et al (1987) Manganese balance and clinical observations in young men fed a manganese-deficient diet. J Nutr 117:133–143

63. Erway L, Hurley LS, Fraser A (1966) Neurological defect: manganese in phenocopy and prevention of a genetic abnormality of the inner ear. Science 152:1766–1768

64. Klimis-Tavantzis DJ, Taylor PN, Wolinsky I (1994) Manganese, lipid metabolism, and atherosclerosis. In Klimis-Tavantzis DJ (ed), Manganese in health and disease. CRC Press, Boca Raton, FL, pp 87–100

65. Carl GF, Critchfield JW, Thompson JL, et al (1990) Genetically epilepsy prone rats are characterized by altered tissue trace element concentrations. Epilepsia 31:247–252

66. Carl GF, Keen CL, Gallagher BB, et al (1986). Association of low blood manganese concentrations with epilepsy. Neurology 36:1584–1587

67. Lombeck I, Wendel U, Versieck J, et al (1986) Increased manganese content and reduced arginase activity in erythrocytes of a patient with prolidase deficiency (iminodipeptiduria). Eur J Pediatr 144:571–573

68. National Research Council (1989) Recommended dietary allowances, 10th ed. National Academy Press, Washington, DC

69. Pennington JAT, Young BE (1991) Total diet study nutritional elements, 1982–1989. J Am Diet Assoc 91:179–183

70. Freeland-Graves J (1994) Derivation of manganese estimated safe and adequate daily dietary intakes. In Mertz W, Abernathy CO, Olin SS (eds), Risk assessment of essential elements. ILSI Press, Washington DC, pp 237–252

71. Cooper WC (1984) The health implications of increased manganese in the environment resulting from the combustion of fuel additives: a review of the literature. J Toxicol Environ Health 14:23–46

72. Roels H, Lauwerys R, Buchet J, et al (1987) Epidemiological survey among workers exposed to manganese: effects on lung, central nervous system, and some biological indices. Am J Ind Med 11:307–327

73. Iregren A (1990) Psychological test performance in foundry workers exposed to low levels of manganese. Neurotoxicol Teratol 12:673–675

74. Banta G, Markesbery WR (1977) Elevated manganese levels associated with dementia and extrapyramidal signs. Neurology 27:213–216

75. Kondakis XG, Makris N, Leotsinidis M, Prinous M, Papapetropoulos T (1989) Possible health effects of high manganese concentration in drinking water. Arch Environ Health 44:175–178

76. Velazuez SF, Du JT (1994) Derivation of the reference dose for manganese. In Mertz W, Abernathy CO, Olin SS (eds), Risk assessment of essential elements. ILSI Press, Washington, DC, pp 253–266

77. Sanchez DJ, Domingo JL, Llobet JM, Keen CL (1993) Maternal and developmental toxicity of manganese in the mouse. Toxicol Lett 69:45–52

78. Kihira T, Mukoyama M, Ando K, et al (1990) Determination of manganese concentrations in the spinal cords from amyotrophic lateral sclerosis patients by inductively coupled plasma emission spectroscopy. J Neurosci 98:251–258

79. Nelson K, Golnick J, Korn T, Angle C (1993) Manganese encephalopathy: utility of early magnetic resonance imaging. Br J Ind Med 50:510–513

80. Dvenyi AG, Barron TF, Mamourian AC (1994) Dystonia, hyperintense basal ganglia, and high whole blood manganese levels in Alagille's syndrome. Gastroenterology 106:1068–1071

81. Mirowitz SA, Westrich TJ (1992) Basal ganglia signal intensity alterations: reversal after discontinuation of parenteral manganese administration. Radiology 185:535–536

82. Hauser RA, Zesiewica TA, Rosemurgy AS, et al (1994) Manganese intoxication and chronic liver failure. Ann Neurol 36:871–875

83. Reynolds AP, Kiely E, Meadows N (1994) Manganese in long term paediatric parenteral nutrition. Arch Dis Child 71:529–531

84. Lloyd RV (1995) Mechanism of the manganese-catalyzed autoxidation of dopamine. Chem Res Toxicol 8:111–116

85. Clegg MS, Lonnerdal B, Hurley LS, Keen CL (1986) Analysis of whole blood manganese by flameless atomic absorption spectrophotometry and its use as an indicator of manganese status in animals. Anal Chem 157:12–18

Chapter 34

Chromium

Barbara J. Stoecker

In 1957 Schwarz and Mertz[1] reported that a compound termed "glucose tolerance factor," which was extracted from porcine kidney, restored impaired glucose tolerance in rats. Chromium was identified as the essential element that potentiated insulin action.[2] Subsequently, malnourished children with impaired glucose tolerance were given oral supplements of 250 μg chromium as $CrCl_3 \cdot 6H_2O$, and improvement in glucose removal rate was noted in children presumed to be chromium-deficient.[3] Since that time, chromium supplementation has been reported to correct chromium depletion in three patients receiving total parenteral nutrition.[4–6] Chromium supplementation generally, but not always, has relieved impaired glucose tolerance in humans.[7] Chromium metabolism has been reviewed by several investigators.[8–15]

Chromium is present in biological tissues in very low concentrations, making it crucial to avoid contamination of specimens obtained in a clinical setting.[16,17] Over the years, the reported concentration of chromium in serum and urine has decreased by at least three orders of magnitude. The lower values reflect improvements in analytical instrumentation and greater attention to the myriad sources of chromium contamination in sample collection and analysis.[16,17]

Chemistry

Chromium is a transition element that can occur in a number of valence states, with 0, +2, +3, and +6 being the most common.[18,19] Cr^{3+} is the most stable form in biological systems.[8,19,20] Cr^{6+} is a strong oxidizing agent that comes primarily from industrial sources.[21] Cr^{6+} consumed in small amounts is reduced to Cr^{3+} in the acidic environment of the stomach.[8,22] There are major differences in solubility of chromium salts.[22] Various organic complexes help to prevent formation of biologically inert chromium oxides and help to retain solubility at the pH of intestinal contents.[8,19] These chromium complexes have a slow rate of ligand exchange and vary in biological activity.[8,23]

Absorption, Transport, Storage, and Turnover

Absorption. Intestinal absorption of trivalent chromium is low. Estimates of absorption in fasted rats range from <0.5% to 2–3%.[8,24,25] In rats, only a small amount of intravenously or orally administered $^{51}CrCl_3$ is excreted via the bile.[26,27]

In a metabolic balance study, two men consuming an average of 36.8 μg chromium per day had a mean apparent net absorption of chromium of 1.8%.[28] Because of the analytical problems associated with measurement of actual chromium absorption, several researchers have used urinary excretion as an indicator of absorption. Normal subjects given a dose of $^{51}CrCl_3$ had a mean of 0.69% (range, 0.3–1.3%) of the dose in the urine within 72 hours.[29] In adults receiving 200 μg chromium supplements daily, urinary excretion was approximately 0.4%.[30]

Prior chromium status and amount of chromium present in the diet apparently affect chromium absorption.[31,32] In a study of guinea pigs depleted of chromium, there was more ^{51}Cr in blood and liver 3 hours after an oral dose of $^{51}CrCl_3$ than in animals fed diets adequate in chromium.[31] When dietary chromium intake was 10 μg, approximately 2% of that amount was absorbed (estimated as urinary excretion), whereas at chromium intakes of 40 μg, only 0.4–0.5% of the chromium was recovered in urine.[32]

Various dietary components also alter chromium absorption. Using double intestinal perfusion techniques in rats, Dowling and colleagues[33] determined that the presence of amino acids in a test meal enhanced chromium transport into the vascular perfusate. Starch feeding generally increased tissue chromium derived from the diet and from $^{51}CrCl_3$ in obese and control mice compared with mice fed fructose, glucose, and sucrose.[34] Absorption of ^{51}Cr was increased in zinc-deficient rats and was reduced by zinc administration.[35]

Ascorbic acid promotes chromium absorption. In a study with this finding, three women consumed 1 mg chromium as chromium chloride with or without 100 mg ascorbic acid. Plasma chromium concentrations were consistently higher following the chromium given in conjunction with ascorbic acid.[36] Integrated areas under the plasma appearance curves were 144%, 277%, and 448% of the areas obtained when chromium was given without ascorbic acid.[36] Likewise in rats, ^{51}Cr in urine 24 hours after dosing with ascorbic acid and $^{51}CrCl_3$ was significantly higher than in the control group.[37]

Chelation of a mineral may increase or decrease its availability. When oxalate (0.1 mmol/L) and $^{51}CrCl_3$ were mixed together and administered orally, ^{51}Cr levels in the blood, whole body, and urine of rats were markedly increased at 24 hours. The same concentration of phytate caused a much smaller but still significant decrease in ^{51}Cr levels.[38] However, when rats were fed a soy-protein diet containing a somewhat higher phytate-to-chromium ratio, there was no effect on glucose tolerance or fasting plasma insulin.[39] Currently, there is considerable interest in increasing absorption of chromium by chelating chromium with various amino acids or their derivatives.[23,40] However, physiological impacts need clarification.

Common medications apparently enhance or impair chromium absorption. Chelation and changes in cytoprotective factors in the gastrointestinal tract may contribute to these effects. Rats given 40 mg aspirin orally had markedly enhanced absorption of ^{51}Cr from [51]CrCl$_3$ compared with controls.[25] A lower dose of 40 mg aspirin per kilogram of body weight again significantly enhanced ^{51}Cr in blood, tissues, and urine in rats.[41] Intraperitoneal injection of 5 mg indomethacin per kilogram of body weight significantly increased ^{51}Cr in blood, tissues, and urine of rats, indicating that blocking the synthesis of gastrointestinal prostaglandins enhanced chromium absorption.[42] When the rats were given an oral supplement of an analog of prostaglandin E$_2$, this reduced ^{51}Cr in blood and tissues significantly below that of the control group.[42] Single doses of several antacids significantly reduced ^{51}Cr in blood and tissues compared with controls.[25,37]

Transport. In rats that were intubated and fed physiological levels of [51]CrCl$_3$, >99% of the ^{51}Cr in blood was associated with the noncellular component 24 hours after ^{51}Cr administration. When transferrin was precipitated from ^{51}Cr-labeled human serum, 80% of the isotope was present in the precipitate. Iron added to the serum before the addition of ^{51}Cr resulted in a dose-responsive reduction in ^{51}Cr bound to transferrin.[43] Either albumin or apo-transferrin were necessary for normal transport of ^{51}Cr to the vascular perfusate in rats.[44] Human apo-transferrin dissolved in Earle's medium bound chromium in the presence of citric acid, and iron uptake by apo-transferrin was reduced by either aluminum or chromium.[45] Addition of iron to the medium reduced binding of aluminum or chromium to apo-transferrin.[45] Likewise, a study of rats that were injected intraperitoneally with 1 mg/kg chromium as chromium chloride daily for 45 days showed they had significant reductions in serum iron, serum total iron-binding capacity, serum ferritin, and in hemoglobin and hematocrit.[46] It has been hypothesized that iron interferes with the transport of chromium in hemochromatosis.[47,48]

Storage. Studies have shown that after injection or oral dosing of [51]CrCl$_3$ in rats, there was accumulation of ^{51}Cr in liver, kidney, testis, bone, and spleen.[25,26,49,50] In humans, ^{51}Cr accumulated in liver, spleen, soft tissue, and bone.[47] In young Finnish accident victims, mean chromium concentration of the liver was 8 ng/g dry weight and spleen chromium concentration was 15 ng/g dry weight, illustrating low chromium concentrations even in those organs that are known to accumulate chromium.[51]

Turnover. In rats intubated with [51]CrCl$_3$, ^{51}Cr reached a peak in the blood by 1 hour after administration and decreased logarithmically to 20% of the peak value after 24 hours.[43] However, circulating chromium does not appear to be in equilibrium with tissue chromium stores.[8,40,43]

Mertz and coworkers[52] injected rats intravenously with [51]CrCl$_3$ and used whole-body counting to determine ^{51}Cr retention. On the basis of retention rates, they proposed three compartments with half-lives estimated at 0.5, 5.9, and 83.4 days. Onkelinx[53] also proposed a three-compartment model, but suggested different characteristics for the third compartment.

In humans, the distribution of intravenous [51]Cr^{3+} was observed with whole-body scanning, a whole-body counter, and plasma counting in five normal subjects. A model was proposed with a plasma pool in equilibrium with fast ($t_{1/2} = 0.56$ days), medium ($t_{1/2} = 12.7$ days), and slow ($t_{1/2} = 192$ days) compartments.[48] Hemochromatosis altered the rate constants for chromium pools.[48] Subsequently, Do Canto and colleagues[54] injected ^{51}Cr as chromium chloride intravenously in seven adult-onset diabetes patients and compared the data with those of three normal subjects. The average half-life for urinary excretion was 0.97 days for the diabetic group and 1.51 days for normal subjects. A four-compartment model was formulated containing a central compartment, a compartment within the blood pool, and slow- and fast-tissue compartments. The fast-tissue compartment showed the most difference between groups; half-life values for the fast-exchange tissue compartment were 19 hours for normal subjects but only 5 hours for the diabetic subjects ($P < 0.005$). Those authors suggest that this pool would be the best candidate for chromium used in glucose metabolism.

Dietary factors may impact chromium turnover. In one study, 37 subjects consumed high-sugar diets (35% of total calories from simple sugars) for 6 weeks. Twenty-seven of these subjects had increased urinary chromium excretion compared with the period when they consumed only 15% of total calories from simple sugars.[55] Urinary chromium losses were related to the insulinogenic properties of carbohydrates.[56]

Physiologic Functions

Chromium potentiates insulin action. Addition of chromium to epididymal fat tissue from chromium-deficient rats stimulated glucose uptake in the presence of added insulin.[8,57] Exogenous insulin stimulated significantly more uptake of amino acids by heart protein in chromium-supplemented animals than in chromium-depleted ones.[58]

In the early studies of chromium, a factor was extracted from brewers' yeast that improved glucose tolerance of chromium-deficient rats.[8] This factor, which appeared to contain nicotinic acid, glutamic acid, glycine, and a sulfur-containing amino acid, was called glucose tolerance factor. Controversy has continued about the precise structure of glucose tolerance factor because of the difficulty in purifying or synthesizing the active compound.[7] Further research is needed to resolve the questions about function and structure of glucose tolerance factor. However, chromium as found in brewers' yeast and in some other naturally occurring and synthetic complexes is more effective in stimulating glucose use than is chromium chloride or chromium found in torula yeast.[59–63]

Chromium effects on growth. Several studies cited by Mertz[8] reported increases in growth and survival of chromium-supplemented rats and mice. Growth also was impaired in guinea pigs that were fed diets containing <60 μg chromium per kilogram.[64] A significantly increased rate of growth was observed in a group of malnourished children given a chromium supplement compared with a similar group who received no chromium supplementation.[65] Two patients receiving chromium-deficient total parenteral nutrition solutions showed weight loss that was restored with chromium supplementation.[4,5]

Potential effects of chromium on feed efficiency and muscle area have been of interest to the livestock industry. Page et al.[66] noted increased daily gain in weight and percent of muscle in pigs when diets were supplemented with 200 μg chromium as chromium picolinate. However, pigs whose diets were supplemented with porcine pituitary somatotropin, 300 μg chromium per kilogram diet (as picolinate), or both in a 2 × 2 factorial design had improved growth performance with somatotropin but not with chromium.[67]

Chromium effects on glucose tolerance. Effects of chromium supplementation in humans have been reviewed recently. Mertz[7] noted that in 12 of 15 controlled studies, chromium supplementation improved the efficiency of insulin or the blood lipid profiles of subjects. In only three of these studies was there no effect on glucose, insulin, or lipids. As one would expect, subjects with some degree of impaired glucose tolerance were more responsive to chromium supplementation than other subjects.[7,68] In one study, 20 of the 76 subjects had serum glucose concentrations ≥ 5.5 mmol/L (100 mg/dL) 90 minutes after a 1 g/kg body weight glucose challenge. Chromium chloride supplementation (200 μg chromium per day) significantly reduced 90-minute glucose concentration in these 20 subjects.[68] Serum insulin concentrations did not change. In another study, subjects were fed low-chromium diets (<20 μg/day) for 14 weeks. After

4 weeks, 200 μg chromium ($CrCl_3$) or placebo was randomly assigned for 5 weeks in a crossover trial. Chromium supplementation in subjects with normal glucose tolerance had no effect; however, the glucose tolerance of the eight subjects with initially impaired glucose tolerance deteriorated further during the placebo period and improved significantly during chromium supplementation.[69] Less than 20 μg chromium/day was sufficient to prevent impaired glucose tolerance in the control group, but how long normal glucose tolerance could be maintained on such a low chromium intake is unknown.

Chromium effects on lipid metabolism. Data on effects of chromium on serum cholesterol in experimental animals and humans are equivocal. Supplementation of diets of obese mice with 2 mg chromium/kg diet as chromium chloride markedly reduced total hepatic lipid and tended to reduce circulating insulin.[70] In a study of rabbits, daily injection of either potassium chromate or chromium chloride for 135 days produced a marked reduction in aortic cholesterol and in the percentage of aortic intimal surface covered by plaque.[71] Some studies reported decreased total serum cholesterol and increased high-density lipoprotein cholesterol and apolipoprotein A concentrations with chromium supplementation; others showed no effects of chromium supplementation. One contributor to this variability is the inability to determine initial chromium status of the subjects. For a mean of 11 months, Abraham et al.[72] gave daily supplements of either 250 μg chromium as chloride or placebo to 76 patients with established atherosclerotic disease. Serum triacyglycerol levels were lower and high-density lipoprotein cholesterol was higher at the end of supplementation. Among men receiving beta-blockers, supplementation with 600 μg chromium from high-chromium brewers' yeast resulted in significant increases in high-density lipoprotein cholesterol compared with patients receiving placebo.[73] Supplementation with 150 μg chromium as chromium chloride for subjects who had total cholesterol >6.21 mmol/L (240 mg/dL) decreased total serum cholesterol, low-density lipoprotein cholesterol, and apolipoprotein B.[74] Lefavi et al.[75] suggested that a chromium-nicotinic acid complex lowered total serum cholesterol of subjects with initial values in the normal range. In another study, combined supplements of chromium and nicotinic acid significantly reduced total integrated glucose area in a glucose tolerance test.[76]

Chromium interactions with nucleic acids. Chromium in mouse liver was found to be concentrated in the nuclei 48 hours after intraperitoneal injection of 0.005–5 mg chromium chloride/kg body weight.[77] Ohba and colleagues[78] reported that Cr^{3+} bound to DNA in vitro and increased the number of initiation sites, thereby enhancing RNA synthesis. In another study, chromium chloride was administered intraperitoneally (5 mg chromium/kg body weight) to rats that underwent partial hepatectomy 24 hours later. A nucleolar chromium-bound protein of 70 kD was identified that enhanced hepatic nucleolar RNA synthesis in the rats that had undergone partial hepatectomy, but not in normal rats.[79] This research group suggested that the cellular action of chromium may be involved in the regulation of cell growth.

Chromium effects on immune response. A few recent studies have suggested benefits of chromium supplementation in diets of stressed cattle. After market-transit stress, steer calves receiving supplements of 0.4 mg chromium/kg diet had significantly decreased serum cortisol and increased serum immunoglobulin.[80] Two additional studies confirmed an effect of chromium on specific immune responses.[81,82]

Chromium supplementation in diabetics. Effects of chromium supplementation in diabetics have generally been unremarkable. In one study, supplements of 200 µg $CrCl_3$ given to non-insulin-dependent diabetics had no effects on measured lipid parameters, on glucose tolerance, or on fasting serum insulin.[83] In another study, a group of 43 diabetic men (ketosis-prone and ketosis-resistant) and 20 normal subjects were given supplements of chromium chloride, a glucose tolerance factor yeast, a yeast extract without glucose tolerance factor, or a placebo. Fasting plasma glucose and lipids were not significantly altered by any of the treatments.[84] Abraham et al.[72] found no change in blood glucose in persons who received supplements of 250 µg chromium for a mean of 11 months. Sherman et al.[85] found that chromium chloride did not improve hyperglycemia in diabetic patients. Mossop,[86] on the other hand, noted dramatic improvements in fasting blood glucose of 13 diabetics receiving supplements of 600 µg chromium as chromium chloride.

Chromium needs of the elderly. In an early study by Levin and colleagues,[87] chromium supplements of 150 µg/d were given to 10 elderly subjects; glucose tolerance was normalized in four subjects. Mean chromium intakes of the elderly, as well as the young, are below the estimated safe and adequate daily dietary intake.[32,88,89] Despite an increase in the frequency of impaired glucose tolerance with age, total chromium excreted in urine was not related to age.[89] Offenbacher and colleagues[89,90] found that age itself was not a risk factor for chromium deficiency.

Chromium needs in cases of metabolic stress. Studies have shown that trauma patients and persons who exercised strenuously had elevated urinary excretion of chromium.[91,92] In addition, it has been postulated that chromium needs may increase during pregnancy.[93,94] Nielsen[95] has suggested that metabolic stress is a key factor in identifying the essentiality of the ultratrace minerals.

Effects of Chromium Deficiency

Chromium was designated an essential element based on its role in restoring glucose tolerance in rats.[2] However, because chromium is ubiquitous in the environment, it is difficult to produce a clear chromium deficiency in laboratory animals. No chromium-dependent enzyme has been identified. Chromium concentrations in serum or plasma are near the detection limits of currently available instruments and do not appear to be good indicators of actual chromium status.[96] Therefore, studies that seek to reverse a possible chromium-deficiency symptom by supplementation are hampered by inadequate means to assess the initial chromium status of the subjects. Nonetheless, understanding of the physiological functions of chromium is increasing. Metabolic stress may exacerbate the deficient state.[8,91,95,97]

Cellular level. In cell culture, mouse myotubes were differentiated in chromium-adequate or chromium-poor media. In the chromium-poor media, insulin-stimulated uptake of radiolabeled glucose was reduced by almost 50% compared with that in myotubes in chromium-replete media. Physiological concentrations of inorganic chromium restored uptake of glucose. Sensitivity of the cells to insulin was lessened by a reduction in the chromium content of the media and was repleted when chromium was returned to the media.[98] In another study, insulin secretion by the perfused rat pancreas from chromium-supplemented rats was higher than in chromium-depleted animals.[99]

Animal studies. Decreased weight gain has been reported for rats, mice, and guinea pigs whose diets were depleted of chromium.[8,64,100] Obese mice depleted of chromium had significantly elevated hepatic lipid and reduced circulating insulin.[70] Rats given chromium chloride supplements had significantly lower fasting glucose than rats fed chromium-depleted diets.[8,101] In another study, chromium-depleted mice had significantly reduced muscle and cardiac glycogen.[34] Chromium depletion also reduced sperm count in rats.[102]

Human studies. In studies of patients whose total parenteral nutrition solutions contained no chromium or were supplemented with inadequate amounts of chromium, insulin requirements were reduced and glucose intolerance reversed with chromium chloride supplementation.[4-6] Two of these patients had weight loss that was restored with chromium supplementation.[4,5] Peripheral neuropathy was seen in one of the patients and it was reversed with chromium supplementation.[4]

Requirement—Recommended Dietary Allowance

In 1980 a recommendation for dietary chromium appeared as an estimated safe and adequate daily dietary intake in the ninth edition of the *Recommended Dietary Allowances*. The estimated safe and adequate daily dietary intake remained at 50–200 µg/day in the 10th edition in 1989.[103] Because no enzyme has been identified as an indicator of chromium status and because of the very low concentrations of chromium in accessible tissues, it has not been possible to monitor a large group of subjects with variable chromium intakes.

Chromium intakes for many people are below the lower range of the estimated safe and adequate daily dietary intake.[28,32,89,104,105] Otherwise-adequate diets can be formulated with <3.8 µg chromium/MJ (16 µg chromium/1000 kcal).[32,106] High-fat diets apparently have lower chromium than isocaloric low-fat diets.[107] In one study, self-selected diets were composited for seven days and analyzed for chromium content. The mean chromium intake of 10 adult men was 33 µg/d (range, 22–48) and chromium intake for 22 women was 25 µg/d (range, 13–36).[32] Various studies have found 22–100% of the subjects to have chromium intakes <50 µg/d.[32,104,105]

When the original estimated safe and adequate daily dietary intake for chromium was established in 1980, most data on chromium concentrations in food, serum, and urine had been obtained without using the types of background correction currently available on instruments; many early data are too high because of analytical problems and contamination.[9,108,109] Currently available data might suggest a lower estimated safe and adequate daily dietary intake than the current 50–200 µg/d for adults.

As the appropriate chromium intakes for different age groups are considered, the estimated safe and adequate daily dietary intake for infants of 10–40 µg/day is particularly problematic. An infant consuming 750 mL of human milk receives less than 1 µg chromium per day, based on current measurements.[110–113] There is no indication of enhanced absorption of chromium from human milk, which makes the estimated safe and adequate daily dietary intake for this age group appear too high.

Food and Other Sources

In the United States, meat, poultry, fish, and especially dairy products tend to be low in chromium. Fruits and vegetables and grain products have variable chromium concentrations.[106] Pulses, seeds, and dark chocolate may contain more chromium than most other foods.[114] Certain spices such as black pepper contain high concentrations of chromium but contribute little to the usual diet on a per serving basis.[106,115] A number of years ago, large losses of chromium in milling were reported,[116] but a more recent analysis found chromium to have a relatively homogeneous distribution between the grist and mill streams.[117] However, loss of chromium in the process of refining sugar has been noted.[118]

Processing also may add chromium to the food supply. Stainless steel typically contains 11–30% chromium.[119] In one study, chromium was leached from stainless steel containers, particularly when contents were acidic.[120] Another study showed that some brands of beer contain significant amounts of chromium, some of which presumably is exogenous.[121] Processed meats also appear to gain chromium during manufacture.[106]

In addition to the variable chromium concentrations found in foods, there are differences in bioavailability and biological activity of chromium in various complexes.[57,122] The best-known chromium complex is the glucose tolerance factor first identified by Mertz et al.[57] and suggested to contain nicotinic acid, glycine, glutamic acid, and cysteine. A low-molecular-weight chromium-binding material also has been identified in bovine colostrum, but whether such a complex is present in mature milk is not known.[123]

Excess and Toxicity

Intakes of trivalent chromium that are adequate to produce a physiological effect are considered safe[8]; furthermore, the safety of 200-µg chromium supplements given as chromium chloride has been established in a number of studies.[7] Because trivalent chromium is poorly absorbed, high oral intakes would be necessary to attain toxic levels.

One study showed that tannery workers exposed to Cr^{3+} had elevated body loads of chromium, but apparently the chromium is excreted rapidly.[124] Workers handling wet hides had significantly higher serum chromium levels and urinary chromium-creatinine ratios than workers in other areas of the tannery. Hexavalent chromium in air samples was below the detection limit; the authors indicated that the tanning compounds contained trivalent chromium almost exclusively.

Toxic effects of industrial exposure have been attributed primarily to airborne Cr^{6+} compounds.[21,125,126] Toxicity symptoms included allergic dermatitis, skin and nasal septum lesions, and increased incidence of lung cancer.[19,21,22,127,128] A key to the toxicity of Cr^{6+} compounds may be products of its cellular reduction to Cr^{3+}.[20,22,129] Welding of stainless steel generates hexavalent chromium. In a meta-analysis for lung cancer that accounted for asbestos exposure and smoking, a pooled relative risk of 1.94 was found for the welders.[130]

In some areas of the United States, soil contains elevated levels of both trivalent and hexavalent chromium. However, test results indicated that soil levels below 450 ppm Cr^{6+} and 165,000 ppm Cr^{3+} should not pose a hazard of allergic-contact dermatitis for at least 99.99% of exposed persons.[127]

Summary

Chromium analysis remains challenging because of its low levels in biological tissues and because of potential sample contamination.[16,131] Furthermore, chromium concentrations in accessible tissues apparently do not reflect metabolically active chromium pools in the body.[17] The essentiality of chromium has been demonstrated, but further research is necessary to clarify its physiological functions. The inability to accurately assess chromium status hampers study design and interpretation. Many people in the United States consume <50 µg chromium per day.[32,88,89] Long-term consequences of dietary intakes <50 µg/d and of metabolic stressors need to be determined. Clinical tests that identify individuals who are chromium-deficient are clearly needed.

Appropriate chromium supplementation for total parenteral nutrition patients should be carefully evaluated. On the basis of signs of chromium deficiency in total parenteral nutrition patients, an expert panel of the American Medical Association has recommended 10–15 µg chromium per day for adults whose disease condition has stabilized.[132] Initial supplementation with at least 20 µg chromium per day was recently suggested by Frankel.[133] The daily supplementation of total parenteral nutrition with 0.14–0.20 µg chromium per kilogram was recommended for children.[132] If orally and intravenously administered chromium are utilized similarly, an intravenous dose of 15 µg chromium per day is equivalent to a daily oral intake of 3000 or 1500 µg/day at absorption rates of 0.5% or 1%, respectively. Moukarzel et al.[134] reported that children receiving total parenteral nutrition (0.15 µg chromium per kilogram) had serum chromium concentrations 20 times higher than control children (2.1 versus 0.10 µg/L).

Another area to be investigated is the widespread practice of self-supplementation of chromium. One article referred to this phenomenon as the "scam of the hour."[135] Some studies have suggested chromium has an effect on muscle and fat distribution, but chromium supplementation should not have a nutritional effect unless a deficiency exists. Nine weeks of chromium supplementation with 200 µg chromium as picolinate was ineffective in causing changes in body composition or strength of football players during intensive weight-lifting training.[136] Another study suggested that any potential anabolic effects due to enhanced insulin function would likely be marginal.[137] Furthermore, in normal rat kidney (NRK) cells, picolinic acid markedly reduced iron uptake and arrested growth.[138] The efficacy and safety of various forms of chromium supplements need evaluation.[139]

References

1. Schwarz K, Mertz W (1957) A glucose tolerance factor and its differentiation from factor 3. Arch Biochem Biophys 72:515–518

2. Schwarz K, Mertz W (1959) Chromium(III) and the glucose tolerance factor. Arch Biochem Biophys 85:292–295

3. Hopkins LL Jr, Ransome-Kuti O, Majaj AS (1968) Improvement of impaired carbohydrate metabolism by chromium(III) in malnourished infants. Am J Clin Nutr 21:203–211

4. Jeejeebhoy KN, Chu RC, Marliss EB, et al (1977) Chromium deficiency, glucose intolerance, and neuropathy reversed by chromium supplementation in a patient receiving long-term total parenteral nutrition. Am J Clin Nutr 30:531–538

5. Freund H, Atamian S, Fischer JE (1979) Chromium deficiency during total parenteral nutrition. JAMA 241:496–498

6. Brown RO, Forloines-Lynn S, Cross RE, Heizer WD (1986) Chromium deficiency after long-term total parenteral nutrition. Dig Dis Sci 31:661–664

7. Mertz W (1993) Chromium in human nutrition: a review. J Nutr 123:626–633

8. Mertz W (1969) Chromium occurrence and function in biological systems. Physiol Rev 49:163–239

9. Anderson RA (1987) Chromium. In Mertz W (ed), Trace elements in human and animal nutrition, 5th ed. Academic Press, New York, pp 225–244

10. Offenbacher EG, Pi-Sunyer FX (1988) Chromium in human nutrition. Annu Rev Nutr 8:543–563

11. Ducros V (1992) Chromium metabolism: a literature review. Biol Trace Elem Res 32:65–77

12. Anderson RA (1994) Nutritional and toxicologic aspects of chromium intake: an overview. In Mertz W, Abernathy CO, Olin SS (eds), Risk assessment of essential elements. ILSI Press, Washington, DC, pp 187–196

13. Stoecker BJ (1994) Derivation of the estimated safe and adequate daily dietary intake for chromium. In Mertz W, Abernathy CO, Olin SS (eds), Risk assessment of the essential elements. ILSI Press, Washington, DC, pp 197–205

14. Mertz W (1992) Chromium: history and nutritional importance. Biol Trace Elem Res 32:3–8

15. Anderson RA (1993) Recent advances in the clinical and biochemical effects of chromium deficiency. Prog Clin Biol Res 380:221–234

16. Veillon C (1989) Analytical chemistry of chromium. Sci Total Environ 86:65–68

17. Iyengar GV (1989) Nutritional chemistry of chromium. Sci Total Environ 86:69–74

18. Emsley J (1992) The elements. Oxford University Press, Oxford, pp 52–53

19. Losi ME, Amrhein C, Frankenberger WT Jr (1994) Environmental biochemistry of chromium. Rev Environ Contam Toxicol 136:91–121

20. Cohen MD, Kargacin B, Klein CB, Costa M (1993) Mechanisms of chromium carcinogenicity and toxicity. Crit Rev Toxicol 23:255–281

21. Von Burg R, Liu D (1993) Chromium and hexavalent chromium. J Appl Toxicol 13:225–230

22. O'Flaherty EJ (1994) Comparison of reference dose with estimated safe and adequate daily dietary intake for chromium. In Mertz W, Abernathy CO (eds), Risk assessment of essential elements. ILSI Press, Washington, DC, pp 213–218

23. Evans GW, Pouchnik DJ (1993) Composition and biological activity of chromium-pyridine carboxylate complexes. J Inorg Biochem 49:177–187

24. Sayato Y, Nakamuro K, Matsui S, Ando M (1980) Metabolic fate of chromium compounds. I. Comparative behavior of chromium in rat administered with $Na_2{}^{51}CrO_4$ and ${}^{51}CrCl_3$. J Pharmacobiodyn 3:17–23

25. Davis ML, Seaborn CD, Stoecker BJ (1995) Effects of over-the-counter drugs on ^{51}chromium retention and urinary excretion in rats. Nutr Res 15:202–210

26. Hopkins LL Jr (1965) Distribution in the rat of physiological amounts of injected Cr-51(III) with time. Am J Physiol 209:731–735

27. Davis-Whitenack ML, Adeleye BO, Rolf LL, Stoecker BJ (1996) Biliary excretion of [51]chromium in bile-duct cannulated rats. Nutr Res, in press

28. Offenbacher E, Spencer H, Dowling HJ, Pi-Sunyer FX (1986) Metabolic chromium balances in men. Am J Clin Nutr 44:77–82

29. Doisy RJ, Streeten DHP, Souma ML, et al (1971) Metabolism of chromium-51 in human subjects. In Mertz W, Cornatzer WE (eds), Newer trace elements in nutrition. Marcel Dekker, New York, pp 155–168

30. Anderson RA, Polansky MM, Bryden NA, et al (1983) Effects of chromium supplementation of urinary Cr excretion of human subjects and correlation of Cr excretion with selected clinical parameters. J Nutr 113:276–281

31. Seaborn CD, Stoecker BJ (1992) Effects of ascorbic acid depletion and chromium status on retention and urinary excretion of [51]chromium. Nutr Res 12:1229–1234

32. Anderson RA, Kozlovsky AS (1985) Chromium intake, absorption and excretion of subjects consuming self-selected diets. Am J Clin Nutr 41:1177–1183

33. Dowling HJ, Offenbacher EG, Pi-Sunyer FX (1990) Effects of amino acids on the absorption of trivalent chromium and its retention by regions of the small intestine. Nutr Res 10:1261–1271

34. Seaborn CD, Stoecker BJ (1989) Effects of starch, sucrose, fructose, and glucose on chromium absorption and tissue concentrations in obese and lean mice. J Nutr 119:1444–1451

35. Hahn CJ, Evans GW (1975) Absorption of trace metals in the zinc-deficient rat. Am J Physiol 228:1020–1023

36. Offenbacher EG (1994) Promotion of chromium absorption by ascorbic acid. Trace Elem Electrolytes 11:178–181

37. Seaborn CD, Stoecker BJ (1990) Effects of antacid or ascorbic acid on tissue accumulation and urinary excretion of [51]chromium. Nutr Res 10:1401–1407

38. Chen NSC, Tsai A, Dyer IA (1973) Effect of chelating agents on chromium absorption in rats. J Nutr 103:1182–1186

39. Keim KS, Stoecker BJ, Henley S (1987) Chromium status of the rat as affected by phytate. Nutr Res 7:253–263

40. Polansky MM, Bryden NA, Anderson RA (1993) Effects of form of chromium on chromium absorption [abstract]. FASEB J 7:A77

41. Davis ML, Spicer MT, Stoecker BJ, Sangiah S (1992) Alteration of ^{51}Cr absorption and retention by drugs that affect prostaglandins [abstract]. FASEB J 6:A1951

42. Kamath SM, Stoecker BJ, Whitenack MD, et al (1995) Indomethacin and prostaglandin E_2 analogue effects on absorption, retention, and urinary excretion of [51]chromium [abstract]. FASEB J 9:A577

43. Hopkins LL Jr, Schwarz K (1964) Chromium (III) binding to serum proteins, specifically siderophilin. Biochim Biophys Acta 90:484–491

44. Dowling HJ, Offenbacher EG, Pi-Sunyer FX (1990) Effects of plasma transferrin and albumin on the absorption of trivalent chromium. Nutr Res 10:1251–1260

45. Moshtaghie AA, Ani M, Bazrafshan MR (1992) Comparative binding study of aluminum and chromium to human transferrin: effect of iron. Biol Trace Elem Res 32:39–46

46. Ani M, Moshtaghie AA (1992) The effect of chromium on parameters related to iron metabolism. Biol Trace Elem Res 32:57–64

47. Lim TH, Sargent T III, Kusubov N (1983) Kinetics of trace element chromium(III) in the human body. Am J Physiol 244:R445–R454

48. Sargent T III, Lim TH, Jenson RL (1979) Reduced chromium retention in patients with hemochromatosis, a possible basis of hemochromatotic diabetes. Metabolism 28:70–79

49. Jain R, Verch RL, Wallach S, Peabody RA (1981) Tissue chromium exchange in the rat. Am J Clin Nutr 34:2199–2204

50. Wallach S, Verch RL, Berdanier CD (1988) Radiochromium retention and distribution in young and old glucose-intolerant rats. J Trace Elem Exp Med 1:89–94

51. Vuori E, Kumpulainen J (1987) A new low level of chromium in human liver and spleen. Trace Elem Med 4:88–91

52. Mertz W, Roginski EE, Reba RC (1965) Biological activity and fate of trace quantities of intravenous chromium in the rat. Am J Physiol 209:489–494

53. Onkelinx C (1977) Compartment analysis of metabolism of chromium(III) in rats of various ages. Am J Physiol 232:E478–E484

54. Do Canto OM, Sargent T III, Liehn JC (1995) Chromium (III) metabolism in diabetic patients. In Sive Subrananian KN, Wastney ME (eds), Kinetic models of trace element and mineral metabolism. CRC Press, Boca Raton, FL, pp 205–219

55. Kozlovsky AS, Moser PB, Reiser S, Anderson RA (1986) Effects of diets high in simple sugars on urinary chromium losses. Metabolism 35:515–518

56. Anderson RA, Bryden NA, Polansky MM, Reiser S (1990) Urinary chromium excretion and insulinogenic properties of carbohydrates. Am J Clin Nutr 51:864–868

57. Mertz W, Toepfer EW, Roginski EE, Polansky MM (1974) Present knowledge of the role of chromium. Fed Proc 33:2275–2280

58. Roginski E, Mertz W (1969) Effects of chromium(III) supplementation on glucose and amino acid metabolism in rats fed a low protein diet. J Nutr 97:525–530

59. Tuman RW, Bilbo JT, Doisy RJ (1978) Comparison and effects of natural and synthetic glucose tolerance factor in normal and genetically diabetic mice. Diabetes 27:49–56

60. Offenbacher EG, Pi-Sunyer FX (1980) Beneficial effect of chromium-rich yeast on glucose tolerance and blood lipids in elderly subjects. Diabetes 29:919–925

61. Toepfer EW, Mertz W, Polansky MM, et al (1977) Preparation of chromium-containing material of glucose tolerance factor activity from brewer's yeast extracts and by synthesis. J Agric Food Chem 25:162–166

62. Stoecker BJ, Li Y-C, Wester DB, Chan S-B (1987) Effects of torula and brewer's yeast diets in obese and lean mice. Biol Trace Elem Res 14:249–254

63. Evans GW, Bowman TD (1993) Chromium picolinate increases membrane fluidity and rate of insulin internalization. J Inorg Biochem 46:243–250

64. Seaborn CD, Cheng NZ, Adeleye B, et al (1994) Chromium and chronic ascorbic acid depletion effects on tissue ascorbate, manganese and ^{14}C retention from ^{14}C-ascorbate in guinea pigs. Biol Trace Elem Res 41:279–294

65. Gurson CT, Saner G (1973) Effects of chromium supplementation on growth in marasmic protein-calorie malnutrition. Am J Clin Nutr 26:988–991

66. Page TG, Southern LL, Ward TL, Thompson DL Jr (1993) Effect of chromium picolinate on growth and serum and carcass traits of growing-finishing pigs. J Anim Sci 71:656–662

67. Evock-Clover CM, Polansky MM, Anderson RA, Steele NC (1993) Dietary chromium supplementation with or without somatotropin treatment alters serum hormones and metabolites in growing pigs without affecting growth performance. J Nutr 123:1504–1512

68. Anderson RA, Polansky MM, Bryden NA, et al (1983) Chromium supplementation of human subjects: effects on glucose, insulin, and lipid variables. Metabolism 32:894–899

69. Anderson RA, Polansky MM, Bryden NA, Canary JJ (1991) Supplemental-chromium effects on glucose, insulin, glucagon, and urinary chromium losses in subjects consuming controlled low-chromium diets. Am J Clin Nutr 54:909–916

70. Li Y-C, Stoecker BJ (1986) Chromium and yogurt effects on hepatic lipid and plasma glucose and insulin of obese mice. Biol Trace Elem Res 9:233–242

71. Abraham AS, Brooks BA, Eylath U (1991) Chromium and cholesterol-induced atherosclerosis in rabbits. Ann Nutr Metab 35:203–207

72. Abraham AS, Brooks BA, Eylath U (1992) The effects of chromium supplementation on serum glucose and lipids in patients with and without non-insulin-dependent diabetes. Metabolism 41:768–771

73. Roeback JR Jr, Hla KM, Chambless LE, Fletcher RH (1991) Effects of chromium supplementation on serum high-density lipoprotein cholesterol levels in men taking beta-blockers. Ann Int Med 115:917–924

74. Hermann J, Arquitt A, Stoecker BJ (1994) Effect of chromium supplementation on plasma lipids, apolipoproteins, and glucose in elderly subjects. Nutr Res 14:671–674

75. Lefavi RG, Wilson GD, Keith RE, et al (1993) Lipid-lowering effect of a dietary chromium(III)-nicotinic acid complex in male athletes. Nutr Res 13:239–249

76. Urberg M, Zemel MB (1987) Evidence for synergism between chromium and nicotinic acid in the control of glucose tolerance in elderly humans. Metabolism 36:896–899

77. Okada S, Suzuki M, Ohba H (1983) Enhancement of ribonucleic acid synthesis by chromium(III) in mouse liver. J Inorg Biochem 19:95–103

78. Ohba H, Suketa Y, Okada S (1986) Enhancement of in vitro ribonucleic acid synthesis on chromium(III)-bound chromatin. J Inorg Biochem 27:179–189

79. Okada S, Tsukada H, Tezuka M (1989) Effect of chromium (III) on nuclear RNA synthesis. Biol Trace Elem Res 21:35–39

80. Chang X, Mowat DN (1992) Supplemental chromium for stressed and growing feeder calves. J Anim Sci 70:559–565

81. Moonsie-Shageer S, Mowat DN (1993) Effect of level of supplemental chromium on performance, serum constituents, and immune status of stressed feeder calves. J Anim Sci 71:232–238

82. Burton JL, Mallard BA, Mowat DN (1993) Effects of supplemental chromium on immune responses of periparturient and early lactation dairy cows. J Anim Sci 71:1532–1539

83. Uusitupa MIJ, Kumpulainen JT, Voutilainen E, et al (1983) Effect of inorganic chromium supplementation on glucose tolerance, insulin response, and serum lipids in noninsulin-dependent diabetics. Am J Clin Nutr 38:404–410

84. Rabinowitz MB, Gonick HC, Levin SR, Davidson MB (1983) Effects of chromium and yeast supplements on carbohydrate and lipid metabolism in diabetic men. Diabetes Care 6:319–327

85. Sherman L, Glennon JA, Brech WJ, et al (1968) Failure of trivalent chromium to improve hyperglycemia in diabetes mellitus. Metabolism 17:439–442

86. Mossop RT (1983) Effects of chromium III on fasting blood glucose, cholesterol and cholesterol HDL levels in diabetics. Central African J Med 29:80–82

87. Levine RA, Streeten DHP, Doisy RJ (1968) Effects of oral chromium supplementation on the glucose tolerance of elderly human subjects. Metabolism 17:114–125

88. Anderson RA, Bryden NA, Polansky MM (1993) Dietary intake of calcium, chromium, copper, iron, magnesium, manganese, and zinc: duplicate plate values corrected using derived nutrient intake. J Am Diet Assoc 93:462–464

89. Offenbacher EG (1992) Chromium in the elderly. Biol Trace Elem Res 32:123–131

90. Offenbacher E, Rinko C, Pi-Sunyer FX (1985) The effects of inorganic chromium and brewer's yeast on glucose tolerance, plasma lipids, and plasma chromium in elderly subjects. Am J Clin Nutr 42:454–456

91. Borel JS, Majerus TC, Polansky MM, et al (1984) Chromium intake and urinary chromium excretion of trauma patients. Biol Trace Elem Res 6:317–326

92. Anderson RA, Bryden NA, Polansky MM, Deuster PA (1988) Exercise effects on chromium excretion of trained and untrained men consuming a constant diet. J Appl Physiol 64:249–252

93. Saner G (1981) The effect of parity on maternal hair chromium concentration and the changes during pregnancy. Am J Clin Nutr 34:853–855

94. Wallach S, Verch RL (1984) Placental transport of chromium. J Am Coll Nutr 3:69–74

95. Nielsen FH (1988) Nutritional significance of the ultratrace elements. Nutr Rev 46:337–341

96. Anderson RA, Bryden NA, Polansky MM (1985) Serum chromium of human subjects: effects of chromium supplementation and glucose. Am J Clin Nutr 41:571–577

97. Anderson RA, Polansky MM, Bryden NA (1984) Acute effects on chromium, copper, zinc, and selected clinical variables in urine and serum of male runners. Biol Trace Elem Res 6:327–336

98. Morris B, Gray T, MacNeil S (1995) Evidence for chromium acting as an essential trace element in insulin-dependent glucose uptake in cultured mouse myotubes. J Endocrinol 144:135–141

99. Striffler JS, Polansky MM, Anderson RA (1993) Dietary chromium enhances insulin secretion in perfused rat pancreas. J Trace Elem Exp Med 6:75–81

100. Schroeder HA (1966) Chromium deficiency in rats: a syndrome simulating diabetes mellitus with retarded growth. J Nutr 88:439–445

101. Schroeder HA (1969) Serum cholesterol and glucose levels in rats fed refined and less refined sugars and chromium. J Nutr 97:237–242

102. Anderson RA, Polansky MM (1981) Dietary chromium deficiency: effect on sperm count and fertility in rats. Biol Trace Elem Res 3:1–5

103. National Research Council (1989) Recommended dietary allowances. National Academy Press, Washington, DC

104. Bunker VW, Lawson MS, Delves HT, Clayton B (1984) The uptake and excretion of chromium by the elderly. Am J Clin Nutr 39:797–802

105. Gibson RS, Scythes CA (1984) Chromium, selenium, and other trace element intakes of a selected sample of Canadian premenopausal women. Biol Trace Elem Res 6:105–116

106. Anderson RA, Bryden NA, Polansky MM (1992) Dietary chromium intake: freely chosen diets, institutional diets, and individual foods. Biol Trace Elem Res 32:117–121

107. Kumpulainen JT, Wolf WR, Veillon C, Mertz W (1979) Determination of chromium in selected United States diets. J Agric Food Chem 27:490–494

108. Guthrie BE, Wolf WR, Veillon C (1978) Background correction and related problems in the determination of chromium in urine by graphite furnace atomic absorption spectrometry. Anal Chem 50:1900–1902

109. Veillon C, Patterson KY, Bryden NA (1982) Chromium in

urine as measured by atomic absorption spectrometry. Clin Chem 28:2309–2311

110. Casey CE, Hambidge KM (1984) Chromium in human milk from American mothers. Br J Nutr 52:73–77

111. Anderson RA, Bryden NA, Patterson KY, et al (1993) Breast milk chromium and its association with chromium intake, chromium excretion, and serum chromium. Am J Clin Nutr 57:519–523

112. Deelstra H, Van Schoor O, Robberecht H, et al (1988) Daily chromium intake by infants in Belgium. Acta Paediatr Scand 77:402–407

113. Kumpulainen JT (1992) Chromium content of foods and diets. Biol Trace Elem Res 32:9–18

114. Jorhem L, Sundstrom B (1993) Levels of lead, cadmium, zinc, copper, nickel, chromium, manganese, and cobalt in foods on the Swedish market, 1983–1990. J Food Comp Anal 6: 223–241

115. Khan A, Bryden NA, Polansky MM, Anderson RA (1990) Insulin potentiating factor and chromium content of selected foods and spices. Biol Trace Elem Res 24:183–188

116. Schroeder HA (1971) Losses of vitamins and trace minerals resulting from processing and preservation of foods. Am J Clin Nutr 24:562–573

117. Osborne BG, Laal-Khoshab A (1989) Distribution of some essential trace elements in commercial flour-mill streams. J Sci Food Agric 39:95–100

118. Wolf W, Mertz W, Masironi R (1974) Determination of chromium in refined and unrefined sugars by oxygen plasma ashing flameless atomic absorption. J Agric Food Chem 22:1037–1042

119. Kuligowski J, Halperin KM (1992) Stainless steel cookware as a significant source of nickel, chromium, and iron. Arch Environ Contam Toxicol 23:211–215

120. Offenbacher EG, Pi-Sunyer FX (1983) Temperature and pH effects on the release of chromium from stainless steel into water and fruit juices. J Agric Food Chem 31:89–92

121. Anderson R, Bryden NA (1983) Concentration, insulin potentiation, and absorption of chromium in beer. J Agric Chem 31:308–311

122. Toepfer EW, Mertz W, Roginski EE, Polansky MM (1973) Chromium in foods in relation to biological activity. J Agric Food Chem 21:69–73

123. Yamamoto A, Wada O, Suzuki H (1988) Purification and properties of biologically active chromium complex from bovine colostrum. J Nutr 118:39–45

124. Randall JA, Gibson RS (1987) Serum and urine chromium as indices of chromium status in tannery workers. Proc Soc Exp Biol Med 185:16–23

125. International Programme on Chemical Safety (1988) Chromium. Environmental Health Criteria 61. World Health Organization, Geneva

126. Katz SA, Salem H (1993) The toxicology of chromium with respect to its chemical speciation: a review. J Appl Toxicol 13:217–224

127. Nethercott J, Paustenbach D, Adams R, et al (1994) A study of chromium induced allergic contact dermatitis with 54 volunteers: implications for environmental risk assessment. Occup Environ Med 51:371–380

128. Lin S-C, Tai C-C, Chan C-C, Wang J-D (1994) Nasal septum lesions caused by chromium exposure among chromium electroplating workers. Am J Ind Med 26:221–228

129. Bridgewater LC, Manning FCR, Patierno SR (1994) Base-specific arrest of in vitro DNA replication by carcinogenic chromium: relationship to DNA interstrand crosslinking. Carcinogenesis 15:2421–2428

130. Sjogren B, Hansen KS, Kjuus H, Persson P-G (1994) Exposure to stainless steel welding fumes and lung cancer: a meta-analysis. Occup Environ Med 51:335–336

131. Versieck J (1984) Trace element analysis—a plea for accuracy. Trace Elem Med 1:2–12

132. Expert Panel for Nutrition Advisory Group, AMA Department of Foods and Nutrition (1979) Guidelines for essential trace element preparations for parenteral use. JAMA 241:2051–2054

133. Frankel DA (1993) Supplementation of trace elements in parenteral nutrition: rationale and recommendations. Nutr Res 13:583–596

134. Moukarzel AA, Song MK, Buchman AL, et al (1992) Excessive chromium intake in children receiving total parenteral nutrition. Lancet 339:385–388

135. Anonymous (1993) Chromium picolinate: scam of the hour. Obesity Health 7:54

136. Clancy SP, Clarkson PM, DeCheke ME, et al (1994) Effects of chromium picolinate supplementation on body composition, strength, and urinary chromium loss in football players. Int J Sport Nutr 4:142–153

137. Lefavi RG, Anderson RA, Keith RE, et al (1992) Efficacy of chromium supplementation in athletes: emphasis on anabolism. Int J Sport Nutr 2:111–122

138. Fernandez-Pol JA (1977) Iron: possible cause of the G1 arrest induced in NRK cells by picolinic acid. Biochem Biophys Res Commun 78:136–143

139. Stearns DM, Wise JP Sr, Patierno SR, Wetterhahn KE (1995) Chromium (III) picolinate produces chromosome damage in Chinese hamster ovary cells. FASEB J 9: 1643–1649

Chapter 35

Other Trace Elements

Forrest H. Nielsen

All elements that have not been assigned separate chapters in this volume fit into the category of elements that have become known as the ultratrace elements. Ultratrace elements are those with estimated dietary requirements usually <1 µg/g and often <50 ng/g of diet for laboratory animals.[1] At least 18 elements have been suggested to be ultratrace elements: aluminum, arsenic, boron, bromine, cadmium, chromium, fluorine, germanium, iodine, lead, lithium, molybdenum, nickel, rubidium, selenium, silicon, tin, and vanadium. The quality of the experimental evidence supporting the suggestion of nutritional essentiality varies widely among these elements. The evidence for the essentiality of three elements, iodine, molybdenum, and selenium, is quite substantial and noncontroversial; specific biochemical functions have been defined for these elements. Iodine and selenium are discussed in Chapters 36 and 31, respectively; molybdenum will be discussed here. Specific biochemical functions have not been identified for the other 15 elements. Thus, their essentiality is based on circumstantial evidence; that is, a dietary deprivation consistently results in a suboptimal biological function that is preventable or reversible by an intake of physiological amounts of the element in question. The circumstantial evidence for essentiality is substantial for arsenic, boron, chromium, nickel, silicon, and vanadium; thus, except for chromium, which is discussed in Chapter 34, they will be discussed in detail here. The evidence for essentiality of the other elements is generally limited to a few gross observations in one or two species by one or two research groups. Because it was judged premature to discuss these elements in detail here, these elements will be only briefly mentioned in table form at the end of this chapter. However, fluoride, which has a well-known beneficial pharmacologic property (anticariogenic), is discussed in Chapter 32.

Arsenic

History. Although arsenic has been considered synonymous with poison for centuries, its bad reputation did not prevent it from becoming an important pharmaceutical agent. By 1937, the pharmacologic actions of 8000 arsenicals had been recorded. Arsenicals were considered at various times to be specific remedies for the treatment of anorexia and other nutritional disturbances, syphilis, neuralgia, rheumatism, asthma, chorea, malaria, tuberculosis, diabetes, various skin diseases, and numerous hematologic abnormalities.[2] The use of arsenicals for these disorders has either fallen into disrepute or been replaced by more effective alternatives.

Reports describing attempts to produce a nutritional arsenic deficiency first appeared in the 1930s.[3,4] The first substantial evidence for arsenic essentiality was published in 1975 and 1976.[5] Arsenic deprivation signs were described for rats, pigs, and goats. Subsequently, signs also were described for chickens and hamsters. Thus, it is only recently that arsenic has been studied from the biochemical, nutritional, and physiological, and not only the toxicological or pharmacological, points of view.

Chemistry and method of analysis. Both the trivalent and pentavalent states of arsenic exist in biologic material. The most biochemically important organic arsenic compounds are those that contain methyl groups. The methylation of inorganic oxyarsenic anions occurs in organisms ranging from microbial to mammalian. The methylated end products include arsenocholine, arsenobetaine, dimethylarsinic acid, methylarsonic acid, trimethylarsine oxide, and tetramethylarsonium ion.[6]

Other arsenic compounds of interest are those possibly formed when arsenate replaces phosphate in biological molecules. The relatively unstable nature of arsenyl esters apparently is the reason that only indirect evidence exists for compounds such as glucose-6-arsenate and adenosine diphosphate-arsenate. Nonetheless, arsenate ester might be the form of arsenic that performs an essential function.

A comprehensive review of arsenic chemistry and biochemistry has been published.[7] One of the most precise and sensitive methods for the determination of arsenic in biological material involves measuring arsine generated from dry combusted samples by graphite-furnace atomic absorption spectrometry.[8,9]

Absorption, transport, storage, and turnover. Absorption of inorganic arsenic from the gastrointestinal tract correlates well with the solubility of the compound ingested.[10,11] In humans and most laboratory animals, >90% of inorganic arsenate and arsenite fed in a water solution is absorbed. However, only 20–30% of arsenic in arsenic trioxide or lead arsenate, which are only slightly soluble in water, is absorbed by hamsters, rats, and rabbits.

The form of organic arsenic also determines how well it is absorbed. For example, >90% of an oral dose of arsenobetaine was recovered in the urine of hamsters; 70–80% of an oral dose of arsenocholine was recovered in the urine of mice, rats, and rabbits; and 45% of an oral dose of dimethylarsinic acid was recovered in the urine of hamsters.[12–14] In contrast, >90% of an oral dose of sodium-p-N-glycolylarsenilate was recovered in the feces of rats or humans within 3 days of administration; urinary excretion accounted for only 4–5% of the dose.[15] Also, most orally administered arsenosugars are not absorbed from the gastrointestinal tract.[6]

Arsenate and phosphate, despite structural similarities, do not share a common transport pathway in the duodenum.[16] The absorption of arsenate can be separated into two components. First, arsenate becomes sequestered primarily in or on the mucosal tissue. Eventually, the sites of sequestration become filled, with concomitant movement of arsenate into the body. The absorption of arsenate apparently involves a simple movement down a concentration gradient. In rats, some forms of organic arsenic are absorbed at rates directly proportional to their intestinal concentration over a 100-fold range.[17] This finding suggests that organic arsenicals are absorbed mainly by simple diffusion through lipoid regions of the intestinal boundary.

Once absorbed, inorganic arsenic is transferred to liver, where it is methylated. Thus, blood contains both inorganic (probably protein bound) and methylated forms of arsenic. In 56 healthy volunteers consuming a diet high in organic arsenic, mean blood total arsenic was 7.3 μg/L and was 73% trimethylated arsenic, 14% dimethylated arsenic, and 9.6% inorganic arsenic.[18] Before arsenate is methylated, it is reduced to arsenite via the use of glutathione.[19,20] Methylation takes place in liver with S-adenosylmethionine as the methyl donor.[20,21] In humans, the final product, dimethylarsinic acid, results from the methylation of the monomethylarsenic acid precursor formed from arsenite.[22] The methylation of arsenic can be modified by changing the glutathione, methionine, and choline status of the animal.[23,24]

The fate of absorbed organic arsenic depends on its form. For example, arsenobetaine passes through the body into the urine without biotransformation.[25] Some orally ingested arsenocholine appears in the urine, and some is incorporated into body phospholipids similarly to choline; however, most is biotransformed to arsenobetaine before being excreted in urine.[13]

If the ingestion of arsenic is low, no tissue has significant accumulation of arsenic.[26] The highest amounts of arsenic are usually found in skin, hair, and nails, probably the result of arsenite binding to SH groups of proteins that are relatively plentiful in these tissues.[10]

The metabolism of arsenic in some animal species is quite unusual. For example, rats, unlike other mammals, concentrate arsenic in their erythrocytes.[27] Marmoset monkeys are unable to methylate arsenite, which is a major reaction in the elimination of arsenic from the body for most animals.[28,29] Studies with rabbits, hamsters, and chicks seem to give findings on the metabolism of arsenic most applicable to humans.

The excretion of ingested arsenic is rapid, principally in urine. Only minor amounts are removed through sweat, loss of hair and skin, and bile.[10] A reported example of the proportions of the forms of arsenic in human urine after an oral dose of inorganic arsenic is 51% dimethylarsinic acid, 21% monomethylarsonic acid, and 27% inorganic arsenic.[30] The proportions are quite different, however, with the consumption of organic arsenic. For example, an analysis of urine from 102 Japanese students who consumed luxuriant amounts of organic arsenic in seafood revealed 9.4% inorganic arsenic, 3.0% monomethylarsonic acid, 28.9% dimethylarsinic acid, and 58.2% trimethylated arsenic compound.[31] Similar findings were obtained in another study of 56 healthy volunteers.[18]

Physiological (biochemical) function. The evidence suggesting that arsenic is essential does not clearly define its biochemical function. Recent findings suggest that arsenic affects the formation of various metabolites from methionine (e.g., S-adenosylmethionine, S-adenosyl homocysteine, cysteine, and taurine) and arginine (e.g., putrescine, spermidine, and spermine) or affects labile methyl-group metabolism.[32] Arsenic deprivation depressed the concentrations of putrescine, spermidine, and spermine in liver of rats fed marginal amounts of methionine and depressed the taurine concentration in the plasma of hamsters.

Perhaps arsenic has a role in some enzymatic reactions.[5] As an enzyme activator, arsenic as arsenate probably substitutes for phosphate. As an inhibitor, arsenic as arsenite apparently affects enzymes by reacting with sulfhydryl groups.

Arsenic may also regulate gene expression. Arsenite can induce the cellular production of certain proteins known as heat-shock or stress proteins.[33,34] The production of these proteins in response to arsenite apparently is controlled at the transcriptional level and may involve changes in the methylation of core histones.[33] Recent findings have shown that arsenic deprivation in the rat, chick, and hamster affects labile methyl metabolism.[32,35] Also, arsenic enhances DNA synthesis in unsensitized human lymphocytes[36] and in those stimulated by phytohemagglutinin.[37]

Deficiency signs. Arsenic deprivation has been induced in chickens, hamsters, goats, miniature pigs, and rats.[5,32,38] In goats, miniature pigs, and rats, the most consistent signs of arsenic deprivation were depressed growth and abnormal reproduction characterized by impaired fertility and elevated perinatal mortality. Other notable signs of deprivation in goats were depressed serum triacylglycerol concentrations and death during lactation. Myocardial damage was also present in lactating goats. The organelle of myocardium most affected was the mitochondrion, which was affected at the membrane level;[39] in advanced stages, the membrane actually ruptured. Other signs of arsenic deprivation have been reported. Listing these signs is problematic because studies with chicks, rats, and hamsters have revealed that the nature and severity of the signs of arsenic deprivation are affected by several dietary manipulations, including variations in the concentrations of zinc, arginine, choline, methionine, taurine, and guanidoacetic acid (a methyl-depleting agent). The signs of arsenic deprivation were changed and generally enhanced by nutritional stressors that affected sulfur amino acid or labile methyl-group metabolism. However, some recently reported responses to arsenic deprivation that may be significant are decreased glutathione S-transferase activity and increased kidney calcium concentrations in female rats fed the AIN-76 diet.[40]

In humans, decreased serum arsenic concentrations in people undergoing hemodialysis treatment were correlated to injuries of the central nervous system, vascular diseases, and cancer.[41]

Requirement. Only data from animal studies are available for estimating the arsenic need of humans. An arsenic requirement of <50 ng/g and probably ≈25 ng/g was suggested for growing chicks and rats fed an experimental diet containing 20% protein, 9% fat, 60% carbohydrate, 11% fiber, minerals, and vitamins.[42,43] Thus, the arsenic requirement is apparently between 6.25 and 12.5 μg/4.18 MJ (6.25 and 12.5 μg/1000 kcal). From these data a possible arsenic requirement for humans eating 8.37 MJ (2000 kcal) would be ≈12–25 μg/day.[42,43] A safe upper limit of arsenic intake most likely will be 140–250 μg/day.[42,43]

Food and other sources. The reported arsenic content of diets from various parts of the world indicates that the average daily intake of arsenic is generally 12–40 μg.[44-46] However, the dietary arsenic intake by a typical Japanese person (high-seafood diet) was found to be 195 μg/day (range 16–1039 μg/day).[18] Fish, grain, and cereal products contribute most of the arsenic to the diet.

Excess (toxicity). Because of mechanisms for the homeostatic regulation of arsenic, its toxicity through oral intake is relatively low; it is actually less toxic than selenium, an ultratrace element with a well-established nutritional value. Toxic quantities of inorganic arsenic generally are reported in milligrams. For example, the estimated fatal acute dose of arsenic trioxide for humans is 70–180 mg, or ≈0.76–1.95 mg As/kg body weight.[47]

The ratio of the toxic to the nutritional dose for rats apparently is near 1250. Some forms of organic arsenic are virtually nontoxic; for example, a 10 g/kg body weight dose of arsenobetaine (common form of arsenic in food) depressed spontaneous motility and respiration in male mice, but these signs disappeared within 1 hour.[48] Arsenocholine is slightly more toxic than arsenobetaine; a dose of 5.8 g/kg body weight caused death in some rats, but a dose of 4.8 g/kg did not.[49]

Briefly, the signs of subacute and chronic high exposure of arsenic in humans include the development of dermatoses of various types (hyperpigmentation, hyperkeratosis, desquamation, and loss of hair); hematopoietic depression; liver damage characterized by jaundice, portal cirrhosis, and ascites; sensory disturbances; peripheral neuritis; anorexia; and weight loss.[50-52]

Results of numerous epidemiologic studies have suggested an association between chronic arsenic overexposure and the incidence of some forms of cancer. Although the role of arsenic in carcinogenesis remains controversial, arsenic does not seem to act as a primary carcinogen and is either an inactive or extremely weak mutagen.[53]

Summary. Until more is known about the biochemical and physiological functions of arsenic, it is inappropriate to associate specific disorders with deficient arsenic nutriture. At present, it is important to recognize the likelihood that arsenic is essential for humans. Thus, the belief that any form or amount of arsenic is unnecessary, toxic, or carcinogenic is unrealistic, if not potentially harmful.

Boron

History. In the 1870s it was discovered that pharmacological amounts of borax and boric acid could be used to preserve foods. For about the next 50 years, borates were considered some of the best preservatives for extending the palatability of foods such as fish, meat, cream, and butter. In 1904, however, Wiley[54] reported that human volunteers consuming >500 mg of boric acid per day for 50 days displayed disturbed appetite, digestion, and health. Subsequent to this report, the opinion that boron posed a risk to health gained momentum; by the middle 1950s boron was essentially forbidden throughout the world as a food preservative.

In 1923 Warrington[55] showed that boron is an essential element for plants. About 15 years later, attempts to demonstrate boron essentiality for higher animals began; these attempts were unsuccessful.[56-60] Thus, before 1980, students of biochemistry and nutrition were taught that boron was a unique element because it was essential for plants but not for higher animals. In 1981 it was reported that boron stimulated growth and partially prevented leg abnormalities present in cholecalciferol-deficient chicks.[61] Since then, evidence has been accumulating indicating that boron is an essential nutrient for higher animals including humans.

Chemistry and methods of analysis. Boron exists in biological material mainly bound to oxygen. Thus, boron biochemistry is essentially that of boric acid. Dilute aqueous boric acid solutions comprise $B(OH)_3$ and $B(OH)_4^-$ species at the pH of blood (7.4); because the pK_a of boric acid is 9.2, the abundance of these two species should be 98.4% and 1.6%, respectively.[62]

Boric acid forms ester complexes with hydroxyl groups of organic compounds; this preferably occurs when the hydroxyl groups are adjacent and *cis*.[63] Among the hydroxylated substances of biological interest with which boron complexes are adenosine-5-phosphate, pyridoxine, riboflavin, dehydroascorbic acid, and pyridine nucleotides. Formation of these complexes may be biologically important because, in vitro, it results in the competitive inhibition of some enzymes.[62] These include oxidoreductases that require *cis*-hydroxyl–containing pyridine or flavin nucleotides as cofactors.

The added stabilization of hydrogen bonding between hydroxyls bound to boron and hydrogen of imidazole or amido groups allows complexes to be formed between borate and compounds containing single hydroxyl groups. Through forming this type of complex, borate and boronic acid derivatives can form transition analogues that inhibit the activity of some enzymes.[64] For example, serine hydrolases are inhibited when a tetrahedral complex is formed between the serine hydroxyl group and boron, with hydrogen bonding to an imidazole ring of an adjacent histidine adding stabilization.[62]

Two naturally occurring organoboron compounds have been identified; they contain boron bound to four oxygen groups. These compounds are aplasmomycin, a novel ionophoric macrolide antibiotic isolated from strain ss-20 of *Streptomyces griseus,* and boromycin, an antibiotic synthesized by *Streptomyces antibioticus*.[65,66] Boromycin can encapsulate alkali metal cations and increase the permeability of the cytoplasmic membrane to potassium ions.

Only recently have methods been developed that can determine low concentrations of boron in biological substances with acceptable accuracy. Development of such methods has been difficult because many boron compounds volatilize at temperatures far below those required for most dry or wet ashing procedures, and most forms of glassware and chemical reagents contain significant amounts of boron. Procedures that have been developed to digest biological substances with minimal boron loss or contamination include a low-temperature wet digestion in semiclosed teflon tubes and a teflon bomb digestion in a microwave oven.[67,68] Inductively coupled argon plasma spectroscopy is generally used to determine the boron content of the digestates.[67,68]

Prompt gamma activation analysis and neutron activation–mass spectrometry (NA-MS) techniques have been developed that can accurately measure the usual or normal concentration of boron in biomaterials.[69] One major advantage of these techniques is that they do not require the destruction of the organic matrix containing boron. For example, with NA-MS, a freeze-dried sample is irradiated to generate ^{4}He from ^{10}B; the ^{4}He is measured by mass spectrometry. The sophistication and cost of the equipment precludes either of these methods from becoming of general laboratory use.

Absorption, transport, storage, and turnover. Sodium borate, boric acid, and possibly food boron are rapidly absorbed and are excreted largely in the urine. Because there is no usable radioisotope of boron, the study of its metabolism has been made difficult. However, it is likely that most ingested boron is converted to $B(OH)_3$, the normal hydrolysis end product of most boron compounds and the dominant inorganic species at the pH of the gastrointestinal tract. It is postulated that boron is absorbed and excreted mainly as undissociated $B(OH)_3$. The mechanism by which boron is transported through the body has not been defined. Recently, an inductively coupled plasma–mass spectrometry method using the ratio of the two stable isotopes, ^{11}B/^{10}B, was developed to study boron metabolism.[70] This method was used to show that boron in broccoli, intrinsically enriched with ^{10}B, was absorbed as well as extrinsic boron ^{10}B in boric acid from a test meal by rats. When 20 μg of ^{10}B isotope were fed to rats, 95% of this isotope was detected in the urine and 4% in the feces after 3 days. This agrees with other urinary recovery findings indicating that >90% of ingested boron is usually absorbed.[71,72]

Boron is distributed throughout soft tissues and fluids of animals and humans at concentrations mostly between 0.015 and 0.6 μg/g fresh tissue.[62,73–75] Bone, fingernails, hair, and teeth usually contain several times these concentrations.

Evidence showing that boron is homeostatically controlled includes the rapid urinary excretion of absorbed boron, the lack of accumulation of boron in tissues, and the relatively narrow range of boron concentrations in blood of apparently healthy individuals. In a group of 50 blood samples collected from hospitals and clinics in the United Kingdom, the serum boron concentration ranged from 0.77 to 4.45 μmol/L (8.4 to 48.1 ng/mL), with a median of 2.06 μmol/L (22.3 ng/mL).[75] In postmenopausal women, an increase in dietary boron from 0.36 mg/day (probably deficient) to 3.3 mg/day (luxuriant) did not increase plasma boron concentrations when dietary magnesium was 340 mg/day; however, a 2.4-fold increase occurred when dietary magnesium was 109 mg/day (C.D. Hunt and F.H. Nielsen, unpublished data, 1987). Increasing dietary boron from 0.465 (deficient) to 2.465 (luxuriant) mg/kg diet increased the plasma boron concentration by only 50% in cholecalciferol-deficient chicks.[76,77] As with other mineral elements, overcoming homeostatic mechanisms by high boron intakes will elevate tissue boron concentrations.

Physiological (biochemical) function. A biochemical function for boron has not been elucidated, even for plants for which boron has been known for 70 years to be essential and for which boron deficiency has a multiplicity of effects.[78,79] Two hypotheses recently advanced for the biochemical function of boron in higher animals accommodate a large and varied response to boron deprivation and the known biochemistry of boron. Hunt[77] proposed that boron is a metabolic regulator through complexing with a variety of substrate or reactant compounds in which there are hydroxyl groups in favorable positions. On the basis of the knowledge that two classes of enzymes are competitively inhibited in vivo by borate or its derivatives and his findings showing dietary boron can alter the in vivo activity of a number of these enzymes, Hunt hypothesized that the metabolic regulation by boron is mainly negative; that is, boron controls a number of metabolic pathways by competitively inhibiting some key enzyme reactions. Nielsen[80] hypothesized that boron has a role in cell membrane function or stability such that it influences the response to hormones by modulating transmembrane signaling or transmembrane movement of regulatory cations or anions. This hypothesis is supported by the recent findings that boron influences the transport of extracellular calcium and the release of intracellular calcium in rat platelets activated by thrombin and that boron influences redox actions involved in cellular membrane transport in plants.[79,81]

Deficiency signs. The listing of the signs of boron deficiency is difficult because most boron-deficiency studies have used stressors to enhance the response to changes in dietary boron. Thus, it has been found that the response to boron deprivation varies as the diet varies in its content of nutrients such as calcium, phosphorus, magnesium, potassium, and cholecalciferol.[82] However, although the nature and severity of the changes may vary with dietary composition, many findings indicate that boron deprivation impairs calcium and energy metabolism. For example, a boron supplement of 3 μg boron/g alleviated the cholecalciferol-deficiency-induced distortion of marrow sprouts of chick proximal tibial epiphyseal plate and elevated the number of osteoblasts within the marrow sprouts.[76] Boron also substantially alleviated or corrected cholecalciferol-deficiency-induced elevations in plasma glucose, changes in energy substrate use, and depressions in growth.[77]

Brain composition and function are also affected by dietary boron. Boron deprivation was found to systematically influence brain electrical activity assessed by an electrocorticogram in mature rats; the principal effect was on the frequency distribution of electrical activity.[83] In this study, brain copper concentrations were higher in boron-deprived than in boron-supplemented rats. Furthermore, calcium concentrations in total brain and in brain cortex, as well as the phosphorus concentration in the cerebellum, were found to be higher in boron-deprived

than in boron-supplemented rats fed a cholecalciferol-deficient diet.[84]

Some of the preceding findings may reflect an effect of dietary boron on macromineral metabolism. The apparent absorption and balance of calcium, magnesium, and phosphorus were found to be higher in boron-supplemented (2.72 μg boron/g diet) than in boron-deprived (0.158 μg boron/g diet) rats fed a cholecalciferol-deficient diet.[84]

Findings involving boron deprivation of humans have come mainly from two studies in which men over the age of 45, postmenopausal women, and postmenopausal women on estrogen therapy were fed a low-boron diet (0.25 mg/8.37 MJ [0.25 mg/2000 kcal]) for 63 days and then fed the same diet supplemented with 3 mg boron/day for 49 days.[81,85–89] These dietary intakes were near the low and high values in the range of dietary boron intakes (0.5–3.1 mg/day) found in a limited number of surveys.[90] In the first experiment the diet was low in magnesium (115 mg/8.37 MJ) and marginally adequate in copper (1.6 mg/8.37 MJ) throughout the study.[85,86] In the second experiment the diet provided 300 mg magnesium and only 1.7 mg copper/8.37 MJ for the first 32 days; from day 33 onward, the diet was supplemented to contain 2.4 mg copper/8.37 MJ.[87,88] Thus, the major differences between the two experiments were the intakes of copper and magnesium; in one experiment they were marginal or inadequate, in the other they were adequate. Among the effects of boron supplementation after 63 days of boron depletion in these experiments were the following: an effect on macromineral and electrolyte metabolism evidenced by increased serum 25-hydroxycholecalciferol and decreased serum calcitonin (with low dietary magnesium and copper);[86,88] an effect on energy substrate metabolism suggested by decreased serum glucose (with low dietary magnesium and copper) and increased serum triglycerides (with adequate dietary magnesium and copper);[85,88] an effect on nitrogen metabolism indicated by decreased blood urea nitrogen and serum creatinine and increased urinary hydroxyproline excretion;[81,85,87,88] an effect on oxidative metabolism indicated by increased erythrocyte superoxide dismutase and serum ceruloplasmin;[81,85] and an effect on erythropoiesis and hematopoiesis suggested by (all with adequate dietary magnesium and copper) increased blood hemoglobin and mean corpuscular hemoglobin content but decreased hematocrit, platelet number, and erythrocyte number.[87] Boron supplementation after depletion also enhanced the elevation in serum 17ʙ-estradiol and plasma copper caused by estrogen ingestion, altered electroencephalograms such that they suggested improved behavioral activation (e.g., less drowsiness) and mental alertness, and improved psychomotor skills and the cognitive processes of attention and memory.[88,89]

Requirement. For normal development, chicks apparently require ≈1 μg boron/g diet.[91] In the human studies just described, the subjects responded to a boron supplement after consuming a diet supplying only ≈0.25 mg boron/8.37 MJ for 63 days. Thus, humans apparently have a dietary boron requirement >0.3 mg/day and, on the basis of animal studies, probably closer to 1 mg/day.

Food and other sources. The daily intake of boron by humans can vary widely depending on the proportions of various food groups in the diet.[90,92,93] Foods of plant origin, especially noncitrus fruits, leafy vegetables, nuts, and legumes, are rich sources of boron. Wine, cider, and beer are also high in boron. Meat, fish, and dairy products are poor sources of boron. A limited number of surveys indicate that average daily intakes of boron range between 0.5 and 3.1 mg.[69,90,93,94]

Excess (toxicity). Boron has a low order of toxicity when administered orally. Toxicity signs in animals generally occur only after dietary boron exceeds 100 μg/g. When boron was 150 mg/L in drinking water, rats exhibited depressed growth, lack of incisor pigmentation, aspermia, and impaired ovarian development.[95] When boron was 300 mg/L in drinking water, rats exhibited depressed plasma triacylglycerols, protein, and alkaline phosphatase and depressed bone fat and calcium.[96] Pigs fed 8 mg boron/kg body weight per day exhibited an osteoporosis associated with a reduction in parathyroid activity.[97] Boron toxicity was a focus of a recent symposium.[98]

In humans, the signs of acute toxicity include nausea, vomiting, diarrhea, dermatitis, and lethargy.[99] In addition, high boron intake induces riboflavinuria.[100] The signs of chronic boron toxicity through dietary intake have not been clearly defined. As mentioned previously, Wiley[54] found that humans consuming >500 mg boric acid/day for 50 days displayed disturbed appetite, digestion, and health. Two infants who had their pacifiers dipped into a preparation of borax and honey for a period of several weeks exhibited scanty hair, patchy dry erythema, anemia, and seizures.[101] The seizures stopped and the other abnormalities were alleviated when the use of the borax and honey preparation was discontinued.

Summary. Knowledge about boron nutrition, biochemistry, and metabolism is growing, but more is needed before clinical disorders can be attributed to subnormal boron nutrition or a recommended dietary allowance can be established. Boron clearly is, however, a biologically dynamic ultratrace element that affects macromineral metabolism in higher animals, including humans. Thus, there is an urgent need to identify the specific biochemical role of boron to conclusively establish its essentiality and to help determine its practical nutritional importance.

Molybdenum

History. Evidence for the essentiality of molybdenum first appeared in 1953 when xanthine oxidase was iden-

tified as a molybdenum metalloenzyme.[102,103] Subsequently, attempts to produce molybdenum deficiency in rats and chicks were successful only when the diet contained massive amounts of tungsten, an antagonist of molybdenum metabolism.[102] These studies showed that the dietary requirement for maintaining normal growth of animals was <1 μg molybdenum/g diet, an amount substantially lower than requirements for other trace elements recognized as essential at the time. Thus, molybdenum was not considered to be of practical importance in animal and human nutrition. Consequently, relatively little effort has been devoted to the study of the metabolism and nutrition of molybdenum in monogastric animals or humans.

Chemistry and methods of analysis. Molybdenum is a transition element that readily changes its oxidation state and can thus act as an electron transfer agent in oxidation-reduction reactions. In the oxidized form of molybdoenzymes, molybdenum is probably present in the 6+ state. Although enzymes during electron transfer are probably reduced to the 5+ state, other oxidation states of reduced enzymes have been found. Molybdenum apparently is present at the active site of molybdoenzymes in a small nonprotein cofactor containing a pterin nucleus.[103–106] More than 40% of molybdenum not attached to an enzyme in liver exists as this cofactor bound to the mitochondrial outer membrane.[103] This form can be transferred to an apoenzyme of xanthine oxidase or sulfite oxidase, which transforms it into an active enzyme molecule. In addition to the molybdenum cofactor and "enzymatic" molybdenum, the other important form of molybdenum is molybdate.[107] Evidence suggests that molybdenum in blood and urine exists mainly as the molybdate ion (MoO_4^{2-}).

Inductively coupled plasma emission spectrometric methods have produced accurate measurements of molybdenum in biological material.[108]

Absorption, transport, storage, and turnover. Molybdenum (except as MoS_2) in foods and in the form of soluble complexes is readily absorbed. In one study, humans fed ammonium molybdate contained in a liquid-formula component of a diet absorbed 88–93% of the molybdenum.[109] Molybdenum absorption in rats occurs rapidly in the stomach and throughout the small intestine, the rate of absorption being higher in the proximal than in the distal parts of the small intestine.[107] Whether an active or a passive mechanism is most important in the absorption of molybdenum is uncertain. One study indicated that, at low concentrations, molybdenum absorption is carrier mediated and active.[110] Another study showed that in vivo absorption rates were essentially the same over a 10-fold range of molybdenum concentrations, which suggests that molybdate was absorbed by diffusion only.[111] The possibility exists that molybdate is moved both by diffusion and by active transport, but at high concentrations the relative contribution of active transport to molybdenum flux is small.[107] The absorption and retention of molybdenum are influenced strongly by interactions between molybdenum and various dietary forms of sulfur.[102]

Molybdate absorbed into the blood is loosely attached to erythrocytes and tends to bind specifically to A_2-macroglobulin.[112] Molybdate in food and water apparently is not chemically changed by absorption and transport in the blood. The organs that retain the highest amounts of molybdenum are liver and kidney.[102,107,112,113] The molybdenum in liver is entirely present in macromolecular association, partly as known molybdoenzymes and the remainder as molybdenum cofactor.[103]

After absorption, most molybdenum is turned over rapidly and eliminated as molybdate through the kidney; thus, excretion rather than regulated absorption is the major homeostatic mechanism for molybdenum.[109] Significant amounts of this element are excreted in bile.[112]

Physiological (biochemical) function. Molybdenum functions as an enzyme cofactor.[102–106] Molybdoenzymes catalyze the hydroxylation of various substrates.[114] Aldehyde oxidase oxidizes and detoxifies various pyrimidines, purines, pteridines, and related compounds. Xanthine oxidase/dehydrogenase catalyzes the transformation of hypoxanthine to xanthine, and xanthine to uric acid. Sulfite oxidase catalyzes the transformation of sulfite to sulfate.

Molybdate may also be involved in stabilizing the steroid-binding ability of the unoccupied glucocorticoid receptor. During isolation procedures, molybdate protects steroid hormone receptors, particularly the glucocorticoid receptor, against inactivation.[115] It is hypothesized, however, that molybdate affects the glucocorticoid receptor because it mimics an endogenous compound called "modulator."[116]

Deficiency signs. The signs of molybdenum deficiency were reviewed by Mills and Bremner.[117] In rats and chickens, molybdenum deficiency aggravated by excessive dietary tungsten results in the depression of molybdenum enzymes, disturbances in uric acid metabolism, and increased susceptibility to sulfite toxicity. Under field conditions a molybdenum-responsive syndrome was found in hatching chicks. This syndrome was characterized by a high incidence of late embryonic mortality, mandibular distortion, anophthalmia, and defects in leg bone development and feathering. Skeletal lesions, subsequently detected in older birds, included separation of the proximal epiphysis of the femur, osteolytic changes in the femoral shaft, and lesions in the overlying skin that were ultimately attributed to intense irritation in these areas. The incidence of this syndrome was particularly high in commercial flocks reared on diets containing high concentrations of copper (a molybdenum antagonist) as a growth stimulant. These apparently dissimilar pathologic changes were suggested to be caused by a defect in sulfur metabolism.

Deficiency uncomplicated by high dietary tungsten or copper was produced in goats and pigs fed diets containing <24 ng molybdenum/g.[118] Deficiency signs were depressed feed consumption, depressed growth, and impaired reproduction characterized by infertility and elevated mortality in both mothers and offspring.

Recognition of the role of molybdenum as a component of sulfite oxidase and that sulfite oxidase deficiency markedly deranges cysteine metabolism has resulted in the recognition of a human disorder caused by the lack of functioning molybdenum. A genetic deficiency of sulfite oxidase was identified in humans; this deficiency is characterized by severe brain damage, mental retardation, and dislocation of ocular lenses and results in increased urinary output of sulfite, S-sulfocysteine, and thiosulfate and a marked decrease in sulfate output.[103] A patient receiving prolonged total parenteral nutrition therapy acquired a syndrome described as acquired molybdenum deficiency.[119] This syndrome, exacerbated by methionine administration, was characterized by hypermethioninemia, hypouricemia, hyperoxypurinemia, hypouricosuria, and very low urinary sulfate excretion. In addition, the patient suffered mental disturbances that progressed to coma. The symptoms were indicative of a defect in sulfur amino acid metabolism at the level of sulfite oxidation to sulfate (sulfite oxidase deficiency) and a defect in uric acid production at the level of xanthine and hypoxanthine transformation to uric acid (xanthine oxidase deficiency). Supplementation of the patient with ammonium molybdate improved the clinical condition, reversed the sulfur handling defect, and normalized uric acid production.

Requirement. Attempts to determine the minimum dietary molybdenum requirements for animals and humans have been made recently. Goats apparently require 50–100 µg/kg diet.[118] The requirement of rats fed the AIN-76 diet was estimated to be 200 µg/kg diet.[120] The minimum requirement of healthy young men was concluded to be slightly >22 µg/day.[109,118]

The current United States estimated safe and adequate daily dietary intakes for molybdenum are the following (in µg): infants aged 0–0.5 years, 15–30 µg, and aged 0.5–1.0 years, 20–40 µg; children and adolescents aged 1–3 years, 25–50 µg, aged 4–6 years, 30–75 µg, aged 7–10 years, 50–150 µg, and aged 11 years and older, 75–200 µg; and adults, 75–250 µg.[121] Data to support these estimates are scant. These values apparently were set by using balance data, which may be questionable, and through the reasoning that usual dietary intakes are within this range and do not result in signs of deficiency or toxicity.

Food and other sources. As with other elements, the daily intake of molybdenum varies depending upon the composition of the diet. Recent surveys indicate that the daily intake of molybdenum is 50–350 μg.[122–125] However, most diets apparently supply ≈50–100 μg molybdenum/day; thus, many diets do not meet the minimum level of the suggested safe and adequate intake. The richest food sources of molybdenum include milk and milk products, dried legumes, organ meats (liver and kidney), cereals, and baked goods. The poorest sources of molybdenum include vegetables other than legumes, fruits, sugars, oils, fats, and fish.[123,126]

Excess (toxicity). Large oral doses are necessary to overcome the homeostatic control of molybdenum. Thus, molybdenum is a relatively nontoxic element; in nonruminants an intake of 100–5000 mg/kg of food or water is required to produce clinical toxicity symptoms.[102,107] Ruminants are more susceptible to elevated dietary molybdenum. The mechanisms of molybdenum toxicity are uncertain. Most signs are similar or identical to those of copper deficiency (i.e., growth depression and anemia) or indicate abnormal sulfur metabolism.[102,107] In humans, both occupational and high dietary exposure to molybdenum have been linked through epidemiologic methods to elevated uric acid in blood and increased incidence of gout.

Summary. The essentiality of molybdenum is unquestioned. Biochemical functions have been defined for molybdenum, and signs and symptoms of molybdenum deficiency have been described. However, except for the molybdenum-responsive patient with "acquired molybdenum deficiency" resulting from long-term use of total parenteral nutrition, there is no indication that molybdenum is clinically important. The search for possible molybdenum-responsive syndromes in humans is still warranted because situations may be occurring where molybdenum nutriture is important. For example, low dietary molybdenum might be detrimental to human health and well-being through an effect on the detoxification of xenobiotic compounds. Molybdenum deprivation depresses the activity of the molybdenum hydroxylases without any apparent overall detrimental effect in animals; perhaps the same phenomenon occurs in humans. Low molybdenum hydroxylase activity may have undesirable consequences when a person or animal is stressed by high intakes of xenobiotics. The molybdenum hydroxylases apparently are as important as the microsomal monooxygenase system in the metabolism of drugs and foreign compounds.[114]

Nickel

History. Although nickel was first suggested to be nutritionally essential in 1936, strong evidence for essentiality did not appear until 1970. Studies between 1970 and 1975, however, gave inconsistent signs of nickel deprivation, probably because of suboptimal experimental conditions.[1,127,128] Since 1975, diets and environments that allow optimal growth and survival of laboratory animals have been used in studies of nickel nutrition and metabolism. Thus, most of the significant biochemical, nutritional, and physiological studies of nickel have appeared subsequent to 1975.

Chemistry and method of analysis. Monovalent, divalent, and trivalent forms of nickel apparently are important in biochemistry. Like other ions of the first transition series, Ni^{2+} can complex, chelate, or bind with many substances of biological interest.[127] The binding of divalent nickel by various ligands, including amino acids (especially histidine and cysteine), proteins (especially albumin), and a macroglobulin called nickeloplasmin, probably is important in the extracellular transport, intracellular binding, and urinary and biliary excretion of nickel.[129–131] Ni^{2+}, in a tightly bound form, is required for the activity of urease, an enzyme found in plants and microorganisms.[132,133] In the microbial enzyme, methyl coenzyme M reductase, nickel is present in a chromophore called factor F_{430}.[133–135] Coenzyme M, which is involved in methane formation in anaerobic bacteria, is 2,2'-dithiodiethane sulfonic acid. Factor F_{430} is a tetrapyrrole similar in structure to vitamin B-12, and the formation of factor F_{430} also requires the presence of Ni^{2+}.

Ni^{3+} apparently is essential for enzymatic hydrogenation, desulfurization, and carboxylation reactions in mostly anaerobic microorganisms.[134,135] In some of these reactions, the redox action of nickel may involve the 1+ oxidation state, especially in that of methyl-coenzyme M reductase. Nickel also acts as a structural component in some enzymes.

The determination of nickel in biological material after appropriate collection and preparation is most precisely done with great analytical sensitivity through the use of electrothermal atomic absorption spectrometry.[136]

Absorption, transport, storage and turnover. When nickel in water is ingested after an overnight fast, as much as 50% but usually closer to 20–25%, of the dose is absorbed.[137,138] This high absorption is depressed by certain foodstuffs and simple substances, including milk, coffee, tea, orange juice, ascorbic acid, and ethylene diamine tetraacetic acid (EDTA).[137] Foods such as those found in a typical Guatemalan meal or in a North American breakfast suppress the absorption of nickel to <1%.[137] Thus, nickel is often poorly absorbed (<10%) when ingested with typical diets.[130,137] Nickel absorption is enhanced by iron deficiency, pregnancy, and lactation.[138–141] Pigs were found to absorb >19% of nickel ingested from day 21 of pregnancy until parturition.[140]

The mechanisms involved in the transport of nickel through the gut have not been conclusively established. Becker et al.[142] reported that the transport of nickel across the mucosal epithelium apparently is an energy-driven process rather than simple diffusion and suggested that nickel ions use the iron transport system located in the proximal part of the small intestine. On the other hand, Foulkes and McMullen[143] presented evidence that indicates no existence of a specific nickel carrier mechanism at the brush-border membrane; thus, nickel absorption probably depends upon the efficiency of mucosal trapping through charge neutralization on the membrane. This suggests that nickel crosses the basolateral membrane through passive leakage or diffusion, perhaps as part of an amino acid or other low-molecular-weight complex. The passage as a lipophilic complex is a possibility because nickel affects the absorption of ferric ions, which probably traverse biomembranes as lipophilic complexes.[144] Oral intakes of lipophilic nickel-pyridinethione complexes markedly increased the concentrations of nickel in tissues of mice.[145]

The extracellular transport of nickel is probably through a variety of ligands; however, the principal ligand in blood apparently is serum albumin.[131] The remaining nickel in serum is associated with the amino acid L-histidine and with α_2-macroglobulin.[131,146]

No tissue significantly accumulates orally administered physiological doses of nickel. Recently reported reference values for nickel concentrations in some human tissues are (mean µg/kg dry weight) lung, 173; thyroid, 141; adrenal, 132; kidney, 62; heart, 54; liver, 50; brain, 44; spleen, 37; and pancreas, 34.[147] The physiological significance of the relatively high nickel concentrations in thyroid and adrenal glands is unknown.

Although fecal nickel excretion (mostly unabsorbed nickel) is 10–100 times as great as urinary excretion, the small fraction of nickel absorbed from the intestine and transported to the plasma is rapidly excreted via the kidney as urinary low-molecular-weight complexes. In human renal cytosol the low-molecular-weight fraction contains two nickel-binding components; these are anionic oligosaccharides that bind 70% of the nickel and an acidic peptide that binds the remaining 30%.[148] High-molecular-weight proteins ranging from 10 to 13 kDa were also fractionated from renal cytosol and microsomes.[149] The role of these proteins in the renal handling of nickel needs clarification.

Although urine is the major excretory route of absorbed nickel, significant amounts are lost through sweat and bile.[130,147,150] The nickel content of sweat is high, which indicates active nickel secretion by the sweat glands.[150] The loss of nickel through the bile has been estimated at 2-5 µg/day.[147]

Physiological (biochemical) function. A defined biochemical function for nickel in higher animals, and thus humans, has not been described. Recently, however, functional roles for nickel have been defined for bacteria, fungi, plants, and invertebrates. These roles may provide clues as to the nature of the biological function of nickel in higher animals; thus, some of them are described here.

Since the discovery in 1975 that jackbean urease is a nickel-containing enzyme, evidence has accumulated indicating that nickel is a universal component of ureases (urea amidohydrolases, EC 3.5.1.5).[132] Nickel has been found in ureases from bacteria, mycoplasma, fungi, yeast, algae, higher plants, and invertebrates. Highly purified urease contains two Ni^{2+} ions per 96.6-kDa subunit. An elegant model proposed for the urease mechanism of action involves the polarization of the urea carbonyl by one nickel ion that allows nucleophilic attack by an activated hydroxyl anion associated with the second nickel ion.[132]

The hydrogenases are an extremely heterogeneous group of enzymes.[151] All known hydrogenases contain iron-sulfur clusters. In addition, some hydrogenases also contain nickel, or a nickel-selenocysteine bond; these have been designated as (NiFe) hydrogenases and (NiFeSe) hydrogenases. Hydrogenases containing nickel have been identified for over 35 species of bacteria, including methanogenic, hydrogen-oxidizing, sulfate-reducing, phototrophic, and aerobic N_2–fixing bacteria. Nickel may be a common constituent of hydrogenases that function physiologically to oxidize rather than to evolve H_2. The oxidation state of nickel in hydrogenase is a point of controversy. However, all parties in the controversy agree that nickel is redox active and apparently interacts with the substrate.

In addition to its redox role, nickel also has a regulatory role in the production of hydrogenase. Evidence has been presented that nickel is required for the synthesis of the hydrogenase mRNA in *Bradyrhizobium japonicum*.[152] For the hydrogenase gene to be expressed, O_2 and H_2, when diffused into the cell, affect the redox state of the nickel bound to a nickel-containing, DNA-binding protein, which in turn leads to transcriptional regulation of the hydrogenase message.

Carbon monoxide dehydrogenase (carbon monoxide: [acceptor] oxidoreductase, EC 1.2.99.2; CODH), which oxidizes CO to CO_2, is a nickel enzyme that has been found in acetogenic, methanogenic, phototrophic, and sulfate-reducing anaerobic bacteria.[153,154] In addition to oxidizing CO to CO_2, CODH in acetogenic bacteria catalyzes the reduction of CO_2 to CO and the synthesis and degradation of acetyl-CoA, and thus can also be designated as an acetyl-CoA synthase.

Methyl-S-coenzyme-M reductase is the terminal enzyme in the conversion of CO_2 to methane in methanogenic bacteria.[133–135] The enzyme catalyzes the reductive cleavage of CH_3SCoM to methane and coenzyme M. The enzyme contains factor F_{430}, which is thought to be the site of substrate reduction. Factor F_{430} has been called a tetrahydrocorphin because of its hybrid relationship to corrin and porphyrin macrocytic structures; nickel-corphin has been suggested to be a missing link between iron porphyrin and cobalt corrin systems.

Another nickel porphynoid, tunichlorin, was isolated from the Caribbean tunicate *Trididemnum solidum*.[155] Tunichlorin is a blue-green pigment and is identified as nickel(II) 2-devinyl-2-hydroxymethylpyropheophorbide A. The function of tunichlorin is unknown but it is suspected to be involved in a reductive process similar to that occurring with methyl-S-coenzyme-M reductase.

Thus, nickel participates in hydrolysis and redox reactions, regulates gene expression, and, possibly, stabilizes certain structures. In these roles, nickel forms ligands with sulfur, nitrogen, and oxygen and exists in oxidation states of 3+, 2+, 1+, and perhaps 0 and 4+. Because nickel is so dynamic in lower forms of life, it most likely has an essential functional role in higher forms of life, including humans. Supporting this supposition is the response of experimental animals when they are deprived of dietary nickel. Findings indicate that vitamin B-12 status affects signs of nickel deprivation in rats and that vitamin B-12 must be present for optimal nickel function.[35,156,157] Nickel may have a function in higher animals that involves a pathway using vitamin B-12.

Deficiency signs. The reported signs of nickel deprivation for six animal species—chickens, cows, goats, pigs, rats, and sheep—are extensive and have been listed in several reviews.[127,140,158,159] Unfortunately, the described signs probably will have to be redefined because recent studies indicate that many of the reported signs of nickel deprivation may be manifestations of pharmacological actions of nickel.[128,160] That is, high dietary nickel was alleviating an abnormality caused by something other than nickel deficiency, or changing a variable that was not necessarily subnormal.

The suggestion that some of the reported signs of nickel deprivation are misinterpreted manifestations of a pharmacological action does not necessarily detract from the conclusion that nickel is an essential element. Several studies that apparently examined nickel physiologically indicate that signs of nickel deprivation include depressed growth, reproductive performance, and plasma glucose concentrations. Nickel deprivation also affects the distribution and proper functioning of other nutrients, including calcium, iron, zinc, and cobalamin (vitamin B-12). Also, the nature and severity of nickel deprivation signs are affected by diet composition and nutritional stressors. For example, vitamin B-12 deprivation seemed to depress growth in nickel-supplemented rats but enhanced growth in rats depressed by nickel deprivation. As a result, there was no difference in growth between nickel-deprived and -supplemented rats fed a diet deficient in vitamin B-12.[156] This and other similar findings suggest that in higher animals, vitamin B-12 is necessary for the optimal expression of the biological role of nickel.[157]

Requirement. Because of the strong circumstantial evidence indicating that nickel is essential for several animals, a reasonable hypothesis is that nickel is also required by humans. Some animal studies provide some idea about the amount of nickel possibly required by humans. Most monogastric animals have a dietary nickel requirement of <200 µg/kg diet. If it is assumed that adult humans consume 500 g of a mixed diet daily (dry basis), then the dietary nickel requirement of humans would be <100 µg/day. A nickel requirement for humans of 25–35 µg/day has been suggested.[161]

Food and other sources. Total dietary nickel intakes of humans vary greatly with the amounts and proportions of foods of animal (nickel-low) and plant (nickel-high) origin consumed. Rich sources of nickel include chocolate, nuts, dried beans and peas, and grains;[123,161–163] diets high in these foods could supply >900 µg nickel/day. Conventional diets, however, often provide <100 µg/day. Examples of reported intakes are 69–162 µg/day in the United States and 130 µg/day (range 60–260) in Denmark.[123,163]

Excess (toxicity). Life-threatening toxicity of nickel through oral intake is unlikely. Because of excellent homeostatic regulation, nickel salts exert their toxic action mainly by gastrointestinal irritation and not by inherent toxicity. Generally, ≥250 µg nickel/g diet is required to produce signs of nickel toxicity (such as depressed growth) in rats, mice, chickens, rabbits, and monkeys.[164,165] If animal data can be extrapolated to humans, a daily dose of 250 mg of soluble nickel would produce toxic symptoms in humans.

Some findings, however, suggest that oral intake of nickel in moderate doses could adversely affect health under certain conditions. Moderate amounts of dietary nickel exacerbate signs of severe iron deficiency and copper deficiency in rats.[127,128,159,160] Nickel may act similarly in humans. Some evidence suggests that the ingestion of small amounts of nickel may be more important than external contacts in maintaining eczema caused by nickel allergy. An oral dose as low as 0.6 mg nickel as nickel sulfate given with water to fasting subjects (thus nickel was highly available) produced a positive reaction in some nickel-sensitive individuals.[166] This dose is only a few times higher than the human daily requirement postulated from animal studies.

Summary. A biochemical function for nickel in higher animals has not been defined. However, multiple defined functions in lower forms of life, the response of experimental animals to low dietary intakes, and nickel's dynamic stimulation in vitro of some enzymes strongly suggest that nickel has an essential functional role in higher animals, including humans.

Silicon

History. In 1901 it was reported that high concentrations of silicon were present in tendons, aponeuroses, and eye tissues.[167] As early as 1911, researchers suggested that silicon might have an antiatheroma action.[168] Until 1972, however, silicon was generally considered nonessential, except in some lower classes of organisms (diatoms, radiolarians, and sponges) in which silica serves a structural role. In that year, the first substantial evidence was published that silicon is an essential element for chickens and rats.[169] Most of the limited studies on the biochemical, nutritional, and physiologic roles of silicon have been published since 1974.

Chemistry and method of analysis. The chemistry of silicon is similar to that of carbon, its sister element.[170] Silicon forms silicon-silicon, silicon-hydrogen, silicon-oxygen, silicon-nitrogen, and silicon-carbon bonds. Thus, organosilicon compounds are analogues of organocarbon compounds. The substitution of silicon, however, for carbon, or vice versa, in organocompounds results in molecules with different properties because silicon is larger and less electronegative than carbon.

In animals, silicon is found both free and bound. Silicic acid probably is the free form. The bound form has never been rigorously identified. Silicon may be present in biologic material as a silanolate, an ether (or ester-like) derivative of silicic acid. R_1-O-Si-O-R_2 or R_1-O-Si-O-Si-O-R_2 bridges may play a role in the structural organization of some mucopolysaccharides.[171]

Inductively coupled argon plasma emission and graphite-furnace atomic absorption spectrometric methods have been used to obtain apparently accurate measures of silicon in biological material.[172–174]

Absorption, transport, storage and turnover. Little is known about the metabolism of silicon.[90] Increasing silicon intake increases urinary excretion up to fairly well-defined limits in humans, rats, and guinea pigs. However, the upper limits of urinary silicon excretion apparently are not determined exclusively by the excretory ability of the kidney because urinary excretion can be elevated above these limits by peritoneal injections of silicon.[175] Thus, the upper limits apparently are set by the rate and extent of silicon absorption from the gastrointestinal tract.

The form of dietary silicon determines whether it is well absorbed. In one study, humans absorbed only ≈10% of a large single dose of an alumina-silicate compound but absorbed >70% of a single dose of methylsilanetriol salicylate, a drug used to treat circulatory ischemias and osteoporosis.[176] Further evidence that some forms of silicon, including those in food, are well absorbed is that in rats and humans urinary excretion can be a high percentage (close to 50%) of daily silicon intake.[177] Silicon absorption is affected in rats by age, sex, and the activity of various endocrine glands.[90] The mechanisms involved in the intestinal absorption of silicon are unknown.

Connective tissue (including aorta, trachea, tendon, bone, and skin) and its appendages contain much of the silicon that is retained in the body.[178] The high silicon content of connective tissues may be the result of its presence as an integral component of the glycosaminoglycans and their protein complexes that contribute to structural framework.

Silicon is not protein bound in plasma; it is believed to exist in plasma almost entirely in the undissociated monomeric silicic acid form, $Si(OH)_4$.[169,179] The elimination of absorbed silicon is mainly via the urine, where it probably exists as magnesium orthosilicate.[169,179]

Physiological (biochemical) function. The distribution of silicon and the biochemical changes caused by silicon deprivation in bone indicate that silicon influences bone formation by affecting cartilage composition and ultimately cartilage calcification. Silicon is localized in the active growth areas or the osteoid layer and within the osteoblasts in young bone of mice and rats.[169,180,181] In bone of silicon-deficient animals, hexosamine (glycosaminoglycans) and collagen concentrations are depressed whereas macromineral composition of bone mineral is not markedly affected. Extraction and purification procedures have shown silicon to be chemically combined with the glycosaminoglycan fraction of several types of connective tissues.[169,180,181] Silicon is required for maximal bone prolylhydroxylase activity, which is important for collagen formation.[169] Additionally, silicon was suggested to be involved with phosphorus in the organic phase in the series of events leading to calcification.[180] Silicon may be involved in allowing an association between phosphoprotein-mucopolysaccharide macromolecules and collagen, which play a role in the initiation of calcification and the regulation of crystal growth.

The finding that silicon affects gene expression in some diatoms suggests that a similar role may also exist in higher animals.[182]

Deficiency signs. Most of the signs of silicon deficiency in chickens and rats indicate aberrant metabolism of connective tissue and bone.[169,180,181] Chicks fed a semisynthetic silicon-deficient diet exhibited skull structure abnormalities associated with depressed collagen content in bone and long-bone abnormalities characterized by small, poorly formed joints and defective endochondral bone growth. Tibias of silicon-deficient chicks exhibit depressed contents of articular cartilage, water, hexosamine, and collagen. In optimally growing chickens, growth is not significantly retarded by silicon deficiency. In rats, humerus hexose is increased and hydroxyproline is decreased, plasma amino acid and bone mineral composition is altered, and femur alkaline and acid phosphatase are decreased by silicon deprivation.[183–186] Growth of rats is not markedly affected by silicon deprivation.[184,185] Signs of silicon deprivation can be influenced by low dietary calcium and high dietary aluminum.[185,187] Rats fed a diet low in calcium and silicon and high in aluminum accumulated high amounts of aluminum in brain.[187]

Requirement. Although a biochemical function for silicon is unknown, animal findings strongly suggest that silicon is required by humans. However, postulating a silicon requirement for humans is difficult because no appropriate human data and only limited usable animal data are available. Rats fed about 4.5 mg silicon/kg diet, mostly as the very available sodium metasilicate, do not differ from rats fed about 35 mg silicon/kg diet; both prevent, equally well, silicon deficiency signs exhibited by rats fed $\approx$1.0 mg silicon/kg diet.[183] Animal diets contain $\approx$4000 kcal/kg. The food an average person consumes daily often contains between 8.37 and 10.46 MJ (2000 and 2500 kcal). Thus, if dietary silicon is highly available, on the basis of animal data, the human requirement for silicon is quite small, perhaps in the range of 2–5 mg/day. However, silicon as found in most diets probably is not absorbable or as available as sodium metasilicate; significant amounts probably occur as aluminosilicates and silica from which silicon is not readily available.[188] Factors such as aging and low estrogen status apparently decrease the ability to absorb silicon.[189] Thus, the recommended intake of silicon may be found to be between 5 and 10 mg/day.

Food and other sources. Total dietary silicon intake of humans varies greatly with the amount and proportions of foods consumed and the amounts of refined and processed foods in the diet.[1,90,190,191] Normally, refining reduces the silicon content of foods. However, in recent years, silicate additives have been increasingly used in prepared foods and confections as anticaking or antifoaming agents.[192] Although this increases total dietary silicon, most of it is not bioavailable. The silicon content of drinking water, and beverages made thereof, shows geographical variation; silicon is high in hard-water and low in soft-water areas. The richest sources of silicon are unrefined grains of high fiber content, cereal products, and root vegetables.[90,190,191]

Average daily intakes of silicon apparently range from $\approx$20 to 50 mg/day. The calculated silicon content of the FDA total diet was 19 mg/day for women and 40 mg for men.[191] A human balance study indicated that the oral intake of silicon could be $\approx$21-46 mg/day.[177] The average British diet was estimated to supply 31 mg silicon/day.[190]

Excess (toxicity). Most silicon compounds are essentially nontoxic when taken orally. Magnesium trisilicate, an over-the-counter antacid, has been used by humans for >40 years without obvious deleterious effects. Other silicates are food additives used as anticaking or antifoaming agents.[192] However, antioxidant enzymes, including superoxide dismutase, catalase, and glutathione peroxidase, were reduced in rats fed high amounts of sodium metasilicate.[193] Additionally, ruminants consuming plants with a high silicon content may develop siliceous renal calculi. Renal calculi in humans may also contain silicates.[169]

Summary. Ample circumstantial evidence exists to indicate that silicon is an essential nutrient for higher animals, including humans. Findings from animals indicate that silicon nutriture affects macromolecules such as glycosaminoglycans, collagen, and elastin. Although more should be known about the physiological or biochemical function and requirement for silicon before doing so, speculation has materialized on the possible involvement of silicon deprivation in the occurrence of several human disorders, including atherosclerosis, osteoarthritis, osteoporosis, hypertension, and Alzheimer's disease.[90,194] This speculation indicates the need for more work to clarify the consequences of silicon deficiency in humans.

Vanadium

History. In 1876, Priestley and Gamgee reported on the toxicity of sodium vanadate in frogs, pigeons, guinea pigs, rabbits, dogs, and cats.[195] However, the paper considered to be the classic for pharmacological and toxicological actions of vanadium appeared in 1912.[196] It was also at this time that high vanadium concentrations were discovered in the blood of ascidian worms.[197,198] A surge of interest in vanadium started in 1977 when Cantley et al.[199] reported that vanadate, which inhibits ATPases, was a contaminant of commercially available ATP. The interest was maintained subsequently by the finding in the early 1980s that vanadium is an insulin mimetic agent.[200] The first vanadium-containing enzyme, a bromoperoxidase from the marine alga *Ascophyllum nodosum*, was isolated in 1984.[201] These in vitro, pharmacological, and lower-life-form findings have stimulated speculations about the nutritional importance of vanadium.

The hypothesis that vanadium has an essential role in higher animals has had a long and inconclusive history. Findings reported between 1971 and 1974 by four different research groups led many to conclude that vanadium is an essential nutrient.[202] However, many of these findings may have been the consequence of high vanadium supplements (10–100 times the amount normally found in natural diets) that induced pharmacologic changes in animals fed imbalanced diets.[128,202–204] The most substantive evidence for vanadium essentiality has appeared only since 1987.

Chemistry and methods of analysis. The chemistry of vanadium is complex because the element can exist in at least six oxidation states and can form polymers. In higher animals, the tetravalent and pentavalent valence states apparently are the most important forms of vanadium.[205,206] The tetravalent state appears most simply as the vanadyl cation, VO^{2+}. The vanadyl cation behaves like a simple divalent aquo ion and competes well with Ca^{2+}, Mn^{2+}, Fe^{2+}, etc., for ligand binding sites. Thus VO^{2+} easily forms complexes with proteins, especially those associated with iron, such as transferrin or hemoglobin, which stabilize vanadyl against oxidation. The pentavalent state of vanadium is known as vanadate ($H_2VO_4^-$ or more simply VO_3^-). Vanadate forms complexes with other biological substances, including those that result in it being a phosphate transition-state analogue, and thus competes with or replaces phosphate in many biochemical processes. Vanadate is easily reduced by ascorbate, glutathione, or NADH. For example, with certain cells (e.g., adipocytes), vanadate enters through nonspecific anionic channels and is reduced and complexed by glutathione.[207–209]

Another form of vanadium has been discussed as being responsible for many biological actions of vanadium, including its insulin mimetic action and haloperoxidase role; this is the peroxo form.[209–211] Vanadate can interact with $O_2^{\bullet-}$ formed by NADPH oxidase to generate peroxovanadyl [V(IV)-OO]. Peroxovanadyl can in turn remove hydrogen from NADPH to yield vanadyl hydroperoxide [V(IV)-OOH]. Peroxo (hetero-ligand) vanadate adducts have been suggested to represent a useful model for the active-site vanadium involved in bromide oxidation in haloperoxidases.[211]

Heydorn[212] reviewed analytical methods for the determination of vanadium in the low amounts found in tissues, blood, and urine. For this task, especially for human plasma and serum, methods using atomic emission spectrometry, particle-induced x-ray emission, flame atomic absorption spectrometry, and catalysis were found to be inadequate. Methods that apparently can determine vanadium accurately in low amounts are electrothermal atomic absorption spectrometry (ETAAS), neutron activation analysis with radiochemical separation (RNAA), and neutron activation with preirradiation separation (NAA).[213–216] RNAA and NAA are methods not available to most laboratories; thus, ETAAS is the method of choice for analysis of samples that have been dry-ashed, wet-digested, or bomb-digested in a microwave.[212–214,216] As with all trace elements, contamination of samples is a concern, but apparently for vanadium this is not as much of a concern as it is for some other trace elements.[212,214–216]

Absorption, transport, storage, and turnover. Most ingested vanadium is unabsorbed and is excreted in the feces. Because very low concentrations of vanadium, generally <0.8 μg/L, are found in urine, compared with the estimated daily intake of 12–30 μg and the fecal content of vanadium, apparently <5% of vanadium ingested is normally absorbed.[214,217,218] Byrne

and Kosta[217] estimated that ≤1% of vanadium normally ingested with the diet is absorbed. Curran et al.[219] reported that ≈0.1–1.0% of vanadium in 100 mg of very soluble diammonium oxytartarovandate was absorbed by the human gastrointestinal tract. Animal studies generally support the concept that vanadium is poorly absorbed.[220–222] However, two studies with rats indicated that vanadium absorption can exceed 10%.[223,224] These studies suggest caution in assuming that ingested vanadium always will be poorly absorbed from the gastrointestinal tract. Factors such as fasting and dietary composition probably had an influence on the percentage absorbed from the intestine in these studies.

Kinetic modeling of whole-body vanadium metabolism in sheep indicates that much of vanadium absorbed is absorbed in the upper gastrointestinal tract.[225] Most ingested vanadium probably is transformed in the stomach to VO^{2+} and remains in this form as it passes into the duodenum.[226] However, in vitro studies suggest that vanadate can enter cells through phosphate or other anion transport systems. This may be the reason that VO_3^- is absorbed 3 to 5 times more effectively than VO^{2+}. Thus, the different absorbability rates, the effect of other dietary components on the forms of vanadium in the stomach, and the speed at which it is transformed into VO^{2+} apparently markedly affect the percentage of ingested vanadium absorbed.[226] Supporting this concept are the reviewed findings showing that a number of substances can ameliorate vanadium toxicity, including ascorbic acid, EDTA, chromium, protein, ferrous iron, chloride, and aluminum hydroxide.[204]

Based on studies using intravenous or intraperitoneal injections of the element in animals, vanadium is rapidly removed from the blood plasma and is retained in highest amounts in the kidney, liver, testes, bone, and spleen. For example, at 96 hours, 30–46% of an intravenous dose of ^{48}V was found in the urine and 9–10% was found in the feces of rats.[227,228] Thirty minutes after an intraperitoneal injection of ^{48}V, rats retained 7.2% in the kidney and 2.1% in bone; at 48 hours, the kidney retained 1.6% and bone 3.45% of the dose.[222]

Much evidence suggests that the binding of the vanadyl ion to iron-containing nonheme proteins is important in vanadium metabolism. For example, vanadium in milk of lactating rats injected with ^{48}V was found mainly in the protein fraction and apparently was associated with a transferrin-like protein, perhaps lactoferrin.[229] Nursing pups absorbed a significant amount of the ^{48}V in the milk; this suggests that a lactoferrin-vanadium complex is important in vanadium metabolism in suckling rat pups. In older rats, vanadium apparently is converted into vanadyl-transferrin and vanadyl-ferritin complexes in plasma and body fluids.[226,227,230,231] One study showed that 1 day after intravenous administration of $^{48}VO^{2+}$, 29% of ^{48}V incorporated in rat liver cytosol existed as a vanadium low-molecular-weight complex (<5000 mol wt).[232] By day 9, however, the low-molecular-weight complex had disappeared and vanadium was present only as vanadyl-ferritin (15%) and vanadyl-transferrin (85%) in rat liver cytosol. It remains to be determined whether vanadyl-transferrin can transfer vanadium into cells through the transferrin receptor or whether ferritin is a storage vehicle for vanadium.

Under normal conditions, the body burden of vanadium is low (≈100µg); most tissues contain <10 ng vanadium/g wet weight.[204] However, tissue vanadium is markedly elevated in animals fed high dietary vanadium. In rats, liver vanadium increased from 10 to 55 ng vanadium/g wet weight when dietary vanadium was increased from 0.1 to 25 µg/g.[223] In sheep, bone vanadium increased from 220 to 3320 ng/g dry weight when dietary vanadium was increased from 10 to 270 µg/g.[233] Thus, bone apparently is a major sink for excessive retained vanadium.

On the basis of studies in which vanadium is administered parenterally, urine is the major excretory route for absorbed vanadium.[224,227,228] Both high- and low-molecular-weight complexes have been found in urine;[227,228] one of these may be transferrin. A significant portion of absorbed vanadium may be excreted through the bile. Byrne and Kosta[217] found 0.65, 0.55, and 1.85 ng vanadium/g of human bile. In two studies, 8–10% of an injected dose of [48]V was found in the feces of rats.[224,228] The form of vanadium in bile apparently has not been determined.

Physiological (biochemical) function. A defined biochemical function for vanadium in higher animals, and thus humans, has not been described. Numerous biochemical and physiological functions for vanadium have been suggested on the basis of its in vitro and pharmacological actions; these have been discussed in several reviews and are too extensive to discuss in detail here.[206,207,234,235] In vitro studies with cells and pharmacological studies with animals have shown that vanadium has insulin-mimetic properties; numerous stimulatory effects on cell proliferation and differentiation; effects on cell phosphorylation-dephosphorylation; inhibitory effects on the motility of sperm, cilia, and chromosomes; effects on glucose and ion transport across plasma membranes; interfering effects on intracellular ionized calcium movement; and effects on oxidation-reduction processes. In vitro cell-free systems have shown that vanadium inhibits numerous ATPases, phosphatases, and phosphoryl transfer enzymes.[234] The pharmacological action of vanadium receiving the most attention recently is its ability to mimic insulin.[200] Functional roles for vanadium were recently defined for some algae, lichens, fungi, and bacteria. These roles may provide clues as to the nature of the actual biochemical role of vanadium in humans; thus, they are briefly described here.

Haloperoxidases catalyze the oxidation of halide ions by hydrogen peroxide, thus facilitating the formation of a carbon-halogen bond. In 1984, vanadium was found essential to enzymatic activity of a bromoperoxidase from the brown algae *Ascophyllum nodosum*.[201] Since then, vanadium-dependent bromoperoxidases have been found in a number of marine brown algae, marine red algae, and a terrestrial lichen.[201,236] Vanadium-dependent iodoperoxidases were also detected in brown seaweeds, and a chloroperoxidase was identified in the fungus *Curvularia inaequalis*.[201,236,237]

The mechanism of action of vanadium in the haloperoxidases has not been firmly established. However, findings to date do not favor a mechanism in which V^{5+} is reduced to V^{4+} or V^{3+} and reoxidized to V^{5+} by H_2O_2. Rather, in the bromoperoxidases, H_2O_2 reacts with vanadium as V^{5+} to form a dioxygen species, which reacts with bromide to yield an oxidized bromine species, the intermediate that forms the carbon-halogen bond.[238]

Conversion of atmospheric nitrogen to ammonia by nitrogen-fixing microorganisms is catalyzed by the enzyme nitrogenase. Vanadium-dependent nitrogenases were recently reviewed.[239] The reduction of dinitrogen by nitrogenase involves the sequential MgATP-dependent transfer of electrons from an iron-protein to a vanadium-iron-cofactor center at the substrate-binding site in nitrogenase.

Vanadium is found in high concentrations in some species of the mushroom genus *Amanita*. The isolation and structure determination of a vanadium-containing compound found in mushrooms and named amavadin was reviewed.[240] The physiological function of amavadin is unknown but has been suggested to be a cofactor with a protective oxidase or peroxidase action.[211] The electrochemistry of amavadin is such that it may function in electron-transfer reactions through a V^{5+}/V^{4+} redox couple.[241]

Deficiency signs. Between 1971 and 1985 several research groups described possible signs of vanadium deficiency for some animals.[202] However, most of the early studies were performed with animals fed unbalanced diets which resulted in suboptimal health and growth. The diets used often had widely varied contents of protein, sulfur-containing amino acids, ascorbic acid, iron, copper, and perhaps other nutrients that affected, or were affected by, vanadium metabolism.[202] Thus, pharmacological responses may have been induced by the high-vanadium supplements fed. As a result, it is difficult to determine whether the deficiency signs in early experiments with questionable diets were true deficiency signs, indirect changes caused by an enhanced need for vanadium in some metabolic function, or manifestations of a pharmacological action of vanadium. Vanadium deficiency signs for humans have not been described.

Table 1. Ultratrace elements needing further study to confirm nutritional importance

Element	Reported deficiency signs	Apparent deficient dietary intake	Other apparent beneficial or physiological action	Dietary sources for humans
Aluminum (Al)	Goat: Increased spontaneous abortions, depressed growth, incoordination and weakness in hind legs, and decreased life expectancy[250] Chick: Depressed growth[251]	Goat: 162µg/kg Chick: not given	Activates adenylate cyclase;[252] enhances calmodulin activity;[253] stimulates DNA synthesis in cell cultures;[254] stimulates osteoblasts to form bone through activating a putative G-protein coupled cation sensing system[255]	Baked goods prepared with chemical leavening agents (e.g. baking powder) processed cheese, grains, vegetables, herbs, tea, antacids, buffered analgesics[256]
Bromine (Br)	Goat: Depressed growth, fertility, milk fat production, hematocrit, hemoglobin and life expectancy, and increased spontaneous abortions[257,258]	Goat: 0.8 mg/kg	Alleviates growth retardation caused by hyperthyroidism in mice and chicks;[259,260] substitutes for part of chloride requirement for chicks;[261] insomnia exhibited by many hemodialysis patients associated with bromide deficit[262]	Grains, nuts, fish[263]
Cadmium (Cd)	Rat: Depressed growth[264,265] Goat: Depressed growth[266]	Rat: <4µg/kg Goat: 20µg/kg	Has transforming growth factor activity or stimulates growth of cells in soft agar[267]	Shellfish, grains—especially those grown on high-cadmium soils, leafy vegetables[268]
Fluorine (F)	Rat: Depressed growth and incisor pigmentation[269] Goat: Depressed growth and life span,[270] histological changes in kidney and endocrine organs[271]	Rat: 0.04–0.46 mg/kg Goat: <0.3 mg/kg	High dietary fluoride improves fertility, hematopoiesis and growth in mice and rats;[272,273] is anticariogenic;[274] can be antiosteoporotic,[274] prevents phosphorus-induced nephrocalcinosis[275,276]	Fish, tea, fluoridated water[274]
Germanium (Ge)	Rat: Altered bone and liver mineral composition, and decreased tibial DNA[184]	Rat: 0.7 mg/kg	Reverses changes in rats caused by silicon deprivation;[184] some organic germanium compounds have antitumor activity[277,278]	Wheat bran, vegetables, leguminous seeds[263]
Lead (Pb)	Rat: Depressed growth, anemia, disturbed iron metabolism, decreased liver glucose, triglycerides, LDL-cholesterol phospholipids, glutamic-oxalic transaminase activity and glutamic-pyruvate transaminase activity, increased liver cholesterol and alkaline phosphatase activity, increased serum ceruloplasmin, and decreased blood catalase[279-282]	Rat: 200 µg/kg[279] Rat: 18–45 µg/kg[280-282]	Alleviates iron deficiency signs in young rats[284]	Seafood, plant foodstuffs grown under high-lead conditions[285]

Table continues on next page

Table 1. *Continued*

Element	Reported deficiency signs	Apparent deficient dietary intake	Other apparent beneficial or physiological action	Dietary sources for humans
	Pig: Depressed growth, and elevated serum cholesterol, phospholipids, and bile acids[283]	Pig: 30–32 µg/kg		
Lithium (Li)	Goat: Depressed fertility, birth weight, life span, liver monoamine oxidase activity, and serum isocitrate dehydrogenase, malate dehydrogenase, aldolase, and glutamate dehydrogenase activities, and increased serum creatine kinase activity[286]	Goat: <1.5 mg/kg	Stimulates growth of some cultured cells;[289] exhibits insulinomimetic action;[290] incidence of violent crimes higher in areas with low-lithium drinking water;[291] hair lithium low in violent criminals, learning-disabled subjects, and heart disease patients[292]	Eggs, meat, processed meat, fish, milk, milk products, potatoes, vegetables (content varies with geological origin)[286]
	Rat: Depressed fertility, birth weight, litter size, and weaning weight[287,288]	Rat: 0.6–15 µg/kg		
Rubidium (Rb)	Goat: Depressed food intake, growth, and life expectancy, and increased spontaneous abortions[293]	Goat: 180 µg/kg	Factor R, which prevents hind leg paralysis, swelling of abdomen and death may be rubidium[294]	Coffee, black tea, fruits and vegetables (especially asparagus), poultry, fish[295]
Tin (Sn)	Rat: Depressed growth, alopecia, response to sound, feed efficiency, heart zinc and copper, tibial copper and manganese, muscle iron and manganese, spleen iron, kidney iron and lung magnesium; increased lung calcium[296,297]	Rat: 17 µg/kg	Influences heme oxygenase activity;[298,299] associated with thymus immune and homeostatic function[300]	Canned foods[301]

The uncertainty about vanadium deficiency signs stimulated new efforts to produce deficiency signs in animals fed diets apparently containing adequate and balanced amounts of all known nutrients. Anke et al.[242] found that, when compared with controls fed 2 µg vanadium/g diet, goats fed <10 ng vanadium/g diet exhibited a higher rate of spontaneous abortion, and animals that delivered offspring produced less milk during the first 56 days of lactation. Forty percent of kids from vanadium-deprived goats died between days 7 and 91 of lactation, with some deaths preceded by convulsions; only 8% of kids from vanadium-supplemented goats died during this time. Vanadium-deficient goats had only 55% the life span of control goats. Also, skeletal deformations were seen in the forelegs, and forefoot tarsal joints were thickened.

Uthus and Nielsen[243] reported that, when compared with controls fed 1 µg vanadium/g diet, vanadium deprivation (2 ng vanadium/g diet) increased thyroid weight and the ratio of thyroid weight to body weight and tended to decrease growth of rats. Vanadium deprivation also depressed erythrocyte glucose-6-phosphate dehydrogenase and cecal total carbonic anhydrase.[244] Uthus and Nielsen[243] also found that, as dietary iodine increased from 0.05 to 0.33 to 25 µg/g, thyroid peroxidase activity decreased, and the decrease was more marked in the vanadium-supplemented than the vanadium-deprived rats. Also, as dietary iodine increased, plasma glucose increased in the vanadium-deprived rats but decreased in the vanadium-supplemented rats. These vanadium-deprivation studies probably have found some true deficiency signs. It is unlikely the diets lacked any nutrient that caused such marked deficiency signs, which were prevented by pharmacological action of the small vanadium supplements used.

Requirement. If vanadium is essential for humans, its requirement most likely is small. The diets used in animal deprivation studies contained only 2–25 ng V/g; these often did not markedly affect the animals. Vanadium deficiency has not been identified in humans, yet diets generally supply <30 µg vanadium/day and most supply only 15 µg/day.[122,123,217,218] Thus, a daily dietary intake of 10 µg of vanadium probably will meet any postulated vanadium requirement.

Food and other sources. Foods rich in vanadium include shellfish, mushrooms, parsley, dill seed, black pepper, and some prepared foods.[90,213,217] Beverages, fats and oils, and fresh fruits and vegetables contain the least vanadium (<1 to 5 µg/g).

Excess (toxicity). Vanadium is a relatively toxic element. The threshold level for toxicity apparently is near 10–20 mg/day, or 10–20 µg/g of diet; this is supported by animal findings[195,196,245] and the following human findings. Schroeder et al.[246] fed 15 patients 4.5 and 9 mg vanadium/day as diammonium oxytartarovanadate for 6–16 months without apparent detrimental effect. However, serum cholesterol was reduced slightly by the treatment, so the vanadium supplement was not inactive. Curran et al.[219] fed each of five subjects 13.5 mg/day in three divided doses as diammonium oxytartarovanadate for 6 weeks; no sign of intolerance or toxicity was found. Somerville and Davies[247] gave each of 12 patients 13.5 mg vanadium/day for 2 weeks and then 22.5 mg vanadium/day for 5 months; five patients exhibited gastrointestinal disturbances and five patients exhibited green tongue. Dimond et al.[248] gave ammonium vanadyl tartrate orally to six subjects for 6–10 weeks in amounts ranging from 4.5 to 18 mg vanadium/day; green tongue, cramps, and diarrhea were observed at the larger doses.

From their in-depth study of vanadium toxicity, Proescher et al.[249] concluded that vanadium is a neurotoxic and hemorrhagic-endotheliotoxic poison with nephrotoxic, hepatotoxic, and probably leukocytotoxic components. Thus, it is not surprising that a variety of toxicity signs exist and that they can vary among species and with dosage. Some of the more consistent signs include depressed growth, diarrhea, depressed food intake, and death.

Summary. Although it has numerous in vitro and pharmacological properties that suggest essentiality, the importance of vanadium in nutrition remains to be determined. Identification of a specific biochemical role for vanadium is necessary to disentangle pharmacological from nutritional observations to assess the nutritional importance of vanadium and to determine its safe and adequate intakes. Because vanadium is so pharmacologically active, a beneficial pharmaceutical role for this element may be found.

Other Elements

As indicated in the introduction, the evidence for essentiality of aluminum, bromine, cadmium, fluorine, germanium, lead, lithium, rubidium, and tin is quite limited. Findings that have led to some researchers suggesting that these elements are essential are summarized in Table 1.

References

1. Nielsen FH (1984) Ultratrace elements in nutrition. Annu Rev Nutr 4:21–41
2. Gorby MS (1994) Arsenic in human medicine. In Nriagu JO (ed), Arsenic in the environment, Part II: Human health and ecosystem effects. Wiley, New York, pp 1–16
3. Coulson EJ, Remington RE, Lynch KM (1935) Metabolism in the rat of the naturally occurring arsenic in shrimp as compared with arsenic trioxide. J Nutr 10:255–270
4. Hove E, Elvehjem CA, Hart EB (1938) Arsenic in the nutrition of the rat. Am J Physiol 124:205–212
5. Nielsen FH, Uthus EO (1984) Arsenic. In Frieden E (ed),

Biochemistry of the essential ultratrace elements. Plenum, New York, pp 319–340

6. Shiomi K (1994) Arsenic in marine organisms: chemical forms and toxicological aspects. In Nriagu JD (ed), Arsenic in the environment, Part II: Human health and ecosystems effects. Wiley, New York, pp 261–282

7. Dhubhghaill OMN, Sadler PJ (1991) The structure and reactivity of arsenic compounds: biological activity and drug design. Struct Bond 78:129–190

8. Uthus EO, Collings ME, Cornatzer WE, Nielsen FH (1981) Determination of total arsenic in biological samples by arsine generation and atomic absorption spectrometry. Anal Chem 53:2221–2224

9. Wang WJ, Hanamura S, Winefordner JD (1986) Determination of arsenic by hydride generation with a long absorption cell for atomic absorption spectrometry. Anal Chim Acta 184:213–218

10. Vahter M (1983) Metabolism of arsenic. In Fowler BA (ed), Biological and environmental effects of arsenic. Elsevier, Amsterdam, pp 171–198

11. Marafante E, Vahter M (1987) Solubility, retention, and metabolism of intratracheally and orally administered inorganic arsenic compounds in the hamster. Environ Res 42:72–82

12. Yamauchi H, Kaise T, Yamamura Y (1986) Metabolism and excretion of orally administered arsenobetaine in the hamster. Bull Environ Contam Toxicol 36:350–355

13. Marafante E, Vahter M, Dencker L (1984) Metabolism of arsenocholine in mice, rats and rabbits. Sci Total Environ 34:223–240

14. Yamauchi H, Yamamura Y (1984) Metabolism and excretion of orally administered dimethylarsinic acid in the hamster. Toxicol Appl Pharmacol 74:134–140

15. McChesney EW, Hoppe JO, McAuliff P, Banks WF Jr (1962) Toxicity and physiological disposition of sodium p-N-glycolylarsanilate. I. Observations in mouse, cat, rat and man. Toxicol Appl Pharmacol 4:14–23

16. Fullmer CS, Wasserman RH (1985) Intestinal absorption of arsenate in the chick. Environ Res 36:206–217

17. Hwang SW, Schanker LS (1973) Absorption of organic arsenical compounds from the rat small intestine. Xenobiotica 3:351–355

18. Yamauchi H, Takahashi K, Mashiko M, et al (1992) Intake of different chemical species of dietary arsenic by the Japanese, and their blood and urinary arsenic levels. Appl Organomet Chem 6:383–388

19. Vahter M, Envall H (1983) In vivo reduction of arsenate in mice and rabbits. Environ Res 32:14–24

20. Thompson DJ (1993) A chemical hypothesis for arsenic methylation in mammals. Chem Biol Interact 88:89–114

21. Marafante E, Vahter M (1984) The effect of methyltransferase inhibition on the metabolism of (⁷⁴As) arsenite in mice and rabbits. Chem Biol Interact 50:49–57

22. Buchet JP, Lauwerys R (1985) Study of inorganic arsenic methylation by rat liver in vitro: relevance for the interpretation of observations in man. Arch Toxicol 57:125–129

23. Buchet JP, Lauwerys R (1987) Study of factors influencing the in vivo methylation of inorganic arsenic in rats. Toxicol Appl Pharmacol 91:65–74

24. Vahter M, Marafante E (1987) Effects of low dietary intake of methionine, choline or proteins on the biotransformation of arsenite in the rabbit. Toxicol Lett 37:41–46

25. Vahter M, Marafante E, Dencker L (1983) Metabolism of arsenobetaine in mice, rats and rabbits. Sci Total Environ 30:197–211

26. Yamauchi H, Yamamura Y (1983) Concentration and chemi-

cal species of arsenic in human tissue. Bull Environ Contam Toxicol 31:267–270

27. Lanz H Jr, Wallace PC, Hamilton JG (1950) The metabolism of arsenic in laboratory animals with As⁷⁴ as a tracer. Univ Calif Publ Pharmacol 2:263–282

28. Vahter M, Marafante E, Lindgren A, Dencker L (1982) Tissue distribution and subcellular binding of arsenic in marmoset monkeys after injection of ⁷⁴As-arsenite. Arch Toxicol 51:65–77

29. Vahter M, Marafante E (1985) Reduction and binding of arsenate in marmoset monkeys. Arch Toxicol 57:119–124

30. Tam GKH, Charbonneau SM, Bryce F, et al (1979) Metabolism of inorganic arsenic (⁷⁴As) in humans following oral ingestion. Toxicol Appl Pharmacol 50:319–322

31. Yamato N (1988) Concentrations and chemical species of arsenic in human urine and hair. Bull Environ Contam Toxicol 40:633–640

32. Uthus EO (1992) Evidence for arsenic essentiality. Environ Geochem Health 14:55–58

33. Desrosiers R, Tanguay RM (1986) Further characterization of the posttranslational modifications of core histones in response to heat and arsenite stress in Drosphilia. Biochem Cell Biol 64:750–757

34. van Bergen en Henegouwen PMP, Linnemans WAM (1987) Heat shock gene expression and cytoskeletal alterations in mouse neuroblastoma cells. Exp Cell Res 171:367–375

35. Nielsen FH (1988) Possible future implications of ultratrace elements in human health and disease. In Prasad AS (ed), Essential and toxic trace elements in human health and disease. Current Topics in Nutrition and Disease, Vol 18. Liss, New York, pp 277–292

36. Meng Z, Meng N (1994) Effects of inorganic arsenicals on DNA synthesis in unsensitized human blood lymphocytes in vitro. Biol Trace Elem Res 42:201–208

37. Meng Z (1993) Effects of arsenic on DNA synthesis in human lymphocytes stimulated by phytohemagglutinin. Biol Trace Elem Res 39:73–80

38. Anke M (1986) Arsenic. In Mertz W (ed), Trace elements in human and animal nutrition, Vol 2. Academic Press, Orlando, FL, pp 347–372

39. Schmidt A, Anke M, Groppel B, Kronemann H (1984) Effects of As-deficiency on skeletal muscle, myocardium and liver. A histochemical and ultrastructural study. Exp Pathol 25:195–197

40. Uthus EO (1994) Diethyl maleate, an in vivo chemical depletor of glutathione, affects the response of male and female rats to arsenic deprivation. Biol Trace Elem Res 46:247–259

41. Mayer DR, Kosmus W, Pogglitsch H, et al (1993) Essential trace elements in humans. Serum arsenic concentrations in hemodialysis patients in comparison to healthy controls. Biol Trace Elem Res 37:27–38

42. Uthus EO, Nielsen FH (1993) Determination of the possible requirement and reference dose levels for arsenic in humans. Scand J Work Environ Health 19(suppl 1):137–138

43. Uthus EO (1994) Estimation of safe and adequate daily intake for arsenic. In Mertz W, Abernathy CO, Olin SS (eds), Risk assessment of essential elements. ILSI Press, Washington, DC, pp 273–282

44. Evans WH, Sherlock JC (1987) Relationships between elemental intakes within the United Kingdom total diet study and other adult dietary studies. Food Addit Contam 4:1–8

45. Buchet JP, Lauwerys R, Vandevoorde A, Pycke JM (1983) Oral daily intake of cadmium, lead, manganese, copper, chromium, mercury, calcium, zinc, and arsenic in Belgium: a duplicate meal study. Food Chem Toxicol 21:19–24

46. Mykkänen H, Räsänen L, Ahola M, Kimppa S (1986) Dietary intakes of mercury, lead, cadmium, and arsenic by Finnish children. Hum Nutr Appl Nutr 40A:32–39

47. Vallee BL, Ulmer DD, Wacker WEC (1960) Arsenic toxicology and biochemistry. AMA Arch Ind Health 21:132–151

48. Kaise T, Watanabe S, Itoh K (1985) The acute toxicity of arsenobetaine. Chemosphere 14:1327–1332

49. Kaise T, Horiguchi Y, Fukui S, et al (1992) Acute toxicity and metabolism of arsenocholine in mice. Appl Organometal Chem 6:369–373

50. Squibb KS, Fowler BA (1983) The toxicity of arsenic and its compounds. In Fowler BA (ed), Biological and environmental effects of arsenic. Elsevier, Amsterdam, pp 233–269

51. Ishinishi N, Tsuchiya K, Vahter M, Fowler BA (1986) Arsenic. In Friberg L, Nordberg GF, Vouk V (eds), Handbook on the toxicology of metals, 2nd ed. Elsevier, Amsterdam, pp 43–83

52. Morton WE, Dunnette DA (1994) Health effects of environmental arsenic. In Nriagu JO (ed), Arsenic in the environment, Part II: Human health and ecosystem effects. Wiley, New York, pp 17–34

53. Goldman M, Dacre JC (1991) Inorganic arsenic compounds: are they carcinogenic, mutagenic, teratogenic? Environ Geochem Health 13:179–191

54. Wiley HW (1904) Influence of food preservatives and artificial colors on digestion and health. I. Boric acid and borax. US Department of Agriculture Bulletin No. 84, Pt. 1. Government Printing Office, Washington, DC

55. Warrington K (1923) The effect of boric acid and borax on the broad bean and certain other plants. Ann Bot 37:629–672

56. Hove E, Elvehjem CA, Hart EB (1939) Boron in animal nutrition. Am J Physiol 127:689–701

57. Orent-Keiles E (1941) The role of boron in the diet of the rat. Proc Soc Exp Biol Med 44:199–202

58. Teresi JD, Hove E, Elvehjem CA, Hart EB (1944) Further study of boron in the nutrition of rats. Am J Physiol 140:513–518

59. Skinner JT, McHargue JS (1945) Response of rats to boron supplements when fed rations low in potassium. Am J Physiol 143:385–390

60. Follis RH Jr (1947) The effect of adding boron to a potassium-deficient diet in the rat. Am J Physiol 150:520–522

61. Hunt CD, Nielsen FH (1981) Interaction between boron and cholecalciferol in the chick. In McC Howell J, Gawthorne JM, White CL (eds), Trace element metabolism in man and animals, TEMA-4. Australian Academy of Science, Canberra, Australia, pp 597–600

62. Woods WG (1994) An introduction to boron: history, sources, uses and chemistry. Environ Health Perspect 102(suppl 7):5–11

63. Zittle CA (1951) Reaction of borate with substances of biological interest. Adv Enzymol 12:493–527

64. Lindquist R, Terry C (1974) Inhibition of subtilisin by boronic acids, potential analogs of tetrahedral reaction intermediates. Arch Biochem Biophys 160:135–144

65. Chen TSS, Chang C-J, Floss HG (1980) Biosynthesis of the boron-containing antibiotic aplasmomycin. Nuclear magnetic resonance analysis of aplasmomycin and desboroaplasmomycin. J Antibiotics 33:1316–1322

66. Dunitz JD, Hawley DM, Miklos D, et al (1971) Structure of boromycin. Helv Chim Acta 54:1709–1713

67. Hunt CD, Shuler TR (1989) Open-vessel, wet-ash, low-temperature digestion of biological materials for inductively coupled argon plasma spectroscopy (ICAP) analysis of boron and other elements. J Micronutr Anal 6:161–174

68. Ferrando AA, Green NR, Barnes KW, Woodward B (1993) Microwave digestion preparation and ICP determination of boron in human plasma. Biol Trace Elem Res 37:17–25

69. Iyengar GV, Clarke WB, Downing RG (1990) Determination of boron and lithium in diverse biological matrices using neutron activation-mass spectrometry (NA-MS). Fresenius J Anal Chem 338:562–566

70. Vanderpool RA, Hoff D, Johnson PE (1994) Use of inductively coupled plasma-mass spectrometry in boron-10 stable isotope experiments with plants, rats and humans. Environ Health Perspect 102(suppl 7):13–20

71. Kent NL, McCance RA (1941) The absorption and excretion of "minor" elements by man. I. Silver, gold, lithium, boron, and vanadium. Biochem J 35:837–844

72. Jansen JA, Schou JS, Aggerbeck B (1984) Gastro-intestinal absorption and in vitro release of boric acid from water-emulsifying ointments. Food Chem Toxicol 22:49–53

73. Havercroft JM, Ward NI (1991) Boron and other elements in relation to rheumatoid arthritis. In Momčilović B (ed), Trace elements in man and animals 7. IMI, Zagreb, pp 8.2–8.3

74. Shuler TR, Pootrakul P, Yarnsukon P, Nielsen FH (1990) Effect of thalassemia/hemoglobin E disease on macro, trace, and ultratrace element concentrations in humans tissues. J Trace Elem Med 3:31–43

75. Abou-Shakra FR, Havercroft JM, Ward NI (1989) Lithium and boron in biological tissues and fluids. Trace Elem Med 6:142–146

76. Hunt CD (1989) Dietary boron modified the effects of magnesium and molybdenum on mineral metabolism in the cholecalciferol-deficient chick. Biol Trace Elem Res 22:201–220

77. Hunt CD (1994) The biochemical effects of physiologic amounts of dietary boron in animal nutrition models. Environ Health Perspect 102(suppl 7):35–43

78. Loomis WD, Durst RW (1992) Chemistry and biology of boron. BioFactors 3:229–239

79. Blevins DG, Lukaszewski KM (1994) Proposed physiologic functions of boron in plants pertinent to animal and human metabolism. Environ Health Perspect 102(suppl 7):31–33

80. Nielsen FH (1991) Nutritional requirements for boron, silicon, vanadium, nickel and arsenic: current knowledge and speculation. FASEB J 5:2661–2667

81. Nielsen FH (1994) Biochemical and physiologic consequences of boron deprivation in humans. Environ Health Perspect 102(suppl 7):59–63

82. Nielsen FH (1991) The saga of boron in food: from a banished food preservative to a beneficial nutrient for humans. Curr Top Plant Biochem Physiol 10:274–286

83. Penland JG (1990) Dietary boron affects brain function in mature Long-Evans rats. Proc ND Acad Sci 44:78

84. Hegsted M, Keenan MJ, Siver F, Wozniak P (1991) Effect of boron on vitamin D deficient rats. Biol Trace Elem Res 26:243–255

85. Nielsen FH (1989) Dietary boron affects variables associated with copper metabolism in humans. In Anke M, Baumann W, Bräunlich H, et al (eds), 6th International Trace Element Symposium, 1989, Vol 4. Friedrich-Schiller-Universitat, Jena, pp 1106–1111

86. Nielsen FH, Mullen LM, Gallagher SK (1990) Effect of boron depletion and repletion on blood indicators of calcium status in humans fed a magnesium-low diet. J Trace Elem Exp Med 3:45–54

87. Nielsen FH, Mullen LM, Nielsen EJ (1991) Dietary boron affects blood cell counts and hemoglobin concentrations in humans. J Trace Elem Exp Med 4:211–223

88. Nielsen FH, Gallagher SK, Johnson LK, Nielsen EJ (1992) Boron enhances and mimics some effects of estrogen therapy in postmenopausal women. J Trace Elem Exp Med 5:237–246

89. Penland JG (1994) Dietary boron, brain function, and cognitive performance. Environ Health Perspect 102(suppl 7):65–72

90. Nielsen FH (1988) The ultratrace elements. In KT Smith (ed), Trace minerals in foods. Marcel Dekker, New York, pp 357–428

91. Hunt CD (1988) Boron homeostasis in the cholecalciferol-deficient chick. Proc ND Acad Sci 42:60.

92. Hunt CD, Shuler TR, Mullen LM (1991) Concentration of boron and other elements in human foods and personal-care products. J Am Diet Assoc 91:558–568

93. Anderson DL, Cunningham WC, Lindstrom TR (1994) Concentrations and intakes of H, B, S, K, Na, Cl, and NaCl in foods. J Food Comp Anal 7:59–82

94. Clarke WB, Gibson RS (1988) Lithium, boron, and nitrogen in 1-day diet composites and a mixed-diet standard. J Food Comp Anal 1:209–220

95. Green GH, Lott MD, Weeth HJ (1973) Effects of boron-water on rats. Proc West Sec Am Soc Anim Sci 24:254–258

96. Seal BS, Weeth HJ (1980) Effect of boron in drinking water on the male laboratory rat. Bull Environ Contam Toxicol 25:782–789

97. Franke J, Runge H, Bech R, et al (1985) Boron as an antidote to fluorosis? Part 1. Studies of the skeletal system. Fluoride 18:187–197

98. Health effects of boron. (1994) Environ Health Perspect 102(suppl 7)

99. Linden CH, Hall AH, Kulig KW, Rumack BH (1986) Acute ingestions of boric acid. Clin Toxicol 24:269–279

100. Pinto J, Huang YP, McConnell RJ, Rivlin RS (1978) Increased urinary riboflavin excretion resulting from boric acid ingestion. J Lab Clin Med 92:126–134

101. Gordon AS, Prichard JS, Freedman MH (1973) Seizure disorders and anemia associated with chronic borax intoxication. Can Med Assoc J 108:719–721

102. Mills CF, Davis GK(1987) Molybdenum. In Mertz W (ed), Trace elements in human and animal nutrition, Vol 1. Academic Press, San Diego, pp 429–463

103. Rajagopalan KV (1988) Molybdenum: an essential trace element in human nutrition. Annu Rev Nutr 8:401–427

104. Rajagopalan KV (1984) Molybdenum. In Frieden E (ed), Biochemistry of the essential ultratrace elements. Plenum, New York, pp 149–174

105. Rajagopalan KV (1988) Molybdopterin—problems and perspectives. BioFactors 1:273–278

106. Wootton JC, Nicolson RE, Cock JM, et al (1991) Enzymes depending on the pterin molybdenum cofactor: sequence families, spectroscopic properties of molybdenum and possible cofactor-binding domains. Biochim Biophys Acta 1057:157–185

107. Winston PW (1981) Molybdenum. In Bronner F, Coburn JW (eds), Disorders of mineral metabolism, Vol. 1, Trace minerals. Academic Press, New York, pp 295–315

108. Ward AF, Marciello LF, Carrara L, Luciano VJ (1980) Simultaneous determination of major, minor, and trace elements in agricultural and biological samples by inductively coupled argon plasma spectrometry. Spect Lett 13:803–831

109. Turnlund JR, Keyes WR, Pfeiffer GL (1993) A stable isotope study of the dietary molybdenum requirement of young men. In Anke M, Meissner D, Mills CF (eds), Trace elements in man and animals, TEMA-8. Verlag Media Touristik, Gersdorf, pp 189–193

110. Cardin CJ, Mason J (1976) Molybdate and tungstate transfer by rat ileum. Competitive inhibition by sulphate. Biochim Biophys Acta 455:937–946

111. Kosarek LJ, Winston PW (1977) Absorption of molybdenum-

99 (Mo-99) as molybdate with various doses in the rat [abstract]. Fed Proc 36:1106

112. Lener J, Bibr B (1984) Effects of molybdenum on the organism (a review). J Hyg Epidemiol Microbiol Immunol 28:405–419

113. Grace ND, Martinson PL (1985) The distribution of Mo between the liver and other organs and tissues of sheep grazing a ryegrass white clover pasture. In Mills CF, Bremner I, Chesters JK (eds), Trace elements in man and animals, TEMA 5. Commonwealth Agricultural Bureaux, Farnham Royal, pp 534–536

114. Beedham C (1985) Molybdenum hydroxylases as drug-metabolizing enzymes. Drug Metab Rev 16:119–156

115. Blanchardie P, Lustenberger P, Orsonneau JL, et al (1984) Influence of molybdate, ionic strength and pH on ligand binding to the glucocorticoid receptor. Steroids 44:159–174

116. Bodine PV, Litwack G (1988) Evidence that the modulator of the glucocorticoid-receptor complex is the endogenous molybdate factor. Proc Natl Acad Sci U S A 85:1462–1466

117. Mills CF, Bremner I (1980) Nutritional aspects of molybdenum in animals. In Coughlan MP (ed), Molybdenum and molybdenum-containing enzymes. Pergamon, Oxford, pp 517–542

118. Anke M, Risch MA (1989) Importance of molybdenum in animal and man. In Anke M, Baumann W, Bräunlich H, et al (eds), 6th International Trace Element Symposium, Molybdenum, Vanadium. Friedrich-Schiller-Universitat, Jena, pp 303–321b

119. Abumrad NN, Schneider AJ, Steel D, Rogers LS (1981) Amino acid intolerance during prolonged total parenteral nutrition reversed by molybdate therapy. Am J Clin Nutr 34:2551–2559

120. Wang X, Oberleas D, Yang MT, Yang SP (1992) Molybdenum requirement of female rats. J Nutr 122:1036–1041

121. National Research Council (1989) Recommended dietary allowances, 10th ed. National Academy Press, Washington, DC

122. Evans WH, Read JI, Caughlin D (1985) Quantification of results for estimating elemental dietary intakes of lithium, rubidium, strontium, molybdenum, vanadium, and silver. Analyst 110:873–877

123. Pennington JAT, Jones JW (1987) Molybdenum, nickel, cobalt, vanadium, and strontium in total diets. J Am Diet Assoc 87:1644–1650

124. Shiraishi K, Yamagami Y, Kameoka K, Kawamura H(1988) Mineral contents in model diet samples for different age groups. J Nutr Sci Vitaminol (Tokyo) 34:55–65

125. Glei M, Anke M, Müller M, Lösch E (1994) Molybdänaufnahme und Molybdänbilanz Erwachsener in Deutschland. In Anke M, Meissner D, Bergmann H, et al (eds), Defizite und Überschüsse an Mengen-und Spurenelementen in der Ernährung. 14. Arbeitstagung Mengen-und Spurenelemente 1994. Verlag Harald Schubert, Leipzig, pp 251–256

126. Anke M, Lösch E, Glei M, et al (1993) Der Molybdängehalt der Lebensmittel und Getränke Deutschlands. In Anke M, Bergmann H, Bitsch R, et al (eds), Mengen-und Spurenelemente. 13. Arbeitstagung 1993. Verlag MTV Hammerschmidt, Gersdorf, pp 537–553

127. Nielsen FH (1984) Nickel. In Frieden E (ed), Biochemistry of the essential ultratrace elements. Plenum, New York, pp 293–308

128. Nielsen FH (1985) The importance of diet composition in ultratrace element research. J Nutr 115:1239–1247

129. Sunderman FW Jr (1977) A review of the metabolism and toxicology of nickel. Ann Clin Lab Sci 1:377–398

130. Nieboer E, Tom RT, Sanford WE (1988) Nickel metabolism in man and animals. In Sigel H, Sigel A (eds), Metal ions in

biological systems, Vol 23, Nickel and its role in biology. Marcel Dekker, New York, pp 91–121

131. Tabata M, Sarkar B (1992) Specific nickel (II)-transfer process between the native sequence peptide representing the nickel (II)-transport site of human albumin and L-histidine. J Inorg Biochem 45:93–104

132. Andrews RK, Blakely RL, Zerner B (1988) Urease—a Ni (II) metalloenzyme. In Lancaster JR Jr (ed), The bioinorganic chemistry of nickel. VCH, New York, pp 141–165

133. Walsh CT, Orme-Johnson WH (1987) Nickel enzymes. Biochemistry 26:4901–4906

134. Thauer RK (1985) Nickelenzyme im Stoffwechsel von methanogenen Bakterien. Biol Chem Hoppe Seyler 366:103–112

135. Hausinger RP (1987) Nickel utilization by microorganisms. Microbiol Rev 51:22–42

136. Sunderman FW Jr, Hopfer SM, Crisostomo MC (1988) Nickel analysis by electrothermal atomic absorption spectrometry. Methods Enzymol 158:382–391

137. Solomons NW, Viteri F, Shuler TR, Nielsen FH (1982) Bioavailability of nickel in man. Effects of foods and chemically-defined dietary constituents on the absorption of inorganic nickel. J Nutr 112:39–50

138. Sunderman FW Jr, Hopfer SM, Swift T, et al (1988) Nickel absorption and elimination in human volunteers. In Hurley LS, Keen CL, Lönnerdal B, Rucker RB (eds), Trace elements in man and animals 6. Plenum, New York, pp 427–428

139. Nielsen FH (1983) Studies on the interaction between nickel and iron during intestinal absorption. In Anke M, Baumann W, Braünlich H, Brückner C (eds), 4 Spurenelement-Symposium. Friedrich-Schiller-Universitat, Jena, pp 11–18

140. Kirchgessner M, Roth-Maier DA, Schnegg A (1981) Progress of nickel metabolism and nutrition research. In McHowell J, Gawthorne JM, White CL (eds), Trace element metabolism in man and animals, TEMA 4. Australian Academy of Science, Canberra, Australia, pp 621–624

141. Kirchgessner M, Roth-Maier DA, Spörl R (1983) Spurenelementbilanzen (Cu, Zn, Ni, und Mn) laktierender Sauen. Z Tierphysiol Tierernhr Futtermittelkd 50:230–239

142. Becker G, Dörstelmann U, Frommberger U, Forth W (1980) On the absorption of cobalt (II)- and nickel (II)-ions by isolated intestinal segments in vitro of rats. In Anke M, Schneider H-J, Brückner C (eds), 3 Spurenelement-Symposium, Nickel. Friedrich-Schiller-Universitat, Jena, pp 79–85

143. Foulkes EC, McMullen DM (1986) On the mechanism of nickel absorption in the rat jejunum. Toxicology 38:35–42

144. Nielsen FH (1980) Effect of form of iron on the interaction between nickel and iron in rats: growth and blood parameters. J Nutr 110:965–973

145. Jasim S, Tjälve H (1986) Effect of sodium pyridinethione on the uptake and distribution of nickel, cadmium, and zinc in pregnant and non-pregnant mice. Toxicology 38:327–350

146. Nomoto S, Sunderman FW Jr (1988) Presence of nickel in alpha-2 macroglobulin isolated from human serum by high performance liquid chromatography. Ann Clin Lab Sci 18:78–84

147. Rezuke WN, Knight JA, Sunderman FW Jr (1987) Reference values for nickel concentrations in human tissue and bile. Am J Ind Med 11:419–426

148. Predki PF, Whitfield DM, Sarkar B (1992) Characterization and cellular distribution of acidic peptide and oligosaccharide metal-binding compounds from kidneys. Biochem J 281:835–841

149. Sunderman FW Jr, Mangold BLK, Wong SHY, et al (1983) High-performance size-exclusion chromatography of ^{63}Ni-constituents in renal cytosol and microsomes from ^{63}NiCl$_2$-treated rats. Res Commun Chem Pathol Pharmacol 39:477–492

150. Cohn JR, Emmett EA (1978) The excretion of trace metals in human sweat. Ann Clin Lab Sci 8:270–275

151. Przybyla AE, Robbins J, Menon N, Peck HD Jr (1992) Structure-function relationships among the nickel-containing hydrogenases. FEMS Microbiol Rev 88:109–136

152. Kim H, Yu C, Maier RJ (1991) Common cis-acting region responsible for transcriptional regulation of Bradyrhizobium japonicum hydrogenase by nickel, oxygen, and hyrogen. J Bacteriol 173:3993–3999

153. Diekert G (1988) Carbon monoxide dehydrogenase of acetogens. In Lancaster JR Jr (ed), The bioinorganic chemistry of nickel. VCH, New York, pp 299–309

154. Ragsdale SW, Wood HG, Morton TA, et al (1988) Nickel in CO dehydrogenase. In Lancaster JR Jr (ed), The bioinorganic chemistry of nickel. VCH, New York, pp 311–332

155. Bible KC, Buytendorp M, Zierath PD, Rinehart KL (1988) Tunichlorin: A nickel chlorin isolated from the Caribbean tunicate Trididemnum solidum. Proc Natl Acad Sci USA 85:4582–4586

156. Nielsen FH, Zimmerman TJ, Shuler TR, et al (1989) Evidence for a cooperative metabolic relationship between nickel and vitamin B$_{12}$ in rats. J Trace Elem Exp Med 2:21–29

157. Nielsen FH, Uthus EO, Poellot RA, Shuler TR (1993) Dietary vitamin B$_{12}$, sulfur amino acids, and odd-chain fatty acids affect the response of rats to nickel deprivation. Biol Trace Elem Res 37:1–15

158. Anke M, Groppel B, Kronemann H, Grün M (1984) Nickel—an essential element. In Sunderman FW (ed), Nickel in the human environment. International Agency for Research of Cancer, Lyon, pp 339–365

159. Spears JW (1984) Nickel as a "newer trace element" in the nutrition of domestic animals. J Anim Sci 59:823–835

160. Nielsen FH, Shuler TR, McLeod TG, Zimmerman TJ (1984) Nickel influences iron metabolism through physiologic, pharmacologic and toxicologic mechanisms in the rat. J Nutr 114:1280–1288

161. Anke M, Angelow L, Müller M, Glei M (1993) Dietary trace element intake and excretion of man. In Anke M, Meissner D, Mills CF (eds), Trace elements in man and animals, TEMA 8. Verlag Media Touristik, Gersdorf, pp 180–188

162. Flyvholm M-A, Nielsen GD, Andersen A (1984) Nickel content of food and estimation of dietary intake. Z Lebensm Unters Forsch 179:427–431

163. Veien NK, Anderson MR (1986) Nickel in Danish food. Acta Derm Venereol (Stockh) 66:502–509

164. Kirchgessner M, Reichlmayr-Lais A, Maier R (1985) Ni retention and concentrations of Fe and Mn in tissues resulting from different Ni supply. In Mills CF, Bremner I, Chesters JK (eds), Trace elements in man and animals, TEMA 5. Commonwealth Agricultural Bureaux, Farnham Royal, pp 147–151

165. Nielsen FH (1977) Nickel toxicity. In Goyer RA, Mehlman MA (eds), Advances in modern toxicology: Toxicology of trace elements, Vol 2. Wiley, New York, pp 129–146

166. Cronin E, Di Michiel AD, Brown SS (1980) Oral challenge in nickel-sensitive women with hand eczema. In Brown SS, Sunderman FW Jr (eds), Nickel toxicology. Academic Press, New York, pp 149–152

167. Schulz H (1901) Uber den Kieselsaüregehalt menschlicher und thierischer Gewebe. Pflugers Arch Ges Physiol 84:67–100

168. Gouget MA (1911) Athérome expérimental et silicate de soude. La Presse Medicale 97:1005–1006

169. Carlisle EM (1984) Silicon. In Frieden E (ed), Biochemistry of the essential ultratrace elements. Plenum, New York, pp 257–291

170. Wannagat U (1978) Sila-pharmaca. Nobel Symp 40:447–472
171. Schwarz K (1973) A bound form of silicon in glycosaminoglycans and polyuronides. Proc Natl Acad Sci U S A 70:1608–1612
172. Berlyne GM, Caruso C (1983) Measurement of silicon in biological fliuds in man using flameless furnace atomic absorption spectrophotometry. Clin Chim Acta 129:239–244
173. Zhuoer H (1994) Silicon measurement in bone and other tissues by electrothermal atomic absorption spectrometry. J Anal Atomic Spect 9:11–15
174. Lichte FE, Hopper S, Osborn TW (1980) Determination of silicon and aluminum in biological matrices by inductively coupled plasma emission spectrometry. Anal Chem 52:120–124
175. Sauer F, Laughland DH, Davidson WM (1959) Silica metabolism in guinea pigs. Can J Biochem Physiol 37:183–191
176. Allain P, Cailleux A, Mauras Y, Renier JC (1983) Etude de l'absorption digestive du silicium aprés administration unique chez l'homme sous forme de salicylate de méthyl silane triol. Therapie 38:171–174
177. Kelsay JL, Behall KM, Prather E (1979) Effect of fiber from fruits and vegetables on metabolic responses of human subjects. II. Calcium, magnesium, iron and silicon balances. Am J Clin Nutr 32:1876–1880
178. Adler AJ, Etzion Z, Berlyne GM (1986) Update, distribution, and excretion of [31]silicon in normal rats. Am J Physiol 251:E670–E673
179. Berlyne GM, Adler AJ, Ferran N, et al (1986) Silicon metabolism. I. Some aspects of renal silicon handling in normal men. Nephron 43:5–9
180. Carlisle EM (1981) Silicon in bone formation. In Simpson TL, Volcani BE (eds), Silicon and siliceous structures in biological systems. Springer, New York, pp 69–94
181. Carlisle EM (1988) Silicon as a trace nutrient. Sci Tot Environ 73:95–106
182. Reeves CD, Volcani BE (1985) Role of silicon in diatom metabolism. Messenger RNA and polypeptide accumulation patterns in synchronized cultures of Cylindrotheca fusiformis. J Gen Microbiol 131:1735–1744
183. Seaborn CD, Nielsen FH (1993) Silicon: A nutritional beneficence for bones, brains and blood vessels? Nutr Today 28:13–18
184. Seaborn CD, Nielsen FH (1994) Effects of germanium and silicon on bone mineralization. Biol Trace Elem Res 42:151–164
185. Seaborn CD, Nielsen FH (1994) High dietary aluminum affects the response of rats to silicon deprivation. Biol Trace Elem Res 41:295–304
186. Seaborn CD, Nielsen FH (1994) Dietary silicon affects acid and alkaline phosphatase and [45]calcium uptake in bone of rats. J Trace Elem Exp Med 7:11–18
187. Carlisle EM, Curran MJ (1987) Effect of dietary silicon and aluminum on silicon and aluminum levels in the rat brain. Alzheimer Dis Assoc Disorders 1:83–89
188. Benke GM, Osborn TW (1979) Urinary silicon excretion by rats following oral administration of silicon compounds. Food Cosmet Toxicol 17:123–127
189. Charnot Y, Pérès G (1971) Contribution à l' étude de la régulation endocrinienne du métabolisme silicique. Ann Endocrinol 32:397–402
190. Bowen HJM, Peggs A (1984) Determination of the silicon content of food. J Sci Food Agric 35:1225–1229
191. Pennington JAT (1991) Silicon in foods and diets. Foods Addit Contam 8:97–118
192. Villota R, Hawkes JG (1986) Food applications and the toxicological and nutritional implications of amorphous silicon dioxide. CRC Crit Rev Food Sci Nutr 23:289–321
193. Najda J, Goss M, Gminski J, et al (1994) The antioxidant enzymes activity in the conditions of systemic hypersilicemia. Biol Trace Elem Res 42:63–70
194. Eisinger J, Clairet D (1993) Effects of silicon, fluoride, etidronate and magnesium on bone mineral density: a retrospective study. Magnes Res 6:247–249
195. Priestley J, Gamgee A (1876) On the physiological action of vanadium. Philos Trans R Soc Lond [Biol] 166:495–556
196. Jackson DE (1912) The pharmacological action of vanadium. J Pharmacol 3:477–514
197. Henze M (1911) Untersuchungen über das Blut der Ascidien. I. Mitt. Die Vanadiumverbindung der Blutkörperchen. Hoppe Seylers Z Physiol Chem 72:494–501
198. Henze M (1912) Untersuchungen über das Blut der Ascidien. Hoppe Seylers Z Physiol Chem 79:215–228
199. Cantley LC Jr, Josephson L, Warner R, et al (1977) Vanadate is a potent (Na,K)-ATPase inhibitor found in ATP derived from muscle. J Biol Chem 252:7421–7423
200. Orvig C, Thompson KH, Battell M, McNeill JH (1995) Vanadium compounds as insulin mimics. In Sigel H, Sigel A (eds), Metal ions in biological systems, Vol 31, Vanadium and its role in life. Marcel Dekker, New York, pp 575–594
201. Vilter H (1995) Vanadium-dependent-haloperoxidases. In Sigel H, Sigel A (eds), Metal ions in biological systems, Vol 31, Vanadium and its role in life. Marcel Dekker, New York, pp 325–362
202. Nielsen FH, Uthus EO (1990) The essentiality and metabolism of vanadium. In Chasteen ND (ed), Vanadium in biological systems. Physiology and biochemistry. Kluwer Academic, Dordrecht, Netherlands, pp 51–62
203. Nechay BR, Nanninga LB, Nechay PSE, et al (1986) Role of vanadium in biology. Fed Proc 45:123–132
204. Nielsen FH (1995) Vanadium in mammalian physiology and nutrition. In Sigel H, Sigel A (eds), Metal ions in biological systems, Vol 31, Vanadium and its role in life. Marcel Dekker, New York, pp 543–573
205. Kustin K, Macara I (1982) The new biochemistry of vanadium. Comments Inorg Chem 2:1–22
206. Boyd DW, Kustin K (1984) Vanadium: a versatile biochemical effector with an elusive biological function. Adv Inorg Biochem 6:311–365
207. Nechay BR (1984) Mechanisms of action of vanadium. Annu Rev Pharmacol Toxicol 24:501–524
208. Degani H, Gochin M, Karlish SJD, Schechter Y (1981) Electron paramagnetic resonance studies and insulin-like effects of vanadium in rat adipocytes. Biochemistry 20:5795–5799
209. Liochev SI, Fridovich I (1990) Vanadate-stimulated oxidation of NAD(P)H in the presence of biological membranes and other sources of O_2^-. Arch Biochem Biophys 279:1–7
210. Fantus IG, Kadota S, Deragon G, et al (1989) Pervanadate [peroxide(s) of vanadate] mimics insulin action in rat adipocytes via activation of the insulin receptor tyrosine kinase. Biochemistry 28:8864–8871
211. Wever R, Kustin K (1990) Vanadium: a biologically relevant element. Adv Inorg Chem 35:81–115
212. Heydorn K (1990) Factors affecting the levels reported for vanadium in human serum. Biol Trace Elem Res 26/27:541–551
213. Myron DR, Givand SH, Nielsen FH (1977) Vanadium content of selected foods as determined by flameless absorption spectroscopy. Agric Food Chem 25:297–300
214. Ishida O, Kihira K, Tsukamoto Y, Marumo F (1989) Improved determination of vanadium in biological fluids by

electrothermal atomic absorption spectrometry. Clin Chem 35:127–130

215. Byrne AR, Versieck J (1990) Vanadium determination at the ultratrace level in biological reference materials and serum by radiochemical neutron activation analysis. Biol Trace Elem Res 26/27:529–540

216. Byrne AR, Kučera J (1991) New data on levels of vanadium in man and his diet. In Momčilović B (ed), Trace elements in man and animals 7. IMI, Zagreb, pp 25.18–25.20

217. Byrne AR, Kosta L (1978) Vanadium in foods and in human body fluids and tissues. Sci Total Environ 10:17–30

218. Myron DR, Zimmerman TJ, Shuler TR, et al (1978) Intake of nickel and vanadium by humans. A survey of selected diets. Am J Clin Nutr 31:527–531

219. Curran GL, Azarnoff DL, Bolinger RE (1959) Effect of cholesterol synthesis inhibition in nomocholesteremic young men. J Clin Invest 38:1251–1261

220. Hansard SL II, Ammerman CB, Henry PR (1982) Vanadium metabolism in sheep. II. Effect of dietary vanadium on performance, vanadium excretion and bone deposition in sheep. J Anim Sci 55:350–356

221. Parker RDR, Sharma RP (1978) Accumulation and depletion of vanadium in selected tissues of rats treated with vanadyl sulfate and sodium orthovanadate. J Environ Pathol Toxicol 2:235–245

222. Roschin AV, Ordzhonikidze EK, Shalganova IV (1980) Vanadium—toxicity, metabolism, carrier state. J Hyg Epidemiol Microbiol Immunol 24:377–383

223. Bogden JD, Higashino H, Lavenhar MA, et al (1982) Balance and tissue distribution of vanadium after short-term ingestion of vanadate. J Nutr 112:2279–2285

224. Wiegmann TB, Day HD, Patak RV (1982) Intestinal absorption and secretion of radioactive vanadium ($^{48}VO_3^-$) in rats and effect of $Al(OH)_3$. J Toxicol Environ Health 10:233–245

225. Patterson BW, Hansard SL II, Ammerman CB, et al (1986) Kinetic model of whole-body vanadium metabolism: studies in sheep. Am J Physiol 251:R325–R332

226. Chasteen ND, Lord EM, Thompson HJ (1986) Vanadium metabolism. Vanadyl (IV) electron paramagnetic resonance spectroscopy of selected tissues in the rat. In Xavier AV (ed), Frontiers in bioinorganic chemistry. VCH Verlagsgesellschaft, Weinhein, pp 133–141

227. Sabbioni E, Marafante E (1978) Metabolic patterns of vanadium in the rat. Bioinorg Chem 9:389–407

228. Hopkins LL Jr, Tilton BE (1966) Metabolism of trace amounts of vanadium 48 in rat organs and liver subcellular particles. Am J Physiol 211:169–172

229. Edel J, Sabbioni E (1989) Vanadium transport across placenta and milk of rats to the fetus and newborn. Biol Trace Elem Res 22:265–275

230. Sabbioni E, Marafante E (1981) Relations between iron and vanadium metabolism: in vivo incorporation of vanadium into iron proteins of the rat. J Toxicol Environ Health 8:419–429

231. Harris WR, Friedman SB, Silberman D (1984) Behavior of vanadate and vanadyl ion in canine blood. J Inorg Biochem 20:157–169

232. E Sabbioni, E Marafante (1981) Progress in research on newer trace elements: the metabolism of vanadium as investigated by nuclear and radiochemical techniques. In McC Howell J, Gawthorne JM, White CL (eds), Trace element metabolism in man and animals (TEMA-4). Australian Academy of Science, Canberra, pp 629–631

233. Hansard SL II, Ammerman CB, Fick KR, Miller SM (1978) Performance and vanadium content of tissues in sheep as influenced by dietary vanadium. J Anim Sci 46:1091–1095

234. Willsky GR (1990) Vanadium in the biosphere. In Chasteen ND (ed), Vanadium in biological systems. Physiology and biochemistry. Kluwer, Dordrecht, Netherlands, pp 1–24

235. Stern A, Yin X, Tsang S-S, et al (1993) Vanadium as a modulator of cellular regulatory cascades and oncogene expression. Biochem Cell Biol 71:103–112

236. Wever R, Krenn BE (1990) Vanadium haloperoxidases. In Chasteen ND (ed), Vanadium in biological systems. Physiology and biochemistry. Kluwer, Dordrecht, Netherlands, pp 81–97

237. van Schijndel JWPM, Vollenbroek EGM, Wever R (1993) The chloroperoxidase from the fungus Curvularia inaequalis; a novel vanadium enzyme. Biochim Biophys Acta 1161:249–256

238. Soedjak HS, Butler A (1991) Mechanism of dioxygen formation catalyzed by vanadium bromoperoxidase from Macrocystis pyrifera and Fucus distichus: steady state kinetic analysis and comparison to the mechanism of V-BrPO from Ascophyllum nodosum. Biochim Biophys Acta 1079:1–7

239. Eady RR (1995) Vanadium nitrogenases of Azotobacter. In Sigel H, Sigel A (eds), Metal ions in biological systems, Vol 31, Vanadium and its role in life. Marcel Dekker, New York, pp 363–405

240. Bayer E (1995) Amavadin, the vanadium compound of Amanitae. In Sigel H, Sigel A (eds), Metal ions in biological systems, Vol 31, Vanadium and its role in life. Marcel Dekker, New York, pp 407–421

241. Frausto da Silva JJR (1989) Vanadium in biology—the case of the Amanita toadstools. Chem Spec Bioavail 1:139–150

242. Anke M, Groppel B, Gruhn K, et al (1989) The essentiality of vanadium for animals. In Anke M, Baumann W, Bräunlich H, et al (eds), 6th International Trace Element Symposium, 1989, Vol 1. Friedrich-Schiller-Universitat, Jena, pp 17–27

243. Uthus EO, Nielsen FH (1990) Effect of vanadium, iodine and their interaction on growth, blood variables, liver trace elments and thyroid status indices in rats. Magnesium Trace Elem 9:219–226

244. Poellot RA, Seaborn CD, Uthus EO (1992) The effect of vanadium deprivation in thyroxine replete-thyroidectomized rats. Proc ND Acad Sci 46:75

245. Nielsen FH (1987) Vanadium. In Mertz W (ed), Trace elements in human and animal nutrition, Vol 1. Academic Press, San Diego, pp 275–300

246. Schroeder HA, Balassa JJ, Tipton IH (1963) Abnormal trace metals in man—vanadium. J Chronic Dis 16:1047–1071

247. Somerville J, Davies B (1962) Effect of vanadium on serum cholesterol. Am Heart J 64:54–56

248. Dimond EG, Caravaca J, Benchimol A (1963) Vanadium. Excretion, toxicity, lipid effect in man. Am J Clin Nutr 12:49–53

249. Proescher F, Seil HA, Stillians AW (1917) A contribution to the action of vanadium with particular reference to syphillis. Am J Syph 1:347–405

250. Angelow L, Anke M, Groppel B, et al (1993) Aluminum: an essential element for goats. In Anke M, Meissner D, Mills CF (eds), Trace elements in man and animals, TEMA 8. Verlag Media Touristik, Gersdorf, pp 699–704

251. Carlisle EM, Curran MJ (1993) Aluminum: an essential element for the chick. In Anke M, Meissner D, Mills CF (eds), Trace elements in man and animals, TEMA 8. Verlag Media Touristik, Gersdorf, pp 695–698

252. Sternweis PC, Gilman AG (1982) Aluminum: a requirement for activation of the regulatory component of adenylate cyclase by fluoride. Proc Natl Acad Sci USA 79:4888–4891

253. Johnson NE, Zierold C, Dunn MA (1991) Aluminum enhances

calmodulin activity. In Momčilovič B (ed), Trace elements in man and animals 7. IMI, Zagreb, pp 17:15–17:16

254. Smith JB (1984) Aluminum ions stimulate DNA synthesis in quiescent cultures of Swiss 3T3 and 3T6 cells. J Cell Physiol 118:298–304

255. Quarles LD, Hartle JE II, Middleton JP, et al (1994) Aluminum-induced DNA synthesis in osteoblasts: mediation by a G-protein coupled cation sensing mechanism. J Cell Biochem 56:106–117

256. Greger JL (1993) Aluminum metabolism. Annu Rev Nutr 13:43–63

257. Anke M, Groppel B, Arnhold W, Langer M (1988) Essentiality of the trace element bromine. In Braetter P, Schramel P (eds), Trace element analytical chemistry in medicine and biology. Walter de Gruyter, Berlin, pp 618–626

258. Anke M, Groppel B, Angelow L, et al (1993) Bromine: an essential element for goats. In Anke M, Meissner D, Mills CF (eds), Trace elements in man and animals, TEMA 8. Verlag Media Touristik, Gersdorf, pp 737–738

259. Huff JW, Bosshardt DK, Miller OP, Barnes RH (1956) A nutritional requirement for bromine. Proc Soc Exp Biol Med 92:216–219

260. Bosshardt DK, Huff JW, Barnes RH (1956) Effect of bromine on chick growth. Proc Soc Exp Biol Med 92:219–221

261. Leach RM Jr, Nesheim MC (1963) Studies on chloride deficiency in chicks. J Nutr 81:193–199

262. Oe PL, Vis RD, Meijer JH, et al (1981) Bromine deficiency and insomnia in patients on dialysis. In McC Howell J, Gawthorne JM, White CL (eds), Trace element metabolism in man and animals, TEMA-4. Australian Academy of Science, Canberra, pp 526–529

263. Nielsen FH (1986) Other elements: Sb, Ba, B, Br, Cs, Ge, Rb, Ag, Sr, Sn, Ti, Zr, Be, Bi, Ga, Au, In, Nb, Sc, Te, Tl, W. In Mertz W (ed), Trace elements in human and animal nutrition, Vol 2. Academic Press, Orlando, FL, pp 415–463

264. Schwarz K, Spallholz JE (1979) The potential essentiality of cadmium. In Bolck F, Anke M, Schneider H-J (eds), Kadmium-Symposium. Friedrich-Schiller Universitat, Jena, pp 188–194

265. Reeves PG, Johnson PE, Rossow KL (1994) Absorption and organ accumulation of cadmium in male rats fed diets containing sunflower kernels [abstract]. FASEB J 8:A196

266. Anke M, Hennig A, Groppel B, et al (1978) The biochemical role of cadmium. In Kirchgessner M (ed), Trace element metabolism in man and animals-3. Tech Univ Munchen, Freising-Weihenstephen, pp 540–548

267. Barham SS, Tarara JE, Enger MD (1985) Cadmium as a transforming growth factor [abstract]. Fed Proc 44:520

268. Kostial K (1986) Cadmium. In Mertz W (ed), Trace elements in human and animal nutrition, Vol 2. Academic Press, Orlando, pp 319–345

269. Schwarz K, Milne DB (1972) Fluorine requirement for growth in the rat. Bioinorg Chem 1:331–338

270. Anke M, Groppel B, Krause U (1991) Fluorine deficiency in goats. In Momčilovič B (ed), Trace elements in man and animals 7. IMI, Zagreb, pp 26:28–26:29

271. Avtsyn AP, Anke M, Zhavoronkov AA, et al (1993) Pathological anatomy of the experimentally-induced fluorine deficiency in she-goats. In Anke M, Meissner D, Mills CF (eds), Trace elements in man and animals, TEMA 8. Verlag Media Touristik, Gersdorf, pp 745–746

272. Messer HH, Armstrong WD, Singer L (1974) Essentiality and function of fluoride. In Hoekstra WG, Suttie JW, Ganther HE, Mertz W (eds), Trace element metabolism in animals-2. University Park Press, Baltimore, pp 425–437

273. Wegner ME, Singer L, Ophaug RH, Magil SG (1976). The

interrelation of fluoride and iron in anemia. Proc Soc Exp Biol Med 153:414–418

274. Jenkins GN (1990) The metabolism and effects of fluoride. In Priest ND, Van De Vyver FL (eds), Trace metals and fluoride in bones and teeth. CRC Press, Boca Raton, FL, pp 141–173

275. Grooten HNA, Ritskes-Hoitinga J, Mathot JNJJ, et al (1991) Dietary fluoride prevents phosphorus-induced nephrocalcinosis in female rats. Biol Trace Elem Res 29:147–155

276. Fransbergen AJ, Lemmens AG, Beynen AC (1991) Dietary fluoride, unlike bromide or iodide, counteracts phosphorus-induced nephrocalcinosis in female rats. Biol Trace Elem Res 31:71–78

277. Sato I, Yuan BD, Nishimura T, Tanaka N (1985) Inhibition of tumor growth and metastasis in association with modification of immune response by novel organic germanium compounds. J Biol Response Mod 4:159–168

278. Suzuki F, Brutkiewicz RR, Pollard RB (1986) Cooperation of lymphokine(s) and macrophages in expression of antitumor activity of carboxyethylgermanium sesquioxide (Ge-132). Anticancer Res 6:177–182

279. Schwarz K (1975) Potential essentiality of lead. Arh Hig Rada Toksikol 26(suppl):13–28

280. Kirchgessner M, Reichlmayr-Lais AM (1981) Lead deficiency and its effects on growth and metabolism. In McC Howell J, Gawthorne JM, White CL (eds), Trace element metabolism in man and animals, TEMA 4. Australian Academy of Science, Canberra, pp 390–393

281. Reichlmayr-Lais AM, Kirchgessner M (1985) Newer research on lead essentiality. In Mills CF, Bremner I, Chesters JK (eds), Trace elements in man and animals, TEMA 5. Commonwealth Agricultural Bureaux, Farnham Royal, pp 283–286

282. Reichlmayr-Lais AM, Kirchgessner M (1991) Lead—an essential trace element. In Momčilovič B (ed), Trace elements in man and animals, 7. IMI, Zagreb, pp 35:1–35:2

283. Kirchgessner M, Plass DL, Reichlmayr-Lais AM (1991) Lead deficiency in swine. In Momčilovič B (ed), Trace elements in man and animals, 7. IMI, Zagreb, pp 11:20–11:21

284. Uthus EO, Nielsen FH (1988) Effects in rats of iron on lead deprivation. Biol Trace Elem Res 16:155–163

285. Müller M, Anke M, Thiel C, Hartmann E (1993) Exposure of adults to lead from food estimated by analysis and calculation—comparison of methods. In Anke M, Meissner D, Mills CF (eds), Trace elements in man and animals, TEMA 8. Verlag Media Touristik, Gersdorf, pp 241–242

286. Anke M, Arnhold W, Groppel B, Krause U (1990) The biological importance of lithium. In Schrauzer GN, Klippel K-F (eds), Lithium in biology and medicine. VCH Publishers, Weinheim, pp 148–167

287. Patt EL, Pickett EE, O'Dell BL (1978) Effect of dietary lithium levels on tissue lithium concentrations, growth rate, and reproduction in the rat. Bioinorg Chem 9:299–310

288. Pickett EE, O'Dell BL (1992) Evidence for dietary essentiality of lithium in the rat. Biol Trace Elem Res 34:299–319

289. Rybak SM, Stockdale FE (1981) Growth effects of lithium chloride in BALB/c 3T3 fibroblasts and Madin-Darby canine kidney epithelial cells. Exp Cell Res 136:263–270

290. Rossetti L, Giaccari A, Klein-Robbenhaar E, Vogel LR (1990) Insulinomimetic properties of trace elements and characterization of their in vivo mode of action. Diabetes 39:1243–1250

291. Schrauzer GN, Shrestha KP (1990) Lithium in drinking water and the incidence of crimes, suicides, and arrests related to drug addictions. Biol Trace Elem Res 25:105–113

292. Schrauzer GN, Shrestha KP, Flores-Arce MF (1992) Lithium in scalp hair of adults, students, and violent criminals. Ef-

fects of supplementation and evidence for interactions of lithium with vitamin B-12 and with other trace elements. Biol Trace Elem Res 34:161–176

293. Anke M, Angelow L, Schmidt A, Gürtler H (1993) Rubidium: an essential element for animal and man? In Anke M, Meissner D, Mills CF (eds), Trace elements in man and animals, TEMA 8. Verlag Media Touristik, Gersdorf, pp 719–723

294. Eisa O, Yudkin J (1989) Mineral elements in unrefined sugar, and rat reproduction. Int J Vitam Nutr Res 59:77–79

295. Angelow L, Anke M (1994) Rubidium in der Nahrungskette. In Anke M, Meissner D, Bergmann H, et al (eds), Defizite und Überschüsse an Mengen-und Spurenelementen in der Ernährung. 14. Arbeitstagung Mengen-und Spurenelemente 1994. Verlag Harald Schubert, Leipzig, pp 285–300

296. Schwarz K, Milne DB, Vinyard E (1970) Growth effects of tin compounds in rats maintained in a trace element-con-trolled environment. Biochem Biophys Res Commun 40:22–29

297. Yokoi K, Kimura M, Itokawa Y (1990) Effect of dietary tin deficiency on growth and mineral status in rats. Biol Trace Elem Res 24:223–231

298. Kappas A, Drummond GS, Simionatto CS, Anderson KE (1984) Control of heme oxygenase and plasma levels of bilirubin by a synthetic heme analogue, Tin-protoporphy-rin. Hepatology 4:336–341

299. Kappas A, Drummond GS (1984) Control of heme and cy-tochrome P-450 metabolism by inorganic metals, organo-metals and synthetic metalloporphyrins. Environ Health Perspect 57:301–306

300. Cardarelli N (1990) Tin and the thymus gland: a review. Thymus 15:223–231

301. Greger JL (1988) Tin and aluminum. In Smith KT (ed), Trace minerals in foods. Marcel Dekker, New York, pp 291–323

Chapter 36

Iodine Deficiency and the Iodine Deficiency Disorders

John B. Stanbury

The only role that iodine plays in the economy of the body is that of an essential component of the thyroid hormones. Thyroid hormone is essential to development. The principal secretion product of the thyroid gland is thyroxine, which contains four iodine atoms. It is largely converted in the periphery to the principal metabolically active species, triiodothyronine, which is identical except for the removal of one iodine atom from the 5′ position on the outer ring.

The thyroid gland removes iodine from the blood, concentrates it, and attaches it to tyrosyl residues in peptide linkage to form mono- and diiodotyrosine, which in turn are formed into thyroxine through linkage of the two benzyl groups through an ether bridge to form the finished hormone. This is stored in the colloid of the thyroid follicles, from whence the hormone is mobilized and secreted as required. The 5′ iodine is removed through action of a deiodinase that is present in many tissues, especially the liver.

The thyroid hormones circulate noncovalently bonded to carrier proteins. Triiodothyronine interacts with the genome through specific receptors. Both hormones are degraded through a complex set of pathways, and the iodine is excreted almost entirely in inorganic form in the urine.

Absorption, Transport, Storage, and Turnover

Iodide in inorganic form is rapidly and almost completely absorbed in the stomach and upper small bowel. Organic forms of iodine are variably degraded in the gut and the released iodide is absorbed, while others may be absorbed intact. About 80% of thyroxine is absorbed without change and the remainder is lost in the feces. The iodinated substances used in visualization of the gall bladder are readily absorbed. Iodate, a form of iodine commonly used in the fortification of salt for the prevention of the iodine deficiency disorders, is rapidly reduced in the gut and the iodide is immediately absorbed. Iodate is also rapidly reduced to iodide in blood.

Absorbed iodide enters a distribution space approximately equal to that of the extracellular fluid volume. It appears in the blood in free and dialyzable form. It is not bound to the proteins of the blood, but is rapidly picked up by the thyroid and kidney. Concentration in the plasma depends on supply and on clearance rates. The kidney clears approximately 30 mL of plasma per minute of iodide, whereas the clearance by the thyroid depends on the history of iodine intake. If iodine supply has been abundant, only about 10% or less of the iodine absorbed by the gut may appear in the thyroid, but with long-standing iodine deficiency the fraction cleared into the thyroid may approach 80% or more. Small amounts of iodide are secreted by the salivary glands and very small amounts appear in the choroid plexus, tears, and sweat. Action of the thyroid in removal of iodide from the blood and synthesis and storage of the thyroid hormones is controlled by the thyrotropic hormone from the pituitary, which in turn is controlled by the level of circulating thyroid hormone. Thus the thyroid system is orchestrated by a set of complex feedback interactions among iodine supply, hormone synthesis and secretion, pituitary secretion of thyrotropin, and secretion of the thyrotropin-releasing hormone from the hypothalamus. Control is not exerted at the level of absorption from the gut or iodide excretion by kidney.[1-5]

Virtually the only storage site of iodide is the thyroid gland, where it appears almost entirely as mono- and diiodotyrosine and thyroxine, with a small component of triiodothyronine. Normally 80% or more is found in the iodotyrosine fraction. Small amounts of iodohistidine have been detected also in the gland. The quantity of iodine in any form in the peripheral tissues is exceedingly small, but that which is present in hormonally active form is critically important. While most tissues respond to thyroxine or triiodothyronine, the brain depends on thyroxine and metabolizes it locally to triiodothyronine.[6]

Large amounts of iodine are stored in the thyroid as hormone or hormone precursors. When iodine supply has been abundant, 10–20 mg of iodine may be present, while with chronic iodine deficiency the supply may be highly variable. Thus if deficiency has been prolonged and unrelieved, the content of the thyroid may be reduced to 200 µg or less, whereas occasional episodes of iodide exposure may enable the deficient thyroid to store large amounts of iodine. The iodine-deficient gland may store large fractions of iodine for several weeks before it finally shuts down. This is the presumed cause of the paradox of a normal or high iodine content of a goiter in a region of iodine deficiency.[7]

The iodide of the blood is turned over rapidly with a rate that is largely governed by the uptake by the thyroid. Under normal circumstances it is cleared from the plasma with a half-time of approximately 10 hours, but this may be reduced if the thyroid is overactive as in thyrotoxicosis or iodine deficiency.

Turnover of the thyroid hormones is relatively slow. The normal half-life of thyroxine is about 7 days, while that of triiodothyronine is about 1.5–3 days.[8]

Physiologic Function

Thyroid hormone has multiple functions as a regulator of cell activity and growth. It crosses the placental barrier very early in human embryonic life to have presently undefined effects before the embryonic thyroid begins to function.[9] It influences neuronal cell growth, migration, and dendritic spine development.[10–12] It also promotes growth and maturation of peripheral tissues, perhaps most obviously visible in skeletal radiographs showing delayed bony development in the hormone-deficient human embryo and in the iodine-deficient sheep model.[13] There is no evidence that iodine per se has any role in growth, development, or physiological function except through the mediation of thyroid hormone.

Postnatal statural growth and bone maturation depend on a normal flow of thyroid hormone. These are retarded when the supply of iodine is low. Thyroid hormone is also principally involved in the metabolic energy flow of most of the cells of the body. The most familiar indicator of this is the basal metabolic rate. A series of characteristic changes occur when iodine deficiency impairs hormone production. These include skin changes, enlargement of the tongue, subcuticular deposits of mucopolysaccharides, hoarsening of the voice, slowness of movements, delayed reflex relaxation times, rises in lipid content of the plasma, and when advanced, to cardiac insufficiency, fluid accumulation in body cavities and pericardial sac, and increased sensitivity to some drugs, such as morphine.

The cellular function of thyroid hormone, mediated through triiodothyronine, is directed to the genome, where it attaches to thyroid response elements that, through a series of interactions at several gene sites, serve to turn on or off the activity of specific genes involved in synthesis of specific messenger ribonucleic acids, which in turn control synthesis or inhibition of particular proteins involved in the function of cells.[14,15]

Deficiency

A deficiency of iodine in animals and man has important consequences to both embryonic and postnatal development.[16] These have been subsumed under the term "iodine deficiency disorders." These disorders are among the most important and prevalent of the diseases of mankind and are highly significant in animal husbandry. Indeed, iodine deficiency is the most prevalent cause of preventable mental retardation in the world.[17] The reason for this prevalence is that iodine is deficient in soils in most parts of the world, and is especially deficient in soils leached by glacial run-off and in flood plains. The prevalence of iodine deficiency in mountain regions has been dramatized in the literature of the field, but some of the most severely depleted areas with the highest prevalence of iodine deficiency disorders are flatlands from which the iodine has long since disappeared through rainfall or sublimation. For examples, the Gangetic plain of northeastern India and the Tacloman Desert of central western China are major sites of severe iodine deficiency disorders. In the latter region, supplementation with iodine in feeds has sharply improved sheep survival and substantially increased economic benefits (DeLong, personal communication).

The thyroid gland of the normal human subject receiving an ample supply of iodine weighs between 15 and 20 g. When iodine is in reduced supply there is a compensatory increase in iodine clearance by the gland mediated by increased secretion of thyrotropin and thyroid growth. If the deficient state continues, growth continues, and this may be readily detected by the experienced examiner; when severe, it may be readily visible, even at a distance. In some cases these growths become grotesque. With continued growth, thyroid follicles may fuse and become encapsulated as thyroid nodules.[18] The significance of a nodular thyroid is that it represents a long period of iodine deficiency. Further, some of these nodules and the paranodular tissue under continuing stimulation and growth become autonomous of pituitary control and may secrete thyroid hormone independent of hormonal needs if sufficient iodine becomes available in the diet or through excessive supplementation.

Goiter may be cosmetically unattractive or unacceptable, may also cause obstruction to trachea and esophagus, and may damage the recurrent laryngeal nerves to cause hoarseness. It may be the site of malignant change, although this is a controversial issue. The surgery that is often performed has its own risks, and after surgery such subjects may become hypothyroid and require replacement medication, which is often unavailable in many regions of the world.

While iodine deficiency alone is a necessary and a sufficient cause for goiter, there may be other dietary factors that accentuate the effects of the deficiency.[19] The most thoroughly researched of these is the thioglycoside linamarin, a constituent of cassava, one of the most widely consumed foods in the developing countries.[20] Many other dietary items also contain goitrogenic substances, among them the commonly consumed millet, sweet potato, various beans, and certain polluting industrial products related to resorcinol, phthalic acid, and others.[19] Goitrogens have also been detected in certain well waters in Colombia. When cassava is insufficiently soaked or not cooked enough, it is hydrolyzed in the gut to release cyanide, which in turn is metabolized to thiocyanate, and the latter inhibits uptake of iodide by the thyroid. High intake of improperly prepared cassava has been implicated as an ancillary factor in the pathogenesis of endemic cretinism, especially the myxedematous type.[21]

It should be emphasized that while the dietary goitrogens may potentiate the impact of iodine deficiency, they do not produce goiter when iodine intake is sufficient.

The fetus, iodine deficiency, and cretinism. The fetus is particularly vulnerable to iodine deficiency, and particularly so if the mother is limited in her own production of thyroid hormone because of iodine deficiency. The impact of the deficiency probably begins in early fetal life, but becomes most apparent during the second trimester.[22] Iodine supplements given early in the second trimester overcome most of the damage, but given later the neonate may be permanently damaged in growth, and especially in neuromuscular and cognitive attainment. Iodine deficiency in both animals and man is accompanied by reduced fertility and increased fetal and perinatal mortality.[23]

"Cretinism" is a term that embraces the most severe forms of damaged persons resulting from iodine deficiency. Two distinct varieties of cretinism have been described, the more common being that with predominantly neurological deficits that are distinctive and include spastic diplegia with sparing of the distal extremities. Another form is seen most frequently in central Zaire, but also elsewhere, with the predominant findings of long and severe hypothyroidism.[24,25] Both forms exhibit severe mental retardation. The latter, or myxedematous form, have all the laboratory and clinical manifestations of profound hypothyroidism, and characteristically but not universally have only modest enlargement of the thyroid. While the differences between the two forms of cretinism are striking, it is generally conceded that they are the extreme ends of a spectrum of the disorders that arise from severe iodine deficiency in mother and child. The reasons for the differences are largely speculative in nature.[26]

The prevalence of cretinism varies widely and is related to the severity and duration of iodine deficiency. It customarily happens in children of mothers who themselves are iodine-deficient and frequently goitrous. The prevalence in some remote communities is remarkably high: rates as high as 12% in the total population have been recorded, which is a remarkable figure in view of the poor survival of a cadre of persons among whom infant and childhood mortality is high.[27]

Cretinism may occur independently of iodine deficiency for congenital or genetic causes. It occurs in about 1 in 4000 live births in iodine-replete regions, and is largely or probably entirely reversible if proper treatment is begun early.[28]

Iodine deficiency and endemic retardation. In addition to overt cretinism, chronic iodine deficiency is responsible for cognitive and neuromuscular impairment in many children at risk. This is evident in school performance and in the results of formalized tests adapted to the local environment where they are administered.[17] This is in part due to permanent impairment of development and in part to the chronically impeded performance resulting from endemic hypothyroidism. The latter is correctable by administration of iodine. Endemic retardation from this cause is doubtless a factor in regional social and economic development. This derives in part from the impaired energy and work productivity of the human population, but also from the lowered fertility and survival of livestock. Iodine is not a factor in growth of agricultural products such as maize, potatoes, beans, and so on.

Requirements for Iodine

The normal human thyroid can tolerate wide fluctuations in iodine supply. Its activity in removing iodine from the blood and secreting hormone is regulated in large part by the pituitary secretion of thyroid-stimulating hormone in such a balance that when there is more iodine than needed, the thyroid signals the pituitary to slow down to maintain balance. Thus, exceedingly large amounts of iodine can be consumed without substantial increase in hormone secretion.

This framework of control does not apply when the thyroid is abnormal, as from chronic thyroiditis, prior surgery, or radioiodine therapy, when the gland is inhibited by iodide in amounts greater than needed for normal metabolism. Neither does it apply, on the other hand, when there are autonomous elements in the gland such as may be induced by chronic iodine insufficiency, when iodide in excess may induce thyrotoxicosis.

The customarily accepted optimal level of iodine in the diet, as reflected in urinary iodide excretion, is about 150 µg per 24 hours. It is usually not practical to collect 24-hour specimens in the field, so that concentration per deciliter or per gram creatinine in the urine is generally accepted as surrogates for 24-hour collections. Creatinine is being abandoned as a poor and unreliable base for calculations.

The recommended daily allowance for iodine was set in 1989 at 40–120 μg for children up to age 10 and 150 μg for adults. These levels apply when there is no iodine deficiency.[29] When iodine deficiency exists, these recommended doses are almost surely too high (see the following discussion).

Salt has become the customary and recommended vehicle for the provision of iodine in countries where there is iodine deficiency. The experience in Switzerland, where there was earlier severe endemic goiter, has been excellent for over half a century[30] in eliminating this nutritional deficiency, as it has in many other countries, including the United States.

Field studies around the world, especially in regions of endemic goiter, have led to the general conclusion that when the mean value of iodine in urine in representative samples is less than 5 μg/dL, the community is at risk of iodine deficiency disorders. When the value is less than 2 μg/dL there is serious risk of children being born with typical cretinism. The upper limit of tolerance when there is no endemic goiter is not well established, but is certainly as high as a milligram per day.

Values for the sodium or potassium salts of iodide or iodate for purposes of prophylaxis or treatment of iodine deficiency are identical when calculated on the basis of iodine content.

Iodine needs may be met by oral or intramuscular iodinated oil. The product of Laboratoire Guerbet in Paris is that most commonly used. It is available as Lipiodol UF for intramuscular use or as an oral preparation, Oriodol. The dosage is presently controversial, and partly depends on the frequency with which the dose may be repeated because of logistical reasons. Generally the recommended dosage is 1 mL by either route, but it would generally be necessary to repeat the oral dose every 6 months.[31–33] One investigation has indicated that 0.2 mL is sufficient for a year.[34]

The oral preparation is degraded in the gut to give a surge in plasma inorganic iodide, which may have consequences as described in a following discussion.

Iodine is widely but sparsely distributed in nature. Generally, the content of foods of both animal and vegetable origin are related to the soil on which they are grown. An exception, of course, is the thyroid of animals, which may contain huge amounts of iodine. Iodine in organic form is also found in certain seaweeds.

Iodine is a constituent of many medications, such as vitamin tablets or capsules. It is often used in bread-making as a dough conditioner, and as iodophors for cleansing milk cans and teats.

Excess and Toxicity

Except for unusual and rare instances of hypersensitivity to iodide, the human subject is remarkably tolerant of high levels of iodine intake. Many patients have used it in gram amounts daily for the treatment of viscous bronchial secretions, as in asthma.

The situation is quite different when there has been substantial iodine deficiency; such persons are at risk for thyrotoxicosis if the iodine intake is increased in the course of preventive programs for iodine deficiency disorders. This phenomenon is known as "jodbasedow," and has been recognized for a century or more. When it occurs it is almost universally in persons in the older age groups who have nodular goiter, but it must be recalled that nodules may be difficult or impossible to palpate. Toxic nodular goiter is subtle in its manifestations and different in many respects from Graves' disease. These patients do not have the ophthalmopathy of Graves' disease, and its symptoms are more subtle in their development. Clinical signs such as weight loss, tachycardia, muscle weakness, or skin warmth may escape detection or be overlooked. Toxic nodular goiter may be dangerous when superimposed on underlying heart disease.

Increases in frequency of hospital admissions for thyrotoxicosis have been observed in the United States, several European countries, Zimbabwe, and Zaire, and are particularly well documented in Tasmania and Austria.[35] Generally, this epidemic has died down after a few years, but has risen again in iodine-deficient regions when the level of iodine in salt has been raised. This observation is consistent with the contention that once autonomy develops in the thyroid, in either nodular or paranodular locations, it never resumes normal control.[18]

The fact of jodbasedow should never be construed as an argument against the iodization of salt; rather, these fortification programs should be continued and extended vigorously so that instances of newly susceptible persons, and especially developmentally damaged children, disappear from the scene. The change that seems indicated is a reduction in the level of iodine in iodized salt and improvement in the packaging and delivery of iodized salt so that what leaves the plant arrives in the kitchen. In the opinion of the present author, iodine in salt at 20–50 ppm is sufficient when there is no iodine deficiency disorder; however, if there is iodine deficiency disorder of any degree, the level should begin at 10 ppm, and not be increased for at least a half decade. Meanwhile, there should be monitoring of hospital or community incidence of iodine deficiency disorders, especially of unexpected abnormalities of cardiac function.

Summary

Iodine is sparsely distributed in the soil and water of the earth. It is an essential component of the thyroid hormones, which are required for normal statural, cognitive, and neuromotor development.

- Iodine is present in small amounts in water and in plants, and in animals surviving on these. The concentration varies widely around the world. Deficiency of iodine in soil and water primarily occurs in mountainous regions, but there is also iodine deficiency in many flood plain areas and areas of glacial run-off.
- The disorders arising from iodine deficiency are among the most common of mankind. These include goiter, cognitive and neuromuscular impairment, increased embryonal and postnatal mortality, deaf-mutism, and impaired fertility. They may be responsible for reduced economic productivity. The most severe form of the iodine deficiency disorders is cretinism, with markedly impaired mentation and neural disorders. All these disorders vanish among newborns when iodine is introduced prophylactically before the third trimester of pregnancy.
- Iodine deficiency of long standing induces thyroid enlargement and nodule formation. Some elements of the thyroid under this circumstance become autonomous of normal control, and this loss of control may be permanent.
- In developed countries, iodine finds its way into the food chain through many paths, including water, milk, bread, and many medications. In a number of countries, including the United States, the intake of iodine is far in excess of minimal needs.
- A most important public health measure is the introduction or continuation of iodine prophylaxis wherever iodine deficiency exists. While the normal thyroid can tolerate large amounts of iodine because of an intact control system, the gland with autonomy may respond to excessive iodine by secreting more thyroid hormone than needed, and thyrotoxicosis may result. This is usually a relatively trivial problem, but when it continues for a long time, or when there are complicating disorders such as heart disease, the health effects may be serious.

References

1. Braverman LE, Utiger RD, eds (1991) The thyroid. Lippincott, Philadelphia
2. Hetzel BS (1989) The story of iodine deficiency: an international challenge to nutrition. Oxford Univeristy Press, Oxford
3. DeGroot LJ, Larsen PR, Refetoff S, Stanbury JB (1984) The thyroid and its diseases, 5th ed. Wiley, New York
4. Hetzel BS, Dunn JT, Stanbury JB, eds (1987) The prevention and control of iodine deficiency disorders. Elsevier, Amsterdam
5. Dunn JT, Pretell EA, Daza CH, Viteri FE, eds (1986) Toward the eradication of endemic goiter, cretinism and iodine deficiency. Pan American Health Organization, Washington, DC
6. Crantz FR, Larsen PR (1980) Rapid thyroxine to 3,5,3' triiodothyronine conversion binding in rat cerebral cortex and cerebellum. J Clin Invest 65:935–938
7. Stanbury JB, Brownell GL, Riggs DS, et al (1954) Endemic goiter: the adaptation of man to iodine deficiency. Harvard University Press, Boston
8. Oppenheimer JH, Schwartz HL, Surks MI (1975) Determination of common parameters of iodothyronine metabolism and distribution in man by noncompartmental analysis. J Clin Endocrinol Metab 41:319–324
9. Morreale de Escobar S, Obregon MJ, Escobar del Rey F (1988) Transfer of thyroid hormones from the mother to the fetus. In Delange F, Fisher DA, Glenoer D (eds), Research in congenital hypothyroidism. Plenum Press, New York, p 15
10. Balazs R, Richter D (1973) Effects of hormones on the biochemical maturation of the brain. In Himivich W (ed), Biochemistry of the developing brain. Dekker, New York, p 253
11. Ferreiro B, Bernal J, Potter BJ (1987) Ontogenesis of thyroid hormone receptor in foetal lambs. Acta Endocrinol (Copenh) 116:205–210
12. Porterfield SP, Hendrich CE (1993) The role of thyroid hormone in prenatal and neonatal neurological development—current perspectives. Endocr Rev 14:94–106
13. Potter BJ, McIntosh GH, Mano MT, et al (1986) The effect of maternal thyroidectomy prior to conception on fetal brain development in sheep. Acta Endocrinol (Copenh) 112:93–99
14. Refetoff S, Weiss RE, Usala SJ (1993) The syndromes of resistance to thyroid hormone. Endocr Rev 14:348–398
15. Stein SA (1994) Molecular and neuroanatomical substrates of motor and cerebral cortex abnormalities in fetal thyroid hormone disorders. In Stanbury JB (ed), The damaged brain of iodine deficiency. Cognizant Communication Corp, New York, p 67
16. Delange F (1994) The disorders induced by iodine deficiency. Thyroid 4:107–128
17. Stanbury JB, ed (1994) The damaged brain of iodine deficiency. Cognizant Communication Corp, New York
18. Studor H, Gerber H (1991) Pathogenesis of nontoxic diffuse and nodular goiter. In Braverman LE, Utiger RD (eds), The thyroid. Lippincott, Philadelphia, p. 1107
19. Gaitan E (1989) Environmental goitrogenesis. CRC Press, Boca Raton, FL
20. Delange F, Iteke FB, Ermans AM, eds (1982) Nutritional factors involved in the goitrogenic action of cassava. International Development Research Centre, Ottawa, Ontario
21. Ermans AM, Moulameko NM, Delange F, Alhuwalia R, eds (1980) Role of cassava in the aetiology of endemic goiter and cretinism. International Development Research Centre, Ottawa, Canada
22. DeLong GR (1987) Neurological involvement in iodine deficiency disorders. In Hetzel BS, Dunn JT, Stanbury JB (eds), The prevention and control of iodine deficiency disorders. Elsevier, Amsterdam, p 49
23. McMichael AJ, Potter JD, Hetzel BS (1980) Iodine deficiency, thyroid function, and reproductive failure. In Stanbury JB, Hetzel BS (eds), Endemic goiter and endemic cretinism. Wiley, New York, p 445

24. Dumont JE, Ermans AM, Bastenie PA (1963) Thyroid function in a goiter endemic. IV. Hypothyroidism and endemic cretinism. J Clin Endocrinol Metab 23:325–335

25. Choufoer JC, van Rhijn M, Querido A (1965) Endemic goiter in western New Guinea. II. Clinical picture, incidence and pathogenesis of endemic cretinism. J Clin Endocrinol Metab 25:385–402

26. Vanderpas J, Bourdoux P, Lagasse R, et al (1984) Endemic infantile hypothyroidism in a severe endemic goiter area of Central Africa. Clin Endocrinol 20:327–340

27. Ibbertson HK, Gluckman PD, Croxson MS, Strang LJW (1974) Goiter and cretinism in the Himalayas: a reassessment. In Dunn JT, Medeiros-Neto GA (eds), Endemic goiter and cretinism: continuing threats to world health. Pan American Health Organization, Washington, DC, p 129

28. Klein AH, Meltzer S, Kenney FH (1972) Improved prognosis in congenital hypothyroidism treated before age 3 months. J Pediatr 81:912–915

29. National Research Council (1989) Recommended dietary allowances, 10th ed. National Academy Press, Washington, DC

30. Burgi HM, Supersaxo Z, Selz B (1990) Iodine deficiency diseases in Switzerland one hundred years after Theodor Kocher's survey: a historical review with some new goitre prevalence data. Acta Endocrinol (Copenh) 123: 577–590

31. Chaouki M, Benmiloud M (1994) Prevention of iodine deficiency disorders by oral administration of lipiodol during pregnancy. Eur J Endocrinol 130:547–551

32. Phillips DIW, Osmond C (1989) Iodine supplementation with oral or intramuscular iodized oil: a two-year follow-up of a comparative trial. Int J Epidemiol 18:907–910

33. Eltom FA, Karlsson AM, Kamal AM, et al (1985) The effectiveness of oral iodized oil in the treatment and prophylaxis of endemic goiter. J Clin Endocrinol Metab 61:1112–1117

34. Tonglet R, Bourdoux P, Minga T, Ermans A-M (1992) Efficacy of low oral doses of iodized oil in the control of iodine deficiency in Zaire. N Engl J Med 326:236–241

35. Connolly RJ, Vidor GI, Stewart JC (1970) Increase in thyrotoxicosis in endemic goitre area after iodation of bread. Lancet i:500–502

Chapter 37

Pregnancy and Lactation

Mary Frances Picciano

Improving maternal and infant health is a national priority in the United States, with measurable health promotion and disease prevention objectives for the year 2000.[1] Many of these objectives are based on nutrition research that offers promise for enhancing reproductive outcome. Evidence is accumulating from assessment of public health nutrition programs and nutrient-specific intervention trials that maternal nutritional modifications can and do produce desirable health advantages that are also cost-effective.[2-4]

Nutritional requirements are increased during pregnancy and lactation for the support of fetal and infant growth and development along with associated changes in maternal structure and metabolism. Total nutrient requirements are not necessarily the sum of those accumulated in maternal tissues and products of pregnancy and lactation and those attributable to maintenance of nonreproducing women, although this approach is often used to derive estimates of recommended nutrient intakes. Maternal metabolism is adjusted through the use of hormones as mediators, redirecting nutrients to highly specialized maternal tissues specific to reproduction (i.e., placenta and mammary gland), and transferring nutrients to the developing fetus or infant. In this chapter, I review the physiological adjustments and nutritional requirements of pregnant and lactating women.

Physiological Adjustments of Pregnancy

Hormonal profile of pregnancy. Figure 1 shows the levels of some key reproductive hormones in plasma of pregnant women. Plasma levels of human chorionic gonadotropin (hCG) begin to increase immediately on implantation of the ovum; the hormone is detectable in urine within 2 weeks of implantation. It reaches a peak at ≈8 weeks of gestation and then declines to a stable plateau until birth. hCG maintains corpus luteum function for 8-10 weeks. Human placental lactogen (also called human chorionic somatomammotropin, or hCS) has a structure that closely resembles growth hormone, and its rate of secretion appears to parallel placental growth and may be used as a measure of placental function. At its peak, the rate of secretion of placental lactogen

is 1-2 g/day, far in excess of the production of any other hormones. Placental lactogen stimulates lipolysis, antagonizes insulin actions, and may be important in maintaining a flow of substrates to the fetus. Placental lactogen along with prolactin from the pituitary may promote mammary gland growth. After delivery, placental lactogen rapidly disappears from the circulation.

The placenta becomes the main source of steroid hormones at weeks 8-10 of gestation. Before that time, progesterone and estrogens are synthesized in the maternal corpus luteum. These hormones play essential roles in maintaining the early uterine environment and development of the placenta. The placenta takes over progesterone production, which increases throughout pregnancy. Progesterone, known as the hormone of pregnancy, stimulates maternal respiration; relaxes smooth muscle, notably in the uterus and gastrointestinal tract; and may act as an immunosuppressant in the placenta, where its levels can be 50 times those in plasma. Progesterone may promote lobular development in the breast and is responsible for the inhibition of milk secretion during pregnancy.

The secretion of estrogens from the placenta is complex. Estradiol (E_2) and estrone (E_1) are synthesized from the precursor dehydroepiandrosterone sulfate (DHEA-S), which is derived from both maternal and fetal blood. The synthesis of estriol (E_3) is from fetal 16-α-hydroxy-dehydroepiandrosterone sulfate (16-OH-DHEA-S). The fetus is unable to synthesize pregnenolone, the precursor of DHEA-S and 16-OH-DHEA-S, and must get the precursor from the placenta. The placental secretion of estrogens also increases manyfold with the progression of pregnancy. The functions of high estrogen levels in pregnancy include stimulation of uterine growth, enhancement of uterine blood flow, and possibly promotion of breast development. Because estrogen precursors originate in the fetus, maternal estrogen levels can be used as a measure of fetal viability.

The increased amount of estrogens during pregnancy also stimulates a population of cells (somatotrophs) in the maternal pituitary to become mammotrophs or prolactin-secreting cells. The increased prolactin secretion probably helps promote mammary development. In addition, the

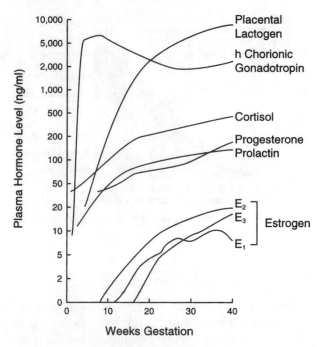

Figure 1. Levels of some reproductive hormones in maternal plasma during pregnancy. E_1, estrone; E_2, estradiol; E_3, estriol.

increased number of pituitary mammotrophs at the end of pregnancy provides the large amounts of prolactin necessary to initiate and maintain lactation.

Another maternally derived hormone that increases in plasma during pregnancy is cortisol. Plasma elevation of cortisol is due both to an increase in its binding protein that is stimulated by estrogens and to an increase in free hormone. Cortisol is antagonistic to insulin and stimulates glucose synthesis from amino acids.

Blood volume and composition. The patterns of change in blood volume, plasma volume, red cell mass, and hematocrit in pregnant women are presented in Figure 2. The increase in blood volume expressed as a percentage of the nonpregnant value is ≈35–40% and is due principally to the expansion of plasma volume by ≈45–50% and of red cell mass by ≈15–20% as measured in the third trimester. Because the expansion of red cell mass is proportionally less than the expansion of plasma, hemoglobin concentration and hematocrit values fall in parallel with red cell volume. Hemoglobin and hematocrit values are at their lowest in the second trimester of pregnancy and rise again in the third trimester.[5] For these reasons, trimester-specific values for hemoglobin and hemotocrit are proposed for screening for anemia in pregnant women.[6]

The concentration of total plasma proteins falls from ≈7 to 6 g/100 mL due largely to a fall in albumin concentration from ≈4 to 2.5 g/100 mL near term. The several globin fractions behave differently. Plasma concentrations of α_1-, α_2-, and β-globulins increase by ≈60, 50,

and 35%, respectively, whereas the γ-globulin fraction decreases by ≈13%.[7] This spectrum of changes in plasma proteins is brought about by estrogens because it can be reproduced by administration of estradiol to nonpregnant women. Plasma levels of most lipid fractions, including triacylglycerol, very-low-density lipoproteins, low-density lipoproteins, and high-density lipoproteins, increase during pregnancy.

Renal function. During pregnancy, renal function is altered dramatically, presumably to facilitate the clearance of nitrogenous and other waste products of fetal and maternal metabolism. The effective renal plasma flow (ERPF), glomerular filtration rate (GFR), and filtration fraction change during pregnancy. The increase in effective renal plasma flow of ≈75% as determined by clearance of *p*-aminohippurate is one of the earliest physiological adjustments of pregnancy. The glomerular filtration rate similarly increases in early pregnancy but not as dramatically (≈50%). Because the glomerular filtration rate is raised in pregnancy by a proportion smaller than the effective renal plasma flow, the filtration fraction (GFR/ERPF) decreases early in pregnancy and returns to nonpregnant values in the third trimester. Changes in renal function are associated with marked urinary excretion of glucose, amino acids, and water-soluble vitamins. Glucose excretion is unrelated to blood glucose concentrations and can increase more than 10-fold. Similarly, plasma profiles of individual

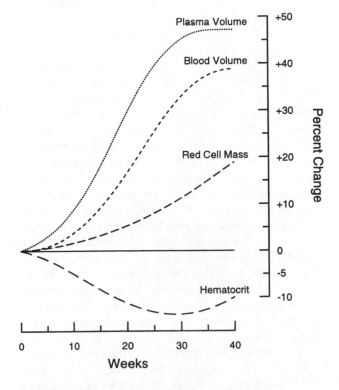

Figure 2. Relative changes in maternal plasma volume, blood volume, red cell mass, and hematocrit during pregnancy.

amino acids are unrelated to excretion patterns that vary from two- to sevenfold, with daily total losses averaging ≈2 g/day. Urinary excretion of folate doubles during pregnancy, and although average excretions of 10–15 µg/day are not large, some women excrete as much as 50 µg/day.[8]

Weight gain and its components. The average weight gained by "healthy primigravidae eating without restriction" is 12.5 kg (27.5 lb).[7] This weight gain represents two major components: 1) the products of conception: fetus, amniotic fluid, and the placenta, and 2) maternal accretion of tissues: expansion of blood and extracellular fluid, enlargement of uterus and mammary glands, and maternal stores (adipose tissue).

Mean values for the components of maternal weight gained during pregnancy are shown in Figure 3. Average weight gain was derived from an analysis of 3868 British primigravidas who experienced no major obstetrical complications such as preeclampsia, prenatal death, or low birth weight. Comparable longitudinal data for multigravidas are not available but Hytten and Leitch[7] suggest that a gain lower by ≈0.9 kg (2 lb) could be expected. For each quarter of pregnancy, the curve presented in Figure 3 corresponds to the following rates of gain (kg/week): 0.065 from 0 to 10 weeks, 0.335 from 10 to 20 weeks, 0.45 from 20 to 30 weeks, and 0.335 from 30 to 40 weeks. In deriving this "normal" curve for weight gain and its components, Hytten and Leitch[7] were careful to point out that wide variations ranging from weight loss to more than twice the average gain are compatible with successful pregnancy. However, the risk of pregnancy complications increases at both extremes.

Low weight gain is associated with increased risk of intrauterine growth retardation and perinatal mortality. High weight gain is associated with high birth weight and secondarily with increased risk of complications related to fetopelvic disproportion. A large body of epidemiologic evidence is now available to show convincingly that maternal prepregnancy weight-for-height is a determinant of fetal growth above and beyond gestational weight gain. At the same gestational weight gain, thin women give birth to infants smaller than those born to heavier women. Because higher birth weights present lower risk for infants, current recommendations for weight gain during pregnancy are higher for thin women than for women of normal weight and lower for short overweight and obese women.[5] These recommendations are summarized in Table 1. They were formulated in recognition of the need to balance the benefits of increased fetal growth against the risks of labor and delivery complications and of postpartum maternal weight retention. The target range for desirable weight gain in each prepregnancy weight-for-height category is that associated with delivery of a full-term infant weighing between 3 and 4 kg.

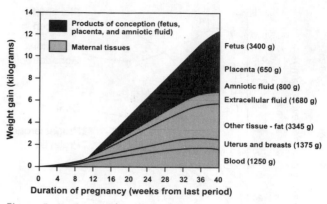

Figure 3. Pattern and components of average weight gain during pregnancy.

Nutritional Needs During Pregnancy

Determination of nutrient needs during pregnancy is complicated because nutrient levels in tissues and fluids available for evaluation and interpretation are normally altered by hormone-induced changes in metabolism, shifts in plasma volume, and changes in renal function and patterns of urinary excretion.[5] Nutrient concentrations in blood and plasma are often decreased because of expanding plasma volume, although total circulating quantities can be greatly increased. Individual profiles vary widely, but in general, water-soluble nutrients and metabolites are present in lower concentrations in pregnant compared with nonpregnant women, whereas fat-soluble nutrients and metabolites are present in similar or higher concentrations. Homeostatic control mechanisms are not well understood and abnormal alterations are ill-defined.

Table 2 presents the recommended dietary allowances for pregnant and lactating women in comparison with those of adult, nonreproducing women.[9] The recommended intakes for pregnant adolescents generally would

Table 1. Recommended total weight gain ranges for pregnant women by prepregnancy body mass index (BMI)

Weight-for-height category	Recommended total gain, kg (lb)
Low (BMI<19.8)	12.5–18 (28–40)
Normal (BMI 19.8–26.0)	11.5–16 (25–35)
High[a] (BMI>26–29)	7–11.5 (15–25)

Young adolescent and African American women should strive for gains at the upper end of the recommended range. Short women (<157 cm, or 62 in) should strive for gains at the lower end of the range. BMI is weight in kg/(height in meters)[2].

[a]The recommended target weight gain for obese women (BMI >29.0) is ≥6 kg (15 lb).

Table 2. Recommended dietary allowances of adult women, pregnant women, and lactating women: percentage increase over allowances of nonreproducing adult women

	Adult women (25–49 years)	Pregnant women (third trimester)	Lactating women[a]	Percentage increase over nonreproducing adult women	
				Pregnancy (%)	Lactation (%)
Energy (kJ)	9205	10,460	11,297	14	23
Protein (g)	50	60	65	20	30
Vitamin A (RE)	800	800	1300	0	33
Vitamin D (µg)	5	10	10	100	100
Vitamin E (TE, mg)	8	10	12	25	50
Vitamin C (mg)	60	70	95	16	58
Thiamin (mg)	1.1	1.5	1.6	35	45
Riboflavin (mg)	1.3	1.6	1.8	23	38
Niacin (NE, mg)	15	17	20	14	33
Vitamin B-6 (mg)	1.6	2.1	2.1	31	31
Folate (µg)	(180)[b]	400	(280)[b]	—	—
Vitamin B-12 (µg)	2	2.2	2.6	10	30
Calcium (mg)	800	1200	1200	50	50
Phosphorus (mg)	800	1200	1200	50	50
Iron (mg)[c]	15	30[c]	15	100	0
Zinc (mg)	12	15	19	25	58
Iodine (µg)	150	175	200	16	33
Selenium (µg)	55	65	75	20	36

[a]During the first 6 months of lactation.
[b]Current recommendation from the U.S. Public Health Service is 400 µg/day for women of childbearing age.
[c]The increased iron requirement for pregnancy cannot always be met by the usual American diet or from body stores; thus, a supplement of 30 mg elemental iron is recommended.

be increased by an amount proportional to the incomplete maternal growth at conception. The percentage increase in estimated energy requirement is small (14%) relative to the estimated increased need for most other nutrients. Accordingly, the nutrient density of foods selected by pregnant women should assume enhanced importance.

Energy. Energy needs during pregnancy are based on estimates of the energy equivalents of protein (21.67 MJ, or 5180 kcal) and fat (152.03 MJ, or 36,337 kcal) in maternal and fetal compartments and the increment in energy expenditure (109.8 MJ, or 26,244 kcal) brought about by these added maternal and fetal tissues.[7] The cumulative total net energy need from these estimates is 283.51 MJ (67,761 kcal). This net energy need was then increased by 10% to account for the cost of converting food energy to metabolizable energy, resulting in a total cumulative energy need for pregnancy of 311.86 MJ (74,537 kcal). In deriving the current recommended dietary allowance, this value was rounded up to ≈335 MJ (80,000 kcal), then divided by the 250 days of pregnancy following the first month to arrive at a recommended intake of 1255 kJ/day (300 kcal/day) (after rounding down from 320 kcal/day) for the 2nd and 3rd trimesters of pregnancy.[9] This value may overestimate energy needs during pregnancy because of energy savings due to decreased activity. Durnin et al.[10,11] estimated that the total energy cost of pregnancy is 288.7–292.88

MJ (69,000–70,000 kcal) and that an increased daily intake of no more than 418–628 MJ (100–150 kcal) is compatible with a normal weight gain. Discrepancies among estimates of energy needs during pregnancy may stem from under- or overestimation of maternal fat stores, alterations in activity patterns and energy efficiency during pregnancy, or both.[12–14]

Protein. Additional protein is needed during pregnancy to cover the estimated 925 g protein deposited in fetal, placental, and maternal tissues. Daily protein increments during each successive quarter of pregnancy are estimated to be 0.6, 1.8, 4.8, and 6.1 g.[7] Assuming that protein utilization is ≈70%, the average pregnant woman would need an additional 8.5 g protein/day at the time of peak requirement. If a coefficient of variability of 15% for pregnancy protein gain is used, the recommended intake is increased by 10 g/day to cover the needs of virtually all healthy women during pregnancy.[9] Women of reproductive age select diets providing mean protein intakes of about 70 g/day, a value well above theoretical need during pregnancy.[15]

Vitamins and minerals. The assessment of vitamin and mineral status during pregnancy is hampered by the general lack of pregnancy-specific laboratory indexes of nutritional evaluation. Plasma concentrations of many vitamins and minerals exhibit a slow, steady decline with the progression of gestation, which is possibly due to hemodilution; however, other vitamins and minerals are unaffected or increased because of pregnancy-induced changes in levels of carrier molecules.[16] When these patterns are unaltered by elevated maternal intakes, it is easy to conclude that they represent a normal physiological adjustment to pregnancy rather than increased needs or deficient intakes. Even when enhanced maternal intake does induce a change in an observed pattern, interpretation of such a change is difficult unless it can be related to some functional consequence.[17] For these reasons, much of our knowledge is based on observational studies and intervention trials in which low or high maternal intakes are associated with adverse or favorable pregnancy outcomes. Available data on vitamin and mineral metabolism and requirements during pregnancy are fragmentary at best, and it is exceedingly difficult to determine consequences of seemingly deficient or excessive intakes in human populations. Yet, animal data show convincingly that maternal vitamin and mineral deficiencies can cause fetal growth retardation and congenital anomalies. Similar associations in humans are rare. I discuss here vitamins and minerals that are likely to be limiting or excessive in the diets of pregnant women—vitamins A, D, and B-6; folate; calcium; iodine; iron; and zinc—and their association with pregnancy outcome.

There is significant placental transport of vitamin A between mother and fetus; low maternal vitamin A status is associated with preterm birth, intrauterine growth retardation, and low birth weight in underprivileged communities.[18,19] Overt vitamin A deficiency is not apparent in the United States; instead, the concern during pregnancy is about excess intake, from either supplements or pharmaceutical preparations of the vitamin A analogue isotretinoin, which is used in the treatment of severe cystic acne. Ingestion of isotretinoin in the early months of pregnancy can produce spontaneous abortions and major congenital defects.[20] The major features of isotretinoin-induced defects include abnormalities of the central nervous system, cardiovascular abnormalities, and facial anomalies. Large doses of vitamin A ($\approx$20,000–50,000 IU) may produce similar defects, but comparable doses of carotenoids do not appear to be toxic. Physicians have been warned about the possible ill effects of high prenatal doses of vitamin A and its analogues.[21] Product labels for isotretinoin now carry warning labels and many prenatal supplements furnish a portion of the vitamin A activity as β-carotene.

The main circulating form of vitamin D in plasma, 25-hydroxycholecalciferol, is responsive to increased maternal intake and falls with maternal deficiency. The biologically active form of the vitamin, 1,25-dihydroxycholecalciferol, circulates in bound and free forms and both are elevated in pregnancy.[22] All forms of vitamin D are transported across the placenta to the fetus. Vitamin D deficiency during pregnancy is associated with several disorders of calcium metabolism in both the mother and her infant, including neonatal hypocalemia and tetany, infant hypoplasia of tooth enamel, and maternal osteomalacia.[23-25] Supplementation of 10 μg (400 IU)/day in affected women lowered the incidence of neonatal hypocalcemia and tetany and maternal osteomalacia, whereas higher amounts (25 μg/d) increased weight and length gains in infants postnatally.[26] The prevalence of vitamin D deficiency is high in pregnant Asian women in England and in pregnant women in other European countries at northern latitudes, where the amount of ultraviolet light reaching the earth's surface is not sufficient for synthesis of vitamin D in the skin during winter months. Under these circumstances, food sources of vitamin D assume great importance. In the United States, vitamin D–fortified milk represents the most significant food source, and its widespread availability and usage undoubtedly account for the lack of similar findings even in the most northern states. However, supplementation with vitamin D should be considered for strict vegetarians and for women who voluntarily restrict their intake of milk.[5] When supplementation is indicated, doses that are known to be safe, 5–10 μg/day, are recommended for pregnant women in the United States.

Compared with nonpregnant women, pregnant women exhibit significantly reduced plasma values for vitamin B-6 and its active metabolite, pyridoxal phosphate (PLP). Additionally, other functional measures of vitamin B-6 status are diminished during pregnancy.[27] The mechanism of placental transport of vitamin B-6 is unknown. The fetus maintains significantly higher circulating levels of PLP than does the mother, a consistent observation that led to the belief that PLP was actively transported from maternal to fetal compartments. Recent evidence suggests that vitamin B-6 is transferred principally as pyridoxine by passive diffusion and that fetal conversion to PLP traps the vitamin in the fetal compartment.[28] High dietary levels of vitamin B-6 (>10 mg/day) are needed to prevent a decrease in plasma PLP and to normalize other functional measures of vitamin B-6 status during pregnancy.[27] Because amounts of vitamin B-6 >10 mg/day cannot be furnished from foods, and raising maternal plasma PLP concentration and other indexes of vitamin B-6 status are without demonstrable improvements in pregnancy outcomes, low levels of PLP are viewed as normal physiological adjustments rather than as evidence of inadequate vitamin B-6 intake. An additional 0.6 mg vitamin B-6 is recommended during pregnancy for a total intake of 2.2 mg/day.[9] Typical vitamin B-6 intakes of pregnant women are consistently lower than the recommended amount.[5] Despite the wide use of large doses (75 mg/d) of vitamin B-6 to treat pregnancy-induced nausea and vomiting, such treatment is only completely effective in severe cases. Supplemental vitamin

B-6 (2.0 mg/day) is recommended for pregnant women at high risk for inadequate intake, i.e., substance abusers, pregnant adolescents, and women bearing twins.[5]

Compromised maternal folate intake or status is associated with several negative pregnancy outcomes including low birth weight, abruptio placentae, and neural tube defects.[29] In developing countries of the world, megaloblastic anemia during pregnancy is a common finding. Blood folate levels (plasma and erythrocytes) normally fall during the course of pregnancy, presumably as the result of expansion of blood volume and increased urinary excretion. Folate absorption is not altered. Fetal blood folate is maintained at a high concentration, often at maternal expense. The placenta is rich in folate-binding proteins that may serve as membrane receptors for uptake, but the mechanism of placental folate transport is not known. Amounts of dietary folate needed during pregnancy are 280, 660, and 470 µg/day in the first, second, and third trimesters, respectively.[29] These requirements are based on estimates of metabolic turnover as measured by urinary excretion of folate catabolites. Folic acid supplementation is associated with increased birth weight and reduced numbers of infants with low birth weights in both developing and developed countries.[30,31] The relationship between neural tube defects and low folate intake was first suspected >30 years ago. There are now no fewer than 10 studies showing that folate intake is an important determinant of risk for neural tube defects. About 2500 infants are born with neural tube defects each year in the United States, and an estimated 1500 fetuses affected by these birth defects are aborted.[4]

Periconceptional folic acid supplementation prevents both the occurrence and recurrence of neural tube defects in most but not all cases.[29] The effective intake is believed to be 400 µg/day. Malformations occur during the first 28 days of pregnancy when most women are unaware that they are pregnant. Typical intakes of U.S. women of reproductive age are only ≈200–250 µg/day, and recommendations to increase folate intakes when pregnancy is planned will not be wholly effective because >50% of U.S. pregnancies are unplanned.[32] The Centers for Disease Control and Prevention recommend that all women capable of becoming pregnant should consume 400 µg folate/day to reduce their risk of having a pregnancy affected with neural tube defects.[4] Strategies to increase folate intake include education to increase awareness of the need to routinely ingest folate-rich foods or daily use of a supplement containing 400 µg folate, both of which are difficult to implement and require long-term compliance to be effective. The Food and Drug Administration has proposed requiring the addition of folate to enriched cereal-grain products.[33] Fortification could enhance folate intakes of women in a continuous and passive manner, but a major concern is that nontargeted

groups will receive high intakes (>1 mg/day). High intakes of folate can mask the hematological signs of vitamin B-12 deficiency and will delay treatment while irreversible neurological damage progresses. The mechanism by which folate prevents neural tube defects is not known. Blood folate concentrations of women with affected pregnancies are not different from those of women with unaffected pregnancies. These and other observations suggest that a genetic defect rather than folate deficiency is responsible and that high folate intakes modify expression of the defect.

Calcium metabolism is dramatically altered during pregnancy via a complex interplay of poorly understood hormonal mechanisms that include increased absorption and retention of calcium, elevated plasma concentrations of 25-hydroxycholecalciferol and 1,25-dihydroxycholecalciferol, and unchanged plasma concentrations of parathyroid hormone.[12,34] Total circulating calcium in pregnant women decreases progressively to 5% below values in nonpregnant women. Values increase again shortly near term.[16,34] Calcium is transported across the placenta against a concentration gradient by an energy-dependent process that may involve vitamin D–dependent calcium-binding protein.[35] The fetus accumulates ≈30 g calcium at a rate of ≈7 mg/day in the first trimester and 110 mg/day in the second trimester, reaching 350 mg/day near term. The recommended calcium intake during pregnancy is 1200 mg/day, which represents an increase of 400 mg/day for women aged >25 years and no increase for younger women. Calcium intakes of pregnant women are often below the recommended level. Low calcium intakes during pregnancy are not associated with poor maternal or fetal outcomes. Whether low calcium intakes negatively affect bone mineral content of young mothers (<25 years) and increase their risk of developing osteoporosis later in life has not been established. Calcium supplementation of 600 mg/day is recommended for women aged <25 years who choose diets low in calcium (≈600 mg/day).[5]

The long-held belief that the fetus is an effective parasite with respect to iron even in the face of maternal deficiency severe enough to produce anemia is now being challenged.[6] The belief was based on data showing that infants born to mothers with iron deficiency were not anemic and had normal iron stores. There is now a large body of evidence linking iron-deficiency anemia in early pregnancy with prematurity and low birth weight, the most common causes of infant morbidity and mortality.[16] Iron-deficiency anemia is also associated with inadequate weight gain during pregnancy. Data from NHANES III indicate that 4–10% of women of reproductive age in the United States have iron-deficiency anemia. National prevalence data on iron-deficiency anemia in pregnant women are not available; however, data are available on low-income women from the Pregnancy Nutrition Surveillance of the Centers for Disease Control and Prevention. These data show prevalences of iron-deficiency anemia of 10, 14, and 33% in the first, second, and third trimesters of pregnancy, respectively. Surveillance data further indicate that the high prevalence of maternal iron-deficiency anemia in low-income populations has remained stable from 1979 to 1990.[36]

The total iron cost of pregnancy is estimated at 1040 mg, of which 200 mg are retained by the woman when blood volume decreases after delivery and 840 mg are permanently lost.[9] Iron is transferred to the fetus ($\approx$300 mg) and used for the formation of the placenta (50–75 mg), expansion of red cell mass ($\approx$450 mg), and blood loss during delivery ($\approx$200 mg). Hemoglobin concentration declines during pregnancy along with serum iron, percentage saturation of transferrin, and serum ferritin. Although these decreases reflect hemodilution to a large extent, transferrin levels actually increase from mean nonpregnant values of 300 μg/100 mL to 500 μg/100 mL in the last trimester of pregnancy, perhaps to facilitate iron transfer to the fetus. The transport of iron across the human placenta is accomplished via specific transferrin-binding receptors and possibly micropinocytosis of the iron-transferrin complex.[12] Enhanced intestinal iron absorption (two- to threefold) is an important physiological adjustment that assists pregnant women in meeting the requirement for absorbed iron, which is estimated to be $\approx$3 mg/day. To preserve maternal stores and to prevent the development of iron deficiency, the recommended iron intake during pregnancy is increased by 15 mg to a total of 30 mg/day.[9] This level cannot normally be obtained from foods, and a supplement providing 30 mg iron/day (beginning after 12 weeks of pregnancy) is recommended.[5] The routine use of iron supplements during pregnancy, however, is not universally endorsed, because both high and low hemoglobin values are associated with adverse pregnancy outcomes (premature birth and low birth weight). High levels of hemoglobin probably reflect an unphysiologically low expansion of plasma volume and not iron status.

Maternal iodine deficiency leading to fetal hypothyroidism results in cretinism, for which severe mental retardation is the hallmark feature.[3] Thyroid hormones are critical for normal brain development and maturation. Manifestation of other features of cretinism (deaf-mutism, short stature, and spasticity) depends on the stage of pregnancy when hypothyroidism develops. When it develops late in pregnancy, the neurological damage is not as severe compared with when it exists early in pregnancy. Cretinism is prevented by correcting maternal iodine deficiency before or during the first 3 months of pregnancy. The World Health Organization estimates that 20 million people worldwide have brain damage due to maternal iodine deficiency that could be prevented by iodine supplementation.[37] The recommended iodine intake is 175 μg/day during pregnancy.[9] The mean intake of U.S. women of childbearing age is $\approx$170 μg/day, excluding iodine from iodized salt.[5]

Animal studies provide a wealth of information concerning the importance of adequate maternal zinc intake for achieving normal fetal growth and preventing malformations.[38] Human studies on the role of maternal zinc status as a mediator of pregnancy outcome have produced mixed results.[39] Of 41 investigations from various parts of the world, the association between infant birth weight and maternal zinc status as assessed from laboratory or dietary measures was positive in roughly half of the studies, whereas in the remainder no relationship was found.[38] Similarly, results of nine intervention trials with maternal zinc supplementation of 4.6–45 mg/day are inconclusive. The reasons for the conflicting data from human studies are unknown but may include small sample size, variable conditions among studies, and the lack of sensitive and specific laboratory measures of zinc status. In the most recent trial, Goldenberg et al.[40] enrolled U.S. low-income women at high risk for low infant birth weight who were selected on the basis of low plasma zinc concentrations. The provision of 25 mg zinc/day elevated plasma zinc and significantly increased infant birth weight, head circumference, arm and femur lengths, and subscapular skinfold thickness.

Plasma zinc, 75% of which is bound to albumin and 25% to α_2-macroglobulin, begins to decline in concentration early in pregnancy and continues to decline until term, when it is $\approx$35% below concentrations in nonpregnant women. There are discrepancies concerning the rate of decline, which may reflect varying zinc status among women studied. The plasma ratio of fetal to maternal zinc is $\approx$1.5. Placental zinc transfer to the fetus, presumably via an active transport process, reaches a rate of $\approx$0.6–0.8 mg/day in the third trimester. The total zinc retained in maternal and fetal tissues during pregnancy is estimated to be 100 mg, of which $\approx$53 mg is contained in the fetus.[41,42] An additional 3 mg zinc, for a total of 15 mg/day, is recommended to cover the increased need during pregnancy, assuming 20% absorption to allow for poor bioavailability of dietary zinc.[9] Typical zinc intakes of U.S. pregnant women are 9–11 mg/day and intakes of vegetarians are usually much lower.[38] Pregnant women are reported to be in positive zinc balance when consuming diets containing 9 mg/day;[43,44] yet the women studied by Goldenberg et al.,[40] a population that displayed improved reproductive performance with zinc supplementation, had customary intakes of 13 mg/day. Currently, zinc supplementation (15 mg/day) is recommended for pregnant women who ordinarily consume an inadequate diet or who are at great risk for poor reproductive outcomes, i.e., heavy smokers, drug abusers, and women carrying multiple fetuses. Because therapeutic doses of iron (>30 mg/day) may interfere with zinc absorption, zinc supplementation (15 mg/day) also is recommended for women being treated for iron-deficiency anemia during pregnancy.[5]

Nutrition-related Problems During Pregnancy

Diabetes. Regulation of maternal plasma glucose is of utmost importance for successful pregnancy outcome in women with diabetes mellitus and in those with gestational diabetes. When maternal plasma glucose is high, it is similarly high in the fetus and stimulates fetal insulin secretion and increases the need for oxygen to metabolize the glucose load. Elevated blood glucose during the first 6–8 weeks of pregnancy, as in mothers with diabetes mellitus, is associated with a 4 to 10 times greater risk of congenital malformations. Increased blood glucose later in pregnancy is associated with macrosomia (infants weighing >4000 g), infant hypoglycemia, perinatal mortality, and prematurity. High fetal insulin acts as a growth factor resulting in macrosomia. The relative hypoxia produced by enhanced glucose oxidation stimulates erythoropoietin secretion, which in turn increases red blood cell mass leading to polycythemia and hyperbilirubinemia. Recently, it has become clear that these effects (including congenital anomalies) can be prevented if plasma glucose is aggressively controlled throughout pregnancy with diet and insulin therapy. Oral hypoglycemia drugs are contraindicated during pregnancy. All pregnant women should be screened for gestational diabetes between 24 and 28 weeks of pregnancy, because selective screening has proved inadequate.[45]

Pregnancy-induced hypertension. Previously termed "toxemia," pregnancy-induced hypertension includes preeclampsia (hypertension with proteinuria, edema, or both in a previously normotensive woman) and eclampsia (the development of grand mal seizure in preeclampsia). The causes of pregnancy-induced hypertension are unknown, but many nutritional factors are implicated, including maternal obesity, high intake of sodium, and inadequate intakes of vitamin B-6, zinc, calcium, magnesium, and protein. Maternal obesity does place a woman at increased risk for pregnancy-induced hypertension, but salt intake is not related to the development of this disorder. Salt restriction, use of diuretics, and restricting weight gain are no longer recommended as prophylactic measures, because they are ineffective. Data linking other nutrients to pregnancy-induced hypertension are inconclusive.

Alcohol. Each year in the United States, ≈1200 infants are born with fetal alcohol syndrome, a pattern of malformations including prenatal and postnatal growth retardation, central nervous system abnormalities, facial anomalies, and increased incidence of other birth defects.[46] The incidence of fetal alcohol syndrome

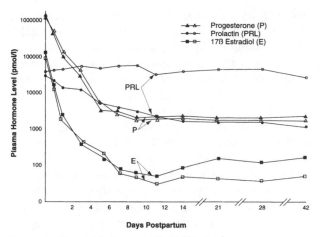

Figure 4. Changes in hormonal profiles in the postpartum period. Levels of estrogens and progesterone fall markedly in both lactating and nonlactating women. Prolactin remains elevated In lactating women.

is 10% in women consuming 1.5–8 drinks/week and 30–40% in women consuming >8 drinks/week. A standard drink is defined as 355 mL (12 oz) beer, 148 mL (5 oz) wine, or 44 mL (1.5 oz) 80-proof distilled spirits, each containing ≈17 g (0.6 oz) absolute alcohol. The U.S. Surgeon General recommends that pregnant women abstain completely from alcohol. Occasional small doses of alcohol but not binge drinking are viewed as safe during pregnancy by some professional groups, but the safest option is complete abstinence.

Caffeine. The Food and Drug Administration recommends that pregnant women limit their coffee intake or, if possible, avoid coffee altogether because of the teratogenic effects of caffeine in animals. In humans, coffee and caffeine do not appear to be teratogenic, but high levels (>300 mg/day) may reduce birth weights.[47] Pregnant women are advised to limit their caffeine consumption to <300 mg/day. Typical caffeine sources and contents include brewed coffee (125 mg in 237 mL, or 8 ounces), instant coffee (90 mg), tea (70 mg), cocoa or hot chocolate (25 mg), and cola drinks (50 mg).[48]

Endocrine Regulation of Lactation

The establishment and maintenance of human lactation are under the influence of complex neuroendocrine control mechanisms.[49] Immediately after parturition, the withdrawal of estrogens and progesterone in the presence of sustained, elevated levels of prolactin (Figure 4) results in the onset of milk secretion (lactogenesis). For milk secretion to occur, the breasts must have undergone appropriate growth and development that began during puberty and was completed during pregnancy. Infant suckling is not required for initiation of lactogenesis, but lactation cannot be maintained unless the infant is put to the breast by 3 or 4 days. For the first 3–5 days postpartum the mammary secretion is termed "colostrum." This thick straw-colored fluid is rich in sodium, chloride, and immune factors (i.e., lactoferrin and secretory immunoglobulin A) but low in lactose and total protein. The concentration of lactose increases and that of sodium and chloride decrease as secretory activity is enhanced and tight junctions between alveolar (mammary epithelial) cells close. By 10 days postpartum, the milk has assumed the characteristics of mature milk.

Once lactation is established, maintenance of milk production (galactopoiesis) is dependent on prolactin. In response to suckling, prolactin is released to the circulation from mammotrophs in the anterior pituitary. Prolactin release via suckling is mediated by a transient decline in the secretion of dopamine from the hypothalamus, which normally inhibits prolactin secretion. Galactopoiesis continues as long as the infant continues to suckle more than once a day. The daily milk volume transferred to the infant increases from ≈50 mL on day 1, to 500 mL by day 5, to ≈650 mL by 1 month, and to 750 mL at 3 months of lactation. In most women, there is a capacity to secrete considerably more milk than is needed by a single infant. Milk secretion is a continuous process, but the amount produced is mainly regulated by infant demand. Suckling also initiates a neuroendocrine response essential for milk removal from the gland. Suckling causes neural impulses to reach the hypothalamus that trigger oxytocin release from the posterior pituitary. Oxytocin circulates to the mammary galnd, where it causes contraction of myoepithelial cells that surround mammary alveoli and ducts, forcing milk into ducts and sinuses close to the nipple so that it can be removed by the suckling infant. This response is termed "milk ejection" or "let-down" and can be initiated by the mere sight of the infant or by hearing the infant cry. Let-down can also be inhibited by emotional distress. Continuation of lactation and associated hyperprolactinemia inhibit ovarian activity by suppressing the pulsatile release of luteinizing hormone and by interfering with the secretion of gonadotropin-releasing hormone. This provides 98% protection from pregnancy during the first 6 months of lactation if the mother is breast-feeding only and remains amenorrheic.[50] In the absence of suckling or milk removal, milk production ceases within 24–48 hours.

Nutritional Needs During Lactation

The nutritive demands of lactation are considerably greater than those of pregnancy. In the first 4–6 months of the postpartum period, an infant doubles his or her birth weight accumulated during the 9 months of pregnancy. The milk secreted in 4 months represents an amount of energy roughly equivalent to the total energy cost of pregnancy. However, some of the energy and many of the nutrients stored during pregnancy are available to support milk production.

The recommended intakes for energy and specific nutrients during lactation are summarized in Table 2. Most of these recommended intakes are based on our knowledge of the amount of milk produced during lactation, its energy and nutrient contents, and the amounts of maternal energy and nutrient reserves. Recommended intakes during lactation are based on even less quantitative data than recommendations during pregnancy. Lactation is viewed as successful when the fully breast-fed infant is growing well and maintaining appropriate biochemical indexes of nutritional status. The quantity of milk consumed by the infant and the nutrient composition of human milk under these circumstances are often used as proxies to assess maternal nutritional adequacy during lactation. In very few studies have specific measures of nutritional status been applied to the lactating mother.

Human milk feeding is adequate as the sole source of nutrition for the first 4–6 months of life. Whether human milk feeding alone can provide sufficient nutrients after this period is a matter of controversy. Analysis of human milk reveals considerable variation in nutrient content, not only between different women but also in the same woman at different times. Amounts of some nutrients can vary with the time of day, in addition to longer-term variations. Also, the milk secreted first in anyone nursing, known as "foremilk," often differs from the "hindmilk" secreted at the end of nursing. These wide variance patterns are nonetheless compatible with successful lactation. The reader is referred to *The Handbook of Milk Composition* for complete data on human milk composition and factors capable of altering it.[51] Human milk not only provides nutrients in highly bioavailable forms, it also furnishes several important bioactive components including enzymes, hormones, growth factors, host-resistant factors, immune-regulating substances, and anti-inflammatory agents. The role of these bioactive components is just beginning to be explored.

Available information on nutrients whose abundance in milk may be affected by maternal nutrition is summarized in Table 3. Also identified are those nutrients that have been associated with recognizable deficiencies in breast-fed infants. The Subcommittee on Nutrition During Lactation of the Committee on Nutritional Status During Pregnancy and Lactation[52] reviewed the literature concerning the effects of maternal nutrition on the composition of human milk; its findings are summarized as follows:

1. Even if the usual dietary intake of a macronutrient is less than that recommended in the *Recommended Dietary Allowances*,[9] there will be little or no effect on the total amount of that nutrient in the milk. However,

the proportions of the different fatty acids in human milk vary with maternal dietary intake.

2. The concentrations of major minerals (calcium, phosphorus, magnesium, sodium, and potassium) in human milk are not affected by diet. Maternal intakes of selenium and iodine are positively related to con-

Table 3. Possible influences of maternal intake on the nutrient composition of human milk and nutrients for which clinical deficiency is recognizable in breast-fed infants

Nutrient or nutrient class	Effects of maternal intake on milk composition[a]	Recognizable nutritional deficiency in breast-fed infants
Macronutrients		
Proteins	+	Unknown[b]
Lipids	+[c]	Unknown
Lactose	o	Unknown
Minerals		
Calcium	o	Unknown
Phosphorus	o	Unknown
Magnesium	o	Unknown
Sodium	o	Unknown
Potassium	o	Unknown
Chlorine	o	Unknown
Iron	o	Yes[d]
Copper	o	Unknown
Zinc	+,o	Unknown
Manganese	+	Unknown
Selenium	+	Unknown
Iodine	+	Yes
Fluoride	−	Unknown
Vitamins		Yes
Vitamin C	+	Yes
Thiamin	+	Unknown
Riboflavin	+	Unknown
Niacin	+	Yes
Pantothenic acid	+	Yes
Vitamin B-6	+	Yes
Biotin	+	Yes
Folate	+	Yes
Vitamin B-12	+	Yes
Vitamin A	+	Yes
Vitamin D	+	Yes
Vitamin E	+	Yes
Vitamin K	+	Yes[e]

[a]"+" denotes a positive effect of intake on nutrient content of milk. The magnitude of the effect varies widely among nutrients; "o" denotes no known effect of intake on nutrient content of milk; "−" denotes a negative effect.

[b]Evidence is not sufficiently conclusive to categorize as "no."

[c]Effect appears to be on type of fatty acids present but not on total content of triacylglycerol or cholesterol in the milk.

[d]Deficiency is not related to maternal intake.

[e]Maternal intake is not the primary determinant of infant vitamin K status.

centrations of these minerals in human milk, but there is no convincing evidence that the concentrations of other trace elements in human milk are affected by maternal diet.

3. The vitamin content of human milk is dependent on the mother's current vitamin intake and her vitamin stores, but the strength of the relationship varies with the vitamin. Chronically low maternal intakes of vitamins may result in milk that contains low amounts of these essential nutrients.

4. The content of at least some nutrients in human milk may be maintained at a satisfactory level at the expense of maternal stores. This applies particularly to folate and calcium.

5. Increasing the mother's intake of a nutrient to levels above the recommended dietary amount ordinarily does not result in unusually high levels of the nutrient in her milk; exceptions are vitamin B-6, iodine, and selenium. Studies have not been conducted to evaluate the possibility that high levels of nutrients in milk are toxic to the infant.

6. Some studies suggest that poor maternal nutrition is associated with decreased concentrations of certain host resistance factors in human milk, whereas other studies do not suggest this association.

The additional energy required to sustain lactation is proportional to the amount of milk produced. The average energy content of human milk is 280–293 kJ (67–70 kcal)/100 mL, and the energy efficiency of milk synthesis by the mother is assumed to be 80% (range of estimates, 76–94%). Thus, it is estimated that 356 kJ (85 kcal) is needed for each 100 mL milk produced.[9] Average milk secretion is $\approx$750 mL/day during the first 6 months of lactation and 600 mL/day in the second 6 months. Fat stores accumulated during pregnancy can theoretically provide 418–837 kJ/day (100–200 kcal/day). The recommended intake is an additional 2092 kJ (500 kcal) throughout lactation. Women with adequate energy reserves can apparently maintain successful lactation even with seemingly low energy intakes. Lactating women typically lose $\approx$0.5–1 kg/month, but some maintain weight and others gain weight. Lactating women are advised not to lose more than 2 kg/month.[52]

As is the case during pregnancy, nutrient density of the maternal diet assumes great importance during lactation because the estimated increase in energy needs is less than estimated increases in needs for other nutrients. At energy intakes less than recommended (11.30 MJ/day, or 2700 kcal/day), maternal intakes of calcium, magnesium, zinc, vitamin B-6, and folate are likely to be correspondingly low. The extent to which low intakes of these and other nutrients affect the success of lactation and long-term maternal and infant health has not been examined except when a distinct nutritional deficiency is evident in the nursing infant, for example, in vitamins D and B-12. A supplement of vitamin D (10 µg/day) is recommended for women who avoid milk and other foods fortified with vitamin D. Similarly, a supplement of vitamin B-12 (2.6 µg/day) is recommended for lactating women who are complete vegetarians.[52]

Acknowledgment. I express gratitude to M. C. Neville from the University of Colorado School of Medicine for providing resource materials on the physiology of human pregnancy and lactation that were used in the preparation of this chapter.

References

1. National Center for Health Statistics (1993) Health United States, 1992. Public Health Service, Hyattsville, MD
2. Rush D (1988) The national WIC evaluation: evaluation of the special supplemental food program for women, infants and children. Am J Clin Nutr 48:389–519
3. Hetzel BS, Dunn JT (1989) The iodine deficiency disorders: their nature and prevention. Annu Rev Nutr 9:21–38
4. Centers for Disease Control (1992) Recommendations for the use of folic acid to reduce the number of cases of spina bifida and other neural tube defects. MMWR 41:1–7
5. Institute of Medicine/Subcommittee on Nutritional Status and Weight Gain During Pregnancy (1990) Nutrition during pregnancy. National Academy Press, Washington, DC
6. Institute of Medicine, Earl R, Woteki CE, eds (1993) Iron deficiency anemia: recommended guidelines for the prevention, detection, and management among U.S. children and women of childbearing age. National Academy Press, Washington, DC.
7. Hytten FE, Leitch I (1971) The physiology of human pregnancy, 2nd ed. Blackwell Scientific Publications, Oxford, United Kingdom
8. Landon MJ, Hytten FE (1971) The excretion of folate in pregnancy. J Obstet Gynaecol Br Commonw 78:769–775
9. National Research Council (1989) Recommended dietary allowances, 10th ed. National Academy Press, Washington, DC
10. Durnin JVGA (1991) Energy requirements of pregnancy. Acta Paediatr Scand 373(Suppl):33–42
11. Durnin JVGA, McKillop FM, Grant S, et al (1987) Energy requirements of pregnancy in Scotland. Lancet 2:895–896
12. Rosso P (1990) Nutrition and metabolism in pregnancy: mother and fetus. Oxford University Press, New York
13. Forsum E, Sadurskis A, Wager J (1988) Resting metabolic rate and body composition of healthy Swedish women during pregnancy. Am J Clin Nutr 47:942–947
14. Van Raaij JMA, Schouk CM, Vermaat-Viedema SH, et al (1989) Body fat mass and basal metabolic rate in Dutch women before, during and after pregnancy: a reappraisal of energy cost of pregnancy. Am J Clin Nutr 49:765–772
15. McDowell MA, Briefel RR, Alaimo K, et al (1994) Energy and macronutrient intakes of persons ages 2 months and over in the United States: NHANES III, phase 1, 1988–91. Advance Data from Vitae and Health Statistics, no 255. National Center for Health Statistics, Hyattsville, MD
16. Institute of Medicine, Committee on Nutrition of the Mother and Preschool Child (1978) Laboratory indices of nutritional status in pregnancy. National Academy of Sciences, Washington, DC
17. King JC, Bronstein MN, Fitch WL, et al (1987) Nutrient utilization during pregnancy. World Rev Nutr Diet 52:71–142
18. Donoghue S, Richardson DW, Sklan D, et al (1985) Placental transport of retinal in ewes fed high intakes of vitamin A. J Nutr 115:1562–1571
19. Shah RS, Rajalakshmi R (1984) Vitamin A: status of the newborn in relation to gestational age, body weight, and maternal nutritional status. Am J Clin Nutr 40:794–800
20. Life Science Research Office, Federation of American Societies for Experimental Biology (1989) Nutritional monitoring in the United States—an update report on nutrition monitoring. US Government Printing Office, Washington, DC
21. Teratology Society Position Paper (1987) Recommendations for vitamin A use during pregnancy. Teratology 35:269–275
22. Paulson SK, DeLuca HF (1986) Vitamin D metabolism during pregnancy. Bone 7:331–336
23. Paunier L, Lacourt G, Pilloud P, et al (1978) 25-Hydroxyvitamin D and calcium levels in maternal, cord and infant serum in relation to maternal vitamin D intake. Helv Paediatr Acta 33:95–103
24. Purves RJ, Barrie WJ, Mackay GS, et al (1973) Enamel hypoplasia of the teeth associated with neonatal tetany: a manifestation of maternal vitamin D deficiency. Lancet 2:811–814
25. Brooke OG, Brown IRF, Bone CDM, et al (1980) Vitamin D supplements in pregnant Asian women: effects on calcium status and fetal growth. Br Med J 280:751–754
26. Brooke OG, Butters F, Wood C (1981) Intrauterine vitamin D nutrition and postnatal growth in Asian infants. Br Med J 283:1024
27. Smolen A (1995) Vitamin B-6 metabolism and the maternal-fetal relationship. In Raiten DJ (ed), Vitamin B-6 metabolism in pregnancy, lactation, and infancy. CRC Press, Boca Raton, FL, pp 93–108
28. Schenker S, Johnson RF, Mahuren JD, et al (1992) Human placental vitamin B-6 (pyridoxal) transport: normal characteristics and effects of ethanol. Am J Physiol 262:966–974
29. Bailey L, ed (1995) Folate in health and disease. Marcel Dekker, New York
30. Iyengar L, Rajalakshmi K (1975) Effect of folic acid supplement on birth weight of infants. Am J Obstet Gynecol 122:332–336
31. Goldenberg RL, Tamura T, Cliver SP, et al (1992) Serum folate and fetal growth retardation: a matter of compliance? Obstet Gynecol 79:719–722
32. Alaimo K, McDowell MA, Briefel RR, et al (1994) Daily intakes of vitamins, minerals, and fiber of persons ages 2 months and over in the United States: NHANES III, phase 1, 1988–91. Advance Data from Vital and Health Statistics, no 258. National Center for Health Statistics, Hyattsville, MD
33. Food and Drug Administration (1993) Proposed rule. Food standards: amendments of the standards of identity for enriched grain products to require addition of folic acid. Fed Register 58:53305–53312
34. Cross NA, Hillman LS, Allen SH, et al (1995) Calcium homeostasis and bone metabolism during pregnancy, lactation, and postweaning: a longitudinal study. Am J Clin Nutr 61:514–523
35. Lester GE (1986) Cholecalciferol and placental calcium transport. Fed Proc 45:2524–2527
36. Kim I, Hungerford R, Yip SA, et al (1992) Pregnancy nutrition surveillance system—United States, 1979–1990. MMWR 41:26–42
37. Xue-Yi C, Xin-Min J, Zhi-Hong D, et al (1994) Timing of vulnerability of the brain to iodine deficiency in endemic cretinism. N Engl J Med 331:1739–1744

38. Apgar J (1992) Zinc and reproduction: an update. J Nutr Biochem 3:266–278

39. Tamura T, Goldenberg RL (1995) Zinc nutriture and pregnancy outcome. Nutr Res 16:139–181

40. Goldenberg RL, Tamura T, Neggers N, et al (1995) The effect of zinc supplementation on pregnancy outcome. JAMA 274:463–468

41. Swanson CA, King JC (1987) Zinc and pregnancy outcome. Am J Clin Nutr 46:763–771

42. Widdowson EM, Spray CM (1951) Chemical development in utero. Arch Dis Child 26:205–214

43. Topper LJ, Oliva JT, Ritchey SF (1985) Zinc and copper retention during pregnancy: the adequacy of prenatal diets with and without dietary supplementation. Am J Clin Nutr 41:1184–1192

44. Campbell DM (1988) Trace element needs in human pregnancy. Proc Nutr Soc 47:45–55

45. American Diabetes Association (1991) Position statement: gestational diabetes mellitus. Diabetes Care 14:5–6

46. Lewis DD, Woods SE (1994) Fetal alcohol syndrome. Am Fam Physician 50:1025–1032

47. Nehlig A, Debry G (1994) Consequences on the newborn of chronic maternal consumption of coffee during gestation and lactation: a review. J Am Coll Nutr 13:6–21

48. Fenster L, Eskenaz B, Windham G, et al (1991) Caffeine consumption during pregnancy and fetal growth. Am J Public Health 81:458–461

49. Picciano MF, Lönnerdal B, eds (1992) Mechanisms regulating lactation and infant nutrient utilization. Wiley-Liss, New York

50. Kennedy KI, Rivera R, McNeilly AS (1989) Consensus statement on the use of breastfeeding as a family planning method. Contraception 39:477–496

51. Jensen RG (1995) Handbook of milk composition. Academic Press, San Diego

52. Institute of Medicine, Subcommittee on Nutrition During Lactation (1991) Nutrition during lactation. National Academy Press, Washington, DC

Chapter 38

Nutritional Requirements During Infancy

William C. Heird

During the first year of life, a normal infant triples its weight and doubles its length. At the same time, organ function and body composition show dramatic developmental changes. These rapid rates of growth and development impose unique nutritional needs upon the already relatively high maintenance requirements of infants. In addition, the young infant's lack of teeth and immature digestive and metabolic processes mandate availability of easily digestible products to provide the special nutrient needs. Questions also have been raised about the impact of early diet on later development and health.

Despite the unique nutritional requirements of infancy, recommended dietary allowances (RDAs) for most nutrients have been established. The most recent recommendations[1] for both the 0–6-month-old and the 6–12-month-old infant are summarized in Table 1. These recommendations as well as other aspects of nutrition for each age group are discussed briefly as are the issues of breast versus formula feeding and using formula versus bovine milk after 6 months of age.

Requirements and Recommended Allowances

At the outset, it is important to distinguish between requirement and recommended allowance. The former is the amount of a specific nutrient required to achieve some physiological end point. In infants, requirement is usually equated to the amount necessary to maintain a satisfactory rate of growth and development or prevent development of specific signs of deficiency. The requirement of a specific nutrient is usually defined experimentally, often using a small, homogeneous study population. Recommended allowance, on the other hand, is the intake of an essential nutrient deemed by a scientifically knowledgeable group of individuals to be adequate to meet the requirement of all healthy members of a population. In general, if the requirement of a specific population is normally distributed, the recommended allowance is set at the mean requirement of the population plus two standard deviations. Since the requirements of most nutrients are not normally distributed, other considerations of population variability are frequently necessary.

The 0–6-Month-Old Infant

Energy. The RDA for energy represents an exception to the general rule for establishing recommended allowances. Since an energy intake that is adequate for all individuals is likely to result in obesity in individuals with a low or an average requirement, the RDAs for energy reflect the mean energy requirement for each population.

Expressed per unit of body weight, the normal newborn infant requires 3–4 times more energy per day than the adult, i.e., 376.2–501.6 kJ/kg (90–120 kcal/kg) for an infant versus 125.4–167.2 kJ/kg (30–40 kcal/kg) for an adult. The greater energy requirement of the infant reflects primarily the higher metabolic rate of the infant and the special needs for growth and development. Inefficient intestinal absorption contributes only minimally to the higher energy requirement of the infant fed human milk or modern infant formulas.

There is no evidence that either carbohydrate or fat is a superior source of energy. Sufficient carbohydrate is required to prevent ketosis and hypoglycemia (<5.0 g/kg) as is enough fat to avoid development of essential fatty acid deficiency (0.5–1.0 g/kg of linoleic acid daily plus a smaller amount of linolenic acid). Currently, there is concern that infants also may require long-chain, polyunsaturated n–3 and, perhaps, n–6 fatty acids. This issue with respect to the normal term infant is far from clear and will not be discussed. In toto, the specific daily needs for carbohydrate and fat amount to 125.4 kJ (<30 kcal/kg), or only approximately a third of the infant's total energy need.

Protein. The protein requirement of the normal infant also is greater per unit of body weight than that of the adult, and the infant requires a higher proportion of

Table 1. Recommended dietary allowances of nutrients for normal infants[a]

Nutrient	Recommended intake per day	
	0–6 Months weight = 6 kg	6–12 Months weight = 9 kg
Energy (kJ[kcal])	2717 [650]	3553 [850]
Fat (g)		
Carbohydrate		
Protein (g)	13	14
Electrolytes and minerals		
Calcium (mg)	400	600
Phosphorus (mg)	300	500
Magnesium (mg)	40	60
Sodium (mg)[b]	120	200
Chloride (mg)[b]	180	300
Potassium (mg)[b]	500	700
Iron (mg)	6	10
Zinc (mg)	5	5
Copper (mg)[c]	0.4–0.6	0.6–0.7
Iodine (µg)	40	50
Selenium (µg)	10	15
Manganese (µg)[c]	0.3–0.6	0.6–1.0
Fluoride (mg)[c]	0.1–0.5	0.2–1.0
Chromium (µg)[c]	10–40	20–60
Molybdenum (µg)	15–30	20–40
Vitamins		
Vitamin A (µg RE)	375	375
Vitamin D (µg)	7.5	10
Vitamin E (mg α-TE)	3	4
Vitamin K (µg)	5	10
Vitamin C (mg)	30	35
Thiamin (mg)	0.3	0.4
Riboflavin (mg)	0.4	0.5
Niacin (mg NE)	5	6
Vitamin B-6 (mg)	0.3	0.6
Folate (µg)	25	35
Vitamin B-12 (µg)	0.3	0.5
Biotin (µg)[c]	10	15
Pantothenic Acid (mg)[c]	2	3

[a]Data from *Recommended Dietary Allowances,* 10th ed. (reference 1).

[b]Minimum requirements (mg/day) rather than recommended.

[c]Estimated safe and adequate daily intake.

essential amino acids than the adult. In addition to the amino acids recognized as essential (or indispensable) for the adult (leucine, isoleucine, valine, threonine, methionine, phenylalanine, tryptophan, lysine, and histidine), infants also are thought to require cysteine and tyrosine. The need for cysteine is thought to be secondary to delayed development of hepatic cystathionase activity; this key enzyme in conversion of methionine to cysteine does not reach adult levels until at least 4 months of age.[2,3] The reason for the apparent need for tyrosine is not clear; the hepatic activity of phenylalanine hydroxylase, the rate-limiting enzyme for conversion of phenylalanine to tyrosine, is at or near adult levels early in gestation.[4]

In general, human milk protein and all proteins currently used in infant formulas contain adequate amounts of all essential amino acids, including cysteine and tyrosine. Even the sum of the highest estimates of the requirement of each amino acid is only a third to a half of the overall protein requirement. Thus, total protein intake probably is more important than the amino acid pattern of the particular protein. Obviously, however, the required intake of a specific protein depends upon its quality, that is, how closely its amino acid pattern resembles that of human milk. The overall quality of a specific protein can be improved by supplementing it with the limiting essential amino acid(s). Native soy protein, for example, has insufficient methionine; however, when fortified with methionine, its quality approaches or equals that of bovine milk protein.[5]

Although the amino acid composition of human milk protein is considered ideal, the total protein content of human milk, though quite variable, averages only ≈10 g/L. On average, 180–200 mL/kg must be ingested daily to meet the RDA for protein (2.0–2.2 g/kg). This fact has led some to question the validity of the RDA and others to question the adequacy of the protein content of human milk. However, it is clear that few breast-fed infants develop protein deficiency, because the high quality and easy digestibility of human milk protein compensate for any quantitative deficiency.

Bovine milk protein and modern preparations of soy protein, the protein sources of most infant formulas, also are very high quality proteins. If properly processed, these proteins are utilized nearly as well as human milk protein; thus the actual requirement for these proteins may be little, if at all, higher than the requirement for human milk protein.[6]

Electrolytes, minerals, and vitamins. The normal infant's requirements for electrolytes, minerals, and vitamins are not as well defined as those for energy and protein. Nonetheless, RDAs, minimal requirements, and estimated safe and adequate intakes have been established for most (Table 1), and infants who receive these intakes experience few problems. In recent years, the concept that limitation of sodium intake may decrease the incidence of hypertension later in life has received some attention; however, there are few hard data on which to base a definitive conclusion.[7]

The normal newborn infant is thought to have sufficient stores of iron to meet requirements for 4–6 months. Nonetheless, iron deficiency is the most common nutrient deficiency syndrome in infancy. This probably is related to the facts that iron stores at birth as well as the absorption of iron are quite variable. Interestingly, although human milk contains less iron than most formulas, iron deficiency is less common in breast-fed infants. To prevent iron deficiency, routine iron supplementation of formula-fed infants is recommended.[8] In fact, increased use of iron-fortified formulas over the past decade has dramatically reduced the incidence of iron deficiency.

If protein intake is adequate, vitamin deficiencies are rare; if not, deficiencies of nicotinic acid and choline, which are synthesized, respectively, from tryptophan and methionine, may develop. In contrast, if bovine milk and bovine milk formulas were not supplemented with vitamin D, hypovitaminosis D would be endemic among formula-fed infants, particularly those with limited exposure to sunlight. Breast-fed infants may not be as susceptible to development of vitamin D deficiency as formula-fed infants,[9] but vitamin D supplementation is recommended.

Routine perinatal administration of vitamin K is recommended as prophylaxis against hemorrhagic disease of the newborn. Thereafter, deficiency of this vitamin is uncommon except in infants with conditions associated with fat malabsorption.

Water. The normal infant's absolute daily requirement for water probably is 75–100 mL/kg. However, because of higher obligate renal, pulmonary, and dermal water losses as well as a higher metabolic rate, the infant is more likely to develop dehydration, particularly with vomiting and diarrhea, than the older child or adult. Thus, daily provision of 150 mL/kg is recommended. The typical breast-fed infant as well as the typical formula-fed infant usually consumes at least this volume for the first several weeks of life.

The 6–12-Month-Old Infant

The nutritional needs of the infant during the last half of the first year of life are not as firmly based on experimental data as those of the younger infant. In fact, the RDAs for most nutrients for this age group (Table 1) rely heavily on data obtained in younger infants. These recommendations take into account the developmental differences between younger and older infants as well as the greater level of activity and somewhat slower rate of growth after 6 months of age. Despite the lack of experimental data concerning the nutrient needs of this age group, few participants in a recent symposium on the nutritional needs of the 6–12-month-old infant felt that the RDAs for this age group require extensive revision.[10]

One exception was the RDA for energy, which is higher than the energy intake of many apparently normal infants.[11] Although the rates of weight gain as well as the rates of increase in skinfold thickness of infants receiving the lower intakes are lower than the National Center for Health Statistics (NCHS) standards, rates of increase in length and head circumference are at least equal to NCHS standards. Thus, proponents of a lower RDA for energy (355.3 versus 397.1 kJ/kg, or 85 ver-

sus 95 kcal/kg) argue that the growth of modern infants ingesting the lower energy intake is adequate and, moreover, reflects the current concepts of parents regarding appropriate body size and proportions. It also is argued that the growth of infants fed lower energy intakes better reflects current feeding practices (a higher incidence of breast-feeding and delayed introduction of solid foods) than the NCHS growth standards. More data are needed, but there is no evidence that the lower energy intake of many modern infants is harmful.

By 6 months of age, the infant's capacity to digest and absorb a variety of dietary components as well as to metabolize, utilize, and excrete the absorbed products of digestion is near adult capacity.[12] Moreover, teeth are beginning to erupt and the infant is more active and is beginning to explore his/her surroundings. With the eruption of teeth, the role of diet in development of dental caries must be considered.[13] Consideration of the long-term effects of inadequate or excessive intakes during infancy also assumes greater importance as does consideration of the psychosocial role of foods during development.

These considerations, rather than concerns about delivery of adequate amounts of nutrients, are the basis for many feeding practices that are advocated during the second 6 months of life. While it is clear that all nutrient needs during this period can be met with reasonable amounts of currently available infant formulas, the addition of weaning foods is usually recommended after the child reaches an age of 4–6 months. These should be introduced in a stepwise fashion, beginning about the time the infant is able to sit unassisted. Cereals are usually the first such foods given. Vegetables and fruits are introduced next, followed shortly by meats and, finally, eggs. Multivitamin supplements are usually recommended when breast milk or formula intake begins to decrease.

By ≈1 year of age, most infants have graduated successfully to table food and are content with three or four meals daily. Once a few teeth have erupted and tolerance of solid foods has been demonstrated, weaning should have been completed.

Weaning or follow-up formulas have been popular in Europe for some time and have recently been introduced in the United States. These formulas contain somewhat more protein (usually bovine milk protein) than standard infant formulas. Their fat content may be somewhat lower and their carbohydrate content somewhat higher. The types of fat and carbohydrate present are similar to those of standard infant formulas (vegetable oils and lactose plus corn syrup solids).

Aside from the association of bottle feeding with dental caries,[13] little is known about the various issues related to the nonnutritional role of diet during the second half of the first year of life. Most recent surveys indicate that

Table 2. Composition (amount/100 kcal) of standard formulas for normal infants

Component	Similac[a]	Enfamil[b]	SMA[c]	Gerber[d]	Good Start[e]
Protein (g)	2.14 (Bovine milk)	2.2 (Bovine milk; whey)	2.2 (Bovine milk; whey)	2.2 (Bovine milk)	2.4 (Whey)
Fat (g)	5.4 (Soy and coconut oils)	5.6 (Palm-olein, soy, coconut, and high-oleic safflower oils)	5.3 (Oleo, coconut, high-oleic safflower, and soy oils)	5.4 (Palm-olein, coconut, soy and high-oleic safflower oils)	5.1 (Palm-olein, high-oleic safflower, soy, and coconut oils)
Carbohydrate (g)	10.7 (Lactose)	10.3 (Lactose)	10.6 (Lactose)	10.7 (Lactose)	11.0 (Lactose; malto dextrin)
Electrolytes and minerals					
Calcium (mg)	73	69	63	75	64
Phosphorus (mg)	56	47	42	58	36
Magnesium (mg)	6	7.8	7	6	6.7
Iron (mg)	0.22(1.8)[f]	0.16(1.88)[f]	0.2(1.8)[f]	0.48(1.8)[f]	1.5
Zinc (mg)	0.75	0.78	0.8	0.75	0.75
Manganese (μg)	5	15.6	15	5	7
Copper (μg)	90	94	70	90	80
Iodine (μg)	14	10.2	9	8	8
Selenium (μg)	2.2	1.77	1.8	—	—
Sodium (mg)	27	27	22	33	24
Potassium (mg)	120	108	83	108	98
Chloride	64	63	55.5	70	59
Vitamins					
Vitamin A (IU)	300	310	300	300	300
Vitamin D (IU)	60	63	60	60	60
Vitamin E (IU)	3.0	3.1	1.4	3	2
Vitamin K (μg)	8	8.6	8	8	8.2
Thiamin (μg)	100	78	100	100	60
Riboflavin (μg)	150	156	150	150	135
Vitamin B-6 (μg)	60	63	62.5	60	75
Vitamin B-12 (μg)	0.25	0.23	0.2	0.25	0.22
Niacin (μg)	1050	1250	750	1050	750
Folic acid (μg)	15	15.6	7.5	15	9
Pantothenic acid(μg)	450	470	315	450	450
Vitamin C (mg)	9	8.1	8.5	9	8
Biotin (μg)	4.4	2.3	2.2	4.4	2.2
Choline (mg)	16.0	15.6	15.0	16	12
Inositol (mg)	4.7	4.7	4.7	4.7	18

[a]Ross Laboratories, Columbus, Ohio.
[b]Mead-Johnson Nutritionals, Evansville, Indiana.
[c]Wyeth-Ayerst Laboratories, Philadelphia, Pennsylvania.
[d]Gerber Products Company, Fremont, Michigan.
[e]Carnation Nutritional Products, Glendale, California.
[f]Content of iron-fortified formula shown in parentheses.

infants fed according to current practices receive the RDAs for most nutrients.[14]

Human Milk and Artificial Formula

The ready availability and safety of human milk coupled with the possibility that it may enhance intestinal development, resistance to infection, and bonding between the mother and infant have led most to conclude that human milk is the perfect food for the normal infant.[15] However, there are some theoretical as well as practical concerns about breast-feeding that deserve consideration.

The major nutritional concern is not that human milk contains too little protein (see above) but that its low content of calcium and phosphorus may not support optimal skeletal development. In this regard, breast-fed infants have a less well mineralized skeleton throughout the early months of life than formula-fed infants. However, since there are no major differences in bone density of older formerly breast-fed and formula-fed infants, the lower calcium and phosphorus intakes of breast-fed infants do not seem to be detrimental.

Hyperbilirubinemia is more common in breast-fed than in formula-fed infants. It is usually a transient phenomenon limited to the first few days or weeks of life, and most experts feel that proscription of breast-feeding is not necessary unless hyperbilirubinemia persists or plasma bilirubin concentration is excessively high. Even in these situations, substituting formula at every other feeding or for only 1 or 2 days usually is sufficient to resolve the problem.

Certain noxious or infectious agents (chemicals, drugs, foreign proteins, viruses) may be present in breast milk.[16] However, the risk of infection secondary to mode of feeding is far greater in formula-fed than breast-fed infants, particularly if the artificial formula is prepared under less than optimal hygienic conditions.

As has been publicized recently in the lay press,[17] it cannot automatically be assumed that maternal milk supply will be adequate and constant. It is essential that breast-fed infants, particularly first-born infants, be followed closely over the first few days or weeks of life in order to ensure that growth and development are proceeding normally. With proper counseling, most problems can be corrected or avoided.

In large part, the historical problems associated with artificial feeding have been solved. In fact, the safety and easy digestibility of modern infant formulas approach the safety and digestibility of breast milk. Further, the clear economic advantages and microbiological safety of breast-feeding are less important for affluent, developed societies with ready access to a clean water supply than for less developed, less affluent societies. A reasonable and conservative approach for health care professionals is to allow the mother to make an informed choice of how she wishes to feed her infant and support her in that decision. As stated by Fomon:[18]

> . . . in industrialized countries, any woman with the least inclination toward breast feeding should be encouraged to do so, and all assistance possible should be provided by nurses, physicians, nutritionists, and other health workers. At the same time, there is little justification for attempts to coerce women to breast feed. No woman in an industrialized country should be made to feel guilty because she elects not to breast feed her infant.

Breast-fed infants in affluent societies have fewer common and serious infections during early life than formula-fed infants. If this difference is attributable to breast-feeding rather than to myriad other factors (socioeconomic status), the current emphasis on promoting breast-feeding clearly is warranted.

A number of formulas are available for feeding the normal infant. The composition of the most commonly used ones is shown in Table 2. Most are available in both a ready-to-use and a concentrated liquid form. Powdered products, which are usually lower in cost, also are available and are being used with increasing frequency; these products often are the only ones available in many other parts of the world.

The most commonly used formulas contain either unmodified or modified bovine milk protein. The protein concentration of all is about 15 g/L. Thus, the infant whose daily formula intake is 150–180 mL/kg receives a protein intake of 2.25–2.7 g/kg. This is ≈50% more than the intake of the breast-fed infant and ≈25% more than the current RDA for protein. Unmodified bovine milk protein has a whey:casein ratio of 18:82, whereas modified bovine milk protein has a whey:casein ratio of 60:40. Products containing the latter protein are prepared from either a mixture of bovine milk protein and bovine milk whey proteins or a mixture of bovine milk whey proteins and caseins. For the normal term infant, modified and unmodified bovine milk proteins appear to be equally efficacious. Formulas containing soy protein as well as formulas containing partially hydrolyzed bovine milk proteins are available for feeding infants who are intolerant of bovine milk or soy protein (Table 3).

Although lactose-free bovine milk formulas have recently been introduced, the major carbohydrate of the most commonly used bovine milk formulas is lactose. The most commonly used soy protein formulas contain either sucrose or a glucose polymer. Soy formulas or lactose-free bovine milk protein formulas are useful for the infant with either transient or congenital lactase deficiency.

The fat content of both bovine milk and soy protein formulas usually supplies ≈50% of nonprotein energy. In general, the blend of vegetable oils present in most formulas is quite easily absorbed; most studies suggest that intestinal absorption is at least 90%.

The electrolyte, mineral, and vitamin contents of most formulas are similar, and when fed in adequate daily amounts (150–180 mL/kg), all provide the RDAs for these nutrients. Both iron-supplemented (≈12 mg/L, recommended) and nonsupplemented (≈1 mg/L) formulas are available.

The goal of both breast-feeding and formula-feeding is to deliver enough nutrients to support adequate growth. As a rule of thumb, the normal term infant's weight should double by 4–5 months of age and triple by 12 months of age. Demand feeding is considered preferable, particularly during the early weeks of life. However, most infants easily adjust to a schedule of every 3 or 4 hours and, after the age of 2 months, rarely demand night feedings.

Infant Formula and Bovine Milk

Although current recommendations are to limit the intake of bovine milk and to avoid low-fat or skimmed milk until the infant is >1 year old, surveys suggest that a sizable percentage of 6–12-month-old infants are fed bovine milk rather than infant formula.[19–21] More important, almost half of these infants are fed low-fat or

Table 3. Composition of soy and hydrolyzed protein formulas

Component	Isomil[a]	Prosobee[b]	Nursoy[c]	Nutramigen[b]	Pregestimil[b]	Alimentum[a]
Protein (g)	2.66 (soy protein isolate and L-methionine)	3 (soy protein isolate and L-methionine)	3.1 (soy protein isolate and L-methionine)	2.8 (casein hydrolysate, cystine, tyrosine and tryptophan)	2.8 (casein hydrolysate, cystine, tyrosine and tryptophan)	2.75 (casein hydrolysate, cystine, tyrosine and tryptophan)
Fat (g)	5.46 (soy and coconut oils)	5.3 (palm-olein, soy, coconut, and high-oleic safflower oils)	5.3 (oleo coconut, high-oleic safflower, and soy oils)	3.9 (corn and soy oils)	5.6 (medium-chain triglycerides; corn and high oleic safflower oils)	5.54 (medium-chain triglycerides; safflower and soy oils)
Carbohydrate (g)	10.1 (corn syrup sucrose)[d]	10 (corn syrup solids)	10.2 (sucrose)	13.4 (corn syrup solids and modified corn starch)	10.3 (corn syrup solids, modified corn starch, and dextrose)	10.2 (sucrose and modified tapioca starch)
Electrolytes and minerals						
Calcium (mg)	105	94	90	94	94	105
Phosphorus (mg)	75	74	63	63	63	75
Magnesium (mg)	7.5	10.9	10	10.9	10.9	7.5
Iron (mg)	1.8	1.88	1.7	1.88	1.88	1.8
Zinc (mg)	0.75	0.78	0.8	0.78	0.94	0.75
Manganese (μg)	30	25	30	31	31	30
Copper (μg)	75	94	70	94	94	75
Iodine (μg)	15	10.2	9	7	8	15
Selenium (μg)	2.1	2.3	1.0	2.3	2.3	2.8
Sodium (mg)	44	36	30	47	39	44
Potassium (mg)	108	122	105	109	109	118
Chloride	62	83	56.5	86	86	80
Vitamins						
Vitamin A (IU)	300	310	300	310	380	300
Vitamin D (IU)	60	63	60	63	75	45
Vitamin E (IU)	3.0	3.1	1.4	3.1	3.8	3.0
Vitamin K (IU)	15	15.6	15.	15.6	18.8	15
Thiamine (μg)	60	78	100	78	78	60
Riboflavin (μg)	90	94	150	94	94	90
Vitamin B-6 (μg)	60	63	62.5	63	63	60
Vitamin B-12 (μg)	0.45	0.31	0.3	0.31	0.31	0.45
Niacin (μg)	1350	1250	750	1250	1250	1350
Folic acid (μg)	15	15.6	7.5	15.6	15.6	15
Pantothenic acid (μg)	750	470	450	470	470	750
Biotin (μg)	4.5	7.8	5.5	7.8	7.8	4.5
Vitamin C (mg)	9	8.1	8.5	8.1	11.7	9.0
Choline (mg)	8	7.8	13.0	13.3	13.3	8
Inositol (mg)	5	4.8	4.1	4.7	4.7	8

[a]Ross Laboratories, Columbus, Ohio.
[b]Mead-Johnson Nutritionals, Evansville, Indiana.
[c]Wyeth-Ayerst Laboratories, Philadelphia, Pennsylvania.
[d]Isomil-SF (sucrose free) has similar composition with the exception that glucose polymers are substituted for corn syrup and sucrose.

skimmed milk often, interestingly, on the advice of their physician.

The consequences of this practice are not known with certainty. However, infants fed bovine milk, on average, ingest roughly three times the RDA for protein and ≈50% more sodium than the upper limit of the safe range of intake of this mineral but only about two-thirds of the RDA for iron and only half of the RDA for linoleic acid. The protein and sodium intakes of infants fed skimmed rather than whole bovine milk are even higher, the iron intake is equally low, and most important, the intake of

linoleic acid is very low. Ironically, while the most common reason for substituting low-fat or skimmed milk for whole milk or formula is to reduce fat and energy intakes, the total energy intake of infants fed skimmed milk is not necessarily lower than that of infants fed whole milk or formula.[21] It appears that they compensate for the lower energy density of low-fat or skimmed milk by increasing intake of other foods.

Whether the high protein and sodium intakes of infants fed either whole or skimmed milk are desirable is not known with certainty. Clearly the low iron intake is not desirable, but medicinal iron supplements should prevent iron deficiency. The low intake of linoleic acid may be more problematical. While signs or symptoms of essential fatty acid deficiency appear to be uncommon in infants fed either whole or skimmed milk, an exhaustive search for such symptoms has not been made. Moreover, because essential fatty acid deficiency develops in both younger and older infants fed formulas providing an equally low linoleic acid intake, it would be very surprising if a search did not uncover a reasonably high incidence of essential fatty acid deficiency. On the other hand, infants fed formulas with a high linoleic acid content before they are 6 months old may have sufficient body stores to limit the consequences of a low intake between 6 and 12 months of age. Because essential fatty acid deficiency in animals is associated with long-term deleterious effects on development, it is wise to be cautious about the consequences of a biochemical essential fatty acid deficiency that is without clinically detectable symptoms.[22]

Practical as well as health reasons demand a resolution of the issues concerning the use of bovine milk in feeding the 6–12-month-old infant. Since the cost of bovine milk is considerably less than that of infant formula, replacing formula with homogenized bovine milk would obviously offer important economic advantages for most families, particularly those with limited income. In addition, if the federal food assistance programs could provide homogenized bovine milk rather than formula to infants over 6 months of age, the programs' current funds would permit expansion of benefits to many more of the country's most needy infants. This, of course, cannot be considered without data on the safety of bovine milk during the second 6 months of life.

The increasingly common practice of substituting skimmed or low-fat milk for whole milk or formula raises a number of more complex questions. For example, the suggestion that infants fed skimmed milk increase their intake of other foods to maintain the same energy intake raises the important question of whether the amount of food intake during infancy may, in some way, imprint intake patterns throughout life. If so, this apparent attempt to improve longevity, or at least cardiovascular health, paradoxically, is likely to be more detrimental to both than a less prudent diet during infancy.

Acknowledgments

This work is a publication of the USDA/ARS Children's Nutrition Research Center, Department of Pediatrics, Baylor College of Medicine, Houston, Texas, and has been funded in part by funds from the U.S. Department of Agriculture, Agricultural Research Service under Cooperative Agreement No. 38-6250-1-003. The contents of this publication do not necessarily reflect the views or policies of the U.S. Department of Agriculture, nor does the mention of trade names, commercial products, or organizations imply endorsement by the United States Government.

References

1. Subcommittee on the Tenth Edition of the RDAs, Food and Nutrition Board, Commission on Life Sciences, National Research Council (1989) Recommended dietary allowances, 10th ed. National Academy Press, Washington, DC
2. Sturman JA, Gaull GA, Räihä NCR (1970) Absence of cystathionase in human liver: is cystine essential? Science 169: 74–76
3. Gaull GE, Sturman JA, Räihä NCR (1972) Development of mammalian sulfur metabolism: absence of cystathionase in human fetal tissues. Pediatr Res 6:538–547
4. Räihä NCR (1973) Phenylalanine hydroxylase in human liver during development. Pediatr Res 7:1–4
5. Fomon SJ, Thomas LN, Filer LJ, et al (1973) Requirements of protein and essential amino acids in early infancy: studies with a soy-isolate formula. Acta Paediatr Scand 62:33–45
6. Räihä NCR (1985) Nutritional proteins in milk and the protein requirements of normal infants. Pediatrics 75:136–141
7. Holliday MA (1991) Do dietary factors in the 6 to 12 month period of life affect blood pressure later in life? In Heird WC (ed), Nutritional needs of the six to twelve month old infant. Raven Press, New York, pp 283–295
8. American Academy of Pediatrics Committee on Nutrition (1976) Iron supplementation for infants. Pediatrics 58: 765–768
9. Lakdewala DR, Widdowson EM (1977) Vitamin D in human milk. Lancet 1:167–168
10. Heird WC, ed (1991) Nutritional needs of the six to twelve month old infant. Raven Press, New York
11. Whitehead RG, Paul AA (1991) Dietary energy needs from 6 to 12 months of age. In Heird WC (ed), Nutritional needs of the six to twelve month old infant. Raven Press, New York, pp 135–148
12. Montgomery RK (1991) Functional development of the gastrointestinal tract: the small intestine. In Heird WC (ed), Nutritional needs of the six to twelve month old infant. Raven Press, New York, pp 1–17
13. Mandel ID (1991) The nutritional impact on dental caries. In Heird WC (ed), Nutritional needs of the six to twelve month old infant. Raven Press, New York, pp 89–107
14. Purvis GA, Bartholmey SJ (1988) Infant feeding practices: commercially prepared baby foods. In Tsang R, Nichols B (eds), Nutrition during infancy. Hanley & Belfus, Philadelphia, pp 399–417
15. Committee on Nutrition, American Academy of Pediatrics (1982) The promotion of breast feeding. Pediatrics 69: 654–661
16. Goldfarb J (1985) Breastfeeding: AIDS and other infectious diseases. Clin Perinatol 20:225–243
17. Wall Street Journal (1994) July 22, page 1
18. Fomon SJ (1993) Recommendation for feeding normal infants. In Fomon SJ (ed), Nutrition of normal infants. Mosby, St Louis, pp 455–458
19. Committee on Nutrition, American Academy of Pediatrics (1992) The use of whole cow's milk in infancy [policy statement]. AAP News 8:18–22
20. Ryan AS, Martinez GA, Kreiger FW (1987) Feeding low-fat milk during infancy. Am J Phys Anthropol 73:539–548

21. Martinez GA, Ryan AS, Malec DJ (1985) Nutrient intakes of American infants and children fed cow's milk or infant formula. Am J Dis Child 139:1010–1018

22. Crawford MA, Stassam AG, Stevens PA (1981) Essential fatty acid requirements in pregnancy and lactation with special reference to brain development. Prog Lipid Res 20:31–40

Chapter 39

Adolescence

Johanna T. Dwyer

Growth during the second decade of life requires abundant nutrients. The recommended dietary allowances (RDAs) for adolescents may be inappropriate in some individual cases.[1] Standards for over- and underweight assessment are examined, the prevalence of obesity is reviewed, and associations between obesity, energy intakes, and outputs, and problems involving physical activity and fitness, are described. Differences between adolescents' reported intakes and recommended dietary patterns are considerable for foods, food energy, and other nutrients. Some other major nutrition-related problems are iron deficiency and iron-deficiency anemia, inadequate calcium intakes, hyperlipidemia, hypertension, and alcohol abuse. Recommendations for dietary improvement are summarized for adolescent pregnancy, for adolescents who lead very sedentary or very physically active lifestyles, or who have other disorders. Special problems of athletes (such as the nutritional consequences of steroid use), nutrition-related amenorrhea and reproductive disorders, problems associated with special needs, handicaps, unusual dietary habits, and disease are also addressed.

Nutrient Needs of Adolescents

Nutritional needs of adolescents correlate closely with biological maturation and are extensively reviewed elsewhere.[2-5] In affluent countries the age at which physical maturation occurs is determined primarily by genetics. Males mature ≈2 years later than females, although differences of several years are seen among those of the same sex. Environmental factors such as malnutrition and disease may delay the onset of puberty.

Nutrient needs of males and females of the same age differ little in childhood but diverge after the onset of the pubertal growth spurt.[3] After puberty, differences in nutrient needs persist. The reasons for the sex differences in nutrient recommendations after the age of 10 include the earlier maturation of females, considerable variability in the age of puberty within each sex, and variations in physiological needs for some nutrients by sex and biological age. These differences become particularly striking in later adolescence because of sex-related differences in body composition and functions.

Compared with adults, adolescents in the pubertal growth spurt need a higher ratio of many nutrients to energy if they are to sustain the needs of growth and the accretion of lean tissues. Once growth has ceased and greater size is achieved, mineralization of the skeleton and maintenance of a larger body keep many nutrient needs higher than they were in childhood. Changes in physiology associated with reproductive capacity also alter needs for some nutrients, such as that for iron in menstruating and pregnant females.

Changes in life-style also alter adolescent nutrient needs. Adolescents need more food energy than they did when they were younger and smaller because their bodies are larger. However, adolescents are not necessarily more physically active and their energy needs per unit weight do not rise above those of childhood.

The RDAs are the standard for planning dietary intakes.[1] Except for energy, they represent recommendations that are adequate for the needs of all healthy people, with a generous margin of safety above requirements.

From birth to 10 years of age, the RDAs for males and females are similar for most nutrients. From the age of 10 onward, separate RDAs are provided for males and females because sex affects age of puberty, evolving activity patterns, and body composition and function. The current RDAs are stated by chronological ages: 11–14, 15–18, and 19–24 years. For adolescents, data are often interpolated between data collected in adults and children, rather than being based on actual experimental evidence.

Energy recommendations are minimum average requirements because the body cannot store a plethora of food energy without gaining fat tissue, and excess adiposity has adverse health effects. The present RDAs for energy reflect estimates of minimal average population requirements for each age group, but they are very imprecise and apply only if the assumptions with respect to weight and energy output stated in the RDA are met. These recommendations will not suffice without adjustment for adolescents who are at the extremes with respect to maturation or physical activity.

On average, during most chronological and biological ages of adolescence, males have higher energy needs

Table 1. Prevalence of overweight among adolescents in the Second and Third National Health and Nutrition Examination Surveys

Sex and survey	Sample size	%	95% confidence interval
Male			
NHANES II	1351	15	12.9–16
NHANES III	717	20	15.3–24.6
Female			
NHANES II	1241	15	12.1–17.3
NHANES III	739	22	18.4–26.3
Total			
NHANES II	2562	15	13.1–16.4
NHANES III	1456	21	17.5–24.6

Note: Obesity is defined as BMI (body mass index) equal to or >23.0 in males 12–14 years, 25.8 for males 15–17 years, and 26.8 for males 18–19 years. For females similar limits were 23.4, 24.8, and 25.7.

Source: Prevalence of Overweight Among Adolescents, United States, 1988–1991. *Morbidity and Mortality Weekly Report* 43(1994):819

than females have. Among females, those who are pregnant and lactating have higher food energy needs than their nonpregnant peers have.

Weights for children are relatively easy to assess using weight-for-height, weight-for-age, and height-for-age growth charts. In contrast, appropriate weights for adolescents are more difficult to establish because sexual maturity varies, especially early in adolescence. Therefore, chronological age-based standards are not a good guide.[6] A better approach is to use body mass index (BMI), which is calculated from weight in kilograms divided by height in meters squared. Such standards are helpful for evaluating over- and underweight in adolescents. BMI is well correlated with subcutaneous and total body fat in adolescents. Individuals with a BMI >95th percentile for age and sex or whose BMI is >30 (whichever is smaller) are classified as overweight, and those <5th percentile as underweight.[7,8]

Energy Needs and Obesity

Obesity is becoming more rather than less prevalent, despite major national efforts to prevent and treat it. This trend is evident in Table 1, which contrasts the most recent data from the 1988–1991 Third National Health and Nutrition Examination Survey (NHANES III) with the earlier 1976–1980 survey (NHANES II), which used similar techniques.[9] A national health objective is that by the year 2000 the prevalence of overweight should not exceed 15% among adolescents (12–19 years old). However, the existing prevalence exceeds this target, and rates appear to be increasing rather than decreasing.

Early obesity tends to persist. For example, 26–41% of obese preschoolers become obese adults, and for obese preschoolers the risk of adult obesity is 2–2.6 times that of their nonobese peers in most studies. By school age, from 42% to 63% of obese children (depending on the group in question) go on to become obese adults, and the risk of adult obesity rises to 3.9–6.5 times that of their lean peers. Adolescent obesity is predictive of adult obesity.[9,10] Adolescent fatness is fraught with risk of later obesity, particularly for women. In one study, 30% of all obese women but only 10% of obese men were fat as adolescents. When obesity begins in adolescence it is highly associated with morbidity and mortality.[11,12] Excessive fatness in childhood and adolescence is a major health concern because it is associated with immediate as well as longer-term health problems that include hypertension, abnormal glucose tolerance, and hyperlipidemia.[13,14]

Energy intakes and obesity. Dietary intakes of energy and other nutrients from records or recalls are usually underestimated, often by as much as 15–30% depending on the method.[15,16] Serious reporting biases exist by weight status: heavier individuals report less energy intake than do people of more normal weight.[17]

Table 2 presents intakes of food energy by adolescents as reported in NHANES III.[18,19] These intakes are lower than recommendations, probably in part because they were underestimated. Compared with dietary records or recalls, energy intakes inferred from well-standardized doubly labeled water estimates are more accurate. Such estimates suggest that current recommendations from later infancy to 5 years of age are too high.[20,21] In contrast, for some subgroups of adolescents the estimates may be too low, because it is known that energy expenditures and intakes of some nonobese, and occasionally obese, adolescents exceed current recommendations.[22,23]

Energy output and obesity. The causes of obesity in adolescence are not due to lower resting energy expenditure or thermic effects of food but primarily to physical inactivity. Resting energy expenditure is not different in obese and nonobese children. Values for energy expenditure per unit fat-free mass are lower among obese children because body build characteristics and environmental influences are such that bone mass tends to be higher and muscle mass lower among them than among the nonobese.[24] Thermic effects of food do not differ between obese and nonobese adolescents although they do between obese and nonobese adults.[25–28]

Table 2. Mean energy intakes of children and adolescents by age and sex in the Third National Health and Nutrition Examination Survey 1988–1991 in kJ (kcal)

Age (years)	Males	Females
6–11	8519 (2036)	7335 (1753)
12–15	10,786 (2578)	7690 (1838)
16–19	12,958 (3097)	8192 (1958)

Physical activity influences growth and development of skeletal bone, muscle, and fat in adolescence. Some investigators find no differences in physical activity between lean and obese children, others find low activity, and a few find very high levels of physical activity in the obese.[29-37] These differences in energy output are attributable to different methods of measurement, to whether subjects were weight stable or in dynamic periods of weight gain when measured, and to heterogeneity among the obese with respect to physical activity. Doubly labeled water measurements demonstrate an inverse association between physical activity and body fat mass. The association between fatness and the ratio of total to resting energy expenditure (an index of physical activity) persists after adjustment for body size in obese children.[24,38,39] The ratio of total to resting energy expenditure declines as body fat increases. However, total energy expenditure may be normal or even high among the obese because resting energy expenditure and the energy costs of most activities increase with body size. In weight-stable obese children, total energy expenditure for physical activity appears to be normal to high, whereas the duration of total movement and vigorous activity is normal or low according to doubly labeled water techniques, which ascertain energy outputs.[40] Finally, energy intakes also vary at differing levels of physical activity.

Problems Involving Physical Activity and Fitness

At puberty, linear growth and body mass increase, and physiological changes (increased aerobic and anaerobic power, and tolerance to heat and cold) improve physical and athletic ability. Levels of physical activity do not necessarily rise during adolescence, and low levels are commonly reported.[41] Adolescents are almost certainly less physically active, probably less fit than they were several decades ago, and certainly less fit than they should be.[42] Several lines of evidence support such a contention. Recommendations for the reference adolescent's RDAs for energy stated on a body weight basis have declined since the first RDAs were published in the 1940s.[43] Relatively little of the decrease in energy recommendations is due to a larger size at each age, because of the secular trend toward earlier puberty and hence a larger size at a given age. The more likely explanation for the decline in recommendations is that American children and adolescents are becoming more sedentary. Sedentary activities, such as television viewing, are often associated not only with decreased energy output but with increased energy intake. Some studies report a positive association between television viewing and body fatness while others fail to find an association, probably because study populations also vary in their overall levels of physical activity and in their food intakes.[32,44,45] Adolescents may become obese because they watch more television, and not simply because they are obese to begin with.[45] There is also suggestive evidence from other sources. Enrollment in and participation in daily physical education classes decrease in late adolescence. Participation in physical education classes declines sharply in high school, and only ≈30% of students participate in daily physical education in the 12th grade. Moreover, only ≈20% of the time in these classes is spent in moderate or vigorous physical activity. The consensus among experts is that trends that currently encourage a sedentary lifestyle, such as sedentary entertainment, an emphasis on the "star" system in child athletic events, and cutbacks in government-sponsored physical education programs, need to be reversed. Several excellent references are now available on sports nutrition.[46-48]

Many older adolescent girls, the obese, and those with certain psychosocial characteristics are especially likely to be physically inactive.[41] Adolescents suffering from chronic illness or disabilities such as mental retardation, blindness, motor problems, and extreme obesity are likely to be unfit and in need of special help.[49]

Underweight. Data on the prevalence of underweight among adolescents from NHANES III is not yet available. Earlier surveys found that adolescents (14-17 years old) living in poverty were shorter but not necessarily leaner for their age and sex than their more affluent peers.[50]

Undernutrition during adolescence may result not only from inadequate food intake, but from inappropriate reducing diets, excessive competitive athletic training, eating disorders, and certain chronic illnesses such as gastrointestinal diseases that modify absorption and appetite.[51-55] The consequences and possible remedies for these problems are reviewed elsewhere in greater depth.[56]

Differences Between Adolescents' Intakes and Recommendations

Food intakes. The U.S. Department of Agriculture's (USDA's) most recent Continuing Survey of Food Intake of Individuals (CSFII) found that some changes in diets of children and teenagers, such as increased intakes of cereals and reduced intakes of dietary fat, between the 1977-1978 and 1989-1990 surveys were in line with *Dietary Guidelines for Americans.*[57] Other trends, such as decreased intakes of vegetables, were not. It is not clear whether the decrease in vegetable intakes was the result of poor reporting because vegetables were being eaten as part of mixtures rather than by themselves or whether intakes actually declined. The *Dietary Guidelines* recommend consumption of at least two servings of fruits a day, yet substantial proportions of children and teenagers ate no fruit during the 3 days of the survey.

Table 3. Sources of food energy in males and females, Third National Health and Nutrition Examination Survey 1988–1991

Percent of energy from:	Age 6–11 males	Age 6–11 females	Age 12–15 males	Ages 12–15 females	Age 16–19 males	Age 16–19 females
Protein	14	15	14	14	14	14
Fat	34	34	33	34	35	34
Saturated fat	13	13	12	12	13	12
Polyunsaturated fatty acids	6	6	6	7	6	7
Monounsaturated fatty acids	13	13	13	13	13	13
Carbohydrate	54	53	54	54	50	52
Alcohol	0	0	0	0	3	1
Cholesterol, mg	234	215	293	202	372	210
Fiber, g	13	12	15	11	17	13

Energy intakes. Table 2 shows that energy intakes in NHANES III were consistently higher for males than for females over all ethnic groups. Food energy intakes tended to peak in later adolescence and declined thereafter. From the standpoint of ethnicity, white non-Hispanic males over the age of 12 and black females in both childhood and adolescence had the highest energy intakes. Intakes were lower than the RDA for most groups, yet rates of overweight are high. Probably reports were underestimates of true intakes, and respondents' physical activity levels were lower than those specified in the RDA.

The percentages of food energy from various sources in diets surveyed over a 3-day period among individuals 6–19 years old in the 1989–1990 CSFII were 35% of energy from fat, 15% from protein, and 51% from carbohydrate, compared with 39%, 16%, and 46%, respectively, in a similar survey conducted in 1977–1978.[58] Sources of food energy in children and adolescents surveyed with 24-hour recalls in NHANES III are shown in Table 3. These data agree closely with CSFII data. Taken together, these surveys suggest that dietary fat intakes are declining, but are still in excess of recommendations. In particular, fat and saturated fat intakes exceed the *Dietary Guidelines.*

Other nutrients. Table 4 presents intakes of other nutrients reported in NHANES III.[18,19] Adolescents' intakes of protein, as well as of vitamins A and C, thiamine, riboflavin, niacin, vitamin B-6, folic acid, and vitamin B-12, met or nearly met the RDA in both the CSFII and NHANES III. Clinical evidence of deficiencies in these nutrients is rare, and although intakes may fail to meet recommended levels for certain subgroups, in general their dietary status appears to be good.

Magnesium intakes in the CSFII expressed as a percentage of the RDA exceeded the RDA for both males (137%) and females (128%) 6–11 years of age, but adolescents 12–19 years old had mean intakes that failed to meet recommendations (males 91%, females 71%). Intakes of magnesium in NHANES III were also low. Zinc intakes also failed to meet the RDA for both

younger children aged 6–11 years (89% males, 85% females) and adolescents aged 12–19 years (93% RDA males, 78% females) in the CSFII; intakes in NHANES III were also low. However, the effects of these shortfalls on nutritional status are not clear. Intakes of other nutrients of major concern are discussed below.

Dietary factors and coronary artery and cardiovascular disease risk. Risks of these diseases already evident in adolescence include sedentary life-styles, smoking, and diet. The National Cholesterol Education Program has recently issued guidelines for attaining and maintaining appropriate serum cholesterol levels in children and adolescents.[59] Similar documents have been published on blood pressure control in children and adolescents.[60]

Iron intakes and iron-deficiency anemia. Both NHANES III (see Table 4) and other recent surveys of dietary intake such as the CSFII suggest that although iron intakes suffice for most adolescent boys, intakes in older adolescent girls are low compared with recommendations. For example, intakes as a percentage of the 1989 RDA for 3 days in 1989–1990 in the USDA's CSFII were 119% for 6–11-year-old boys and 147% for 12–19-year-old males, whereas for 6–11-year-old females they were 114% but only 77% for 12–19-year-olds.[58]

Iron deficiency is the most prevalent dietary deficiency disease today in children and adolescents, even though it is less common now than before cereals were fortified with higher levels of iron and before oral contraceptive agents, which decrease menstrual iron losses, were widely used by adolescent girls. Groups of adolescents who are at special risk are older adolescent girls (owing to increased iron need and low dietary intake), pregnant adolescents (who have greatly increased needs), and female athletes such as runners (who may lose iron through occult gastrointestinal bleeding). Young pubertal adolescent boys sometimes have anemias that are physiological because of their rapid growth, but the anemias usually disappear when growth velocity slows. Anemia is of concern because it decreases exercise capacity, may impair body temperature

Table 4. Intakes of selected nutrients, Third National Health and Nutrition Examination Survey 1988–1991

Nutrient	Age 6–11 males	Age 6–11 females	Age 12–15 males	Age 12–15 females	Age 16–19 males	Age 16–19 females
Iron, mg	15	13	20	12	19	13
Calcium, mg	1007	867	1136	796	1274	822
Magnesium, mg	243	218	291	206	340	230
Phosphorus, mg	1274	1132	1517	1079	1825	1152
Sodium, mg	3138	2852	4018	2927	4763	3097
Potassium, mg	2110	1968	2361	2080	2761	1984
Zinc, mg	10	10	15	10	16	10
Vitamin A, retinol equivalents (RE)	931	823	1231	738	959	816
Carotene, RE	270	275	283	255	323	400
Folic acid, µg	278	235	382	220	333	234
Vitamin B-12, µg	4.37	4.26	6.77	4.09	6.80	3.93
Ascorbic acid, mg	4.5	3.1	8.4	6.2	8.9	8.4
Vitamin E, mg, α-tocopherol equivalents	7	7	15	7	10	8

regulation, lower resistance to infection, and possibly affect attention, if severe.

Calcium intakes and growth. Achieving peak bone mass is critical to decreasing later risks of osteoporosis. Optimizing bone accretion during childhood and adolescence is therefore desirable.[61] Nonetheless, many children and adolescents fail to reach peak bone mass.[62] In part this may be due to dietary choices. Data from NHANES III provide evidence that calcium intakes in adolescent females are lower than recommendations, as is suggested by other data. In the 1989–1990 CSFII, calcium intakes over 3 days in males aged 6–11 years were 115% and in males aged 12–19 years were 98% of the RDAs, whereas for females aged 6–11 years they were 113%, dropping to 65% for 12–19-year-olds. Milk or milk products were consumed by 90% of male and 80% of female teenagers on these days, although two or three servings of milk, milk products, or alternates are suggested.[58] Average intakes of milk by teenagers were consistent with the survey of a decade earlier, but in the more recent survey skim and low-fat milk intakes increased and whole-milk intakes decreased. However, intakes of milk and milk products for younger children were lower than during previous years. This is a matter of concern for the future, because soft drinks and fruit juices provide no calcium to speak of. Calcium intakes are strongly associated with peak bone mass in Americans, and therefore milk or some other good, highly available source of calcium is recommended.[63,64] Calcium absorption is enhanced by estrogens and inhibited when amenorrhea is present; for this reason calcium nutriture is often adversely affected in eating disorders or in other conditions associated with anovulation and amenorrhea. Other factors, such as low intakes of calcium or vita-

min D or consumption of nonbioavailable forms of the mineral, also adversely affect calcium nutrition. For this reason vegan or vegetarian diets need to be carefully planned to ensure that calcium needs are met.

Alcohol. Alcohol intakes are poorly reported in most dietary survey data on adolescents, yet intakes of alcohol are of importance because the major causes of death in adolescents and young adults today are alcohol-connected unintentional injuries and homicides. More than one-half of motor vehicle crashes (78% of unintentional injury deaths) are associated with alcohol, and a substantial proportion of homicides are associated with alcohol and other drug abuse.[65] Although alcohol intakes are relatively low among adolescents as a group, some adolescents abuse alcohol with fatal results. Therefore, abstinence is best, and moderation is essential if adolescents do use alcohol.

Recommendations

The *Surgeon General's Report on Nutrition and Health* suggests that adolescent females increase consumption of calcium-rich foods, including low-fat dairy products.[66] Adolescents and women of childbearing age, especially those in low-income families, should increase their consumption of foods that are good sources of iron. Adolescents should limit the amount and frequency of foods high in sugars and carbohydrate-rich starchy or sugary foods that are retained in the mouth, and use fluoridated water to lessen vulnerability to dental caries.

The diet and health report of the National Academy of Sciences[67] suggests a dietary pattern that is suited to adolescents as well as to adults. The recommended pattern is to keep fat intake to not >30% of energy, saturated fat to not >10% of energy, and dietary cholesterol to not >300 mg/day. Salt intake recommendations are not >6 g/day, protein no more than twice RDA levels, optimal levels of fluorides, and nutrient supplements at no more than the RDA, if they are used. The pattern emphasizes a plant-based diet with six or more servings of breads, cereals, legumes, and other starches, and five or more servings of fruits and vegetables a day. Alcohol is not recommended; for adults, not more than 30 mL (1 ounce) of absolute alcohol a day is suggested. The use of high-carbohydrate, moderate-fat dietary patterns needs to be balanced with other nutrient needs, especially problem nutrients such as calcium, iron, and possibly magnesium, which are likely to be low in the diets of children and adolescents.[68]

Other Nutritional Problems of Adolescents

Adolescent pregnancy. One out of 10 young women in the 15–19-year-old age group becomes pregnant.[69] Pregnancy is common in adolescence and although many pregnancies are aborted, birth rates to teenagers continue to be high and appear to be on the rise rather than the decline. Between 1986 and 1991, birth rates for younger teens 15–17 years of age increased 27%, and those for older teens (18–19 years old) increased 19%.[70] In 1991 birth rates for 15–17-year-olds were 38.7 per thousand and 94.4 for 18–19-year-olds. Live birth rates in adolescents 10–14 years old did not increase as rapidly, but were 1.4 per thousand in 1991.

For adolescent pregnancies that are carried to term, nutritional considerations are paramount. Nutrient needs rise considerably during pregnancy, particularly during adolescence. Adequate food energy, calcium, and iron are of particular concern because intakes before pregnancy may have been low and needs increase as the pregnancy progresses. Childbearing in very young adolescents who may still be growing themselves, and whose social environmental circumstances are poor, is fraught with nutritional risk. Young women who are poor or otherwise disadvantaged and who conceive out of wedlock appear to be at particular risk of poor outcomes.[71] Adequate nutrition is also important when the pregnant woman is unusually physically active; some limitations may be in order if she engages in very competitive sports.

Nutritional problems of very sedentary adolescents. A major problem faced by very sedentary adolescents is the difficulty of obtaining all the needed nutrients from food sources, especially iron, copper, vitamin B-6, and zinc, at levels approximating the RDA when energy intakes are low. Second, sedentary life-styles may lead to obesity and lack of fitness, which have their own negative implications for health.

Nutritional problems of very physically active adolescents. Energy needs increase with vigorous training, especially when the activity involves moving the body and lifting. These nutrient needs may not be met because appetite may not keep up, a lean physique is required for aesthetic reasons, or because inappropriate training diets are used. The end result may be weight loss or leanness almost to the point of emaciation.

Vigorous exercise increases fluid needs, and if they are not met, there is risk of dehydration. The usual rule of thumb is 1 mL/4.184 kJ (1 mL/1 kcal) of energy needs. Adequate fluid is essential to prevent heat stress and to make up for losses in sweat. Intentional dehydration is sometimes used by athletes to "weigh in" at a lower weight and to thus gain an advantage in weight classification. Excessive sweating, limiting fluid intakes, and use of diuretics for the purpose of temporary weight loss may adversely affect performance.

If food guides such as the USDA food pyramid are followed, the likelihood is small that the diets of very active adolescents will be inadequate in nutrients, because so much food must be eaten to meet energy needs.[72] Problems more likely to develop are mineral deficiencies, particularly of iron and calcium, but these are usually confined to trained athletes engaged in competition.

Megadose vitamin and mineral use can be overdone. There is no performance advantage to taking vitamins, minerals, single amino acids, or other nutrients in levels above the RDA.

Nutritional consequences of steroid use in athletes. The use of anabolic steroids and ergogenic drugs to enhance athletic performance and body image may have adverse effects on health as well as nutrition.[73,74] The drugs are widely available and widely used. Students are aware that anabolic steroids and ergogenic drugs have negative effects, but they are often so intent on winning that the negative effects are ignored. Among the nutritional consequences of steroid use are endocrine effects, including accelerated maturation and premature closure of the epiphyses, decreased HDL (high-density-lipoprotein) and increased LDL (low-density-lipoprotein) cholesterol, hypertension, clotting abnormalities, feminization (males), and masculinization (females).[75] If short stature and cardiac damage ensue, they are not reversible. Some girls engaged in athletics use androgenic steroids to manipulate their menstrual cycles. The problem is that this may cause amenorrhea or increased serum testosterone.

At least 25% of steroid users, especially the heavy users, may become addicted. Anticipatory guidance that emphasizes the issue of decision making and problem solving works better than warnings against the side effects of steroids. Winning and appearance are two values fostered by the larger society and need less emphasis if steroid use is to decline. Random drug testing programs with penalties for drug use also help students to reconsider steroid use.

Nutrition-related amenorrhea and reproductive disorders in female athletes. As more girls participate in competitive sports and ideal body types become leaner, the incidence of various disorders of menstruation has increased.[76] Delayed menarche in athletes is not due solely to the preselection of girls with thin body types and familial late puberty; excessive training and athletic activity also play a role. Pubertal delay in females is usually defined as no pubertal changes occurring by age 13 (two standard deviations over the mean age of stage 1 of sexual maturity). The rule of thumb is that for every 1 year of extensive competitive training before menarche, menarche is delayed by 5 months. Amenorrhea is considered to be present if six or more cycles are missed after it has been established or if the individual has one period or less per year.

Delays in pubertal development are most common in thin athletes who begin training premenarcheally and do so competitively. In some fields like ballet and gymnastics, staying lean is helpful because the low body fat gives the person a greater strength-to-weight ratio. The adolescent may diet or take other steps to stay thin, delaying menarche. The ultimate nutritional effects associated with long-delayed menarche or chronic secondary amenorrhea include scoliosis and stress fractures, health hazards to avoid.[77]

Dietary factors play a part in causing secondary amenorrhea. Chief among the factors are deficient energy intakes, due either to eating less food or eating poorly planned vegetarian or very-low-fat diets that are coupled with low energy intakes. Occasionally zinc deficiency is suggested as a causative factor, but little evidence exists.[78–81] Secondary amenorrhea is not inevitable with heavy exercise (that is, exercise of >1 hour a day). There is nothing inherently harmful about exercise; problems emerge only with excessive exercise.[82]

Ballet dancers, runners, and gymnasts most often show amenorrhea and oligomenorrhea. Swimmers, cyclists, and racquetball players are less likely to do so. Competitive running (>20 miles per week) can induce amenorrhea in some women, but individual tolerance varies widely. In others, the stress of going away to camp or college, heavy training, or the consumption of unusual and inadequate diets may be involved. Low weight-for-height, lean build, or decreased body fat are signs of possible amenorrhea.

The Committee on Sports Medicine of the American Academy of Pediatrics has issued detailed advice about amenorrhea in athletes and its treatment.[83] Amenorrheic athletes within 3 years of menarche should be counseled to decrease intensity of exercise and improve their nutritional intakes, especially with respect to calcium and protein, if they are undernourished in these respects. Hormone therapy is not advised. Older, mature amenorrheic athletes (>3 years postmenarche or >16 years old) and who are hypoestrogenic may be helped by estrogen supplements, possibly with low-dose contraceptives.

All thin adolescents, even if they are menstruating, need counseling to avoid amenorrhea and stress factors, with emphasis on calcium and protein intakes. Hypoestrogenic amenorrheic athletes need very high calcium intakes (1500 mg daily), and even then they are at risk of osteoporosis.

If there is concern about bone mineral density in an adolescent female athlete, levels can now be determined relatively inexpensively with dual-emission x-ray absorptiometry (DEXA). Young women with low bone density are sometimes treated with estrogen and progesterone or oral contraceptives, and seem to gain back bone mineral density, so osteoporosis is not inevitable. However, if deficits go on too long, bone mineral levels become subnormal and cannot be restored.

Other disorders of reproductive status, including oligomenorrhea, dysmenorrhea, and failure to ovulate with irregular cycles are not amenable to manipulation through diet. Dysmenorrhea is not effectively treated by dietary measures. In some patients antiprostaglandins are helpful, and in others a congenital defect is present. Premenstrual syndrome, if accompanied by fluid retention, is not amenable to preventive or curative dietary alterations.[84] Oral contraceptives are helpful in relieving symptoms. Some young women athletes attempt to alter their menstrual cycles by the use of oral contraceptives, continuing the pill beyond 21 days for an extra 5–8 days to delay their period for a competitive event. This method is preferable to attempts to control cycles through diet or by use of steroids.

Adolescents with special needs and handicaps. The special nutritional needs of adolescents who are ill or have other handicaps are discussed elsewhere.[85] Less commonly considered are their needs for physical activity. Today, special health problems with nutritional implications are rarely a cause for excluding adolescents from sports and athletics, and there are many opportunities for adolescents with chronic diseases or disabilities to participate in sports.[86] The American Academy of Pediatrics has published guidelines to degrees of strenuousness and the potential for contact in various athletic activities.[87] Special health conditions such as diabetes mellitus may need additional nutritional adaptations for physical activity and exercise.[88] Diabetes is not a reason for exclusion, but complications such as hypoglycemia (either during exercise or several hours later) because of inadequate carbohydrate or insulin during sports participation is a risk, as is ketoacidosis if blood sugar is high before the competition. Therefore it is vital that the adolescent monitor blood sugars and keep them at 5.55–13.88 mmol/L (100–250 mg/dL), and modify eating habits, insulin, and site of injection if needed.[89] Similarly, in sickle-cell anemia particular attention must be paid to avoiding dehydration and heat stress to prevent complications such as vaso-occlusive phenomena and hemolysis. Trauma resulting from sports injuries also may alter nutritional needs secondary to enforced immobility.[90] The guiding principle today is that there is some sport that each adolescent can participate in, even those with health problems.

Vegetarianism. Vegetarianism during adolescence is relatively common.[91] It need not be a problem if eating patterns are planned carefully so that benefits of the vegetarian diet are balanced by attention to adequate intakes of energy, protein, calcium, iron, and other nutrients that are less available in plant foods.[92]

Eating disorders. Eating disorders common in adolescence include anorexia, bulimia, and bulimia nervosa. Dietary, societal, and cultural factors may increase the risk, but in essence they are psychiatric problems and are discussed extensively elsewhere.[93]

The medical complications of anorexia and bulimia are numerous, including metabolic, renal, gastroenterological, cardiovascular, pulmonary, endocrine, neurological, hematological, immunological, dental, and dermatological damage.[94] Amenorrhea is common in females, possibly from undernutrition alone, or from undernutrition in addition to underlying neurotransmitter abnormalities. The amenorrhea gives rise to both hypoestrogenemia and osteopenia.[95]

The treatment of eating disorders is essentially psychiatric; nutritional measures are adjunctive rather than curative. Treatment is difficult and often not rapidly successful. Because both nutritional as well as psychiatric issues must be addressed for a long-term cure, both mental health and nutrition professionals should be involved in the treatment.[96,97]

References

1. National Research Council (1989) Recommended dietary allowances, 10th ed. National Academy Press, Washington, DC

2. Carruth BR (1990) Adolescence. In Brown ML (ed), Present knowledge in nutrition. International Life Sciences Institute, Washington, DC, pp 325–332

3. Gong EJ, Heald FP (1988) Diet, nutrition and adolescence. In Shils ME, Young VR (eds), Modern nutrition in health and disease, 7th ed. Lea and Febiger, Philadelphia, pp 969–981

4. Congress of the United States, Office of Technology Assessment (1991) Adolescent health, vol. 1, Summary and policy options [OTA H 468]. US Government Printing Office, Washington, DC

5. Gans JE, Blyth DA, Elser AB, Gaveras LL (1990) America's adolescents: how healthy are they? American Medical Association Profiles of Adolescent Health, vol. 1. American Medical Association, Chicago

6. Rolland-Cachera MF (1993) Body composition during adolescence: methods, limitations, and determinants. Horm Res 39(suppl 3):25–40

7. Must A, Dallal GE, Dietz WH (1991) Reference data for obesity: 85th and 95th percentiles of body mass index

(wt/ht²) and triceps skinfold thickness. Am J Clin Nutr 53:839–846

8. Himes JH, Dietz WH (1994) Guidelines for overweight in adolescent preventive services: recommendations from an expert committee. Am J Clin Nutr 59:307–316

9. Anonymous (1994) Prevalence of overweight among adolescents, United States, 1988–91. MMWR 43:819–821

10. Braddon FEM, Rodgers B, Wadsworth MEJ, Davies JMC (1986) Onset of obesity in a 36 year birth cohort study. Br Med J 293:299–303

11. Must A, Jacques PF, Dallal GE, Bajema CJ, Dietz WH (1992) Long term morbidity and mortality of overweight adolescents. N Engl J Med 327:1350–1355

12. Nieto FJ, Szklo M, Comstock GW (1992) Childhood weight and growth rate as predictors of adult mortality. Am J Epidemiol 136:201–213

13. Serdula MK, Ivery D, Coates RJ, et al (1993) Do obese children become obese adults? a review of the literature. Prev Med 22:167–177

14. Bandini LG (1992) Obesity in the adolescent. Adolesc Med State Art Rev 3(3):459–472

15. Howat PM, Mohan R, Champagne C, et al (1994). Validity and reliability of reported dietary intake data. J Am Diet Assoc 94:169–173

16. Kasdoun MC, Johnson RK, Goran MI (1994) Comparison of energy intake by semiquantitative food frequency questionnaire with total energy expenditure by the doubly labeled water method in young children. Am J Clin Nutr 60:1–5

17. Lindroos AK, Lissner L, Sjostrom L (1993) Validity and reproducibility of a self administered dietary questionnaire in obese and non-obese subjects. Eur J Clin Nutr 47:461–481

18. McDowell MA, Briefel RR, Alaimo K, et al (1994) Energy and macronutrient intakes of persons ages 2 months and over in the United States: Third National Health and Nutrition Examination Survey, Phase 1, 1988–91. Advance data from vital and health statistics, no. 255. National Center for Health Statistics, Hyattsville, MD, pp 1–24

19. Alaimo K, McDowell MA, Briefel RR, et al (1994) Dietary intake of vitamins, minerals, and fiber of persons ages 2 months and over in the United States: Third National Health and Nutrition Examination Survey, Phase 1, 1988–91. Advance data from vital and health statistics, no. 258. National Center for Health Statistics, Hyattsville, MD, pp 1–4

20. Prentice AM, Lucas A, Vasquez-Velasquez L, et al (1988) Are current dietary guidelines for young children a prescription for overfeeding? Lancet 2:1066–1068

21. Fontvielle AM, Harper IT, Spraul M, Ravusin E (1993) Daily energy expenditure by five year old children measured by doubly labeled water. J Pediatr 123:200–207

22. Bandini LG, Schoeller DA, Dietz WH (1990) Energy expenditure in obese and nonobese adolescents. Pediatr Res 27:198–203

23. Wong WW (1994) Energy expenditure of female adolescents. J Am Coll Nutr 13:332–337

24. Roberts SB, Vinken AG (1995) Energy and substrate regulation in obesity. In Walker WA (ed), Nutrition in pediatrics. Neville Press, Charlestown, SC

25. Molnar D, Varga P, Rubecz I, et al (1985) Food induced thermogenesis in obese children. Eur J Pediatr 144:27–31

26. Bandini LG, Schoeller DA, Edwards J, et al (1989) Energy expenditure during carbohydrate overfeeding in obese and nonobese adolescents. Am J Physiol 256:E357–E367

27. Maffeis C, Schutz Y, Pinelli L (1992) Postprandial thermogenesis in obese children before and after weight reduction. Eur J Clin Nutr 46:577–583

28. Segal KR, Lacayanga I, Dunaif A, et al (1989) Impact of body

fat mass and percent fat on metabolic rate and thermogenesis in men. Am J Physiol 256:E573–E579

29. Stefanik PA, Heald FP, Mayer J (1959) Caloric intake in relation to energy output of obese and nonobese adolescent boys. Am J Clin Nutr 7:55–62

30. Wilkinson PW, Pearlson J, Parkin J, et al (1977) Obesity in childhood: a community study in Newcastle upon Tyne. Lancet 350–352

31. Klesges RC, Shelton ML, Klesges LM (1993) Effects of television on metabolic rate: potential implications for childhood obesity. Pediatrics 91:28l–286

32. Wolf AM, Gortmaker SL, Cheung L, et al (1993) Activity, inactivity and obesity: racial, ethnic and age differences among schoolgirls. Am J Public Health 83:1625–1627

33. Waxman M, Stunkard AJ (1980) Caloric intake and expenditure of obese boys. J Pediatr 96:187–193

34. Berkowitz RI, Agras WS, Korner AF, et al (1985) Physical activity and adiposity: a longitudinal study from birth to childhood. J Pediatr 106:734–738

35. Unnegardh J, Bratteby LE, Hagma U, Samuelson G (1986) Physical activity in relation to energy intake and body fat in 8 and 13 year old children in Sweden. Acta Paediatr Scand 75:955–963

36. Eck LH, Klesges RC, Hanson CL, Slawson D (1992) Children at familial risk for obesity: an examination of dietary intake, physical activity and weight status. Int J Obes 16:71–78

37. Gazzaniga JM, Burns TL (1993) Relationship between diet composition and body fatness with adjustment for resting energy expenditure and physical activity in preadolescent children. Am J Clin Nutr 58:21–28

38. Goran MI, Carpenter WH, Poehlman ET (1993) Total energy expenditure in 4–6 yr old children. Am J Physiol 264:E706–E711

39. Schoeller DA, Fjeld C (1991) What have we learned from the doubly labeled water method? Annu Rev Nutr 11:355–375

40. Roberts SB, Heyman MB, Evans WJ, et al (1991) Dietary energy requirements of young adult men determined by using the doubly labeled water method. Am J Clin Nutr 54:499–505

41. Dwyer JT (1991) Nutrition and fitness problems: prevention and services. In Office of Technology Assessment, Congress of the United States. Adolescent health, vol. II: Background and the effectiveness of selected prevention and treatment services [OTA H 466]. U.S. Government Printing Office, Washington, DC, pp 193–228

42. Raunikar RA, Strong WB (1991) The status of adolescent physical fitness. Adolesc Med State Art Rev 2(1):65–76

43. Dwyer JT (1981) Nutritional requirements of adolescence. Nutr Rev 31(2):56–72

44. Dietz WH, Gortmaker SL (1985) Do we fatten our children at the television set? obesity and television viewing in children and adolescents. Pediatrics 75:807–812

45. Robinson TN, Hammer LD, Killen JD, et al (1993) Does television viewing increase obesity and reduce physical activity? cross sectional and longitudinal analyses among adolescent girls. Pediatrics 91:273–280

46. Dyment PG, ed (1991) Sports and the adolescent. Adolesc Med State Art Rev 2(1):1–251

47. Marriott BM, ed, and Committee on Military Nutrition Research, Food and Nutrition Board (1994) Fluid replacement and heat stress. National Academy Press, Washington, DC

48. Marriott BM, ed, and Committee on Military Nutrition Research, Food and Nutrition Board (1993) Nutritional needs in hot environments: applications for military personnel in field operations. National Academy Press, Washington, DC

49. Meredith CN, Frontera WR (1992) Adolescent fitness. Adolesc Med State Art Rev 3(3):391–404

50. Joint Nutrition Monitoring Evaluation Committee (1986) Nutrition monitoring in the United States: a progress report from the Joint Nutrition Monitoring Evaluation Committee [DHHS publication no. 86-1255]. US Department of Health and Human Services and US Department of Agriculture, Washington, DC

51. National Adolescent Student Survey (1988) Highlights of the survey. Health Educ, Aug/Sept, pp 4–8

52. Pugliese M, Recker B, Lifshitz F (1988) A survey to determine the prevalence of abnormal growth patterns in adolescents. J Adolesc Health Care 9:181–187

53. Meredith CN, Dwyer JT (1991) Nutrition and exercise: effects on adolescent health. Annu Rev Public Health 12:309–33

54. Herzog DM, Copeland PM (1985) Eating disorders. N Engl J Med 313(5):295–303

55. Booth IW (1991) The nutritional consequences of gastrointestinal disease in adolescence. Acta Pediatr Scand Suppl 373:91–102

56. Story M, Heald F, Dwyer JT (1990) Adolescent nutrition: trends and critical issues for the 1990's. In Sharbaugh CN, Egan MC (eds) Call to action: better health for mothers and children. National Center for Maternal and Child Health, Washington, DC, pp 281–317

57. US Department of Agriculture, US Department of Health and Human Services (1989) Dietary guidelines for Americans, 4th ed. US Government Printing Office, Washington, DC

58. Reed DA, Mickle SJ, Tippett KS (1994) Diets of school age children 1989–90. Survey notes: nationwide food surveys. US Department of Agriculture, Hyattsville, MD, p 7

59. National Institutes of Health, National Cholesterol Education Program (1991) Report of the Expert Panel on Blood Cholesterol Levels in Children and Adolescents [NIH Publication No. 91-2732]. US Department of Health and Human Services, Public Health Service, Washington, DC

60. Task Force on Blood Pressure Control in Children (1987) Report of the Second Task Force on Blood Pressure Control in Children. Pediatrics 79:1–25

61. Matkovic V (1992) Calcium and peak bone mass. J Intern Med 231:151

62. Chan GM (1991) Dietary calcium and bone mineral status of children and adolescents. Am J Dis Child 145: 631

63. Sandler RB, Slemenda CW, LaPorte RE, et al (1985) Postmenopausal bone density and milk consumption in childhood and adolescence. Am J Clin Nutr 42:270

64. Fehily AM, Coles RJ, Evans WD, Elwood PC (1992). Factors affecting bone density in young adults. Am J Clin Nutr 56:579

65. Office of Disease Prevention and Health Promotion, Public Health Service (1994) Prevention '93: federal programs and progress. US Department of Health and Human Services, US Government Printing Office, Washington, DC, p 17

66. Office of the Assistant Secretary for Health (1988) Surgeon General's report on nutrition and health. US Government Printing Office, Washington, DC

67. Committee on Diet and Health (1989) Diet and health: implications for reducing chronic degenerative disease risk. National Academy Press, Washington, DC

68. McBean LD (1995) Child and adolescent nutrition: nutrient adequacy and a low fat diet. In Miller GD, Jarvis JK, McBean LD (eds), Handbook of dairy foods and nutrition. CRC Press, Boca Raton, FL, pp 223–254

69. Rees JM, Lederman SA (1992) Nutrition for the pregnant adolescent. Adolesc Med State Art Rev 3(3):439–458

70. National Center for Health Statistics (1994) Health United States 1993. Public Health Service, Hyattsville, MD, pp 11, 64

71. McAnarney ER (1987) Young maternal age and adverse neonatal outcome. Am J Dis Child 141:1053–1059

72. US Department of Agriculture (1992) The food guide pyramid [publication HG252]. Human Nutrition Information Service, Hyattsville, MD

73. Foldy JD, Schydlower M (1993) Anabolic steroid and ergogenic drug use by adolescents. In Schydlower M, Rogers PD (eds), Adolescent substance abuse and addictions. Adolesc Med State Art Rev 4(2):341–352

74. Soderstrom CA, Dearing-Stuck BA (1993) Substance misuse and trauma: clinical issues and injury prevention in adolescents. In Schydlower M, Rogers PD (eds), Adolescent substance abuse and addictions. Adolesc Med State Art Rev 4(2):423–438

75. Johnson MD (1991) Steroids. Adolesc Med State Art Rev 2(3l):79–92

76. Gidwani GP (1991) The athlete and menstruation. Adolesc Med State Art Rev 2(1):27–46

77. Warren MP, Brooks Gunn J, Hamilton LH, et al (1986) Scoliosis and fractures in young ballet dancers. N Engl J Med 314:1348–1353

78. Deuster PA, Kylem SB, Moster PB, et al (1986) Nutritional intakes and status of highly trained amenorrheic and eumenorrheic women runners. Fertil Steril 46:636–643

79. Marcus R, Cann C, Mading P, et al (1985) Menstrual function and bone mass in elite women distance runners. Ann Intern Med 102:158–163

80. Pirke KM, Schewiger U, Laessle W (1986) Dieting influences the menstrual cycle: vegetarian versus nonvegetarian diet. Fertil Steril 46:1083

81. Drinkwater BL, Nelson K, Chestnut CH III, et al (1984) Bone mineral content of amenorrheic and eumenorrheic athletes. N Engl J Med 311:277–281

82. Wilson C, Emans SJ, Mansfield J, et al (1984) The relationship of calculated percent body fat, sports participation, age, and place of residence on menstrual patterns in healthy adolescent girls at an independent New England high school. J Adolesc Health Care 5:248–253

83. Committee of Sports Medicine (1989) Recommendations: American Academy of Pediatrics. Pediatrics 2:394–396

84. Casey V, Dwyer JT (1987) Premenstrual syndrome: theories and evidence. Nutr Today, November-December, pp 4–12

85. Suskind RM, ed (1981) Textbook of pediatric nutrition. Raven Press, New York

86. Nelson MA (1991) Medical exclusion from sport. Adolesc Med State Art Rev 2(1):13–26

87. Committee on Sports Medicine (1988) Recommendations for participation in competitive sports: American Academy of Pediatrics. Pediatrics 81:737–739

88. Friedenberge GR, Orr DP (1993) Adolescents with insulin dependent diabetes. In Ludwig S, Jay MS (eds) Emergency care of adolescents. Adolesc Med State Art Rev 4(1):115–148

89. Horton ES (1989) Exercise and diabetes in youth. In Gisolfi CV, Lamb DR (eds), Perspectives in exercise science and sports medicine: youth exercise and sport. Benchmark Press, Carmel, IN, pp 539–574

90. Schwarz D (1993) Adolescent trauma: epidemiologic approach. In Ludwig S, Jay MS (eds), Emergency care of adolescents. Adolesc Med State Art Rev 4(1):11–22

91. Johnston PK, Haddad E, Sabate J (1992) Adolesc Med State Art Rev 3(3):417–438

92. Dwyer JT, Loew FM (1994) Nutritional risks of vegan diets to women and children: are they preventable? J Agric Environ Ethics 7(1):87–109

93. Nussbaum MP, Dwyer JT, eds (1992) Adolescent nutrition and eating disorders. Adolesc Med State Art Rev 3(3):377–559

94. Fisher M (1992) Medical complications of anorexia and bulimia nervosa. Adolesc Med State Art Rev 3(3):487–502

95. Golden NH, Shenker IR (1992) Amenorrhea in anorexia nervosa: etiology and implications. Adolesc Med State Art Rev 3(3):503–518

96. Kreipe RE, Uphof M (1992) Treatment and outcome of adolescents with anorexia nervosa. Adolesc Med State Art Rev 3(3):519–540

97. Schebendach J, Nussbaum MP (1992) Nutrition management in adolescents with eating disorders. Adolesc Med State Art Rev 3(3):541–558

Chapter 40

Aging and Nutrition

Philip J. Garry and Bruno J. Vellas

Life expectancy at birth in the United States is now 75.4 years, compared with about 47 years at the beginning of this century.[1] The average age and the proportion of the older population are also increasing. Individuals over age 65 now comprise 12% of the population, compared with 4% in 1900. This percentage is expected to rise to 20.1% by the year 2030. According to projections from the U.S. Census Bureau,[1] the population over age 65 will be approximately 60 million by the middle of the 21st century. This increased life expectancy for older Americans is resulting in an even more rapid growth of the population over age 85, increasing sixfold to 18 million.

The lack of a satisfactory definition of "old" is a problem. When does one become old? Clearly, physiological age is not the same as chronological age. On the other hand, numerous attempts to determine a simple and accurate indicator of physiological age have not yet yielded a satisfactory instrument. When using simple chronological cutoffs, one must remember that there is tremendous heterogeneity within the populations over 65, over 75, and over 85. However, the term "older" generally refers to individuals over age 65.

Aging is a complex phenomenon that includes molecular, cellular, physiological, and psychological changes.[2] Health problems and physiological decline develop gradually, and partly result from a lifetime of poor health habits. Direct effects from the aging process seem to be less important than previously reported, and some very old individuals can stay healthy with good nutritional status. However, year after year an increasing proportion of elderly persons become frail, with some diminution of visual function, increase of cognitive impairments, or gait and balance disorders that affect mobility and may decrease an old person's ability to purchase and prepare food. Moreover, decrease of appetite due to decreased physical activity, dental and oral problems, or mood disorders with increased age results in overall lower energy intake, which can lead to lowered intakes of essential nutrients. At this stage, the elderly often show a rapid decline of health and nutritional status resulting from stress and loss of independence.

Assessing dietary intakes against some standard, for example, the recommended dietary allowances,[3] may help to identify individuals at risk for malnutrition. However, it should be remembered that the recommended dietary allowances were established for healthy persons, not taking into account the presence of chronic disease, handicap, or acute illnesses often present in elderly persons.[4]

Even in presumably healthy elderly individuals, deficiencies have been reported for vitamin B-6 (low intake and higher requirements for the elderly), vitamins B-12 and folate (low intakes and malabsorption), vitamin D (lack of exposure to sunlight, low intakes, age-related decreased synthesis), calcium (low intake), and zinc (low intake related to low energy intakes).[5] In clinical practice, dietary requirements for the elderly should be based on the following health categories: 1) healthy elderly persons, for whom the requirements are similar to young adults (with the exception of vitamin D and calcium); 2) acutely ill elderly persons, with increased requirements in response to hypercatabolism due to the stress of an acute or chronic illness (e.g., Alzheimer's disease); and 3) frail elderly persons who have poor appetites, low dietary intake, and an increased need for specific nutrients.[5]

As noted, aging is accompanied by a variety of physiological, psychological, economic, and social changes that may compromise nutritional status. In recent years there have been a number of book chapters summarizing age-related physiological, psychological, and socioeconomic changes that can influence nutritional status of older individuals.[6-9]

The 1988 Surgeon General's Workshop on Health Promotion and Aging addressed nutrition and aging issues.[10] The workshop report regarding nutrition and aging was based on the premise that "good nutritional status is essential for a high quality of life and food contributes to the quality of life through psychological, social, as well as physical mechanisms." The workshop report identified key scientific issues that need to be addressed, and examples in each of these areas are briefly reviewed in this chapter. These issues are effects of aging on nutritional status, evaluation of the nutritional status of the older population, and effects of nutritional deficiencies on the older population.

Effects of Aging on Nutritional Status

Both cross-sectional and longitudinal studies, showing mean values for cohorts, seem to indicate that many organ functions and metabolic parameters decline with age, as does the dietary intake for most nutrients. However, if one follows individual subjects longitudinally, a number of elderly subjects show no decline in functional status with age. Thus, one needs to separate "successful" aging from "usual" aging. In other words, what has been described in cross-sectional and longitudinal studies to date is "usual" aging, incorporating the effects of pathology and life-style (diet, exercise, smoking and drinking habits, and psychosocial events). Selected individuals, especially those free of risk factors such as smoking, hypertension, diabetes, or hyperlipidemia, may show little or no change in organ function with age. It has been suggested that there is a need to examine more carefully what determines "successful" aging so that this kind of life-style and disease prevention can be advocated and promoted. This approach to a longitudinal study with careful analysis of differences in nutritional status and life-style may help to identify those factors that predispose to decreases in organ function and impairment of metabolic functions.

Changes in dietary intakes and plasma lipids with age were studied in a group of healthy elderly men ($n = 65$) and women ($n = 92$) enrolled in the New Mexico Aging Process Study.[11] Dietary intakes and blood lipid levels were assessed in elderly men and women over a 9-year period, 1980–1989. Mean age in 1980 was 70 years (range, 60–84). Energy intakes per kilogram body weight showed no cross-sectional association with age in the men, suggesting that current weight, rather than age, determined energy intakes. Protein intake per kilogram, as well as fat, cholesterol, and carbohydrate intakes, showed slight and statistically insignificant decreases with age. Findings for women were similar.

In contrast, longitudinal analyses showed significant changes in dietary intake over the 9-year period. In the women, there were significant decreases in total fat and cholesterol consumption over time. In the men, in addition to decreases in fat intake, there were decreases in energy and protein intakes, whether expressed as absolute consumption or per kilogram body weight. The decreases in energy intakes did not result in changes in weight, implying that the decreases were balanced by decreases in physical activity or changes in body composition, or both. No significant changes over time were detected in energy or protein intake per kilogram body weight in the women; however, in contrast to the men, there were significant decreases in weight.

There were significant decreases in total, high-density lipoprotein, and low-density lipoprotein plasma cholesterol levels over time in both men and women.

The decreases in total fat and cholesterol intakes were significantly correlated with decreases in total plasma cholesterol.

The finding of longitudinal but not cross-sectional differences indicates that temporal trends, rather than age per se, were primarily responsible for the dietary changes noted over time in this healthy elderly population. The dietary trends noted in this study were probably the result of national educational efforts to reduce the morbidity and mortality associated with coronary heart disease by reducing fat intake. The medical significance of these changes in healthy elderly persons with a low prevalence of other risk factors is unclear.

Evaluation of the Nutritional Status of the Older Population

In the past two decades, a number of geriatric assessment instruments have been developed to diagnose and treat high-risk elderly patients. However, too little attention has been given to identifying those elderly patients who would benefit from early detection of undernutrition. At the present time, the major components of a good geriatric assessment include four major domains—physical health, functional ability, psychological health, and socioenvironmental factors—comprising several subdomains.[12] As noted by Rubenstein,[12] use of the following well-validated instruments that encompass the major assessment domains makes the geriatric assessment more reliable and considerably easier: activities of daily living,[13] instrumental activities of daily living,[14] mini–mental-state examination,[15] geriatric depression scale,[16] Tinetti[17] balance and gait evaluation, and nutritional examination.

Assessing the nutritional status of the older population requires clinical studies to evaluate physical signs of nutritional health or disease, dietary studies to evaluate nutrient intakes with accepted standards, and laboratory investigations to provide data about quantities of particular nutrients in the body or to evaluate certain biochemical functions that depend on an adequate supply of a particular nutrient. Because use of a single measure is rarely sufficient to establish the level of malnutrition in a population, nutritional assessment is best accomplished using a combination of these methods. The greater the number of measurements outside the standard range, the more likely a population is to suffer from poor nutritional status.

Use of valid and reliable instruments to assess nutritional status has, for the most part, been absent from most geriatric assessment programs. The most challenging problem for physicians and other health care providers in geriatric medicine today is to identify those elderly persons who would benefit from dietary intervention, realizing that not every elderly individual seen in a geriatric clinic, hospital, or nursing home needs to have a battery of anthropometric, dietary, and laboratory tests to assess nutritional status.

Until recently, no instruments to evaluate nutritional status have been available. The "Public Awareness Checklist" was developed within the context of the U.S. Nutrition Screening Initiative.[18,19] Its purpose is to increase public awareness of malnutrition in the elderly population and help identify individuals at risk of nutritional problems.[18,20] The checklist used the mnemonic "DETERMINE" to convey basic nutritional information and help users recall the major risk factors and indicators of poor nutritional status. The checklist is not intended to be used as a diagnostic device but rather as an indicator of high risk. Subjects who score poorly on this self-administered instrument are encouraged to take the checklist with them the next time they visit their physicians, dietitians, or other health care providers.

The screening initiative for this checklist is completed by a two-level approach by professionals. Level I is completed by a social service or health care professional, and level II is completed by a physician or other qualified health professional. The purpose is to screen for persons at risk of malnutrition or with poor nutritional status.[19] Level I is used to collect data on weight and weight change, diet, and functional status to refer the person to the appropriate health care professional. Level II is used to collect the same type of data, with use of anthropometric and laboratory data to assess the underlying problem responsible for malnutrition.

To assess nutritional status as part of a geriatric evaluation in elderly patients in clinics, nursing homes, hospitals, or those who are otherwise frail, a single and rapid nutritional assessment, the Mini Nutritional Assessment (MNA), was recently designed and validated.[21] The aim of the MNA is to evaluate the risk of malnutrition to permit early nutritional intervention when needed, without necessitating a specialized nutritional team. The following requirements were considered in developing the test: a reliable scale, definition of thresholds, compatible with the skills of a generalist assessor, minimal bias introduced by the data collector, acceptable to patients, and inexpensive. The MNA instrument is composed of simple measurements and questions to be completed in less than 15 minutes. It includes the following items: anthropometric measurements (weight, height, and weight loss), global assessment (six questions related to life-style, medication, and mobility), dietary questionnaire (six questions related to number of meals, food and fluid intake, and autonomy of feeding), and subjective assessment (self-perception of health and nutrition).

A study designed to evaluate the discrimination potential of the MNA was performed on 155 subjects recruited in the Geriatric Evaluation Unit at the University of Toulouse, France.[21] Besides having the MNA administered, a complete nutritional assessment was made using anthropometric and biochemical markers, as well as a dietary intake and functional geriatric assessment (mini–mental-state examination, activities and instrumental acitivities of daily living). Complementary studies were completed in 350 elderly persons from the New Mexico Aging Process Study.[11] A further study was conducted in another 120 elderly persons from the Toulouse Geriatric Evaluation Unit to study change in MNA over a 3-month period in healthy, frail, and sick elderly subjects.[21]

Discriminant analysis was used to test the MNA by comparing it with the nutritional status classifications set by physicians, using extensive nutritional assessment with complete anthropometric, clinical, biological, and dietary parameters, which served as the nutritional "gold standard." In the Toulouse study, few subjects (2.2%) were misclassified, with 0.8% changing nutritional status from well nourished to malnourished, and 1.4% changing from malnourished to well nourished. Principal component analysis showed that the MNA, even without clinical biochemistry, could be used to screen for nutritional status. In the second Toulouse study, 75% of the elderly were classified as well nourished or undernourished in agreement with the "gold standard," while 25% were assessed as at risk of malnutrition.

The sum of the scores of each part of the MNA (anthropometric, dietary, global, and subjective assessments) distinguishes elderly patients with adequate nutrition from those at risk of malnutrition or those who are frankly malnourished. The MNA instrument is based on the following point system, with a score of 30 being the maximum: ≥ 24 points, at no risk for malnutrition; 17–23.5 points, at risk for malnutrition; <17 points, malnourished.

In conclusion, early detection of malnutrition is very important because it is difficult to correct a person's nutritional status once it has deteriorated. The MNA appears to be a practical, noninvasive instrument allowing for rapid screening of the nutritional status of frail elderly persons. Nutritional assessment using the MNA can easily be completed by health professionals at hospital entry, entry into nursing homes, or by physicians for early detection of risks of malnutrition.

Effects of Nutritional Deficiencies on the Older Population

A number of studies have indicated a high risk of vitamin deficiencies in older persons on the basis of low dietary intakes, but such deficiencies are not always confirmed by biochemical or clinical studies.[22] In addition, interpretation of biochemical parameters is hampered by lack of data on normal standards for the older population.[23] For example, the New Mexico Aging Process

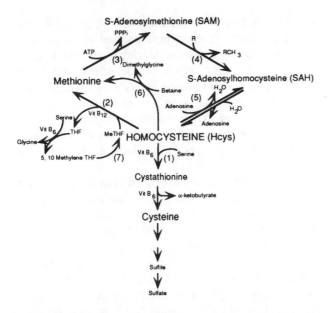

Figure 1. The generation of homocysteine. THF, tetrahydrofolate. See text for details of numbers in parentheses.

Study revealed that more than one-fourth of the older population consumed less than 75% of the recommended dietary allowances for folate and vitamins B-6 and B-12 from diet alone.[24] However, measurement of these vitamins in the blood failed to confirm that these individuals were at risk for developing clinical symptoms associated with low intakes of these vitamins, based on standard cutoff values for plasma levels of these vitamins.[25] This raises a question concerning the sensitivity and specificity of these measurements to detect vitamin deficiencies in elderly subjects, especially folate and vitamin B-12. Some investigators have shown that levels of amino acid metabolites, namely, homocysteine and methylmalonic acid, in serum may be better indicators of folate and vitamins B-6 and B-12 deficiency states than vitamin levels themselves.[26]

As pointed out in a recent review by Selhub and Miller[27] on the pathogenesis of homocysteinemia, the renewed interest in this condition has been spurred by the recognition that moderate homocysteinemia is associated with vascular disease. Elevated plasma homocysteine has been recognized for years as a risk factor for vascular disease, since individuals with homocysteinuria, due to cystathionine β-synthase deficiency, develop premature atherosclerosis and vascular thromboses.[28] Cystathionine β-synthase deficiency is an inherited autosomal recessive disease; approximately 50% of individuals with this condition benefit from large doses of pyridoxine. Homocysteine plasma concentrations are increased in vitamin B-6, folate, and vitamin B-12 deficiency states, while increased methylmalonic acid occurs in vitamin B-12 but not folate deficiency. Thus, the measurement of these two me-

tabolites can distinguish between deficiencies due to vitamin B-12 and folate.

Figure 1 outlines the important pathways in the generation of homocysteine. Homocysteine is the substrate for cystathione β-synthase leading to the formation of cystathionine and cysteine (reaction 1 in Figure 2). Cystathione β-synthase is a pyridoxal 5-phosphate (vitamin B-6)-dependent enzyme condensing homocysteine with serine, thereby forming cystathionine and leading ultimately to sulfite and sulfate. This pathway is generally known as the transsulfuration pathway. Homocysteine is also converted to methionine by methionine synthase, a vitamin B-12–dependent enzyme (reaction 2). The methionine synthase reaction also requires 5-methyltetrahydrofolate (5-MeTHF), which is converted to tetrahydrofolate. In vitamin B-12 deficiency, 5-MeTHF becomes trapped because methionine synthase is the only reaction that can convert 5-MeTHF to tetrahydrofolate. This can result in a shutdown of other metabolic reactions requiring folate, since 5-MeTHF is not in metabolic equilibrium with other forms of folate unless it transfers its methyl group to methionine.

Part of the problem also rests with the fact that the 5,10-methylene tetrahydrofolate reductase reaction, which synthesizes 5-MeTHF from 5,10-methylene tetrahydrofolate, is irreversible (Reaction 7). Methionine is converted to S-adenosylmethionine by adenosyltransferase (reaction 3). S-adenosylmethionine participates in over 100 methyl transfer reactions by a variety of methyltransferases, with S-adenosylhomocysteine (SAH) being the other product of these reactions (reaction 4). The SAH is hydrolyzed by SAH hydrolase to homocysteine. This reaction is reversible, and the equilibrium constant favors the formation of SAH. Because of the low levels of homocysteine due to shunting of homocysteine to methionine by methionine synthase, and because approximately 50% of the homocysteine formed is diverted into the transsulfuration pathway, the low levels of homocysteine allow the SAH hydrolase reaction to favor the formation of homocysteine. Homocysteine can also be

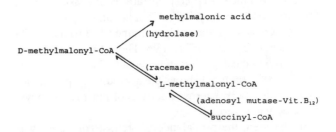

Figure 2. The generation of methylmalonic acid.

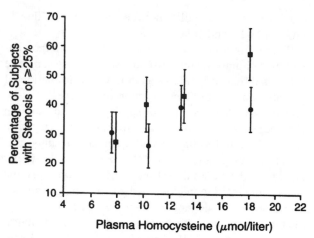

Figure 3. Age-adjusted prevalence of maximal extracranial carotid artery stenosis of ≥25% in men (■) and women (●), according to the quartile of plasma homocysteine concentration. The bars indicate the 95% confidence intervals. The quartiles of homocysteine concentration were ≤9.1, 9.2–11.3, 11.4–14.3, and ≥14.4 μmol/L. The prevalence is plotted at the sex-specific median concentration for each quartile. (Test for linear tread, $P < 0.001$ for men and $P = 0.03$ for women). Reprinted with permission from reference 29.

re-methylated by the enzyme betaine:homocysteine methyltransferase to methionine (reaction 6). It is thought that this enzyme is incapable of converting excess homocysteine formed under abnormal conditions because of its limited tissue distribution. In vitamin B-12 deficiency, L-methylmalonyl-CoA accumulates due to the inability of the adenosyl mutase, a vitamin B-12–dependent enzyme, to convert it to succinyl-CoA, which can then enter the Krebs cycle. As L-methylmalonyl-CoA builds up, it is shunted back to D-methylmalonyl-CoA, which is hydrolyzed to methylmalonic acid. Figure 2 shows the generation of methylmalonic acid.

Although it is not possible to review all of the literautre linking slightly elevated homocysteine levels with risk of vascular disease, several recent studies will be briefly reviewed because they deal specifically with older individuals.

In the study by Selhub et al.,[29] the relation between carotid artery stenosis, as assessed by ultrasonography, and plasma concentrations of homocysteine was examined in the Framingham Heart Study cohort. The investigators also measured concentrations of plasma folate, vitamin B-12, and pyridoxal-5'-phosphate (vitamin B-6). This cross-sectional study examined 418 men and 623 women between ages 67 and 96. The subjects were classified into two categories: stenosis of 0–24% and stenosis of 25–100%. Figure 3 shows the age-adjusted prevalence of stenosis (≥25%) across quartiles of plasma homocysteine concentration.

In the men, the prevalence of stenosis of ≥25% was 27% in the lowest homocysteine quartile and 58% in the highest quartile. In the women, the prevalence of stenosis

of ≥25% in the lowest quartile was 31% and 39% in the highest quartile. Twenty-nine percent of the subjects examined had homocysteine levels greater than 14 μmol/L, the upper limit of normal as determined by the authors. Plasma homocysteine levels were highest in subjects with the lowest plasma levels of folic acid, vitamin B-12, or vitamin B-6. Plasma concentrations of folate and vitamin B-6 were inversely associated with carotid artery stenosis after adjustment for age, sex, and other risk factors.

In 1993, Selhub et al.[30] examined plasma homocysteine levels in the same Framingham population as noted in the study just discussed. They also measured plasma levels of folic acid, vitamins B-12 and B-6, and dietary intakes of these vitamins. Homocysteine levels were highest in individuals with the lowest plasma levels of the three vitamins. Also, plasma homocysteine levels were inversely related to dietary intakes of folate and vitamin B-6, but not vitamin B-12. Lowest levels of homocysteine were achieved when daily intakes of folate approached 400 μg.

In the New Mexico Aging Process Study, variables affecting serum homocysteine were examined in 100 elderly volunteers, aged 68–96, who were consuming or not consuming self-selected supplements of three vitamins (folate and vitamins B-12 and B-6).[31] Compared with the nonsupplemented group, the supplemented group had lower mean serum metabolites (homocysteine and methylmalonic acid) and higher serum vitamin B-12 and serum and erythrocyte folate. A stepwise linear regression model for serum homocysteine explained 61.7% of the variance, and included (in order) serum creatinine, folate, vitamin B-12, albumin, age, and body mass index. Folate did not enter the model for supplemented subjects, supporting the existence of a "threshold effect." Serum homocysteine was inversely related to serum folate in subjects with lower serum folate (nonsupplemented subjects), but at higher serum folate (supplemented subjects) the relationship was flat. These elderly volunteers had generally good folate status. However, improvement in folate status of some subjects might reduce serum homocysteine to within the normal range, provided they do not have a vitamin B-12 deficiency or renal insufficiency.

In summary, since coronary artery disease remains a leading cause of morbidity and mortality in older adults, it remains to be seen whether regular use of vitamin supplements will result in a reduction in serum homocysteine and whether this, in turn, will reduce the incidence of coronary artery disease in this population.

In this chapter we examined some data from recently published studies that address key nutritional research issues related to ongoing attempts to understand how aging affects nutritional status, and vice versa. Research in these areas is necessary to improve the quality of life for older individuals. The key to improving the quality of life for older individuals is a better understanding of the aging process and an ability to identify those individuals whose health status can be improved by nutritional intervention.

References

1. US Bureau of the Census (1994) Statistical abstract of the United States: 1994, 114th ed. US Government Printing Office, Washington, DC

2. Munro HN (1988) Aging. In Kinney JM, Jeejeebhoy KN, Hill GL, Owen OE (eds), Nutrition and metabolism in patient care. WB Saunders, Philadelphia, pp 145–166.

3. National Research Council (1989) Recommended dietary allowances, 10th ed. National Academy Press, Washington, DC

4. Rudman D (1989) Nutrition and fitness in the elderly. Am J Clin Nutr 49:1090–1098

5. Guigoz Y (1994) Recommended dietary allowances (RDA) for the free living elderly. In Facts and research in gerontology (supplement on nutrition and aging). Springer Publishing Co, New York, pp 113–143

6. Department of Health and Human Services (1988) Nutrition and aging. In The Surgeon General's report on nutrition and health. Publication no. 88-50210, DHHS (PHS). Washington, DC, pp 595–627

7. Garry PJ, Hunt WC (1986) Biochemical assessment of vitamin status in the elderly: effects of dietary and supplemental intakes. In Hutchinson M, Munro HN (eds), Nutrition and aging. Academic Press, New York, pp 117–137

8. Koehler KM, Garry PJ (1993) Nutrition and aging. In Labbe RF (ed), Clinics in laboratory medicine: nutrition support. Laboratory management: thoughts on quality for pathology, vol 13. WB Saunders, Philadelphia, pp 433–453

9. Smiciklas-Wright H (1989) Aging. In Present knowledge in nutrition, 6th ed. International Life Sciences Institute, Washington, DC, pp 333–340

10. US Department of Health and Human Services (1988) Surgeon General's workshop on health promotion and aging. DHHS, Washington, DC

11. Garry PJ, Hunt WC, Koehler KM, VanderJagt DJ, Vellas BJ (1992) Longitudinal study of dietary intakes and plasma lipids in healthy elderly men and women. Am J Clin Nutr 55:682–688

12. Rubenstein LZ (1990) Assessment instruments. In Abrams WB, Berkow R (eds), The Merck manual of geriatrics. Merck Sharp & Dohme Research Laboratories, Division of Merck & Co, Rahway, NJ, pp 1189–1200

13. Katz S, Downs TD, Cash HR, et al (1970) Progress in the development of the index of ADL. Gerontology 1:20–30

14. Lawton MP, Brody EM (1969) Assessment of older people: self-monitoring and instrumental activities of daily living. Gerontologist 9:179–186

15. Folstein MF, Folstein S, McHuth PR (1975) Mini-mental state: a practical method for grading the cognitive state of patients for the clinician. J Psychiatr Res 12:189–198

16. Yesavage J, Brink T, RoseT, et al (1983) Development and validation of a geriatric depression screening scale: a preliminary report. J Psychiatr Res 17:37–49

17. Tinetti ME (1986) Performance-oriented assessment of mobility problems in the elderly. J Am Geriatr Soc 36:613–616

18. Nutrition Screening Initiative (1991) Report of nutrition screening, 1: toward a common view. Nutrition Screening Initiative, Washington, DC

19. Posner BM, Jette AM, Smith KW, Miller DR (1993) Nutrition and health risks in the elderly: the nutrition screening initiative. Am J Public Health 83:972–978

20. Rush D (1993) Evaluating the nutrition screening initiative [editor's note]. Am J Public Health 83:944–945

21. Guigoz Y, Vellas BJ, Garry PJ (1994) Mini nutritional assessment: a practical assessment tool for grading the nutritional state of elderly patients. In Facts and research in gerontology (supplement on nutrition and aging). Springer Publishing Co, New York, pp 15–59

22. Garry PJ, Hunt WC (1986) Biochemical assessment of vitamin status in the elderly: effects of dietary and supplemental intakes. Bristol-Myers Nutrition Symposia, 1986. In Nutrition and aging, vol. 5, ed. Hutchinson M and Munro HN. Academic, Orlando, FL

23. Kirsch A, Bidlack WR (1987) Nutrition and the elderly: vitamin status and efficacy of supplementation. Nutrition 3:305–314

24. Garry PJ, Goodwin JS, Hunt WC, et al (1982) Nutritional status in a healthy elderly population: dietary and supplemental intakes. Am J Clin Nutr 36:319–331

25. Garry PJ, Goodwin JS, Hunt WC (1984) Folate and vitamin B-12 status in a healthy elderly population. J Am Geriatr Soc 32:719–726

26. Lindenbaum J, Rosenberg IH, Wilson PWF, Stabler SP, Allen RH (1994) Prevalence of cobalamin deficiency in the Framingham elderly population. Am J Clin Nutr 60:2–11

27. Selhub J, Miller JW (1992) The pathogenesis of homocysteinemia: interruption of the coordinate regulation by S-adenosylmethionine of the remethylation and transsulfuration of homocysteine. Am J Clin Nutr 55:131–138

28. Mudd SH, Skovby F, Levy HL, et al (1985) The natural history of homocysteinura due to cystathionine B-synthase deficiency. Am J Hum Genet 37:1–31

29. Selhub J, Jacques PF, Bostom AG, et al (1995) Association between plasma homocysteine concentrations and extracranial carotid-artery stenosis. N Engl J Med 332:286–291

30. Selhub J, Jacques PF, Wilson PW, et al (1993) Vitamin status and intake as primary determinants of homocysteinemia in an elderly population. JAMA 270:2693–2698

31. Koehler KM, Romero LJ, Liang HC, et al (1995) Vitamin supplementation and other variables affecting serum homocysteine concentration in healthy elderly men and women [abstract]. Am J Clin Nutr 61:910

Chapter 41

Exercise

Elsworth R. Buskirk

This brief review is focused on recent information related to nutrition and exercise, including provocative insights that may well provide worthy pursuits for further research. Coverage of topics is selective rather than all-inclusive. For more complete information, the reader is referred to other sources.[1-3]

General Considerations

Despite expansion of knowledge in the field of nutrition and exercise, a basic premise still appears to hold true—there is little reason for the physically active person's diet to deviate substantially from that of other healthy persons. To this end, all healthy persons would be well advised to consider major contributions of complex carbohydrates to their diet and to lessen their intake of saturated fat. Regarding the latter, there is a need for some dietary fat for endurance-event competitors or athletes who train extremely hard. These athletes may even be forced to consume additional fat from highly energy-dense foods if only to supply sufficient energy to support prolonged hard, exhausting exercise.

There is growing evidence that our population is, in general, sedentary and that a healthy life-style is partially dependent on regular physical activity in addition to appropriate nutrition. A special communication by the American Medical Association entitled "Physical Activity and Public Health" sets forth a position emphasizing the protective effects of exercise against several chronic diseases, including coronary heart disease (CHD), hypertension, non-insulin-dependent diabetes mellitus, osteoporosis, colon cancer, anxiety, and depression.[4] The report cites studies that associate habitual physical inactivity and poor physical fitness with increased all-cause mortality rates. In addition, it relays the information that possibly as many as 250,000 deaths per year in the United States ($\approx 12\%$ of deaths) are attributable to lack of exercise. Regular exercise was identified with improvement in CHD risk factors, including an increase in high-density-lipoprotein cholesterol, a decrease in serum triacylglycerol, decreased blood pressure, enhanced fibrinolysis, and lessened platelet adherence (thereby diminishing the risk of acute thrombosis), enhanced glucose toler-

ance and insulin sensitivity, and lessened myocardial sensitivity to catecholamines, resulting in a reduced risk for cardiac arrhythmias. In addition, other outcomes linked to nutrition and exercise were identified as increased bone density and more desirable body composition. The report contended that most of these health benefits can be achieved by engaging in moderate-intensity physical activities outside of organized physical activity programs, i.e., walking briskly for ≥30 minutes several times a week, mowing the lawn pushing a power mower, playing golf for nine or more holes and pulling a cart or carrying a set of clubs, or continuous swimming at a moderate pace for ≥20 minutes. Pate et al.[4] conclude on the basis of available data that cardiovascular disease incidence and mortality are reduced by regular physical activity in a dose-response relationship and that intermittent bouts of moderate-intensity physical activity, perhaps as brief as 8–10 minutes, but totaling ≥30 minutes on most days, provides improved fitness and better health.

Energy Turnover

Although not new, the doubly labeled water ($^2H_2{}^{18}O$) technique for assessing total-body energy turnover has added to our knowledge of energy needs for diverse types of physical activity. There are important restrictions that limit the application of this technique, namely, isotopic availability, cost for both isotopes and analytical equipment, and technical complications such as accurate sample preparation and analysis. Despite these limitations the technique has become accepted as a useful procedure for assessing free-living 24-hour energy turnover under a variety of conditions.

One problem that has been addressed through use of the doubly labeled water method is whether the relatively low energy intakes reported for runners are real, i.e., whether runners have an enhanced metabolic efficiency compared with more sedentary persons. Edwards et al.[5] found a 32% imbalance between energy expenditure ascertained by the doubly labeled water method and energy intake determined from food diaries. The nine women distance runners were studied over a 7-day interval. The correlation coefficient (r) between energy expenditure and intake was −0.83, whereas the correlation between body weight and energy intake was −0.74. It was concluded that the heavier runners significantly underreported their food intake, which largely accounted for the discrepancy between expenditure and intake. The daily energy demands for the runners averaged ≈13 MJ/day (≈3000 kcal/day) and ranged from 10.42 to 13.18 MJ/day (2490–3150 kcal/day). Thus, the concept of enhanced energy utilization in well-conditioned athletes was not supported.

Earlier, Schulz et al.,[6] investigating a similar group of distance runners, came to essentially the same conclusion: training as a distance runner does not facilitate metabolic adaptations that lower energy needs. The discrepancy between energy expenditure and intake was ≈10%. Average daily energy expenditure was 11.82 ± 1.31 MJ/day (2826 ± 312 kcal/day). By also studying the runners in a respiratory chamber, the investigators calculated that the runners' energy cost for training (daily running) was 4.55 ± 1.02 MJ/day (1087 ± 244 kcal/day). Corrections were made for the thermic effect of food and spontaneous activity under sedentary conditions. Free-living energy expenditure divided by basal metabolic rate yielded an average ratio for the nine women of 1.99 ± 0.30 (range, 1.53–2.48). Here also, food intake records were shown to underestimate energy intake in these women with stable body weights and compositions.

Another question that could be addressed through use of the doubly labeled water method concerns the maximal sustainable energy expenditure by an exercising human. On the basis of animal studies, this value may be ≈50 MJ/day (12,000 kcal/day) for a 70-kg man, which is five to six times sedentary energy turnover estimated at 10 MJ/day (2400 kcal/day).[7] There is some question whether the gastrointestinal tract can handle intakes of this magnitude and whether the assimilation and metabolism of nutrients can keep pace.[8] In an effort to obtain data from an undertaking requiring extreme energy turnover, i.e., preliminary 24-hour bicycle rides as well as actual competition, energy intakes of competitors in the Race Across America were assessed. In addition to normal food, glucose and electrolyte beverages were used to meet the demand for carbohydrates and fluids. The daily totals during competition amounted to 18 kg food and fluid, i.e., 35.27 MJ/day (8429 kcal/day) and approximately 9 L fluid. Energy turnover was estimated at 3.5 times that necessary for sedentary living.[9] The 24-hour qualifying race presumably involved 43.28 MJ/day (10,343 kcal/day). In this endurance situation the doubly labeled water method would have complemented intake assessment.

Concerning studies of high energy turnover at terrestrial altitude, Stager et al.[10] summarized their observations with the doubly labeled water method during climbing expeditions on Denali (Mount McKinley) in Alaska. Weight loss has been commonly observed in climbing expeditions, but use of the doubly labeled water method facilitated calculation of the energy intake deficit after comparison with food intake records.[7] Food intake analysis was as accurate as possible, and the calculated energy deficit averaged 10.20 MJ/day (2439 kcal/day) for the six climbers who ascended from 2190 m (7200 ft) to 6190 m (20,320 ft). Energy expenditure during the climb was 23.37 ± 1.18 MJ/day (5586 ± 282 kcal/day) compared with an energy intake of 13.17 ± 3.98 MJ/day (3147 ± 952 kcal/day). Mean body weight loss was 2.3 kg. Food intake showed considerably more variability than did energy expenditure. Subsequent studies verified the point that inadequate energy intake accounts for the energy balance deficit during strenuous climbing and that climbers can appreciably modify weight loss by maintaining adequate energy intake.[11]

Resting Metabolic Rate

The interest in different types of physical activity as a means of modifying energy balance has increased; serious consideration has been given to strength and weight training programs in an effort to preserve fat-free body mass when diet restriction and weight-loss regimens are undertaken. The obvious solution for producing a negative energy balance is diet reduction, but in addition to loss of fat, fat-free mass is also lost, resulting in a decrease in the resting metabolic rate, the major component of daily energy expenditure.[12,13] Mixed results have been reported regarding the effect of exercise on the thermic effect of food, postexercise oxygen consumption, and the resting metabolic rate. Interindividual differences associated with genetic characteristics, as well as study design and methodological differences, have contributed to the mixed results.

Most exercise studies that included diet restriction used aerobic exercise to alter energy expenditure, but the use of resistance or weight training to preserve or enhance fat-free mass and, thus, resting metabolic rate may be more promising. Ludo et al.[14] investigated the effect of weight training in 21 men for 12 weeks, but chose metabolic rate during sleep rather than resting metabolic rate as the dependent variable, because the two are related. Interestingly, they found that fat-free mass increased and fat mass decreased, but that metabolism during sleep was unchanged. By appraising fat utilization via respiratory quotient changes, they concluded that in several subjects with initially low rates of fat oxidation, these rates increased in association with the training, whereas in subjects with initially high rates of fat oxidation, fat oxidation was lowered with training. Thus, it remains unclear whether exercise clearly modifies resting metabolic rate in a way that is of consequence to weight loss and subsequent maintenance. In the study by Ludo et al.,[14] as in many others, changes in body composition were small, i.e., a gain in fat-free mass of 1.1 ± 1.3 kg and a loss in fat mass of 2.3 ± 1.5 kg. Perhaps such changes are too small to produce significant differences in resting metabolic rate when considering both interindividual biological variability and methodological error.

Substrate Utilization

Carbohydrate. Carbohydrates are readily available for oxidation and contribute significantly to energy turnover when ingested before or during exercise. In general, their oxidation rate increases as overall energy turnover increases with increasing exercise intensity.[15] In an investigation of the relationship between metabolic rate and oxidation rate of exogenous ^{13}C-labeled glucose and fructose, Massicotte et al.[16] studied 18 young men cycling on an ergometer (60% $\dot{V}O_2$max) for 120 minutes. The respective carbohydrate solutions were given in equal portions at 20-minute intervals from 0 to 100 minutes during exercise. The oxidation rate ($mg\cdot kg^{-1}\cdot min^{-1}$) of both glucose and fructose increased linearly with increasing metabolic rate ($W\cdot kg^{-1}\cdot min^{-1}$). Less fructose than glucose was oxidized during the exercise, i.e., ≈9% fructose and 14% glucose. It appears that the rate of absorption and the rate of conversion of fructose to glucose in the liver did not limit oxidation. With respect to fuel utilization during exercise, exogenous glucose was somewhat more efficiently utilized than was fructose.

Over the past 10–15 years, considerable attention has been paid to the formulation of optimal carbohydrate beverages to support physical performance. The efficacy of utilization of carbohydrates such as glucose, fructose, maltose, and glucose polymers has been reported.[17–19] In a recent study it was confirmed that administration of carbohydrate immediately before exercise increased plasma glucose concentrations, enhanced carbohydrate oxidation, and elevated the respiratory quotient.[20] The practical outcome was a significant improvement in time to exhaustion during prolonged cycling on an ergometer at 65% $\dot{V}O_2$max for 90 minutes followed by cycling at 75% $\dot{V}O_2$max for as long as possible. Results were essentially the same whether glucose or maltodextrin (8–12-chain glucose polymer) was consumed. The use of guar gum to attenuate absorption and modify the early insulin response to glucose had no apparent effect. Despite some variation in osmolality, the equality of energy content and volume was apparently responsible for the comparable results. The amount of carbohydrate oxidized was ≈70 g in 90 minutes, a value similar to values found in much of the earlier work. Blood concentrations of epinephrine and norepinephrine were lower, but insulin was elevated early in exercise after carbohydrate ingestion.

It was concluded that carbohydrate supplementation before prolonged exercise is useful, but the type of carbohydrate is unimportant. Regarding the latter, it is important to note that fructose was not included as part of this investigation.

Coleman[21] reviewed the relative importance of the type (solid or liquid) of carbohydrate feeding in relation to exercise. He concluded that solid and liquid forms of carbohydrate are equally effective in raising blood glucose concentrations and enhancing performance during exercise as well as in promoting glycogen synthesis after exercise. He also concluded that these two types of feedings should be studied in more detail with respect to food type, amount, and time of consumption before exercise. Sherman et al.[22] suggested that to avoid possible gastrointestinal distress, the carbohydrate content of a meal should be low if it is fed close to the beginning of exercise. They recommended 1 g/kg given 1 hour before exercise, in contrast to 4.5 g/kg given 4 hours before exercise. The only obvious situation to avoid would be the consumption of a large, solid meal immediately before exercise.

The question of how much carbohydrate can be utilized during the performance of endurance exercise was examined in some detail by Coyle and Montain.[23] They concluded that, depending on the type of exercise and intraindividual idiosyncrasies, from 30 to 60 g carbohydrate/hour consumed as glucose, sucrose, or starch efficiently supports endurance performance.

Although not much has been done to explore the importance of the glycemic index of foods for exercise performance, it appears that such study would be worthwhile. By providing a slower rate of hydrolysis and absorption, the lesser glucose release of low–glycemic index foods would modify the insulin surge and provide a more constant glucose supply to working muscle when consumed just before exercise. On the other hand, high–glycemic index foods might be favored when glycogen stores are low or when glycogen is being replenished after exhausting exercise. Thomas et al.[24] explored the glycemic index question in a preliminary way by feeding lentils (low glycemic index, 1 g carbohydrate/kg) and similar amounts of potato (high glycemic index) and glucose. Endurance time when cycling on an ergometer at ≈70% $\dot{V}O_2$max was 20 minutes longer ($p < 0.05$) for the trial involving lentil consumption than for potato and glucose.

Thomas et al.[25] extended their studies with high– and low–glycemic index foods by feeding them to trained cyclists 60 minutes before they cycled on an ergometer at 65–70% $\dot{V}O_2$max for 90 minutes. Plasma glucose concentrations after 90 minutes of exercise were inversely correlated with the glycemic index of the foods. Endurance times were not different. It was concluded that slower digestion of the foods with a lower glycemic index favors higher concentrations of needed substrates for muscle even after the exercise. Repetition of these studies appears warranted as does extension of glycemic index investigations to other foods, timing of consumption in relation to exercise, and evaluation of substrate utilization.

In an interesting study that may have applicability to people taking inhibitors of adipose tissue lipolysis for the purpose of reducing serum lipids and thus the risk of atherosclerosis and coronary heart disease, Gautier et al.[26] administered Acipimox® (Farmitalia, Carlo Erba, Milan, Italy), an analogue of nicotinic acid that inhibits adipose tissue lipolysis. When Acipimox was given along with glucose to subjects walking for 3 hours on a treadmill at 45% $\dot{V}O_2$max, endogenous carbohydrate reserves were partly spared and performance was improved compared with that in subjects taking Acipimox alone. Thus, the exogenous glucose became an important source of energy, averaging 19% of the total energy requirement. Symptoms of fatigue and leg cramps that occurred in subjects not given glucose were absent with glucose ingestion. Interestingly, there was an almost constant rate of both lipid and carbohydrate oxidation with both treatments even though there was a nearly complete suppression of the increase in fatty acids and glycerol in plasma that normally occurs with exercise.

Fat. The availability of sufficient metabolic substrates plays a significant role in exercise capacity, and the limiting effect of glycogen depletion is well known. Nevertheless, there is an important role of lipid metabolism through the utilization by contracting skeletal muscle of fatty acids derived from adipose tissue and from intramuscular triacylglycerols. Endurance training extends the intensity range of exercise in which lipid constitutes the primary fuel. Depletion of intramuscular triacylglycerols during strenuous exercise illustrates their pivotal role in supplying fatty acids to working muscle.[27] Endurance training also results in greater intramuscular lipid storage as well as utilization of these reserves.[28] Lipid oxidation during exercise is enhanced by metabolic and enzymatic adaptations to a high-fat diet, provided the period of adaptation is long enough.[29] Thus, the capacity to oxidize fatty acid during endurance exercise no doubt plays a more important role than thought previously.[30] There is some evidence that high-intensity exercise overwhelms lipolysis in adipose tissue and that fatty acid availability is impaired.[31] The conclusion is that low stores of triacylglycerol in muscle reduce performance just as glycogen depletion does.

In an effort to understand the fat-carbohydrate metabolic interaction in skeletal muscle, Dyck et al.[32] used triacyglycerol emulsion infusions and muscle biopsies in subjects who cycled on ergometers at 85% $\dot{V}O_2$max. The results indicated that muscle glycogenolysis was reduced after the lipid-induced elevation in fatty acid concentration. Muscle citrate and acetyl-CoA could not account for the reduced glycogenolysis as classically suggested in the glucose–fatty acid cycle. Dyck et al.[32] suggested instead that regulation was at the level of glycogen phosphorylase. This interesting speculation is well worth further research with additional enzymatic analysis. Because the lipid is infused rapidly, both glucose and related hormonal status effects are minimized, thus simplifying somewhat the experimental approach.

To test the hypothesis that endurance training reduces plasma fatty acid turnover and oxidation in relation to total body lipid oxidation, Martin et al.[33] studied 13 subjects participating in a 12-week endurance-training regimen involving cycling on an ergometer at 75% $\dot{V}O_2$max. Observations during a 90–120-minute exercise bout both pre- and posttraining revealed decreased plasma fatty acid turnover and oxidation resulting from a slower rate of fatty acid release from adipose tissue. This slower rate occurred despite the nearly 50% more energy derived from total body fat oxidation. It was concluded that human subjects derive less energy from plasma fatty acids during submaximal exercise when trained than when sedentary but derive more from intramuscular triacylglycerols. Such training-induced reductions in plasma fatty acid oxidation and turnover are consistent with blunted adipose tissue lipolysis brought about by a lesser sympathoadrenal response.

In the resting state, the situation is somewhat different; it has been shown that lipid kinetics are increased during rest after an endurance-training regimen and this increase may enhance the potential for increasing fatty acid oxidation rapidly at the beginning of subsequent exercise. Romijn et al.[34] studied the rates of appearance of glycerol (index of whole-body lipolysis), palmitate (index of fatty acid release), triacylglycerol–fatty acid substrate cycling (index of reesterification of fatty acids released during lipolysis), and fat oxidation in trained cyclists at rest. Stable isotope methodology and indirect calorimetry were used. Glycerol and fatty acid rates of appearance in those who trained were two- to threefold higher than rates in untrained subjects. The total rate of triacylglycerol–fatty acid cycling was fourfold higher in those who trained. Hormones regulating lipid kinetics such as insulin and catecholamines were comparable in both groups. It was concluded that the elevated triacylglycerol-fatty acid cycling may facilitate redistribution of endogenous triacylglycerol and replenish intramuscular triacylglycerol stores utilized during the previous bout of exercise.

To ascertain whether adaptation to a high-fat diet that avoided ketosis, but altered muscle glycogen stores and rates of carbohydrate and lipid oxidation, modifies performance during low- and high-intensity submaximal exercise, endurance-trained athletes were studied after 2 weeks on two different diets.[35] The high-fat diet consisted of 70% fat and 7% carbohydrate and the low-fat diet 12% fat and 74% carbohydrate. The subjects adapted to the respective diets over a 2-week period. Despite a lower muscle glycogen content at the onset of moderate-intensity exercise (60% $\dot{V}O_2$max), exercise time to exhaustion was significantly longer after the high-fat diet, i.e., 79.7 compared with 42.5 minutes for the low-fat diet, and was associated with a lower respiratory-exchange ratio. A decreased rate of carbohydrate oxidation was also observed. Exercise time to exhaustion during high-intensity exercise (90% $\dot{V}O_2$max) was not different between trials nor were the rates of glycogen utilization, even though muscle glycogen content was lower with consumption of the high-fat diet. It was concluded that 2 weeks of adaptation to a high-fat diet can occur without ketosis, can spare endogenous carbohydrate, and can delay fatigue during performance of moderate-intensity exercise. Even though these effects were not found during high-intensity exercise, overall performance was unimpaired by the high-fat diet. Thus, a lengthy period of adaptation to a high-fat diet is key to its effectiveness and so too is the provision of sufficient glucose to avoid the debilitating effects of ketosis. The tendency to reject high-fat diets even when energy needs are extremely high is unreasonable. Further work on the utilization of high-fat diets is warranted, bearing in mind public health considerations for the prevention of chronic diseases including atherosclerosis.

Protein and amino acids. The concept that several amino acids are conducive to improved performance by body builders and resistance or weight trainers has been based on somewhat controversial evidence of stimulated hormone release.[36] Carlson et al.[37] indicated that amino acids may either directly or indirectly affect pituitary hormone release and hypothalamic function. Lemon[38] reported on a series of experiments involving arginine and ornithine dosages up to 20 g/day. Only a few subjects (<10%) showed slight increases in growth hormone release when amino acids were given in conjunction with heavy resistance training. Carli et al.[39] found significantly increased serum testosterone, ratio of testosterone to cortisol, sex hormone–binding globulin, and serum insulin in marathon runners who ran for 60 minutes at a pace that reached their lactate threshold. The runners consumed 12 g milk protein, 29 g carbohydrate, and 10 g branched-chain amino acids 90 minutes before running. It was suggested that branched-chain amino acids in conjunction with relatively intense exercise can modify hormonal release and perhaps reduce some catabolic effects of exercise.

The persisting concept that strength-, resistance-, or weight-training athletes need a greater intake of protein and amino acids has been challenged by several investigators. Tarnopolsky et al.[40] studied body builders who consumed 1.0–2.7 g protein·kg⁻¹·day⁻¹ as part of a diet containing 20.08 MJ/day (4800 kcal/day) while engaged in a regimen of strength and endurance training. Their nitrogen balance became significantly more positive compared with that during consumption of their control diet, but no increase was observed in their fat-free mass. The investigators concluded that excess protein above the recommended dietary allowance (RDA) was unnecessary for these body builders when their energy intake was sufficient to support their activity.[41] Lemon et al.,[42] in a similar study, found that increased protein intake from 1.35 to 2.62 g·kg⁻¹·day⁻¹ was not associated with increasing muscle size or strength during the 4 weeks of intensive weight training. Nitrogen balance was positive with the higher protein intake (2.67 g·kg⁻¹·day⁻¹) and negative at the lower intake (0.99 g·kg⁻¹·day⁻¹). They concluded that nitrogen balance could probably have been achieved at a protein intake of 1.6–1.7 g·kg⁻¹·day⁻¹ in these novice bodybuilders engaged in weight training.

That the issue of possible benefits of protein supplementation has not been settled for weight-training athletes is supported by the investigation of Frontera et al.[43] These investigators supplemented their subjects' regular diets with 2.8 g protein·kg⁻¹·day⁻¹ during a 12-week weight-training regimen. A comparatively increased urinary creatinine excretion (an indicator of increased muscle mass) and enlarged quadriceps muscles were found in the supplemented compared with the control subjects. In addition, Tarnopolsky et al.[44] found that beginning bodybuilders had greater nitrogen retention when consuming >300% of the RDA for protein. Thus, the controversy remains as to the optimal intake of protein and amino acids to enhance performance, optimize body composition, and preserve nitrogen balance in strength-, resistance-, or weight-training athletes. The recommendation of ≈1.5 g protein·kg⁻¹·day⁻¹ appears reasonable on the basis of current evidence.

No recommendations can be made at this time as to the utility of supplementation with individual amino acids for purposes of performance enhancement. Nevertheless, some interesting thoughts and observations in this regard have been brought forward. Blomstrand et al.[45] were interested in the effects of supplementation with branched-chain amino acids on performance in 30- and 40-km runs. Supplementation caused a significant increase in plasma valine, but not in leucine or isoleucine, concentration during the 30-km run but not the 42-km run. All three amino acids were significantly increased compared with concentrations in control subjects given a 5%-carbohydrate solution. In addition, the ratio of free tryptophan to branched-chain amino acids was lowered, and tyrosine, a measure of net protein degradation, was less in the supplemented group. Nevertheless, final run times were unaffected by the supplementation except in the slowest runners. Davis et al.[46] concluded from studies with various carbohydrate drinks during endurance exercise that the carbohydrate attenuated the ratio of tryptophan to branched-chain amino acids and helped delay fatigue, but that protein degradation still occurred, as evidenced by a fall in plasma concentrations of branched-chain amino acids.

Kreider et al.,[36] in interpreting observations of supplementation with branched-chain amino acids during endurance activities, suggested that amounts ≥295 mg leucine/hour, ≥105 mg isoleucine/hour, and ≥150 mg valine/hour may well reduce body protein degradation and improve negative protein balance. They suggested further that the addition of branched-chain amino acids and glutamine to the commonly consumed carbohydrate beverages during prolonged endurance events not only provides substrate fuel but reduces protein degradation. Kreider et al.[36] cite a study in which five triathletes were supplemented with a commercial nutritional system for 17 days. Branched-chain amino acids, glutamine, and carnitine were also added. Serum insulin concentrations and fat oxidation were increased, but protein degradation was reduced. Despite these metabolic changes, final performance times were not improved.

Concerning glycogen storage, Zawadzki et al.[47] found that carbohydrate-protein supplements produced higher serum insulin concentrations than did either carbohydrate or protein alone in endurance cyclists. Glycogen storage was also greater because of enhanced glycogen resynthesis, perhaps because of insulin-mediated glycogen restoration.

In a study of swim training, Kreider et al.[36] found that serum ammonia, cortisol, and the ratio of cortisol to testosterone were lower in swimmers who received amino acids and carnitine in addition to carbohydrate supplements compared with those who received carbohydrate alone. Fat mass was reduced and fat-free mass increased with the combined supplementation. These results were also interpreted as supporting the theory of reduced protein degradation with amino acid inclusion in substrate supplementation. Because results thus far are inconclusive, further research is needed on the physiological and performance effects of the inclusion of protein and amino acid supplements in the dietary patterns of very active people, particularly endurance athletes. Progress, thus far, is both stimulating and encouraging.

Another nutrition-exercise link is an effect on the immune system. Relatively low-intensity exercise has been shown to enhance lymphocyte response to in vitro mitogenic stimulation and increase the number of circulating lymphocytes and natural killer cells. Thus, immune function is enhanced by low-intensity exercise. In contrast, prolonged exercise of high intensity decreases the ratio of CD4+ to CD8+, T lymphocyte response to mitogenic stimulation, and antibody synthesis—all adverse effects.[48] Newsholme,[49] in reviewing the biochemical mechanisms thought to explain the observed immu-

nosuppression, implicated the plasma concentration of glutamine as a "metabolic link" between skeletal muscle and cells of the immune system. Presumably, skeletal muscle synthesizes and stores glutamine. Plasma glutamine is decreased with endurance exercise and overtraining. Thus, if the process of glutamine release is compromised by exercise, the glutamine requirement of the immune cells is not met and immune function is impaired. To elevate plasma concentrations of glutamine, supplementation with branched-chain amino acids appears effective because it significantly modified the drop in plasma glutamine concentrations after a marathon run in overtrained athletes.[50] The mechanism for the decrease in plasma glutamine concentration with overtraining and endurance exercise remains unknown, although the rate of release from skeletal muscle remains a viable path to investigate.

Yoshimura et al.[51] promoted the idea that during the beginning of a resistance-training regimen the protein anabolism in skeletal muscle was derived from breakdown products from plasma proteins, erythrocytes, myoglobin, and perhaps other body tissues. Greater provision of amino acids would then be required to reform myoglobin and other tissue components, synthesize erythrocytes, and replenish enzymes. These investigators' work has not been systematically evaluated with newer tools, nor has their concept of sports-induced amenia been adequately explored.

Special Considerations

Caffeine. Caffeine is commonly utilized by athletes as an ergogenic aid.[52] In addition to its action on adinosine receptors and Ca^{2+}-release channels, caffeine causes increased lipolysis and a sparing of muscle glycogen associated with enhanced fatty acid oxidation. As a consequence of these actions, endurance should be enhanced, particularly when glycogen depletion would limit performance.[53] The story is not clear-cut, however. Essig et al.[54] observed a significant increase in resting intramuscular triacylglycerol stores of ≈18% associated with an increase in plasma concentrations of fatty acids after consumption of 5 mg caffeine/kg. When exercise was performed at 69% $\dot{V}O_2$max for 30 minutes, intramuscular triacylglycerol utilization increased 150%. The respiratory-exchange ratio decreased and total fat utilization was estimated to increase ≈50%. Presumably, an important adaptation to training for endurance events is greater use of intramuscular triacylglycerol. The question of whether the increase in intramuscular triacylglycerol after caffeine ingestion only reflects the greater availability of substrate remains to be answered. The work of Essig et al.[54] has not been duplicated and should be repeated with arteriovenous fatty acid differences and stable-isotope labels.

There is other evidence that caffeine leads to glycogen sparing early in endurance exercise and that this effect is related to changes in the ratio of acetyl CoA to CoA-SH and an elevation in muscle citrate brought about by increased fat oxidation.[55] That caffeine elicits these effects during endurance exercise is suggestive and deserving of further research.

Ethanol. Ethanol has been shown to be a poor substrate for support of energy metabolism during exercise. In a study with ^{13}C labeling of the oxidation of ethanol during prolonged moderate exercise, it was found that ethanol oxidation represented only $5.2 \pm 1.0\%$ of total energy expenditure. Endogenous substrate oxidation was not significantly modified. The exercise involved cycling on an ergometer at $\approx 70\%$ $\dot{V}O_2$max for 90 minutes. Ethanol was ingested at two doses: 0.4 and 0.8 g/kg body weight. The ethanol was diluted in 770 ± 72 mL water. There was no difference in ethanol oxidation during exercise between the two quantities administered. The oxidation of exogenous ethanol was increased during exercise compared with rest, i.e., ≈ 9 g/kg during 90 minutes of exercise and 2.1 g/kg when at rest for 90 minutes.[56] The latter results at rest are comparable with those obtained by Suter et al.,[57] who used direct calorimetry to show that ethanol-induced thermogenesis increased 24-hour energy expenditure by $\approx 5.5\%$ when 95.6 ± 1.8 g ethanol/kg was administered in 1 day as part of three meals. Both studies support the concept of inefficient utilization of energy derived from ethanol. Whether efficiency of utilization changes somewhat as the result of the type, intensity, and duration of exercise remains to be explored. Earlier work by Juhlin-Dannfelt et al.[58] indicated that during 180 minutes of exercise at 30% $\dot{V}O_2$max, splanchnic uptake of exogenous ethanol was 18 g and the utilization of acetate and lactate derived from ethanol constituted 8–10% of total oxidative metabolism.

Ammonia. The effects of low body-glycogen stores induced by restricted carbohydrate feeding (5% carbohydrate, 50% fat, and 45% protein) for 3 days on plasma ammonia concentration and excretion in sweat were ascertained in seven young men before, during, and after exercise. Comparisons were made with a normal mixed diet (60% carbohydrate, 25% fat, and 15% protein); both diets supplied sufficient energy to maintain body weight. Exercise intensity was at 60% $\dot{V}O_2$max and subjects cycled on an ergometer for 1 hour. Plasma ammonia concentration, sweat ammonia concentration, and total ammonia loss was considerably greater after the low-carbohydrate diet.[59] These results are similar to those found by Greenhaff et al.[60] and by Broberg and Sahlin,[61] although the latter investigators studied more exhausting exercise (75% $\dot{V}O_2$max). In such studies, an elevated ammonia production is thought to result from reduced initial carbohydrate stores, principally in muscle.

Sahlin et al.[62] suggested that a reduction in tricarboxylic acid (TCA) intermediates may account for the increased muscle ammonia production. If TCA intermediates are low, a reduced flux through the TCA cycle occurs, which reduces the rate of oxidative phosphorylation and enhances adenosine-5′-monophosphate deamination to inosine-5′-monophosphate and ammonia. The higher plasma ammonia concentration may well be a consequence of modified muscle metabolism and the maintenance of TCA intermediates to ensure complete oxidation of fat.[59]

The degradation of purine nucleotides and oxidation of amino acids may produce ammonia in muscle with decreased carbohydrate availability during exercise.[61] MacLean et al.[63] found that purine nucleotides were not degraded during exercise. They suggested instead that oxidation of branched-chain amino acids is the source of excess plasma ammonia via removal of an amino group by transdeamination catalyzed by amino transferase and glutamate dehydrogenase. Protein catabolism may also be increased by changes in hormonal release and circulation during exercise, i.e., decreases in insulin and increases in glucocorticoids, glucagon catecholamines, and growth hormone. Glycogen depletion before exercise may well enhance protein utilization during exercise.[64]

Interestingly, because ammonia behaves like water with respect to transfer through membranes, the increased plasma concentration of ammonia is thought to provide a sufficient driving force for the appearance of ammonia in sweat. Not taking sweat excretion into account when studying nitrogen balance or protein turnover can lead to underestimates, particularly when exercise is prolonged and carbohydrate intake is low.

Antioxidants. Free radicals are generated by exercise, but their fate has not been resolved, nor has their effect on performance. In the body, various pools of antioxidants exist that, together with antioxidant adaptation to oxidative stress through metabolizing and regenerating systems, complicate interpretation.[65,66] Obtaining an understanding of free radical effects, although difficult, should provide an area of fruitful research. The paradox is obvious—oxygen is needed to support exercise in an intensity-dependent relationship, yet the body needs protection against oxygen reaction products, chiefly free radicals. Free radical effects on living systems were reviewed by Halliwell and Gutteridge,[67] who point to a variety of disease susceptibilities as well as vulnerability during aging.

High doses to megadoses of antioxidants have been recommended or prescribed to counter ostensible negative effects of free radical production during exercise. Vitamin C, β-carotene, and vitamin E in separate or combined doses are the antioxidants commonly prescribed. They are generally considered safe in large doses.[68,69] Herbert[70] cautioned, however, that high doses of antioxidants may well induce oxidant effects. Kanter[71] emphasized that there is evidence supporting antioxidant utilization, but that available data do not justify excessive antioxidant use by very active people, including athletes.

In addition to the nutritionally available antioxidants mentioned above, the following critical antioxidant enzymes should be mentioned: superoxide dismutase, glutathione peroxidase, and catalase. Concentrations of these enzymes, all complements of mammalian cells, are undoubtedly largely genetically determined. Minerals are built into these enzymes, e.g., copper and zinc are part of cytostolic superoxide dismutase, copper is in ceruloplasmin, iron is involved with catalase, manganese is involved with mitochondrial superoxide dismutase, and selenium is involved with glutathione peroxidase. Ostensibly, enzyme formation would be compromised by deficiencies of these minerals.[71] Both Jenkins[65] and Kanter,[71] after reviewing studies dealing with both acute and chronic exercise, found either modest antioxidant enzyme changes in tissues or none at all. Those studies showing increases on the order of 15–50% are contradicted by the observation that oxidative enzyme activity is increased markedly after regular exercise or training, which suggests a decrease in the ratio of antioxidant to oxidant enzymes and a reduction in protection.[72] Such reasoning implies that habitual exercisers might well benefit from use of antioxidant supplements. Nevertheless, it should be restated that results to date are equivocal with respect to the effects of supplementation with antioxidants on lipid peroxidation and tissue damage related to exercise.

β-Carotene, selenium, and coenzyme Q_{10} are other nutrients that have been studied when given either separately or as part of an antioxidant mixture. Findings are mixed regarding the effectiveness of these nutrients on enhancement of performance. β-Carotene has been linked to the detoxification of singlet oxygen species and serves as a precursor of vitamin A. Selenium forms part of the structure of several selenoenzymes, including glutathione peroxidase. Coenzyme Q_{10} operates in electron shuttling between the citric acid cycle and the respiratory chain and possibly as a free radical quencher. Coenzyme Q_{10} has been related importantly to exercise capacity.[71] Snider et al.[73] found that a supplement consisting of 100 mg coenzyme Q_{10}, 500 mg cytochrome c, 100 mg inosine, and 200 IU vitamin E had no effect on the endurance of trained triathletes.

In summary, there may well be a relationship between free radical production during exercise and lipid peroxidation and cellular damage. If so, supplementation with antioxidants may curb adverse exercise-induced effects. More research is needed to understand the types, intensities, and durations of exercise to be avoided; the type and quantity of antioxidants to use; and the appropriate, sensitive methods to detect the magnitude of lipid peroxidation, cellular damage, and free radical production. Current methodologies are inadequate; more sensitive and specific techniques are needed.

References

1. Buskirk ER (1990) Exercise. In Brown ML (ed), Present knowledge in nutrition, 6th ed. International Life Sciences Institute, Washington, DC, pp 341–348
2. Simopoulos AP, Pavlou KN, eds (1993) Nutrition and fitness for athletes, vol 71, part 1, 2nd ed. International conference on nutrition and fitness. S Karger AG, Basel, Switzerland
3. Hickson JR Jr, Wolinsky I, eds (1989) Nutrition in exercise and sport. CRC Press, Boca Raton, FL
4. Pate RR, Prott M, Blair SN, et al (1995) Physical activity and public health. JAMA 273:402–407
5. Edwards JE, Lindeman AK, Mikesky AE, Stager JM (1993) Energy balance in highly trained female endurance runners. Med Sci Sports Exerc 25:1398–1404
6. Schulz LO, Alger S, Harper I, et al (1992) Energy expenditure of elite female runners measured by respiratory chamber and doubly labeled water. J Appl Physiol 72:23–28
7. Stager JM, Lindeman AK, Edwards JE (1992) Energy intake and energy expenditure during a high altitude expedition on Mt McKinley, Alaska [abstract]. Int J Sports Med 13:89
8. Diamond J (1991) Evolutionary design of intestinal nutrient absorption: enough but not too much. News Physiol Sci 6:92–96
9. Lindeman AK (1991) Nutrient intake of an ultraendurance cyclist. Int J Sport Nutr 1:79–85
10. Stager JM, Lindeman A, Edwards J (1995) The use of doubly labelled water in quantifying energy expenditure during prolonged activity. Sports Med 19:166–172
11. Tanner DA, Stager JM (1993) Weight and body composition changes during a mountaineering expedition in Mt McKinley [abstract]. Med Sci Sports Exerc 25:S52
12. Poehlman ET, Horton ES (1989) The impact of food intake and exercise on energy expenditure. Nutr Rev 47:129–137
13. Poehlman ET (1989) A review: exercise and its influence on resting energy metabolism in man. Med Sci Sports Exerc 21:515–525
14. Ludo ML, Van Etten A, Westerterp KR, Verstappen FTJ (1995) Effect of weight-training on energy expenditure and substrate utilization during sleep. Med Sci Sports Exerc 27:188–193
15. Peronnet F, Adopo E, Massicotte D (1992) Exogenous substrate oxidation during exercise: studies using isotopic labelling. Int J Sports Med 13:S123–S125
16. Massicotte D, Peronnet F, Adopo E, et al (1994) Effect of metabolic rate on the oxidation of ingested glucose and fructose during exercise. Int J Sports Med 15:177–180
17. Murray R (1987) The effects of consuming carbohydrate-electrolyte beverages on gastric emptying and fluid absorption during and following exercise. Sports Med 4:322–351
18. Buskirk ER, Puhl S (1989) Nutritional beverages: exercise and sport. In Hickson JR Jr, Wolinsky I (eds), Nutrition in exercise and sport, chapter 9. CRC Press, Boca Raton, FL, pp 201–231
19. Moodley D, Noakes TD, Bosch AN, et al (1992) Oxidation of exogenous carbohydrate during prolonged exercise: the effects of the carbohydrate type and its concentration. Eur J Appl Physiol 64:328–334

20. MacLaren DPM, Reilly T, Campbell IT (1994) Hormonal and metabolic responses to glucose and malto-dextrin ingestion with or without the addition of guar gum. Int J Sports Med 15:466–471

21. Coleman E (1994) Update on carbohydrate: solid vs liquid. Int J Sport Nutr 4:80–88

22. Sherman WM, Peden MC, Wright DA (1991) Carbohydrate feedings 1 hr before exercise improves cycling performance. Am J Clin Nutr 54:866–870

23. Coyle EF, Montain SJ (1992) Benefits of fluid replacement with carbohydrate during exercise. Med Sci Sports Exerc 24(Suppl):S324–S330

24. Thomas DE, Brotherhood JR, Brand JC (1991) Carbohydrate feeding before exercise: effect of glycemic index. Int J Sports Med 12:180–186

25. Thomas D, Brotherhood JR, Miller JB (1994) Plasma glucose levels after prolonged strenuous exercise correlate inversely with glycemic response to food consumed before exercise. Int J Sports Nutr 4:361–373

26. Gautier JF, Pirnay F, Jandrain B, et al (1994) Availability of glucose ingested during muscle exercise performed under Acipimox-induced lypolysis blockade. Eur J Appl Physiol 68:406–412

27. Staron RS, Hikida RS, Murray TF, et al (1989) Lipid depletion and repletion in skeletal muscle following a marathon. J Neurol Sci 94:29–40

28. Hurley BF, Nemeth PM, Martin WH III, et al (1986) Muscle triglyceride utilization during exercise: effect of training. J Appl Physiol 60:562–567

29. Simi B, Sempore B, Mayet M, Favier R (1991) Additive effects of training and high fat diet on energy metabolism during exercise. J Appl Physiol 71:197–203

30. Hagerman FC (1992) Energy metabolism and fuel utilization. Med Sci Sports Exerc 24(Suppl):S309–S314

31. Hodgetts V, Coppack SW, Frayn KN, Hockadag DR (1991) Factors controlling fat mobilization from human subcutaneous adipose tissue during exercise. J Appl Physiol 71:445–451

32. Dyck DJ, Putman CT, Heigenhauser CJF, et al (1993) Regulation of fat-carbohydrate interaction in skeletal muscle during intense aerobic cycling. Am J Physiol 265:E852–E859

33. Martin WH III, Dalsky DP, Hurley BF, et al (1993) Effect of endurance training on plasma free fatty acid turnover and oxidation during exercise. Am J Physiol 265:E708–E714

34. Romijn JA, Klein S, Coyle EF, et al (1993) Strenuous endurance training increases lipolysis and triaglyceride-fatty acid cycling at rest. J Appl Physiol 75:108–113

35. Lambert EV, Speechly DP, Dennis SC, Noakes TD (1994) Enhanced endurance in trained cyclists during moderate intensity exercise following 2 weeks adaptation to a high fat diet. Eur J Appl Physiol 69:287–293

36. Kreider RB, Miriel V, Bertum E (1993) Amino acid supplementation and exercise performance—analysis of the proposed ergogenic value. Sports Med 16:190–209

37. Carlson HE, Miglietta JT, Roginsky MS, Stegink LD (1989) Stimulation of pituitary hormone secretion by neurotransmitter amino acids in humans. Metabolism 28:1179–1182

38. Lemon PWR (1991) Protein and amino acid needs of the strength athlete. Int J Sport Nutr 1:127–145

39. Carli G, Bonifazi M, Lodi L, et al (1992) Changes in exercise-induced hormone response to branched chain amino acid administration. Eur J Appl Physiol 64:272–277

40. Tarnopolsky MA, MacDougall JD, Atkinson SA (1988) Influence of protein intake and training status on nitrogen balance and lean body mass. J Appl Physiol 64:187–193

41. National Research Council (1989) Recommended dietary allowances, 10th ed. National Academy Press, Washington, DC

42. Lemon PR, Tarnopolsky MA, MacDougall JD, Atkinson, SA (1992) Protein requirements and muscle mass/strength changes during intensive training in novice bodybuilders. J Appl Physiol 73:767–775

43. Frontera WR, Meredith CN, Evans, WJ (1988) Dietary effects on muscle strength gain and hypertrophy during heavy resistance training in older men [abstract]. Can J Sport Sci 13:13P

44. Tarnopolsky MA, Lemon PWR, MacDougall JD, Atkinson JA (1990) Effect of body building exercise on protein requirements. Can J Sport Sci 15:225

45. Blomstrand E, Hassmen P, Ekblom B, Newsholme EA (1991) Administration of branch-chain amino acids during sustained exercise—effects on performance and on plasma concentration of some amino acids. Eur J Appl Physiol 63:83–88

46. Davis JM, Baily SP, Woods JA, et al (1992) Effects of carbohydrate feedings on plasma free tryptophan and branched-chain amino acids during prolonged cycling. Eur J Appl Physiol 65:513–519

47. Zawadzki KM, Yaspelkis BB, Ivy JL (1992) Carbohydrate-protein complex increases the rate of muscle glycogen storage after exercise. J Appl Physiol 72:1854–1859

48. Keast D, Cameron K, Morton AR (1988) Exercise and the immune response. Sports Med 5:248–267

49. Newsholme EA (1994) Biochemical mechanisms to explain immunosuppression in well-trained and overtrained athletes. Int J Sports Med 15:S142–S147

50. Newsholme EA, Parry-Billings M, McAndrew N, Budgett R (1991) A biochemical mechanism to explain some characteristics of overtraining. Med Sport Sci 32:79–93

51. Yoshimura H, Inoue T, Yamada T, Shiraki K (1980) Anemia during hard physical training (sports anemia) and its causal mechanism with special reference to protein nutrition. World Rev Nutr Diet 35:1–45

52. Delbeke FT, Debachere M (1984) Caffeine: use and abuse in sports. Int J Sports 5:179–182

53. Tarnopolsky MA (1994) Caffeine and endurance performance. Sports Med 18:109–125

54. Essig D, Costill DL, Van Handel PJ (1980) Effects of caffeine ingestion on utilization of muscle glycogen and lipid during ergometer cycling. Int J Sports Med 1:86–90

55. Spriet LL, MacLean DA, Dyck DJ, et al (1992) Caffeine ingestion and muscle metabolism during prolonged exercise in humans. Am J Physiol 25:E891–E898

56. Massicotte D, Provencher S, Adopo E, et al (1993) Oxidation of ethanol at rest and during prolonged exercise in men. J Appl Physiol 75:329–333

57. Suter PM, Jequier E, Schutz Y (1994) Effect of ethanol on energy expenditure. Am J Physiol 35:R1204–R1212

58. Juhlin-Dannfelt A, Ahlborg G, Hagenfeldt L, et al (1977) Influence of ethanol on splanchnic and skeletal muscle substrate turnover during prolonged exercise in man. Am J Physiol 233:E195–E202

59. Czarnowski D, Langfort J, Pilis W, Gorski J (1995) Effect of a low-carbohydrate diet on plasma and sweat ammonia concentrations during prolonged nonexhausting exercise. Eur J Appl Physiol 70:70–74

60. Greenhaff PL, Leiper JB, Ball D, Maughan RS (1991) The influence of dietary manipulation on plasma ammonia accumulation during incremental exercise in man. Eur J Appl Physiol 63:338–344

61. Broberg S, Sahlin K (1988) Hyperammonemia during prolonged exercise: an effect of glycogen depletion. J Appl Physiol 65:2475–2477

62. Sahlin K, Katz A, Broberg S (1990) Tricarboxylic acid cycle intermediates in human muscle during prolonged exercise. Am J Physiol 2590:C834–C841

63. MacLean DA, Spriet LL, Hultman E, Graham TE (1991) Plasma and muscle amino acid and ammonia responses during prolonged exercise in humans. J Appl Physiol 70:2095–2103

64. Lemon PWR, Mullin JP (1980) Effect of initial muscle glycogen levels on protein catabolism during exercise. J Appl Physiol 48:624–629

65. Jenkins RR (1993) Exercise, oxidative stress, and antioxidants: a review. Int J Sport Nutr 3:356–375

66. Chow CK (1991) Vitamin E and oxidative stress. Free Radic Biol Med 11:215–232

67. Halliwell B, Gutteridge JMC (1989) Free radicals in biology and medicine. Clarendon Press, Oxford

68. Brooks G, Gillam I, Kanter M, Packer L (1992) Proceedings of the panel discussion: antioxidants and the elite athlete. Henkel Fine Chemicals, La Grange, IL, pp 1–21

69. Simon-Schnass I (1993) Vitamin requirements for increased physical activity: vitamin E. In Simopoulos AP, Pavlou KN (eds), Nutrition and fitness for athletes. World Rev Nutr Diet 71:144–153

70. Herbert V (1993) Viewpoint: does mega-C do more good than harm or more harm than good? Nutr Today, Jan/Feb, pp 28–32

71. Kanter MM (1994) Free radicals, exercise and antioxidant supplementation. Int J Sport Nutr 4:205–220

72. Higuchi M, Cartier LJ, Chen M, Holloszy J (1985) Superoxide dismutase and catalase in skeletal muscle: adaptive response to acute exercise. J Gerontol 40:281–286

73. Snider IP, Bazzarre TL, Murdock SD, Goldfarb A (1992) Effects of a coenzyme athletic performance system as an ergogenic aid on endurance performance to exhaustion. Int J Sports Med 2:272–286

Chapter 42

Atherosclerosis

Alice H. Lichtenstein

Arteriosclerosis refers to a group of disorders characterized by a thickening of the arterial wall with resultant loss of elasticity. Frequently, nutrition scientists focus on one type of arteriosclerosis, atherosclerosis. Atherosclerosis is defined as the development of fatty plaque within the intima and media of medium and large arteries. The disease can involve the coronary, cerebral, femoral, and iliac arteries and the aorta. Vessels that have become atherosclerotic are associated with the development of coronary heart disease, stroke, aneurysm, and peripheral vascular disease. The fatty plaque is composed primarily of cholesterol and cholesteryl esters. These lipids are associated with foam cells and macrophages in the arterial wall. More advanced lesions can become calcified and include necrotic debris. These lesions are often covered by a cap composed of fibrous tissue and smooth muscle cells. The resultant lesion protrudes into the lumen of the vessel, causing narrowing and impeding blood flow. If the lesion becomes ulcerated a thrombogenic surface often develops. Resultant thrombi can further impede blood flow or totally occlude the vessel. Hemorrhaging into the plaque can precipitate the formation of thrombi.

Atherosclerotic lesions in coronary arteries result in the development of coronary heart disease (CHD). CHD is characterized by reduced blood flow or stenosis of the coronary arteries. Early manifestations of the disease include angina pectoris (ischemic pain on physical exertion). Of more concern is the high risk of occlusion of an atherosclerotic coronary artery by a thrombosis. The subsequent loss of blood flow to the cardiac muscle causes a myocardial infarct, or heart attack. The ensuing ischemia results in arrhythmia (nonproductive contractile impulse of the heart), which can be fatal to the patient. If the event is nonfatal, ischemic necrosis of the myocardium develops, which can impede normal heart function. Recovery can be protracted and at times incomplete. If the damaged heart cannot pump adequate quantities of blood, congestive heart failure develops.

Atherosclerotic lesions in the cerebral artery can result in interrupted blood flow to the brain. This disorder, which results in ischemic brain necrosis or cerebral infarct, is termed stroke. The clinical manifestations of a cerebral stroke depend on the anatomical location and severity of the infarct. The limited recovery often expected after a nonfatal cerebral stroke is primarily attributed to the inability of the damaged neurons to regenerate themselves.

Atherosclerotic lesions occurring in the abdominal aorta, iliac artery, or femoral artery can result in decreased blood flow to the lower extremities. Intermittent claudication aggravated by physical exertion is the most common manifestation. More advanced atherosclerosis in the affected arteries can result in ischemic necrosis of the extremities or gangrene.

Incidence and Effect of Cardiovascular Disease in the United States

Since 1919 arteriosclerosis has become the leading cause of death and disability in the United States. In 1991 cardiovascular disease accounted for 43% of all deaths in men and women. Although age-adjusted death rates from cardiovascular disease fell by 26% during 1981–1991, the actual number of deaths declined by only 6%. It has been estimated that cardiovascular diseases will affect more than one of every five Americans at some point in their lives.[1]

Myocardial infarction is currently the single leading cause of death in the United States. Of those in whom a myocardial infarction develops, about one-third will not survive. Although myocardial infarctions usually occur at a younger age in men than in women, both sexes are eventually affected at about the same rate. Despite the common misconception that women are at a greater risk of death from breast cancer than myocardial infarction, over a lifetime, five times the number of women will die from cardiovascular diseases than from breast cancer.

Stroke is the third leading cause of death in the United States. Incidence rates are ≈60% higher in African Americans than whites. Stroke occurs at slightly higher rates in women than in men and is responsible for about twice as many deaths in women as breast cancer. About one-third of those developing a stroke do not survive. Of those who do survive, many are left with permanent and debilitating disorders.

Lipoprotein Particles: Terminology

Although terms such as low-density lipoprotein (LDL) and high-density lipoprotein (HDL) were once used solely in scientific publications, they now commonly appear in the popular press. There are six major classes of lipoprotein particles: chylomicrons, very-low-density lipoproteins (VLDLs), intermediate-density lipoproteins (IDLs), LDLs, HDLs, and lipoprotein(a) [Lp(a)]. In general, except possibly for Lp(a), when the concentration of lipoprotein particles is expressed, unless otherwise stated it is on the basis of the cholesterol content (e.g., LDL cholesterol). Terminology for the protein component of the lipoprotein particle is also coming into general usage. The specific proteins on lipoprotein subclasses are termed apolipoproteins. Most lipoprotein particles have a number of constituent apolipoproteins; however, only the major ones will be specifically cited.

Chylomicrons. Chylomicrons are intestinally derived lipoprotein particles formed and secreted after the ingestion of fat. Their main function is to provide a mechanism whereby dietary fat (triacylglycerol), cholesterol, and other fat-soluble compounds are carried from the site of absorption (intestine) to other parts of the body for subsequent uptake and potential metabolism or storage. Chylomicron particles are the largest of all the lipoprotein subclasses. The core of the particle is composed primarily of triacylglycerol and a small amount of cholesteryl ester. The surface of the particle contains phospholipid, apolipoproteins, and free cholesterol. The major apolipoprotein on the chylomicron particle is apolipoprotein (apo) B-48, which originates in the intestine. Under normal circumstances the triacylglycerol content of these particles is decreased markedly while in circulation through the action of lipoprotein lipase and hepatic lipase. These triacylglycerol-depleted particles are called chylomicron remnants. The remnant particles are rapidly cleared from circulation by the liver.

VLDLs and IDLs. VLDLs are hepatically derived particles. They are enriched in triacylglycerol derived from chylomicron remnants that are both taken up by and endogenously synthesized in liver. The components of VLDL particles are similar to those of chylomicrons although the proportion of triacylglycerol is less; the major differences between the two particles are their sites of origin and apolipoprotein contents. The major apolipoproteins on VLDL are apo B 100 and apo E. Again, similar to the fate of chylomicron particles, VLDLs once in circulation are depleted of triacylglycerol by lipases. At this point the metabolism of chylomicron and VLDL particles diverges.

As a result of the gradual loss of triacylglycerol from the VLDL particles and transfer of some of the apolipoprotein components, the particles shift from those rich in triacylglycerol to those rich in cholesterol. As this process progresses, the density of the particle increases because of the loss of lipid. These particles are reclassified as IDLs and, after subsequent loss of lipid and apolipoproteins, eventually LDLs. IDLs are a heterogeneous class of lipoprotein particles that normally do not accumulate in plasma.

LDLs. LDLs are the major cholesterol-carrying lipoprotein particles in circulation. Levels of LDL cholesterol have been associated with increased risk of atherosclerosis.[2] Apo B 100 is the major and possibly sole apolipoprotein on LDL. LDL can be removed from circulation by receptor-dependent and receptor-independent mechanisms. Uptake of LDL particles by the receptor-mediated process provides a mechanism for inhibiting endogenous cholesterol synthesis via inhibition of the rate-limiting enzyme in cholesterol synthesis, HMG CoA reductase. The system is delicately balanced to meet the critical cholesterol needs of the cell and to avoid excess intracellular cholesterol accumulation. Unfortunately, for reasons that are not altogether clear, this delicate balance is often lost, the clinical manifestations of which are seen in the development of the various forms of arteriosclerosis. Of all the subclasses of lipoprotein particles, LDLs are by far most strongly and positively correlated with the risk of developing atherosclerosis.

HDLs. HDL is a subclass of lipoprotein particles originating from intestine, liver, and the surface of chylomicron remnants. They are the densest subclass of lipoprotein particles. HDL particles are thought to be involved with reverse cholesterol transport, the only process by which cholesterol in peripheral tissues is transported to liver for metabolism or excretion from the body. HDL concentrations are negatively correlated with the risk of developing atherosclerosis.[2]

Lp(a). Lp(a) is a unique lipoprotein particle composed of an LDL particle onto which, via a disulfide bridge, a high-molecular-weight glycoprotein termed apo (a) is linked. High concentrations of Lp(a) have been associated with increased risk of cardiovascular disease, possibly because of the homology of apo (a) with plasminogen. Concentrations of Lp(a) are highly heritable and less affected by environmental factors than are other lipoproteins.

Factors Associated with Increased Risk of Developing Cardiovascular Disease

Recommendations about the diagnosis and treatment of hypercholesterolemia have been provided by the National Cholesterol Education Program Expert Panel on Detection, Evaluation, and Treatment of High Blood Cholesterol in Adults.[2] The recommendations stress the importance of risk factors in devising individualized treatment plans. The recommendations identify elevated levels of total and LDL cholesterol as the primary criteria for lipid-lowering regimes; total cholesterol <5.2 mmol/L (200 mg/dL) is desirable, 5.2–6.2 mmol/L (200-240 mg/dL) is borderline high, and >6.2 mmol/L (240 mg/dL) is high. The current list of negative and positive risk factors is shown in Table 1.

Relationship of Cardiovascular Disease and Plasma Cholesterol Concentrations

Cross-cultural comparisons clearly identified a positive relationship between mean plasma cholesterol concentrations and the incidence of CHD.[3] Similar observations were made within the United States.[4,5] Migration patterns accompanied by changes in plasma cholesterol concentrations and incidence of CHD strengthened these observations.[6,7] Primary prevention clinical trials demonstrated that the degree to which plasma cholesterol concentrations are reduced is directly related to reduction of the incidence of both fatal and nonfatal CHD.[8–11] Interest is now centering on the potential for inducing regression of atherosclerotic lesions by lowering plasma cholesterol concentrations via diet, drug therapy, or both.[12–14]

In addition to a relationship between plasma cholesterol concentrations and incidence of CHD, there is also a considerable body of epidemiologic data relating plasma cholesterol concentrations to dietary fat intake.[15–17] Results from the classic Seven Countries Study and more recently the MONICA study suggest that in populations, mean total cholesterol levels correlate with the percent of energy consumed as fat and saturated fat.[3,18]

Relationship of Diet and Plasma Cholesterol Concentrations

The limited work documenting a relationship between an intervention and the incidence of CHD can be attributed, in part, to ineffective long-term dietary intervention and to difficulties in studying the incidence of CHD within the lifetime of the researchers. Hence, much of the work relating to altering the risk of CHD is based on the effect of the intervention on plasma cholesterol concentrations.

Two independent reports published in the 1960s involving a series of clinical trials indicated that consumption of saturated fatty acids and dietary cholesterol increased plasma cholesterol, polyunsaturated fatty acids decreased plasma cholesterol, and monounsaturated fatty acids had no effect on plasma cholesterol levels.[19,20] A more recent report derived from a meta-analysis of 27 feeding studies concluded that under isocaloric metabolic-ward conditions, replacement of saturated fatty acids with unsaturated fatty acids with no decrease in total fat intake resulted in the most favorable lipoprotein risk profile.[21] Additionally, replacement of carbohydrates with fat lowered serum triacylglycerol concentrations.

Table 1. Risk factors other than low-density lipoprotein cholesterol for cardiovascular disease[a]

Positive risk factors
- Age: males ≥ 45 years; females ≥55 years or premature menopause without estrogen replacement therapy
- Family history of premature coronary heart disease (myocardial infarction or sudden death before 55 years of age in father or other male first-degree relative or before 65 years of age in mother or other female first-degree relative)
- Current cigarette smoking
- Hypertension (blood pressure ≥140/90 mm Hg, or taking antihypertensive medication)
- Low HDL cholesterol (≤0.9 mmol/L [35 mg/dL])
- Diabetes mellitus

Negative risk factor
- High HDL cholesterol (≥1.6 mmol/L [60 mg/dL])

[a]Adapted from reference 2.

Dietary fat. Altering the fatty acid composition of the diet has consistently been reported to alter plasma cholesterol and lipoprotein concentrations. However, it is difficult to predict the exact magnitude of the change in response to a dietary perturbation for a specific group of individuals. Most likely absolute changes are influenced by the age of the study subjects; their sex; the presence of genetic mutations in apolipoproteins, lipoprotein receptors, or other proteins involved in lipoprotein metabolism; efficiency of absorption; the magnitude of the dietary perturbation; the length of study period; the habitual diet before entering the experimental protocol; whether different fatty acids are substituted for each other or replaced by carbohydrate; and possibly initial plasma lipid concentrations of the study subject. The National Cholesterol Education Program's most recent recommendations for individuals with total cholesterol >5.2 mmol/L is to limit total fat intake to ≤30% of energy.[2] This recommendation has been extended by the Surgeon General of the United States to all people older than 2 years living in the United States.

Saturated fatty acids. Saturated fatty acids have no double bonds in the carbon chain. One of the most consistent observations with respect to the effect of diet on plasma lipid levels is that the consumption of foods relatively high in saturated fatty acids (henceforth referred to as saturated fat) results in an increase in plasma cholesterol concentrations.[22] The increased plasma concentration observed is accounted for by increases in the concentration of both LDL and HDL cholesterol. A decreased removal rate of LDL from plasma has been suggested as a possible mechanism for the observation.[23] The consumption of saturated fat has not been shown to have a consistent effect on plasma triacylglycerol concentrations. This issue is complicated when the level of specific fatty acids is altered by the substitution of carbohydrate, because carbohydrate tends to increase plasma triacylglycerol concentrations independent of the fatty acid composition of the diet.

Although consumption of saturated fat generally results in increased plasma cholesterol concentrations, this is not true for all saturated fatty acids. In general, the short-chain fatty acids (6–10 carbons) and stearic acid (18 carbons) have little effect on plasma cholesterol concentrations.[23] Lauric (12 carbons), myristic (14 carbons), and palmitic acids (16 carbons) raise plasma cholesterol concentrations. Some variability with respect to the effect of different fatty acids on plasma cholesterol levels has been reported, especially when animals are used as the experimental model. Differences in the total diet dictated by the nutritional needs of the species and genetic differences are likely to account for much of the variability. The total absence of cholesterol in some of the animal diets also complicates interpretation of the data. Unless chemically defined formula diets are consumed, it is difficult to formulate a diet that contains only saturated fatty acids that are neutral with regard to cholesterol but avoids the hypercholesterolemic saturated fatty acids. The National Cholesterol Education Program's most recent recommendations limit saturated fat intake initially to <10% of energy and, if an inadequate response on plasma cholesterol is observed, to <7% of energy.[2]

Monounsaturated fatty acids. Monounsaturated fatty acids are a class of fatty acids that have one double bond in the carbon chain. Until recently, more emphasis was given to the ratio of dietary polyunsaturated to saturated fatty acids than to the intake of the specific fatty acid classes. This occurred, in part, because early work suggested that consumption of monounsaturated fatty acids is neutral with regard to plasma cholesterol levels.[19,20] Investigators reconsidering the effects of polyunsaturated and monounsaturated fatty acids on plasma lipids and lipoproteins have generally found that the replacement of saturated fatty acids with either of these fatty acid classes has a hypocholesterolemic effect.[24–27]

A more refined methodology to monitor individual lipoprotein concentrations revealed that the decrease in plasma cholesterol concentrations resulting from decreased consumption of saturated fat and increased consumption of polyunsaturated fat was attributable to decreases in both LDL- and HDL-cholesterol concentrations.[24–27] Some reports suggest that consumption of diets relatively high in monounsaturated fatty acids compared with polyunsaturated fatty acids had the advantage of selectively decreasing LDL cholesterol while minimizing the decrease in HDL cholesterol.[28,29] However, a recent meta-analysis of the available work suggests that the effect of consuming polyunsaturated fat and monounsaturated fat is similar and results in a decrease in both LDL and HDL cholesterol.[30] Current

recommendations are that monounsaturated fat intake compose 5–15% of the total dietary energy. Interestingly, a possible mechanism for the lack of a cholesterol-raising effect of the saturated fatty acid stearic acid is that after ingestion, it is rapidly converted to oleic acid (18 carbons, one double bond).[23]

In addition to the effects of dietary monounsaturated fatty acids on plasma lipid and lipoprotein concentrations, interest has also centered on the susceptibility of LDL to oxidation when isolated from individuals consuming different types of fatty acids. The atherogenicity of LDL has been reported to be increased after the postsecretory oxidation of the lipoprotein particle.[31,32] Consumption of diets rich in monounsaturated fatty acids compared with polyunsaturated fatty acids results in a decreased susceptibility to oxidative modification.[33,34] This is most likely attributable to the decreased total number of double bonds in the dietary fat. Further work is necessary to better define the relationship between the levels of antioxidants in specific dietary fat sources and in the actual lipoproteins and how these factors influence the susceptibility of lipoproteins to oxidation. Also important will be work on defining the relationship between in vitro measures of susceptibility of LDL to oxidation and the in vivo development of the lesion in the arterial wall.

Polyunsaturated fatty acids. Polyunsaturated fatty acids are a class of fatty acids that have two or more double bonds in the carbon chain. They are a very heterogeneous group of fatty acids and occur in a wide variety of foods. The nomenclature for describing the location of the double bond in polyunsaturated fatty acids depends on which end of the carbon chain, carboxyl or methyl, the carbon atoms are numbered. Classically, when describing the position of the double bonds, numbering starts from the carboxyl end of the carbon chain. In recent years there has been more emphasis on describing classes of polyunsaturated fatty acids according to the location of the first double bond from the methyl end; those with the first double bond at carbon 6 are classified as n–6 (ω6) fatty acids, and those with the first double bond at carbon 3 are classified as n–3 (ω3) fatty acids. Different biological functions have been reported for fatty acids of the n–3 and n–6 series.

Linoleic acid (18 carbons, 2 double bonds, n–6: 18:2n–6) is an essential fatty acid because it cannot be synthesized in the body in adequate amounts. Therefore, it needs to be supplied from dietary sources. A subsequent metabolic product of linoleic acid is arachidonic acid (20:4). When linoleic acid is provided in inadequate amounts, arachidonic acid can partially substitute for the linolenic acid requirement. The issue of whether α-linolenic acid (18:3n–3) is also an essential fatty acid has only recently been resolved. Alpha-linolenic acid can be elongated and desaturated to produce eicosapentaenoic

Table 2. Common fatty acids

Symbol	Common name	Code
Saturated fatty acids		
12:0	Lauric acid	$CH_3(CH_2)_{10}COOH$
14:0	Myristic acid	$CH_3(CH_2)_{12}COOH$
16:0	Palmitic acid	$CH_3(CH_2)_{14}COOH$
18:0	Stearic acid	$CH_3(CH_2)_{16}COOH$
Monosaturated fatty acids		
cis-16:1n-7	Palmitoleic acid	$CH_3(CH_2)_5CH=(c)CH(CH_2)_7COOH$
cis-18:1n-9	Oeic acid	$CH_3(CH_2)_7CH=(c)CH(CH_2)_7COOH$
trans-18:1n-9	Elaidic acid	$CH_3(CH_2)_7CH=(t)CH(CH_2)_7COOH$
Polyunsaturated fatty acids		
cis-18:2n-6,9	Linoleic acid	$CH_3(CH_2)_4CH=(c)CHCH_2CH=(c)CH(CH_2)_7COOH$
cis-18:3n-3,6,9	α-Linolenic acid	$CH_3CH_2CH=(c)CHCH_2CH=(c)CHCH_2CH=(c)CH(CH_2)_7COOH$
cis-18:3n-6,9,12	γ-Linolenic acid	$CH_3(CH_2)_4CH=(c)CHCH_2CH=(c)CHCH_2CH=(c)CH(CH_2)_4COOH$
cis-20:4n-6,9,12,15	Arachidonic acid	$CH_3(CH_2)_4CH=(c)CHCH_2CH=(c)CHCH_2CH=$ $(c)CHCH_2CH=(c)CH(CH_2)_3COOH$
cis-20:5n-3,6,9,12,15	Eicosapentaenoic acid	$CH_3(CH_2CH=(c)CH)_5(CH_2)_3COOH$
cis-22:6n-3,6,9,12,15,18	Docosahexaenoic acid	$CH_3(CH_2CH=(c)CH)_6(CH_2)_2COOH$

acid (20:6n–3) and docosahexaenoic acid (22:5n–3). Current evidence suggests that fatty acids of the n–3 series cannot completely substitute for linoleic acid.

Essential fatty acids are precursors of the biologically active class of compounds collectively termed eicosanoids. Eicosanoids include prostaglandins, thromboxanes, and leukotrienes. The precursor fatty acid from either the n–3 or n–6 series determines the specific product; the precursors often compete with each other for enzyme systems. Eicosanoids, in turn, are involved in a wide range of regulatory processes. The inability of humans to synthesize certain fatty acids is attributed to the lack of the δ-12 dehydrogenase enzyme, which inserts a double bond after the ninth carbon from the carboxyl end of the chain. No specific essential fatty acid requirements have been set. Safe intakes are frequently quoted as 1–2% of energy, although higher estimates have found their way into the literature. A list of the major fatty acids is included in Table 2.

The major n–6 polyunsaturated fatty acid consumed in the U.S. diet is linoleic acid (18:2). Current National Cholesterol Education Program recommendations are that polyunsaturated fat intake should be ≤10% of energy.[2]

Soon after the hypocholesterolemic effects of vegetable oils were reported, similar effects were reported for oils derived from fish and marine mammals. However, it was not until reports appeared of low rates of CHD in Greenland Eskimos[35] and the inverse relationship between fish consumption and mortality from CHD[36] that the area received expanded attention. It is unclear whether the benefit of fish in the diet is due to substitution for foods higher in saturated fat or whether it has some independent protective qualities. In addition to the cholesterol-

lowering effect of n–3 and n–6 fatty acids relative to saturated fatty acids, other positive factors with respect to CHD have been attributed specifically to n–3 fatty acids, including decreases in triacylglycerol levels, platelet aggregation, and blood pressure.[37–39] Of some concern is a recent report suggesting that high levels of fish consumption result in decreased immune response.[40] The practical significance of this finding is unclear. No specific recommendations for n–3 fatty acid consumption have been made. At present it seems prudent to recommend moderate intakes of foods containing high levels of n–3 fatty acids.

Trans *fatty acids*. A relatively new concern with respect to dietary fat is *trans* fatty acid intake.[41] *Trans* fatty acids are so termed on the basis of the conformation of a double bond in the acyl chain. Except for fatty acids formed in the rumen of animals, most naturally occurring unsaturated fatty acids are in the *cis* configuration. The hydrogenation process, which is used to convert liquid oils into semisolid fats (e.g., transforming vegetable oil to margarine or vegetable shortening), results in formation of *trans* double bonds. As a result of the increased consumption of hydrogenated fat, the intake of *trans* fatty acids has increased in the United States since 1900. The difference between double bonds in the *cis* and *trans* configuration has to do with the angle of the carbon atoms around the double bond in the fatty acid chain. Double bonds with a *cis* configuration have a conformation with a greater bond angle or kink in the carbon chain than do those containing double bonds with a *trans* configuration. The latter tend to resemble saturated fatty acids in conformation. Therefore, increasing the *trans* fatty acid content of a fat results in closer packing or aligning of the fatty acid chains (due to fewer kinks), resulting in decreased fluidity of the fat. Early work on the effects of *trans* fatty acid consumption in humans on plasma lipids was inconclusive.[42-44] However, recent studies reported a negative effect on plasma lipoproteins of consuming products enriched in elaidic acid (*trans*-18:1) or hydrogenated fat as compared with oleic acid (*cis*-18:1) or the liquid oil.[41,45-47] Recent epidemiologic studies have reported a positive association between *trans* fatty acid intake and plasma cholesterol concentration or incidence of cardiovascular disease, whereas other studies have reported no association between adipose tissue *trans* fatty acid content (used as a measure of long-term dietary intake) and incidence of cardiovascular disease.[48]

Dietary cholesterol. Most data have confirmed observations originally made in animals that increasing dietary cholesterol results in higher plasma cholesterol levels[49,50] and is associated with increased CHD risk.[51-53] Less clear are the modulating effects of the fatty acid composition of the diet and the characteristics of the study subjects in response to dietary cholesterol. Additionally, although dietary cholesterol is discussed separately, naturally occurring foods rich in saturated fat also tend to contain cholesterol (notable exceptions include coconut, palm, and palm kernel oils). Although a vast literature exists on the effect of dietary cholesterol on plasma lipids, the area remains somewhat controversial because of the inconsistent nature of the observations.[49,50,54,55] Factors that may partially account for the variable results reported include the form of dietary cholesterol (egg yolk or crystalline), the type of diet (natural foods or formula), the amount of supplemental cholesterol (within the range of common intake or above), the fat content and composition of the background diet, and whether the supplemental cholesterol was added to diets of free-living subjects or incorporated into defined diets provided by a metabolic kitchen. Also complicating the picture is the variable response of individuals, even at times the same individual, to a dietary cholesterol challenge. However, increasing the level of dietary cholesterol usually results in increased plasma cholesterol concentrations.

The current recommendations are that dietary cholesterol intake be limited to ≤300 mg/day. If an individual is hyperlipidemic and an inadequate response is observed, intake is restricted further, to ≤200 mg/day.

Summary

Arteriosclerosis is a term that refers to a group of disorders characterized by thickening and loss of elasticity of the arterial wall and frequently by compromised blood flow. Accumulation of fatty plaque composed primarily of cholesterol and cholesteryl esters is the hallmark of the disease. Arteriosclerosis can include a variety of vessels, including coronary, cerebral, femoral, and iliac arteries and aorta. It is the leading cause of death and disability in the United States despite the data indicating that during the 1980s, the age-adjusted death rates from cardiovascular disease decreased by 26%. A major risk factor for the development of arteriosclerosis is elevated levels of LDL cholesterol. Other risk factors associated with the development of arteriosclerosis include age, family history, current cigarette smoking, hypertension, and diabetes mellitus. Levels of HDL cholesterol have been negatively associated with risk of developing arteriosclerosis. One approach to decreasing plasma cholesterol levels is to reduce the amount of cholesterol and total and saturated fat in the diet. The value of this approach is supported by animal, metabolic, and epidemiologic research. The current dietary recommendation for the general population is to reduce total fat to ≤30% of energy, saturated fat to <10% of energy, and cholesterol to <300 mg/day. For hyperlipidemic individuals for whom such a diet does not provide adequate blood cholesterol lowering, a reduction of saturated fat to <7% of energy and cholesterol to <200 mg/day is recommended.

References

1. American Heart Association (1994) Research facts—update. Facts about cardiovascular diseases. American Heart Association, Dallas
2. Expert Panel on Detection, Evaluation, and Treatment of High Blood Cholesterol in Adults (1993) Summary of the second expert panel of the National Cholesterol Education Program (NCEP) Expert Panel on Detection, Evaluation, and Treatment of High Blood Cholesterol in Adults (Adult Treatment Panel II). JAMA 269:3015–3023
3. Keys A, Menotti A, Karvonen MJ, et al (1986) The diet and 15-year death rate in the Seven Countries Study. Am J Epidemiol 124:903–915
4. Shekelle RB, Shryock AM, Paul O, et al (1981) Diet, serum cholesterol, and death from coronary heart disease: the Western Electric Study. N Engl J Med 304:65–70
5. Pekkanen J, Linn S, Heiss G, et al (1990) Ten-year mortality from cardiovascular disease in relation to cholesterol level among men with and without preexisting cardiovascular disease. N Engl J Med 322:1700–1707
6. Kushi LH, Lew RA, Stare FJ, et al (1985) Diet and 20-year mortality from coronary heart disease: the Ireland-Boston Diet-Heart Study. N Engl J Med 312:811–818
7. Nichaman MZ, Hamilton HB, Kagan A, et al (1975) Epidemiological studies of coronary heart disease and stroke in Japanese men living in Japan, Hawaii and California: distribution of biochemical risk factors. Am J Epidemiol 102:491–501
8. Dayton S, Pearce ML, Goldman H, et al (1968) Controlled trial of a diet high in unsaturated fat for prevention of atherosclerotic complications. Lancet 2:1060–1062
9. Lipid Research Clinics (1984) The Lipid Research Clinics Coronary Primary Prevention Trial results. I. Reduction in incidence of coronary heart disease. JAMA 251:351–364
10. Lipid Research Clinics (1984) The Lipid Research Clinics Coronary Primary Prevention Trial results. II. The relation-

ship of reduction in incidence of coronary heart disease to cholesterol lowering. JAMA 251:365–374

11. Multiple Risk Factor Intervention Trial Research Group (1982) Multiple risk factor intervention trial: risk factor changes and mortality results. JAMA 248:1465–1477

12. Blankenhorn DH, Johnson RL, Mack WJ, et al (1990) The influence of diet on the appearance of new lesions in human coronary arteries. JAMA 263:1646–1652

13. Waters D, Lespérance J (1991) Regression of coronary atherosclerosis: an achievable goal? Review of results from recent clinical trials. Am J Med 91;1B(Suppl):10S–17S

14. Watts GF, Lewis B, Brunt JNH, et al (1992) Effects on coronary artery disease of lipid-lowering diet, or diet plus cholestyramine, in the St Thomas' Atherosclerosis Regression Study (STARS). Lancet 339:563–569

15. Keys A (1957) Diet and the epidemiology of coronary heart disease. JAMA 164:1912–1919

16. Keys A, Menotti A, Karvonen MJ, et al (1986) The diet and 15-year death rate in the Seven Countries Study. Am J Epidemiol 124:903–915

17. Kahn HA, Medalie JH, Neufeld HN, et al (1969) Serum cholesterol: its distribution and association with dietary and other variables in a survey of 10,000 men. Isr J Med Sci 5:1117–1127

18. Tunstall-Pedoe H, Kuulasmaa K, Amouyel P, et al (1994) Myocardial infarction and coronary deaths in the World Health Organization MONICA project: registration procedures, event rates, and case-fatality rates in 38 populations from 21 countries in four continents. Circulation 90:583–612

19. Hegsted DM, McGandy RB, Myers ML, Stare FJ (1965) Quantitative effects of dietary fat on serum cholesterol in man. Am J Clin Nutr 17:281–295

20. Keys A, Anderson JT, Grande F (1965) Serum cholesterol response to changes in the diet. I. Iodine value of dietary fat versus 2S-P. Metabolism 14:747–758

21. Mensink RP, Katan MB (1992) Effect of dietary fatty acids on serum lipids and lipoproteins: a meta-analysis of 27 trials. Arterioscler Thromb 12:911–919

22. Schaefer EJ, Lichtenstein AH, Lamon-Fava S, et al (1995) Lipoproteins, nutrition, aging, and atherosclerosis. Am J Clin Nutr 61:726S–740S

23. Grundy SM, Denke MA (1990) Dietary influences on serum lipids and lipoproteins. J Lipid Res 31:1149–1172

24. Ginsberg HN, Barr SL, Gilbert A (1990) Reduction of plasma cholesterol levels in normal men on an American Heart Association Step I diet or a Step I diet with added monounsaturated fat. N Engl J Med 322:574–579

25. Berry EM, Eisenberg S, Haratz D, et al (1991) Effects of diet rich in monounsaturated fatty acids on plasma lipoproteins—the Jerusalem Nutrition Study: high MUFAs vs high PUFAs. Am J Clin Nutr 53:899–907

26. Wardlaw GM, Snook JT, Lin M-C, et al (1991) Serum lipid and apolipoprotein concentrations in healthy men on diets enriched in either canola oil or safflower oil. Am J Clin Nutr 54:104–110

27. Lichtenstein AH, Ausman LM, Carrasco W, et al (1993) Effects of canola, corn, and olive oils on fasting and postprandial plasma lipoproteins in humans as part of a National Cholesterol Education Program Step 2 diet. Arterioscler Thromb 13:1533–1542

28. Mattson FH, Grundy SM. (1985) Comparison of effects of dietary saturated, monounsaturated, and polyunsaturated fatty acids on plasma lipids and lipoproteins in man. J Lipid Res 26:194–202

29. Mata P, Garrido JA, Ordovas JM, et al (1992) Effect of dietary monounsaturated fatty acids on plasma lipoproteins and apolipoproteins in women. Am J Clin Nutr 56:77–83

30. Gardner CD, Kraemer HC (1995) Mono- versus polyunsaturated dietary fat and serum lipids: a meta-analysis. Arterioscler Thromb Vasc Biol 15:1917–1927

31. Ylä-Herttuala S, Palinski W, Rosenfeld ME, et al (1989) Evidence for the presence of oxidatively modified low density lipoprotein in atherosclerotic lesions of rabbit and man. J Clin Invest 84:1086–1095

32. Steinberg D, Parthasarathy S, Carew TE, et al (1989) Beyond cholesterol: modifications of low-density lipoprotein that increase its atherogenicity. N Engl J Med 320:915–924

33. Reaven PD, Grasse BJ, Tribble DL (1994) Effects of linoleate-enriched and oleate-enriched diets in combination with α-tocopherol on the susceptibility of LDL and LDL subfractions to oxidative modification in humans. Arterioscler Thromb 14:557–566

34. Parthasarathy S, Khoo JC, Miller E, et al (1990) Low density lipoprotein rich in oleic acid is protected against oxidative modification: implications for dietary prevention of atherosclerosis. Proc Natl Acad Sci USA 87:3894–3898

35. Bang HO, Dyerberg J (1985) Fish consumption and mortality from coronary heart disease. N Engl J Med 313:822–823

36. Kromhout D, Bosschieter EB, Coulander CL (1985) The inverse relationship between fish consumption and 20-year mortality from coronary heart disease. N Engl J Med 312:1205–1209

37. Nestel PJ, Connor WE, Reardon MF, et al (1984) Suppression by diets rich in fish oil of very low density lipoprotein production in man. J Clin Invest 74:82–89

38. van Schacky C, Weber PC (1985) Metabolism and effects on platelet function of the purified eicosapentaenoic and docosahexanenoic acids in humans. J Clin Invest 76:2446–2450

39. Knapp HR, FitzGerald GA. (1989) The antihypertensive effects of fish oil. N Engl J Med 320:1037–1043

40. Meydani SN, Lichtenstein AH, Cornwall S, et al (1993) Immunological effects of National Cholesterol Education Panel Step 2 diets with and without fish-derived n-3 fatty acid enrichment. J Clin Invest 192:105–113

41. Mensink RP, Katan MB (1990) Effect of dietary trans fatty acids on high density and low density lipoprotein cholesterol levels in healthy subjects. New Engl J Med 323:439–445

42. Erickson BA, Coots RH, Mattson FH, Kligman AM (1964) The effect of partial hydrogenation of dietary fats, of the ratio of polyunsaturated to saturated fatty acids, and of dietary cholesterol upon plasma lipids in man. J Clin Invest 43:2017–2025

43. Mattson FH, Hollenbach EJ, Kligman AM (1975) Effect of hydrogenation fat on the plasma cholesterol and triglyceride levels of man. Am J Clin Nutr 28:726–731

44. Vergroesen AJ (1972) Dietary fat and cardiovascular disease: possible modes of action of linoleic acid. Proc Nutr Soc 31:323–329

45. Zock PL, Katan MB (1992) Hydrogenation alternatives: effects of trans fatty acids and stearic acid versus linoleic acid on serum lipids and lipoproteins in humans. J Lipid Res 33:399–410

46. Lichtenstein AH, Ausman LM, Carrasco W, et al (1993) Hydrogenation impairs the hypolipidemic effect of corn oil in humans. Arterioscler Thromb 13:154–161

47. Judd JT, Clevidence BA, Muesing RA, et al (1994) Dietary trans fatty acids: effects on plasma lipids and lipoproteins of healthy men and women. Am J Clin Nutr 59:861–868

48. Expert Panel on Trans Fatty Acids and Coronary Heart Disease (1995) Trans fatty acids and coronary heart disease risk. Am J Clin Nutr 62:655S–708S

49. Connor WE, Stone DB, Hodges RE (1964) The interrelated effects of dietary cholesterol and fat upon human serum lipid levels. J Clin Invest 43:1691–1696

50. Hopkins PN (1992) Effects of dietary cholesterol on serum cholesterol: a meta-analysis and review. Am J Clin Nutr 55:1060–1070

51. Armstrong BK, Mann JI, Adelstein AM, Eskin F (1975) Commodity consumption and ischemic heart disease mortality, with special reference to dietary practices. J Chronic Dis 28:455–469

52. Stamler J, Stamler R, Shekelle RB (1970) Regional differences in prevalence, incidence, and mortality from atherosclerotic coronary heart disease. In deHaas JH, Hemker HC, Snellen HA (eds), Ischaemic heart disease. Leiden University Press, Leiden, The Netherlands, pp 84–127

53. Kromhout D, de Lezenne Coulander C (1984) Diet, prevalence and 10-year mortality from coronary heart disease in 871 middle-aged men: the Zutphen Study. Am J Epidemiol 119:733–741

54. Katan MB, Beynen AC, DeVries JHM, Nobels A (1986) Existence of consistent hypo and hyperresponders to dietary cholesterol in man. Am J Epidemiol 123:221–234

55. McNamara DJ, Kolb R, Parker TS, et al (1987) Heterogeneity of cholesterol homeostasis in man: response to changes in dietary fat quality and cholesterol quantity. J Clin Invest 79:1729–1739

Chapter 43

Nutritional Aspects of Hypertension

Howard R. Knapp

Considerable evidence has accumulated that suggests that nutritional factors, in combination with genetics, play a major role in the development of hypertension in humans. It has been difficult, however, to isolate the specific nutrients responsible for differences in the prevalence of hypertension between populations. Instead of attempting to critically assess all of the controversies in the area, this summary will review the dietary components most often studied for their effects on human blood pressure and discuss the limitations of the epidemiologic and experimental data that have led to confusion in the literature. It is hoped that with an increased appreciation for these issues, the reader will be better equipped to evaluate both existing work and the many papers that will be devoted to this expanding subject in the near future.

In a number of recent surveys, patients with mild essential hypertension (most hypertensive patients) have not been found to derive a cardiac benefit from drug therapy.[1,2] In fact, the health risk of some drugs used to treat mild hypertension probably outweighs the marginal benefit that many patients in this group would obtain, particularly since up to one-third of these individuals have been found to be normotensive when away from the physician's office. Therefore, dietary and other non-pharmacological therapies for hypertension are being avidly sought for this large number of patients, with the hope of increased benefit and decreased risk and cost.[3,4] Prior to a discussion of the actual studies relating diet and blood pressure, however, a description of hypertension study design and methods will illustrate how misleading results can be generated in studies that fail to take these well-established characteristics of blood pressure measurement into account.

Dietary Experiments on Volunteers

Studying outpatient blood pressure in a meaningful way requires careful attention to study design, subject selection, and observer bias. Similar issues arise in per-forming metabolic ward–type studies, but in addition, one is faced with the issue of how applicable the findings are to the blood pressures of patients in the everyday world performing their normal daily tasks. The recent advent of ambulatory blood pressure monitoring has revealed considerable differences between subjects' blood pressures obtained in the clinic, at work, and at home.[5] This discrepancy can be in either direction, depending on the circumstances. For instance, about one-third of patients believed to have mild hypertension on the basis of clinic blood pressure measurements are found to be normotensive away from the doctor's office. On the other hand, patients believed to be receiving adequate antihypertensive therapy on the basis of supine blood pressure readings, obtained after 5 minutes of rest, may be found to lack significant blood pressure control when assessed with ambulatory monitors during their routine, stressful activities. Obviously, the latter values are more pertinent in producing end-organ damage and morbidity from elevated blood pressure. It has been shown, too, that blood pressure values obtained with ambulatory monitors correlate with left ventricular hypertrophy much better than do clinic blood pressures.[6]

Although ambulatory monitors can provide useful data if one is practiced in evaluating their performance, it is possible to use random-zero sphygmomanometers to at least eliminate observer bias in pressure measurement. Blood pressure is highly variable in both normotensive and hypertensive subjects, and it is essential to take into account a number of well-known problems in assessing changes in it. The blood pressures of most subjects entering studies will fall as they become accustomed to having their pressures measured. Also, since blood pressure is changing continuously during the day, subjects selected for inclusion in a study on the basis of a high (for them) pressure measurement will exhibit a better picture of their true (lower) mean pressure with repeated measurement. These effects of habituation and regression on the mean require that diet–blood pressure studies must have run-in periods that are long enough (up

Table 1. Problems in studying hypertension

Problem	Solution
Measurement errors and bias	Ambulatory monitors Random-zero sphygmomanometer
Marked variability of blood pressure	Multiple measurements
Effects of multiple dietary changes	Adequate controls, careful dietary change assessment
Habituation and regression on the mean effects	Run-in and recovery periods
Season and environment effects	Parallel, randomized controls

to 6 weeks) and have enough pressure measurements taken so that the subjects' true mean pressures are revealed. It has been shown, for example, that in a randomized, crossover study, several weeks of placebo treatment caused actual decreases in urinary catecholamine excretion and 10 mm Hg drops in blood pressure.[7] This degree of blood pressure reduction is larger than that reported in most dietary intervention studies. Such observations also raise the issue of needing appropriate placebo control groups during these types of studies.

Another study design feature almost never employed in nutritional intervention studies of blood pressure is the posttreatment recovery period. If true baseline pressures have been achieved prior to the dietary intervention, and a diet-related change is then observed, one would expect the blood pressures to return to baseline after the patients return to their usual diets, unless a permanent cure of their hypertension is anticipated. When such measurements are taken, it is sometimes obvious that the subjects' blood pressures never go back up toward the presumed baseline, and that the observed reduction was only a habituation effect occurring during the treatment period, that is, the run-in was inadequate. Other issues not usually addressed by studies in this area include blinding of subjects to the dietary intervention when possible, and actually assessing the subjects' diets during the study to see whether the intended dietary change has provoked unanticipated alterations in the subjects' eating patterns because of gastrointestinal objections to the trial diet. Such evaluation of personal habits should also include documenting the use of alcohol, nonsteroidal anti-inflammatory agents, and other drugs that may alter blood pressure or other parameters (for example, prostaglandins and plasma lipids) being measured.[8] In addition, one must appreciate how difficult it is to change one dietary component in isolation, and that eating more of one type of food means that less of something else must be consumed to avoid weight changes, which can alter blood pressure.[9,10]

Finally, study design issues that are routine in clinical pharmacology often seem to be unappreciated or ignored in nutrition intervention trials. These issues include randomization of subjects in both treated and control groups, and matched parallel control groups, to account for environmental or seasonal changes and to avoid crossover effects. Statistical power calculations are notably rare as well, and would give some assurance that the experiment has enough subjects to have a reasonable chance of detecting a biologically meaningful change in blood pressure. A summary of some problems encountered in studying outpatient blood pressure is presented in Table 1.

Epidemiologic Studies

There are a number of problems in the interpretation of data relating diet and blood pressure in populations. It is rare to find two groups of people eating diets that differ in only one dietary component. Most groups eating diets with a high fish content, for example, also have a high intake of salt, which could obscure any hypotensive influence of fish. Also, the consumption of an unusual type of food over many generations may result in genetic adaptation to some components, which would, therefore, have different effects in different population groups. It is possible, for instance, that a high intake of n–3 fatty acids by Eskimos on a marine diet may have fewer or different long-term effects for them than the same amounts of these compounds being consumed as dietary supplements by Americans.

Many nutrients have a high degree of association in foodstuffs, and it is important to remember that people eat food, not specific nutrients as individual items. It is, therefore, very difficult to isolate the health effects of particular dietary components. Many dietary habits that are believed to have a direct influence on blood pressure are also related to other personal characteristics that are known to affect it, such as alcohol intake, body size, physical activity, and obesity. It has been noted, for instance, that total energy intake is intimately related to the consumption of all major nutrients and is driven by physical activity level. Schoolchildren found to have lower blood pressures, for example, were also found to have a higher intake of all nutrients, primarily because

Table 2. Problems in diet–blood pressure epidemiology

Lack of standardized blood pressure measurements
Inaccuracy of nutrient intake estimates
Confounding effects of environment and social factors
Possible genetic differences in response to nutrients
Comparisons of noncontemporaneous populations, with different levels of public health measures and infections

they were more active.[4] As a result, it would be difficult to interpret any inverse associations found between particular nutrients and blood pressure. An additional problem in population studies is estimating nutrient intake accurately and being sure that standardized methods of blood pressure measurement were used in the different groups being compared. Because of these numerous difficulties in interpretation, epidemiologic studies are useful in finding associations and generating hypotheses, but these must be tested in carefully controlled dietary intervention studies. Some of the issues confounding epidemiologic studies of diet-blood pressure relationships are summarized in Table 2.

Alcohol and Vascular Function

Although an entire chapter of this volume is devoted to the nutritional aspects of alcohol, it must be mentioned as a confounding variable in population studies on vascular disease and blood pressure. Mediterranean populations have a lower incidence of vascular disease than those of Northern Europe, and this is frequently ascribed to differences in the amount and type of lipid in their diets.[11] The dietary component that correlated most strongly with a healthy vasculature in the famous Seven Countries Study, however, was red wine intake.[12] The percent of total calories that populations consume as alcohol is highly variable, and seems to be frequently overlooked in studies of hypertension and atherosclerosis. In the United States, it has been estimated that excess alcohol intake is responsible for about 10% of hypertension, especially in middle-aged men.[3,13] As a result, excess alcohol intake is the leading cause of secondary hypertension in this group. On a statistical basis, individuals who regularly consume over 60 mL of ethanol per day have a higher prevalence of hypertension, and a reduced consumption is recommended for hypertensive patients.[13] Since the hypertensive effects of even small doses of alcohol have been well documented, it is difficult to see how dietary intervention studies on blood pressure could be conducted without taking this into account.[3]

Obesity and Weight Loss

The effect of obesity on blood pressure appears to be independent of dietary components other than alcohol,

with which it has an additive effect.[3,4] It is now known that a male obesity pattern, with excess weight predominantly in the upper body and abdomen, is more strongly correlated with hypertension than is the female pattern, where excess weight is mainly in the buttocks and thighs.[14] In the United States, there has been a strong and consistent association between obesity and hypertension, especially in men under age 45.[15,16] This influence must be appreciated when comparing data across populations, as well as between different subgroups within a country. It has long been considered that an increase in blood pressure with age was a hallmark of populations eating a diet high in salt.[17] There is some evidence, however, that this phenomenon is actually related to the increase in weight with age in most acculturated societies, and it is rarely seen in populations without such a weight increase. In addition, the responses of obese hypertensive patients to dietary manipulations may not be the same as those of lean subjects, so it is important that the subjects' weights be taken into account in study design. This would include setting study inclusion criteria for body mass index (height/weight^2), as well as being sure that the randomization process produces comparable numbers of similar patients in the different study groups.

The effects of weight loss on blood pressure have been studied extensively, but with controversial results.[8,18] Calorie-restricted diets are usually low in sodium as well, but a number of well-designed trials in hypertensive subjects have found a significant lowering of blood pressure that was attributable to weight loss.[18,19] It is important, therefore, that dietary interventions are designed with such effects in mind, and that the subjects' weights are actually measured during the study. Since achieving ideal body weight will nearly normalize the blood pressures of many obese male (and some female) hypertensive patients, this is a first step in management of their condition.

Sodium

There have been a number of observations that hypertension is virtually nonexistent in primitive societies with a diet low in salt.[17] This topic has been the subject of much controversy, but there is some consensus that a diet high in calories, fat, and sodium and low in potassium is associated with the development of hypertension.[3,4]

People in primitive societies are, for the most part, physically active throughout their lives and lean vegetarians who are not exposed to alcohol, so the dietary components actually responsible for the development of hypertension are unclear.[4] The role of sodium itself in causing hypertension is difficult to study within a population since there may not be a sufficiently diverse intake of sodium; that is, the dose-response relationship between sodium and blood pressure may be flat over the range of intake in a population. Studies of migrations and recruitment of primitive people into modern armies in Africa, however, have lent support to the importance of chronically high sodium intake in increased blood pressure. Major criticisms of the available epidemiologic data include the difficulty in measuring sodium intake and the lack of standardization of blood pressure measurement.[3,4,20]

Clinical trials of sodium restriction in hypertensive subjects have been reviewed, and there is reasonable evidence that such restriction will lower blood pressure in many patients and reduce their need for antihypertensive drugs.[21] Although the blood pressure response to sodium restriction is quite heterogeneous, there is no known hazard to a moderate sodium restriction; it will benefit the salt-sensitive subset of patients. From a practical standpoint, reducing sodium intake in the American diet would most likely also lead to a reduction in dietary fat content, which is considered desirable from several health standpoints.[11] If dietary sodium were a major factor in the development of hypertension in industrialized countries, however, one would expect that increased intake would increase blood pressure in normotensive subjects, especially those with strong family histories of hypertension, who are at increased risk of developing hypertension themselves. However, this has not been found to be the case. In addition, the fact that strict vegetarians or thin nondrinkers can have a low prevalence of hypertension and a high sodium intake has suggested that sodium by itself has a minor role in the development of hypertension.[4]

Potassium

It has been proposed that primitive societies lack hypertension because of their high potassium, rather than low sodium, intake.[22] As is the case with sodium, the epidemiologic data have many limitations. A number of investigators, however, believe that the dietary potassium-sodium ratio is an important predictor of the tendency to blood pressure elevation; studies have reported an inverse correlation between blood pressure and the ratio of these electrolytes in urine where there was no correlation with the excretion of either electrolyte alone.[3,4]

Trials of dietary potassium supplementation have all involved small numbers of patients for a short duration, and this information has been summarized.[3,4,23] Such supplements have no effect on the blood pressures of normotensive subjects, although it has been shown recently that potassium depletion of normal individuals causes sodium retention and increased blood pressure both at baseline and in response to a saline infusion.[24] The effects of potassium supplements on hypertensive individuals also appear to involve a natriuresis and depend on the subjects' sodium status. If the patients have a low potassium intake and have not been treated with sodium restriction, then additional potassium seems to have a moderate hypotensive effect.[23]

Calcium, Magnesium, and Trace Elements

During the last few years, there has been considerable discussion of the role of dietary calcium in the prevention and management of hypertension. On the basis of an extensive population survey, it was suggested that calcium intake had a potent blood pressure–lowering effect, and some small clinical trials have reported positive results.[25] After the epidemiologic data were reanalyzed to account for the confounding effects of age, income, alcohol consumption, and obesity, the effects of calcium were less clear-cut.[4,26] Also, several well-designed intervention trials performed more recently have been negative, and it has been shown that the intake of calcium, mainly derived from dairy products, is strongly associated with that of potassium and protein.[4] Some bias in the population survey data may also have been introduced by the fact that social class and activity level strongly influence both dairy product consumption and blood pressure. Not only have intervention trials given conflicting results, but even those that are considered by the authors to show a hypotensive effect of calcium supplements reveal a heterogeneous response, with substantial increases in blood pressure in some subjects. This, plus the reports of increased urinary calcium excretion or altered calcium metabolism in hypertensive patients, makes a confusing picture.[27,28] A recent National Institutes of Health consensus conference on dietary calcium and blood pressure suggested that recommending changes in dietary calcium for the purpose of lowering blood pressure was premature.[29]

While magnesium sulfate has effective hypotensive properties when rapidly infused, there is little direct evidence for its role in blood pressure regulation. Results in properly designed clinical trials showed that dietary magnesium supplements had no effect on blood pressure of hypertensive patients, except in those patients whose potassium levels had been depleted by diuretics.[30,31] There have been a number of observations correlating lower urinary magnesium excretion or low erythrocyte magnesium levels with higher blood pressure in population groups, but this has not been corroborated by other workers.[32] These sorts of data suffer from the disadvantage of small numbers of subjects and the fact that negative findings are less likely to be published. Perhaps future work will clarify the relationship between dietary magnesium, other cations, blood pressure, and renin, as has been speculated.[33]

Combinations of Dietary Metals

In addition to discussing the possible role of individual dietary metals in blood pressure control, it should be mentioned that, as with many groups of nutrients, it is unusual for dietary changes to result in altered intake of one particular component. Therefore, it is of interest that a lowering of blood pressure has been detected in some studies incorporating changes in the intake of several metals. One recent report claimed a reduction in blood pressure with a dietary combination of low sodium, high potassium, and high magnesium intakes.[34] The subjects were 100 men, aged 55–75, with mild to moderate hypertension; the study was performed over a 24-week treatment period. This study also included a 25-week posttreatment phase, during which the lowered blood pressures returned to their pretreatment values. Such a well-designed clinical trial will no doubt serve as a stimulus for further work to define optimal intakes of sodium, potassium, and magnesium in our increasingly elderly population.

A major portion of trace element intake is via drinking water. Blood pressure elevation has been demonstrated in studies of animals given clearly toxic amounts of cadmium and in humans poisoned chronically with cadmium, lead, mercury and thallium, but there is no epidemiologic evidence relating the intake of these elements to hypertension in the general population.[35,36] However, work in this area—the epidemiology of the health effects of trace metal ingestion—is continuing.[37] A direct involvement of selenium, copper, zinc, and other essential trace elements in blood pressure regulation in man has not been suggested by clinical or animal studies thus far.

Lipids

The association of obesity and a high-fat diet with hypertension in population studies was made more clinically plausible by the reported correlation between dietary saturated fat, plasma cholesterol, and atherosclerotic vascular disease.[9,11,17] Since dietary polyunsaturated (at the expense of saturated) fat has been determined to benefit atherosclerotic vascular disease, it seemed reasonable to hypothesize that the ratio of dietary polyunsaturated-to-saturated fat would influence blood pressure regulation. More recently, it has been found that the two biochemical classes of polyunsaturated fatty acids have different metabolic effects in humans, so the concept of the polyunsatured-to-saturated fat ratio as an important dietary index requires some modification.

Briefly, nature constructs fatty acids from the non-carboxyl (omega) end, and mammals are not able to produce long-chain fatty acids with unsaturations beyond the ninth carbon from the omega end. Fatty acids that we can make with such an unsaturation are referred to as being in the omega–9 (or n–9) class, and the monounsaturate oleic acid is one example. Humans must obtain polyunsaturated fatty acids through their diets. There are two major classes of polyunsaturated fatty acids that we cannot interconvert. These are the n–6 class, long regarded as "essential " for mammals, and the more recently studied n–3 class. The former are present in large amounts in the vegetable oils most widely used in the United States (such as corn, sunflower, safflower oils), while the latter are primarily found in marine oils. Some terrestrial sources of 18-carbon n–3 fatty acids exist (for example, linseed and canola oil), but it does not appear that these acids can be rapidly converted in humans to the longer chain (20 and 22 carbons) acids found in marine oils. The epidemiologic data relating either of these polyunsaturated fatty acid classes to human blood pressure are confounded by the many variables discussed above that are present in such types of data.[38,39]

Unlike many dietary lipid components, a small fraction of the polyunsaturated fatty acids ingested each day are converted in the body to local hormone-like compounds that exert a wide variety of potent biological activities.[39] Since the precursor acids for these substances (such as prostaglandins, thromboxanes, prostacyclin, and leukotrienes) have 20 carbons (that is, they are eicosanoic acids), these autocoids are often called eicosanoids, and they are known to be involved in numerous processes regulating blood pressure in humans. As a result, any physiological changes taking place during supplementation studies of polyunsaturated fatty acids have been ascribed to alterations in the types or amounts of eicosanoids produced in vivo. Very few studies have directly addressed this hypothesis, however, and the many problems in this field have been reviewed.[39]

Intervention studies have been performed with both n–6 and n–3 fatty acid supplements in both normotensive and hypertensive subjects. The literature on dietary n–6 fatty acids and blood pressure has recently been summarized.[38] In a number of the studies where a lowering of blood pressure was observed with increased dietary n–6 fatty acids, several dietary components (for example, total fat, sodium) were changed simultaneously, making it difficult to ascribe the hypotensive effect to an altered dietary polyunsaturated-to-saturated fat ratio alone. In fact, more recent work that carefully controlled total dietary fat, calories, and other components found no effect of greatly increased n–6 fatty acid intake.[40] The

Table 3. Status of dietary factors in hypertension management

Dietary Factor	Benefit
Achieving ideal body weight	Always recommended
Reducing alcohol intake (<60 mL/day)	Always recommended
Reduced sodium intake (<2 g/day)	Usually recommended
Increased potassium intake	Appears worthwhile
Increased calcium	Not clearly indicated
Increased magnesium	Not clearly indicated
Increased n–6 polyunsaturates	Not beneficial
Increased n–3 polyunsaturates	Benefit under study

opposite experiment, that of practically eliminating saturated fat from the diet of normotensive subjects to increase the polyunsaturated-to-saturated fat ratio, also failed to show any change in blood pressure.[41]

Much enthusiasm for exploring the vascular benefits of n–3 fatty acids from marine oils has been shown in recent years. Epidemiologic data, however, do not reveal lower blood pressures in populations with a high fish consumption. In fact, Eskimos have the same age-related increase in blood pressure as do Europeans, and Oriental groups with a large intake of fish have some of the highest prevalences of hypertension in the world, perhaps because of their high salt intake.[39] Numerous intervention trials have claimed a hypotensive effect of fish oils, while only several negative studies have been published. Generally, poor study design and lack of attention to basic principles of hypertension research make much of this literature uninterpretable. Despite this, two recent meta-analyses have concluded that n–3 fatty acid supplements do lower blood pressure in patients with hypertension, but not necessarily in normotensive individuals.[42,43] It appears likely, however, that the mechanism for lowering the blood pressure is not simply one of altered eicosanoid formation.[44] The amount of n–3 fatty acids needed to achieve the effect in a short time would be essentially impossible to obtain by dietary means (several pounds of oily fish per day would be required). This area has also been reviewed.[39]

Currently, studies with highly enriched n–3 fatty acid preparations (>80%, as opposed to fish oils containing <30% n–3 acids) are in progress to determine the mechanisms and dose-response relationship of their hypotensive effect. Such preparations would also avoid the large caloric load of long-term, high-dose fish oil supplements. Since the duration of the effect, necessary dose, and possible complications of long-term n–3 fatty acid supplements have not yet been explored, it is not possible at this time to make a recommendation for fish oil or n–3 fatty acids as a therapy for hypertension.[44] There is much current research being done in this area, however, so the data necessary to define the therapeutic role (if any) of these compounds should be available shortly. An important aspect of this role would be how such supplements would fit into the American diet, and whether other dietary modification (for example, lower total fat, salt restriction) would allow a hypotensive effect to be revealed at a more easily achievable dose of n–3 acids.

Summary

It seems clear that much of the hypertension in acculturated societies is related in part to dietary habits. The majority of hypertensive patients have only mild blood pressure elevations, and can benefit significantly from dietary management alone.[45] A summary of dietary changes that would possibly benefit blood pressure is presented in Table 3. Unfortunately, many patients are not able to modify their dietary habits, so drug therapy will continue to be necessary for subjects with moderately elevated blood pressure (diastolic pressure >100 mm Hg). Achieving ideal body weight and reducing excess consumption of salt and alcohol can be recommended to lower blood pressure. From a practical standpoint, this also means lowering dietary fat and increasing potassium, which are likely to be beneficial dietary changes. Increased dietary n–6 fatty acid intake does not appear to lower blood pressure, while n–3 fatty acids do have hypotensive properties. The nutritional role of the latter group, and how it fits together with recommendations for intake of other nutrients, remains to be defined.

Acknowledgments

This work was supported in part by grants from the National Institutes of Health (HL-48877 and HL-49264).

References

1. Freis ED (1982) Should mild hypertension be treated? N Engl J Med 307:306–330
2. Medical Research Council Working Party (1985) MRC trial of treatment of mild hypertension: principal results. Br Med J 291:97–104
3. Stamler J, Stamler R, Neaton JD (1993) Blood pressure, systolic and diastolic, and cardiovascular risks: US population data. Arch Intern Med 153:598–615

4. Beilin LJ (1987) Diet and hypertension: critical concepts and controversies. J Hypertens 5(suppl 5):S447–S457

5. Pickering TG, Harshfield GA, Devereux RB, Laragh JH (1985) What is the role of ambulatory blood pressure monitoring in the management of hypertensive patients? Hypertension 7:171–177

6. Devereux RB, Pickering TG, Harshfield GA, et al (1983) Left ventricular hypertrophy in patients with hypertension: importance of blood pressure response to regularly recurring stress. Circulation 68:470–476

7. Hossman V, FitzGerald GA, Dollery CT (1981) Influence of hospitalization and placebo therapy on blood pressure and sympathetic function in essential hypertension. Hypertension 3:113–118

8. Johnson AG, Nguyen TV, Day RO (1994) Do nonsteroidal anti-inflammatory drugs affect blood pressure? a meta-analysis. Ann Intern Med 121:289–300

9. Hovell MF (1982) The experimental evidence for weight-loss treatment of essential hypertension: a critical review. Am J Public Health 72:359–368

10. Tuck ML, Sowers J, Dornfield L, Kledzik G, Maxwell M (1981) The effect of weight reduction on blood pressure, plasma renin activity, and plasma aldosterone levels in obese patients. N Engl J Med 304:930–933

11. Stallones RA (1983) Ischemic heart disease and lipids in blood and diet. Annu Rev Nutr 3:155–185

12. St Leger AS, Cochrane AL, Moore F (1979) Factors associated with cardiac mortality in developed countries, with particular reference to the consumption of wine. Lancet 1:1017–1020

13. Friedman GD, Klatsky AL, Siegelaub AB (1983) Alcohol intake and hypertension. Ann Intern Med 98:846–849

14. Weisner RL, Norris DJ, Birch R, et al (1985) The relative contribution of body fat and fat pattern to blood pressure level. Hypertension 7:578–585

15. Chiang BN, Perlamn LV, Epstein FH (1969) Overweight and hypertension: a review. Circulation 39:403–421

16. MacMahon S, Cutler J, Brittain E, Higgins M (1987) Obesity and hypertension: epidemiological and clinical issues. Eur Heart J 8(suppl B):57–70

17. Dahl LK (1958) Salt intake and salt need. N Engl J Med 258:1152–1157

18. Wing RR, Caggiula AW, Norwalk MP, et al (1984) Dietary approaches to the reduction of blood pressure: the independence of weight and sodium/potassium interventions. Prev Med 13:233–244

19. Reisin E, Abel R, Modan M, et al (1978) Effect of weight loss without salt restriction on the reduction of blood pressure in overweight hypertensive patients. N Engl J Med 298:1–6

20. Luft C (1989) Salt and hypertension: recent advances and perspectives. J Lab Clin Med 114:215–221

21. Prineas RJ, Blackburn H (1985) Clinical and epidemiologic relationships between electrolytes and hypertension. In Horan MJ, Blaustein M, Dunbar JB, et al (eds), NIH workshop on nutrition and hypertension: proceedings from a symposium. Biomedical Information Corp, New York, pp 63–85

22. Tobian L (1988) Potassium and hypertension. Nutr Rev 46:273–282

23. Suki WN (1988) Dietary potassium and blood pressure. Kidney Int 34(suppl 25):S175–S176

24. Krishna GG, Miller E, Kapoor S (1989) Increased blood pressure during potassium depletion in normotensive men. N Engl J Med 320:1177–1182

25. McCarron DA, Morris CD, Henry HJ, Stanton JL (1984) Blood pressure and nutrient intake in the United States. Science 224:1392–1398

26. Zawada ET, Brautbar N (1985) Calcium supplement therapy of hypertension—has the time come? Nephron 41:129–131

27. Kestleloot H, Geboers J, Van Hoof R (1983) Epidemiological study of the relationship between calcium and blood pressure. Hypertension 5(suppl II):52–56

28. Resnick LM (1989) Calcium metabolism in the pathophysiology and treatment of clinical hypertension. Am J Hypertens 2:179S–185S

29. National Institutes of Health (1994) Optimal calcium intake. NIH consensus statement 1994. National Institutes of Health, Bethesda, MD

30. Cappuccio FP, Markandu ND, Beynon GW, et al (1985) Lack of effect of oral magnesium on high blood pressure: a double-blind study. Br Med J 291:235–238

31. Dyckner T, Wester PO (1983) Effect of magnesium on blood pressure. Br Med J 286:1847–1849

32. Whelton PK, Klag MJ (1989) Magnesium and blood pressure: review of the epidemiologic and clinical trial experience. Am J Cardiol 63:26G–30G

33. Resnick LM, Laragh JH, Sealley JE, Alderman MH (1983) Divalent cations in essential hypertension: relations between serum ionized calcium, magnesium, and plasma renin activity. N Engl J Med 309:888–891

34. Geleijnse JM, Witteman JC, Bak AA, den Breeijen JH, Grobbee DE (1994) Reduction in blood pressure with a low sodium, high potassium, high magnesium salt in older subjects with mild to moderate hypertension. Br Med J 309:436–440

35. Saltman P (1983) Trace elements and blood pressure. Ann Intern Med 98:823–827

36. Sparrow D, Sharrett AR, Garvey AJ, Craun GF, Silbert JE (1984) Trace metals in drinking water: lack of influence on blood pressure. J Chron Dis 371:59–65

37. Mertz W (1985) Trace metals and hypertension. In Horan MJ, Blaustein M, Dunbar JB, et al (eds), NIH workshop on nutrition and hypertension: proceedings from a symposium. Biomedical Information Corp, New York, pp 271–276

38. Sacks FM (1989) Dietary fats and blood pressure: a critical review of the evidence. Nutr Rev 47:291–300

39. Knapp HR (1989) Omega-3 fatty acids, endogenous prostaglandins, and blood pressure regulation in humans. Nutr Rev 47:301–313

40. Margetts BM, Beilin LJ, Armstrong BK, et al (1985) Blood pressure and dietary polyunsaturated and saturated fats: a controlled trial. Clin Sci 69:165–177

41. Sacks FM, Wood PG, Kass EH (1984) Stability of blood pressure in vegetarians receiving dietary protein supplements. Hypertension 6:199–201

42. Appel LJ, Miller ER, Seidler AJ, Whelton PK (1993) Does supplementation of diet with "fish oil" reduce blood pressure? a meta-analysis of controlled clinical trials. Arch Intern Med 153:1429–1438

43. Morris MC, Sacks F, Rosner B (1993) Does fish oil lower blood pressure? a meta-analysis of controlled trials. Circulation 88:523–533

44. Knapp HR, FitzGerald GA (1989) The antihypertensive effects of fish oil: a controlled study of polyunsaturated fatty acid supplements in essential hypertension. N Engl J Med 320:1037–1043

45. Stamler J, Farinaro E, Mojonnier LM, et al (1980) Prevention and control of hypertension by nutritional-hygienic means: long-term experience of the Chicago coronary prevention evaluation program. JAMA 243:1819–1823

Chapter 44

Diabetes Mellitus

Edward S. Horton and Raffaele Napoli

Diabetes mellitus is not a single disease but a group of disorders of varying etiology and pathogenesis that are characterized by an elevated blood glucose concentration; insulin deficiency or decreased insulin action; abnormalities of glucose, lipid, and protein metabolism; and the development of both acute and long-term complications. Acute complications of diabetes include severe hyperglycemia leading to polyuria, increased thirst, dehydration, weight loss, blurred vision, fatigue, and occasionally hyperosmotic nonketotic coma. In severe insulin deficiency ketoacidosis may occur. People with diabetes who are not treated adequately may be more prone to infection and may demonstrate poor wound healing. Long-term complications include the development of microvascular abnormalities leading to retinopathy and nephropathy, the development of peripheral neuropathy and other neuropathic disorders, premature cataract formation, and accelerated macrovascular disease leading to coronary artery disease, cerebrovascular disease, and peripheral vascular disease.

Because of its acute and long-term complications, diabetes is a major cause of morbidity and mortality. It is increasing in prevalence in many populations around the world; in the United States today there are estimated to be >16 million people with diabetes mellitus, ≈6% of the total population. However, about one-half of those with diabetes have not yet been diagnosed. This is because the symptoms are often absent and not very specific in the most common form of the disease, non-insulin-dependent diabetes mellitus (NIDDM). Early diagnosis and treatment are important because there is now strong evidence that the development of the long-term complications of diabetes can be significantly decreased by proper treatment. In addition, the onset of diabetes itself in those who are genetically susceptible may be prevented or delayed by appropriate changes in diet, exercise, and other life-style habits.

Classification of Diabetes Mellitus

Diabetes mellitus is currently classified into four clinically different types: insulin-dependent diabetes mellitus (IDDM or type I), NIDDM or type II, gestational diabetes mellitus (GDM), and diabetes secondary to or associated with other diseases that damage the pancreas or produce severe insulin resistance. Diabetes can be diagnosed when a random plasma glucose value is >11.1 mmol/L (>200 mg/dL) and the patient has the classic signs and symptoms. Alternatively, a fasting plasma glucose value ≥7.8 mmol/L (≥140 mg/dL) on at least two occasions or a fasting plasma glucose value <7.8 mmol/L (<140 mg/dL) along with sustained, elevated plasma glucose concentrations (>11.1 mmol/L, or 200 mg/dL) during at least two oral glucose-tolerance tests (OGTTs) is enough to establish a diagnosis of diabetes. If the fasting plasma glucose is <7.8 mmol/L (<140 mg/dL), the 2-hour OGTT plasma glucose is between 7.8 and 11.0 mmol/L (140–199 mg/dL), and an intervening plasma glucose is >11.1 mmol/L (>200 mg/dL), impaired glucose tolerance (IGT) can be diagnosed. IGT is not considered a class of diabetes, although ≈30% of people with IGT will progress to NIDDM over a period of 10 years.

Insulin-dependent diabetes mellitus. Patients with IDDM have severe insulinopenia and are absolutely dependent on exogenous insulin to prevent ketoacidosis and death. At the onset these patients are often lean and frequently have experienced recent weight loss. IDDM is more common in white than in nonwhite populations and is estimated to account for only 5–10% of all known cases of diabetes mellitus. Onset is most frequently during childhood, although IDDM may occur at any age.

The primary defect in IDDM is inadequate insulin secretion due to an autoimmune process that destroys the pancreatic β cells. Clinical onset of symptoms is usually preceded by an asymptomatic period of months to years during which the β cells are progressively destroyed by a T lymphocyte–mediated process in genetically susceptible individuals. The evolving process of β cell destruction, with progressive insulin loss, gives rise to a predictable pattern of glucose homeostasis both before and for some time after diagnosis of diabetes. Antibodies to islet cells and insulin can be detected in the plasma and defective insulin secretion in response to a glucose load is present before clinical diabetes develops. Overt glucose intolerance emerges when insulin secretory reserves are decreased to <20% of normal. At this point all phases of the insulin secretory response are reduced so that glucose uptake by peripheral tissues is impaired and hepatic glucose production becomes excessive, resulting in fasting hyperglycemia and abnormal glucose tolerance. Once metabolic derangements are corrected by insulin therapy, significant residual insulin secretion can often be demonstrated, indicating that some β cell function remains. This period is called the honeymoon period, and some individuals may temporarily cease to require insulin. It is unusual for the honeymoon period to last for more than several months to 1 year, when the need for exogenous insulin replacement becomes inevitable. Current research is directed toward identification of genetically susceptible individuals who have evidence of autoimmune β cell destruction but who have not yet developed clinical diabetes. Various treatments to suppress the immune response and thus prevent diabetes from developing, or to prolong the honeymoon phase in those who do develop diabetes, are being developed and tested.

Non-insulin-dependent diabetes mellitus. NIDDM is by far the most common form of diabetes, accounting for 90% of cases worldwide. It is a heterogeneous disorder characterized by a genetic predisposition and interaction between insulin resistance and decreased β cell function. Patients with NIDDM may have few or none of the classic symptoms of diabetes mellitus when the disease is first discovered. They are not absolutely dependent on exogenous insulin for survival and are not prone to the development of ketoacidosis except during conditions of severe stress such as those caused by infections, trauma, or surgery. In Western countries there is a strong association between the presence of obesity and low levels of physical exercise and the development of NIDDM. However, NIDDM may also develop in lean individuals. It is usually diagnosed after the age of 30 years and the incidence increases significantly with increasing age.

Compared with prevalence in whites, there is an increased prevalence of NIDDM in blacks, Hispanics, Asians, and American Indians in the United States. On the basis of the second National Health and Nutrition Examination Survey (NHANES II), which included blacks and non-Hispanic whites, and the Hispanic Health and Nutrition Examination Survey (HHANES), which included Mexican Americans, Puerto Ricans, and Cubans, the overall prevalence of NIDDM in U.S. populations is 6.6% in the age range of 20–74 years and is as high as 17.7% in those aged 65–74 years.[1-4] Compared with that in whites, rates in Hispanics are more than twofold greater and rates in blacks are increased by 50–60%.[5] The prevalence of NIDDM is also increased in Asian Americans.[6,7] The highest rates of NIDDM in the U.S. population were observed in American Indians; the highest rates in this group occur in the Pima Indians of southwest Arizona, in whom NIDDM occurs in 35% of adults.[8]

Although the pathogenesis of NIDDM is not fully understood, it is clear that at least three factors are important: a genetic predisposition to the disease; a decrease in the action of insulin in insulin-sensitive tissues, including adipose tissue, skeletal muscle, and liver; and a defect in pancreatic β cell function.[9] Conditions associated with the development of insulin resistance increase the risk of NIDDM greatly. Chief among these are obesity, advancing age, and physical inactivity. Insulin resistance and hyperinsulinemia are also associated with hypertension, hypertriglyceridemia, decreased high-density-lipoprotein (HDL) cholesterol and increased risk of atherosclerosis and cardiovascular disease.[10-16]

It is well documented that moderate degrees of weight reduction in obese individuals and increased levels of physical activity and physical training are associated with decreases in fasting and postprandial insulin concentrations, improved insulin sensitivity, and improved plasma glucose concentrations in individuals with NIDDM.[17-22] Weight reduction and increased physical activity are also associated with improvement of several other cardiovascular risk factors including decreased blood pressure and improvement in lipid profiles.[23-25] Physical inactivity, on the other hand, is associated with the development of insulin resistance and decreased glucose tolerance.[26] Recently, prospective studies of the development of NIDDM in both males and females demonstrated that regular physical activity has a protective effect on the development of NIDDM.[27-29] These data suggest that lifestyle interventions to decrease the development of obesity and increase physical activity may be beneficial in individuals who are at increased risk of developing NIDDM.[30]

Gestational diabetes mellitus. The term "gestational diabetes mellitus" is used to describe glucose intolerance that has its onset or is first detected during pregnancy. Women with diagnosed diabetes before conception are not classified as having GDM. GDM occurs in ≈2% of pregnant women, usually during the second and third trimesters, when levels of insulin-antagonist hormones increase and insulin resistance normally occurs. After parturition, patients with GDM should be reclassified on the basis of plasma glucose testing. In most cases, glucose tolerance returns to normal after parturition, although over time a significant percentage of women with a history of GDM will develop overt NIDDM.

It is important to identify women with GDM by performing screening tests in all pregnant women between the 24th and 28th week of gestation. A plasma glucose level ≥7.8 mmol/L (≥140 mg/dL) 1 hour after a 50-g oral glucose load is a positive screening test and should be followed by a 100-g OGTT. The upper limits of normalcy during pregnancy are 5.8, 10.6, 9.2, and 8.1 mmol/L (105, 190, 165, and 145 mg/dL) for the fasting, 1-, 2-, and 3-hour samples, respectively. If present, GDM can usually be treated effectively by diet and increased physical activity, although in some cases insulin may be required.

GDM is a powerful predictor of the development of NIDDM, with cumulative prevalence ranging from 6%

to as high as 62% depending on the duration of follow-up.[31] The increase in risk for NIDDM associated with a history of GDM has been demonstrated in geographic locations throughout the world, strongly suggesting that this is a widespread phenomenon.

The precise influence of race as a risk factor for GDM has not been well defined. Black and Hispanic populations have been shown to have increased relative risks of GDM of 8.81 and 2.45, respectively, after adjustment for maternal age and percentage of ideal body weight.[32] Another study showed an increased risk for GDM in a Chinese population.[33] In parallel with this increased prevalence of GDM, the increase in risk of subsequent diabetes mellitus appears to cross racial lines as well, as demonstrated by studies based in Trinidad and Los Angeles and by a study of Pima Indians.[34-36]

The ability to describe a precise assessment of long-term risk for the development of NIDDM is hampered by the high likelihood that the testing of GDM during pregnancy is detecting women who already had NIDDM or IGT that was undiagnosed until pregnancy. For example, Harris[37] found that 3.8% of 817 nonpregnant American women of childbearing age had OGTTs that would have met the criteria for GDM had they been pregnant. In addition, Kjos et al.[38] performed 2-hour OGTTs 5–8 weeks postpartum in >200 women with a recent history of GDM and found incidences of IGT and diabetes mellitus of 19% and 9%, respectively. These studies support the idea that many women with GDM are already glucose intolerant in the nonpregnant state, and further support the diagnosis of GDM as yielding a population with a high prevalence of already impaired glucose tolerance and a high risk for future development of NIDDM. The mechanism whereby GDM appears to predict the future development of diabetes is thought to involve an unmasking of the tendency for diabetes as a result of hormonal changes of pregnancy.

Despite the positive predictive value of GDM for the development of NIDDM, little has been done in terms of formal studies to decrease the future development of NIDDM. Women with a history of GDM who go on to develop NIDDM have been shown in some studies to have greater body mass indexes (BMIs), although another recent study showed no such relationship.[39,40] Weight reduction is a common clinical recommendation for women with a history of GDM, and these studies raise the importance of clarifying whether weight reduction is actually beneficial in decreasing the long-term risk of diabetes. The finding of greater insulin resistance postpartum in women with a history of GDM also raises the possibility of pharmacological intervention to increase insulin sensitivity.[41]

Other types of diabetes. Various conditions that damage the pancreatic islets or produce severe insulin resistance may result in the development of diabetes mellitus. These include pancreatitis, subtotal or total pancreatectomy, hemochromatosis, exposure to pancreatic toxins, and, in rare cases, the presence of antibodies to insulin receptor or insulin. Depending on the severity of the defect, patients with these disorders may require treatment with diet, oral hypoglycemic agents, or insulin.

Impaired glucose tolerance. IGT as defined by either the National Diabetes Data Group (NDDG) or the World Health Organization (WHO) also has a high prevalence in the U.S. population.[1,42] In NHANES II the identified rates were 4.6% with the use of NDDG criteria and 11.2% with WHO criteria.[3] If the latter definition is accepted, i.e., fasting plasma glucose <7.8 mmol/L (<140 mg/dL) and glucose 2 hours after a 75-g glucose challenge between 7.8 and 11.0 mmol/L (140 and 199 mg/dL), the prevalence of IGT is about twice that of NIDDM in the U.S. population. In addition to the above-mentioned risk factors for NIDDM, the presence of IGT and a history of GDM significantly increase the risk of subsequent development of NIDDM.[37]

As with NIDDM, the prevalence of IGT increases with increasing age and with obesity.[43] It is also increased in minority populations and when there is a family history of diabetes.[6] The progression of IGT to NIDDM has been studied in several white populations in the United States, Great Britain, and Europe, and it was shown that 1–5% of patients developed NIDDM per year.[44-47] Data from NHANES II indicate that the characteristics of people with IGT (age, plasma glucose, past obesity, family history of diabetes, and physical inactivity) are intermediate between subjects with NIDDM and those with normal glucose tolerance, suggesting that IGT may be an intermediate step in the development of overt NIDDM.[3] Furthermore, it has been observed that IGT may be transient or intermittent in some individuals and does not inevitably proceed to NIDDM.[46,47] Factors such as weight gain; the development of hyperinsulinemia, or insulin resistance, or both; and physical inactivity may be important and modifiable factors in the progression of IGT to NIDDM.[48] Because there are no established treatments for IGT, regular screening for IGT is not common and little is known about interventions that may prevent or delay the progression to NIDDM in high-risk populations. At present, a large, multicenter, randomized, prospective, controlled clinical trial is being conducted in the United States to determine whether progression of IGT to NIDDM can be prevented or delayed. Epidemiologic data suggest that the prevention of obesity and increased levels of physical activity have a protective effect.

Treatment of Diabetes Mellitus

The overall goals of therapy for diabetes mellitus are to achieve normal or near-normal carbohydrate, lipid, and protein metabolism; to avoid acute complications such as severe hypoglycemia, hyperglycemia, or ketoacidosis; and to prevent long-term complications of diabetes including microvascular disease causing damage to the eyes and kidneys, neuropathy, and macrovascular disease leading to cardiac, cerebral, and peripheral vascular insufficiency. Currently, diabetes mellitus is the leading cause of new-onset blindness, the most prevalent condition requiring dialysis or kidney transplantation for end-stage renal disease, and the most common cause of nontraumatic amputation of lower extremities in the United States, all potentially preventable complications. In addition, >50% of men and women with diabetes mellitus die from coronary artery or myocardial disease.

There is now overwhelming evidence that good glycemic control plays a major role in reducing the microvascular and neuropathic complications of diabetes. The recently completed Diabetes Control and Complications Trial, a large, multicenter study conducted by the National Institutes of Health and carried out in 29 diabetes centers in the United States and Canada, examined whether intensive treatment of patients with IDDM, with the goal of maintaining blood glucose concentrations as close to the normal range as possible, could decrease the long-term complications of diabetes.[49] A total of 1441 patients with IDDM were followed for up to 9 years and monitored closely for the development or worsening of diabetic retinopathy, nephropathy, neuropathy, hyperlipidemia, and macrovascular disease. Patients were assigned randomly to intensive therapy either with an external pump or by three or more daily insulin injections, guided by frequent blood glucose monitoring and diabetic team support, or to conventional therapy with one or two daily insulin injections and less-stringent monitoring.

Intensive therapy reduced the adjusted mean risk for the development of retinopathy by 76% compared with conventional therapy. In patients with mild retinopathy at the start of the study, intensive therapy slowed the progression of this complication by 54% and reduced the development of proliferative or severe nonproliferative retinopathy by 47%. Intensive therapy also reduced the occurrence of microalbuminuria (urinary albumin excretion of ≥40 mg/24 hours) by 39%, that of clinical albuminuria (urinary albumin excretion of ≥300 mg/24 hours) by 54%, and that of clinical neuropathy by 60%. Modest improvements in hypercholesterolemia and hypertriglyceridemia were also observed in the intensively treated groups, but these changes were not statistically significant. The chief adverse event associated with intensive therapy was a two- to threefold increase in severe hypoglycemic reactions. A lesser problem of intensive therapy was a somewhat greater gain in weight of ≈5 kg (≈10 lb) compared with weight gain in patients receiving conventional therapy. Throughout the study the intensively treated group maintained an average glycosylated hemoglobin (HbA$_{1C}$) and average daily blood glucose profiles that were significantly lower than those in the conventionally treated group. The mean (± SD) value for all glucose profiles in the intensive-therapy group was 8.6 ± 1.7 mmol/L (155 ± 30 mg/dL) compared with 12.8 ± 3.1 mmol/L (231 ± 55 mg/dL) in the conventional therapy group and HbA$_{1C}$ levels were ≈2% lower (mean of 7.1% compared with 9.1%). This study demonstrated conclusively that intensified therapy and improved glycemic control in patients with IDDM has a major effect on the development of long-term complications of diabetes, decreasing significantly the development and progression of retinopathy, nephropathy, and neuropathy.

Although this study was confined to patients with IDDM, it is well documented that hyperglycemia is also associated with the presence or progression of long-term complications in patients with NIDDM, and there is now good evidence that improved glycemic control in patients with NIDDM will also reduce the development or progression of retinopathy, nephropathy, neuropathy, and perhaps macrovascular disease. In the Wisconsin Epidemiological Study of Diabetic Retinopathy, which included both IDDM and NIDDM subjects, there was an inverse correlation between HbA$_{1c}$ concentrations and 10-year incidence of proliferative diabetic retinopathy in subjects with both types of diabetes.[50] In addition, in a recently completed prospective study in Japan on the relationships between glycemic control and the development of long-term complications in patients with NIDDM, lower average glucose and HbA$_{1C}$ levels were associated with a marked reduction in the rate of complications.[51]

Good IDDM treatment requires an appropriate balance among good nutrition and food intake, physical activity, and insulin administration. To achieve this a team approach to management is necessary. The patient must be educated about diabetes and trained in the skills needed for self-management, including diet, exercise, blood glucose monitoring, and insulin dosing and administration. This requires a coordinated effort among the physician, nutritionist, nurse educator, exercise physiologist, behaviorist, and, of course, the patient.

The approach to the management of NIDDM is similar to that of IDDM, although more emphasis on weight management and life-style modification is often needed. In general, it is best to take a stepped approach to the treatment of NIDDM, starting with nonpharmacological interventions to improve diet, achieve weight reduction in obese patients, and increase physical activity. If these measures are inadequate to achieve good metabolic control, oral antidiabetic medications should be added. Various sulfonylureas, metformin, α-glucosidase inhibitors, and thiazolidinedione compounds are now available in many countries, providing an array of medications that can be used, either alone or in combination, to lower blood glucose concentrations. Finally, many patients with NIDDM require insulin therapy.

Nutrition Therapy of Diabetes Mellitus

Periodically, the American Diabetes Association (ADA) appoints a panel of experts to review the current state of knowledge and to update the recommendations for nutritional management of diabetes mellitus and related complications. The most recent review and recommendations were published in May 1994 and provide an excellent source of detailed information, including an extensive bibliography of original research papers.[52,53] In this chapter, we summarize the major recommendations and principles of nutritional management for people with diabetes. The overall goal of nutrition therapy is to assist people with diabetes to achieve and maintain improved metabolic control, to reduce the risk of both acute and long-term complications of diabetes, and to improve general health through good nutrition. More specific goals, as recommended by the ADA, are summarized in Table 1.[53]

In the treatment of IDDM, the goal should be to provide a healthy diet with appropriate energy content and nutrient composition to meet established standards for normal growth and development. It is necessary to coordinate food intake, particularly carbohydrate intake, with insulin injections and physical activity to maintain blood glucose concentrations in an acceptable range and avoid severe hypo- or hyperglycemia. This requires patients to monitor their own blood glucose and to be trained to make appropriate adjustments in diet, exercise, and insulin dosage. Insulin therapy with multiple daily injections or an insulin infusion pump provides greater flexibility for the patient to adjust patterns of eating and exercise in daily life and is now recommended for most patients with IDDM.

The emphasis for medical nutrition therapy in NIDDM should be placed on achieving appropriate blood glucose and lipid, blood pressure, and body weight goals. It has been known for many years that obesity is associated with insulin resistance, hyperinsulinemia, NIDDM, hyperlipidemia, hypertension, and premature atherosclerosis, leading to increased morbidity and mortality from coronary artery disease, stroke, and peripheral vascular disease. This cluster of associated diseases has been termed the "insulin resistance syndrome" or "syndrome X," and treatment of the multiple abnormalities is a central focus of diabetes management.[54] Weight reduction associated with a decrease in total body and intra-abdominal fat results in a marked improvement in insulin resistance and in blood glucose and lipid profiles. Several studies have shown significant beneficial effects of weight loss in the range of 6–20 kg, even if ideal body

Table 1. Goals of nutrition therapy for diabetes mellitus

1. Maintenance of blood glucose levels at as near to normal as possible by balancing food intake with insulin or oral glucose-lowering medications and physical activity.
2. Achievement of optimal serum lipid levels.
3. Provision of adequate energy for maintaining or achieving reasonable weights for adults, normal rates of growth and development in children and adolescents, and optimal nutrition during pregnancy and lactation or recovery from catabolic illnesses.
4. Prevention and treatment of the acute complications of diabetes such as severe hypo-or hyperglycemia.
5. Prevention and treatment of the long-term complications of diabetes such as renal disease, autonomic neuropathy, hypertension, hyperlipidemia, and cardiovascular disease.
6. Improvement in overall health through optimal nutrition.

Adapted from reference 53.

weight is not achieved, in patients with NIDDM. These beneficial effects include improved glycemic control and reduced plasma concentrations of triacylglycerols, very-low-density lipoproteins (VLDLs), apoprotein B, and total cholesterol.[55-57] Thus, moderate weight loss should be recommended in most patients with NIDDM. This weight loss should be achieved by decreasing energy intake and increasing physical activity to reach a daily negative energy balance of −2092 to −4184 kJ/day (−500 to −1000 kcal/day) until the target weight is reached. Often, reduction in the total fat content of the diet will be useful in reaching these goals.

Recommendations for Protein, Fat, and Carbohydrate Intake

The recommended composition of the diet for people with diabetes has changed dramatically over the past 75 years. Before the discovery of insulin in 1921, people with IDDM were kept alive for months or a few years by starvation diets that were low in energy and contained very little carbohydrate. After insulin treatment became available, starvation was no longer needed for survival and patients regained normal body weights. However, carbohydrate continued to be restricted to only 20% of energy until 1950, when the dietary guidelines for diabetes were revised to a recommendation of 40% of energy from carbohydrate, 40% from fat, and 20% from protein. In 1971 the recommendations were modified further to allow 45% of energy from carbohydrate and 35% from fat; the recommendation for protein was kept at 20%. In 1986 the ADA guidelines were again revised to reduce the fat content of the diet to 30% of energy, with saturated fats comprising no more than 10% of energy.[58] This change was made because of the recognition of the high prevalence of dyslipidemia and macrovascular disease in people with diabetes and the desire to bring the guidelines into agreement with those of the American Heart Association for prevention of coronary artery disease.

During the past 10 years a dilemma has developed regarding the most beneficial balance between fat and carbohydrate in the diabetic diet. The debate has centered around the effects of dietary composition on glycemic control and serum lipids, particularly VLDL triacylglycerols, total cholesterol, low-density-lipoprotein (LDL) cholesterol, HDL cholesterol, and various apoproteins. As a result, the current ADA guidelines do not make a single dietary recommendation for people with diabetes, but require that patients be evaluated on an individual basis with nutrition therapy based on specific abnormalities and treatment goals. Thus, there is no longer a single "diabetic diet," but a series of guidelines to assist the nutritionist and the patient in planning the most beneficial diet for optimal medical therapy and prevention of long-term complications of diabetes.[53]

Protein

Protein intake needs to be sufficient to ensure normal growth, development, and maintenance of body functions. For adults the current recommended dietary allowance (RDA) is 0.8 g/kg body weight, which is ≈10% of daily energy requirements.[59] Average dietary protein intake in the United States exceeds the RDA and is in the range of 14–18% of total energy, with about two-thirds coming from animal sources and one-third from vegetables.[59,60] Although some studies have suggested that low-protein diets may prevent or slow the progression of renal disease in diabetes mellitus, others have not demonstrated a protective effect in the absence of established renal failure.[61] Protein intakes <0.8 g/kg body weight are associated with negative nitrogen balance and are not recommended. Thus, the recommended protein intake for people with diabetes is 10–20% of total daily energy under most circumstances. In the presence of renal failure, protein intake should be restricted to 0.8 g/kg body weight, and in conditions requiring additional protein to maintain nitrogen balance, such as treatment of obesity with very-low-energy diets, pregnancy, growth during childhood and adolescence, catabolic diseases, or very high levels of physical activity, protein intake may need to be as high as ≥20% of energy.

Fat and Carbohydrate

If dietary protein intake comprises 10–20% of energy, the remaining 80–90% must be divided between carbohydrate and fat. To reduce risks of coronary artery disease (CAD) and atherosclerosis it is generally recommended that no more than 30% of energy come from fat, with no more than 10% from saturated fat. Dietary cholesterol should not exceed 300 mg/day. Because diabetes is associated with a three- to fourfold increase in the risk of CAD, nutrition recommendations for people with diabetes followed these guidelines from 1986 to 1994.[58] This meant that recommended carbohydrate intakes were 50–60% of energy. In some patients this was associated with increased VLDL production, hypertriglyceridemia, and low HDL-cholesterol levels.[62,63]

Poor glycemic control in people with IDDM is frequently associated with hyperlipidemia, but adequate insulin therapy usually restores plasma lipids to normal.[64] However, people with NIDDM have a two- to threefold increase in the prevalence of dyslipidemia compared with age- and sex-matched nondiabetic control subjects.[65] The most frequent abnormalities are hypertriglyceridemia, increased VLDL cholesterol, and decreased HDL cholesterol. Increased plasma concentrations of total and LDL cholesterol are of the same order of magnitude as those in nondiabetic populations, but may occur in as many as 40% of people with NIDDM.[65] Increased levels of small, dense LDL particles, which may be associated with increased risk of CAD, are also more frequent in people with NIDDM.[66]

Studies of risk factors for CAD in nondiabetic people have clearly shown that LDL cholesterol is a major risk factor and that HDL cholesterol is protective.[67,68] Whether hypertriglyceridemia is a significant risk factor is still not clear. Although few studies have been done in people with diabetes, hypertriglyceridemia and hyperinsulinemia have been identified as risk factors for cardiovascular morbidity and mortality in diabetic men.[69,70] These findings suggest that there are differences in cardiovascular risks associated with different lipid profiles in normal and diabetic people. Thus, nutritional recommendations must be individualized to include a mix of dietary carbohydrate and fat that will minimize the metabolic abnormalities seen in this population.

Although the most common recommendation is to restrict total fat to 30% of energy and saturated fat to 10% of energy, short-term controlled diet studies in people with NIDDM showed that diets containing 60% carbohydrate and 20–25% fat may increase hypertriglyceridemia, reduce HDL cholesterol, and increase postprandial glucose and insulin concentrations, but have no effect on or do not reduce LDL-cholesterol levels.[63,64] Increased plasma triacylglycerol, glucose, and insulin concentrations have been associated with increased risk of CAD in people with diabetes, although the same epidemiologic studies suggest that relatively high-carbohydrate, low-fat diets are also associated with a reduced incidence of cardiovascular disease.[71,72]

Because of this dilemma, some investigators have studied the effects of using monounsaturated fats instead of carbohydrates to compensate for restricted saturated fats in the diet and to thus avoid the adverse effects of high-carbohydrate diets.[63,73] In one study, subjects with NIDDM were randomly assigned to one of three diets: a weight-maintenance diet; a high-carbohydrate, high-fiber diet; or a modified lipid diet containing 36% fat and 45% carbohydrate. Both the high-carbohydrate, high-fiber diet and the modified lipid diet, in which monounsaturated fats were substituted for saturated fats, resulted in similar improvements in LDL cholesterol and glycemic control as measured by HbA_{1c} concentrations.[74]

The recommended distribution of energy from fat and carbohydrate will vary among individuals according to nutritional assessment and treatment goals. The percentage of energy from fat is determined by the desired outcomes for blood glucose, lipids, and body weight. For people with normal lipid levels and acceptable body weights, the guidelines of 30% of total energy from fat and ≤10% from saturated fat can be implemented. If weight loss is desired, a decrease in dietary fat intake is an effective way to decrease energy intake and, when combined with increased physical activity, will promote weight loss.

If increased LDL cholesterol is a significant problem, the National Cholesterol Education Program Step 2 diet guidelines are appropriate: saturated fat should be reduced to ≤7% of energy, total fat to ≤30% of energy, and cholesterol to <200 mg/day.[75] If hypertriglyceridemia and increased VLDL cholesterol are a significant problem, restriction of total energy and weight loss should be tried first. Then, dietary carbohydrates can be restricted, providing 10% of energy each from saturated and polyunsaturated fats and up to 20% of energy from monounsaturated fats. Frequent monitoring of glycemic control and plasma lipids is necessary to evaluate and adjust the treatment plan.

Complex Compared with Simple Carbohydrates

Postprandial hyperglycemia is a major concern in the management of diabetes mellitus, and much attention has been paid to the effects of specific foods or food combinations on the blood glucose response. For many years it was assumed that complex carbohydrates would result in a lesser increase in blood glucose than would glucose, sucrose, or other simple carbohydrates because of the time required for digestion and absorption of complex carbohydrates. That this is not the case was first demonstrated by Crapo et al.[76] in 1976, who found that the glycemic responses produced by equivalent amounts of glucose and carbohydrates from other sources such as bread, rice, or potatoes were not substantially differ-

ent. Numerous studies have confirmed these findings in both normal and diabetic subjects when the carbohydrate challenge is given as a single test meal or drink. However, when combined with other foods containing fat, protein, or dietary fiber, rates of gastric emptying and absorption of glucose vary considerably. This led Jenkins et al.[77,78] to propose the concept of the "glycemic index" as a method of assessing and classifying the glycemic response to carbohydrate-containing foods. Initially, glucose was used as the reference meal, but this was later changed to white bread of known composition. The glycemic index is now defined as the incremental blood glucose area after ingestion of the test food divided by the corresponding area after ingestion of a portion of white bread containing an equal amount of carbohydrate, expressed as a percentage. Although this method has been useful for research purposes, it has not been widely accepted for clinical practice. The main reasons for this are the large variations observed in individual responses, the large effects of physical form and preparation of single foods, and the large effects of mixing carbohydrate with protein and fat in a wide variety of meals.

Another approach has been to study the effects of sucrose and other simple carbohydrates on glycemic control in people with diabetes when substituted isocalorically for complex carbohydrates in the diet. There are now many studies comparing the glycemic effects of isocaloric amounts of sucrose and starch in diabetic subjects, given either as single meals or incorporated into the diet for up to 4 weeks. Five studies assessing the effects of single meals containing from 12% to 25% of energy as sucrose all found no adverse effect of sucrose on glycemia.[79–83] Other studies providing as much as 38% of energy as sucrose for 4 weeks also found no adverse effects on glycemia.[84–88] On the basis of these studies, the ADA panel concluded that restriction of sucrose in the diabetic diet because of concern about adverse effects on glycemia could not be justified, and removed this restriction from the dietary guidelines.[53]

It is less clear whether higher sucrose intakes may have adverse effects on lipemia in diabetes. In one study in subjects with NIDDM, a high-sucrose diet (16% of energy) resulted in an increase in plasma cholesterol and triacylglycerol compared with a sucrose-free diet fed for 15 days.[89] In contrast, other studies found no differences in serum cholesterol or triacylglycerol when high-sucrose (19% of energy) and high-starch (>30% of energy) diets were fed for 4 weeks.[87,88] To resolve these questions more studies are needed with larger numbers of subjects and longer durations of dietary intervention.

Fructose has long been considered to be a potential substitute for sucrose or glucose in the diabetic diet because of its lower effect on blood glucose and the fact that insulin is not required for its uptake and metabolism. Several studies found that when fructose was substituted for other carbohydrates in the diet, postprandial glucose responses decreased.[84,90,91] However, high fructose intakes have been associated with adverse effects on serum lipids, especially increased LDL cholesterol, when compared with sucrose (which contains glucose and fructose).[91-94] Fructose was found to have no adverse effects on serum total cholesterol or triacylglycerol.[84,90,91,95] On the basis of these data the current recommendations are that moderate amounts of fructose in natural foods such as fruits, vegetables, and honey are all right, but that use of added fructose as a sweetener has no overall advantage over other nutritive sweeteners.

Sweeteners

Nutritive sweeteners other than sucrose and fructose are commonly used by people with diabetes as part of their normal diet. These include corn sweeteners, fruit juice concentrates, honey, molasses, dextrose, maltose, and sugar alcohols. These sweeteners all provide energy and must be included in calculations of energy intake. However, none appear to have any advantage over sucrose regarding glycemic control of diabetes.

Currently, several high-intensity sweeteners that provide insignificant amounts of energy are used in diabetic diets in various countries throughout the world. These include aspartame, saccharin, acesulfame K, sucrolose, alitame, and cyclamates. The main purpose of these agents is to provide sweetness to foods and beverages without providing energy or increasing blood glucose concentrations. In the United States these compounds are regulated by the Food and Drug Administration and are approved only if they have been rigorously tested and proven safe for general use. There are no restrictions on their use by people with diabetes and they may be useful in planning low-energy diets for weight reduction and for providing convenient foods and beverages that do not increase blood glucose concentrations in people with diabetes.

Fiber

Extensive studies have been done on the effects of dietary fiber, both soluble and insoluble, on lipid and carbohydrate metabolism in people with diabetes mellitus. These were reviewed by Nuttall[96] and the ADA panel on nutrition guidelines.[53] Consumption of large amounts, usually >20 g/day, of certain soluble fibers such as oat bran, various gums, and psyllium are effective in lowering serum total and LDL cholesterol and triacylglycerol.[97-103] However, many of the studies are difficult to interpret because of lack of appropriate controls for variables such as body weight, total energy, and energy distribution of the diets. Nevertheless, there are some well-conducted trials that show that chronic consumption of soluble fiber of ≥20 g/day, when combined with a high-carbohydrate diet, can marginally reduce total- and LDL-cholesterol while maintaining HDL-cholesterol levels in people with NIDDM beyond the effects of decreasing dietary saturated fat and cholesterol.[104-106] However, it is difficult to achieve such intakes of fiber from foods alone and fiber supplements are needed.

Soluble fibers might be expected to improve glycemic control in people with diabetes because of decreased rates of carbohydrate absorption from the small intestine, effects on secretion of various gastrointestinal hormones, or other effects on metabolism. Guar and oat gums have been shown to decrease the rate of glucose absorption and to reduce both fasting and postprandial glucose concentrations when added to the diet.[96] However, these effects occur at high doses and are probably not significant enough to justify prescribing dietary supplements of fiber. The recommendations for dietary fiber intake for people with diabetes are the same as for nondiabetic individuals. People with diabetes should incorporate foods naturally rich in total fiber into their diet to reach a daily intake of 25–30 g from a variety of food sources including vegetables, legumes, grains, and fruits.[107]

Ethanol

Under normal circumstances, moderate use of alcoholic beverages will not cause any problems with glycemic control or lipid metabolism in people with diabetes. However, ingestion of ethanol in the fasting state may cause hypoglycemia by decreasing hepatic glucose production. In patients treated with insulin or sulfonylureas, alcohol should always be ingested with food to avoid this problem. Large amounts of alcohol or chronic alcohol consumption may also result in hyperglycemia and poor diabetes control; certain medical conditions in people with diabetes should be considered as contraindications to alcohol use. These include pancreatitis, hypertriglyceridemia, neuropathy, myocardiopathy, and renal failure.

Vitamins and Minerals

The nutritional requirements of people with diabetes do not differ from those of the population at large. However, people with diabetes have an increased prevalence of diseases requiring special consideration such as hypertension, renal failure, and congestive heart failure; additionally, use of diuretics and other medications may affect requirements for vitamins and minerals. NIDDM is most common in older populations in whom general nutrition may not be adequate.

Summary

The goals of nutritional therapy in people with diabetes mellitus are to assist in achieving and maintaining blood glucose concentrations as close to normal as possible and to reduce or treat the long-term complications of the disease. Because atherosclerosis and cardiovascular disease are significantly increased in diabetes, particular attention must be paid to reducing associated risk factors, including obesity, hyperinsulinemia, hypertension, and hyperlipidemia. Energy restriction to achieve moderate weight loss, sodium reduction to treat hypertension, and appropriate adjustment in the relative amounts and forms of fat and carbohydrate in the diet to treat hyperlipidemia are the cornerstone of nutrition therapy.

At present, there are insufficient data to support low-protein diets for the prevention of renal disease in diabetes. However, if renal failure develops, protein should be restricted, but not below the RDA of 0.8 g/kg body weight.

There is no one "diabetic diet" that should be prescribed for everyone with diabetes. Individual assessment by a trained nutritionist and establishment of specific treatment goals by the health care team are necessary steps in patient management. Dietary recommendations should take into account requirements for normal growth and development and general health, as well as treatment of the metabolic abnormalities associated with diabetes and its complications.

References

1. Harris MI, Hadden WC, Knowler WC, Bennett PH (1987) Prevalence of diabetes and impaired glucose tolerance and plasma glucose levels in the US population aged 20–74. Diabetes 36:523–534
2. Fiegal KM, Ezzati TM, Harris MI, et al (1991) Prevalence of diabetes in Mexican Americans, Cubans and Puerto Ricans from the Hispanic Health and Nutrition Examination Survey, 1982–1984. Diabetes Care 14:628–638
3. Harris MI (1989) Impaired glucose tolerance in the US population. Diabetes Care 12:464–474
4. Harris MI (1991) Epidemiological correlates of NIDDM in Hispanics, Whites, and Blacks in the US population. Diabetes Care 14:639–648
5. Haffner SM, Hazuda HP, Mitchell BD, et al (1991) Increased incidence of type II diabetes mellitus in Mexican Americans. Diabetes Care 14:102–108
6. Fujimoto WY, Leonetti DL, Kinyoun JL, et al (1987) Prevalence of diabetes mellitus and impaired glucose tolerance among second-generation Japanese-American men. Diabetes 36:721–729
7. Tsunehara CH, Leonetti DL, Fujimoto WY (1990) Diet of second-generation Japanese-American men with and without non-insulin dependent diabetes. Am J Clin Nutr 52:731–738
8. Knowler WC, Pettitt DJ, Saad MF, Bennett PH (1990) Diabetes mellitus in the Pima Indians: incidence, risk factors and pathogenesis. Diabetes Metab Rev 6:1–27
9. DeFronzo RA (1989) The triumvirate β-cell, muscle, liver: a collusion responsible for NIDDM. Diabetes 37:667–687
10. Kissebah AH, Vydelingum N, Murray R, et al (1982) Relation of body fat distribution to metabolic complications of obesity. J Clin Endocrinol Metab 54:254–260
11. Falko JM, Parr JH, Simpson RN, Wynn V (1987) Lipoprotein analyses in varying degrees of glucose tolerance: comparison between non-insulin-dependent diabetic, impaired glucose tolerant, and control populations. Am J Med 83:641–647
12. Modan M, Halkin H, Almog S, et al (1985) Hyperinsulinemia: a link between hypertension obesity and glucose intolerance. J Clin Invest 75:809–817
13. Modan M, Karasik A, Halkin H, et al (1986) Effect of past and concurrent body mass index on prevalence of glucose intolerance and type 2 (non-insulin-dependent) diabetes and on insulin response. Diabetologia 29:82–89
14. Vaccaro O, Rivellese A, Riccardi G, et al (1984) Impaired glucose tolerance and risk factors for atherosclerosis. Arteriosclerosis 4:592–597
15. Wingard DL, Barret-Connor E (1987) Family history of diabetes and cardiovascular disease risk factors and mortality among euglycemic, borderline hyperglycemic, and diabetic adults. Am J Epidemiol 125:948–958
16. Zavaroni I, Dall'Aglio E, Bonora E, et al (1987) Evidence that multiple risk factors for coronary artery disease exist in persons with abnormal glucose tolerance. Am J Med 83:609–912
17. Bjorntorp P, deJounge K, Sjostrom L, Sullivan L (1973) Physical training in human obesity. II. Effects of plasma insulin in glucose-intolerant subjects without marked hyperinsulinemia. Scand J Clin Lab Invest 32:41–45
18. Horton ES (1986) Exercise and physical training: effects on insulin sensitivity and glucose metabolism. Diabetes Metab Rev 2:1–17
19. Horton ES (1988) Role and management of exercise in diabetes mellitus. Diabetes Care 11:201–211
20. Hughes TA, Gwynne JT, Witzer BR, et al (1984) Effects of caloric restriction and weight loss on glycemic control, insulin release and resistance, and atherosclerotic risk in obese patients with type II diabetes mellitus. Am J Med 77:7–17
21. Pi-Sunyer FX (1993) Short term medical benefits and adverse effects of weight loss. Ann Intern Med 119:722–726
22. Wing RR, Marcus MD, Salata R, et al (1991) Effects of a very-low calorie diet on long term glycemic control in obese type 2 diabetic subjects. Arch Intern Med 151:1334–1340
23. Brownell KD, Bachorik PS, Ayeric RS (1982) Changes in plasma lipid and lipoprotein levels in men and women after a program of moderate exercise. Circulation 65:477–484
24. Krotkiewski M, Mandroukis K, Sjostrom L, et al (1979) Effects of long term physical training on body fat, metabolism and blood pressure in obesity. Metabolism 28:650–658
25. Haskell WL (1986) The influence of exercise training on plasma lipids and lipoproteins in health and disease. Acta Med Scand Suppl 711:25–37
26. Borstein R, Polychronakos C, Toess CJ, et al (1985) Acute reversal of the enhanced insulin action in trained athletes: association with insulin receptor changes. Diabetes 34:756–760
27. Helmrich SP, Ragland DR, Leung RW, Paffenbarger RS (1991) Physical activity and reduced occurrence of non-insulin-dependent diabetes mellitus. N Engl J Med 325:147–152
28. Manson JE, Rimm EB, Stampfer MJ, et al (1991) Physical activity and incidence of non-insulin dependent diabetes mellitus in women. Lancet 338:774–778
29. Manson JE, Nathan DM, Krolewski AS, et al (1992) A prospective study of exercise and incidence of diabetes among US male physicians. JAMA 268:63–67
30. Eriksson KF, Lindgarde F (1991) Prevention of type 2 (non-insulin-dependent) diabetes mellitus by diet and physical

exercise: the 6-year Malmo feasibility study. Diabetologia 34:891–898

31. O'Sullivan JB (1993) Diabetes mellitus after GDM. Diabetes 40(suppl 2):131–135

32. Dooley SL, Metzger BE, Cho NH (1991) Gestational diabetes mellitus: influence of race on disease prevalence and perinatal outcome in a US population. Diabetes 40 (suppl 2):25–29

33. Green JR, Dawson IG, Schumacher LB, et al (1990) Glucose tolerance in pregnancy: ethnic variation and influence of body habits. Am J Obstet Gynecol 163:86–92

34. Ali Z, Alexis SD (1990) Occurrence of diabetes mellitus after gestational diabetes mellitus in Trinidad. Diabetes Care 13:527–529

35. Mestman JH, Anderson GV, Guadalupe V (1972) Follow-up study of 360 subjects with abnormal carbohydrate metabolism during pregnancy. Obstet Gynecol 39:421–425

36. Pettit DJ, Knowler WC, Baird HR, Bennett PH (1980) Gestational diabetes: infant and maternal complications of pregnancy in relation to third-trimester glucose tolerance in the Pima Indians. Diabetes Care 3:458–464

37. Harris MI (1988) Gestational diabetes may represent discovery of pre-existing glucose intolerance. Diabetes Care 11:402–411

38. Kjos SL, Buchanan TA, Greenspoon JS, et al (1990) Gestational diabetes mellitus: the prevalence of glucose intolerance and diabetes mellitus in the first two months postpartum. Am J Obstet Gynecol 163:93–98

39. O'Sullivan JB (1982) Body weight and subsequent diabetes mellitus. JAMA 248:949–952

40. Damm P, Kuhl C, Bertelsen A, Molsted-Pedersen L (1992) Predictive factors for the development of diabetes in women with a previous history of gestational diabetes mellitus. Am J Obstet Gynecol 167:607–616

41. Catalano PM, Bernstein IM, Wolfe RR, et al (1986) Subclinical abnormalities of glucose metabolism in subjects with previous gestational diabetes. Am J Obstet Gynecol 155:1255–1262

42. National Diabetes Data Group (1979) Classification and diagnosis of diabetes mellitus and other categories of glucose intolerance. Diabetes 28:1039–1057

43. Harris MI (1990) Epidemiology of diabetes mellitus among the elderly in the United States. Clin Geriatr Med 6:703–719

44. Birmingham Diabetes Survey Working Party (1976) Ten-year follow-up report of the Birmingham diabetes survey of 1961. Br Med J 2:35–37

45. Jarrett RJ, Keen H, Fuller H, McCartney M (1984) The Whitehall study: ten-year follow-up report on men with impaired glucose tolerance with reference to worsening to diabetes and predictors of death. Diabetic Med 1:279–283

46. Keen H, Harrett RJ, McCartney P (1982) The ten-year follow-up of the Bedford survey (1962–72): glucose tolerance and diabetes. Diabetologia 22:73–78

47. Sartor G, Schersten B, Carlstrom S, et al (1980) Ten-year follow-up of subjects with impaired glucose tolerance: prevention of diabetes by tolbutamide and diet regulation. Diabetes 29:41–49

48. Saad MF, Knowler WC, Pettit DJ, et al (1988) The natural history of impaired glucose tolerance in the Pima Indians. N Engl J Med 319:1500–1506

49. The Diabetes Control and Complications Trial Research Group (1993) The effect of intensive treatment of diabetes on the development and progression of long term complications of insulin dependent diabetes mellitus. N Engl J Med 329:977–986

50. Klein R, Blein BE, Moss SE, Cruickshanks KJ (1994) The Wisconsin Epidemiologic Study of diabetic retinopathy: ten-year incidence and progression of diabetic retinopathy. Arch Ophthalmol 112:1217–1228

51. Ohkubo Y, Kishikawa H, Araki E, et al (1995) Intensive insulin therapy prevents the progression of diabetic microvascular complications in Japanese patients with non-insulin-dependent diabetes mellitus: a randomized prospective 6-year study. Diabetes Res Clin Pract 28:103–117

52. Franz MJ, Horton ES, Bantle JP, et al (1994) Nutrition principles for the management of diabetes and related complications. Diabetes Care 17:490–518

53. American Diabetes Association (1994) Nutrition recommendations and principles for people with diabetes mellitus. Diabetes Care 17:519–522

54. Reaven GM (1988) Role of insulin resistance in human disease. Diabetes 39:1595–1607

55. Wing RR, Koeske R, Epstein LH, et al (1987) Long term effects of modest weight loss in type II diabetic patients. Arch Intern Med 147:1749–1753

56. Liu G, Coulston AM, Lardinois CK, et al (1985) Moderate weight loss and sulfonylurea treatment on non-insulin-dependent diabetes mellitus. Arch Intern Med 145:665–669

57. Reaven GM (1985) Beneficial effect of moderate weight loss in older patients with non-insulin-dependent diabetes mellitus poorly controlled with insulin. J Am Geriatr Soc 33:93–95

58. American Diabetes Association (1987) Nutritional recommendations and principles for individuals with diabetes mellitus. Diabetes Care 10:126–132

59. National Research Council (1989) Recommended dietary allowances, 10th ed. National Academy Press, Washington, DC, pp 52–77

60. Committee on Diet and Health, National Research Council (1989) Diet and health: implications for reducing chronic disease risk. National Academy Press, Washington, DC, pp 259–631

61. Henry RR (1994) Protein content of the diabetic diet. Diabetes Care 17:1502–1513

62. Coulston AM, Hollenbeck CB, Swislocki ALM, et al (1987) Deleterious metabolic effects of high carbohydrate, sucrose containing diets in patients with NIDDM. Am J Med 82:213–220

63. Garg A, Bonanome A, Grundy SM, et al (1988) Comparison of a high-carbohydrate diet with high-monounsaturated-fat diet in patients with non-insulin-dependent diabetes mellitus. N Engl J Med 391:829–834

64. Kern P (1987) Lipid disorders in diabetes mellitus. Mt Sinai J Med 54:245–252

65. Stern MP, Patterson JK, Haffner SM, et al (1989) Lack of awareness and treatment of hyperlipidemia in type II diabetes in a community survey. JAMA 262:360–364

66. Feingold KR, Grunfeld C, Pang M, et al (1992) LDL subclass phenotypes and triglyceride metabolism in non-insulin-dependent diabetes. Arteriosclerosis 12:1496–1502

67. Kannel WB, Castelli WP, Gordon T, McNamara PM (1971) Serum cholesterol, lipoprotein, and the risk of coronary heart disease. Ann Intern Med 74:1–12

68. Castelli WP, Doyle JT, Gordon T, et al (1977) HDL cholesterol and other lipids in coronary heart disease: cooperative lipoprotein phenotyping study. Circulation 55:767–772

69. Fontbonne A, Eschwege E, Cambien F, et al (1989) Hypertriglyceridemia as a risk factor of coronary heart disease mortality in subjects with impaired glucose tolerance or diabetes. Diabetologia 32:300–304

70. Austin MA (1989) Plasma triglyceride as a risk factor for coronary heart disease: the epidemiologic evidence and beyond. Am J Epidemiol 129:249–259

71. Stout RW (1990) Insulin and atheroma: 20-yr perspective. Diabetes Care 13:631–654
72. Reaven GM (1992) The role of insulin resistance and hyperinsulinemia in coronary heart disease. Metabolism 41:16–19
73. Parillo M, Rivellese AA, Ciardullo AV, et al (1992) A high-monounsaturated-fat/low-carbohydrate diet improves peripheral insulin sensitivity in non-insulin-dependent diabetic patients. Metabolism 41:1371–1378
74. Milne RM, Mann JI, Chisholm AW, Williams SM (1994) Long-term comparison of three dietary prescriptions in the treatment of NIDDM. Diabetes Care 17:74–80
75. Expert Panel on Detection, Evaluation, and Treatment of High Blood Cholesterol in Adults (1993) Summary of the second report of the National Cholesterol Education Program (NCEP) Expert Panel on Detection, Evaluation, and Treatment of High Blood Cholesterol in Adults (Adult Treatment Panel II). JAMA 269:3015–3023
76. Crapo PA, Reaven G, Olefsky J (1976) Plasma glucose and insulin responses to orally administered simple and complex carbohydrates. Diabetes 25:741–747
77. Jenkins DJA, Wolever TMS, Taylor RH, et al (1981) Glycemic index of foods: a physiological basis for carbohydrate exchange. Am J Clin Nutr 34:362–366
78. Jenkins DJA, Wolever TMS, Jenkins AL (1988) Starchy foods and glycemic index. Diabetes Care 11:149–159
79. Bantle JP, Laine DC, Castle GW, et al (1983) Postprandial glucose and insulin responses to meals containing different carbohydrates in normal and diabetic subjects. N Engl J Med 309:7–12
80. Slama G, Haardt MJ, Jean-Joseph P, et al (1984) Sucrose taken during mixed meal has no additional hyperglycemic action over isocaloric amounts of starch in well-controlled diabetics. Lancet 2:122–125
81. Bornet F, Haardt MJ, Costagliola D, et al (1985) Sucrose or honey at breakfast have no additional acute hyperglycemic effect over an isoglucidic amount of bread in type II diabetic patients. Diabetologia 28:213–217
82. Forlani G, Galuppi V, Santacroce G, et al (1989) Hypoglycemic effect of sucrose ingestion in IDDM patients controlled by artificial pancreas. Diabetes Care 12:296–298
83. Peters AL, Davidson MB, Eisenberg K (1990) Effect of isocaloric substitution of chocolate cake for potato in type I diabetic patients. Diabetes Care 13:888–892
84. Bantle JP, Laine CW, Thomas JW (1986) Metabolic effects of dietary fructose and sucrose in type I and II diabetic subjects. JAMA 256:3241–3246
85. Wise JE, Keim KS, Huisinga JL, Willmann PA (1989) Effect of sucrose-containing snacks on blood glucose control. Diabetes Care 12:423–426
86. Loghmani E, Richard K, Washburne L, et al (1991) Glycemic response to sucrose-containing mixed meals in diets of children with insulin-dependent diabetes mellitus. J Pediatr 119:531–537
87. Abraira C, Derler J (1988) Large variations of sucrose in constant carbohydrate diets in type II diabetes. Am J Med 84:193–200
88. Bantle JP, Swanson JE, Thomas W, Laine DC (1993) Metabolic effects of dietary sucrose in type II diabetic subjects. Diabetes Care 16:1301–1305
89. Coulston AM, Hollenbeck CB, Donner CC, et al (1985) Metabolic effects of added dietary sucrose in individuals with non-insulin-dependent diabetes mellitus (NIDDM). Metabolism 34:962–966
90. Crapo PA, Kolterman OG, Henry RR (1986) Metabolic consequence of two-week fructose feeding in diabetic subjects. Diabetes Care 9:111–119
91. Bantle JP, Swanson JE, Thomas W, Laine DC (1992) Metabolic effects of dietary fructose in diabetic subjects. Diabetes Care 15:1468–1476
92. Hallfrisch J, Reiser S, Prather ES (1983) Blood lipid distribution of hyperinsulinemic men consuming three levels of fructose. Am J Clin Nutr 37:740–748
93. Reiser S, Powell AS, Scholfield DJ, et al (1989) Blood lipids, liproproteins, apoproteins, and uric acid in men fed diets containing fructose or high-amylose cornstarch. Am J Clin Nutr 49:832–839
94. Swanson JE, Laine DC, Thomas W, Bantle JP (1992) Metabolic effects of dietary fructose in healthy subjects. Am J Clin Nutr 55:851–856
95. Thorburn AW, Crapo PA, Beltz WF, et al (1989) Lipid metabolism in non-insulin-dependent diabetes: effects of long term treatment with fructose-supplemented mixed meals. Am J Clin Nutr 50:1015–1022
96. Nuttall FQ (1993) Dietary fiber in the management of diabetes. Diabetes 42:503–508
97. Lepre F, Crane S (1992) Effect of oat bran on mild hyperlipidemia. Med J Aust 157:305–308
98. Ripsin CM, Keenan JM, Jacobs DR Jr, Elmer PJ (1992) Oat products and lipid lowering: a meta-analysis. JAMA 267:3317–3325
99. Jenkins DJA, Hegele RA, Jankins AL, et al (1993) The apolipoprotein E gene and the serum low-density lipoprotein cholesterol response to dietary fiber. Metabolism 42:585–593
100. Kay RM (1977) Dietary fiber. Nutr Rev 35:6–11
101. Anderson JW, Riddel-Mason S, Gustafson NJ, et al (1992) Cholesterol-lowering effects of psyllium-enriched cereal as an adjunct to a prudent diet in the treatment of mild to moderate hypercholesterolemia. Am J Clin Nutr 56:93–98
102. Vinik AL, Jenkins DJA (1986) Dietary fiber in management of diabetes. Diabetes Care 11:160–173
103. Anderson JW, Ward K (1978) Long-term effects of high-carbohydrate, high-fiber diets on glucose and lipid metabolism: a preliminary report on patients with diabetes. Diabetes Care 1:77–82
104. Aro A, Uusitupa M, Voutilainen E, et al (1981) Improved diabetic control and hypocholesterolemia effect induced by long term dietary supplementation with guar gum in type II (insulin-independent) diabetes. Diabetologia 21:29–33
105. Lalor BC, Chatnager D, Winocour PH, et al (1990) Placebo-controlled trial of the effects of guar gum and metformin on fasting blood glucose and serum lipids in obese, type II diabetic patients. Diabetic Med 7:242–252
106. Uusitupa M, Sutonen O, Savolainen K, et al (1989) Metabolic and nutritional effects of long term use of guar gum in the treatment of non-insulin-dependent diabetes of poor metabolic control. Am J Clin Nutr 49:345–351
107. American Diabetes Association (1993) Health implications of dietary fiber (position statement). J Am Diet Assoc 93:1446–1447

Chapter 45

Nutritional Advances in Osteoporosis and Osteomalacia

MaryFran Sowers

Nutritional studies continue to be an important element in advancing our understanding of the causes and prevention of metabolic bone disease and osteoporosis. This is particularly evident in considering the advances in three areas. First, there have been advances in our understanding of the importance of calcium intake on bone mineralization of adolescents. Second, we have come to a much more complete understanding of the interaction of the calcium demands of pregnancy, lactation, and bone. Third, the availability and use of new calcium supplements has renewed the interest in dietary and supplementary calcium intake in the elderly for slowing the progression of bone demineralization. This has been accompanied by investigations indicating that bone disease in elderly people may not only be osteoporosis, but also osteomalacia, vitamin D deficiency of adults. Such studies indicate the need to address the vitamin D status, not just the calcium status, of people with little sunlight exposure, such as elderly people.

This chapter addresses the role of nutrition, particularly calcium intake, as it affects bone mineral density associated with the development of peak bone mass through adolescence, the maintenance of peak bone mass through the reproductive years of young adulthood, and the age-related bone loss of elderly people, with the attendant expression of osteopenia and fracture.

Calcium Intake and Adolescent Bone Mineralization

The role of nutrition, particularly calcium nutrition, in the mineralization of bone in preadolescence and adolescence has been minimally investigated for the past 20 years; however, recently, that trend has been reversed. Much of the impetus for this current work is based on the belief that modest increases in bone mineralization during adolescence will be maintained into young adulthood when bone mass is at its peak. It is further hypothesized that this greater peak bone mass

will be translated into a greater bone mass at menopause and through the subsequent years of aging. Ultimately, with this greater sustained bone density, fracture risk will be reduced.

Over the past 5 years, three approaches have been used to evaluate the role of dietary calcium intake in adolescence as it may influence bone density. These approaches include calcium balance studies, examination of variation in diet as it relates to variation in bone density measured in populations, and the use of calcium supplementation in clinical trials. For example, two investigators have reexamined 487 reported calcium balance studies in children aged <18 years conducted from 1922 to 1947.[1-2] These investigators suggested that the threshold for achieving calcium balance exceeds the level of calcium intake currently suggested by the recommended dietary allowances.

The cross-sectional studies of bone density in preadolescence and adolescence consistently report associations of bone density with age, weight, height, and pubertal status.[3-10] In addition, Mora et al.[11] suggested that the determinants of cortical bone density throughout growth are mechanical and weight-bearing stressors, whereas the determinants of cancellous bone density, as measured by quantitative tomography, are more likely to be associated with hormonal changes in late adolescence.

Although the role of age, weight, height, and pubertal status are consistently reported, the association with dietary calcium intake during adolescence with bone density has been mixed. Studies of diet and bone density, measured concurrently during adolescence, report both positive associations[12-14] or no association,[3,15] particularly after controlling for the influence of pubertal status.[5,16] Some studies report an association between historical adolescent diet and current bone density measured in adulthood.[17-18]

Two longitudinal studies of adolescents examined the relation of dietary calcium with bone density. In a 10-year study of 264 Finnish youth, aged 9–18 years at

Table 1. Clinical trials of calcium supplementation in preadolescent and adolescent girls[a]

Study	Technology, site	Frequency of observation	Sample size	Amount and type of supplement	Findings
Matkovic et al., 1990[21][b]	SPA, radius; DPA, spine	0, 10, 18, 24 months	8 control subjects, 10 supplemented with milk, 10 with $CaCO_3$	Diet ≈850 mg/day, supplemented 4 cups milk, 1000 $CaCO_3$	No difference; type II error?
Johnston et al., 1992[22]	SPA, radius; DPA, spine, femoral neck	0.6 month, 1,2,3 years	n=22 pairs prepubertal twins, n=23 pairs of pubertal twins	Diet ≈950 mg/day, supplemented CCM ≈1000 mg/day	Significant ↑ in prepubertal twin, no benefit in postpubertal twin
Lloyd et al., 1993[23]	DEXA, spine; TBBMD	0, 6, 12, 18 months	n=94 females aged 11.9±0.5 years	Diet ≈960 mg/day, supplemented CCM ≈350 mg/day	Significant ↑ in lumbar spine, marginal ↑ in TBBMD

[a]SPA, single photon absorptiometry; DPA, dual-photon absorptiometry; DEXA, dual-energy x-ray absorptiometry; TBBMD, total-body bone mineral density; $CaCO_3$, calcium carbonate; CCM, calcium citrate maleate.
[b]Study was neither blinded nor placebo-controlled.

baseline, a significant role for variation in calcium intake was not identified in relation to bone mineral density of the spine and femoral neck.[19] However, significant associations with bone density were identified for smoking and exercise.[19] Similarly, in a cohort of Dutch youth who were followed for 15 years to age 27, no significant association of dietary calcium intake with bone density was identified. In this group of 84 males and 98 females, physical activity was identified as being associated with greater bone density.[20]

Three clinical trials assessed the role of calcium supplementation (Table 1). In a trial with additional calcium provided to 10 adolescents by milk or by calcium carbonate, Matkovic et al.[21] showed no difference in bone measurements when comparing the supplemented group to the control group. The investigators suggest that the limited sample size prevented them from being able to detect an existing difference. Johnston et al.[22] supplemented one member of monozygotic twin pairs, aged 6–14 years at baseline, while providing placebo to the other member of the twin pair. They found that calcium supplementation was associated with a significant increase in bone measurements when the twin pairs were prepubertal; however, there was no evidence of effect when the twin pairs were pubertal. Lloyd et al.[23] studied 12-year-old females, some of whom were supplemented with calcium citrate maleate, and reported significant increases in bone mineral density of the lumbar spine and marginal changes in total-body bone mineral density of those given supplemental calcium.

It is difficult to interpret these studies in children and adolescents because of the many factors that may influence the outcome. For example, variation in the type of calcium supplement may alter absorption. Miller et al.[24] reported that calcium salts provided as calcium citrate maleate had an increased fractional absorption relative to calcium carbonate (36% versus 26%), but sample size was not adequate in these clinical trials to stratify subjects by previous dietary calcium intake (low versus high).[21–23] Low calcium intakes before the calcium supplementation period may influence both the rate of calcium absorption and bone turnover, which is particularly important in short-term clinical trials. Finally, detection of modest and sustained differences in bone mineral density attributable to calcium supplements or dietary calcium intake may be hampered by the more prominent effect of changes in hormone levels, body weight, smoking behavior, and physical activity patterns.

The clinical trial data and reanalysis of calcium balance studies have provided the momentum for considering the upward revision of recommended calcium intakes for adolescents. The suggestion by a recent National Institutes of Health Consensus Conference Panel[25] was that calcium intake in the range of 1200–1500 mg/day might result in higher peak adult bone mass. The panel also recommended additional research including longitudinal studies and clinical trials with different calcium supplementations and doses.

Pregnancy and Lactation

Pregnancy and lactation are hypothesized to significantly affect the achievement and maintenance of peak bone mass. During pregnancy and lactation substantial

Table 2. Prospective studies of bone mass measured before or concurrently with pregnancy, with a follow-up measurement in the postpartum

Study	Measurement technology	Number	Times of measurement	Results
Sowers et al. 1991[32]	DPA	32 cases, 32 controls	Preconception and postpartum	No change at the femoral neck
Drinkwater and Chesnut 1991[33]	SPA, DPA	6 cases, 25 controls	Preconception and postpartum	Loss in radius and femoral neck, increase in tibia
Kent et al. 1993[34]	SPA	37 cases, no controls	14 and 36 weeks	No change

amounts of calcium are transferred from the mother to the fetus or infant. Both pregnancy and lactation are accompanied by alterations in the maternal endocrinological environment, particularly levels of estrogen and prolactin, which have been associated with changes in bone density. Levels of circulating maternal estrogen rise during pregnancy because the placenta produces large quantities of estradiol, and lactation is a hypoestrogenic state with elevated prolactin levels.[26-28] The demands of fetuses and breast-feeding infants may outstrip the calcium available from intestinal absorption, particularly in women whose calcium intake is limited, potentially resulting in increased risk for maternal osteoporosis and fracture or poor fetal growth or rate of weight gain during breast-feeding.

Pregnancy. During a full-term pregnancy, ≈30 g of calcium is transferred to the fetus.[29] This calcium demand can be addressed by increased intestinal absorption of calcium or decreased urinary excretion of calcium. If absorption efficiency could be doubled from 20% to 40% and women consumed moderate calcium intakes, the skeletal needs of fetuses could be met without accessing calcium stored in the maternal skeleton. If maternal bone mineral was the sole source of this calcium, the mother's skeleton would lose ≈3% (30 g/1000 g) of its mineral per pregnancy. However, bone mass might increase because of the greater estrogen levels in the last trimester of pregnancy and because of the increased bone-loading with weight gain in pregnancy.

Studies that have examined the bone density changes during pregnancy, particularly studies with a cross-sectional design, produced inconsistent results on bone loss with a pregnancy. In the 1970s, two prospective studies were reported, one showing no change in bone density with pregnancy and the other showing change in trabecular bone but not in cortical bone.[30-31] There were no further prospective studies reported until the 1990s, when three new investigations were published. The two investigations with the largest sample size reported no change with pregnancy, whereas the third investigation reported

detectable change but only at sites including both cortical and trabecular bone (Table 2).[32-34]

These studies have limitations from both technical and nutritional perspectives. Technically, there should be controls because of the error associated with bone density measurement. There also must be an adequate sample size. Usually, at least 25–30 persons per group are required to detect differences of 3% in bone mineral density. These studies do not address the issue of inadequate maternal calcium intake or the effect of adolescent pregnancy, yet there is evidence from three epidemiologic studies that adolescent pregnancy, requiring the skeleton of both fetus and mother to mature and mineralize simultaneously, may result in lower bone density and increased risk of perimenopausal bone loss.[35-36]

The effect of pregnancy should be more evident after multiple pregnancies. However, studies are inconsistent. Some reports show an increase in bone mass, and others show no association between parity and bone density.[37-42] Generally, these studies do not consider whether the association with parity is because of differences in weight gained during and subsequently retained after pregnancy. Findings from studies of fracture rate in relation to parity are examples of the inconsistencies. A longitudinal study and a case-control study suggested a protective effect of parity with regard to hip fracture,[43-44] whereas three more recent studies showed no detectable association.[45-47]

It was reported that, as a result of the increase in 1,25-dihydroxyvitamin D levels during pregnancy and the accompanying increase in calcium absorptive efficiency, a state of positive calcium balance exists during pregnancy, including adolescent pregnancy.[48-51] Higher circulating levels of 1,25-dihydroxyvitamin D levels and greater intestinal absorption efficiency appear to be major mechanisms for meeting fetal calcium needs. These findings suggest that there is no substantial bone loss with pregnancy. The associations of parity with greater bone mass or lower fracture risk are partly a function of the effect of weight gain on weight bearing during pregnancy.

Table 3. Longitudinal studies of lactation with bone density characterized during the lactation time interval

Study	Measurement technology	Frequency and time frame	Sample size	Findings
Chan et al. 1982[58]	SPA	2 weeks, 16 weeks	23 cases, 11 controls	Loss of 10% BMC
Hayslip et al. 1989[59]	SPA, DPA	2 days postpartum, 6 months	12 cases, 7 controls	6.5% loss at spine, no loss at radius
Kent et al. 1990[60]	SPA	6 months postpartum, postweaning	40 cases, 40 controls	7% loss; recovery
Drinkwater and Chesnut 1991[33]	SPA, DPA	6 weeks, after 6 months	6 cases, 25 controls	3% loss at hip, no change at other six sites
Sowers et al. 1993[61]	DEXA	2 weeks; 2, 4, 6, 12, and 18 months	64 full cases, 24 partial cases; 20 controls	5% loss hip and spine; recovery

Lactation. There is significant calcium demand during lactation, with the degree of calcium demand related to the amount of breast milk produced and the duration of breast-feeding. Thus, maternal mobilization of calcium from the skeleton could be more variable than mobilization in pregnancy. An estimated cost to the maternal skeleton with 6 months of full lactation would approximate 4–6% of skeletal calcium. If no compensatory mechanisms existed for increasing calcium absorption, this amount would have to be mobilized from the skeletal depot.

Calcium is transferred directly from serum to breast milk. Approximately 600 mL milk/day is produced at 3 months after parturition (168 mg calcium/day), and 1 L milk/day is produced at 6 months after parturition (280 mg calcium/day). A comparison of calcium concentration in milk from West African and British women showed that a very low calcium intake can result in a lower calcium content of human milk.[52] Several studies, but not all, have identified that increased absorption efficiency is not evident during lactation.[53-54]

Prolactin levels are higher and estrogen levels are lower during lactation.[55-56] Similar hormone changes have been associated with lower bone mass in prolactin-secreting adenomas and during menopause.

As with pregnancy, the cross-sectional and retrospective studies of bone mineral content and fracture risk in women who have breast-fed have been highly inconsistent. In the 1970s, Atkinson and West[57] and Lamke et al.[31] measured prospectively a small number of breast-feeding women and reported bone loss. There were no additional prospective studies reported for almost 20 years, a time during which bone measurement technology advanced significantly. With this newer technology,

investigators in five longitudinal studies confirmed that there is significant bone loss with extended lactation (Table 3).[33,58-61] These findings were supported by two additional investigations that indicated more intense activity of markers of bone turnover in breast-feeding women than in control subjects.[62,63]

Although there is convincing evidence that substantial bone loss occurs with lactation, two recent studies also showed that there is recovery of bone mineral mass.[60,61,63] Sowers et al.[61,63] showed that recovery is related to reestablishment of menses: calcium intake is not predictive of bone mineral recovery. Thus, there is an initial rapid bone loss with extended lactation and subsequent recovery of bone mineral with weaning and with reestablishment of menses. This recovery appears to continue during a subsequent pregnancy.[64]

The pattern of bone loss and recovery during lactation would be obscured in cross-sectional studies or short-term longitudinal studies. Epidemiologic studies, which determine breast-feeding retrospectively, might observe no effect because by the time of assessment of bone density, recovery of bone mass may have occurred. Studies in postmenopausal women would include the influence of menopause. Furthermore, any study in which the lactation exposure is classified as "ever versus never" is likely to misclassify the calcium demand. Breast-feeding duration of <4–6 months appears unlikely to generate a calcium demand sufficient to create a bone loss detectable with current technology.

These studies still leave important issues unaddressed. Foremost among these issues is the influence of limited dietary calcium intake, or of outright vitamin D deficiency, occurring prominently in much of the world. Furthermore, these studies do not address breast-feeding by adolescents (with one exception) or breast-feeding at obstetric maturity.

In summary, there appears to be little ultimate loss of mineral from the maternal skeleton with the pregnancy or lactation of well-nourished women if during or after lactation consistent menstrual cycling is reestablished within a reasonable length of time. The evidence suggests that the acute skeletal loss associated with extended lactation occurs despite high dietary calcium intakes. Variation in the calcium intake of well-nourished women does not appear to be related to either the amount of bone loss or its recovery. The time of return of menses was consistently associated with the time of bone mineral recovery. Evidence is insufficient to evaluate whether maternal skeletal loss may be occurring in women with lower dietary calcium intakes (<600 mg/day).

Presently, much is to be learned about the mechanisms associated with both the rapid loss during lactation as well as the rapid recovery of bone mineral that follows weaning. Understanding these mechanisms could possibly be extrapolated and lead to greater understanding of mechanisms of other bone-loss processes, including those associated with menopause, and assist in developing ways to facilitate bone mineral recovery.

Vitamin D and Calcium in Elderly People

Vitamin D. The nutritional focus of bone studies in elderly people has usually been on dietary calcium intake; however, vitamin D levels in blood are typically lower in older than in younger people. Aksnes et al.[65] showed that serum concentrations of 25-dihydroxy-vitamin D and 24,25-dihydroxyvitamin D were less in elderly adults than in younger and middle-aged adults (aged 22–59 years). Furthermore, a gradient of serum concentrations was found in elderly people, with the more active individuals having higher serum levels than did those confined to home or health care facilities. Komar et al.[66] found that 86% of persons admitted to nursing home residency had circulating levels of 25-hydroxy-vitamin D <50 nmol/L and 41% had values <25 nmol/L, values which were considered to be low to low-normal. In addition, 16% of the residents had high circulating levels of parathyroid hormone, considered an indicator of increased bone mobilization.

Serum vitamin D levels are more likely to correlate with exposure to sunlight in younger women and with dietary intake (principally from fortified milk) in older women.[67] Thus, Meuleman[68] recommended that 400–600 IU/day of vitamin D should be given to elderly subjects who do not get significant exposure of their skin to sunlight. Despite these observations, less attention has been paid to this area than to calcium supplementation.

Several clinical trials assessed the effect of vitamin D supplementation on fracture frequency or bone density in elderly subjects.[69–71] Heikinheimo et al.[69] conducted a 4-year trial of vitamin D using a dose of 150,000–300,000 IU annually. The supplement was given intramuscularly in autumn to elderly Finnish participants. The investigators reported a substantial reduction in fractures from 6.1% in the control group to 2.9% in the treated group. Dawson-Hughes et al.[71] reported that bone mineral density, as measured by dual-energy x-ray densitometry, improved significantly more in a group treated for 1 year with 400 IU/day than in the control group. Two other trials that included large doses of vitamin D as well as calcium are reported in the next section.

There is a growing appreciation of the need for adequate vitamin D nutriture in elderly person, including those who may not manifest gross deficiency. However, there have been no initiatives to monitor more closely the adequacy of foods fortified with vitamin D, to provide more universal supplementation with vitamin D, or to increase the recommended dietary allowance for vitamin D.

Dietary calcium. Although adequate calcium is acknowledged to act as an antiresorptive agent in bone, controversy exists about the effectiveness of supplemental calcium in retarding the rate of bone loss in postmenopausal women. The controversy about effectiveness appears to include at least three factors: 1) the age or stage in life of the woman to whom the supplement is provided (Heaney[72] has stressed the importance of evaluating the role of calcium in the diet and from supplementation in women who are clearly advanced in age so as not to include menopause with its inevitable bone loss), 2) the usual dietary calcium intake (the assumption being that the effect of supplementation is likely to be more substantial in women whose usual intake is low), and 3) the type of calcium salt used as the supplement (Table 4).

The importance of these factors is well illustrated in the clinical trial reported by Dawson-Hughes et al.[73] The study included 112 women whose usual calcium intake, as estimated by food frequency, was <400 mg/day and an additional 124 women whose usual calcium intake was <650 mg/day. Statistical analysis was used to isolate the effect of menopause (within 5 years). The study indicated a significant retardation of bone mineral density loss at the spine, femoral neck, and radius with calcium citrate maleate supplementation in women with usual dietary intakes <400 mg/day. Supplementation with either calcium carbonate or calcium citrate maleate was not effective in women with usual intakes between 400 and 650 mg/day. The number of women in the early postmenopausal group was too small to establish a dose response.

Reid et al.[74] evaluated the effect of calcium supplementation in women with greater than usual dietary

Table 4. Recent clinical trials of calcium supplementation in elderly people[a]

Study	Age or stage of life	Usual dietary calcium intake	Amount, type of supplement	Findings
Dawson-Hughes et al. 1990[73]	Early menopause late menopause	<650 mg	500 mg CaCO₃, 500 mg CCM	CCM supplementation of late menopausal women with low calcium intake is beneficial
Chapuy et al. 1992[70]	84 years	≈500 mg/day	1.2 g tricalcium phosphate and 800 IU vitamin D	Reduction in fractures in the supplemented group
Reid et al. 1993[74]	3 years postmenopause	Mean intake 750 mg/day	Calcium lactate, calcium gluconate	Beneficial effect calcium supplements
Chevalley et al. 1994[75]	72 years for BMD, 78 years for fracture	≈600 mg/day	800 mg CaCO₃, osseino-mineral complex, 300,000 IU vitamin D	Supplements retarded femoral BMD loss and vertebral factures

[a]CaCO₃, calcium carbonate; CCM, calcium citrate maleate; BMD, bone mineral density.

calcium intakes (mean 750 mg/day) who were at least 3 years postmenopause. Calcium lactate or calcium gluconate provided 1000 mg calcium/day. The investigators concluded that the supplementation regimen significantly slowed bone loss at both axial and appendicular sites.

Two clinical trials evaluated the combination of calcium and vitamin D supplementation. The largest trial, reported by Chapuy et al.,[70] included 1634 women receiving tricalcium phosphate (1.2 g of elemental calcium) and 800 IU of vitamin D daily compared with 1636 women receiving placebo. The participants were nursing home residents who were followed for 18 months. The investigators reported a 50% reduction in the number of fractures among the supplemented residents. Further, in subgroups evaluated for bone density, the supplemented group had an increase of 2.6% in bone mineral density as compared with a decline of 4.6% in the control subjects.

In a trial with fewer participants that was not placebo-controlled, Chevalley et al.[75] evaluated two calcium salts, calcium carbonate and an "osseino-mineral complex." Bone mineral density was measured in 82 healthy elderly women and in 63 women with a recent hip fracture. In addition to the calcium supplement, all participants received a single dose of 300,000 IU of vitamin D at the onset of the trial. The study found that calcium supplementation prevented a decline in femoral bone mineral density, as measured by dual-photon absorptiometry, and reduced the vertebral fracture rate, as measured by a six-point vertebral height measurement performed on radiographs. The impact of this later trial is difficult to evaluate because all women, both treated and control subjects, received vitamin D supplementation and no women in the hip fracture group were administered a placebo. Additionally, sample size was too small to evaluate the effect of each calcium salt separately.

Women have been the target of almost all studies. However, Orwoll et al.[76] reported that men with relatively high calcium intakes (≈1150 mg/day) did not experience retardation of bone loss from the spine or radius when supplemented with 1000 mg/day of calcium and vitamin D.

In light of these studies, a recent NIH consensus conference recommended that a calcium intake of 1500 mg/day would be prudent in men and women older than 65.[25] The consensus statement stopped short of making a recommendation regarding vitamin D but did acknowledge the possibility of vitamin D insufficiency in homebound elderly people and in residents of long-term care facilities.

Summary

The importance of calcium and vitamin D nutrition cannot be minimized in relation to the prevention of osteoporosis and attendant fractures, in part because increased intake of these two nutrients is readily implementable, relatively inexpensive interventions that are safe for most of the population. In the past 5 years there has been a growing appreciation that low bone mineral density is not exclusively a calcium-deficiency disease. Indeed, calcium intake is only one of many factors, including hormonal status, age, weight, and physical activity as well as efficiency of calcium absorption, that affect mineral density of bone. Studies of calcium supplementation have demonstrated that the effectiveness of supplementation on bone depends on the level of usual calcium intake, hormone status, and absorptive efficiency of the calcium salt.

References

1. Matkovic V (1991) Calcium metabolism and calcium requirements during skeletal modeling and consolidation of bone mass. Am J Clin Nutr 54:245S–260S
2. Matkovic V, Heaney RP (1992) Calcium balance during human growth: evidence for threshold behavior. Am J Clin Nutr 55:992–996
3. Dhuper S, Warren MP, Brooks-Gunn J, Fox R (1990) Effects of hormonal status on bone density in adolescent girls. J Clin Endocrinol Metab 71:1083–1088
4. Ponder SW, McCormick DP, Fawcett HD, et al (1990) Spinal bone mineral density in children aged 5.00 through 11.99 years. Am J Dis Child 144:1346–1348
5. Grimston SK, Morrison K, Harder JA, Hanley DA (1992) Bone mineral density during puberty in western Canadian children. Bone Miner 19:85–96
6. Bonjour JP, Theintz G, Buchs B, et al (1991) Critical years and stages of puberty for spinal and femoral bone mass accumulation during adolescence. J Clin Endocrinol Metab 73:555–563
7. Lloyd T, Rollings N, Andon MB, et al (1992) Determinants of bone density in young women. I. Relationships among pubertal development, total body bone mass, and total body bone density in premenarchal females. J Clin Endocrinol Metab 75:383–387
8. Katzman DK, Bachrach LK, Carter DR, Marcus R (1991) Clinical and anthropometric correlates of bone mineral acquisition in healthy adolescent girls. J Clin Endocrinol Metab 73:1332–1339
9. Lu PW, Briody JN, Ogle GD, et al (1994) Bone mineral density of total body, spine, and femoral neck in children and young adults: a cross-sectional and longitudinal study. J Bone Miner Res 9:1451–1458
10. De Schepper J, Derde MP, Van den Broeck M, et al (1991) Normative data for lumbar spine bone mineral content in children: influence of age, height, weight, and pubertal stage. J Nucl Med 32:216–220
11. Mora S, Goodman WG, Loro ML, et al (1994) Age-related changes in cortical and cancellous vertebral bone density in girls: assessment with quantitative CT. AJR Am J Roentgenol 162:405–409
12. Turner JG, Gilchrist NL, Ayling EM, et al (1992) Factors affecting bone mineral density in high school girls. N Z Med J 105:95–96
13. Rubin K, Schirduan V, Gendreau P, et al (1993) Predictors of axial and peripheral bone mineral density in healthy children and adolescents, with special attention to the role of puberty. J Pediatr 123:863–870
14. Kristinsson JO, Valdimarsson O, Steingrimsdottir L, Sigurdsson G (1994) Relation between calcium intake, grip strength and bone mineral density in the forearms of girls aged 13 and 15. J Intern Med 236:385–390
15. Kroger H, Kotaniemi A, Vainio P, Alhava E (1992) Bone densitometry of the spine and femur in children by dual-energy x-ray absorptiometry. Bone Miner 17:75–85
16. Glastre C, Braillon P, David L, et al (1990) Measurement of bone mineral content of the lumbar spine by dual energy x-ray absorptiometry in normal children: correlations with growth parameters. J Clin Endocrinol Metab 70:1330–1333
17. Nieves JW, Golden AL, Siris E, et al (1995) Teenage and current calcium intake are related to bone mineral density of the hip and forearm in women aged 30–39 years. Am J Epidemiol 141:342–351
18. Tylavsky FA, Anderson JJ, Talmage RV, Taft TN (1992) Are calcium intakes and physical activity patterns during adolescence related to radial bone mass of white college-age females? Osteoporos Int 2:232–240
19. Valimaki MJ, Karkkainen M, Lamberg-Allardt C, et al (1994) Exercise, smoking, and calcium intake during adolescence and early adulthood as determinants of peak bone mass: Cardiovascular Risk in Young Finns Study Group. Br Med J 309:230–235
20. Welten DC, Kemper HC, Post GB, et al (1994) Weight-bearing activity during youth is a more important factor for peak bone mass than calcium intake. J Bone Miner Res 9:1089–1096
21. Matkovic J, Fontana D, Tominac C, et al (1990) Factors that influence peak bone mass formation: a study of calcium balance and the inheritance of bone mass in adolescent females. Am J Clin Nutr 52:878–888
22. Johnston CC Jr, Miller JZ, Slemenda CW, et al (1992) Calcium supplementation and increases in bone mineral density in children. N Engl J Med 327:82–87
23. Lloyd T, Andon MB, Rollings N, et al (1993) Calcium supplementation and bone mineral density in adolescent girls. JAMA 270:841–844
24. Miller JZ, Smith DL, Flora L, et al (1988) Calcium absorption from calcium carbonate and a new form of calcium (CCM) in healthy male and female adolescents. Am J Clin Nutr 48:1291–1294
25. NIH Consensus Development Panel on Optimal Calcium Intake (1994) Optimal calcium intake. JAMA 272:1942–1948
26. Reddy GS, Norman AW, Willis DM, et al (1983) Regulation of vitamin D metabolism in normal human pregnancy. J Clin Endocrinol Metab 56:363–370
27. Jaffe RB, Dell'Acqua S (1985) The endocrine physiology of pregnancy and the peripartal period. Raven Press, New York
28. Speroff L, Glass RH, Kase NG (1989) Clinical gynecology, endocrinology and infertility. Williams and Wilkins, Baltimore
29. Givens MH, Macy IG (1933) The chemical composition of the human fetus. J Biol Chem 102:7–17
30. Christiansen C, Rodbro R, Heinild B (1976) Unchanged total body calcium in normal human pregnancy. Acta Obstet Gynecol Scand 55:141–143
31. Lamke B, Brundin J, Moberg P (1977) Changes of bone mineral content during pregnancy and lactation. Acta Obstet Gynecol Scand 56:217–219
32. Sowers MF, Crutchfield M, Jannausch M, et al (1991) A prospective evaluation of bone mineral change in pregnancy. Obstet Gynecol 77:841–845
33. Drinkwater BL, Chesnut III CH (1991) Bone density changes during pregnancy and lactation in active women: a longitudinal study. Bone Miner 14:153–160
34. Kent GN, Price RI, Gutteridge DH, et al (1993) Effect of pregnancy and lactation on maternal bone mass and calcium metabolism. Osteoporos Int 3(Suppl 1):S44–S47
35. Sowers MFR, Clark MK, Hollis B, et al (1992) Radial bone mineral density in pre- and perimenopausal women: a prospective study of rates and risk factors for loss. J Bone Miner Res 7:647–657
36. Fox KM, Magaziner J, Sherwin R, et al (1993) Reproductive correlates of bone mass in elderly women. J Bone Miner Res 8:901–908

37. Nilsson BE (1969) Parity and osteoporosis. Surg Gynecol Obstet 129:27–28

38. Melton III LJ, Bryant SC, Wahner HW, et al (1993) Influence of breastfeeding and other reproductive factors on bone mass later in life. Osteoporos Int 3:76–83

39. Laitinen K, Valimaki M, Keto P (1991) Bone mineral density measured by dual-energy x-ray absorptiometry in healthy Finnish women. Calcif Tissue Int 48:224–231

40. Cox ML, Khan SA, Gau DW, et al (1991) Determinants of forearm bone density in premenopausal women: a study in one general practice. Br J Gen Pract 41:194–196

41. Kritz-Silverstein D, Barrett-Connor E, Hollenbach KA (1992) Pregnancy and lactation as determinants of bone mineral density in postmenopausal women. Am J Epidemiol 136:1052–1059

42. Bauer DC, Browner WS, Cauley JA, et al (1993) Factors associated with appendicular bone mass in older women. Ann Intern Med 118:657–665

43. Paganini-Hill A, Chao A, Ross RK, Henderson BE (1991) Exercise and other factors in the prevention of hip fracture: the Leisure World Study. Epidemiology 2:16–25

44. Hoffman S, Grisso JA, Kelsey JL, et al (1993) Parity, lactation and hip fracture. Osteoporos Int 3:171–176

45. Kreiger N, Gross A, Hunter G (1992) Dietary factors and fracture in postmenopausal women: a case-control study. Int J Epidemiol 21:953–958

46. Ribot C, Tremollieres F, Pouilles JM, et al (1993) Risk factors for hip fracture. Bone 14:S77–80

47. Cumming RG, Klineberg RJ (1993) Breastfeeding and other reproductive factors and the risk of hip fractures in elderly women. Int J Epidemiol 22:684–691

48. Kent GN, Price RI, Gutteridge DH, et al (1991) The efficiency of intestinal calcium absorption is increased in late pregnancy but not in established lactation. Calcif Tissue Int 48:293–295

49. Duggin GG, Dale NE, Lyneham RC, et al (1974) Calcium balance in pregnancy. Lancet 2:926–927

50. Heaney RP, Skillman TG (1971) Calcium metabolism in normal human pregnancy. J Clin Endocrinol 33:661–670

51. Shenolikar IS (1970) Absorption of dietary calcium in pregnancy. Am J Clin Nutr 23:63–67

52. Laskey MA, Prentice A, Shaw J, et al (1990) Breast-milk calcium concentrations during prolonged lactation in British and rural Gambian mothers. Acta Paediatr Scand 79:507–512

53. Thomas ML (1991) Calcium uptake duodenal epithelial cells increased during lactation. Proc Soc Exp Biol Med 196:214–217

54. Specker BL, Vieira NE, O'Brien KO, et al (1994) Calcium kinetics in lactating women with low and high calcium intakes. Am J Clin Nutr 59:593–599

55. Baird DT, McNeilly AS, Sawers RS, Sharpe RM (1979) Failure of estrogen-induced discharge of luteinizing hormone in lactating women. J Clin Endocrinol Metab 49:500–506

56. Zarate A, Canales ES (1987) Endocrine aspects of lactation and postpartum infertility. J Steroid Biochem 27:1023–1028

57. Atkinson PJ, West RR (1970) Loss of skeletal calcium in lactating women. J Obstet Gynaecol Br 77:555–560

58. Chan GM, Slater P, Ronald N, et al (1982) Bone mineral status of lactating mothers of different ages. Am J Obstet Gynecol 144:438–441

59. Hayslip CC, Klein TA, Wray HL, Duncan WE (1989) The effect of lactation on bone mineral content in healthy postpartum women. Obstet Gynecol 73:588–592

60. Kent GN, Price RI, Gutteridge DH, et al (1990) Human lactation: forearm trabecular bone loss, increased bone turnover, and renal conservation of calcium and inorganic phosphate with recovery of bone mass following weaning. J Bone Miner Res 5:361–369

61. Sowers MF, Corton G, Shapiro B, et al (1993) Changes in bone density with lactation. JAMA 269:3130–3135

62. Specker BL, Tsang R, Ho ML (1991) Changes in calcium homeostasis over the first year postpartum: effect of lactation and weaning. Obstet Gynecol 78:56–62

63. Sowers MF, Eyre D, Hollis BW, et al (1995) Biochemical markers of bone tunover in lactating and non-lactating postpartum women. J Clin Endocrinol Metab 80:2210–2216

64. Sowers MF (1995) Bone mass in pregnancy after extended lactation. Obstet Gynecol 85:285–290

65. Aksnes L, Rodland O, Odegaard OR, et al (1989) Serum levels of vitamin D metabolites in the elderly. Acta Endocrinol (Copenh) 121:27–33

66. Komar L, Nieves J, Cosman F, et al (1993) Calcium homeostasis of an elderly population upon admission to a nursing home. J Am Geriatr Soc 41:1057–1064

67. Sowers MF, Wallace RB, Hollis BW, Lemke JH (1986) Parameters related to 25-OH-D levels in a population-based study of women. Am J Clin Nutr 43:621–628

68. Meuleman J (1989) Osteoporosis and the elderly. Med Clin North Am 73:1455–1470

69. Heikinheimo RJ, Inkovaara JA, Harju EJ, et al (1992) Annual injection of vitamin D and fractures of aged bones. Calcif Tissue Int 51:105–110

70. Chapuy MC, Arlot ME, Duboeuf F, et al (1992) Vitamin D3 and calcium to prevent hip fractures in the elderly women. N Engl J Med 327:1637–1642

71. Dawson-Hughes B, Dallal GE, Krall EA, et al (1991) Effect of vitamin D supplementation on wintertime and overall bone loss in healthy postmenopausal women. Ann Intern Med 115:505–512

72. Heaney RP (1993) Nutritional factors in osteoporosis. Annu Rev Nutr 13:287–316

73. Dawson-Hughes B, Dallal GE, Krall EA, et al (1990) A controlled trial of the effect of calcium supplementation on bone density in postmenopausal women. N Engl J Med 323:878–883

74. Reid IR, Ames RW, Evans MC, et al (1993) Effect of calcium supplementation on bone loss in postmenopausal women. N Engl J Med 328:460–464

75. Chevalley T, Rizzoli R, Nydegger V, et al (1994) Effects of calcium supplements on femoral bone mineral density and vertebral fracture rate in vitamin-D-replete elderly patients. Osteoporos Int 4:245–252

76. Orwoll ES, Oviatt SK, McClung MR, et al (1990) The rate of bone mineral loss in normal men and the effects of calcium and cholecalciferol supplementation. Ann Intern Med 112:29–34

Chapter 46

Renal Disease

Saulo Klahr

The hallmark of chronic renal disease is a decrease in glomerular filtration rate (GFR). This decrease may occur through three major mechanisms: 1) a decrease in single-nephron filtration rate (the filtration rate per nephron in humans is 60 nL/minute for a total GFR of 120 mL/minute, assuming 1 million nephrons in each of the two kidneys); 2) a decrease in the number of functional nephrons; or 3) a combination of these two events, which is most likely. The progressive loss of nephrons affects most of the functions of the kidney (Table 1). As GFR falls, solutes that are excreted by the kidney preferentially by filtration (urea, creatinine) accumulate in body fluids and concentrations in plasma increase.[1] Indeed, the plasma concentrations of urea and creatinine provide a crude measurement of the decrease in GFR. As GFR falls to values <25% of normal (≈30 mL/minute), other solutes that are filtered and either reabsorbed or secreted by the renal tubules may accumulate in body fluids.[1,2] These solutes include phosphate, sulfate, uric acid, magnesium, and hydrogen and result in the development of metabolic acidosis. Finally, other compounds are retained in body fluids when renal disease is far advanced. These compounds include phenols, guanidines, organic acids, indoles, a number of metabolic products, and certain peptides. Some of these solutes may be toxic at certain concentrations and could contribute to the symptoms and signs of advanced chronic renal insufficiency (uremia).

As renal function decreases, the ability of patients to respond rapidly to changes in dietary intake, particularly of sodium, potassium, and water, is markedly restricted.[1,2] Although the excretion of solute and water per nephron increases as renal function decreases, the fewer the number of functional nephrons, the smaller is the range of solute or water excretion achievable by the composite nephron population. Thus, the upper and lower limits of excretion for many solutes and for water are less in patients with renal insufficiency than in normal subjects. As renal disease progresses there is decreased flexibility in response to changes in the intakes of sodium, other solutes, and water.[1,2] Therefore, the volume and composition of the extracellular fluid compartment may change as renal function decreases.

A decrease in renal function also imposes restrictions on the dose and frequency of administration of certain drugs, particularly those in which metabolism is greatly dependent on renal excretion.[3,4] Drug interactions also may be modified in patients with uremia.[3]

The loss of synthetic functions of the kidney also contributes to the abnormalities seen in renal insufficiency. For example, decreased production of erythropoietin, a hormone synthesized in the kidney that plays a key role in the maturation of erythrocyte precursors in bone marrow, is a major cause of the anemia seen in patients with renal disease.[5,6] Decreased synthesis of 1,25-dihydroxycholecalciferol (calcitriol), the active metabolite of cholecalciferol, by the diseased kidney results in decreased serum concentrations of this compound and may lead to decreased calcium absorption from the gastrointestinal tract.[7] Decreased concentrations of calcitriol also contribute to the development of hyperparathyroidism in patients with renal disease.[8]

The kidney is the main site of degradation of several peptides (β_2 microglobulin, light chains), proteins, and peptide hormones including insulin, glucagon, growth hormone, and parathyroid hormone.[9] The kidney also is involved in gluconeogenesis (the synthesis of glucose from noncarbohydrate precursors) and lipid metabolism.[9] Failure of the kidneys, therefore, leads to multiple abnormalities that may have a marked effect on

Table 1. Principal functions of the kidney

Excretion of metabolic waste products (i.e., urea, creatinine, uric acid)
Maintenance of volume and ionic composition of body fluids
Elimination and detoxification of drugs and toxins
Regulation of systemic blood pressure
Production of erythropoietin
Control of mineral metabolism via endocrine synthesis (1,25-dihydroxycholecalciferol and 24,25-dihydroxycholecalciferol)
Degradation and catabolism of peptide hormones (e.g., insulin, glucagon, parathyroid hormone) and small-molecular-weight proteins (β_2 microglobulin and light chains)
Regulation of metabolism (gluconeogenesis, lipid metabolism)

intermediary metabolism, concentrations of circulating hormones, and absorption of certain nutrients. In addition, as renal failure progresses, anorexia, nausea, and vomiting may develop, which may further compromise adequate nutrient and energy intake. Specific abnormalities affecting nutritional status and changes requiring diet modifications for patients with progressive renal disease are outlined below.

Phosphate and Calcium

Phosphate excretion changes little as GFR falls, because there is a progressive decrease in tubular reabsorption of phosphate, which is mediated mainly by increased plasma concentrations of parathyroid hormone.[10] However, when GFR falls below 30 mL/minute, even a marked decrease in tubular reabsorption of phosphate is not enough to overcome the substantial decrease in the filtered load, and phosphate accumulates. Hyperphosphatemia, therefore, is seen commonly in patients with GFRs of ≤25 mL/minute unless dietary phosphate is restricted.[10] Changes in serum calcium concentration also occur at this level of GFR and presumably are related to three factors: 1) An increase in serum phosphate produces a reciprocal decrease in serum ionized calcium. 2) Calcitriol concentration decreases at GFR values <30 mL/minute because of decreased calcitriol production, which decreases absorption of calcium from the gastrointestinal tract, a phenomenon documented in patients with this level of GFR.[11] 3) The removal of calcium from bone by parathyroid hormone may be impaired, and such skeletal resistance to the action of this hormone may also contribute to the development of hypocalcemia.[12] Acidosis tends to increase the fraction of plasma calcium that is in the ionized form and, thus, prevents some of the clinical consequences of hypocalcemia. Rapid correction of acidosis may decrease the concentrations of ionized calcium and cause acute manifestations of hypocalcemia, including tetany and convulsions in patients with chronic renal disease.

A reduction in phosphorus intake in patients with mild renal insufficiency reduces the concentrations of parathyroid hormone and improves the skeletal response to the hormone.[13] Phosphorus absorption from the gastrointestinal tract can be decreased by the use of phosphate binders. Until the past decade aluminum salts (hydroxide, carbonate) were used as phosphate binders. However, aluminum is absorbed and may accumulate in plasma and tissues.[14] Because aluminum accumulation is toxic,[14] other phosphate-binding agents, such as calcium carbonate, were introduced.[15] When prescribed as a phosphate binder, calcium carbonate should be administered with meals. Dietary phosphorus can be decreased to 600–900 mg/day by reducing protein intake, particularly by avoiding meats and dairy products, which are the major sources of dietary phosphorus.

Such protein-restricted diets often restrict calcium intake, resulting in negative calcium balance in patients with renal insufficiency. Therefore, calcium supplements of 500–1500 mg/day are recommended for such patients. Calcium supplements should be administered between meals to increase calcium absorption; the amount required depends on the size of the individual, the concentrations of serum calcium, and the gastrointestinal absorption of calcium. Several calcium salts (carbonate, gluconate, lactate, citrate, and chloride) have been used as calcium supplements. In hypocalcemic patients with GFR values <30 mL/minute, administration of small doses of calcitriol may be necessary to increase serum calcium. Administration of calcitriol may reduce the plasma concentrations of parathyroid hormone in patients with renal insufficiency by increasing serum calcium concentration and by inhibiting the synthesis of parathyroid hormone in the parathyroid gland.[11]

In summary, the goals of calcium and phosphorus therapy in patients with renal insufficiency are to maintain plasma concentrations of phosphorus and ionized calcium within normal limits; prevent the development of secondary hyperparathyroidism or to decrease the concentrations of parathyroid hormone when hyperparathyroidism is already established; and prevent or reverse skeletal disease, soft tissue calcification, pruritus, and other manifestations of abnormal calcium-phosphorus homeostasis.

Magnesium

Clinically significant hypermagnesemia is rare in patients with chronic renal insufficiency. Although the kidney is the major route of magnesium excretion, decreased magnesium reabsorption per nephron as renal failure progresses prevents marked increases in plasma concentrations of magnesium.[16] In far-advanced renal insufficiency, mild hypermagnesemia is common. Protein-restricted diets may decrease the total amount of magnesium ingested to ≈200 mg/day. Clinically important hypermagnesemia (serum magnesium concentrations >1.7–2.1 mmol/L) does not occur unless additional magnesium is taken in the form of antacids, enemas, or laxatives with a high magnesium content.[17] Such magnesium-containing preparations should be avoided by patients with marked renal insufficiency.

Water Excretion

Renal disease causes a progressive decrease of the capacity to concentrate urine.[18] In healthy individuals urine osmolality may be as high as 1200 mmol/kg of water, but during renal insufficiency the maximum urine osmolality approaches that of plasma (300 mmol/kg). If total solute excretion by uremic subjects remains at 600 mmol/day and maximal urine osmolality is ≤300 mmol/kg water, an

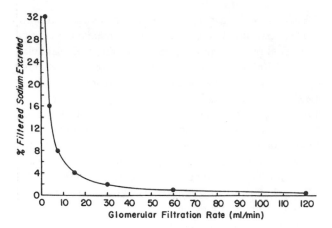

Figure 1. The pattern of sodium excretion at different glomerular filtration rates in subjects with normal renal function or chronic renal disease ingesting 7.0 g sodium chloride/day. Reproduced with permission from reference 1.

obligatory water excretion of 2 L/day is necessary to eliminate the osmolar load. This obligatory excretion restricts the capacity of patients with renal insufficiency to decrease water excretion to that seen in normal individuals.

The upper limit of water excretion is also decreased in patients with renal insufficiency.[19] Although the ability to dilute the urine is well preserved in patients with renal disease (free water generation calculated per 100 mL of GFR is preserved), the total amount of free water that can be excreted decreases as GFR decreases. For example, if water diuresis is induced in a normal person and a uremic patient and both excrete 10 mL free water/100 mL GFR, urine volume will increase in both but by different amounts. The normal person (GFR = 120 mL/minute) can increase urine volume from 2 L isosmotic urine/day to 19.3 L dilute urine/day, whereas the uremic patient (GFR = 4 mL/minute) can increase urine volume from 2 to only 2.6 L/day.

The obligatory increase in water excretion in the patient with chronic renal disease may lead to polyuria and result in the development of nocturia, a manifestation of late renal insufficiency. Occasionally, particularly when extra fluids containing dextrose and water are administered in an effort to flush the kidneys, hyponatremia can occur because of the inability of the patient with chronic renal failure to increase appropriately the excretion of water.

Sodium Excretion

As renal disease progresses fractional sodium excretion increases in a manner that is adequate to maintain external balance (Figure 1). This adaptation occurs until very late in the course of renal disease so that normal extracellular fluid volume is preserved. However, when sodium intake changes, the fractional excretion of sodium must change substantially to maintain sodium balance in the patient with chronic renal failure.[1] For example, in a normal individual, doubling sodium intake from 3.5 to 7 g/day necessitates a change in fractional excretion of sodium from 0.25% to 0.5%. The same increment in salt intake requires a change in fractional sodium excretion from 8% to 16% in a patient with a GFR of 4 mL/minute. Hence, the patient with chronic renal disease can vary sodium excretion only over a rather restricted range, and this range narrows as GFR declines.[1,20] With chronic renal disease an upper and a lower limit of sodium excretion develop. The lower limit is important because it limits the ability of patients with chronic renal disease to conserve sodium maximally, and a low-salt diet can result in a negative sodium balance with loss of a corresponding volume of water. Extracellular fluid volume, plasma volume, and GFR all decrease.

Patients with advanced renal insufficiency also cannot tolerate high intakes of sodium. If excessive sodium is ingested, sodium retention with expansion of the extracellular fluid may occur and may produce or aggravate preexisting hypertension, edema, fluid overload, congestive heart failure, and pulmonary edema. Thus, the loss of flexibility for both sodium and water excretion must be carefully considered in the dietary management of patients with renal insufficiency.

Potassium

Normally, ≈90–95% of ingested potassium is excreted in the urine; the remainder is excreted in the stool.[21] In chronic renal failure a greater fraction of ingested potassium is excreted in the stool, with 20–50% of the ingested amount appearing in the stool when the GFR falls below 5 mL/minute.[22] Potassium excretion per nephron also increases, and potassium excretion approaches and may even surpass the filtered load of potassium. In chronic renal failure, aldosterone and other factors, such as increased flow of fluid through the distal nephron, are the major mediators of increased potassium secretion in the distal tubule. Therefore, adjustments in renal mechanisms that increase potassium excretion in addition to increased stool excretion are sufficient to maintain a normal concentration of potassium in plasma until the GFR reaches <10 mL/minute, even when the intake of potassium is normal (100 mmol/day).

Plasma potassium concentration may increase in chronic renal disease as acidosis develops because of redistribution of potassium between intracellular and extracellular compartments.[23] Intracellular potassium leaves the cells and is replaced by hydrogen and sodium. In addition, hormonal deficiencies such as low aldosterone concentrations in hyporeninemic patients may result in hyperkalemia earlier in the course of renal insufficiency. Lack of insulin may cause patients with insulin-dependent diabetes to also develop hyperkalemia earlier in the course of chronic renal disease.[24] Finally, at very low GFRs, the secretory rate of potassium may be near maximal to maintain the steady state. Thus, very little functional reserve remains to respond to sudden changes in potassium intake. Conditions such as oliguria, a sudden increase in potassium intake, and a sudden development of metabolic acidosis or catabolic states can result in life-threatening hyperkalemia in patients with advanced renal insufficiency.

Despite the tendency for hyperkalemia to develop in advanced chronic renal failure, total body potassium may in fact be decreased. This apparent paradox results from most body potassium being located intracellularly. Decreased intake, increased catabolism, and decreased extrusion of sodium from cells in advanced uremia can lead to decreased intracellular potassium, leading to some degree of potassium depletion despite an elevation of potassium in extracellular fluid.

Emergency therapy for life-threatening hyperkalemia includes stimulation of cellular uptake of potassium by the administration of glucose and insulin or sodium bicarbonate and removal of potassium by the use of intestinal cation-exchange resins (kayexalate) or dialysis.[23] Patients with advanced chronic renal failure should be advised to restrict the intake of foods rich in potassium, such as citrus fruits, avocados, beans, figs, and bananas. Patients on low-sodium diets and using salt substitutes may develop hyperkalemia from the high potassium content of some salt substitutes.

Acid-Base Balance

The contribution of the kidneys to the preservation of acid-base balance in normal individuals requires the reabsorption of the daily filtered load of ≈ 4000 mmol of bicarbonate and the excretion of 50–100 mmol of hydrogen ions in the form of ammonium and titratable acid (H^+ bound to phosphate and other buffer ions).[25] In acid-base regulation, as with many other nephron functions, there are remarkable compensatory responses by the residual functioning kidney mass as overall renal function declines. Except for a small group of patients with hyperchloremic acidosis, most subjects with renal disease do not have significant acidemia attributable to renal disease per se until the GFR falls below $\approx 20\%$ of normal.[25] Although plasma bicarbonate concentration may be depressed at higher GFRs, blood pH remains normal or is only barely depressed because of ventilatory compensation. Even when GFR falls below 20 mL/minute, the degree of acidosis is highly variable. Causes of this variability include the nature of the renal disease, diet, intake of acidic ion salts, extracellular volume status, potassium balance, and efficiency of respiratory compensation.[25]

Because metabolism of proteins is the major source of hydrogen, dietary protein restriction or efforts to de-

crease endogenous catabolism, if present, will markedly decrease the generation of hydrogen.[26] Phospholipids contribute to a smaller degree to the generation of hydrogen. Bicarbonate salts may be administered orally to correct the metabolic acidosis of renal insufficiency. Low plasma phosphate concentrations may lead to decreased titratable acid excretion and aggravation of the metabolic acidosis of uremia.

Nitrogen Metabolism and Protein Intake

In the early 1900s it was noted that ingestion of protein aggravated the clinical symptoms of patients with renal failure. L'Ambard[27] observed that uremic individuals were often wasted and did poorly particularly after ingesting a meal containing meat. These initial clinical correlations suggested that uremic toxicity could be ameliorated by reducing the amount of protein in the diet. Volhard[28] noticed that "in patients with chronic renal insufficiency a reduction in nitrogen intake to levels of 3–5 grams per day (about 20–30 grams of protein) prevents the rise in blood urea for long periods of time; . . . considerably elevated urea, indican and xanthoprotein values decrease and initial signs of uremic intoxication disappear." These and subsequent observations clearly established that restriction of dietary protein in patients with advanced renal insufficiency improves many of the uremic symptoms. In the past decade or so there has also been a great deal of interest in the potential effect of low-protein diets on renal function and on the progression of renal disease in humans.[29] However, definitive evidence that dietary protein restriction ameliorates or halts the progression of renal disease in humans is still lacking.

Blood urea concentrations and, particularly, urea production (usually measured as the total excretion of urea nitrogen in a 24-hour urine collection) have been used to estimate protein intake. However, increased tissue catabolism and degradation of endogenous protein may also increase urea production. Inadequate energy intake, acidosis, intercurrent infections, sodium depletion, or excess glucocorticoid secretion may result in increased urea nitrogen in patients with renal insufficiency. Metabolic acidosis may account for the abnormal metabolism of branched-chain amino acids in uremia.[30,31] Metabolic acidosis significantly decreased the concentrations of branched-chain amino acids in plasma and muscle and increased the oxidation of valine and leucine. Correction of the acidosis by sodium bicarbonate administration diminishes protein catabolism and the altered metabolism of branched-chain amino acids observed in uremia.[31,32]

It has not been clearly established at what point during progressive renal insufficiency protein restriction should be initiated. It seems prudent to restrict protein to prevent an elevation of blood urea nitrogen >35.7

mmol/L, and values <25 mmol/L perhaps should be the goal.[33] Certainly, in patients with GFR values <20–25 mL/minute, some degree of protein restriction should be recommended to ameliorate symptoms of uremia. Protein intake should be restricted to ≈0.6 g protein/kg standard body weight. However, in patients with GFR values <10 mL/minute, some clinicians have used diets providing ≈0.3 g protein/kg body weight supplemented with keto acids or amino acids. Protein restriction alone may not prevent uremic symptoms in patients with GFR values <5 mL/minute. The potential problem of inducing malnutrition by prolonged protein restriction should be considered, and the nutritional status of patients should be carefully evaluated at periodic intervals.[34]

Severe protein malnutrition is less common today than three decades ago when dialysis facilities were in short supply. A combination of inadequate energy intake because of anorexia and rigid reduction of protein intake over many months yielded patients with marked wasting. Patients were often 15–30% below customary weight during the early phase of dialysis after edema fluid had been removed. The nutritional status of patients with end-stage renal disease and those treated by dialysis no doubt has been greatly improved in recent years because of early initiation of dialysis and better application of nutritional knowledge. However, several observations indicate that a lesser but still significant degree of protein malnutrition still may be prevalent.[35] Extravascular pools of albumin may be reduced even though serum albumin concentration remains normal. Serum concentrations of transferrin, possibly a more sensitive indicator of protein malnutrition, has been found to be low in many patients with moderate to advanced renal failure and was also subnormal in a group of patients on chronic dialysis despite their ingestion of 1 g protein/kg.[36] Although inadequate protein, inadequate energy intake, or both may be the major cause of malnutrition in chronic renal failure, the possibility that renal failure per se disturbs one or more steps in the complex process of protein synthesis has not received sufficient study.[37] This possibility is supported by the finding of reduced alkali-soluble protein in muscle from patients with only moderate renal failure.

Energy Needs

The energy expenditure and requirements of patients with chronic renal failure are similar to those of normal subjects. However, energy intake in patients with renal disease tends to decrease because of a gradual onset of anorexia when GFR is <25 mL/minute, and energy malnutrition is common in patients with chronic renal failure. A high-energy intake enhances the use of protein in patients prescribed low-protein diets. An intake of 150 kJ·kg body weight^{-1}·day^{-1} (35 kcal·kg body weight^{-1}·day^{-1}) is recommended for most patients with chronic renal failure; for individuals older than 60 years, a 130 kJ·kg body weight^{-1}·day^{-1} (30 kcal·kg body weight^{-1}·day^{-1}) diet may be adequate. A higher intake of energy is appropriate for patients who engage in vigorous physical activity.

The protein and energy requirements of patients with end-stage renal disease undergoing maintenance dialysis are somewhat different.[38,39] It has been suggested that patients on maintenance hemodialysis should receive 1.2 g protein/kg body weight. Patients on continuous ambulatory peritoneal dialysis who have protein and amino acid losses into the dialysate should receive diets containing ≈1.5 g protein/kg body weight. Energy intakes in these individuals are usually adequate because glucose dialysate solutions are used and enough glucose is absorbed from the peritoneal cavity. In general, hemodialysis patients and predialysis patients with chronic renal failure[40] should receive 150 kJ·kg body weight^{-1}·day^{-1} (35 kcal·kg body weight^{-1}·day^{-1}).

Lipid Metabolism

Lipid abnormalities are common in patients with chronic renal disease, particularly those with nephrotic syndrome.[41] This syndrome is characterized by heavy proteinuria (mainly albuminuria), hypoalbuminemia, high concentration of serum cholesterol, and variable degrees of edema. Hyperlipidemia type IV, with low concentration of high-density lipoproteins, is common in patients with chronic uremia and in patients undergoing maintenance hemodialysis.[42-44] Cardiovascular disease is a major cause of death in long-term hemodialysis patients. Most of the known risk factors for the development of atherosclerosis and coronary artery disease are present in these patients, including hypertension, cigarette smoking, reduced concentrations of high-density-lipoprotein cholesterol, elevate triacylglycerol concentrations, hyperinsulinemia, glucose intolerance, stress, and a sedentary life-style.

Elevated triacylglycerol concentrations are the most common lipid abnormality in patients with chronic renal failure.[44,45] Patients exhibit increased very-low-density-lipoprotein triacylglycerol, reduced high-density-lipoprotein cholesterol, and an increased ratio of low-density-lipoprotein to high-density-lipoprotein cholesterol. The primary defect is a reduction in the removal of triacylglycerol-rich lipoproteins caused by reductions in lipoprotein lipase and hepatic lipase activities. Reduction in dietary carbohydrate and increase in the ratio of polyunsaturated to saturated fatty acids are effective in lowering plasma triacylglycerol concentrations.[43] However, lipid-lowering drugs such as clofibrate or carnitine may be required. In patients with nephrotic syndrome and hypercholesterolemia, lovastatin administration effectively reduces serum cholesterol concentrations.[46] Exercise training also ameliorated hyperlipidemia in patients with chronic renal insufficiency, whereas sedentary control subjects during the same period showed a deterioration in serum lipid profile.[47]

Disorders of Carbohydrate Metabolism

Carbohydrate tolerance is impaired in uremia. This is evident after oral or intravenous glucose loads. The abnormal glucose metabolism of chronic renal failure is characterized by fasting euglycemia, abnormal glucose tolerance, delayed glucose response to insulin, hyperinsulinemia, and hyperglucagonemia.[48,49] Although some studies suggest that the abnormal glucose tolerance is caused by resistance of peripheral tissues to insulin,[50,51] the presence of insulin resistance in skeletal muscle has not been clearly established;[52,53] there may be a circulating factor that induces insulin resistance in muscle.[54] Increased growth hormone concentrations in uremia also may contribute to the resistance of peripheral tissues to insulin.

Diabetic patients who develop progressive renal disease require diminishing doses of insulin as the disease progresses. Reduced energy intake and weight loss plus a reduced degradation of insulin probably play a role in this decreased insulin requirement.

Vitamins

There is only limited information concerning vitamin nutrition in end-stage renal disease.[55-57] Evaluation of published reports is complicated by the frequent omission of information on dietary intake of protein, use of vitamin supplements, time of sampling in relation to dialysis treatment, and intake of drugs that may affect vitamin metabolism. Reduced concentrations of several water-soluble vitamins in serum, erythrocytes, and leukocytes were reported. Hematological evidence of folate deficiency was found at some treatment centers but not at others, probably reflecting variations in dietary intake and use of vitamin supplements.[55,56] In one report patients not receiving vitamin supplements had low plasma and leukocyte concentrations of vitamin C, and a few patients had signs suggestive of mild scurvy.[57] The plasma concentrations of other water-soluble vitamins were normal in most reports.[58] Because the kidney is one route of elimination of water-soluble vitamins and their metabolites, decreased elimination by the kidney may be a protective mechanism, especially for patients on hemodialysis, which may remove water-soluble vitamins. The serum concentrations of retinol (vitamin A) and retinol-binding protein are increased in patients with renal failure.[59-61]

Trace Elements

During renal failure the metabolism of trace elements is altered.[56] The mechanisms underlying this alteration have not been established and the contribution of trace element toxicity or deficiency to the symptoms of advanced renal insufficiency is not known. Highly protein-bound elements such as copper and zinc are lost in excessive amounts with increased proteinuria. There are no data to support a recommendation that trace elements be given routinely to patients with chronic renal failure. There is some evidence to support the supplementation of selenium, zinc, and iron but only after the adequacy of the energy and protein content of the diet has been evaluated. Trace element supplements should be carefully monitored to avoid toxicity, especially with selenium, which has a small therapeutic range. Infections and steroid therapy lower the concentration of zinc in plasma; consequently, these conditions should be excluded before zinc supplementation is prescribed.

Aluminum accumulation, particularly caused by the administration of phosphate binders containing aluminum, may occur in patients with chronic renal failure.[62-65] This may cause bone disease, encephalopathy, and other manifestations.[63,65]

Acknowledgments

Support was provided by NIDDK grant 09976.

References

1. Bricker NS, Klahr S, Lubowitz H, Slatopolsky E (1971) The pathophysiology of renal insufficiency: on the functional transformation in the residual nephrons with advancing disease. Symposium on pediatric nephrology. Pediatr Clin North Am 18:595–611
2. Suki WN, Eknoyan G (1995) Pathophysiology and clinical manifestations of chronic renal failure and the uremic syndrome. In Jacobson H, Striker G, Klahr S (eds), The principles and practice of nephrology, 2nd ed. Mosby, St Louis, pp 603–614
3. Gambertoglio JE, Aweeka FJ, Blythe WB (1993) Use of drugs in patients with renal failure. In Schrier RW, Gottschalk CW (eds), Diseases of the kidney, 5th ed. Boston, Little, Brown, pp 3211–3268
4. Bennett WM, Aronoff GR, Golper TA (1993) Drug prescribing in renal failure: dosing guidelines for adults. American College of Physicians, Philadelphia
5. Eschbach JW (1989) The anemia of chronic renal failure: pathophysiology and the effects of recombinant erythropoietin. Kidney Int 35:134–148
6. Eschbach JW, Egrie JC, Downing MR, et al (1987) Correction of the anemia of end-stage renal disease with recombinant human erythropoietin: results of a combined phase I and II clinical trial. N Engl J Med 316:73–78
7. Wilson L, Felsenfeld A, Drezner MK, Llach F (1985) Altered divalent ion metabolism in early renal failure: role of 1,25(OH)2D. Kidney Int 27:565–573
8. Madsen S, Olgaard K, Ladefoged J (1981) Suppressive

effect of 1,25-dihydroxyvitamin D3 on circulating parathyroid hormone in renal failure. J Clin Endocrinol Metab 53:823–827

9. Klahr S (1983) Nonexcretory functions of the kidney. In Klahr S (ed), The kidney and body fluids in health and disease. Plenum Medical, New York, pp 65–90

10. Delmez J, Slatopolsky E (1992) Hyperphosphatemia: its consequences and treatment in patients with chronic renal disease. Am J Kidney Dis 19:303–317

11. Feinfeld DA, Sherwood LM (1988) Parathyroid hormone and 1,25(OH)2D3 in chronic renal failure. Kidney Int 33:1049–1058

12. Llach F, Massry SF, Singer FR, et al (1975) Skeletal resistance to endogenous parathyroid hormone in patients with early renal failure. J Endocrinol Metab 41:339–345

13. Somerville PJ, Kaye M (1979) Evidence that resistance to the calcemic action of parathyroid hormone in rats is caused by phosphate retention. Kidney Int 16:552–560

14. Alfrey AC (1984) Trace metals. In Eknoyan G, Knochel JP (eds), The systemic consequences of renal disease. Grune and Stratton, Orlando, FL, pp 443–460

15. Slatopolsky E, Weerts C, Lopez-Hilker S, et al (1986) Calcium carbonate as a phosphate binder in patients with chronic renal failure undergoing dialysis. N Engl J Med 315:157–161

16. Steele TH, Wen SF, Evenson MA, Rieselbach RE (1968) The contribution of the chronically diseased kidney to magnesium homeostasis in man. J Lab Clin Med 71:455–463

17. Randall RE, Cohen MD, Spray CC, Rossmeisl (1964) Hypermagnesemia in renal failure: etiology and toxic manifestations. Ann Intern Med 61:73–88

18. Baldwin DJ, Berman JH, Heinemann HO, Smith HW (1955) The elaboration of osmotically concentrated urine in renal disease. J Clin Invest 34:800–807

19. Kleeman CR, Adams DA, Maxwell MH (1961) An evaluation of maximal water diuresis in chronic renal disease. J Lab Clin Med 58:169–184

20. Klahr S, Slatopolsky E (1973) Renal regulation of sodium excretion. Arch Intern Med 131:780–791

21. Wright FS, Giebisch G (1985) Regulation of potassium excretion. In Seldin DW, Giebisch G (eds), The kidney: physiology and pathophysiology. Raven, New York, pp 1223–1249

22. Schultze RG (1973) Recent advances in the physiology and pathophysiology of potassium excretion. Arch Intern Med 131:885–897

23. Allon M (1993) Treatment and prevention of hyperkalemia in end-stage renal disease. Kidney Int 43:1197–1209

24. Bia MJ, DeFronzo RT (1981) Extrarenal potassium homeostasis. Am J Physiol 240:F257–F268

25. Hamm LL, Klahr S (1984) Alterations of acid-base balance. In Klahr S (ed), Differential diagnosis in renal and electrolyte disorders, 2nd ed. Appleton-Century-Crofts, Norwalk, CT, pp 231–250

26. Relman A, Lennon EJ, Lemman J Jr (1961) Endogenous production of fixed acid and the measurement of the net balance of acid in normal subjects. J Clin Invest 40:1621–1630

27. Ambard L (1920) Physiologie normale et pathologique des reins. Masson et Cie, Paris

28. Volhard F (1918) Die doppelseitigen hämatogenen Nierenerkrankungen (Bright'sche Krankheit). In Mohr L, Staehelin R (eds), Handbuch der Inneren Medizin. Springer, Berlin, pp 1149–1172

29. Klahr S, Levey AS, Beck GJ, et al and Modification of Renal Disease Study Group (1994) The effects of dietary protein restriction and blood pressure control on the progression of chronic renal disease. N Engl J Med 330:877–884

30. May RC, Hara Y, Kelly RA, et al (1987) Branched-chain amino acid metabolism in rat muscle: abnormal regulation in acidosis. Am J Physiol 252:E712–E718

31. Hara Y, May RC, Kelly RA, Mitch WE (1987) Acidosis, not azotemia, stimulates branched-chain, amino acid catabolism in uremic rats. Kidney Int 32:808–814

32. Papadoyannakis NJ, Stefanidis CS, McGeown M (1984) The effect of the correction of metabolic acidosis on nitrogen and potassium balance of patients with chronic renal failure. Am J Clin Nutr 40:623–627

33. Kopple JD, Coburn JW (1974) Evaluation of chronic uremia: importance of serum urea nitrogen, serum creatinine and their ratio. JAMA 227:41–44

34. Blumenkrantz MJ, Kopple JD, Gutman RA, et al (1980) Methods for assessing nutritional status of patients with renal failure. Am J Clin Nutr 33:1567–1585

35. Hakim RM, Levin N (1993) Malnutrition in hemodialysis patients. Am J Kidney Dis 21:125–137

36. Ooi BS, Darocy AF, Pollak VE (1972) Serum transferin levels in chronic renal failure. Nephron 9:200–208

37. Kopple JD (1978) Abnormal amino acid and protein metabolism in uremia. Kidney Int 14:340–348

38. Bergstrom J (1993) Nutritional requirements of hemodialysis patients. In Mitch WE, Klahr S (eds), Nutrition and the kidney, 2nd ed. Little, Brown, Boston, pp 263–289

39. Kopple JD, Hirschberg R (1993) Nutrition and peritoneal dialysis. In Mitch WE, Klahr S (eds), Nutrition and the kidney, 2nd ed. Little, Brown, Boston, pp 290–313

40. Maroni BJ (1993) Requirements for protein, calories and fat in the predialysis patient. In Mitch WE, Klahr S (eds), Nutrition and the kidney, 2nd ed. Little, Brown, Boston, pp 185–212

41. Kaysen GA (1993) The nephrotic syndrome: nutritional consequences and dietary management. In Mitch WE, Klahr S (eds), Nutrition and the kidney, 2nd ed. Little, Brown, Boston, pp 213–242

42. Klahr S (1993) Management of lipid abnormalities in the uremic patient. In Mitch WE, Klahr S (eds), Nutrition and the kidney, 2nd ed. Little, Brown, Boston, pp 132–151

43. Okubo M, Tsukamoto Y, Yoneda T, et al (1980) Deranged fat metabolism and the lowering effect of carbohydrate-poor diet on serum triglycerides in patients with chronic renal failure. Nephron 25:8–14

44. Reaven GM, Swenson RS, Sanfelippo ML (1980) An inquiry into the mechanism of hypertriglyceridemia in patients with chronic renal failure. Am J Clin Nutr 33:1476–1484

45. Sanfelippo ML, Swenson RS, Reaven GM (1977) Reduction of plasma triglyceride by diet in subjects with chronic renal failure. Kidney Int 11:54–61

46. Vega GL, Grundy SM (1988) Lovastatin therapy in nephrotic hyperlipidemia: effects on lipoprotein metabolism. Kidney Int 33:1160–1168

47. Goldberg AP (1984) A potential role for exercise training in modulating coronary risk factors in uremia. Am J Nephrol 4:132–133

48. DeFronzo RA, Andres R, Edgar P, Walker WG (1973) Carbohydrate metabolism in uremia: a review. Medicine 52:469–497

49. Horton ES, Johnson C, Lebovitz AE (1968) Carbohydrate metabolism in uremia. Ann Intern Med 68:63–74

50. Hager SR (1989) Insulin resistance of uremia. Am J Kidney Dis 14:272–276

51. Westervelt FB (1969) Insulin effect in uremia. J Lab Clin Med 74:79–84

52. Davis TA, Klahr S, Karl IE (1987) Glucose metabolism in muscle of sedentary and exercised rats with chronic uremia. Am J Physiol 252:F138–F145

53. Garber AJ (1970) Skeletal muscle protein and amino acid metabolism in experimental chronic uremia in the rat: accelerated alanine and glutamine formation and release. J Clin Invest 62:623–632

54. McCaleb ML, Izzo MS, Lockwood DH (1985) Characterization and partial purification of a factor from uremia serum that induces insulin resistance. J Clin Invest 75:391–396

55. Dobbelstein H, Korner WF, Mempel W, et al (1974) Vitamin B6 deficiency in uremia and its implications for the depression of immune responses. Kidney Int 5:233–239

56. Gilmour ER, Hartley GH, Goodship THJ (1993) Trace elements and vitamins in renal disease. In Mitch WE, Klahr S (eds), Nutrition and the kidney, 2nd ed. Little, Brown, Boston, pp 114–131

57. Ihle BU, Gillies M (1983) Scurvy and thrombocytopathy in a chronic hemodialysis patient. Aust NZ J Med 13:523

58. Stein G, Schone S, Sperschneider H, et al (1988) Vitamin status in patients with chronic renal failure. Contrib Nephrol 65:33–42

59. Kopple JD (1981) Nutritional therapy in kidney failure. Nutr Rev 39:193–206

60. Smith FR, Goodman DS (1971) The effects of diseases of the liver, thyroid and kidney on transport of vitamin in human plasma. J Clin Invest 50:2426–2436

61. Vahlquist A, Peterson PA, Wibell L (1973) Metabolism of the vitamin A transporting protein complex. I. Turnover studies in normal persons and in patients with chronic renal failure. Eur J Clin Invest 3:352–362

62. Zumkley H, Bertram HP, Lison A, et al (1979) Aluminum, zinc and copper concentrations in plasma in chronic renal insufficiency. Clin Nephrol 12:18–21

63. Alfrey AC, Legendre GR, Kaehny WD (1976) The dialysis encephalopathy syndrome—possible aluminum intoxication. N Engl J Med 294:184–189

64. Kaysen GA, Schoenfeld PY (1984) Aluminum homeostasis in patients undergoing continuous ambulatory peritoneal dialysis. Kidney Int 25:107–114

65. McGonigle RJ, Parsons V (1985) Aluminum-induced anemia in haemodialysis patients. Nephron 39:1–9

Chapter 47

Nutrition in Liver Disease

Josef E. Fischer and Timothy D. Kane

Liver is the body's central metabolic organ. The anatomic structure, location, and function of liver enable metabolism and clearance of most of the nutrients and toxins presented to it from portal blood. A myriad of endocrine, neural, or cytokinetic processes can stimulate and modulate the ability of liver to metabolize, detoxify, or redistribute these substances to the periphery. Alterations in the normal metabolism of nutrients as manifestations of liver disease produce extremely complex problems in the management of the patient in hepatic failure.

Current options for the management of liver failure include organ transplantation, use of extracorporeal bioartificial liver devices, and general supportive measures. Although liver transplantation has been successful in patients with end-stage cirrhosis and fulminant hepatic failure, organ availability has been the limiting factor for this mode of therapy.[1,2,3] Bioartificial liver technology has been proposed as a bridge to either transplantation or natural recovery of hepatic function, providing temporary support during hepatic failure.[4-6] Although some of the recent experimental reports are exciting, this technology needs further development.

Liver is unique among the visceral organs for its ability to regenerate its entire cell mass approximately every 50 days.[7,8] Therefore, supportive measures remain the major form of therapy for patients in hepatic failure. Of the measures that most affect hepatic regeneration (including use of hepatocyte growth factor, steroids, and growth hormone), nutritional support has been the most manageable therapeutic intervention for patients with liver disease.[9] Not all of these factors are stimulatory; steroids, for example, are permissive.

Issues to be considered in providing nutritional support to patients in hepatic failure include specific disease processes and pathophysiology of liver failure, alterations in metabolic processes in the diseased liver, and the goals and effects of providing nutritional support in hepatic failure.

Pathophysiology of Liver Failure

The liver is the largest internal organ of the human body, weighing between 1200 and 1500 g.[10] It receives its blood supply from two sources: The portal vein provides 65–75% of total hepatic blood flow but only 25–40% of hepatic oxygen delivery. The hepatic artery supplies 25–35% of blood flow but delivers 60–75% of oxygen. Portal blood contains nutrients, toxins, and other substances absorbed from the gut; it is relatively oxygen-poor until mixing occurs with arterial blood at the level of the hepatic sinusoids. The hepatic architecture is such that all hepatocytes have direct access to the sinusoids.[10] The portal triad consists of a portal venule, a hepatic arteriole, and a bile duct, which drains into the hepatic sinusoids. Blood passes from the portal to the central regions, where substrates are removed and metabolic products are added to the sinusoidal blood.[10,11] These substrates and metabolic products may induce the synthesis of enzyme systems within the hepatocytes and modulate the function of the hepatic lobular cells.

Hepatic failure can be described as either acute or chronic, with some patients demonstrating a combination of both disease states. Fulminant hepatic failure, which has an acute and progressive course, is usually caused by viral or toxic hepatitis and involves patients who previously had normal nutrition and liver function.[12] Although the prognosis for survival is extremely poor, the problem of nutritional support must be addressed in these patients because it may be potentially helpful before transplantation, decreasing protein depletion and improving posttransplant immunologic status.

Chronic liver diseases such as alcoholic hepatitis require prolonged nutritional support to improve survival.[13] Aggressive nutritional support has been shown to improve survival for this group of patients.[14] Cirrhosis is often the underlying disease in patients who develop acute-on-chronic hepatic failure secondary to an acute insult such as gastrointestinal bleeding, infection, starvation, or surgical manipulation. Nutritional support is most beneficial for these patients and may result in improved survival.

The phenomenon of multisystem organ failure is becoming increasingly recognized as a cause of death in surgical patients. During this hypermetabolic state, one hypothesis for the etiology of hepatic failure is that gluconeogenesis becomes sustained at the expense of structural and functional proteins in the vital organs, especially liver, in response to prolonged and excessive stress (e.g., sepsis).[15] Therefore, patients with sepsis and acute-on-chronic hepatic failure require vigorous and aggressive nutritional support.

In the presence of repeated insults to liver from either alcohol or malnutrition, the normal lobular architecture becomes distorted as a result of piecemeal necrosis, bridging necrosis, and collapse and eventual replacement of necrotic hepatic parenchyma by fibrous tissue. The orderly access of single plates of hepatocytes to both arterial and portal flow becomes altered.[16] Regenerating nodules fail to acquire portal blood supply, which makes cirrhotic liver especially vulnerable to systemic changes in blood flow from the hepatic artery.[11,17] Profound vasoconstriction resulting from dehydration, anesthesia, shock, or sepsis may lead to rapid embarrassment of hepatic arterial flow, with subsequent acute deterioration of the regenerating nodules.[3,18] Hepatic necrosis and failure are manifested by elevated bilirubin and decrease in hepatic synthetic capacity. Prolonged prothrombin time and partial thromboplastin time are indices associated with increased mortality in hepatic failure. The causes of decreased serum albumin are multifactorial and are related not only to cytokine-mediated synthesis inhibition[19] but also to a greater percentage of extravascular albumin, which increases degradation.

In addition to serving as the body's metabolic powerhouse, liver serves as a filter for potentially harmful products from the gut, including bacteria, spores, and endotoxin. Liver disease (leading to the inability to provide metabolic regulatory activity) allows amino acids, whose concentrations the liver usually regulates, to escape into the circulation, with various consequences.[20] Hepatocytes in regenerative areas of a diseased liver demonstrate varying functional capacity. Depending upon the extent of hepatic disease, hepatocytes may manifest any degree of normal function, dysfunction, or necrosis. Thus, the inability of dead or dying hepatocytes to metabolize various substances that are normally cleared as the portal blood percolates through the sinusoids has profound metabolic and physiologic effects on the entire organism.

Physiological shunting of blood around liver is seen in both portasystemically shunted patients and in patients who have developed portal hypertension secondary to disrupted hepatic architecture that is a result of liver disease.[21] As the percentage of shunting increases to a level at which portal blood flow is directed away from liver (hepatofugal), clearance of portal substances (e.g., glucose, amino acids, insulin, glucagon, or endotoxin) is not achieved; as a result, toxic or abnormal systemic plasma concentrations of these products occur.

Portal hypertension represents a homeostatic process by which the body attempts to maintain blood flow to liver in the face of increased resistance. Thus, plasma volume expansion, probably secondary to increased aldosterone and antidiuretic hormone and decreased sensitivity to atrial natriuretic factor,[22] may be viewed as an attempt to increase perfusion pressure and flow. Paradoxically, normalization of portal pressure with shunting procedures performed to prevent death by hemorrhage leads to a decrease in hepatic flow and may ultimately contribute to long-term hepatic failure, which often occurs following these procedures. Finally, nutritional restriction secondary to hepatic encephalopathy results in further liver damage because sufficient protein and energy for healing the damaged parenchyma are no longer available.[23,24]

Alterations in Metabolic Processes

Before nutritional support for patients with liver disease is discussed, a review of the disordered metabolism of carbohydrate, fat, and protein as these relate to patients with hepatic failure is necessary.

Carbohydrate metabolism involves the interaction of the storage hormone insulin and the catabolic hormone glucagon. It has been shown that in compromised hepatic function, diminished degradation of glucagon and insulin results in persistent elevation of both of these hormones.[25-27] Portal hypertension decreases hepatocellular exposure to portal venous glucose, leading to aberrant glucose tolerance.[28] Hyperglucagonemia has been associated with portasystemic shunting; it is likely that hyperinsulinemia results from the same mechanism.[25,26] In patients with cirrhosis, there is a tendency toward catabolism in the classic glucagon-insulin imbalance scenario, where the effective insulin-glucagon ratio is decreased as a result of glucagon predominance, cellular insensitivity to insulin, or both.[27] In experimental animals, the decreased insulin-glucagon ratio becomes more prominent as the liver progressively fails.[29] Ziparo et al. have shown that in humans, as hepatic failure and coma supervene, glucagon levels increase markedly, whereas insulin levels either remain stable or fall.[30] In these studies, true alpha-cell hyperfunction suppressible by somatostatin occurred in postshunt patients, especially those with hepatic encephalopathy.

The source of hyperglucagonemia is unclear, but one may presume that it is directed at increasing glucose production by a failing liver or mobilizing and releasing hepatic fat for peripheral energy. Glucagon responds to a variety of influences, including ammonia and several amino acids (the aromatic amino acids in particular) that are present in excess concentrations in blood[31]. Sherwin et al. have proposed that hyperglucagonemia against a background of increased epinephrine and increased steroid levels (probably resulting from decreased degradation) produces a state of sustained gluconeogenesis.[25]

Hypoglycemia is rare but may occur in cases of massive hepatocellular loss, as in fulminant hepatic failure, or in the alcoholic (the model of chronic malnutrition), where inadequate glycogen stores can result in hypoglycemia after only short periods of fasting.[11] The cirrhotic liver fails to store glucose but hepatic gluconeogenesis is active. It is probably assisted by renal gluconeogenesis such as occurs in prolonged starvation. Other energy sources lessen the requirement for glucose production by the failing liver. Lipolysis liberates both glycerol (which contributes to gluconeogenesis) and fatty acids, which are utilized directly or oxidized to ketones. The latter pathway may be impaired in patients with hepatic failure.[33] Skeletal muscle proteolysis generates branched-chain amino acids; at least one carbon atom is oxidized locally, whereas the amino groups and possibly some members of the carbon skeleton generate pyruvate, which forms alanine (glucose-alanine cycle).[34]

In cirrhotic patients, glucose intolerance occurs after both oral and intravenous glucose and is associated with an exaggerated insulin response. The latter is probably caused by shunting; however, the hyperglycemia may be multifactorial. The peripheral uptake of glucose is insulin-dependent; although hepatocellular uptake of glucose is independent of insulin, hepatocellular metabolism of glucose is also insulin-dependent. The decreased insulin-glucagon ratio may therefore account for this hyperglycemia.

The primary hepatic responsibilities in carbohydrate metabolism are producing and storing glucose and maintaining a steady fuel concentration and therefore a stable plasma osmolarity. In summary, the cirrhotic liver fails only in glucose storage while maintaining adequate capacity for the other functions. However, with superimposed acute hepatic failure, gluconeogenesis may ultimately fail, resulting in hypoglycemia. Profound hypoglycemia usually portends a fatal outcome. Hepatic uptake of substrates for this pathway ceases, leading to gross hyperamino-acidemia and lactic acidemia.

Abnormalities in lipid metabolism extend to the subject of fatty acids. Under normal conditions, during resting starvation, lipolysis is a major source of energy, accounting for approximately 75–85% of normal energy expenditure.

Liver plays a major role in the metabolism of long-chain fatty acids to ketone bodies, a major source of peripheral energy, as well as maintaining normal plasma levels of short-chain fatty acids. One current hypothesis implicates short-chain fatty acids, together with ammonia and methane thiols, as one of the prominent substances involved in hepatic encephalopathy.[12] However, some investigators have administered relatively large amounts of these substances without ill effects.[35] Moreover, in conditions such as coma of congenital origin or those involving hypoglycin A, in which short-chain fatty acids have been implicated, the concentrations of short-chain fatty acids are hundreds of times higher than those seen in patients with hepatic encephalopathy.[36,37]

Protein malnutrition can result in fatty changes in liver when lipid availability for export is greater than the supply of protein precursors for lipoprotein synthesis.[7] Excess supply is the basis of fatty liver seen in pregnancy, obesity, steroid use, diabetes, and total parenteral nutrition with excessive glucose.[11] Drugs or toxins such as tetracycline or carbon tetrachloride inhibit protein synthesis and result in fatty changes because of inability to synthesize very-low-density lipoprotein.[10]

Finally, nonesterified fatty acids circulate in the bloodstream at least partially bound to albumin. Nonesterified fatty acids are important with respect to hepatic encephalopathy because of their displacement of bound tryptophan from albumin.[38] Thus, unbound tryptophan increases with lipid mobilization and subsequent increase in nonesterified fatty acids within the circulation, making more tryptophan available for transport across the blood-brain barrier.[39] In summary, the overall effect of liver failure on lipid metabolism is to deprive the body of a source of energy, thus making the organism turn to gluconeogenesis as a primary energy source.

Protein and amino acid metabolism of large amounts of dietary-derived proteins facilitates protein synthesis in liver and other tissues. Amino acids from peripheral tissues are also recycled by liver for degradation, participation in transamination, or contribution to gluconeogenesis.[40]

In cirrhosis, the tendency toward gluconeogenesis requires an equal capacity for ureagenesis to prevent hyperammonemia. Hepatic and renal ureagenesis facilitates the formation of a nontoxic degradation product of nitrogen metabolism that is easily eliminated from the body.[41] In chronic cirrhotic failure, the reserve capacity for glucose production is usually adequate, depending on the degree of hepatocellular dysfunction, but the reserve capacity for ureagenesis may be less well preserved.

Hyperammonemia resulting from diminished ureagenic capacity is difficult to differentiate from that which results from shunting of gut-derived ammonia. Gut gluconeogenesis from glutamine is active; ammonia from this source, as well as from intraluminal deamination of amino acids, requires successful transport to liver for urea synthesis. Hepatocellular dysfunction and shunting of a critical portion of portal blood would result in persistent elevation of plasma ammonia levels.

Of particular importance is the amino acid pattern that characterizes cirrhosis and acute-on-chronic liver failure. Levels of the branched-chain amino acids (BCAAs)—leucine, isoleucine, and valine—are usually below normal whereas levels of phenylalanine, tyrosine, free tryptophan, methionine, glutamate, aspartate, and to a lesser extent histidine are usually elevated.[42]

The BCAAs represent 60–100% of the splanchnic clearance of amino acids and 60–100% of the peripheral nitrogen accumulation in patients who are in energy and nitrogen balance.[43] With impairment of the production or use of the usual energy substrates (glucose, fatty acids, and ketones), the BCAAs contribute up to 30–40% more in terms of energy needs. Therefore, enhanced peripheral consumption provides a reasonable explanation for decreased plasma concentrations in acute-on-chronic failure. In fulminant hepatic failure, BCAA levels remain relatively normal despite gross elevation of all other amino acids; their concentration is maintained primarily by the periphery with little effect on liver.[42,44]

As previously mentioned, tryptophan is albumin-bound. In acute-on-chronic liver failure, although the concentration remains normal or decreased, the unbound fraction is elevated.[38,39,45,46] Tryptophan is displaced by nonesterified fatty acids and bilirubin, both of which are present in high concentrations. The elevations of phenylalanine, tyrosine, methionine, glutamate, aspartate, and histidine are not as clear. However, the conversion of phenylalanine to tyrosine has been found to be impaired in cirrhosis and correlates well with the estimation of portasystemic shunting.[47] Hepatic amino acid uptake has been shown to be quite variable following single circulatory passage through liver.[48] Histidine, aspartate, glutamate, and the aromatic amino acids are 80–100% cleared after initial passage through a functioning liver. Other amino acids such as alanine, lysine, proline, and arginine demonstrate only 20–40% clearance. This may provide clues as to the selective elevations in cirrhosis and acute-on-chronic liver failure. Amino acids that have especially high uptake indices on initial passage may be the most sharply affected if shunting denies direct access of blood to the sinusoids.

Certain amino acids, including phenylalanine, tyrosine, histidine, methionine, and tryptophan, have been implicated in the control of flux of other amino acids through the hepatocellular membrane in vitro.[49] Enzyme systems within liver, which are inducible by and responsive to markedly increased concentrations in the circulation, constitute the principal site of catabolism of these amino acids.

Extensive muscle proteolysis occurring in the context of acute-on-chronic liver failure, which may be associated with starvation, surgical or traumatic insults, and sepsis, provides a common source of amino acids. In addition to amino acids from the gastrointestinal tract (secondary to blood degradation), these quantities only tend to exacerbate the abnormal pattern that existed prior to the insult.

The plasma ratio of BCAAs to aromatic amino acids ([isoleucine + valine + leucine]/ [phenylalanine + ty-rosine]) has been used as an indicator of abnormalities in protein metabolism during liver disease as well as a guide in the clinical therapy of these patients. In normal individuals, this ratio is 3.5–4.0. In hepatic disease the ratio falls below 2.5, in hepatic coma it drops below 1.2, and in profound coma it is usually <0.8.[50,51]

Hepatic Encephalopathy

From a nutritional standpoint, adequate provision of protein is necessary to support protein synthesis and hepatic regeneration, as well as to provide metabolic substrate for immunologic host defense.[52] However, intolerance to protein imposes severe dietary restriction on patients with hepatic failure or in hepatic coma, because of the dramatic abnormalities in nitrogen metabolism found in these patients.

Various hypotheses have been put forward regarding the etiology of hepatic encephalopathy. The unified hypothesis suggests that a multifactorial etiology is responsible for hepatic encephalopathy, ammonia being merely an indicator of disturbed nitrogen metabolism.[53] The clinical presentation (including mood swings and subtle disturbances in judgment, day-night rhythm, and posture) indicates a disorder of the central and peripheral neurotransmitters, particularly those of the aminergic system. The anatomic relationship among aminergic neurons suggests a regulatory function because the axons and dendrites usually end freely in the matrix instead of forming classic synapses.[54]

According to the unified hypothesis, the etiology of this aminergic disturbance has been linked to the amino acid imbalance characteristic of cirrhosis and acute-on-chronic failure. Neutral pH amino acids such as phenylalanine, tyrosine, unbound tryptophan, methionine, histidine, and the BCAAs are transported across the blood-brain barrier via system L.[55,56] A common carrier is thought to be involved in the process that each amino acid competitively employs. Thus, increased concentrations of these amino acids in the brain (except BCAAs) are a direct result of their high plasma concentrations as well as an indirect result of diminished competition from low plasma BCAA levels. In addition, an intrinsic alteration in the velocity of transport across system L may be involved.[57]

Phenylalanine, tyrosine, tryptophan, methionine, and histidine are all precursors of aminergic neurotransmitters. An imbalance of aminergic products resulting from excessive brain concentrations of these amino acids is the basis of this hypothesis. Both animal and human studies have suggested that decreased norepinephrine and dopamine correlate closely with the presence of hepatic encephalopathy.[58,59] Derangement of the aminergic system is further supported by studies that have shown the presence of 5-hydroxyindoleacetic acid and homovanillic acid in the cerebrospinal fluid (CSF) of patients with hepatic encephalopathy.[60,61]

It is known that hyperammonemia stimulates the release of glucagon, thereby further promoting gluconeogenesis and the requirement for concomitant ureagenesis.[31] However, in the brain, ammonia is represented as glutamine, the product of a rapidly turning-over pool of glutamate.[62] CSF levels of glutamine have correlated well with the level of hepatic encephalopathy.[63] In addition, experiments in animals have demonstrated an excellent correlation between CSF glutamine and the concentrations of phenylalanine, tyrosine, and tryptophan.[64]

Because glutamine is also of neutral pH, transport across the blood-brain barrier occurs via system L. If the brain were to export glutamine in blood-brain fashion, it would be conceivable that the system L carrier would be free to exchange at an increased rate for the other neutral amino acids.[53] Other investigators have shown evidence to support this theory in experiments carried out in both animals and in isolated brain capillaries from shunted and normal animals.[45] Methionine sulfoximine inhibits glutamine synthetase, which inhibits the transport of neutral amino acids across the blood-brain barrier, possibly because of decreased glutamine concentrations within the brain.[65] This may explain why the toxicity of ammonia is decreased when this substance is given to experimental animals.[66]

Consistent with this hypothesis is the relationship between amino acid concentrations in plasma and brain in animals following portocaval shunt. Fernstrom and Faller have developed equations for calculating plasma competition ratios that predict the brain concentrations of various neutral amino acids.[67] It has been shown that in the brains of animals with liver disease these concentrations considerably exceed predicted concentrations but seem to follow linear correlations, as if subjected to another influence. Interestingly, when glutamine is exchanged across the blood-brain barrier for other neutral amino acids, the excess of observed over predicted values correlates well with brain glutamine. Only animals with normal brain glutamine have normal levels of brain-neutral amino acids.[65,68]

In summary, the current unified concept of hepatic encephalopathy provides for ammonia; disturbed balance between insulin and glucagon; and increased plasma concentrations of phenylalanine, tyrosine, unbound tryptophan, methionine, and histidine; as well as decreased plasma levels of their blood-brain barrier competitors, the BCAAs. In addition, the unified hypothesis of hepatic encephalopathy explains the reputed beneficial clinical effects of such diverse compounds as L-dopa, bromocriptine, and the BCAAs, as well as neomycin and lactulose.[69,70,71]

Nutritional Support in Hepatic Failure

Enteral nutritional support has been shown to be physiologically superior to parenteral support in reducing the hypermetabolic state induced by injury.[52] However, in patients with hepatic failure, liver dysfunction and the subsequent risk of encephalopathy preclude the administration of enteral protein loads in these patients. Thus, parenteral nutrition consisting of individual amino acids is used in these situations; it is often better tolerated than equivalent amounts of oral protein.

The first study demonstrating the beneficial effects of BCAA-enriched solutions was reported in 1976.[72] The use of these solutions in patients with liver failure is perhaps the earliest example of nutritional pharmacology. BCAA-enriched solutions may be beneficial for metabolic reasons.

- BCAAs are a useful energy source that can be used directly by muscle, heart, brain, liver, and possibly other tissues. Patients with hepatic failure/encephalopathy have reduced glycogen storage and fat reserves. Although these patients are highly catabolic and glucose resistant, ketogenesis and the use of fatty acids are probably decreased secondary to the impairment of the hepatic mechanism that produces ketone bodies from fatty acids. Normally, BCAAs comprise only 6–7% of energy needs. With hypermetabolism, glucose resistance, and decreased ketogenesis, this percentage could climb to 30% because BCAAs do not permeate glucose.
- BCAAs decrease the amounts of aromatic amino acids in the circulation by effectively decreasing the efflux of other amino acids through the myocyte membrane.
- Leucine decreases muscle proteolysis and increases protein synthesis.[73–76]
- In humans, all amino acids increase hepatic protein synthesis, but leucine may be the most potent in this regard.[77]
- Administration of BCAAs normalizes the plasma amino acid pattern secondary to decreased muscle protein breakdown[43] and increased protein synthesis (using aromatic amino acids). Glucose is better than fat as a source of energy, probably because of the influence of insulin.[78]
- As mentioned previously, BCAAs compete with both neutral and aromatic amino acids for entry through system L across the blood-brain barrier. Because BCAAs provide most of the competition, increasing plasma BCAA concentrations will decrease aromatic amino acid plasma levels as well as prevent their penetration across the blood-brain barrier.
- In hepatectomized animals, administration of BCAAs increases reduced brain levels of norepinephrine in three of seven regions.[79]

- Theoretically, provision of a normal precursor pool will lead to normalization of peripheral catecholamine synthesis.
- BCAAs increase ammonia metabolism by muscle and donate the amino group for glutamine synthesis.[80,81]

BCAA-enriched solutions with low aromatic amino acid content have been available for over 20 years; several studies have used various such solutions in the treatment of patients with liver failure and hepatic encephalopathy.[82,83] The encouraging results of these early studies led to several conclusions about human trials with BCAA-enriched solutions: Up to 125 g of BCAA-enriched solution is well tolerated when administered to patients who have a history or presence of hepatic encephalopathy or who are intolerant of conventional solutions or oral protein.[13] Hepatic encephalopathy diminishes with improvement of mental status, despite high amino acid load. BCAA-enriched solutions are designed for acute-on-chronic hepatic failure and not for fulminant hepatitis, in which case the plasma amino acid pattern is quite different. In fulminant hepatitis, massive hyperaminoacidemia is reflective of a dying liver. However, some investigators have reported a beneficial effect of BCAA-enriched solutions in fulminant hepatitis.[82] Positive or near-positive nitrogen balance is required to achieve the full benefits of BCAAs on brain aromatic amino acid levels and for the resultant effect on hepatic encephalopathy to become apparent. This is probably because of the doubling of normal amino acid requirements that occurs in hepatic failure and represents a hypercatabolic state.[13,84] Given an energy source of 130–150 kJ·kg^{-1}·day^{-1} (30–35 kcal·kg^{-1}·day^{-1}), amino acid requirements increase from 0.55 to 1.1 g·kg^{-1}·day^{-1}.

Seven randomized prospective trials have examined the use of BCAA-enriched solutions in the treatment of hepatic encephalopathy.[85–92] Five of these trials, in which hypertonic glucose was the principal energy source, demonstrated a positive effect.[85–88,90] In the remaining two trials, lipid was used as the primary source of energy;[89,92] although the results were equivocal, this may reflect the energy source and not the amino acid solutions used. Naylor et. al.[93] have shown through a meta-analysis of previous studies that BCAA-enriched solutions have a beneficial effect in the treatment of hepatic encephalopathy. Overall, three kinds of beneficial effects of BCAA-enriched solutions can be identified: wake-up time, nutritional effects, and outcome and survival.

Wake-up from hepatic encephalopathy was at least as good in most patients and more rapid in some receiving BCAA-enriched solutions compared with those receiving the standard medical treatment of lactulose and neomycin and significantly better than in control groups receiving hypertonic dextrose alone.[85–92] The U.S. multicenter trial reported wake-up to grade I encephalopathy in 77% of patients given BCAA-enriched solutions compared with 26% in the neomycin control group.[85] Other trials have demonstrated that after treatment with BCAAs and hypertonic dextrose, patients were awake from hepatic encephalopathy after a shorter time than patients treated with hypertonic glucose or lactulose alone.[88,90] At the end of the treatment period, Fiaccadori et al.[87] demonstrated wake-up rates of 94% and 100% after treatment with either BCAAs alone or BCAAs and lactulose, respectively, versus 56% with lactulose alone. Strauss et al. reported mean wake-up times of 33 hours in patients treated with BCAA-enriched solutions compared with 71 hours in the neomycin control group.[92]

Classically, the effectiveness of any nutritional intervention, including the use of BCAA-enriched solutions in the treatment of hepatic failure, is best measured by nitrogen balance. Unfortunately, in only a few of the aforementioned trials was nitrogen balance measured. The U.S. multicenter trial was the only study to demonstrate that patients receiving BCAA-enriched solutions were close to achieving nitrogen equilibrium.[85] By contrast, one trial reported a negative nitrogen balance (−10 g/24 hours) despite nutritional support.[89] This may explain why the U.S. multicenter trial has had more positive results compared with other trials.

In the two trials using BCAA-enriched solutions in patients with hepatic encephalopathy, survival was improved.[85,87] A recent randomized prospective study examined the efficacy of a 35% BCAA-enriched aromatic amino acid–deficient solution with hypertonic dextrose administered intravenously compared with oral nutrition alone perioperatively in patients undergoing hepatic resection for hepatocellular carcinoma.[94] Both lipid emulsion and dextrose were used as energy sources, with medium-chain triacylglyerols comprising 50% of the lipids. A statistically significant reduction in postoperative morbidity was noted in the preoperative nutrition group compared with the control group (34% versus 55%, $p < 0.05$), primarily because of a lower rate of septic complications (17% versus 37%, $p < 0.05$); decreased requirements for diuretic agent use to control ascites were noted in the preoperative nutrition group (25% versus 50%, $p < 0.05$); the preoperative nutrition group experienced less weight loss than the control group (0 kg versus 1.4 kg, $p = 0.01$); less deterioration of liver function (as measured by the change in rate of indocyanine green clearance) was noted in the preoperative nutrition group (−2.8% versus 4.8%, $p < 0.05$); and no difference in mortality was noted between the preoperative nutrition group and the control group.

Thus, as measured by reduction in overall postoperative morbidity, perioperative parenteral nutrition with BCAA-enriched solutions compared with enteral nutrition improves the outcome in patients with cirrhosis undergoing a hepatic resection. The same conclusion cannot be drawn with regard to mortality; whether a larger group of patients or different measurements would reveal a difference between these groups is uncertain on the basis of this study.

Several studies have tested BCAA-enriched solutions in the form of enterally administered nutrition. Only the larger studies (>20 patients) have shown that these solutions lead to improvement in hepatic encephalopathy and nitrogen balance in patients in hepatic failure.[95–98] On the basis of these studies and the purported efficacy of BCAA-enriched solutions in conjunction with glucose as the energy source in the treatment of hepatic encephalopathy, several criteria have been established for the institution of this therapy: patients with hepatic encephalopathy of grade II or higher; BCAA/aromatic amino acid ratio <2.5 and preexisting liver disease; known hepatic dysfunction in a patient whose mental status is unevaluable (i.e., patient is intubated); and intolerance to >40–50 g of a commercially available amino acid mixture. It is known that 50% of patients requiring parenteral nutrition will not tolerate standard amino acid formulas. Because 40–50 g of protein is insufficient for long-term nutritional support, changing to a BCAA-enriched solution is indicated.

The BCAA-enriched enteral formulation Hepatic-Aid is used via the enteral route whenever possible. If enteral nutrition is contraindicated, Hepatamine, the BCAA-enriched parenteral formulation, is administered. Hepatamine contains 4% amino acids and 25% hypertonic glucose. Patients are started at a rate of 40 mL/hour and increased by increments of 20 mL/hour per day until the targeted energy requirement is attained. This usually provides >75–80 g of amino acids per day. In situations where glucose intolerance occurs, a 15% glucose solution is used.

Hepatorenal Syndrome

Combined liver and renal failure presents a difficult dilemma; nutritional support can pose complex problems in the management of two failing organ systems. Each organ system has requirements or deficiencies that are either satisfied or exacerbated, respectively, by a particular nutritional solution. For example, in patients with renal failure who are unable to tolerate dialysis secondary to decreased peripheral vascular resistance, the hypertonic dextrose–essential amino acid solution Nephramine is useful. However, this solution consists largely of aromatic amino acids with few BCAAs. Consequently, although the rise in blood urea nitrogen (BUN) will be diminished, hepatic encephalopathy (if present) will be aggravated. Treating the hepatic encephalopathy with BCAA-enriched aromatic amino acid–deficient hypertonic dextrose solutions may effectively reduce encephalopathy but lead to sharp elevation of BUN.

The combination of liver and renal failure is often fatal; without improvement in hepatic function, it is impossible to salvage patients with hepatorenal syndrome. Thus, any improvement in survival of these patients is a result of improvement in hepatic function, irrespective of the brand of nutritional support selected.

Liver failure in patients with sepsis and multisystem organ failure poses another difficult challenge for the clinician who must provide nutritional support for these patients. Septic patients have altered mental status. Liver dysfunction may be supported with Hepatamine because some of the metabolic derangements that occur during sepsis are comparable to those that occur during liver failure, including glucose intolerance and decreased use of fat as a source of energy. However, the efficacy of BCAA-enriched solutions has not been established in patients with sepsis.

Septic patients exhibit excessive protein degradation, with amino acids once again being used as an energy source. Unabated, sepsis can lead to the syndrome of multisystem organ failure, with the liver being the central organ involved. This is where the similarity to hepatic failure becomes apparent. Freund et al. have noted that the distinctive plasma amino acid pattern in patients with sepsis and septic encephalopathy has many similarities with the amino acid profile of patients with liver failure.[99] Although plasma levels of phenylalanine, tyrosine, methionine, and cysteine are elevated, BCAA levels are low-normal to normal rather than increased as in hepatic encephalopathy. Some studies have used amino acid patterns to predict septic encephalopathy and survival.[100]

Summary

To entertain any hope of improved survival or decreased morbidity in patients with liver failure, one must consider nutritional support.[101] The hypermetabolic state and doubling of the required protein per day (1.1 $g \cdot kg^{-1} \cdot 24 \ hours^{-1}$) in liver failure patients compared with normal individuals produce the classical clinical quandary concerning nutritional support in general and central nervous system tolerance of administered protein in particular.

Over the past 25 years, nutritional support in patients with liver failure has undergone dramatic improvement. With the proven efficacy of BCAA-enriched solutions and the development of Nephramine, nutritional pharmacology has come of age. As more information is obtained about the physiological control of hepatic function and as the nutritional needs of patients become better understood, even at the molecular level, nutritional pharmacology may become the standard for all future nutritional support.[102]

References

1. Iwatsuki K, Starzl T, Todo S, et al (1988) Liver transplantation in the treatment of bleeding esophageal varices. Surgery 104:697–705

2. Brems J, Hiatt J, Ramming K, et al (1987) Fulminant hepatic failure: the role of liver transplantation as primary therapy. Am J Surg 154:137–141

3. Chapman R, Forman D, Peto R, et al (1990) Liver transplantation for acute hepatic failure? Lancet 335:32–35

4. Rozga J, Podesta L, LePage E, et al (1994) A bioartificial liver to treat severe acute liver failure. Ann Surg 219:538–546

5. Sussman N, Chong M, Koussayer T, et al (1992) Reversal of fulminant hepatic failure using an extracorporeal liver device. Hepatology 16:60–65

6. Chari RS, Collins B, Magee J, et al (1994) Brief report: treatment of hepatic failure with an ex-vivo pig liver perfusion followed by liver transplantation. N Engl J Med 331:234–237

7. Meyers WC, Jones (1990) Physiology. In Meyers WC, Jones RS (eds), Textbook of liver and biliary surgery. JP Lippincott, Philadelphia, pp 39–50

8. Merrell RC (1988) Hepatic physiology. In Miller TA (ed), Physiologic basis of modern surgical care. CV Mosby, St Louis, pp 404–416

9. Nakamura T, Nishizawa T, Hagiya M, et al (1989) Molecular cloning and expression of human hepatocyte growth factor. Nature 342:440–443

10. Fischer JE, Bower RH, Bell RH (1987) Liver, biliary, and pancreatic function. In Drucker WR, Foster RS (eds), Clinical surgery. CV Mosby, St Louis, pp 265–277

11. Howard TK, Billiar TR (1992) The liver and biliary tree. In Simmons RL, Steed DL (eds), Basic science review for surgeons. WB Saunders, Philadephia, pp 246–255

12. Zieve FJ, Zieve L, Doizaki WM, et al (1974) Synergism between ammonia and fatty acids in the production of coma: implications for hepatic coma. J Pharmacol Exp Ther 191:10–16

13. Freund H, Dienstag J, Lehrich JM, et al (1982) Infusion of branched-chain amino acid solution in patients with hepatic encephalopathy. Ann Surg 196:209–220

14. Nasrallah SM, Galambos JT (1980) Amino acid therapy of alcoholic hepatitis. Lancet 2:1276–1277

15. Sax H, Talamini M, Fischer JE (1986) Clinical use of branched-chain amino acids in liver disease, sepsis, trauma and burns. Arch Surg 121:358

16. Sherlock S (1975) Diseases of the liver and biliary system, 5th ed. Blackwell, Oxford, pp 425–444

17. Alison MR (1986) Regulation of hepatic growth. Physiol Rev 66:499–541

18. Saadia R, Schein M, MacFarlane C, et al (1990) Gut barrier function and the surgeon. Br J Surg 77:487–492

19. Mackiewicz A, Ganapathi MK, Schultz D, et al (1987) Monokines regulate glycosylation of acute-phase proteins. J Exp Med 166:253–258

20. Vallance P, Moncada S (1991) Hyperdynamic circulation in cirrhosis: a role for nitric oxide? Lancet 337:776–778

21. Reichen J (1990) Liver function and pharmocologic considerations in pathogenesis and treatment of portal hypertension. Hepatology 11:1066–1078

22. Brunkhorst R, Wrenger E, Malcharzik C, et al (1993) Renal effects of atrial natriuretic peptide in cirrhotic rats with and without captopril treatment. Nephron 64:275–281

23. Baldessarini RJ, Fischer JE (1967) S-adenosyl-methionine following portacaval anastomoses. Surgery 62:311–318

24. Fischer JE (1980) Portal hypertension and bleeding esophageal varices. Am J Surg 140:337–338

25. Sherwin R, Joshi P, Hendler R, et al (1974) Hyperglucagonemia in Laennec's cirrhosis: the role of portal-systemic shunting. N Engl J Med 290:239–242

26. Eigler N, Sacca L, Sherwin RS (1979) Synergistic interactions of physiologic investment of glucagon, epinephrine, and cortisol in the dog: a model for stress induced hyperglycemia. J Clin Invest 63:114–123

27. Soeters PB, Fischer JE (1976) Insulin, glucagon, amino acid imbalance, and hepatic encephalopathy. Lancet 2:880–882

28. Reichen J (1988) Etiology and pathophysiology of portal hypertension. Z Gastroenterol 26:3–7

29. Soeters PB, Weir GC, Ebeid AM, et al (1977) Insulin, glucagon, portal-systemic shunting, and hepatic failure in the dog. J Surg Res 23:183–188

30. Fischer JE, Jeppson B, James JH, et al (1980) A unified hypothesis on hepatic encephalopathy. In Orloff MJ, Stipa S, Ziparo V (eds), Medical and surgical problems of portal hypertension. Academic Press, London, vol 34, pp 205–222

31. Strombeck DR, Rogers Q, Stern JS (1978) Effects of intravenous ammonia infusion on plasma levels of amino acids, glucagon, and insulin in dogs [abstract]. Gastroenterology 74:1165

32. Capocaccia L, Angelico M (1991) Fulminant hepatic failure: clinical features, etiology, epidemiology, and current management. Dig Dis Sci 36:775–779

33. Biebuyck JF, Funovics J, Dedrick DF, et al(1974) Neurochemistry of hepatic coma: alterations in putative transmitter amino acids. In Williams R, Murray-Lyons IM (eds), Artificial liver support (Proceedings of an International Symposium on Artificial Support Systems for Acute Hepatic Failure). Pittman, London, pp 51–60

34. Felig P (1973) The glucose alanine cycle. Metabolism 22:179–207

35. Morgan MH, Bolton CH, Morris JS, et al (1974) Medium-chain triglycerides and hepatic encephalopathy. Gut 15:180–184

36. Budd MA, Tanaka K, Holmes LB, et al (1967) Isovaleric acidemia: clinical features of a new genetic defect of leucine metabolism. N Engl J Med 277:321–327

37. Tanaka K, Isselbacher KF, Shih V. (1972) Isovaleric and alphamethylbutyric acidemias induced by hypoglycin A: mechanism of Jamaican vomiting sickness. Science 175:69–71

38. McMenamy RH, Oncley JL (1958) The specific binding of L-tryptophan to serum albumin. J Biol Chem 233:1436–1447

39. Cummings MG, James JH, Soeters PB, et al (1976) Regional brain study of indoleamine metabolism in the rat in acute hepatic failure. J Neurochem 27:741–746

40. Fischer JE, Hasselgren PO (1991) Cytokines and glucocorticoids in the regulation of the "hepato-skeletal muscle axis" in sepsis. Am J Surg 161:266–271

41. Haussinger D (1990) Liver glutamine metabolism. J Parenteral Enteral Nutr 14:56S–62S

42. Fischer JE, Yoshimura N, James JH, et al (1974) Plasma amino acids in patients with hepatic encephalopathy: effects on amino acid infusions. Am J Surg 127:40–49

43. Felig P (1975) Amino acid metabolism in man. Annu Rev Biochem 44:936–955

44. Rosen HM, Yoshimura N, Hodgman JM, Fischer JE (1977) Plasma amino acid patterns in hepatic encephalopathy of differing etiology. Gastroenterology 72:483–487

45. Cardelli-Cangiano P, Cangiano C, James JH, et al (1981) Uptake of amino acids by brain microvessels isolated from rats after portacaval anastomosis. J Neurochem 36:627–632

46. Ono J, Huston DG, Dombro RS, et al (1978) Tryptophan and hepatic coma. Gastroenterology 74:196–200

47. Levine RJ, Conn HO (1967) Tyrosine metabolism in patients with liver disease. J Clin Invest 46:2012–2020

48. Pardridge WM, Jefferson LS (1975) Liver uptake of amino acids and carbohydrates during a single circulatory passage. Am J Physiol 228:1155–1161

49. Jeejeebhoy KN, Phillips RJ (1976) Isolated mammalian hepatocytes in culture. Gastroenterology 71:1086–1096

50. Fischer JE, Baldessarini RJ (1971) False neurotransmitters and hepatic failure. Lancet 2:75

51. Fischer JE, Funovics JM, Aguirre A, et al (1975) The role of plasma amino acids in hepatic encephalopathy. Surgery 78:276–290

52. Alexander JW, MacMillan BG, Stinnett JD, et al (1980) Beneficial effects of aggressive protein feeding in severely burned children. Ann Surg 192:505–517

53. James JH, Jeppson B, Ziparo V, et al (1979) Hyperammonemia, plasma amino acid imbalance, and blood-brain amino acid transport: a unified theory of portalsystemic encephalopathy. Lancet 2:772–775

54. Dismukes K (1977) A new look at the aminergic nervous system. Nature 269:557–558

55. Olendorf WH (1971) Brain uptake of radiolabelled amino acids, amines and hexoses after arterial injection. Am J Physiol 221:1629–1639

56. Pardridge WM, Oldendorf WH (1975) Kinetic analysis of blood-brain barrier transport of amino acids. Biochim Biophys Acta 401:128–136

57. James JH, Escourou J, Fischer JE (1978) Blood-brain neutral amino acid transport activity is increased after portacaval anastomosis. Science 200:1395–1397

58. Dodsworth JM, Cummings MG, James JH, et al (1974) Depletion of brain norepinephrine in acute hepatic coma. Surgery 75:811–820

59. Faraj BA, Camp VM, Ansley JD (1981) Evidence for central hypertyraminemia in hepatic encephalopathy. J Clin Invest 67:395–402

60. Levy LJ, Losowsky MS (1989) Plasma gamma aminobutyric acid concentrations provide evidence of different mechanisms in the pathogenesis of hepatic encephalopathy in acute and chronic liver disease. Hepato-Gastroenterology 36:494–498

61. Knell AJ, Davidson AR, Williams R, et al (1974) Dopamine and serotonin metabolism in hepatic encephalopathy. Br Med J 1:549–551

62. Berl S, Takagaki G, Clarke DD, et al (1962) Metabolic compartments in vivo: ammonia and glutamic acid metabolism in brain and liver. J Biol Chem 237:2562–2569

63. Hourani BT, Hamlin EM, Reynolds TB (1971) Cerebrospinal fluid glutamine as a measure of hepatic encephalopathy. Arch Intern Med 127:1033–1036

64. Smith AR, Rossi-Fanelli F, Ziparo V, et al (1978) Alterations in plasma and CSF amino acids, amines and metabolites in hepatic coma. Ann Surg 187:343–350

65. Samuels S, Fish F, Freedman LS (1978) Effect of gammaglutamyl cycle inhibitors on brain amino acid transport and utilization. Neurochem Res 3:619–631

66. Warren KS, Schenker S (1964) Effect of an inhibitor of glutamine synthesis (methionine sulfoximine) on ammonia toxicity and metabolism. J Lab Clin Med 64:442–449

67. Fernstrom JD, Faller DV (1978) Neutral amino acids in brain: changes in response to food ingestion. J Neurochem 30:1531–1538

68. Buse MG, Reid M (1975) Leucine, a possible regulation of protein turnover in muscle. J Clin Invest 56:1250–1261

69. Fischer JE, James JH (1972) Treatment of hepatic coma and hepatorenal syndrome: mechanism of L-dopa and aramine. Am J Surg 123:222–230

70. Parkes JD, Sharpstone P, Williams R (1970) Levodopa in hepatic coma. Lancet 2:1341–1343

71. Morgan M, Jakobovits A, Elithorn A (1977) Successful use of bromocriptine in the treatment of patients with chronic portasystemic encephalopathy. N Engl J Med 296:793–794

72. Fischer JE, Rosen EM, Ebeid AM, et al (1976) The effect of normalization of plasma amino acids on hepatic encephalopathy in man. Surgery 80:77–91

73. Butterworth RF, Lavoie J, Giguere JF, et al (1988) Affinities and densities of high affinity [³H]muscimol (GABA-A) binding sites and of central benzodiazepine receptors are unchanged in autopsied brain tissue from cirrhotic patients with hepatic encephalopathy. Hepatology 8:1084–1088

74. Chua B, Siehl D, Morgan H (1980) A role for leucine in regulation of protein turnover in working rat hearts. Am J Physiol 239:E510–E514

75. Chua B, Siehl D, Morgan H (1979) Effect of leucine and metabolites of branched chain amino acids on protein turnover in heart. J Biol Chem 54:8358–8362

76. Goldberg AL, Odessey R (1972) Oxidation of amino acids by diaphragm from fed and fasted rats. Am J Physiol 223:1384–1391

77. Bower RH, Fischer JE (1986) Hepatic indications for parenteral nutrition. In Rombeau J, Caldwell M (eds), Clinical nutrition: parenteral nutrition. WB Saunders, Philadelphia, pp 602–604

78. Gelfand RA, Hendler RS, Sherwin RS (1979) Dietary carbohydrate and metabolism of ingested protein. Lancet 1:65–68

79. Herlin P, James JH, Nachbauer C, et al (1983) Effect of total hepatectomy and administration of branched chain amino acids on regional norepinephrine, dopamine, and amino acids in rat brain. Ann Surg 198:172–177

80. Lockwood AH, McDonald JM, Reiman RE, et al (1979) The dynamics of ammonia metabolism in man: effect of liver disease and hyperammonemia. J Clin Invest 63:449–460

81. Riggio O, James JH, Peters JC, et al (1984) Influence of ammonia on leucine utilization in muscle and adipose tissue in vitro. Surg Forum 35:95–97

82. Fryden A, Weiland O, Martensson J (1982) Successful treatment of hepatic coma with balance solution of amino acids. Scand J Infect Dis 14:180

83. Watanabe A, Takesue A, Hihashi T, et al (1979) Serum amino acids in hepatic encephalopathy: effects of branched chain amino acids on serum amino gram. Acta Hepato-Gastroenterol 26:346–357

84. Marchesini G, Zoli M, Dondi C, et al (1982) Anticatabolic effects of branched-chain amino acid solutions in patients with liver cirrhosis. Hepatology 2:420–425

85. Cerra FB, Cheung NK, Fischer JE, et al (1985) Disease specific amino acid solution (F080) in hepatic encephalopathy: a prospective, randomized, double-blind, controlled study. JPEN 9:288–295

86. Cerra FB, McMillan M, Angelico R, et al (1983) Cirrhosis, encephalopathy and improved results with metabolic support. Surgery 94:612–619

87. Fiaccadori F, Ghinelli F, Pedretti G, et al (1984) Branched chain amino acid enriched solutions in the treatment of hepatic encephalopathy: a controlled trial. In Capocaccia L, Fischer JE, Rossi-Fanelli F (eds), Hepatic encephalopathy in chronic liver failure. Plenum Press, New York, pp 323–333

88. Gluud C, Dejgaard A, Hardt F, et al (1983) Preliminary treatment results with balanced amino acid infusion to patients with hepatic encephalopathy [abstract]. Scand J Gastroenterol 18(suppl 86):19

89. Michel H, Pomier-Layrargues G, Aubin JP, et al (1984) Treatment of hepatic encephalopathy by infusion of a modified

amino acid solution: results of a controlled study of 47 cirrhotic patients. In Capocaccia L, Fischer JE, Rossi-Fanelli F (eds), Hepatic encephalopathy in chronic liver failure. Plenum Press, New York, pp 301–310

90. Rossi-Fanelli F, Riggio O, Cangiano C, et al (1982) Branched chain amino acid vs lactulose treatment of hepatic coma: a controlled study. Dig Dis Sci 27:929–935

91. Wahren J, Denis J, Desurmont P, et al (1983) Is intravenous administration of branched chain amino acids effective in the treatment of hepatic encephalopathy? a multicenter study. Hepatology 3:475–480

92. Strauss E, Santos WR, Cartapatti E, et al (1983) A randomized controlled clinical trial for the evaluation of the efficacy of an enriched branched chain amino acid solution compared to neomycin in hepatic encephalopathy [abstract]. Hepatology 3:862

93. Naylor CD, O'Rourke K, Detsky AS, et al (1989) Parenteral nutrition with branched-chain amino acids in hepatic encephalopathy: a meta-analysis. Gastroenterology 97:1033–1042

94. Fan S-T, Lo C-M, Lai ECS, et al (1994) Perioperative nutritional support in patients undergoing hepatectomy for hepatocellular carcinoma. N Engl J Med 331:1547–1552

95. McGhee A, Henderson JM, Millikan WJ, et al (1983) Comparison of the effects of Hepatic-Aid and a casein modular diet on encephalopathy, plasma amino acids, and nitrogen balance in cirrhotic patients. Ann Surg 197:288–293

96. Egberts SH, Schomerus H, Hamster W, et al (1985) Branched chain amino acids in the treatment of latent portasystemic encephalopthy: a double-blind placebo-controlled crossover study. Gastroenterology 88:887–895

97. Horst D, Grace N, Conn HO, et al (1984) Comparison of dietary protein with an oral branched chain enriched amino acid supplement in chronic portal-systemic encephalopathy: a randomized controlled trial. Hepatology 4:279–287

98. Marchesini G, Dioguardi FS, Bianchi GP, et al (1990) Long-term oral branch chain amino acid treatment of chronic encephalopathy: a randomized double-blind casein-controlled trial. J Hepatol 11:92–101

99. Freund H, Ryan JA, Fischer JE (1978) Amino acid derangements in patients with sepsis: treatment with branched chain amino acid enriched infusions. Ann Surg 188:423–430

100. Freund H, Atamian S, Holroyde J, et al (1979) Plasma amino acids as predictors of the severity and outcome of sepsis. Ann Surg 190:571–576

101. Anderson KE, Conney AH, Kappas A (1982) Nutritional influences on chemical biotransformation in humans. Nutr Rev 40:161–171

102. Andus T, Bauer J, Gerok W (1991) Effects of cytokines on the liver. Hepatology 13:364–375

Chapter 48

Cancer and Diet

Michael C. Archer

An overall scheme describing the chemical induction of cancer is presented in Figure 1.[1,2] Metabolism of carcinogens may lead to detoxified products that are excreted or to highly reactive, electrophilic intermediates that react with various cellular nucleophiles including DNA. Reaction at some sites may cause cell death. DNA containing a carcinogen adduct may be enzymatically repaired, thus leading to a normal cell. However, heritable changes may be produced if the carcinogen-damaged DNA template is replicated before it is repaired. If such damage leads to the activation of an oncogene, an initiated cell is produced. Clonal expansion of these initiated cells to produce focal preneoplastic lesions is stimulated by promoting agents. Most of these lesions regress, but in rare cases, progressive development leads to the appearance of neoplastic cells. Diet may account for in excess of one-third of all human cancer.[3] Dietary factors can potentially play a role in carcinogenesis at any one of the steps illustrated in Figure 1. The following discussion reviews studies that suggest how some of these factors initiate, promote, or inhibit cancer development.

Dietary Carcinogens

Foods that are processed or cooked at high temperatures may contain products of pyrolysis. Carcinogenic polycyclic aromatic hydrocarbons (PAHs) such as benzo[a]pyrene or benz[a]anthracene form whenever organic matter is pyrolyzed.[4] Charcoal broiling of foods rich in fats or carbohydrates typically results in PAH contamination.[5,6] Pyrolysis of protein-rich foods such as meat or fish leads to the generation of heterocyclic amines such as 2-amino-3-methylimidazo[4,5-f]quinoline (IQ) and 2-amino-1-methyl-6-phenylimidazo[4,5-b]pyridine (PhIP).[7,8] These compounds are potent mutagens and in experimental animals can cause a variety of tumors, including those of the colon and breast.[9] Cooking foods at lower temperatures (thermolysis) may also produce oxidative or other changes in protein, fat, and carbohydrate that make them carcinogenic, though these processes are not yet well understood.[10] Carcinogenic nitrosamines such as N-nitrosodimethylamine and N-nitrosopyrrolidine are found in foods, particularly those preserved with sodium nitrite, such as bacon and cured meats.[11] In most cases, nitrosamine formation is inhibited when agents such as ascorbic acid or tocopherol are added to the foods.

PAHs, heterocyclic amines, and nitrosamines generally occur in foods at concentrations of micrograms per kilogram or lower. There is little evidence at present to suggest that these levels are an important cause of human cancer. Furthermore, various other chemicals, such as residues of pesticides and herbicides; drugs given to livestock; chemicals used in food processing, packaging materials, and lubricants; and other chemicals associated with food-processing equipment, may be present in foods at very low levels. However, no association has yet been found between exposure to any of these agents and cancer.

A dietary carcinogen that has been implicated strongly in human cancer causation is aflatoxin B_1. This mycotoxin contaminates certain foods consumed in Southeast Asia and Africa, and epidemiologic studies indicate that aflatoxin exposure together with infection with the hepatitis B virus are risk factors for liver cancer.[12] Furthermore, there are good correlations between levels of albumin-bound aflatoxin in serum, urinary excretion of aflatoxin-DNA adducts, and risk of the disease.[13] Finally, foods, particularly plant foods, contain many naturally occurring carcinogens, though the significance of these compounds in human cancer development is unknown.[14]

Dietary Promoters and Inhibitors

Fat. There are large differences among countries in dietary fat intake that correlate with the incidence of cancers such as those of the breast, colon, and prostate.[15–17] However, although the international correlations can be striking (e.g., ≈ 0.8 for fat and breast cancer), many factors other than intake of fat that are related to levels of economic development could be involved. A recent meta-analysis of 23 case-control and cohort studies of dietary fat and breast cancer risk showed that the association was weak (summary relative risk was 1.12).[18] It has been argued that there were insufficient differences

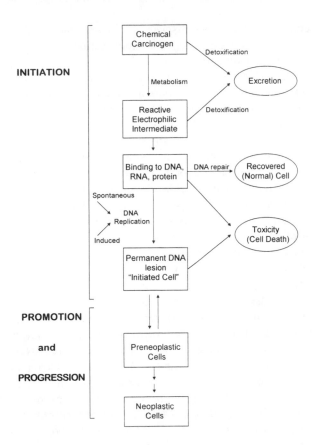

Figure 1. The mechanism of chemical carcinogenesis.

between diets in most of these studies to allow detection of associations.[19] Many, but not all, studies described a positive association between animal fats, or more specifically, saturated fats, and colon cancer incidence.[20] One study showed an association between animal fat consumption and the development of precancerous adenomatous polyps in the colon.[21] However, the association of colon cancer with red meat consumption rather than fat has been more consistent.[22,23]

Studies in experimental animals have consistently shown that diets high in fat enhance the development of chemically induced breast and colon cancers.[24] A promoting effect of n–6 polyunsaturated fatty acids (PUFAs) and an inhibiting effect of n–3 PUFAs have been shown.[25,26] The effects of saturated and monounsaturated fatty acids are less clear-cut. Suggested mechanisms by which dietary fat enhances carcinogenesis differ according to tumor site. In the colon, there is evidence that fats stimulate bile acid release, thereby causing a stimulation of cellular proliferation mediated by protein kinase C.[27,28] Dietary fat may affect breast cancer development by altering profiles of sex hormones.[29] Other proposed mechanisms include effects on the metabolism of arachidonic acid.[30]

Prostate cancer, like breast and colon cancer, occurs at a high rate in affluent countries.[15,31] Associations have been reported between consumption of high levels of dietary fat and prostate cancer.[32] Furthermore, there is some evidence from case-control studies that fat intake is important in cancers of the pancreas and endometrium.[33,34]

Energy intake and carbohydrates. Diets rich in fat have a high energy density, and it is possible that this property is the link between fat intake and cancer. Indeed, it has been known for many years that in rodents, energy restriction leads to a marked decrease in the incidence and growth of both induced and spontaneous tumors.[35] The decrease in tumor incidence is likely caused by the lower mitotic rates and increased apoptosis in preneoplastic cells that are observed in energy-restricted compared with ad libitum–fed rodents.[36] Epidemiologic evidence, although sparse, suggests a role for energy intake in human cancer.[37,38] In a study of pancreatic cancer, the strongest effects were for energy intake, with carbohydrate energy contributing most to the increased risk.[39] High energy intake, as indicated by body weight or obesity, is associated positively with the development of cancer at several sites, whereas high energy expenditure, measured as physical activity, is negatively related to many of the same cancers.[30,40]

Sucrose consumption has been correlated positively with breast cancer mortality, whereas complex carbohydrates tend to be negatively correlated.[41] Rats fed simple sugars developed significantly more dimethylbenzanthracene-induced mammary tumors than rats fed diets containing starches, an effect that was observed at both high and low levels of dietary fat.[41] Two case-control studies found sucrose consumption and sucrose consumption without corresponding fiber consumption to be risk factors for colorectal cancer, whereas consumption of complex carbohydrates was inversely related to disease.[42,43] Sucrose has been shown to enhance the early steps of colon carcinogenesis in mice.[44] It has been hypothesized that postprandial hyperinsulinemia after a high consumption of sugar promotes breast and colon cancer.[45,46]

With respect to polysaccharides, Burkitt[47] first suggested that there might be an inverse relationship between dietary fiber consumption and colorectal cancer. Indeed, in a combined analysis of 13 case-control studies, dietary fiber was found to be protective.[48] Studies in which dietary fiber was measured as nonstarch polysaccharides have shown significant, but weak, negative correlations with colon cancer incidence.[49] Dietary starch has been shown to exert a protective effect.[50]

Animal studies on fiber and colon cancer have given mixed results, although a consistent observation has been an increase in tumor incidence with increasing fat and decreasing fiber content of the diet.[51] This parallels the effects of fat and fiber seen in epidemiologic studies.

A possible mechanism for the action of polysaccharides is that carbohydrates entering the colon are fermented to yield short-chain fatty acids (e.g., acetate, propionate, and butyrate), thereby lowering the pH in the colon and reducing the solubility and toxicity of the secondary bile acids.[52] Starch fermentation yields relatively large amounts of butyrate, which is known to inhibit DNA synthesis and stimulate differentiation.[53]

Fruits and vegetables. The most consistent finding in the cancer epidemiology literature is that daily consumption of fresh fruits and vegetables reduces the risk of most types of cancer.[54] There are several possible mechanisms to account for these protective effects. Although dietary fiber could account for the protective effect against colon cancer, recent evidence suggests that folic acid may account for the reduced risk.[55] Folic acid is required for the synthesis of thymidine and folate deficiency causes chromosomal breaks.[56]

Antioxidants such as ascorbate, tocopherol, carotenoids, and flavonoids in fruits and vegetables may account for some of the protective effects through their inhibition of endogenous oxidative damage to DNA, a process that may contribute to cancer development.[57] Vitamin C also inhibits formation of nitrosamines from nitrite and amines in the stomach, and a protective effect of vitamin C for stomach and esophageal cancers has been suggested.[58,59] Recently, a combination of antioxidant supplements was related to a reduced incidence of gastric cancer in rural China.[60] Several other studies yielded inconsistent results. Thus, vitamins C and E and β-carotene did not reduce the recurrence of adenomatous polyps of the colon.[61] Vitamin E and β-carotene seemed to be unrelated to the risk of lung cancer in a recent large study of heavy smokers, although the duration of this study (6 years) might not have been long enough to see an effect.[62]

Some vegetables, particularly cruciferous vegetables, contain indole compounds that inhibit chemical carcinogenesis by inducing hepatic detoxifying enzymes.[63] Many fruits and vegetables also contain weakly estrogenic lignans that may reduce breast cancer risk.[64]

Protein. Several epidemiologic studies have shown correlations between consumption of total protein, animal protein, or protein-rich foods and several cancers, including those of the colon, breast, pancreas, and kidney.[15,65–68] However, because of the strong correlations between dietary protein and fat and energy intake, it is difficult to establish an independent role for protein. Indeed, the idea that protein intake is simply a marker for other dietary factors is supported by the finding that colon cancer risk is related to consumption of high-fat red meat but not to consumption of low-fat chicken or fish.[69] Limited animal studies suggest that the level of protein in the diet can affect carcinogen metabolism.[70] This increase in colon tumor frequency with increasing dietary protein may be related to the formation of ammonia in the colon via fermentation of amino acids that enter the colon.[71] As discussed in a previous section, protein pyrolysis products, thermolysis products, or both may be carcinogenic.

Alcohol. Alcohol consumption is a risk factor for several types of cancer, particularly those of tissues that come in direct contact with the alcohol, such as the oral cavity and larynx, although other sites such as colorectum, breast, and liver, are also at increased risk.[72–75] At some sites, alcohol acts synergistically with other agents. Thus, the effects of alcohol and tobacco are almost mutiplicative in the development of oral and esophageal cancers.[72] There is also synergy between alcohol consumption and aflatoxin B_1 or hepatitis B virus in the development of liver tumors.[75] Epidemiologic associations between the consumption of specific alcoholic beverages and the development of specific cancers suggest that it is likely that cancer risk may be related not only to the quantity of alcohol consumed, but also to other constituents of the beverages.[76,77] Several mechanisms have been proposed for the effects of alcohol on carcinogenesis; these include DNA adduct formation, free radical generation, and inhibition of DNA repair enzymes by the alcohol metabolite acetaldehyde, as well as effects of alcohol on the enzymes of carcinogen metabolism, excretion, and recirculation of bile acids and on levels of estrogens.[73,75,77,78] Additionally, PAHs and nitrosamines are present in some alcoholic beverages.[79,80]

Miscellaneous factors. Many studies have evaluated the effects of minerals, vitamins, and other minor dietary components on the risk of several cancers. Some of these risk factors are potentially important, and several have already been mentioned. Cancer of the stomach, particularly in Japan, has been associated with excessive salt (sodium chloride) consumption in foods such as salted fish.[81] Salt may act as an irritant, causing degradation of the mucous lining of the stomach, leading to exposure of the epithelial cells to carcinogens in the gastric contents and to increased cell replication.[82,83] Dietary selenium levels may have a protective effect against a variety of cancers, particularly those of the breast and colon.[84] Selenium may exert its protective effect via its role in the activity of glutathione peroxidase, an enzyme that protects against oxidative tissue injury.[85] In contrast to the protective effects of β-carotene, high intakes of vitamin A may increase the risk of several cancers.[86] There is also limited epidemiologic evidence linking vitamin D deficiency with the risk of colorectal cancer.[87] Furthermore, diets that are marginal in riboflavin and nicotinic acid have been associated with risk of esophageal cancer.[88]

Summary

The evidence summarized above suggests that dietary factors have important causative and protective roles in cancer development. Much of our knowledge concerning the specific dietary factors that are involved in carcinogenesis is clearly inconsistent or incomplete. At this point in time, the only consistent finding is that the consumption of fresh fruits and vegetables is associated with a reduced risk of several different cancers. More research is urgently needed to understand the molecular, cellular, and physiological relationships between both macro- and micronutrients and cancer.

Acknowledgment. M.C.A. is the recipient of a Natural Sciences and Engineering Research Council of Canada Industrial Research Chair, and acknowledges support from the member companies of the Program in Food Safety, University of Toronto.

References

1. Archer MC (1992) Chemical carcinogenesis. In Tannock IF, Hill RP (eds), The basic science of oncology. McGraw-Hill, New York, pp 102–118

2. Yuspa SH, Poirier MC (1988) Chemical carcinogenesis: from animal models to molecular models in one decade. Adv Cancer Res 50:25–70

3. Doll R, Peto R (1981) The causes of cancer. J Natl Cancer Inst 66:1191–1308

4. Schmelz I, Hoffmann D (1976) Formation of polynuclear aromatic hydrocarbons from combustion of organic matter. In Freudenthal R, Jones PW (eds), Carcinogenesis—a comprehensive survey, Vol 1, Polynuclear aromatic hydrocarbons, chemistry, metabolism and carcinogenesis. Raven Press, New York, pp 225–239

5. Lijinsky W, Ross AE (1967) Production of carcinogenic polynuclear hydrocarbons in the cooking of food. Food Cosmet Toxicol 5:343–347

6. Grasso P (1984) Carcinogens in food. In Searle CE (ed), Chemical carcinogens, Vol 2, ACS monograph 182. American Chemical Society, Washington, DC, pp 1205–1239

7. Sugimura T (1985) Carcinogenicity of mutagenic heterocyclic amines formed during the cooking process. Mutat Res 150:33–41

8. Felton JS, Knize MG (1990) Heterocyclic amine mutagens/carcinogens in foods. In Cooper CS, Grover PL (eds), Handbook of experimental pharmacology, Vol 94. Springer-Verlag, Berlin, pp 471–502

9. Ito N, Hasegawa R, Sano M, et al (1991) A new colon and mammary carcinogen in cooked food, 2-amino-1-methyl-6-phenylimidazo[4,5-b]pyridine (PhIP). Carcinogenesis 12:1503–1506

10. Bruce WR, Archer MC, Corpet DE, et al (1993) Diet, aberrant crypt foci and colorectal cancer. Mutat Res 290:111–118

11. Tricker AR, Preussmann R (1991) Carcinogenic N-nitrosamines in the diet: occurrence, formation, mechanism and carcinogenic potential. Mutat Res 259:277–289

12. Busby WF Jr, Wogan GN (1984) Aflatoxins. In Searle CE (ed), Chemical carcinogens, Vol 2, ACS monograph 182. American Chemical Society, Washington, DC, pp 945–1136

13. Groopman JD, Kensler TW (1993) Molecular biomarkers for human chemical carcinogen exposures. Chem Res Toxicol 6:764–770

14. Ames BN, Profet M, Gold LS (1990) Dietary pesticides (99–90% all natural). Proc Natl Acad Sci U S A 87:7777–7781

15. Armstrong B, Doll R (1975) Environmental factors and cancer incidence and mortality in different countries, with special reference to dietary practices. Int J Cancer 15:617–631

16. McKeown-Eyssen CE, Bright-See E (1984) Dietary factors in colon cancer: international relationships. Nutr Cancer 6:160–171

17. Higginson J, Sheridan MJ (1991) Nutrition and human cancer. In Alfin-Slater RB, Kritchevsky D (eds), Human nutrition: a comprehensive treatise, vol 7, Cancer and nutrition. Plenum Press, New York, pp 1–50

18. Boyd NF, Martin LJ, Noffel M, et al (1993) A meta-analysis of studies of dietary fat and breast cancer risk. Br J Cancer 68:627–636

19. Goodwin PJ, Boyd NF (1987) Critical appraisal of the evidence that dietary fat intake is related to breast cancer risk in humans. J Natl Cancer Inst 79:473–485

20. Miller AB, Berrino F, Hill M, et al (1994) Diet in the aetiology of cancer: a review. Eur J Cancer 30A:207–220

21. Giovannucci E, Stampfer MJ, Colditz E, Rimm EB, Willett WC (1992) Relationship of diet to risk of colorectal adenoma in men. J Natl Cancer Inst 84:91–98

22. Giovannucci E, Rimm EB, Stampfer MJ, et al (1994) Intake of fat, meat and fiber in relation to risk of colon cancer in men. Cancer Res 54:2390–2397

23. Goldbohm RA, van der Brandt PA, van't Veer P, et al (1994) A prospective cohort study on the relation between meat consumption and the risk of colon cancer. Cancer Res 54:718–723

24. Rogers AE, Longnecker MP (1988) Dietary and nutritional influences on cancer: a review of epidemiologic and experimental data. Lab Invest 59:729–759

25. Fernandes G, Venkatraman JT (1992) Possible mechanisms through which dietary lipids, calorie restriction and exercise modulate breast cancer. Adv Exp Med Biol 322:185–201

26. Zhao LP, Kushi LH, Klein RD, Prentice RL (1991) Quantitative review of studies of dietary fat and rat colon carcinoma. Nutr Cancer 15:169–177

27. McMichael AJ, Potter JD (1985) Host factors in carcinogenesis: certain bile acid metabolic profiles that selectively increase the risk of proximal colon cancer. J Natl Cancer Inst 75:185–191

28. DeRubertis FR, Craven PA (1987) Relationship of bile salt stimulation of colonic epithelial phospholipid turnover and proliferative activity: role of activation of protein kinase C. Prev Med 16:572–579

29. Adlercreutz H (1990) Diet, breast cancer and sex hormone metabolism. Ann NY Acad Sci 595:281–290

30. Simopoulos AP (1987) Nutritional cancer risks derived from energy and fat. Med Oncol Tumor Pharmacother 4:227–239

31. Rose DP, Boyer AP, Synder EL (1986) International comparisons of mortality rates for cancer of the breast, ovary, prostate, and colon and per capita food consumption. Cancer 58:2363–2371

32. Kolonel LN, Yoshizawa CN, Hankin JH (1988) Diet and prostatic cancer: a case-control study in Hawaii. Am J Epidemiol 127:999–1012

33. Ghadivian P, Simard A, Baillargeon J, et al (1991) Nutritional factors and pancreatic cancer in the francophone community in Montreal, Canada. Int J Cancer 47:1–6

34. LaVecchia C, Decarli A, Fasoli M, Gentile A (1986) Nutrition and diet in the etiology of endometrial cancer. Cancer 57:1248–1253

35. Tannenbaum A (1947) Effects of varying caloric intake upon tumor incidence and tumor growth. Ann NY Acad Sci 49:5–17

36. Grasl-Kraupp B, Bursch W, Ruttkay-Nedecky B, et al (1994) Food restriction eliminates preneoplastic cells through

apoptosis and antagonizes carcinogenesis in the liver. Proc Natl Acad Sci USA 91:9995–9999

37. Potter JD, McMichael AJ (1986) Diet and cancer of the colon and rectum: a case-control study. J Natl Cancer Inst 76:557–569

38. Lyon JL, Mahoney AW, West DN, et al (1987) Energy intake: its relation to colon cancer risk. J Natl Cancer Inst 78:853–861

39. Howe GR, Jain M, Miller AB (1990) Dietary factors and the risk of pancreatic cancer: results of a Canadian population-based study. Int J Cancer 45:604–608

40. Albanes D (1987) Caloric intake, body weight and cancer: a review. Nutr Cancer 9:199–218

41. Carroll KK (1991) Carbohydrate and cancer. In Alfin-Slater RB, Kritchevsky D (eds), Human nutrition: a comprehensive treatise, vol 7, Cancer and nutrition. Plenum Press, New York, pp 97–102

42. Bristol JB, Emmett PM, Heaton KW, Williamson RCN (1985) Sugar, fat and the risk of colorectal cancer. Br Med J 291:1467–1470

43. Tuyus AJ, Haelterman M, Kaaks R (1987) Colorectal cancer and the intake of nutrients: oligosaccharides are a risk factor, fats are not: a case-control study in Belgium. Nutr Cancer 10:181–196

44. Stamp D, Zhang X-M, Medline A, et al (1993) Sucrose enhancement of the early steps of colon carcinogenesis in mice. Carcinogenesis 14:777–779

45. Seely S, Horrobin DF (1983) Diet and breast cancer: the possible connection with sugar consumption. Med Hypoth 11:317–327

46. Giovannucci E (1995) Insulin and colon cancer. Cancer Causes Control 6:164–179

47. Burkitt DP (1971) Epidemiology of cancer of the colon and rectum. Cancer 28:3–13

48. Howe GR, Benito E, Castellato R, et al (1992) Dietary intake of fiber and decreased risk of cancers of the colon and rectum: evidence from the combined analysis of 13 case-control studies. J Natl Cancer Inst 84:1887–1896

49. Bingham S, Williams DRR, Cummings JH (1985) Dietary fiber consumption in Britain: new estimates and their relation to large bowel cancer mortality. Br J Cancer 52:399–402

50. Cassidy A, Bingham SA, Cummings JH (1994) Starch intake and colorectal cancer risk: an international comparison. Br J Cancer 6:937–942

51. Angres G, Beth M (1991) Effects of dietary constituents on carcinogenesis in different tumor models: an overview from 1975–1988. In Alfin-Slater RB, Kritchevsky D (eds), Human nutrition: a comprehensive treatise, vol 7, Cancer and nutrition. Plenum Press, New York, pp 337–485

52. Cummings JH (1981) Short chain fatty acids in the human colon. Gut 22:763–779

53. Young GP (1992) Butyrate and the molecular biology of the large bowel (1992) In Roche AF (ed), Short chain fatty acids: metabolism and clinical importance. Ross Laboratories, Columbus, OH, pp 39–45

54. Miller AB, Berrino F, Hill M, et al (1994) Diet in the aetiology of cancer: a review. Eur J Cancer 30A:207–220

55. Glynn SA, Albanes D (1994) Folate and cancer: a review of the literature. Nutr Cancer 22:101–119

56. Everson RB, Wehr CM, Erexson GL, MacGregor JT (1988) Association of marginal folate depletion with increased human chromosonal damage in vivo: demonstration by analysis of micronucleated erythrocytes. J Natl Cancer Inst 80:525–529

57. Ames BN, Gold LS, Willett WC (1995) The causes and prevention of cancer. Proc Natl Acad Sci USA 92:5258–5265

58. Mirvish SS (1986) Effects of vitamins C and E on N-nitroso compound formation, carcinogenesis and cancer. Cancer 58:1842–1850

59. Block G (1991) Vitamin C and cancer prevention: the epidemiological evidence. Am J Clin Nutr 53:2705–2725

60. Blot WJ, Li JY, Taylor PR, et al (1993) Nutrition intervention trials in Linxian, China: supplementation with specific vitamin/mineral combinations, cancer incidence, and disease-specific mortality in the general population. J Natl Cancer Inst 85:1483–1492

61. Greenberg ER, Baron JA, Tosteson TD, et al (1994) A clinical trial of antioxidant vitamins to prevent colorectal adenoma. N Engl J Med 331:141–147

62. Heinonen OP, Huttunen JK, Albanes D, et al (1994) The effect of vitamin E and beta carotene on the incidence of lung cancer and other cancers in male smokers. N Engl J Med 330:1029–1035

63. Wattenberg L (1992) Inhibition of carcinogenesis by minor dietary constituents. Cancer Res 52:2085S–2089S

64. Thompson LU, Robb P, Serraino M, Cheung F (1991) Mammalian lignan production from various foods. Nutr Cancer 16:43–52

65. Drasar BS, Irving D (1973) Environmental factors and cancer of the colon and breast. Br J Cancer 27:167–172

66. Biddi E, Franceschi S, Talamini R, et al (1992) Food consumption and cancer of the colon and rectum in north-eastern Italy. Int J Cancer 50:223–229

67. Baghurst PA, McMichael AJ, Slavotinek AH, et al (1991) A case control study of diet and cancer of the pancreas. Am J Epidemiol 134:167–179

68. Maclure M, Willett WC (1990) A case control study of diet and risk of renal adenocarcinoma. Cancer Causes Control 1:430–440

69. Willett WC, Sampfer MJ, Colditz GA, et al (1990) Relation of meat, fat and fiber intake to the risk of colon cancer in a prospective study among women. N Engl J Med 327:1664–1672

70. Visek WJ, Clinton SK (1991) Dietary protein and cancer. In Alfin-Slater RB, Kritchevsky D (eds), Human nutrition: a comprehensive treatise, vol 7, Cancer and nutrition. Plenum Press, New York, pp 103–126

71. Macfarlane GT, Cummings JH (1991) The colonic flora, fermentation, and large bowel digestive function. In Phillips SF, Pemberton JH, Shorter RG (eds) The large intestine: physiology, pathophysiology, and disease. Raven Press, New York, pp 51–92

72. Tuyns AJ (1991) Aetiology of head and neck cancer: tobacco, alcohol and diet. Adv Otorhinolaryngol 46:98–106

73. Keene GA, Vitetta L (1992) Alcohol consumption and the etiology of colorectal cancer: a review of the scientific evidence from 1957–1991. Nutr Cancer18:97–111

74. Howe G, Rohan T, DeCarli A, et al (1991) The association between alcohol and breast cancer risk: evidence from the combined analysis of six dietary case-control studies. Int J Cancer 47:707–710

75. Rogers AE, Conner MW (1991) Interrelationships of alcohol and cancer. In Alfin-Slater RB, Kritchevsky D (eds), Human nutrition: a comprehensive treatise, vol 7, Cancer and nutrition. Plenum Press, New York, pp 321–336

76. Shottenfeld D (1992) The etiology and prevention of aerodigestive tract cancers. Adv Exp Med Biol 320:1–20

77. Yamada Y, Weller RO, Kleihues P, Ludeke BI (1992) Effects of ethanol and various alcoholic beverages on the formation of O^6-methyldeoxyguanosine from concurrently administerd N-nitrosomethylbenzylamine in rats: a dose-response study. Carcinogenesis 13:1171–1175

78. Reichman ME, Judd JT, Longcope C, et al (1993) Effects of alcohol consumption on plasma and urinary hormone concentrations in premenopausal women. J Natl Cancer Inst 85:722–727

79. Masuda Y, Mori K, Hirohata T, Kuratsune M (1966) Carcinogenesis in the oesophagus. III. Polycyclic aromatic hydrocarbons and phenols in whiskey. Gann 57:549–557

80. Riboli E, Cornee J, Macquart-Moulin G, et al (1991) Cancer and polyps of the colorectum and lifetime consumption of beer and other alcoholic beverages. Am J Epidemiol 134:157–166

81. Forman D (1991) The etiology of gastric cancer. IARC Sci Publ 105:22–32

82. Correa P, Haenszel W, Cuello C, et al (1975) A model for gastric cancer epidemiology. Lancet 2:58–60

83. Correa P (1992) Human gastric carcinogenesis: a multistep and multifactorial process. Cancer Res 52:6735–6740

84. Schrauzer GN, White DA, Schneider CJ (1977) Cancer mortality correlation studies. III. Statistical associations with dietary selenium intakes. Bioinorgan Chem 7:23–31

85. Chow CK (1979) Nutritional influence on cellular antioxidant defense systems. Am J Clin Nutr 32:1066–1081

86. Mayne ST, Graham S, Zheng T (1991) Dietary retinol: prevention or promotion of carcinogenesis in humans? Cancer Causes Control 2:443–450

87. Garland C, Shekelle R, Barrett-Connor B, et al (1985) Dietary vitamin D and calcium and risk of colorectal cancer. Lancet 1:307–309

88. van Rensburg SJ (1981) Epidemiologic and dietary evidence for a specific nutritional predisposition to esophageal cancer. J Natl Cancer Inst 67:243–251

Chapter 49

Gastrointestinal Disease

Linda V. Muir, Kathleen D. Sanders, and Warren P. Bishop

The gut is the most important organ in the body from the viewpoint of nutrition. It has essential functions in digestion, absorption, exclusion, and elimination of ingested substances. It is therefore not surprising that the nutritional health of the organism is very much dependent on normal gut function. Many intestinal diseases will result in disturbance of normal nutrition. We focus on several of the more common of these to illustrate approaches to the nutritional management of disordered digestive and absorptive function. The most striking disturbance of intestinal function is arguably short bowel syndrome, in which insufficient intestinal length is present to allow normal absorption. Because bowel function is affected by the diet, this chapter also will examine gluten enteropathy. Patients with this condition sustain significant mucosal injury when they ingest gluten. Inflammation of the intestine can also lead to impaired function. Chronic inflammatory bowel disease is extensively discussed from the standpoint of both nutritional consequences and nutritional therapy. Many other gastrointestinal conditions can be affected by the diet or interfere with normal absorptive function, but there is not room to cover all such topics in this chapter. However, the basic concepts of gut-nutrient interactions and nutritional therapy of patients with injured or dysfunctional intestines are discussed and are applicable to a wide variety of conditions.

Nutritional Support of Short Bowel Syndrome

In short bowel syndrome the small bowel length is insufficient to allow adequate absorption of nutrients. Diarrhea, weight loss, and malnutrition are the major features of this syndrome. Because the small bowel has a large reserve in absorptive capacity, resections of ≤50% are tolerated without requiring extensive nutritional support. Intestinal losses of >75%, however, result in severe malabsorption.[1-3] Full-term infants normally have ≈250 cm of small bowel, whereas adults have 400–600 cm, depending on measurement technique.[1,2,4] Although resection of >75% of this length results in significant impairment in digestive and absorptive capability, advances in nutritional support have made it possible to survive with only a small fraction of remaining gut. Several reports document that some infants having as little as 10–20 cm of small bowel may eventually be weaned from total parenteral nutrition, usually by 2–3 years of age.[1,2,5-11] The primary causes for gut resection in adults include Crohn's disease unresponsive to medical therapy, bowel infarction, trauma, radiation enteritis, and tumors.[1] In infants, necrotizing enterocolitis and congenital anomalies such as gastroschisis, midgut volvulus, and intestinal atresias are the most frequent causes of extensive intestinal resection.[1,4,5,12,13]

Physiology of bowel resection and malabsorption. The degree and spectrum of the resulting malabsorption depend not only on the extent of resection, but also on the site resected (Table 1).[14] Proximal small bowel has the longest villi and, therefore, the highest hydrolytic activity for disaccharides and peptides as well as the largest absorptive capacity for most nonselectively absorbed nutrients. Hypertrophy of downstream bowel occurs after removal of upstream bowel in an adaptive response to the loss. However, specific nutritional deficits may result from loss of each region of the bowel.

Table 1. Nutritional consequence of short bowel syndrome

Area of resection	Nutritional consequences
Duodenum	Iron, folate, calcium
Jejunum, ileum	Protein-energy, iron, water-soluble vitamins, trace elements, electrolytes
Distal ileum	Vitamin B-12 steatorrhea and deficient fat-soluble vitamins (because of loss of bile acids)
Colon	Water, electrolytes

Complete removal of the most proximal segment of small bowel, the duodenum, could result in deficiencies in calcium, folic acid, and iron because of diminished absorption.[2] Fortunately, duodenectomy is rarely required, even during extensive gut resection.[2]

The jejunum is a site of active sodium absorption coupled to glucose uptake; however, other nutrients are absorbed by passive diffusion. The impact of complete jejunectomy is buffered by the ileum, which adapts and assumes most of the jejunum's absorptive functions. After a jejunectomy, secretion of cholecystokinin and secretin is decreased, causing gall bladder stasis and cholelithiasis. In addition, hormones such as vasoactive intestinal peptide, gastric inhibitory peptide, and serotonin, which are normally released in the jejunum, can no longer exert their inhibitory effects on gastrin release, resulting in gastric hypersecretion.[1,2] Medical therapy to decrease gastric secretion may be necessary.

The ileum is the critical site of bile salt and vitamin B-12 absorption. With loss of the ileum, the unabsorbed bile salts enter the colon in large quantities and cause colonic mucosal irritation. Colonic bacteria deconjugate and dehydroxylate bile salts to bile acids, which induce a secretory diarrhea resulting in large fluid losses. If the net loss of bile salts persists, the body bile salt pool becomes depleted and malabsorption of fat and of the fat-soluble vitamins A, D, E, and K is exacerbated.[1,14]

The ileocecal valve functions as an intestinal brake, slowing intestinal transit time. If the valve is removed, intestinal transit is shortened, causing diarrhea. The valve also acts as a barrier to colonic bacteria, preventing bacterial overgrowth. In its absence, bacteria can reflux back into the small intestine and consume key nutrients, such as vitamin B-12. Other complications of bacterial overgrowth include D-lactic acidosis. Bacteria produce both D- and L-lactic acid, but humans metabolize only the L-lactate. Consequently, D-lactate accumulates, which contributes to acidosis and may cause neurological symptoms.[15,16] Acidosis resulting from this situation and volatile fatty acids produced by bacterial fermentation often require that the patient be supplemented with bicarbonate, citrate, or acetate. Restriction of the carbohydrate load of the diet may help by minimizing availability of substrates for fermentation.[1,2,16]

As material passes through the colon, water, sodium, and potassium are reabsorbed. In the setting of steatorrhea, calcium in the colon combines with unabsorbed fatty acids to form soaps. Normally calcium binds to oxalate in the gut lumen; however, in the presence of the excessive fatty acids this can no longer occur and unbound oxalate is absorbed. Subsequent excretion in the urine can result in oxalate renal stones. Therefore, in the setting of fat malabsorption, a low-oxalate diet may be beneficial.[14,17]

Nutritional therapy of short bowel syndrome. Judicious use of enteral feeding offers several advantages to patients with short bowel syndrome. After small intestinal resection, the remaining small bowel undergoes remarkable adaptation, particularly in the remaining ileum.[11,18–20] Increased proliferation of epithelial cells leads to an increase in mucosal mass. The resulting increase in villous height and crypt depth as well as augmented diameter and length of the remaining bowel lead to increased surface area and absorptive capacity.[4,15] Enteral feedings stimulate this adaptation directly through contact with mucosal cells and indirectly by stimulating secretion of trophic gastrointestinal hormones and secretions.[4,15,18,19,21] Studies to establish the trophic effects of dietary components on the gut have shown that hydrolyzed casein, as well as whole protein, stimulates gut adaptation.[22] In at least one study, long-chain triacylglycerols were more trophic than medium-chain triacylglycerols.[23] Absence of enteral feedings, however, has a deleterious effect on remaining bowel function. Exclusive total parenteral nutrition results in mucosal atrophy, increased risk of catheter-induced sepsis, and risk of cholestatic liver disease.[4,19] Gut adaptation continues more than 2 years after surgery.[24]

During the first few months after surgery, the primary medical goal is to maintain fluid and electrolyte balance in the setting of high intestinal losses. After a major small bowel resection, the patient is at risk of developing dehydration, hyponatremia, hypokalemia, hypomagnesemia, hypocalcemia, and metabolic acidosis.[13,20,24] Careful monitoring of hemodynamic variables as well as electrolytes is necessary. Total parenteral nutrition is often used during this time. Medical management may include vigorous antacid therapy including H2 blockers or omeprazole, and antimotility medications such as codeine or loperamide. Cholestyramine is sometimes used to reduce the secretory diarrhea induced by malabsorption of bile acids after ileal resection.

As the gut recovers, it is critical to begin some degree of enteral feeding to encourage the process of adaptation and to minimize hepatotoxicity of total parental nutrition. Continuous-drip enteral tube feedings are, in general, better absorbed and tolerated than bolus feedings. However, oral feeding has many other advantages over tube feedings. In children, especially, oral feedings are critical to encourage normal development of feeding skills. Delays in introducing oral feeds in infants and small children result in oral aversion and aberrant feeding habits. Nonnutritive stimulation of oral skills directed by a feeding specialist may be helpful when the patient is receiving only parenteral nutrition. In both children and adults the pleasures of eating add significantly to the quality of life and should not be forbidden except under the most unusual circumstances; most foods can be taken orally even with a nasogastric tube in place.

As enteral feedings are gradually advanced, parenteral support should be tapered. Although it is common practice to use elemental diets in short bowel syndrome, their hypertonicity limits the rate at which they are tolerated, and they may not offer any advantage over polymeric feeds.[25,26] Woolf and coworkers have shown that a high fat diet does not increase stomal losses.[27] Although medium-chain triacylglycerols are absorbed directly by the proximal small bowel, long-chain triacylglycerols encourage more trophic adaptation of the gut.[18,23] A low-lactose diet may be necessary if a large portion of the jejunum is resected.[29] Dairy products treated with lactase may be helpful and provide the opportunity for a more normal diet.

Energy intake goals should be adjusted upward to compensate for malabsorbed nutrient losses. Depending upon the degree of malabsorption, energy requirements may be 150–200% of normal.[27–29] Folate and iron should be supplemented if a significant amount of the proximal small bowel has been removed. Vitamin B-12 and the fat-soluble vitamins A, D, E, and K should be monitored and supplemented as required. For patients who have lost the terminal ileum, monthly intramuscular injections of vitamin B-12 ensure adequate delivery of this nutrient. In the absence of adequate bile salt resorption by the ileum, the bile salt pool is depleted and can result in steatorrhea. In this situation, divalent cations bind with unabsorbed fatty acids and are excreted in the stool. Consequently, supplementation of calcium, magnesium, zinc, and other trace minerals is often required.[14,30] Serum levels of calcium, zinc, magnesium, vitamin A, vitamin B-12, and 25-hydroxy vitamin D should be monitored routinely.[1–3,13,20]

Other dietary supplements may aid intestinal adaptation. Pectin is a water-soluble dietary fiber that is fermented in the colon to short-chain fatty acids, a preferred energy source for colonocytes. Animal studies have shown increases in intestinal adaptation to small bowel resection in rats receiving pectin added to their elemental diet. The exact mechanism by which they exert this effect is not known. Short-chain fatty acids have a trophic effect on rat intestinal tract.[30–32] In addition, pectin slows gastrointestinal motility and permits longer contact of luminal contents with mucosal absorptive surface area. This may play a role in its effect.[33–35] Pectin's efficacy in human nutrition support has not been established. Glutamine is a nonessential amino acid and is a vehicle for nitrogen transport between tissues and a precursor for nucleotide synthesis. Some, but not all, studies have shown that it enhances intestinal adaptation with enteral supplementation.[36]

Occasionally, surgical revision is required in the setting of intractable diarrhea after intestinal resection. Insertion of reversed segments of bowel to reverse peristalsis and slow transit time may be performed. Colonic interposition into the small bowel to slow the delivery of nutrients has been tried, as has creation of valves that function as a partial obstruction to slow motor patterns of the small intestine. Several techniques lengthen gut; one of the most commonly used was developed by Bianchi.[37,38] As a last resort, small bowel transplantation may be necessary. Aggressive immunosuppressive therapy is required after this surgery, which is being performed in a limited number of surgical centers with limited success.[15]

Gluten Enteropathy

Gluten enteropathy, also called celiac sprue, is a syndrome of small bowel mucosal injury initiated by gluten, a protein found in certain grains, including wheat, barley, rye, and oats.[39,40] Gluten partitions to the alcohol-soluble fraction (gliadin) in wheat.[41] This disorder classically has its onset in early childhood, soon after wheat gluten is introduced into the diet, but the presentation of symptoms may be delayed even until old age.[42] Since the early 1970s, there appears to be a trend to later onset of illness in many populations.[43,44] The weight of available evidence suggests that the reaction to gluten is a cell-mediated immune response. Direct contact between the mucosa and the injurious substance is required. This interaction results in an inflammatory response in the mucosa that may evolve quickly over hours or, more commonly, over many months.[45]

Pathology and epidemiology of celiac disease. The small bowel injury caused by gluten can vary greatly in severity. Mild cases are characterized by lymphocytes infiltrating the epithelial lining. These intraepithelial T lymphocytes are characterized by an increased proportion (20–35%) bearing surface γ/δ receptors. The most severe lesion is classic sprue, characterized by severe inflammation, total villus atrophy, and crypt hyperplasia.[46,47] Patients with this latter degree of injury have a marked loss of surface area with maldigestion and malabsorption. The mucosal epithelium, particularly in the crypts, increases its expression of human leukocyte antigen class II molecules.[48] Activated T lymphocytes release cytokines that amplify the immune response and recruit other inflammatory cells.[49] The lamina propria of the villi is therefore expanded with lymphocytes, plasma cells, and mast cells as well as eosinophils and neutrophils.[50] Not only is the total surface area of the intestine compromised, but the mucosal enzymes are quantitatively decreased as well.[51] A secondary pancreatic insufficiency may develop because of a diminished cholecystokinin and secretin response of small bowel mucosa to a meal.[52] The result of this injury is a generalized malabsorption of ingested nutrients, the severity of which depends on the length of small bowel involved by the process.[53]

Certain populations are at higher risk for this disorder: Northern European, British, Irish, and Mediterranean

Table 2. Clinical findings in gluten enteropathy

Symptoms	Physical exam
Diarrhea	Weight loss
Vomiting	Poor linear growth
Irritability	Abdominal distention
Abdominal pain	Wasting of extremities
Flatulence	

populations have a higher, though variable, prevalence, whereas among the Chinese, Japanese, and sub-Saharan Africans the condition is rare. The disease has a significant genetic component, being more common among family members of an index case than in the general population, and with a concordance in identical twins of ≈70%.[54] Certain major histocompatibility antigen markers (HLA B8, DQw2, and DR3 or DR5/DR7) are disproportionately found associated with gluten enteropathy. These haplotypes do not, however, inevitably lead to disease so that their contribution, while important, does not completely explain the pathogenesis of the disorder.[55]

Environmental factors almost certainly influence the timing of the onset of the injury as well as the severity of symptoms. The avoidance of wheat exposure in early infancy has been proposed as a protective factor. However, avoidance of wheat may be less protective than breast-feeding. Breast-fed infants have a delayed initiation of this intolerance compared with formula-fed babies.[56] It is unclear whether either of these feeding practices explains why classic gluten enteropathy of early childhood is less common now than in the earlier decades of the twentieth century. Also unknown is whether individuals have been spared the disease entirely or will merely become ill at an older age. Other possible environmental triggers have been postulated. Gliadin shares an amino acid sequence with adenovirus type 12, which may predispose to onset of the disease near the time of this infection, but again, a cause and effect has not been proven.[57]

Gluten enteropathy: clinical features. The clinical severity of gluten enteropathy is variable, determined in part by the age of onset, the period of time the disorder remains untreated, and the length of the small bowel involved by the injury.[58] Clinical manifestations include diarrhea, weight loss, flatulence, abdominal distention, and weakness (Table 2). The number of extraintestinal manifestations that have been described associated with gluten enteropathy continues to increase. Most of these conditions tend to occur as the result of malabsorption of critical nutrients and include refractory anemia, osteopenic bone disease, amenorrhea, and neurologic symptoms.[59] There is an increased incidence of malignancies, particularly lymphomas and squamous cell carcinomas.[60] Screening studies show that a significant number of individuals have histological abnormalities

demonstrable on intestinal biopsy but are asymptomatic. Presumably these individuals are in a latent stage of the disease, may have low-grade malabsorption of nutrients, and may be at risk for the unpredictable worsening of their symptoms.[61] They might therefore benefit from a gluten-free diet, but recommendations for this group are still evolving.

Several disease entities are associated with gluten enteropathy, including dermatitis herpetiformis, type I diabetes mellitus, and selective immunoglobulin A (IgA) deficiency.[62–64] There is a growing list of autoimmune disorders that may be associated with gluten enteropathy as well, including ulcerative colitis and thyroid disease.[65]

The diagnosis of gluten enteropathy is suggested by a history and a physical exam compatible with malabsorption, and a number of tests will document the involvement of various nutrients in the malabsorptive process. The definitive test for celiac disease is still the small bowel biopsy, which reveals the pathological features of mucosal injury and inflammation consistent with the disorder. Symptoms should improve within a matter of weeks after withdrawing all sources of gluten from the diet. Clinical improvement precedes the reversal of the mucosal damage, which may lag by months, but the mucosal abnormalities should eventually revert to normal with thorough gluten restriction. The necessity for a follow-up biopsy may now be individually determined on the basis of the completeness of the response.[66] Strategies for screening people at risk for the disorder include measuring serum antibodies (antigliadin IgG and IgA, antireticulin IgA, antiendomysial IgA) that correlate with active disease. These serological tests have not yet eliminated the small bowel biopsy as the definitive diagnostic test, but their reliability and role continue to be evaluated in different populations.[67]

Dietary therapy of gluten enteropathy. The only treatment of gluten enteropathy is permanent withdrawal from the diet of all foods and drugs containing even minute quantities of gluten. Failure of a patient to respond promptly should lead to a reevaluation of the diagnosis or, more commonly, suggest a problem with compliance or understanding of the diet.[68] Because wheat flour is used as an extender in many manufactured foods, patients must receive detailed dietary counseling and education regarding gluten and its pseudonyms and must read labels on processed foods. The tolerance of patients in remission to ingestion of small amounts of gluten is quite variable, from no clinical symptoms to ongoing malabsorption.[69] However, the goal for all patients, even those with some degree of tolerance, should be total exclusion of gluten from the diet.[70] The commitment to a gluten-free diet must be lifelong to avoid the complications of malabsorption. The benefit of a gluten-free diet in altering the risk of malignancy is still unclear, but there is some indication that strict avoidance may indeed lower the risk.[71] As with all malnourished patients, specific nutritional deficiencies must also be addressed with appropriate supplements.

Inflammatory Bowel Disease

Crohn's disease and ulcerative colitis are chronic inflammatory bowel diseases. These disorders are commonly associated with significant malnutrition; most patients present with substantial weight loss. In childhood, growth failure is a major feature and must be dealt with quickly and effectively before the potential for normal growth is lost. Protein-energy undernutrition must be corrected and its recurrence prevented. Trace element and vitamin deficiencies may be present. Challenges to adequate nutrition include diminished food intake resulting from poor appetite, diminished absorption because of surgical loss of bowel and mucosal injury, losses caused by chronic diarrhea, protein-losing enteropathy, effects of medications, and increased nutritional requirements resulting from fever or catch-up growth. The etiology of Crohn's disease and ulcerative colitis remains unknown. Dietary factors may be involved in triggering the disordered immune response that leads to the chronic intestinal inflammation. Manipulation of dietary factors may be important in directly controlling disease activity.

Diet: a factor in the onset of inflammatory bowel disease? There are many theories about the etiology of inflammatory bowel disease. Various infectious agents, inherited risk factors, and environmental factors have been postulated. The observed increase in incidence of inflammatory bowel diseases in the industrial nations correlates with certain dietary practices in these countries, including fast-service-food consumption, formula feeding during infancy, smoking, and intake of refined sugars.[72–75] Because of the uncontrolled enteric immune response characteristic of inflammatory bowel disease, the role of dietary antigens has been given considerable scrutiny. The institution of a restricted diet followed by sequential introduction of suspected foodstuffs has been used to identify putative causative antigens. In one such study, corn, wheat, eggs, potatoes, tea, coffee, apples, mushrooms, oats, chocolate, dairy products, and yeast were found to be associated with clinical relapses.[66] Patients in this study underwent an elimination diet for 6 weeks followed by staged introduction of suspect foods every 2 days. Patients who avoided foods to which they reacted remained in remission longer than did patients on an unrestricted diet. However, critical analysis of this and other studies reveals that there are problems with interpreting these data.[79] The relapsing nature of inflammatory bowel diseases makes any correlation of symptoms with short-term dietary manipulations difficult and questionable. The very short observation period after each

Table 3. Etiology of malnutrition in inflammatory bowel disease

Decreased intake
Dietary restrictions
Anorexia
Abdominal pain
Increased metabolic rate (fever, etc.)
Malabsorption
Inflammation and injury to mucosa
Surgical loss of bowel
Fistula
Lactose intolerance
Bacterial overgrowth syndrome

dietary addition and the lack of repeat challenge with suspect foodstuffs is of concern. Studies in which the patient and investigators are not blinded to the dietary antigens are subject to bias. Despite these difficulties, this area of investigation does have some promise. For example, elemental diets (i.e., those with crystalline amino acids or oligopeptides) can be of benefit in treatment of Crohn's disease. Nevertheless, the belief that diet triggers inflammatory bowel disease remains unproved, and the use of restricted diets is currently not recommended.

Growth failure associated with inflammatory bowel disease. Growth failure and weight loss occur in as many as 85% of prepubertal children with Crohn's disease and are common in ulcerative colitis as well.[80] Malnutrition is the fundamental cause of this failure to thrive. Weight loss in these individuals occurs as the result of an imbalance between nutritional requirements and needs. Most patients with inflammatory bowel diseases appear to differ little from normal subjects for energy requirements; neither the resting metabolic rate nor the total daily energy expenditures in these patients can be distinguished from those of control subjects.[81] This may not be true in those who suffer from fever and those in whom malabsorption occurs as a result of fistulae or mucosal injury. Such patients may require up to 50% higher daily energy intake to meet their special needs.[82] However, patients with inflammatory bowel disease have been repeatedly shown to have suboptimal energy intakes. Patients in relapse consume between 54% and 80% of their recommended dietary allowance for energy.[80–83] Avoidance of dairy products by those with lactose intolerance eliminates a valuable source of protein, carbohydrate, and fat and in some cases contributes to their poor nutrition. Additional requirements imposed by growth make children more vulnerable to the problem of inadequate intake and make nutritional restitution more difficult.

Growth arrest in children with inflammatory bowel disease is nearly always the result of malnutrition rather than an endocrine disturbance (Table 3). Growth hormone levels are normal when measured by the usual provocation tests.[84,85] The serum levels of insulin-like

Table 4. Nutritional deficiencies in inflammatory bowel disease

---

Protein-energy
Trace elements
  Zinc
  Magnesium
  Selenium
Vitamins
  Vitamin A
  Vitamin E
  Thiamin
  Riboflavin
  Vitamin B-6
  Niacin

---

growth factor I (IGF-I, somatomedin C) tend to be low, reflecting the nutritional status of the patient. This hormone, secreted in response to growth hormone, is an important mediator of growth. Low levels of this hormone in malnourished patients are associated with growth failure and rapidly return to normal with nutritional restitution.[86] Provision of adequate energy for catch-up growth results in rapid reversal of growth failure in these children, whether nutrition is given parenterally or enterally.[87–90]

Specific nutrient deficiencies in inflammatory bowel disease. The combination of inadequate intake because of symptoms, increased enteric losses, malabsorption, and side effects of medications or inadequacy of prescribed special diets may lead to deficiencies of minerals and vitamins (Table 4). Zinc is necessary for normal wound healing, taste sensation, growth, and immune function. Low levels of this essential mineral have been found in the serum of patients with Crohn's disease.[91,92] The loss of appetite and normal ability to taste food because of zinc deficiency could play a significant role in aggravating malnutrition. Diminished zinc stores have also been associated with disordered immune function.[93] Whether such immune effects are related to the immunological injury to the bowel is unclear. Zinc is associated with serum proteins such as albumin, and when low serum protein levels are present because of protein-losing enteropathy or suboptimal nutrition, low total serum zinc levels are also found.[94] When examined in detail, immune defects such as reduced skin test reactivity, diminished response of lymphocytes to mitogens, and impaired phagocyte function correlate better with general measures of malnutrition than with serum or tissue (erythrocyte or leukocyte) zinc status.[95] This evidence suggests that the low serum zinc levels commonly seen in inflammatory bowel disease do not always indicate true zinc deficiency but merely reflect reduced carrying capacity of serum for zinc. A more accurate way to assess zinc status appears to be the measurement of 24-hour zinc excretion in the urine. This value tends to be normal in inflammatory bowel disease patients with low disease activity. In patients with very active disease, however, 24-hour zinc excretion is often reduced, indicating deficiency.[94]

Levels of other trace elements essential to health, including magnesium and selenium, are sometimes also diminished in inflammatory bowel disease. Magnesium deficiency is associated with cramps, fatigue, depression, and impaired healing. As noted for zinc, the serum level of magnesium is insensitive and unreliable as an index of deficiency. Urinary magnesium excretion is the most practical index for clinical use and should be followed in patients with potentially large losses because of diarrhea, significant small bowel resection, or widespread disease.[96] Resection of >200 cm of small bowel has been correlated with selenium deficiency, a potentially dangerous condition with risk of severe cardiomyopathy. Serum or, preferentially, erythrocyte selenium should be monitored in such patients, who should probably receive routine supplementation to prevent deficiency.[97] Measurement of erythrocyte glutathione peroxidase, a selenium-dependent enzyme, may also be a sensitive indicator of deficiency.[97,98]

Deficiencies in the diet and loss of normal bowel function can also lead to vitamin deficiencies. This is particularly true when resection of a significant amount of bowel has occurred (see section on short bowel syndrome). Vitamins A and E are most likely to be significantly depleted in Crohn's disease, with a tendency for lower levels of thiamin, riboflavin, vitamin B-6, and folate as well.[99] This occurs despite evidence of normal absorption of vitamins A and E in these patients.[100] Pellagra (niacin deficiency), perhaps exacerbated by deficiency of riboflavin and vitamin B-6, has also been reported.[101] As with the trace elements, not all low serum vitamin levels necessarily indicate true deficiency. Low levels of retinol-binding protein in patients with active Crohn's disease may lead to falsely low serum levels of vitamin A.[100]

Diet as primary therapy for Crohn's disease. Much excitement and controversy has resulted from observations that dietary manipulation may directly affect the course of Crohn's disease (Table 5). The early observation that total parenteral nutrition (TPN) combined with complete bowel rest was capable of inducing remission

Table 5. Nutritional therapies for inflammatory bowel disease activity

---

Restriction diet
Parenteral nutrition
  Before and after surgery
  Bowel obstruction
  Fistulous disease
Elemental diet
Polymeric diet
Fish oil (experimental)

---

triggered many subsequent studies of nutritional therapy.[102] These have included TPN, elemental enteral diets, and polymeric enteral diets. Although some controversies still exist, the emerging picture is that nutritional repletion has much to offer these patients and can favorably affect the course of the disease. Differences between the types of nutrition offered are probably not significant except in selected circumstances.

Parenteral nutrition is an effective way to induce medical remission. However, comparisons between parenteral and enteral feedings have shown that both are equally effective in effecting clinical remission.[103,104] Enteral feedings are safer than TPN, having fewer side effects and a much lower cost. Therefore, TPN is currently used mostly in Crohn's disease patients with bowel obstruction, postoperative ileus, or other intolerance of enteral feedings.[105,106]

Elemental diets are also useful in Crohn's disease. These formulas are the logical next step after TPN and are used with the idea that dietary antigens may trigger disease activity. Elemental diets, when used with the exclusion of other foods, are capable of inducing remission in about two-thirds of patients, which is somewhat less effective than steroid therapy.[107-109] However, these specialized liquid diets are expensive, have serious problems with palatability, and often have to be given via nasogastric tubes.

Polymeric diets were evaluated recently as alternatives to TPN and elemental diets. Surprisingly, polymeric diets seemed to perform as well as elemental feedings. A recent meta-analysis examined the results of 13 separate trials, comparing these two enteral feeding regimens with steroid therapy.[110] The results show that steroids are more effective than enteral nutrition in the treatment of active Crohn's disease. The data also suggested that elemental diets have no advantage over the less expensive and more palatable polymeric diets.

Taken together, the data for dietary treatment of Crohn's disease show that definite positive effects can be attained by enteral or parenteral nutritional support. Dietary therapy cannot take the place of medical therapy in most patients but is essential to reverse growth failure and correct nutrient deficiencies. Adequate dietary therapy may offer the additional advantage of potentiating medical therapy to ameliorate symptoms of active disease. New dietary therapies hold the promise of additional benefits. The most significant of these is the use of fish oils, rich in n–3 fatty acids to suppress leukotriene synthesis. Several reports have shown some benefits of fish-oil therapy in inflammatory bowel disease, resulting in reduced steroid dose, weight gain, and improved histology of intestinal biopsies.[111-113] The boundaries between diet and drug therapy in inflammatory bowel disease are beginning to become indistinct. Future developments in this field will no doubt continue to benefit patients and generate opportunities for debate and research.

References

1. Shanbhogue LKR, Molenaar JC (1994) Short bowel syndrome: metabolic and surgical management. Br J Surg 81:486–499
2. Dudrick SJ, Latifi R, Fosnocht DE (1991) Management of short-bowel syndrome. Surg Clin North Am 71:625–643
3. ChrisAnderson-Hill D, Heimburger DC (1993) Medical mangement of the difficult patient with short-bowel syndrome. Nutrition 9:536–539
4. Warner BW, Ziegler MM (1993) Management of the short bowel syndrome in the pediatric population. Pediatr Clin North Am 40:1335–1350
5. Goulet OJ, Revillon Y, Jan D, et al (1991) Neonatal short bowel syndrome. J Pediatr 119:18–23
6. Ohkohchi N, Igarashi Y, Tazawa Y, et al (1986) Evaluation of the nutritional condition and absorptive capacity of nine infants with short bowel syndrome. J Pediatr Gastroenterol Nutr 5:198–206
7. Dorney SFA, Ament ME, Berquist WE, et al (1985) Improved survival in very short small bowel of infancy with use of long-term parenteral nutrition. J Pediatr 107:521–525
8. Kurkchubasche AG, Rowe MI, Smith SD (1993) Adaptation in short-bowel syndrome: reassessing old limits. J Pediatr Surg 28:1069–1071
9. Kurz K, Sauer H (1983) Treatment and metabolic findings in an extreme short-bowel syndrome with 11 cm jejunal remnant. J Pediatr Surgery 18:257–263
10. Iacono G, Carroccio A, Montalto G, et al (1993) Extreme short bowel syndrome: a case for reviewing the guidelines for predicting survival. J Pediatr Gastroenterol Nutr 16:216–219
11. Surana R, Quinn FMJ, Puri P (1994) Short-Gut syndrome: intestinal adaptation in a patient with 12 cm of Jejunum. J Pediatr Gastroenterol Nutr 19:246–249
12. Wilmore DW (1972) Factors correlating with a successful outcome following extensive intestinal resection in newborn infants. J Pediatr 80:88–95
13. Vanderhoof JA (1992) Short bowel syndrome: smoothing the road to recovery. Contemporary Pediatr 9:19–34
14. Allard JP, Jeejeebhoy KN (1989) Nutritional support and therapy in the short bowel syndrome. Gastroenterol Clin North Am 18:589–601
15. Vanderhoof JA, Langnas AN, Pinch LW, et al (1992) Short bowel syndrome: invited review. J Pediatr Gastroenterol Nutr 14:359–370
16. Ramakrishnan T, Stokes P (1985) Beneficial effects of fasting and low carbohydrate diet in D-lactic acidosis associated with short-bowel syndrome. J Parenter Enter Nutr 9:361–363
17. Wright JK (1992) Short gut syndrome-options for management. Compr Ther 18:5–8
18. Lentze MJ (1989) Intestinal adaptation in short-bowel syndrome. Eur J Pediatr 148:294–299
19. Feldman EJ, Dowling RH, McNaughton J, et al (1976) Effects of oral versus intravenous nutrition on intestinal adaptation after small resection in the dog. Gastroenterology 70:712–719
20. Purdum PP, Kirby DF (1991) Short-bowel syndrome: a review of the role of nutrition support. West J Med 15:93–101
21. Williamson RCN, Chir M (1978) Intestinal adaptation: mechanisms of control. N Engl J Med 298:1444–1450
22. Vanderhoof JA, Grandjean CJ, Burkley KT, et al (1984) Effect

of casein versus casein hydrolysate on mucosal adaptation following massive bowel resection in infant rats. J Pediatr Gastroenterol Nutr 3:262–267

23. Vanderhoof JA, Grandjean CJ, Kaufmann SS, et al (1984) Effect of high percentage medium chain triglyceride diet on mucosal adaptation following massive bowel resection in rats. J Parenter Enter Nutr 8:685–689

24. Green JH, Heatley RV (1992) Nutritional management of patients with short-bowel syndrome. Nutrition 8:186–190

25. Levy E, Frileux P, Sandrucci S, et al (1988) Continuous enteral nutrition during the early adaptive stage of the short bowel syndrome. Br J Surgery 75:549–553

26. McIntyre PB, Fitchew M, Lennard-Jones JE (1986) Patients with a high jejunostomy do not need a special diet. Gastroenterology 91:25–33

27. Woolf GM, Miller C, Kurian R, et al (1987) Nutritional absorption in short bowel syndrome: evaluation of fluid, calorie and divalent cation requirements. Dig Dis Sci 32:8–15

28. Messing B, Pigot F, Rongier M, et al (1991) Intestinal absorption of free oral hyperalimentation in the very short bowel syndrome. Gastroenterology 100:1502–1508

29. Bernard DKH, Shaw MJ (1983) Principles of nutrition therapy for short-bowel syndrome. Nutr Clin Pract 8:153–162

30. Roediger WEW (1990) The starved colon-diminished mucosal nutrition, diminished absorption and colitis. Dis Colon Rectum 33:858–862

31. Sakata T (1987) Stimulatory effect of short-chain fatty acids on epithelial cell proliferation in the rat intestine: a possible explanation for trophic effects of fermentable fibre, gut microbes and luminal trophic factors. Br J Nutr 58: 95–103

32. Kripke SA, Fox AD, Berman JM, et al (1989) Stimulation of intestinal mucosal growth with intracolonic infusion of short-chain fatty acids. J Parenter Enter Nutr 13(2):109–116

33. Thompson JS (1994) Management of the short bowel syndrome. Gastroenterol Clin North Am 23:403–420

34. Booth IW (1994) Enteral nutrition as primary therapy in short bowel syndrome. Gut 1(suppl):S69–S72

35. Koruda MJ, Rolandelli RH, Settle RG, et al (1986) The effect of a pectin-supplemented elemental diet on intestinal adaptation to massive small bowel resection. J Parenter Enter Nutr 10:343–350

36. Vanderhoof JA, Park JH, Mohammadpour H, et al (1990) Absence of trophic effect of glutamine on intestinal adaptation following massive small bowel resection. J Parenter Enter Nutr 14:85

37. Bianchi A (1980) Intestinal loop lengthening—a technique for increasing small intestinal length. J Pediatr Surg 15:145–151

38. Thompson JS, Pinch LW, Murray N, et al (1991) Experience with intestinal lengthening for the short-bowel syndrome. J Pediatr Surg 26:721–724

39. Dicke WM, Weijers HA, VanderKamer JH (1953) The presence in wheat of a factor having a deleterious effect in cases of Celiac disease. Acta Paediatr 42:34–36

40. Kasarda DD (1981) Proteins and peptides in celiac disease: relation to cereal genetics. In Food nutrition and evolution. Masson Publishing, New York, pp. 201–222

41. Gee S (1888) On the celiac affection. St Bartholomew's Hosp Rep 24:17

42. Langman MJS, McConnell TH, Spegelhalter DJ (1985) Changing pattern of coeliac disease frequency: an analysis of coeliac society membership records. Gut 26:175–178

43. Challacombe DN (1983) The incidence of coeliac disease and early weaning [editorial]. Arch Dis Child 58:326

44. Ciclitra PJ, Ellis HJ (1987) Investigation of cereal toxicity in coeliac disease. Postgrad Med J 63:767–775

45. Kumar P, O'Donoghue DP, Lancaster-Smith M (1979) Cellular changes in the jejunal mucosa following reintroduction of gluten in treated coeliac disease. In Pepys J, Edwards AM (eds.), The mast cell—its role in health and disease. Pitman Medical, Tunbridge Wells, pp 647–656

46. Marsh MN (1992) Gluten, major histocompatibility complex, and the small intestine. Gastroenterology 102:330–354

47. Holm K, Maki M, Savilahti E, et al (1992) Intraepithelial gamma delta T-cell-receptor lymphocytes and genetic susceptibility to coeliac disease. Lancet 339:1500–1503

48. Scott H, Sollid LM, Fausa O, et al (1987) Expression of major histocompatibility complex class II subregion products by jejunal epithelium in patients with coeliac disease. Scand J Immunol 26:563–571

49. Howdle PD, Bullen AW, Losowsky MS (1982) Cell-mediated immunity to gluten within small intestinal mucosa in coeliac disease. Gut 23:115–122

50. Marsh MN, Hinde J (1985) Inflammatory component of coeliac sprue mucosa in mast cells, basophils, and eosinophils. Gastroenterology 89:92–101

51. Peters TJ, Heath JR, Wansbrough-Jones MH, et al (1975) Enzyme activity and properties of lysosomes and brush borders in jejunal biopsies from control subjects and patients with coeliac disease. Clin Sci Molec Med 48:259–267

52. Maton PN, Selden AC, Fitzpatrick ML, et al (1985) Defective gall bladder emptying and cholecystokinen-release in celiac disease: reversal by gluten-free diet. Gastroenterology 88:391–396

53. MacDonald WC, Brandborg LL, Flick AL, et al (1964) Studies of celiac sprue IV response of the whole length of the small bowel to gluten-free diet. Gastroenterology 47:573–578

54. Polanco I, Biemond I, VanLeeuwen A (1981) Gluten-sensibility enteropathy in Spain: genetic and environmental factors. In Genetics of coeliac disease: Proceedings of international symposium (1979). MTP Press, Lancaster, England, pp 211–231

55. Kagnoff MF (1990) Understanding the molecular basis of coeliac disease. Gut 31:497–499

56. Auricchio S, Follo D, DeRitis G (1983) Does breast feeding protect against development of clinical symptoms of coeliac disease in children? J Pediatr Gastroenterol Nutr 2:428–433

57. Kagnoff MF (1989) Celiac disease: adenovirus and alpha gliadin. Curr Top Microbiol Immunol 145:67–78

58. Young WF, Pringle EM (1971) 110 children with coeliac disease, 1950–1969. Arch Dis Child 46:421–436

59. Trier JS (1988) Intestinal malabsorption: differentiation of cause. Hosp Prac 23:195–211

60. Selby WS, Gallagher ND (1979) Malignancy in a 19 year experience of adult celiac disease. Dig Dis Sci 24:684–688

61. Ferguson A, Arranz E, O'Mahony S (1993) Clinical and pathological spectrum of coeliac disease—active, silent, latent, potential. Gut 34:150–151

62. Otley C, Hall RP (1990) Dermatitis herpetiformis. Dermatol Clin 8:759–769

63. Collin P, Salmi P, Hallstrom O (1989) High frequency of coeliac disease in adult patients with type I diabetes. Scand J Gastroenterol 24:81–84

64. Crabbe PA, Heremans JF (1967) Selective IgA deficiency with steatorrhea. Am J Med 42:319–326

65. Trier JS (1991) Celiac sprue. New Engl J Med 325:1709–1719

66. Riordan AM, Hunter JO, Cowan RE, et al (1993) Treatment of active Crohn's disease by exclusion diet: East Anglian multicentre controlled trial. Lancet 342:1131–1134

67. Carrao G, Corazz GR, Andreani ML (1994) Serological screening of coeliac disease: choosing the optimal procedure according to various prevalence values. Gut 35:771–775

68. McNeish AS, Harms HK, Rey J (1979) The diagnosis of celiac disease: a commentary on the current practices of members of the European Society for Paediatric Gastroenterol Nutr (ESPGAN). Arch Dis Child 54:783–786

69. Walker-Smith J (1988) Coeliac disease. In Diseases of the small intestine in childhood. Butterworths, London, United Kingdom, pp. 88–143

70. Shmerling DH, Franckx J (1986) Childhood celiac disease: a long term analysis of relapses in 91 patients. J Pediatr Gastroenterol Nutr 5:565–569

71. Holmes GK, Prior P, Lane MR (1989) Malignancy in coeliac disease—effect of gluten free diet. Gut 30:333–338

72. Persson PG, Ahlbom A, Hellers G (1992) Diet and inflammatory bowel disease: a case-control study. Epidemiology 3:47–52

73. Rigas A, Rigas B, Glassman M, et al (1993) Breast-feeding and maternal smoking in the etiology of Crohn's disease and ulcerative colitis in childhood. Ann Epidemiol 3:387–392

74. Koletzko S, Griffiths A, Corey M, et al (1991) Infant feeding practices and ulcerative colitis in childhood. Biomed J 302:1580–1581

75. Koletzko S, Sherman P, Corey M, et al (1989) Role of infant feeding practices in development of Crohn's disease: an international cooperative study. Scand J Gastroenterol 22:1009–1024

76. Stokes MA (1992) Crohn's disease and nutrition. Br J Surg 79:391–394

77. Katschinski B, Logan RFA, Langman EM (1988) Smoking and sugar intake are separate but interactive risk factors in Crohn's disease. Gut 29:1202–1206

78. Panza E, Franceschi S, La Vecchia C, et al (1987) Dietary factors in the aetiology of inflammatory bowel disease. Ital J Gastroenterol 18:205–209

79. Riordan AM, Hunter JO, Crampton JR, et al (1994) Treatment of active Crohn's disease by exclusion diet. J Pediatr Gastroenterol Nutr 19:135–136

80. Kirschner BS (1990) Growth and development in chronic inflammatory bowel disease. Acta Paediatr 366:98–104

81. Kushner RF, Schoeller DA (1991) Resting and total energy expenditure in patients with inflammatory bowel disease. Am J Clin Nutr 53:161–165

82. Sutton MM (1992) Nutritional needs of children with inflammatory bowel disease. Compr Ther 18:21–25

83. Thomas AG, Taylor F, Miller V (1993) Dietary intake and nutritional treatment in childhood Crohn's disease. J Pediatr Gastroenterol Nutr 17:75–81

84. Tenore A, Berman WF, Parks JS, et al (1977) Basal and stimulated serum growth hormone concentrations in inflammatory bowel disease. J Clin Endocrinol Metab 44:622–628

85. Chong SK, Grossman A, Walker-Smith JA, et al (1984) Endocrine dysfunction in children with Crohn's disease. J Pediatr Gastroenterol Nutr 3:529–534

86. Unterman TG, Vazquez RM, Slas AJ, et al (1985) Nutrition and somatomedin. XIII. Usefulness of somatomedin-C in nutritional assessment. Am J Med 78:228–234

87. Layden T, Rosenberg J, Nemchausky B, et al (1976) Reversal of growth arrest in adolescents with Crohn's disease after parenteral alimentation. Gastroenterology 70:1017–1021

88. Strobel CT, Byrne WJ, Ament ME (1979) Home parenteral nutrition in children with Crohn's disease: an effective management alternative. Gastroenterology 77:272–279

89. Kirschner BS, Klich JR, Kalman SS, et al (1981) Reversal of growth retardation in Crohn's disease with therapy emphasizing oral nutritional restitution. Gastroenterology 80:10–15

90. O'Marain C, Segal AW, Levi AJ (1984) Elemental diet as primary treatment of acute Crohn's disease: a controlled trial. Br Med J 288:1859–1862

91. Solomons NW, Rosenberg IH, Sandstead HH, et al (1977) Zinc deficiency in Crohn's disease. Digestion 16:87–95

92. McClain C, Soutor C, Zieve L (1980) Zinc deficiency: a complication of Crohn's disease. Gastroenterology 78:272–279

93. Van De Wal Y, Van Der Sluys Veer A, Verspaget HW, et al (1993) Effect of zinc therapy on natural killer cell activity in inflammatory bowel disease. Aliment Pharmacol Ther 7:281–286

94. Fleming CR, Huizenga KA, McCall JT, et al (1981) Zinc nutrition in Crohn's disease. Dig Dis Sci 26:865–870

95. Ainley C, Cason J, Slavin BM, et al (1991) The influence of zinc status and malnutrition on immunological function in Crohn's disease. Gastroenterology 100:1616–1625

96. Galland L (1988) Magnesium and inflammatory bowel disease. Magnesium 7:78–83

97. Rannem T, Ladefoged K, Hylander E, et al (1992) Selenium status in patients with Crohn's disease. Am J Clin Nutr 56:933–937

98. Rea HM, Thompson CD, Campbell DR, et al (1979) Relation between erythrocyte selenium concentrations and glutathione peroxidase activities of New Zealand residents and visitors to New Zealand. Br J Nutr 42:201–208

99. Kuroki F, Iida M, Tominaga M, et al (1993) Multiple vitamin status in Crohn's disease. Dig Dis Sci 38:1614–1618

100. Janczewska I, Butruk E, Tomecki R, et al (1991) Metabolism of vitamin A in inflammatory bowel disease. Hepato-Gastroenterology 38:391–395

101. Lifshitz AY, Stern F, Kaplan B, et al (1992) Pellagra complicating Crohn's disease. J Am Acad Dermatol 27:620

102. Fischer JE, Foster GS, Abel RM, et al (1973) Hyperalimentation as primary therapy for inflammatory bowel disease. Am J Surg 125:165–173

103. Gonzalez-Huix F, Fernandez-Banares F, Esteve-Comas M, et al (1993) Enteral versus parenteral nutrition as adjunct therapy in acute ulcerative colitis. Am J Gastroenterol 88:227–232

104. Gonzalez-Huix F, de Leon R, Fernandez-Banares F, et al (1993) Polymeric enteral diets as primary treatment of active Crohn's disease: a prospective steroid controlled trial. Gut 34:778–782

105. Shiloni E, Coronado E, Freund HR (1989) Role of total parenteral nutrition in the treatment of Crohn's disease. Am J Surg 157:180–185

106. Cravo M, Camilo ME, Correia JP (1991) Nutritional support in Crohn's disease: which route? Am J Gastroenterol 86:317–321

107. Teahon K, Smethurst P, Pearson M, et al (1991) The effect of elemental diet on intestinal permeability and inflammation in Crohn's disease. Gastroenterology 101:84–89

108. Gorard DA, Hunt JB, Payne-James JJ, et al (1993) Initial response and subsequent course of Crohn's disease treated with elemental diet or prednisolone. Gut 34:1198–1202

109. Hirakawa H, Fukuda Y, Tanida N, et al (1993) Home elemental enteral hyperalimentation (HEEH) for the maintenance of remission in patients with Crohn's disease. Gastroenterol Jpn 28:379–384

110. Griffiths AM, Ohlsson A, Sherman PM, et al (1995) Meta-analysis of enteral nutrition as a primary treatment of active Crohn's disease. Gastroenterology 108:1056–1067

111. Aslan A, Triadafilopoulos G (1992) Fish oil fatty acid supplementation in active ulcerative colitis: a double-blind, placebo-controlled, crossover study. Am J Gastroenterol 87:432–437

112. Stenson WF, Cort D, Rodgers J, et al (1992) Dietary supplementation with fish oil in ulcerative colitis. Ann Intern Med 116:609–614

113. Hawthorne AB, Daneschmend TK, Hawkey CJ, et al (1992) Treatment of ulcerative colitis with fish oil supplementation: a prospective 12 month randomised controlled trial. Gut 33:922–928

Chapter 50

Estimation of Dietary Intake

Eleanor M. Pao and Yasmin S. Cypel

Dietary intake estimation entails the collection of information on the quantity of individual portions of foods eaten and, using food composition values, the computation of the energy and nutrient content of these foods. Food intake information may be current or from the recent or distant past. Appropriate methods for estimating dietary intake are dictated by the objectives of the study, population or group involved, precision of measurement required, cost, and length of time to be covered.

The estimation of dietary intake serves many purposes. Government, academia, industry, and numerous other groups have a growing need for dietary information for both the overall population and its subgroups. National surveys are a principal means for obtaining descriptions of dietary patterns of the population to use in making policy and program decisions.

Two federal agencies, one in the U.S. Department of Agriculture (USDA) and one in the U.S. Department of Health and Human Services (HHS), conduct dietary surveys of the total diet. The USDA surveys are the Nationwide Food Consumption Survey (NFCS) and the Continuing Survey of Food Intakes by Individuals (CSFII). HHS conducts the Health and Nutrition Examination Survey (NHANES). Table 1 outlines the changes in the dietary intake methodologies used by these agencies since the 1960s. Dietary data collection methodologies have been refined and automation has been introduced. This chapter describes the main methods for obtaining individual food intake information: the food record, 24-hour food recall, food frequency questionnaire, and diet history. Use of the latter two is increasing because they seem more representative of usual dietary intake and are less expensive to carry out. The strengths and weaknesses, the validity and reliability, and the recent developments associated with these methods are reviewed. Data processing, data analysis, and other issues also are presented briefly.

Data Collection Methods

Although four data-collection methods are identified and described here, researchers vary considerably in categorizing and defining each method. The food record, for which foods are weighed or estimated by use of household measures, is used to obtain current intake information; the dietary recall, food frequency questionnaire, and dietary history are used to measure intake that has already taken place. Anderson noted that the 1-day record and 1-day recall are both used to measure quantitative daily consumption of food in a specified time period.[1] To reflect total intake, foods eaten both at home and away from home must be reported. Dietary supplements are sometimes included, but problems have been encountered with quantification because of the extremely large variety of supplements available, their frequent change of formula, and the absence of reliable information about the content of many over-the-counter supplements. Survey questionnaires are used also to collect demographic and personal information about individuals (for example, sex, age, race, income, region, and urbanization of residence) in order to characterize and compare dietary intakes across different groups. Informative reviews of dietary intake methods and related issues are available.[1-16]

Food record. The food record (also called food diary) is kept by the subject or by a designated surrogate (for example, a mother for her child) for a specified time period, usually 1–7 days. Recently, a 2-week estimated food record was used in a study of energy intake by obese and nonobese adolescents.[17] A long period (1 year) has been reported for the weighed record.[18]

In the weighed method food is weighed before eating. Leftovers are weighed and deducted. Foods eaten away from home are usually estimated in household measures. Few large-scale studies or surveys in the United States have used the weighed food record because of high costs, burden on the participants, and difficulty in maintaining a representative sample of the population. Further, habitual eating patterns can be disrupted by the task of weighing, which results in lower reported intakes.[19] To lessen the burden for respondents and researchers, user-friendly computerized systems have been developed for use in the home and for use by multiple subjects.[20] In England, portable electronic tape recorded

Table 1. National dietary intake surveys: methodological changes over time

Year	Survey	Method
		USDA
1965	HFCS	24-hour recall
1977–78	NFCS	24-hour recall + 2 day record, consecutive days
1985–86	CSFII	24-hour recall, 6 at 2 month intervals (1 in person, 5 telephone interviews)
1987–88	NFCS	24-hour recall + 2 day record, consecutive days
1989–91	CSFII	24-hour recall + 2-day record, consecutive days
1994–96	CSFII	2 nonconsecutive 24-hour recalls
		HHS[a]
1965, 1967, 1969	NHES	No dietary data collected
1968–70	Ten State	24-hour recall
1971–73	NHES	"
1974–75	HANES I	24-hour recall + FFQ
1976–80	HANES II	"
1982–84	HHANES	"
1988–94	NHANES III	"

Notes: HFCS is Household Food Consumption Survey. NFCS is Nationwide Food Consumption Survey. CSFII is Continuing Survey of Food Intakes by Individuals. NHES is National Health Examination Survey. NHANES is National Health and Nutrition Examination Survey. HHANES is Hispanic Health and Nutrition Examination Survey. FFQ is food frequency questionnaire.

[a]Sempos et al. (see reference 91).

automated (PETRA) scales make it easier to obtain weighed records.[21]

For the less-burdensome estimated food record respondents are asked to describe foods and amounts eaten. Descriptions of food include kind, preparation, brand name, and main ingredients in mixtures. Several types of measurement varying in accuracy may appear on the estimated record. Standard measuring cups and spoons may be used to report volume of liquids, semisolids, and foods in small pieces and the measures should be level, not rounded or heaping. Solid foods may be measured with a ruler and described by shape (square, rectangle, cylinder, wedge) and dimensions (length, width, height, diameter). Count, such as one egg, and relative size, such as small, medium, or large may be sufficient. Weight or volume measures on labels may be used for foods such as candy bars and beverages in containers. For items such as pies and cakes of which a portion of the whole is eaten, weight or dimensions of the whole and the proportion eaten are appropriate. Reports for meats must indicate whether amounts are for raw or cooked forms, with or without bone, and with or without skin or fat.

In the Nationwide Food Consumption Surveys (NFCSs) conducted in 1977–1978 and in 1987–1988 by the USDA, a set of measuring cups and spoons and a ruler were given to participating households for members to use in keeping 2-day estimated food records. A detailed Food Instruction Booklet was provided to help respondents describe kinds and amounts of food ingested for the 1987–1988 NFCS and 1989–1991 Continuing Survey of Food Intakes by Individuals (CSFII).[22,23]

Interviewers or health professionals working with respondents, clients, or patients provide individuals with food record forms and verbal as well as written instructions for their completion. Some researchers request subjects to use precoded daily food records.[24] Use of measuring devices must be demonstrated, and the individuals should have an opportunity to practice. Arrangements are made for the interviewer's return to collect and review completed records.

Validity refers to whether the method measures what it is supposed to measure. The validity of dietary intakes estimated by food records is especially important because food records are often used as the reference against which other methods are compared. Krall and Dwyer[25] assessed the validity of food diaries by comparing diary reports with weighed portions of food served in a metabolic research unit and found that approximately 9% of all food items were omitted. Another study found that the burden of having to weigh foods before eating resulted in a 13% decrease in caloric intakes, on average, compared with intakes from weekly diary records without weighing.[18,26] When mean food and nutrient intakes obtained from estimated food diaries were compared to those obtained from observed intakes, however, small or no differences between methods were observed for most nutrients.[27] The possibility of systematic error is indicated by the finding that in studies covering multiple days

Table 2. Strengths and weaknesses of food record method

Strengths	Weaknesses
1. Respondent does not rely on memory.	1. Generally, respondents must be literate.
2. Time period is defined.	2. Respondents must be highly cooperative.
3. Portions can be measured or weighed to increase accuracy.	3. Food consumed away from home may be less accurately reported.
4. For elderly people, records may be more accurate than recalls.	4. Habitual eating pattern may be influenced or changed by the recording process.
5. Food intakes are quantified so nutrient contents can be calculated.	5. Requirement for literate respondents may introduce bias as a result of overrepresentation of more highly educated individuals.
6. Multiple days may yield a measure of usual intake for a group.	6. Record keeping increases respondent burden.
7. Two or more days provide data on intra- and interindividual variation in dietary intakes.	7. Increased respondent burden may adversely affect response rates.
8. One-day records kept intermittently over the year may provide an estimate of usual intake by an individual.	8. Self-administered records require more callbacks and editing than interviewer-administered reports.
9. Multiple days provide reliable information about less frequently eaten foods.	9. One-day records provide an inadequate indication of usual intake for groups or individuals.
10. Procedure can be automated.	10. Validity of records may decrease as number of days increases.
	11. Validity of records may be influenced by the level of monitoring.
	12. Substantial underreporting suspected.

of food records, mean food intakes for the first few days often exceed those of later days.[28] In other studies, energy intakes obtained from records are related to estimates of total energy expenditure determined by the doubly labeled water method.[29,30] Large underreporting is evident when individuals' estimates of energy intake are compared with more objective determinations such as the doubly labeled water method.[31]

Reliability often refers to repeatability or reproducibility of results using a particular method. Consumption in two time periods can be compared to appraise reliability. In one study, two sets of 7-day records kept by 127 men during 1 year showed little change during the period; intraclass coefficients based on unadjusted nutrient intakes ranged from 0.50 for vitamin E to 0.90 for vitamin B2.[32]

The food record has several drawbacks. The burden of keeping a diet record may influence a respondent to change usual eating patterns in order to simplify record keeping. Also, the respondent may tire of the task and drop out. Such weaknesses can bias the research results. Table 2 provides a list of the principal strengths and weaknesses of the food record. Comparison of this list with those for the other procedures can yield useful insights.

Twenty-four-hour food recall. A very commonly used method for obtaining food intake information is the 24-hour food recall. In large national dietary intake surveys, as well as smaller studies, this method has been used to estimate dietary intakes of individuals.[23,33,34] However, few studies using 24-hour recalls follow identical procedures. Redesign of the interviewing protocol using

cognitive research procedures may help to improve the quality of information obtained from the 24-hour food recall.[35]

Essentially, the individual is asked to recall and describe the kinds and amounts of all foods (including beverages) ingested during a 24-hour period. Dietary recall questionnaires may be administered in person, by telephone, and in automated interviews.[33,34,36–38] Interviews may be conducted in the home, in a clinic setting, or at some other convenient site.[23,33] The 24-hour food recall takes ≈15–40 minutes to complete.

Usually, the 24-hour and 1-day recall are synonymous, referring to the preceding full day.[23,33] Occasionally, the 24-hour period starts with the last eating event and moves backwards for 24 hours. To obtain an indication of usual intake, six bimonthly 1-day food recalls were obtained from the same individuals during a 1-year panel survey.[38] However, more than half the individuals in the survey dropped out before providing the six recalls requested.

Because individuals vary in their ability and willingness to recall, describe, and quantify foods eaten, interviewers are trained to ask probing questions that encourage and help organize the individual's memories about eating events. Probes to clarify or check information must be neutral and vary with the kind of food. Forgetting may lead to underestimation of intake.[6,39,40] To obtain adequate descriptions of foods, interviewers usually ask about type (e.g., whole or skim milk), preparation (e.g., broiled or fried chicken), brand name (e.g., for ready-to-eat cereal), main ingredients in mixtures, and other special features (such as low calorie or low sodium). In automated interviews response options

Table 3. Strengths and weaknesses of 24-hour food recall methods

Strengths	Weaknesses
1. Administration time is short.	1. Respondent recall depends on memory.
2. Time period is defined.	2. Portion size is difficult to estimate accurately.
3. Food intake can be quantified.	3. Intakes tend to be underreported compared with other methods.
4. Procedure does not alter individual's habitual dietary patterns.	4. Usual intake of an individual cannot be assessed from one day's intake.
5. Interviewer administration allows probing for omitted foods or incomplete information and requires fewer callbacks.	5. Trained interviewers are required.
6. Response rates are relatively high.	6. Interviewer variability may offset standardized procedures.
7. A single contact is required.	7. Procedure may be more difficult for certain population groups (e.g., young children).
8. Procedure is often used to evaluate dietary intakes of large groups.	
9. Two or more days provide data on intra- and interindividual variation in dietary intakes.	
10. Multiple days are necessary to provide reliable data on less frequently eaten foods.	
11. Multiple days may yield a measure of usual intake.	
12. Repeated recalls over a year may provide an estimate of usual intake by an individual.	
13. Respondent does not rely on long-term memory.	
14. Procedure can be administered by telephone.	
15. Procedure can obtain specific details on foods eaten and their methods of preparation.	
16. Procedure can be automated.	

appear on the computer screen, reminding interviewers to provide essential information.[33]

As in estimated food record surveys, a measurement aid (abstract or realistic, two or three dimensional) is usually selected as a common reference to help individuals estimate portion sizes for the 24-hour recall survey. Examples of measurement aids include standard household measuring cups and spoons, rulers, abstract and realistic food models and shapes, two-dimensional food model charts, and others.[23,33,41] Accuracy of portion size estimates using the different approaches has yet to be adequately tested.

Validity of the 24-hour food recall has been assessed in numerous studies by comparing recalled intakes with observed intakes or with intake records obtained by other methods. Investigators found that recalled intakes compared with weighed intakes tend to be overestimated when intakes are low and underestimated when intakes are high.[40,42] Mullenbach et al.[34] concluded that a 24-hour recall conducted by telephone provides valid group-based estimates of nutrient intake. A similar conclusion was drawn for a 24-hour recall administered in person and validated by observation.[43] Still others contend that the accuracy of the 24-hour recall may be overestimated because comparisons between nutrient intakes across methods may conceal differences in food intakes.[44] These studies provide evidence that reporting errors occur, but indications of their direction or extent are not consistent from study to study or from nutrient to nutrient.

Sources of error that affect the reliability of the 24-hour recall have been examined.[45,46] Some focus has been placed on the reliability of nutrient intake estimates obtained from parents of preschool children using 24-hour recall administered over varying numbers of days.[47] Strengths and weaknesses of the 24-hour food recall are outlined in Table 3.

Food frequency questionnaires. The use of food frequency questionnaires to provide a measure of "usual" intake by an individual in epidemiological studies of diet and health relationships has expanded markedly.[13,48] Usual dietary intake over an extended period is more pertinent in assessing the relationship of nutrition to chronic disease than is diet on a recent specific day or week.[49] The method often is used to rank individuals by food or nutrient intake so that characteristics, including disease status, of those with high and low intakes may be compared. The questionnaires vary as to the foods listed, the length of time covered by the reference period, the response intervals for specifying frequency, the procedure for estimating portion size, the nutrient composition database, as well as in the manner the questionnaire is administered. Food frequency questionnaires may be viewed more accurately as a family of methods because specific procedures vary greatly and perform differently in different populations.

The types of foods listed vary depending on whether the researcher is interested in specific nutrients or the total diet.[50] The food lists may include only items high in a specified nutrient, such as calcium, or attempt to represent the total diet.[33,51-53] To derive nutrient intake estimates, these methods require assignment of a nutrient value for each food group listed. The value may be based on the predominant food in the group, on weighting each food in the group by usage, or on some other similar system.

Qualitative food frequency questionnaires generally obtain only the usual number of times each food is eaten during a specified period, such as the past month; information on portion size is not collected.[33] However, information on portion size is necessary for calculations of nutrient intakes and sometimes an average portion size is estimated to allow for nutrient intakes to be calculated.[54] Quantitative methods require subjects to report the amount of food eaten, usually with the use of measurement aids.[52,55] For semiquantitative methods, researchers often provide standard (or average) portion size categories for subjects to respond to.[53]

Reference time periods vary from as short as a few days, 1 week, 1 month, or 3 months to ≥1 year. For example, in a semiquantitative questionnaire with a list of 131 food items, respondents indicated how often during the past year, on average, they had eaten a commonly used portion size.[32] Nine response categories ranged from never or less than once per month to six or more times per day. Food frequency questionnaires may be administered in person, be self-administered, or be administered by a combination of methods.[32,55,56] Computerized versions have also been developed.[57-59] Optical scanning technology has been used to expedite data processing.[60] The many food frequency questionnaires engender considerable discussion about their current use and future development.[13,48,50,60-64]

The validity of various food frequency instruments has been evaluated by comparing results with those from alternative methods. Pietinen et al found generally comparable some nutrient values derived from a 44-item qualitative food frequency questionnaire and from 12 diet records each kept for 2 days.[54] Krall and Dwyer[25] administered a semiquantitative food frequency questionnaire to volunteers in a metabolic study using weighed portions and found that their food frequency questionnaire underestimated values for energy and nutrients. Rimm and coworkers[32] compared results obtained from two administrations of a 131-item semiquantitative food frequency questionnaire with data from two 1-week food records. For data collected from 127 men, they found that Pearson correlation coefficients calculated between the second questionnaire and the average of the two 1-week food records ranged from 0.28 (iron, without supplements) to 0.87 (vitamin E). Stein and coworkers[53] found poor agreement and poor relative validity between two administrations of a semiquantitative food frequency questionnaire and four administrations of a 24-hour food

recall to a sample composed mainly of Hispanic children. (Parents reported their children's intake.) The food frequency questionnaires yielded mean energy and nutrient intakes which were 1.4–1.9 times greater than those obtained from the recalls. This study suggests that this type of food frequency questionnaire may not work well for Hispanics or young children.[53]

In one study, two different food frequency questionnaires were compared to the same set of reference data (16 days of recall/records collected across all seasons and days of the week).[56] When compared to the estimates derived from the recall/records, one questionnaire yielded energy and nutrient intake estimates which were similar to the reference values and the other produced estimates which were higher. Findings from an earlier study indicated that food frequency questionnaires yielded higher energy and nutrient estimates than recall/records.[65]

Reliability of the food frequency questionnaire was assessed in terms of the correlation between two administrations of the questionnaire. The reproducibility of a questionnaire can be affected by several factors such as the amount of time which has elapsed between repeated administrations, the adequacy of instructions for subjects, and the available range of response options and portion sizes.[66] Pietinen et al demonstrated good reproducibility (correlations of 0.48–0.86) for nutrients in three administrations of a food frequency questionnaire to a fairly homogeneous group of Finnish middleaged men.[54] More recently, researchers found that a mailed selfadministered food frequency questionnaire shows adequate reproducibility when used with adult males.[32] Poorer performance was shown by a group of older children and adolescents (mean age = 14 years).[67] Strengths and weaknesses of the food frequency questionnaires are listed in Table 4.

Diet history method. The diet history method was developed originally by Burke[68] to obtain information at regular intervals about dietary habits and the usual diet for use in longitudinal studies of human growth and development. The method incorporated three components: an interview about usual eating patterns, a food list with amounts and usual frequency of eating, and a 3-day food record.[13,68] More recently, modifications of the diet history were designed by epidemiologists to study associations between diet and the onset of such chronic illnesses as cancer and heart disease.[69-73] Individuals are often asked to recall their food intake for the past month, several months, or one year. For design of dietary questionnaires Block et al[74] recommends a data-based approach which uses data previously collected from the target population to construct the food list, portion sizes, and nutrient content of food items. A frequency-type diet history used in the National Health Interview Survey (NHIS) 1987 provides estimates of usual and customary intake.[75] To date, no single method has been accepted for collecting diet history and many variations appear in the literature.

Table 4. Strengths and weaknesses of food frequency questionnaires

Strengths	Weaknesses
1. An indication of usual dietary intake may be obtained.	1. Memory of food patterns in the past is required.
2. Highly trained interviewers are not required.	2. Period of recall may be imprecise.
3. Method can be interviewer administered or self-administered.	3. Quantification of food intake may be imprecise because of poor estimation or recall of portions or use of standard sizes.
4. Administration may be simple and less costly.	4. Respondent burden is governed by number and complexity of foods listed and quantification procedure.
5. Customary eating patterns are not affected.	
6. Individuals may be ranked or classified by food intake.	5. Recall of past diets may be biased by current diets.
7. Response rates are high.	6. Heterogeneity of population influences the reliability of the method.
8. Respondent burden is usually light.	7. Suitability is questionable for certain segments of the population who may not consume foods on the list.
9. Relationship between diet and disease may be examined in epidemiological studies.	
10. Data on the total diet can be obtained or data on selected foods or nutrients.	8. Intakes tend to be overestimated compared with some other methods.
11. Procedure can be administered by mail.	9. Specific descriptions of foods are not usually obtained.
12. Procedure can be automated.	10. Validation of the method is difficult.

The diet history generally obtains the usual intake of foods in terms of frequencies and quantities ingested and often is similar to quantitative food frequency questionnaires. Diet histories may obtain information about food preparation (e.g., removal of skin from poultry) and consumption practices (e.g., use of salt) in the habitual diets of the subjects under study.[70] A diet history usually focuses on foods in the total diet but some have focused on specific dietary constituents.[71,76] The Coronary Artery Risk Factor Development in Young Adults (CARDIA) study uses a diet history which was modeled after an earlier study of coronary heart disease, the Western Electric Study.[70,77] The CARDIA instrument has now been computerized, as have diet histories developed by other researchers.[15,78]

Although highly trained interviewers with backgrounds in nutrition are most often required, interviewers who are not nutritionists or dietitians can be trained as procedures become more standardized.[79] Hankin[80] suggests collecting frequency and quantitative data on foods consumed by a population group as a basis for developing a suitable diet history questionnaire—a data-based approach. To increase accuracy of reported portion sizes, she uses photographs of small, medium, and large servings of each food. Byers et al.[73] also used pictures of food to help recall, others have used models.[71] Jain[71] described in detail a method used by an epidemiology unit in Canada.

Some researchers who assess the validity of diet histories have found that those covering a 1-year period produce higher estimates of intakes than do food records.[69] Also, the CARDIA diet history produced higher estimates of nutrient intake when compared to mean estimates that resulted from a series of 24-hour recalls administered by telephone.[70] Using 24-hour urine nitro-

gen excretion as a validation method, a diet history covering a 1-month period produced no group based differences between nitrogen intake and excretion.[81] Repeated administrations of the diet history indicated that reproducibility was acceptable.[82,83] Strengths and weaknesses of the diet history method are listed in Table 5.

Combination of methods. Sometimes a combination of two or more methods provides greater accuracy; the shortcomings of one method are counterbalanced by the strengths of another.[2,14] For example, as presented in Table 1, the NFCSs 1977–1978 and 1987–1988 conducted by the USDA used a combination of a 1-day food recall and 2-day food record.[7]

Number of days. The number of days for which food intake is obtained by food recall or food record contributes to how the dietary intake estimates can be used.[1,45] One-day dietary intakes from a large sample provide reliable estimates of mean intakes for the group but not for an individual in the group. Intraindividual variation is greater in 1-day dietary data and may conceal relationships between diet and disease.[46] An expert committee considered 1-day data to be less preferable than data from multiple days for such studies.[1]

Collecting many days of dietary information using either the recall or record method decreases intraindividual variation and increases precision of intake estimates.[1] Beaton et al.[46] demonstrated that the width of a confidence interval for estimating the mean of the group is decreased by increasing either sample size or number of intake days. Each additional day of intake information provides an increasingly smaller increment of independent information.[1] A statistical method has been developed for the estimation of the distribution of usual nutrient intakes in a population when at least two independent recalls are available.[84]

Table 5. Strengths and weaknesses of diet history methods

Strengths	Weaknesses
1. Method yields a more representative pattern of usual intakes in the past than other methods. 2. Measurement of usual diet is useful in epidemiological studies of disease states that develop slowly over time. 3. For interviewer-administered methods, respondent literacy is not required. 4. Generally, method is designed to assess total diet.	1. Highly trained interviewers are usually required. 2. Recall period is difficult to conceptualize accurately. 3. Respondents must be highly cooperative. 4. Respondent and interviewer burden may be heavy. 5. Method may require considerable time and cost. 6. The method tends to overestimate intakes compared with other methods. 7. Recall of diets in the past may be biased by current diets.

Measurement error. Dietary intake measures can have both random and systematic errors. Measurement error may originate from the dietary method, the interviewer, the respondent, or the coding process.[4] For example, measurement error can occur when food intakes are based on reports by respondents who describe the kinds and amounts of foods with an unknown degree of precision. Another source of error is in the use of food composition tables which consist of values representative of foods across the nation and across the seasons, but may not be specific for the food items eaten by an individual. Gibson has discussed the impact of these and other errors on estimation of dietary intakes.[4]

Interviewers. The good performance of interviewers is crucial for obtaining reliable and valid data in surveys as well as in special studies. Consequently, interviewers' qualifications, training, and supervision must be given careful attention. Ideally, interviewers should have skill in interviewing techniques and knowledge of food preparation. Training courses provide standardized preparation and practice. Use of reference manuals promotes consistency in performance across time and among interviewers to assure the collection of high-quality data[33] (USDA, "What We Eat in America 1994–1996," unpublished interviewer manual). Computer-assisted interviews may require additional training time. Field work is monitored to ensure that procedures are followed uniformly and problems are handled promptly. Telephone interviewers usually work in a central location, which simplifies supervision.

Advances are being made in the automation of the collection and processing of dietary data for both large and small-scale studies.[15,20,22,33,58,59,78,85,86] Weeks[87] discusses several variations of telephone, face-to-face, and self-administered computerized procedures that have been used in survey research. Some contend that automation could improve the accuracy of data and the costs associated with data collection and processing.[85,88,89] The advantages suggested are improved standardization of probing questions, use of skip patterns, data editing and print-out capabilities, linkage to other data sets, and collection of sensitive information.[57,58,86,89] Birkett, found, however, that a computer-based method resulted in longer interview times and had some hardware-based limitations (e.g., display was difficult to read).[86] Other limitations may involve the level of computer literacy required and the level of ease experienced by system users.[58]

Data Processing and Analysis

Data processing and analysis are included in the planning of a survey or study in order to ensure that required information is collected in usable form. After food intake information has been collected, it must be processed to provide variables and data for analyses that fulfill the objectives of the study. Generally, questionnaires from large surveys are processed in a central office. They are reviewed, edited, and coded immediately upon arrival in case additional information is necessary. Coding is the assignment, either by hand tally or by computer, of numbers to responses for the purpose of data reduction and categorization. Food codes are used to organize food groups according to the system design.

Survey Net, a computer-assisted food coding and nutrient calculation system, is being used to process food intake data for the current USDA nationwide dietary intake survey. The data bases which support Survey Net include food descriptions, household measures and portion size descriptions and weights, recipes, food composition values, and nutrient retention factors. Survey Net capabilities include rapid and effective data entry and retrieval of food intake data, on-line editing features which allow users to modify existing recipes, and translation of food intake data into nutrient intake data. USDA is also developing a computerized system to monitor changes in consumption trends which takes into account improvements that occur in the food composition and other Survey Net data bases.

A major use of dietary intake surveys is estimating the food and nutrient intakes of population groups categorized by sex, age, income, region, and other characteristics. Mean food and nutrient intakes among population subgroups are compared to determine the most commonly eaten foods and variations in eating patterns. Food intakes from the different food groups can be reported.[23] Food consumption data can be converted to servings per day to compare food intakes to dietary guidance recommendations.[90]

Conclusions

Many factors are considered when a procedure for estimating individual dietary intake is chosen. No one method is suitable for all purposes, and all methods have strengths and weaknesses that require tradeoffs. Although four categories of data collection methods are described, numerous variations of each method or a combination of methods can accommodate the special circumstances of particular studies. However, each change in method can affect its validity and reliability. Short-term daily quantitative measures or estimates of intake obtained with food recalls or food records differ substantially in concept from longer term usual intake measures, or estimates of intake obtained with food frequencies or diet histories. Equally important to achievement of study goals is the processing of data from the food intake questionnaires, the review, editing, coding, and adequacy of databases, as well as careful analysis and interpretation of results. Moreover, researchers and users of study results must recognize the limitations of the data and the implications for interpretation.

References

1. Anderson SA, ed (1986) Guidelines for use of dietary intake data. Life Sciences Research Office, Federation of American Societies for Experimental Biology, Bethesda, MD
2. Burk MC, Pao EM (1976) Methodology for large-scale surveys of household and individual diets. Home Economic Research Report No. 40, US Government Printing Office, Washington, DC
3. Bingham SA, Nelson M, Paul AA, et al (1988) Methods for data collection at an individual level. In Cameron ME, Van Staveren WA (eds), Manual on methodology for food consumption studies. Oxford University Press, New York, NY, pp 53–106
4. Gibson RS (1987) Sources of error and variability in dietary assessment methods: a review. J Can Diet Assoc 48:150–155
5. Medlin C, Skinner JD (1988) Individual dietary intake methodology: a 50-year review of progress. J Am Diet Assoc 88:1250–1257
6. Block G, Hartman AM (1989a) Dietary assessment methods. In Moon TE, Micozzi MS (eds), Nutrition and cancer prevention: investigating the role of micronutrients. Marcel Dekker, Inc., New York, NY, pp 159–180
7. Pao EM, Sykes KE, Cypel YS (1989) USDA methodological research for large-scale dietary intake surveys, 1975–88. Home Economics Research Report No. 49, US Government Printing Office, Washington, DC
8. Samet JM (1989) Surrogate measures of dietary intake. Am J Clin Nutr 50:1139–1144
9. Willett W (1990) Nutritional epidemiology. Oxford University Press, New York, NY
10. Fox TA, Heimendinger J, Block G (1992) Telephone surveys as a method for obtaining dietary information: a review. J Am Diet Assoc 92:729–732
11. Hankin JH (1992) Dietary intake methodology. In Monsen ER (ed), Research: successful approaches. American Dietetic Association, Chicago, IL, pp 173–194
12. Sempos CT, Flegal KM, Johnson CL, et al (1993) Issues in the long-term evaluation of diet in longitudinal studies. J Nutr 123:406–412
13. Thompson FE, Byers T (1994) Dietary assessment resource manual. J Nutr 124(suppl):2245S–2317S
14. Dwyer JT (1994) Dietary assessment. In Shils ME, Olson JA, Shike M (eds), Chapter 52, Modern nutrition in health and disease, 8th ed, Vol 1. Lea & Febiger, Philadelphia, pp 842–860
15. Kohlmeier L (1994) Gaps in dietary assessment methodology: meal- vs list-based methods. Am J Clin Nutr 59(suppl):175S–179S
16. Kohlmeier L (1993) Overview of validity, quality control and measurement error issues in nutritional epidemiology. Eur J Clin Nutr 47(suppl 2):S1–S5
17. Bandini LG, Schoeller DA, Cyr HN, Dietz WH (1990) Validity of reported energy intake in obese and nonobese adolescents. Am J Clin Nutr 52:421–425
18. Kim WW, Mertz W, Judd JT, et al (1984) Effect of making duplicate food collections on nutrient intakes calculated from diet records. Am J Clin Nutr 40:1333–1337
19. Dop MC, Milan C, Milan C, N'Diaye AM (1994) Use of the multiple-day weighed record for Senegalese children during the weaning period: a case of the "instrument effect." Am J Clin Nutr 59(suppl):266S–268S
20. Kretsch MJ, Fong AKH (1990) Validation of a new computerized technique for quantitating individual dietary intake: the Nutrition Evaluation Scale System (NESS) vs the weighed food record. Am J Clin Nutr 51:477–484
21. Bingham SA (1991) Limitations of the various methods for collecting dietary intake data. Ann Nutr Metab 35:117–127
22. US Department of Agriculture (1993) Food and nutrient intakes by individuals in the United States, 1, 1987–88. Nationwide Food Consumption Survey 1987–88, NFCS Rep. No. 87-I-1. US Government Printing Office, Washington, DC
23. US Department of Agriculture (1995) Food and nutrient intakes by individuals in the United States, 1, 1989–91. Continuing Survey of Food Intakes by Individuals 1989–91, NFS Rep. No. 91-2. US Government Printing Office, Washington, DC
24. Sempos CT, Johnson NE, Smith EL, Gilligan C (1984) A two-year dietary survey of middle-aged women: repeated dietary records as a measure of usual intake. J Am Diet Assoc 84:1008–1013
25. Krall EA, Dwyer JT (1987) Validity of a food frequency questionnaire and a food diary in a short-term recall situation. J Am Diet Assoc 87:1374–1377
26. Mertz W, Tsui JC, Judd JT, et al (1991) What are people really eating? the relation between energy intake derived from estimated diet records and intake determined to maintain body weight. Am J Clin Nutr 54:291–295
27. Karvetti RL, Knuts LR (1992) Validity of the estimated food diary: comparison of 2-day recorded and observed food and nutrient intakes. J Am Diet Assoc 92:580–584
28. Gersovitz M, Madden JP, Smiciklas-Wright H (1978) Validity of the 24-hr dietary recall and seven-day record for group comparisons. J Am Diet Assoc 73:48–55
29. Livingstone MBE, Prentice AM, Coward WA, et al (1992) Validation of estimates of energy intake by weighed dietary record and diet history in children and adolescents. Am J Clin Nutr 56:29–35
30. Black AE, Prentice AM, Goldberg GR, et al (1993) Measurements of total energy expenditure provide insights into the

validity of dietary measurements of energy intake. J Am Diet Assoc 93:572–579

31. Mertz W (1992) Food intake measurements: is there a "gold standard"? J Am Diet Assoc 92:1463–1465

32. Rimm EB, Giovannucci EL, Stampfer MJ, et al (1992) Reproducibility and validity of an expanded self-administered semiquantitative food frequency questionnaire among male health professionals. Am J Epidemiol 135:1114–1126

33. US Department of Health and Human Services (1994) Plan and operation of the Third National Health and Nutrition Examination Survey, 1988–94. National Center for Health Statistics, Vital Health Stat 1(32), (PHS) 94-1308. US Government Printing Office, Washington, DC

34. Mullenbach V, Kushi LH, Jacobson C, et al (1992) Comparison of 3-day food record and 24-hour recall by telephone for dietary evaluation in adolescents. J Am Diet Assoc 92:743–745

35. DeMaio TJ, Ciochetto S, Davis WL (1993) Research on the Continuing Survey of Food Intakes by Individuals. In Proceedings of the Section on Survey Research Methods, ASA, Vol 2. American Statistical Association, Alexandria, VA, pp 1021–1025

36. Achterberg C, Pugh MA, Collins S, et al (1991) Feasibility of telephone interviews to collect dietary recall information from children. J Can Diet Assoc 52:226–228

37. Dubois S, Boivin JF (1990) Accuracy of telephone dietary recalls in elderly subjects. J Am Diet Assoc 90:1680–1687

38. US Department of Agriculture (1987) Continuing survey of food intakes by individuals: women 19–50 years and their children 1–5 years, 4 days, 1985. NFCS, CSFII Report No. 85-4. US Government Printing Office, Washington, DC

39. Dwyer JT, Krall EA, Coleman KA (1987) The problem of memory in nutritional epidemiology research. J Am Diet Assoc 87:1509–1512

40. Madden JP, Goodman SJ, Guthrie HA (1976) Validity of the 24-hr recall. J Am Diet Assoc 68:143–147

41. Posner BM, Smigelski C, Duggal A, et al (1992) Validation of two-dimensional models for estimation of portion size in nutrition research. J Am Diet Assoc 92:738–741

42. Linusson EEI, Sanjur D, Erickson EC (1974) Validating the 24-hour recall method as a dietary survey tool. Arch Latinoam Nutr 24:277–294

43. Karvetti RL, Knuts LR (1985) Validity of the 24-hour dietary recall. J Am Diet Assoc 85:1437–1442

44. Baranowski T, Sprague D, Baranowski JH, Harrison JA (1991) Accuracy of maternal dietary recall for preschool children. J Am Diet Assoc 91:669–674

45. Beaton GH, Milner J, McGuire V, et al (1983) Source of variance in 24-hour dietary recall data: implications for nutrition study design and interpretation: carbohydrate sources, vitamins, and minerals. Am J Clin Nutr 37:986–995

46. Beaton GH, Milner J, Corey P, et al (1979) Sources of variance in 24-hour dietary recall data: implications for nutrition study design and interpretation. Am J Clin Nutr 32:2546–2559

47. Treiber FA, Leonard SB, Frank G, et al (1990) Dietary assessment instruments for preschool children: reliability of parental responses to the 24-hour recall and food frequency questionnaire. J Am Diet Assoc 90:814–820

48. Willett WC (1994) Future directions in the development of food-frequency questionnaires. Am J Clin Nutr 59(suppl): 171S–174S

49. Sampson L (1985) Food frequency questionnaires as a research instrument. Clin Nutr 4:171–178

50. Zulkifli SN, Yu SM (1992) The food frequency method for dietary assessment. J Am Diet Assoc 92:681–685

51. Angus RM, Sambrook PN, Pocock NA, Eisman JA (1989) A simple method for assessing calcium intake in Caucasian women. J Am Diet Assoc 89:209–214

52. Frank GC, Nicklas TA, Webber LS, et al (1992) A food frequency questionnaire for adolescents: defining eating patterns. J Am Diet Assoc 92:313–318

53. Stein AD, Shea S, Basch CE, et al (1992) Consistency of the Willett semiquantitative food frequency questionnaire and 24-hour dietary recalls in estimating nutrient intakes of preschool children. Am J Epidemiol 135:667–677

54. Pietinen P, Hartman AM, Haapa E, et al (1988) Reproducibility and validity of dietary assessment instruments. II. A qualitative food frequency questionnaire. Am J Epidemiol 128:667–676

55. Clapp JA, McPherson RS, Reed DB, Hsi BP (1991) Comparison of a food frequency questionnaire using reported vs standard portion sizes for classifying individuals according to nutrient intake. J Am Diet Assoc 91:316–320

56. Block G, Thompson FE, Hartman AM, et al (1992) Comparison of two dietary questionnaires validated against multiple dietary records collected during a 1-year period. J Am Diet Assoc 92:686–693

57. Vailas LI, Blankenhorn DH, Selzer RH, Johnson RL (1987) A computerized quantitative food frequency analysis for the clinical setting: use in documentation and counseling. J Am Diet Assoc 87:1539–1543

58. Suitor CW, Gardner JD (1992) Development of an interactive, self-administered computerized food frequency questionnaire for use with low-income women. J Nutr Educ 24:82–86

59. Block G, Coyle LM, Hartman AM, Scoppa SM (1994) Revision of dietary analysis software for the Health Habits and History Questionnaire. Am J Epidemiol 139:1190–1196

60. Kushi LH (1994) Gaps in epidemiologic research methods: design considerations for studies that use food-frequency questionnaires. Am J Clin Nutr 59(suppl):180S–184S

61. Liu K (1994) Statistical issues related to semiquantitative food-frequency questionnaires. Am J Clin Nutr 59(suppl):262S–265S

62. Rimm EB, Giovannucci EL, Stampfer MJ, et al (1992) Authors' response to "invited commentary: some limitations of semiquantitative food frequency questionnaires." Am J Epidemiol 135:1133–1136

63. Sempos CT (1992) Invited commentary: some limitations of semiquantitative food frequency questionnaires. Am J Epidemiol 135:1127–1132

64. Briefel RR, Flegal KM, Winn DM, et al (1992) Assessing the nation's diet: limitations of the food frequency questionnaire. J Am Diet Assoc 92:959–962

65. Larkin FA, Metzner HL, Thompson FE, et al (1989) Comparison of estimated nutrient intakes by food frequency and dietary records in adults. J Am Diet Assoc 89:215–223

66. Block G, Hartman AM (1989b) Issues in reproducibility and validity of dietary studies. Am J Clin Nutr 50:1133–1138

67. Rockett HRH, Wolf AM, Colditz GA (1995) Development and reproducibility of a food frequency questionnaire to assess diets of older children and adolescents. J Am Diet Assoc 95:336–340

68. Burke BS (1947) The dietary history as a tool in research. J Am Diet Assoc 23:1041–1046

69. Hankin JH, Wilkens LR, Kolonel LN, Yoshizawa CN (1991) Validation of a quantitative diet history method in Hawaii. Am J Epidemiol 133:616–628

70. McDonald A, Van Horn L, Slattery M, et al (1991) The CARDIA dietary history: development, implementation, and evaluation. J Am Diet Assoc 91:1104–1112

71. Jain M (1989) Diet history: questionnaire and interview

techniques used in some retrospective studies of cancer. J Am Diet Assoc 89:1647–1652

72. Bloemberg BPM, Kromhout D, Obermann-De Boer GL, Van Kampen-Donker M (1989) The reproducibility of dietary intake data assessed with the cross-check dietary history method. Am J Epidemiol 130:1047–1056

73. Byers T, Marshall J, Anthony E, et al (1987) The reliability of dietary history from the distant past. Am J Epidemiol 125:999–1011

74. Block G, Hartman AM, Dresser CM, et al (1986) A data-based approach to diet questionnaire design and testing. Am J Epidemiol 124:453–469

75. Block G, Subar AF (1992) Estimates of nutrient intake from a food frequency questionnaire: the 1987 National Health Interview Survey. J Am Diet Assoc 92:969–977

76. Howe GR, Harrison L, Jain M (1986) A short diet history for assessing dietary exposure to N-nitrosamines in epidemiologic studies. Am J Epidemiol 124:595–601

77. Shekelle RB, Shryock AM, Paul O, et al (1981) Diet, serum cholesterol, and death from coronary heart disease—the Western Electric Study. N Engl J Med 304:65–70

78. Slattery ML, Caan BJ, Duncan D, et al (1994) A computerized diet history questionnaire for epidemiologic studies. J Am Diet Assoc 94:761–766

79. Hankin JH (1986) 23rd Lenna Frances Cooper Memorial Lecture: a diet history method for research, clinical, and community use. J Am Diet Assoc 86:868–875

80. Hankin JH (1989) Development of a diet history questionnaire for studies of older persons. Am J Clin Nutr 50:1121–1127

81. Van Staveren WA, de Boer JO, Burema J (1985) Validity and reproducibility of a dietary history method estimating the usual food intake during one month. Am J Clin Nutr 42:554–559

82. Hankin JH, Yoshizawa CN, Kolonel LN (1990) Reproducibility of a diet history in older men in Hawaii. Nutr Cancer 13:129–140

83. Jain M, Howe GR, Harrison L, Miller AB (1989) A study of repeatability of dietary data over a seven-year period. Am J Epidemiol 129:422–429

84. Nusser SM, Carriquiry AL, Dodd KW, Fuller WA (1995) A semiparametric transformation approach to estimating usual daily intake distributions. Dietary Assessment Research Series Report 2, Staff Report 95-SR 74. Center for Agricultural and Rural Development, Iowa State University, Ames, IA

85. Levine JA, Madden AM, Morgan MY (1987) Validation of a computer based system for assessing dietary intake. Br Med J 295:369–372

86. Birkett NJ (1988) Epidemiologic programs for computers and calculators: computer-aided personal interviewing, a new technique for data collection in epidemiologic surveys. Am J Epidemiol 127:684–690

87. Weeks MF (1992) Computer-assisted survey information collection: a review of CASIC methods and their implications for survey operations. Journal of Official Statistics 8:445–465

88. Kretsch MJ (1989) New computerized techniques for assessing food intake. In Livingston GE (ed), Chapter 10, Nutritional status assessment of the individual. Food and Nutrition Press, Inc., Trumball, CT, pp 105–112

89. Arab L (1985) Computer-assisted dietary assessment. In Taylor TG, Jenkins NK (eds), Proceedings of the XIII International Congress of Nutrition. John Libbey, London, pp 702–706

90. Krebs-Smith SM, Cook DA, Subar AF, et al (1995) US adults' fruit and vegetable intakes, 1989 to 1991: a revised baseline for the Healthy People 2000 objective. Am J Public Health 85:1623–1629

91. Sempos CT, Briefel RR, Johnson C, Woteki CE (1992) Process and rationale for selecting dietary methods for NHANES III. In Dietary methodology workshop for the Third National Health and Nutrition Examination Survey. National Center for Health Statistics, Vital Health Stat 4(27), Hyattsville, MD, pp 85–90

Chapter 51

Nutritional Epidemiology

Valerie Tarasuk

Epidemiology is the health science that deals with the distribution and determinants of health and illness in populations. Although nutritional epidemiology has a distinct methodology, the field is interwoven with other branches of nutrition research. Through epidemiology, diet-disease relationships observed in basic research can be examined at the level of free-living populations and clinically defined subgroups. Similarly, the interpretation of epidemiological findings is strengthened by the integration of knowledge derived from other branches of nutrition research. In this chapter, I present an overview of epidemiological methods commonly applied to nutrition research. Three issues of particular importance in nutritional epidemiology are discussed: the measurement of dietary exposures, the role of epidemiological data in the determination of causal relationships between diet and disease states, and the development of dietary recommendations from epidemiological findings. For a more comprehensive discussion of this vast, complex, and ever-expanding field, readers are referred to selected texts in epidemiology and nutritional epidemiology.[1-3]

Epidemiological studies can be divided into two broad categories: descriptive and analytical studies, and experimental studies. Descriptive and analytical epidemiology describes the distribution and determinants of specific dietary intake patterns and disease outcomes. Study designs include cross-sectional surveys, ecological comparisons, cohort studies, and case-control studies. Experimental epidemiological investigations identify contributors to specific health or disease phenomena through the implementation of classic experimental methods to test specifically defined hypotheses.

Epidemiological research elucidates risk factors for disease that apply across whole groups or populations. Two key concepts underpin conventional epidemiological methods: "caseness" and "exposure." Caseness refers to the determination of the presence or absence of the particular disease or health outcome variable of interest, resulting in the designation of "case" or "control" status. Exposure refers to the measurement of variables believed to be associated with the presence or absence of disease. In nutritional epidemiology, the primary exposure of interest is dietary intake. Studies are designed to estimate the disease risk associated with a particular exposure by comparing disease incidence and exposure levels across groups. Between-group comparisons yield insight into factors underlying disease incidence, but this is distinct from understanding what causes any individual to become a case. Because the unit of analysis is groups or populations, the findings are also at this level. This focus on populations or subpopulations rather than on individuals distinguishes epidemiology from other biomedical sciences. What follows is an overview of study designs characteristic of descriptive and analytical epidemiology and experimental epidemiology. (Practical illustrations of these designs can be found in the accompanying citations.)

Descriptive and Analytical Epidemiology

Cross-sectional surveys. Perhaps the best example of cross-sectional surveys in nutritional epidemiology are the periodic national population surveys of food and nutrient consumption patterns and health and nutritional status indicators conducted in the United States and some other countries.[4] Such surveys provide descriptive epidemiological data on nutrition at a single point in time, identifying nutritional needs in the population and forming a basis for health promotion and disease prevention programs. Repeated surveys become the basis for monitoring population trends in nutrition. When cross-sectional surveys include measures of health or disease status, nutrition and food consumption patterns across the population are analyzed to identify associations with these indicators. The interpretation of associations identified through such analyses is limited, however, because of the contemporaneous measurement of disease status and dietary exposures necessitated by this study design.

Ecological studies. More commonly, cross-sectional population data on food and nutrient consumption patterns are used in ecological comparisons (also termed correlation studies). In these studies, population groups are most commonly defined geographically and population data on diet and disease are compared across countries.[5-7] Food consumption is expressed per capita, with intake estimates often derived from national food disappearance data. This method yields only a crude estimate of actual food consumption and gives no indication of the distribution of food within the population.[8] The strength of ecological comparisons in nutrition lies in the fact that variation in food consumption tends to be greater between than within countries, and national averages tend to be more stable than individual consumption patterns over time.[9] Random errors in the measurement of dietary variables and disease incidence or mortality rates do not bias the estimates of national averages, which form the basis for ecological comparisons.

Ecological studies may also compare indicators of diet and health or disease within a single population over time to look for secular trends or to compare the disease incidence rates and dietary intake patterns of migrant groups with those of comparable populations in the original and new country.[10] Comparisons of cancer rates among successive generations of Japanese immigrants in California, Japanese living in Japan, and white Californians born in the United States provide an early example of this approach.[11] Migrant and secular trend studies are important for examining the role of genetic factors in disease etiology and for differentiating between genetic and environmental influences.

Ecological comparisons have been important in hypothesizing diet and disease relationships.[5,12] Studies of this type, however, have been criticized because an observed relationship between dietary patterns and morbidity or mortality rates measured at the population level may not indicate a similar relationship at the individual level. For example, a correlation may be observed between per capita fat consumption and breast cancer incidence, but it cannot be inferred that the fat intakes of individual women with breast cancer are the same as the per capita estimate. The logical fallacy inherent in drawing causal inferences from group data to individual behaviors is commonly labeled the "ecological fallacy." A second major criticism of ecological studies is that the design does not allow for the adjustment for other known risk factors operating at the individual level (for example, age at menarche, parity, smoking, and obesity). These criticisms do not negate the value of ecological comparisons, however. Schwartz[13] argued that the group-level comparisons found in ecological studies should not be viewed simply as poor proxies for individual-level data. Ecological comparisons offer insight into environmental, contextual, or sociological influences on disease etiology and health-related behaviors that may not be discernible from individual data but which may have important policy implications.[7]

Cohort studies. In cohort studies, subjects are identified on the basis of their exposure to factors of possible etiologic or prognostic importance, followed over time, and then compared on the basis of their disease status at some future date. Cohort studies are most commonly longitudinal or prospective, with subjects being followed

forward in time over some predefined time period to assess disease onset. They may also be retrospective, with groups identified on the basis of exposure sometime in the past and then followed from that time to the present to establish presence or absence of disease. Applying the simplest of analytical approaches to this design, the risk of disease associated with a given exposure is expressed as a relative risk. Multivariate modeling techniques are used to examine diet-disease associations while controlling for the effects of other known risk factors.

Because exposure is ascertained before disease onset, cohort studies enable determination of the timing and directionality of events and thus provide insight into causal relationships between exposures and disease outcomes. Such studies can be very expensive, however, requiring large sample sizes and lengthy follow-up to study the occurrence of disease states that are relatively rare, have lengthy time periods between exposure and detection, or both. Both conditions hold for most cancers. Although cancers are a major cause of death, the malignancy rates for most sites are relatively low, and the time lag between exposure to causal agents and clinical diagnosis of the disease may be several years.[14] Hebert and Miller[14] note that a cohort of 18,000 40-year-old women followed for 10 years would be required to assess a doubling of risk of breast cancer with 95% confidence and 80% power, comparing those in the highest quintile of nutrient intake with those in the lowest quintile. The research costs associated with cohort study designs mean that such studies are far less common than cross-sectional surveys and case-control studies.

Case-control studies. Subjects are identified and recruited into a case-control study on the basis of the presence or absence of the disease or health outcome variable of interest. Ideally, the controls are randomly selected from the same study base as the cases, and identical inclusion and exclusion criteria are applied to each group.[15] The presence of specific dietary exposures or other factors of etiologic interest in subjects is generally established using surveys or medical record reviews. The measurement of exposures may be cross-sectional or retrospective, depending on the research question. An association between the disease and a specific factor is inferred if the frequency of its occurrence is greater in the cases than in the controls. In its simplest form, this association is expressed as an odds ratio.

Within the general framework for case-control studies are several options for study design and control selection.[15-17] For example, controls may be matched with cases at an individual level on the basis of age, sex, or other variables believed to affect disease risk. Matching eliminates variability between cases and controls with respect to the matching variables and thus controls for the confounding effects of these risk factors on the observed relationship. The feasibility of matching cases and controls on the basis of one or more variables depends on the size of the pool from which study subjects can be drawn. The more exact the match, the larger the pool of potential subjects required.

Case-control studies are by far the most logistically feasible of the analytical study designs in epidemiology, but their application to questions of interest to nutritionists is limited by the particular nature of diet-disease relationships. The role of diet in the etiology of chronic diseases is generally believed to be most important before disease onset or in its early stages—likely before it is clinically observable. The insight to be gained from a cross-sectional comparison of dietary exposures between cases and controls is limited by the possibility that the subjects' dietary patterns have changed since the time that diet was most important to the disease process. Retrospective case-control studies attempt to overcome this limitation by measuring past diet using food-frequency or diet history methods.[18] Much has been written about the accuracy with which individuals recall past intake patterns, and the methods of measuring past diet continue to be refined.[19-21] One concern is that recall of past diet by cases may be influenced by their present disease status.[14,19] If such recall bias is present, it will result in the differential misclassification of cases by levels of exposure to specific dietary factors and bias the estimate of disease risk associated with diet. The few studies of recall bias in the reporting of past dietary practices do not suggest that differential misclassification of cases is a major problem, but more research is warranted.[21]

Nested case-control studies sometimes provide an alternative to the retrospective measurement of dietary intake. As the name suggests, these are case-control studies nested within ongoing prospective cohort studies. Subjects diagnosed with a particular condition or disease state at some time after being enrolled in the cohort become "incident cases" for the study. Exposures originally measured as part of the cohort study are compared between the incident cases and a control group also sampled from the cohort. The design overcomes problems of recall bias because the exposures to be analyzed were measured before the diagnosis. Because both cases and controls are drawn from the same cohort, this study design has the added advantage of being able to match individuals on the basis of time of disease onset and thus control for this confounding effect.[17] Although nested case-control studies are constrained by the sampling design and baseline data collection of the cohort studies into which they are inserted, nesting is an economical way to address some nutrition questions.[22]

Experimental Epidemiology

The experimental epidemiologist, like any basic scientist, tries to conduct controlled studies. Human studies, however, unlike animal studies, involve much that the investigator cannot control, particularly when they are conducted on a free-living population. The control of potentially confounding variables in experimental epidemiology is largely achieved through the random allocation of study subjects to groups that receive different exposures to the variable of interest. Indicators of health or disease status are compared across the groups to identify relationships between exposure levels and indicators of disease outcome. For ethical and economic reasons, premorbid endpoints are usually chosen as the outcome variables of interest. Random allocation is intended to ensure that potential confounding variables are randomly distributed across the study groups and thus will not bias study results. Two study designs dominate this area of epidemiology: randomized control trials and crossover studies.

Randomized control trials. In these studies subjects are randomly assigned to either an exposed or nonexposed group, commonly referred to as the treatment group and the control or placebo group. The use of a placebo indistinguishable from the treatment enables both subjects and investigators to be blinded to the treatment. Blinding eliminates the possibility of systematic differences between the exposed and nonexposed groups on the basis of subject or investigator awareness of the groupings. Changes in indicators of health or disease status are compared between the two groups at the end of the experiment to identify the effect of the exposure.

Crossover studies. Crossover designs in epidemiology operate on the same principles as the repeated-measures designs common to basic science research. All study subjects receive the treatment and the placebo for equal periods of time, with a washout period in between. The order in which treatments and placebos are administered is randomized for each study subject. An indicator of health or disease status is measured at the beginning and end of each period, and paired analyses are conducted whereby each subject acts as his or her own control to assess the effect of the treatment. Crossover designs are appropriate only for studies of treatments that have no lasting effects, a feature that limits their utility in nutritional epidemiology.

In general, experimental epidemiological study designs are well suited to the identification of causal relationships between specific exposures and indicators of health or disease status. Application of these methods is limited, however, by the difficulty in controlling exposures and by the enormous expense associated with population-based intervention trials aimed at modifying risk of chronic diseases. It is difficult to effect the sizable and sustained changes in the eating behavior of a free-living adult sample that are required for a controlled intervention study. Attempts to study the effects of more moderate changes in diet and other health-related behaviors have sometimes been compromised by unexpected changes in risk factors among members of the control group, owing in part to changes in the public's awareness of diet-disease relationships and subsequent dietary modifications.[23,24] It is perhaps more feasible to apply experimental study designs to contrast the effects of pharmacological doses of specific nutrient or food components because placebos can be manufactured for these treatments and exposures can be controlled. Studies of the effects of pharmaceuticals, however, may lack generalization and applicability to free-living populations insofar as their relationships to dietary intake patterns are not readily apparent.

In summary, the field of epidemiology encompasses a variety of study designs, including experimental as well as descriptive and analytical studies. The application of these methods to nutrition questions plays a crucial role in learning about diet-disease relationships. Three particular challenges underpin nutritional epidemiology: the measurement of dietary exposures, the determination of causal relationships from epidemiological data, and the derivation of dietary recommendations from epidemiological findings.

Measurement of Dietary Exposures

The application of epidemiological research methods to examine relationships between dietary factors and disease occurrence is compounded by the particular nature of food consumption. As noted earlier, the epidemiological concept of exposure refers to the key variable or variables to be examined for association with the presence or absence of a disease. In nutritional epidemiology, the primary exposure of interest is dietary intake. Diet is not one exposure, however, but a complex set of exposures. Furthermore, the nature of dietary exposures varies over time. Estimation of chronic or continuing levels of exposure to specific dietary variables (i.e., usual intake patterns) is complicated by the within-subject variation in food consumption from one day to the next. The intercorrelation of dietary variables complicates the study of effects associated with individual factors. Furthermore, dietary effects on disease or health outcomes can only be observed if sufficient variation in the dietary exposures of interest is present in the study population. The lack of heterogeneity in the consumption of some nutrients within populations presents a major obstacle to the study of their relationships to disease. Each issue is now examined in more detail.

Measuring usual intake. In studies of diet-disease relationships, continuing or chronic exposure to a dietary factor is generally the measurement of interest. The exception would be in a situation where a single or irregular acute exposure to high levels of a dietary variable might initiate an outcome. This might hold, for example, with a carcinogenic compound. More commonly, however, it is the chronic or usual level of exposure that is thought to be important in disease processes. In this model, day-to-day variations in intake are not of etiologic interest and represent deviations from the variable of real interest, the average or usual level of intake persisting over moderate periods of time (weeks, months, and years).

In epidemiological studies, usual intake is commonly measured using repeated 24-hour dietary recalls, multiple food records, or a food-frequency questionnaire. (See Thompson and Byers[18] for a review of these methods.) The choice of dietary assessment methods is a function of the particular nutrients or food components of interest, the level of precision required for the analyses, and the cost associated with data collection. Semi-quantitative food-frequency questionnaires are often favored over diet histories or repeated 24-hour recalls because they can be self-administered and are far less expensive to code and analyze than the other methods. Some concern has been expressed, however, about the ability of food-frequency methods to adequately capture the intake practices of diverse cultural groups.[25,26]

It is important to recognize that all methods of dietary intake assessment measure intake with error, and error can hamper the identification of associations between dietary exposures and disease occurrence.[27–33] In recent years, much attention has been devoted to the study of sources of error in dietary assessment, including error in the collection, coding, analysis, and interpretation of intake data. (A comprehensive review of this work can be found in Beaton.[34]) The nature and magnitude of measurement errors appear to differ across assessment methods and depend on the particular dietary exposure under study.[29,35] This implies that even within a single study, the ability to detect significant associations between dietary exposures and disease occurrence will vary, depending in part on the accuracy with which the individual exposures were measured.[29]

Measurement errors can be considered under two broad categories: random error and bias or systematic error. Random error in the classification of subjects according to their usual intakes has the effect of biasing risk estimates towards the null, lessening the likelihood that a significant association between diet and disease will be observed. Bias refers to systematic under- or overreporting of intake in an individual or group, and it may be a function of the reporting process or a result of errors in the food composition databases used to code intake data.[34] Bias in dietary data does not affect ability to detect an association (i.e., the statistical power of the study) but can inflate or deflate the risk estimate, depending on the distribution of this error term within the data and on whether it is related to a variable of interest. For example, consider the situation in which both fat intake and obesity are believed to relate to some disease occurrence and overweight subjects systematically underreport their fat intakes (as has been suggested by the results of some studies).[36] The fact that bias in the reporting of fat intake is associated with obesity could have serious consequences for the analysis and interpretation of the association between fat intake and the disease.

Measurement error, whether random or systematic, can have a serious effect on the analysis and interpretation of relationships between dietary exposures and disease occurrence. Although methods are being refined, it is widely acknowledged that measurement error will probably never be entirely eliminated from dietary assessment.[34,37] One means to address the effect of error is to include substudies to enable estimation of the nature and magnitude of the error associated with the particular dietary assessment method being used in the full study. When 24-hour recalls are being used, the data collection can be designed to enable estimation of within-subject variance in intake (e.g., through the repeated measurement of intake on a representative subsample of the study population), and statistical procedures can be applied to minimize this effect on subsequent estimates.[30] Estimation of the error may permit statistical adjustment of distributional data before analysis.[30] Knowledge of the measurement error associated with a particular dietary assessment method can be used to estimate and correct for the effect of this error on correlation and regression coefficients.[3,31,38] Calibration or standardization substudies, in which an alternate dietary assessment method is applied to a representative subsample of the study population, can be used to obtain estimates of the measurement error associated with semiquantitative food-frequency questionnaires.[39] Calibration methods have also recently been proposed as a means to adjust for differences in bias due to errors in dietary exposure estimates across diverse cultural groups in a multicenter cohort study.[40]

The measurement of biochemical markers of dietary exposures has been proposed as one means to overcome the problems associated with the accurate measurement of dietary intake in observational studies.[41] Markers used in recent population-based studies include plasma carotenoids, plasma α-tocopherol levels, and toenail selenium levels. Few currently available biochemical markers, however, appear to provide a good approximation of dietary intake.[14] Physiological levels can be influenced by genetic, clinical, and environmental factors in addition to levels of intake. The precise time period of intake represented by a biochemical marker is often difficult to specify, but it is crucial to the design and interpretation of epidemiological studies. Markers that reflect recent intake, for example, would be uninformative in a case-control study if the goal was to understand the role of dietary factors in disease etiology. Even if bio-chemical levels of a particular food component are associated with increased risk, lack of knowledge about the exact relationship between intake levels and the biochemical marker in question hampers the ability to draw dietary recommendations from the study results.

Intercorrelation of dietary exposures. Intercorrelations between specific nutrients or food constituents within the diet make it difficult to isolate the effects of any one factor. A variable that appears to be important may simply be a proxy for some other, unmeasured exposure that is present in the same foods as the proxy. Analytical and interpretational problems also arise in attempts to separate generic from specific effects of complex food components (e.g., the overall effect of carbohydrate versus the effects of simple and complex carbohydrates, or the effect of total fat intake versus the effects attributable to individual fat components).[42] Several different analytical approaches have been proposed to differentiate the effect of total energy intake from specific macronutrient effects on disease risk.[43–46] Wacholder et al.[42] suggested, however, that it may be impossible to isolate the effects of individual dietary factors in the analysis of intake data from observational studies. Using data from a large Iowa cohort of postmenopausal women, Kushi et al.[47] contrasted the results obtained from four different analytical approaches to control for the effect of total energy intake while examining the relationship between dietary fat and breast cancer. The methods yielded different results. It appears that there are differences in the error structures of the variables derived from these approaches and subtle differences in the biological questions they address.[48] These findings suggest that there is no one right way to differentiate between energy and macronutrient effects in analysis, but that the analytical approach used does influence the interpretation of study findings.

Variation in intakes within populations. An additional consideration in the interpretation of epidemiological investigations of diet-disease relationships is the sometimes limited variation in dietary intake within a population. An association between specific intake patterns or food components and a disease outcome will be imperceptible if insufficient variation exists in the intake practices of interest within the study population. Risk cannot be inferred beyond the range of intake exposures observed in the study. If little or no variation in exposure exists, then studies simply yield markers of individual susceptibility.[49] The current controversy over the interpretation of the largely negative results from recent U.S. and Canadian studies of dietary fat and breast cancer is a case in point.[39] It is not clear whether the absence of a strong association is a function of the lack of contrast in observed dietary fat intakes within these study populations or whether, indeed, no causal link between dietary fat and breast cancer exists.

The likelihood of detecting risk associated with a variable for which a narrow range of intake levels is observed is further limited by inaccuracies in the measurement of individual intakes.[12,14] As noted earlier, random error in intake measurements biases the risk estimate toward the null. Whereas the true risk associated with the upper versus lower ends of a narrow range of intakes is likely small, the observed risk will be even smaller given the attenuation associated with random error in intake measurements. Detection of risk under such circumstances requires an extremely large sample size. Hebert and Miller[14] estimated that if the true risk of breast cancer in 40-year-old women in the United States was doubled (comparing the extreme upper and lower quintiles of some dietary exposure) but inaccuracies in the dietary assessment halved the detectable risk, 30,000 women would need to be followed for 10 years to detect this apparent 50% increase in risk. If the range of intakes within the population was increased so that the true risk was 4.0 between the highest and lowest quintiles of intake, the required sample size would drop to 18,000. If the accuracy of the intake assessments was improved so that the true relative risk of 4.0 was detectable, the sample size could be reduced to 3000 women.

Kushi[39] reviewed three study designs to increase contrast in observed dietary exposures. One option to maximize contrast is to recruit subjects from defined population subgroups who adhere to particular dietary regimens (e.g., vegetarians and religious groups with particular dietary practices). A second is the implementation of a two-stage sampling design in which individuals are screened for intake levels and those at the extreme ends of the distribution are oversampled. Finally, sampling can be spread across countries with different dietary practices. Whereas between-country comparisons were traditionally a feature of ecological comparisons, multicountry cohort and case-control study designs are becoming increasingly popular as a means to maximize the range of observable exposures.[40]

Determination of Causation from Epidemiological Data

In nutritional epidemiology, the determination of causal relationships between dietary exposures and disease outcomes is generally a matter of inference, requiring the meticulous assembly and thoughtful review of evidence from a wide variety of sources.[5,50,51] Numerous criteria have been identified for the inference of causality from epidemiological data.[1] These criteria speak to the importance of observed associations being congruent with other epidemiological, clinical, and laboratory research findings. To be considered causal, an association between a specific dietary exposure and disease occurrence should be observed consistently across several population-based studies, ideally conducted by different research groups in different settings. The association should be biologically plausible as well and supported by research into the disease process. It is also important that the exposure precede the onset of disease. (This highlights the strength of cohort studies and emphasizes the problem inherent in drawing causal inferences from cross-sectional measures.) In addition, the argument for causality is strengthened when the disease outcome is specific to the dietary exposure and a biological gradient (dose-response relationship) is observable, i.e., increased exposure to the putative causal agent is associated with increased risk of disease. It should be recognized, however, that criteria for causality cannot be simplistically applied as a checklist; failure to fulfill specific criteria may not indicate the absence of a causal relationship.

The inference of causality in nutritional epidemiology is compounded by the multifactorial nature of most chronic diseases linked to dietary factors. Dietary patterns are often specific to population subgroups defined by other variables such as smoking behavior, income, region, or ethnicity—variables that may themselves be associated with disease incidence. Such interrelationships confound the interpretation of observed associations between diet and disease, raising the question of whether the dietary variables are merely markers for some other exposure that is the real causal agent. If potentially confounding factors are known at the outset, it may be possible to control them (e.g., by using confounders such as ethnicity as matching variables in a case-control study) or to measure the factors and adjust for their effects using multivariate techniques. Such steps can be taken, however, only if the study is designed with the factors in mind, and this is not always the case.

Just as the determination of causality in nutritional epidemiology is complicated, so is the rejection of hypothesized causal relationships between dietary exposures and disease occurrence. The absence of an observed relationship between diet and disease is not conclusive evidence of the absence of a relationship. As noted earlier, random error in the measurement of intake will bias risk estimates toward the null. Similarly, a lack of variation in intake levels within the study population will render dietary effects imperceptible. If a randomized control trial yields equivocal results, it may be because the trial did not continue long enough or the study population did not include enough susceptible individuals (i.e., individuals with low dietary intakes of the factor under study) to observe an intervention effect. In summary, issues of study design and measurement make it difficult to identify relationships in nutritional epidemiology but also thwart the rejection of hypotheses regarding diet-disease relationships when studies fail to yield significant associations.

Development of Dietary Recommendations

One of the primary goals of nutritional epidemiology is to determine the etiologic importance of dietary factors for major chronic diseases. When causal relationships are established, the translation of epidemiological findings into public health recommendations for disease prevention is an essential next step. This is an area of nutrition marked by considerable controversy and confusion.[52,53] Dietary recommendations may take the form of guidelines that give qualitative advice, or they may be in the form of dietary goals that make quantitative recommendations. The generation of dietary recommendations to reduce risk of chronic disease must be recognized as conceptually and analytically distinct from the process of establishing recommendations for the prevention of nutrient deficiencies.

Two issues should be considered in generating recommendations from epidemiological data on diet-disease relationships: 1) the strength of the observed association between a particular dietary exposure and disease occurrence, and 2) the risk of disease occurrence within the population. Together, the issues indicate the expected effect of dietary change on the disease in question for the population as a whole. Application of these principles in the development of recommendations is far from straightforward, however. The risks of chronic disease associated with specific dietary exposures tend to be small. Perhaps this reflects attenuation in risk estimates because of errors in the measurement of dietary variables, or perhaps it is a function of the lack of variation in dietary exposures present within a population. Alternatively, the small effects may reflect the fact that chronic diseases tend to have multifactorial etiologies, so diet is just one of several risk factors. Against this backdrop, nutritionists are challenged to decide when the evidence is sufficient to warrant specific dietary recommendations.

When consensus about the relationship between specific dietary exposures and disease risk is reached, recommendations often take the form of dietary guidelines (e.g., to reduce consumption of saturated fats or to increase consumption of fresh fruits and vegetables). These guidelines tend to be descriptions of general trends in dietary patterns that have been observed to be associated with lower disease risk. Their nonspecific nature, however, limits their use for assessment, monitoring, and intervention.

Both conceptual and practical difficulties underline the translation of epidemiological data into quantitative recommendations for the population. The development of quantitative recommendations requires the determination of an optimal level or an optimal range of intake to minimize risk of chronic disease. The risk estimates derived from analytical epidemiological studies, however, typically refer to the level of risk associated with a population or group mean level of exposure. They do not indicate absolute levels of danger. Hence the data required to define optimal intake are often incomplete, and the setting of quantitative recommendations becomes a matter of judgment (and debate).[53]

The generation of quantitative dietary recommendations from epidemiological evidence is further complicated when the evidence has been gathered with a food-frequency questionnaire. Food-frequency questionnaires provide information on the usual frequency of consumption of a selected list of foods that is typically used to rank individuals within a group or classify them into divisions of a frequency distribution (such as quartiles or quintiles) according to level of intake. Such relative rankings are sufficient for most analytical epidemiological studies, but they give no information about the levels of intake that confer increased risk to an individual.[54] This represents a major difficulty in the translation of epidemiological data into quantitative dietary recommendations, given the popularity of food-frequency methods in nutritional epidemiology. The problem may be solvable, however, with the inclusion of dietary standardization substudies (also referred to as calibration studies) in studies in which food-frequency methods are used.[39]

Conceptual and analytical difficulties also underpin the development of dietary recommendations for disease prevention applicable at the level of individuals. As noted above, epidemiological studies yield information about disease risk at the level of populations. An understanding of the relationship between intake and disease risk for individuals is required to set recommendations at the level of the individual. The estimation of such recommendations cannot follow the logic used for setting nutrient requirement recommendations because risk of disease is not analogous to risk of deficiency.[55,56] Nutrient requirements vary across individuals, and although our knowledge of the variability in requirements for some nutrients is incomplete, it is clear that as the intake of an essential nutrient declines, the risk of deficiency increases and eventually reaches 100%. All people will experience deficiency if their intake of an essential nutrient falls low enough. The same cannot be said for diet-related diseases because the probability of disease occurrence never reaches 100% for the entire population. Regardless of how strong the evidence is that vitamin A has a protective effect against lung cancer, for example, lung cancer is not guaranteed to all those with low intakes of vitamin A. Thus, the same kinds of probability density functions that depict relationships between nutrient intake levels and risks of nutrient deficiency cannot be applied directly to questions of diet-disease relationships. The appropriate use of epidemiological information in the translation of dietary recommendations generated at the level of populations to recommendations applicable to individuals is an area in need of further conceptual and analytical development.

Future Directions

Dietary methodology is clearly a central issue in nutritional epidemiology. Although refinements to the data collection process continue, Beaton[34,48] has suggested that the future lies in the development of better techniques to estimate error terms and adjust statistically for their effects in epidemiological analyses. Further development of conceptual foundations and analytical methods for generating population dietary recommendations for chronic disease risk reduction and their application at the individual level is also needed.

Another important future direction is the examination of the relationship between dietary patterns and chronic diseases. In light of the multifactorial nature of these diseases and the suggestion that multiple nutrients may relate to disease risk, a more holistic approach to the study of dietary exposures appears warranted. Similarly, more sophisticated approaches to the examination of diet within the context of other risk factors and risk conditions are needed. The importance of social and economic contexts on the interpretation of risk associated with health-related behaviors is an area of increasing attention in epidemiology, and one of particular relevance to nutrition.[13,57-59] The development of new analytical techniques to enable analysis of contextual variables in conjunction with individual-level variables suggests a potential for important new insight into the role of dietary factors in multifactorial conditions.[60]

Acknowledgment

I am grateful to George H. Beaton and Barbara Davis for their insightful comments, but take full responsibility for the material presented.

References

1. Rothman KJ (1986) Modern epidemiology. Little, Brown and Company, Boston
2. Streiner DL, Norman GR, Munroe Blum H (1989) PDQ epidemiology. BC Decker, Toronto, Ontario
3. Willett W (1990) Nutritional epidemiology. Oxford University Press, New York
4. Interagency Board for Nutrition Monitoring and Related Research (1992) Nutrition monitoring in the United States: the directory of federal and state nutrition monitoring activities. DHHS publication no. (PHS) 92-1255-1 US Public Health Service, Hyattsville, MD
5. Doll R, Peto R (1981) The causes of cancer: quantitative estimates of avoidable risks of cancer in the United States today. J Natl Cancer Inst 66:1191–1308
6. Hebert JR, Landon J, Miller DR (1993) Consumption of meat and fruit in relation to oral and esophageal cancer: a cross-national study. Nutr Cancer 19:169–179
7. Hertz E, Hebert JR, Landon J (1994) Social and environmental factors and life expectancy, infant mortality, and maternal mortality rates: results of a cross-national comparison. Soc Sci Med 39:105–114
8. Gibson RS (1990) Principles of nutritional assessment. Oxford University Press, New York, pp 21–25
9. Hebert JR, Wynder EL (1987) Dietary fat and the risk of breast cancer. N Engl J Med 317:165–166
10. United Nations Administrative Committee on Coordination—Subcommittee on Nutrition (1993) Second report on the world nutrition situation, vol II. Administrative Committee on Coordination—Subcommittee on Nutrition, Geneva
11. Dunn JE (1975) Cancer epidemiology in populations in the United States—with emphasis on Hawaii and California—and Japan. Cancer Res 35:3240–3245.
12. Prentice RL, Pepe M, Welf SG (1989) Dietary fat and breast cancer: a quantitative assessment of the epidemiological literature and a discussion of methodologic issues. Cancer Res 49:3147–3156
13. Schwartz S (1994) The fallacy of the ecological fallacy: the potential misuse of a concept and the consequences. Am J Public Health 84:819–824
14. Hebert JR, Miller DR (1988) Methodologic considerations for investigating the diet-cancer link. Am J Clin Nutr 47:1068–1077
15. Wacholder S, McLaughlin JK, Silverman DT, Mandel JS (1992) Selection of controls in case-control studies I. Principles. Am J Epidemiol 135:1019–1028
16. Wacholder S, Silverman DT, McLaughlin JK, Mandel JS (1992) Selection of controls in case-control studies. II. Types of controls. Am J Epidemiol 135:1029–1041
17. Wacholder S, Silverman DT, McLaughlin JK, Mandel JS (1992) Selection of controls in case-control studies. III. Design options. Am J Epidemiol 135:1042–1050
18. Thompson FE, Byers T (1994) Dietary assessment resource manual. J Nutr 124(suppl):2245S–2317S
19. Coughlin SS (1990) Recall bias in epidemiologic studies. J Clin Epidemiol 43:87–91
20. Dwyer JT, Krall EA, Coleman KA (1987) The problem of memory in nutritional epidemiology research. J Am Diet Assoc 87:1509–1512
21. Friedenreich CM, Slimani N, Riboli E (1992) Measurement of past diet: review of previous and proposed methods. Epidemiol Rev 14:177–196
22. Day GL, Shore RE, Blot WJ, et al (1994) Dietary factors and second primary cancers: a follow-up of oral and pharyngeal cancer patients. Nutr Cancer 21:223–232
23. Burr ML, Gehily AM, Rogers S, et al (1989) Diet and reinfarction trial (DART): design, recruitment, and compliance. Eur Heart J 10:558–567
24. Multiple Risk Factor Intervention Trial Research Group (1982) Multiple risk factor intervention trial. JAMA 248:1465–1477
25. Briefel RR, Flegal KM, Winn DM, et al (1992) Assessing the nation's diet: limitations of the food frequency questionnaire. J Am Diet Assoc 92:959–962
26. Liu K (1994) Statistical issues related to semiquantitative food-frequency questionnaires. Am J Clin Nutr 59(suppl):262S–265S
27. Beaton GH, Milner J, Corey P, et al (1979) Sources of variance in 24-hour dietary recall data: implications for nutrition study design and interpretation. Am J Clin Nutr 32:2546–2559
28. Freudenheim JL, Johnson NE, Wardrop RL (1989) Nutrient misclassification: bias in the odds ratio and loss of power in the Mantel test for trend. Int J Epidemiol 18:2332–2338
29. Freudenheim JL, Marshall JR (1988) The problem of profound

mismeasurement and the power of epidemiological studies of diet and cancer. Nutr Cancer 11:243–250

30. Liu K (1994) Statistical issues in estimating usual intake from 24-hour recall or frequency data. In Wright JD, Ervin B, Briefel RR (eds), Consensus workshop on dietary assessment: nutrition monitoring and tracking the Year 2000 objectives. US Department of Health and Human Services, Hyattsville, MD, pp 92–97

31. Liu K (1988) Measurement error and its impact on partial correlation and multiple linear regression analyses. Am J Epidemiol 127:433–444

32. Liu K, Stamler J, Dyer A, et al (1978) Statistical methods to assess and minimize the role of intra-individual variability in obscuring the relationship between dietary lipids and serum cholesterol. J Chronic Dis 31:399–418

33. McGee D, Rhoads G, Hankin J, et al (1982) Within-person variability of nutrient intake in a group of Hawaiian men of Japanese ancestry. Am J Clin Nutr 36:657–663

34. Beaton GH (1994) Approaches to analysis of dietary data: relationship between planned analyses and choice of methodology. Am J Clin Nutr 59(suppl):253S–261S

35. Bingham SA, Gill C, Welch A, et al (1994) Comparison of dietary assessment methods in nutritional epidemiology: weighed records v. 24 h recalls, food-frequency questionnaires and estimated-diet records. Br J Nutr 72:619–643

36. Schoeller DA (1990) How accurate is self-reported dietary energy intake? Nutr Rev 48:373–379

37. Willett WC (1994) Future directions in the development of food-frequency questionnaires. Am J Clin Nutr 59(suppl): 171S–174S

38. Rosner B, Willett WC (1988) Interval estimates for correlation coefficients corrected for within-person variation: implications for study design and hypothesis testing. Am J Epidemiol 127:377–386

39. Kushi LH (1994) Gaps in epidemiologic research methods: design considerations for studies that use food-frequency questionnaires. Am J Clin Nutr 59(suppl):180S–184S

40. Kaaks R, Plummer M, Riboli E, et al (1994) Adjustment for bias due to errors in exposure assessments in multicenter cohort studies on diet and cancer: a calibration approach. Am J Clin Nutr 59(suppl):245S–250S

41. Gey KF, Puska P (1989) Plasma vitamins E and A inversely correlated to mortality from ischemic heart disease in cross-cultural epidemiology. Ann NY Acad Sci 570:268–282

42. Wacholder S, Schatzkin A, Freedman LS, et al (1994) Can energy adjustment separate the effects of energy from those of specific macronutrients? Am J Epidemiol 140: 848–855

43. Howe G (1989) The first author replies. Am J Epidemiol 129:1314–1315

44. Howe G, Miller AB, Jain M (1986) Re: Total energy intake: implications for epidemiologic analyses. Am J Epidemiol 124:157–159

45. Pike MC, Bernstein L, Peters RK (1989) Re: Total energy intake: implications for epidemiologic analyses. Am J Epidemiol 129:1312–1313

46. Willett W, Stampfer MJ (1986) Total energy intake: implications for epidemiologic analyses. Am J Epidemiol 124:17–27

47. Kushi LH, Sellers TA, Potter JD, et al (1992) Dietary fat and postmenopausal breast cancer. J Natl Cancer Inst 84: 1092–1099

48. Beaton GH (1995) Errors in the interpretation of dietary assessments. Am J Clin Nutr (in press)

49. Rose G (1985) Sick individuals and sick populations. Intl J Epidemiol 14:32–38

50. Block G (1992) The data support a role for antioxidants in reducing cancer risk. Nutr Rev 50:207–213

51. Willett WC (1990) Vitamin A and lung cancer. Nutr Rev 48: 201–211

52. Food and Nutrition Board (1986) Recommended dietary allowances: scientific issues and process for the future. J Nutr 116:482–488

53. Southgate DAT, Cannon G, Rolls BA, et al (1990) Dietary recommendations: how do we move forward [editorial]? Br J Nutr 64:301–305

54. Sempos CT (1992) Invited commentary: some limitations of semiquantitative food frequency questionnaires. Am J Epidemiol 135:1127–1132

55. Beaton GH (1991) Human nutrient requirement estimates. Food Nutr Agric 2/3 1:3–15

56. Harper AE (1987) Evolution of recommended dietary allowances—new directions? Annu Rev Nutr 7:509–537

57. Krieger N (1994) Epidemiology and the web of causation: has anyone seen the spider? Soc Sci Med 39:887–903

58. Wing S (1994) Limits of epidemiology. Med Global Survival 1:74–86

59. Davey Smith G, Bartley M, Blane D (1990) The Black report on socioeconomic inequalities in health 10 years on. Br Med J 310:373–377

60. Cebu Study Team (1991) Underlying and proximate determinants of child health: the Cebu longitudinal health and nutrition study. Am J Epidemiol 133:185–201

Chapter 52

Nutrition Monitoring in the United States

Ronette R. Briefel

Nutrition monitoring has been defined as "an on-going description of nutrition conditions in the population, with particular attention to subgroups defined in socioeconomic terms, for purposes of planning, analyzing the effects of policies and program on nutrition problems, and predicting future trends."[1] This chapter provides a brief history and review of past accomplishments of the National Nutrition Monitoring and Related Research Program (NNMRRP) in the United States, considered one of the best nutrition monitoring systems in the world. Also described are current and planned activities of NNMRRP, progress since 1990, and challenges for improving the program in the future.

The NNMRRP was previously referred to as the National Nutrition Monitoring System (NNMS).[2-6] It is composed of interconnected federal and state activities that provide information about the dietary and nutritional status of the U.S. population, conditions existing in the United States that affect the dietary and nutritional status of individuals, and relationships between diet and health. A general conceptual model representing the relationship between food and health among the five measurement components is presented in Figure 1. The five components are nutrition and related health measurements; food and nutrient consumption; knowledge, attitudes, and behavior assessments; food composition and nutrient data bases; and food supply determinations. Nutrition monitoring data collected at the national, state, and local levels are used directly and indirectly to assess the contribution that diet and nutritional status make to the health of the American people and to determine the factors affecting dietary and nutritional status.

Purposes and Uses of Nutrition Monitoring Data

Nutrition monitoring is vital to policy making and research (Figure 2).[1,2,7] Monitoring provides information and a database for public policy decisions related to nutrition education; public health nutrition programs;

federally supported food service and food assistance programs; the regulation of fortification, safety, and labeling of the food supply; and food production and marketing.[2-7] The nutrition monitoring components provide a database for establishing research priorities.[8,9] Nutrition research provides data for policy making and for identifying the nutrition monitoring needs.[8,9] Table 1 provides examples of uses of nutrition monitoring data for public policy and scientific research.

More specifically, data from NNMRRP have been used to develop the *Dietary Guidelines for Americans*[10] and the Thrifty Food Plan;[11] to evaluate progress towards achievement of the health objectives for the nation for 1990 and 2000;[12,13] to develop the recommended dietary allowances (RDAs);[14] to establish guidelines for preventing, detecting, and managing nutritional conditions;[15-17] and to identify areas of nutrition research that are needed to increase the knowledge base and revise the standards of human nutrient requirements.[14] Nutrition monitoring data are used to track trends and progress toward achieving national health objectives and dietary guidelines.

Data have been used by regulatory agencies to examine U.S. food fortification policies,[2,6,18] to provide dietary exposure estimates for nutrient and nonnutrient food components,[19] and as a basis for food labeling.[20] Nutrition monitoring data collected in the third National Health and Nutrition Examination Survey (NHANES III) are being used to investigate folate status of the U.S. population through the use of dietary and hematologic data. These studies are important to the development of policy and for investigation of the etiology of neural tube defects and risk factors for cardiovascular disease.

Data have also been used to provide information about the relationship between diet, nutrition, and health, such as in *The Surgeon General's Report on Nutrition and Health*,[21] the National Academy of Science's report *Diet and Health: Implications for Reducing Chronic Disease Risk*,[22] and *The Third Report on Nutrition Monitoring in the United States*.[23] This information has been used to identify food and nutrition research priorities of

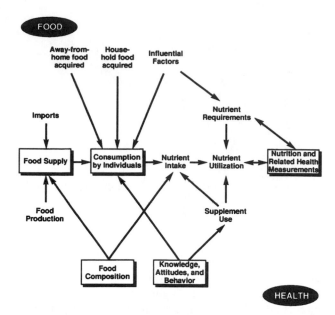

Figure 1. Relationship of food to health. Source: U.S. Department of Health and Human Services and U.S. Department of Agriculture Ten-Year Comprehensive Plan for the National Nutrition Monitoring and Related Research Program.[2]

significance to public health and to evaluate the effect of nutrition initiatives on military feeding systems.[24]

Milestones and Publications

Table 2 provides a chronology of NNMRRP's milestones and publications beginning with its formal establishment in 1977. The Food and Agriculture Act required the Secretaries of the U.S. Department of Agriculture (USDA) and the U.S. Department of Health, Education, and Welfare (currently Health and Human Services [HHS]) to submit to Congress a proposal for a comprehensive nutritional status monitoring system.[25] Details of the subsequent 1981 *Joint Implementation Plan for the NNMS* and the 1987 *Operational Plan for the NNMS* were published.[2,4,5,26] These plans described how the departments intended to achieve the best possible coordination between the two largest components of NNMS, NHANES and the Nationwide Food Consumption Survey (NFCS), and the development of a reporting system to translate the findings from these two national surveys and other monitoring activities into periodic reports to Congress on the nutritional status of the U.S. population. In 1984, a report jointly funded by USDA and HHS and prepared by the National Academy of Sciences described uses of food consumption data and recommendations on survey design that would facilitate wider application of survey data.[27]

The Joint Nutrition Monitoring Evaluation Committee, a federal advisory committee, prepared the first progress report on nutrition monitoring.[28] This 1986 report provided an overview of the dietary and nutritional status of the population and recommendations for improvements in the NNMS.

In 1988, the Interagency Committee on Nutrition Monitoring was established to provide a formal mechanism for improving the planning, coordination, and communication among agencies to facilitate achievement of the system's expanded goals. As a first step, the *Directory of Federal Nutrition Monitoring Activities* was published in 1989[29] and updated and expanded in 1992 to include state surveillance efforts.[30] This publication is extensively used by the public health community, academia, the private sector, and government as a resource for finding nutrition monitoring data, contact persons, and published references.

The second progress report to Congress, published in 1989, was prepared by an expert panel of the Life Sciences Research Office for USDA and HHS.[31] This report updated the dietary and nutritional status information presented in the 1986 report and provided an in-depth analysis of the contributions of NNMS to the evaluation of the relationship of dietary and nutritional factors to cardiovascular disease and to the assessment of iron nutriture.

The National Nutrition Monitoring and Related Research Act (P.L. 101-445) was signed into law on October 22, 1990, after several attempts during 1984–1990 had failed.[32] It was intended ". . . to strengthen national

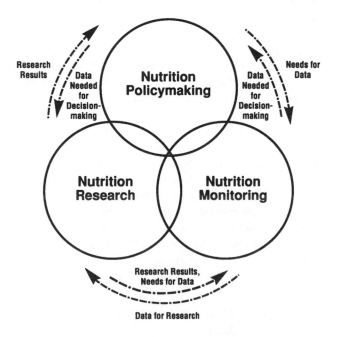

Figure 2. Relationship among nutrition policy making, nutrition research, and nutrition monitoring. Adapted from U.S. Department of Health and Human Services and U.S. Department of Agriculture Ten-Year Comprehensive Plan for the National Nutrition Monitoring and Related Research Program.[2]

Table 1. Uses of nutrition monitoring data[a]

Public policy

Monitoring and surveillance
- Identify high-risk groups and geographical areas with nutrition-related problems to facilitate implementation of public health intervention programs and food assistance programs.
- Evaluate changes in agricultural policy that may affect the nutritional quality and healthfulness of the U.S. food supply.
- Assess progress toward achieving the nutrition objectives in *Healthy People 2000*.[13]
- Evaluate the effectiveness of nutritional initiatives for military feeding systems.
- Recommend guidelines for prevention, detection, and management of nutrition and health conditions.
- Monitor food production and marketing.

Nutrition-related programs
- Develop nutrition education and dietary guidance (*Dietary Guidelines for Americans*).[10]
- Plan and evaluate food assistance programs.
- Plan and assess nutrition intervention programs and public health programs.

Regulatory
- Develop food labeling policies.
- Document the need for and monitor food fortification policies.
- Establish food safety guidelines.

Scientific research
- Establish nutrient requirements (e.g., *Recommended Dietary Allowances*).[14]
- Study diet-health relationships and the relationship of knowledge and attitudes to dietary and health behavior.
- Foster and conduct nutrition monitoring research—national and international.
- Conduct food composition analysis.
- Study the economic aspects of food consumption.
- Inform and assess nutrition education programs.

[a]Adapted from *Ten-Year Plan*.[2]

nutrition monitoring by requiring the Secretary of the Department of Agriculture and the Secretary of the Department of Health and Human Services to prepare and implement a 10-year plan to assess the dietary and nutritional status of the United States population, to support research on, and development of, nutrition monitoring. . . ."[32] The act established several mechanisms to ensure the collaboration and coordination of federal agencies as well as state and local agencies involved in nutrition monitoring.

Federal coordination of the NNMRRP. As specified in the 1990 act, the Secretaries of HHS and USDA have joint responsibility for implementation of the coordinated program and the transmission of required reports to Congress via the President. The Assistant Secretary for Health, HHS, and the Under Secretary for Research, Education, and Economics, USDA, have been delegated the responsibility of implementing NNMRRP and also are joint chairpersons for the Interagency Board for Nutrition Monitoring and Related Research (IBNMRR). The IBNMRR was established in 1991 through the expansion of the function and membership of the Interagency Committee on Nutrition Monitoring to include other agencies that contribute or use NNMRRP data.

Figure 3 provides an overview of the federal structure for coordination of NNMRRP. IBNMRR is the central coordination point for NNMRRP in the federal government. The board coordinates the preparation of the annual budget report on nutrition monitoring and the preparation of biennial reports on progress and policy implications of scientific findings for the president for transmittal to Congress. The board also submits periodic scientific reports that describe the nutritional and related health status of the population to Congress.

In 1993, the board published *Chartbook I: Selected Findings from the National Nutrition Monitoring and Related Research Program* to highlight and update nutrition monitoring data intermediate to the scientific reports.[33] The book includes data in user-friendly graphs and charts with brief narratives. The third progress report on nutrition monitoring was published and sent to Congress in 1995.[23] The board annually reviews progress in accomplishing the 10-year plan and responds to recommendations. In 1997 the board plans to conduct a mid-decade review and revision of the plan with input from outside the program.

Three staff working groups (Survey Comparability, Food Composition Data, and Federal-State Relations and Information Dissemination and Exchange) were established to improve communication and coordination among member agencies on high-priority issues and to provide oversight for 10-year-plan activities. The Survey

Table 2. Milestones and publications of the National Nutrition Monitoring and Related Research Program

1977	Food and Agriculture Act (P.L. 95-113) passed[25]
1978	Proposal for a comprehensive nutritional status monitoring system submitted to Congress
1981	Joint Implementation Plan for a Comprehensive National Nutrition Monitoring System
1983	Joint Nutrition Monitoring Evaluation Committee formed
1986	First progress report on Nutrition Monitoring in the United States published[28]
1987	Operational Plan for the National Nutrition Monitoring System
1988	Interagency Committee on Nutrition Monitoring formed
1989	Second progress report on Nutrition Monitoring in the United States[31] and *The Directory of Federal Nutrition Monitoring Activities* published[29]
1990	National Nutrition Monitoring and Related Research Act (P.L. 101-445) passed[32]
1991	Interagency Board for Nutrition Monitoring and Related Research established through incorporation and expansion of the ICNM
	Proposed Ten-Year Comprehensive Plan for the Nutrition Monitoring and Related Research Program published for comment[35]
1992	National Nutrition Monitoring Advisory Council formed
	The Directory of Federal and State Nutrition Monitoring Activities published[30]
1993	Ten-Year Comprehensive Plan for the National Nutrition Monitoring and Related Research Program published[2]
	Chartbook I: Selected Findings from the National Nutrition Monitoring and Related Research Program published[33]
1995	Third progress report on Nutrition Monitoring in the U.S. published[23]

Comparability Working Group produced the *Report on Comparability of Selected Population Descriptors* in 1992 to standardize the collection and reporting of key socio-economic variables and to enhance data linkages across the program's surveys and surveillance systems. The Federal-State Relations and Information Dissemination and Exchange coordinates the updating of the directories,[29,30] promotes dissemination of information about the NNMRRP and its publications, and fosters communication among national, state, and local nutrition monitoring activities. The Food Composition Data Working Group assesses food composition data needs, coordinates food composition measurement and research, and recommends options for strengthening food composition data to meet NNMRRP needs.

National Nutrition Monitoring Advisory Council. The National Nutrition Monitoring Advisory Council provides scientific and technical guidance to IBNMRR. The council is composed of the co-chairpersons of IBNMRR and nine voting members with expertise in the areas of public health, nutrition monitoring research, and food production and distribution. Five members are appointed by the president on the basis of recommendations by the secretaries of HHS and USDA, and four are appointed by Congress. Appointments are renewed periodically as required by the act.

Since its formation in 1992, the council has evaluated the scientific and technical quality of the 10-year plan and recommended areas for improving NNMRRP in annual reports to the secretaries of HHS and USDA. The council identified six priorities:

1. Identify the best ways to cover high-risk population subgroups.
2. Assess data uses, needs of data users, and the integration of federal, state, and private data needs.
3. Evaluate the mechanism for setting overriding priorities and determining the cost effectiveness of the program.
4. Provide timely dissemination of nutrition monitoring data and information that can be easily linked to decision making.
5. Assess nutrition monitoring research activities that support the program.
6. Define trends in data collected by the program with special emphasis on measures of the food supply available to and consumed by individuals and on knowledge of and attitudes toward nutrition and dietary advice.

Ten-year comprehensive plan. The 10-year plan was developed by the joint HHS-USDA Working Group under the guidance of the IBNMRR, with broad input from the National Nutrition Monitoring Advisory Coun-

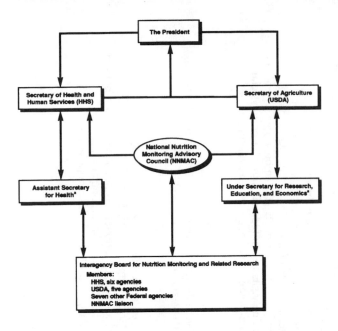

Figure 3. Structure of federal coordination of the National Nutrition Monitoring and Related Research Program.[a] Co-chair, Interagency Board for Nutrition Monitoring and Related Research and Ex-officio, National Nutrition Monitoring Advisory Council.[a]

cil, the public health community, and other users of nutrition monitoring data, including scientific advisors to federal agencies, food and nutrition researchers, economists, the food industry, and academia.

The plan identifies three national objectives critical to the success of the overall goal of a coordinated, comprehensive nutrition monitoring program: provide for a comprehensive NNMRRP through continuous and co-ordinated data collection, improve the comparability and quality of data across NNMRRP, and improve the research base for nutrition monitoring.[2] These objectives expand on the goals delineated in previous plans and are applicable to each of the five measurement components of NNMRRP. The state and local objectives are to strengthen capacity for data collection that complements national surveys, improve the quality of state and local data, and improve methodologies to enhance comparability of NNMRRP data across national, state, and local levels.

The activities in the 10-year plan reflect four areas: requirements of the law,[32] priorities identified by federal agencies responsible for conducting nutrition monitoring surveys and related activities, response to recommendations from scientific experts and organizations[28,31,34] and to public comments on the proposed plan,[35] and recommendations from users of nutrition monitoring data.[27] The plan incorporates accountability by citing federal orga-

nizations as responsible, contributing, and collaborating and by providing time lines for 70 specific activities.[2] A U.S. General Accounting Office review noted that recent progress in planning for a program had been made but that a consistent system was not yet in place and would require close monitoring to ensure the success of the NNMRRP.[36]

Nutrition Monitoring Measurement Components

National dietary surveys were begun in the 1930s. Since then, more than 40 surveys and surveillance systems have evolved in response to the information needs of federal agencies and other nutrition monitoring data users. Chronological listings of past nutrition monitoring surveys and activities have been published.[2,26,37,38] Table 3 lists the major survey and surveillance activities, sponsoring agencies, dates conducted, and coverage of target populations since the 1990 legislation, organized by the five measurement component areas. Brief descriptions of these activities are summarized below and have been described in detail elsewhere.[2,26,30,38]

Nutrition and related health measurements. Nutrition and related health data have a wide variety of policy, research, health and nutrition education, medical practice, and reference standards applications. The cornerstone of the NNMRRP measurement component, NHANES, provides national data on the nutritional status, dietary intake, and numerous health indices of the U.S. population.[2,39] Physical measures such as body measurements, blood pressure, dental examinations, and biochemical and hematological tests allow for studying the relationship between dietary intake, nutritional status, and related health status. NHANES follow-up studies allow epidemiologic investigations of the relationships of nutrition and health to risk of death and disability.

A number of other surveys and surveillance systems, primarily conducted by the Centers for Disease Control and Prevention (CDC), also contribute nutrition-related health information, particularly for low-income pregnant women, infants, and children who participate in publicly funded health, nutrition, and food assistance programs.[30,38,40] These CDC surveillance systems provide data representative of the participating population in participating states. The National Health Interview Survey provides information annually about self-reported health conditions and periodically about special nutrition and health topics such as vitamin and mineral supplement usage and youth behavior.

The continuous collection of objective nutrition and health data is required for generating reference distributions, for monitoring trends over time, and for tracking progress toward achieving national health objectives.[13,41] For example, 1960–1991 NHANES data for

Table 3. Federal nutrition monitoring surveys and surveillance activities since 1990

Date (initiated)	Dept.	Agency	Survey	Target U.S. population
Nutrition and related health measurements				
Continuous (1915)	HHS	CDC/NCHS	National Vital Registration System	Total U.S. population
Annual (1957)	HHS	CDC/NCHS	National Health Interview Survey (NHIS)	Civilian, noninstitutionalized individuals
Periodic (1973)	HHS	CDC/NCHS	National Survey of Family Growth	Women, 15–44 years
Continuous (1973)	HHS	CDC/NCCDPHP	Pregnancy Nutrition Surveillance System	Low-income, high-risk pregnant women
Continuous (1973)	HHS	CDC/NCCDPHP	Pediatric Nutrition Surveillance System	Low-income, high-risk children, birth–17 years
1988–1994	HHS	CDC/NCHS	Third National Health and Nutrition Examination Survey (NHANES III)	Noninstitutionalized, civilian population, 2+ months; oversampling of blacks and Mexican Americans, children 0–5 years, and individuals 60+ years
1990–1991	HHS	IHS	Survey of Heights and Weights of American Indian School Children	American Indian schoolchildren, ages 5–18 years
1991–1992	HHS	IHS	Navajo Health and Nutrition Survey	Persons ages 12+ years residing on or near the Navajo reservation in Arizona, New Mexico, and Colorado
1991	HHS	CDC/NCHS	Longitudinal Followup to the National Maternal and Infant Health Survey	Women from the 1988 National Maternal and Infant Health Survey and live birth cohort at 3 years of age
1992	HHS	CDC/NCHS	NHANES I Epidemiologic Followup Survey	Individuals examined in NHANES I, 25–74 years at baseline (1971–1974)
Continuous (1992)	HHS	CDC/NCHS	NHANES II Mortality Followup Survey	Individuals examined in NHANES II, 35–75 years at baseline (1976–1980)
Continuous (1992)	HHS	CDC/NCHS	Hispanic HANES (HHANES) Mortality Followup Survey	Individuals interviewed in HHANES, 20–74 years at baseline (1982–1984)
Annual (1992)	HHS	CDC/NCHS	National Health Care Survey (integrates: National Home and Hospice Care Survey (1963), National Nursing Home Survey (1963), and Followup (1995), National Hospital Discharge Survey (1965), National Ambulatory Medical Care Survey (1973), National Hospital Ambulatory Medical Care Survey (1992), and National Survey of Ambulatory Surgery (1994)	Record-based health care provider surveys including: visits to hospital emergency and outpatient departments of nonfederal, short-stay, general and specialty hospitals and ambulatory surgical centers; office visits to nonfederal, office-based physicians; and home health agencies and nursing homes
Continuous (1992)	HHS	CDC/NCHS	NHANES III Mortality Followup Survey	Individuals interviewed and examined in NHANES III, 20+ years at baseline (1988–1994)
Food and nutrient consumption				
Continuous (1917)	DOD	USARIEM	Nutritional Evaluation of Military Feeding Systems and Military Populations	Enlisted personnel of the Army, Navy, Marine Corps, and Air Force
Continuous (1980)	DOL	BLS	Consumer Expenditure Survey	Civilian noninstitutionalized population and a portion of the institutionalized population
Continuous (1983)	DOC	FCS	Survey of Income and Program Participation (SIPP)	Civilian, noninstitutionalized population

Dates	Department	Agency	Survey	Population
1995 Supplement	USDA	Census	Supplement on Food Security	See NHANES III listing above.
1988–1994	HHS	CDC/NCHS	NHANES III and Supplemental Nutrition Survey of Older Americans	Individuals ages 50+ years examined in NHANES III with telephones
1989–1991, annual; 1994–1996, annual	USDA	HNIS; ARSa	Continuing Survey of Food Intakes by Individuals (CSFII)	Individuals of all ages residing in households in 48 conterminous states in 1989–1991 and nationwide in 1994–1996; oversampling of individuals in low-income households
1989–1991	HHS	IHS	Strong Heart Dietary Survey	American Indian adults ages 45–74 years in South Dakota, Oklahoma, and Arizona
1991–1992	DOC	NMFS/NOAA	Development of a National Seafood Consumption Survey Model	Individuals residing in eligible households and recreational/subsistence fisherman
1992	USDA	FNS	School Nutrition Dietary Assessment Study	School-aged children in grades 1–12 in 48 conterminous states and Washington, DC
1992	USDA	FNS	Adult Day Care Program Study	Adult day care centers and adults participating in the Child and Adult Care Food Program
Knowledge, attitudes, and behavior assessments				
Continuous (1984)	HHS	CDC/NCCDPHP	Behavioral Risk Factor Surveillance System	Individuals 18+ years residing in households with telephones in participating states
Biennial (1982)	HHS	FDA, NIH/NHLBI	Health and Diet Survey	Civilian, noninstitutionalized individuals in households with telephones, 18+ years
1989–1991, annual; 1994–1996, annual	USDA	HNIS; ARSa	Diet and Health Knowledge Survey	Main-meal planner/preparers in households participating in 1989–1991 and 1994–1996 CSFII
Annual (1990)	HHS	CDC/NCCDPHP	Youth Risk Behavior Survey	Youths attending school in grades 9–12 and 12–21 years of age in households in states; Washington, DC; Puerto Rico; and Virgin Islands
1990	HHS	NIH/NHLBI	Nationwide Survey of Nurses' and Dieticians' Knowledge, Attitudes, and Behavior Regarding Cardiovascular Risk Factors	Registered nurses and registered dietitians currently active in their professions
1990–91	HHS	FDA	Nutrition Label Format Studies	Primary food shoppers, ages 18+ years
1991	HHS	FDA, NIH/NHLBI	Weight Loss Practices Survey	Individuals currently trying to lose weight, 18+ years, in households with telephones
1991	HHS	NIH/NCI	5 a Day Better Health Baseline Survey	Individuals ages 18+ years with telephones
1992	HHS	FDA	Infant Feeding Practices Survey	New mothers and healthy, full-term infants, birth–1 year
1992	HHS	FDA	Consumer Food Handling Practices and Awareness of Microbiological Hazards Screener	Individuals in households with telephones, 18+ years

Table continues on next page

Table 3. *continued*

Date (initiated)	Dept.	Agency	Survey	Target U.S. population
Food composition and nutrient databases				
Continuous (1892)	USDA	ARS[a]	National Nutrient Data Bank Nutrient Composition Laboratory	NA
Annual (1961)	HHS	FDA	Total Diet Study	Representative diets of specific age-sex groups
Continuous (1973)	HHS	FDA	Langual	NA
Biennial (1977)	HHS	FDA	Food Label and Package Survey	NA
Continuous (1977)	USDA	ARS[a]	Survey Nutrient Data Base	NA
Food supply determinations				
Annual (1909)	DOC	NOAA/NMFS	Fisheries of the United States	NA
Annual (1909)	USDA	ERS	U.S. Food and Nutrition Supply Series: Estimates of Food Available	NA
	USDA	ARS[a]	Estimates of Nutrients	
Continuous (1985)	USDA	ERS, FCS	A.C. Nielsen SCANTRACK	NA

Abbreviations: ARS, Agricultural Research Service; BLS, Bureau of Labor Statistics; CDC, Centers for Disease Control and Prevention; DOC, Department of Commerce; DOD, Department of Defense; DOL, Department of Labor; FDA, Food and Drug Administration; ERS, Economic Research Service; FCS, Food and Consumer Service (previously FNS, Food and Nutrition Service); HHS, U.S. Department of Health and Human Services; HNIS, Human Nutrition Information Service; IHS, Indian Health Service; NCCDPHP, National Center for Chronic Disease Prevention and Health Promotion; NCHS, National Center for Health Statistics; NCI, National Cancer Institute; NHLBI, National Heart, Lung, and Blood Institute; NIH, National Institutes of Health; NA—not applicable; NMFS, National Marine Fisheries Service; NOAA, National Oceanic and Atmospheric Administration; USARIEM, U.S. Army Research Institute of Environmental Medicine; USDA, U.S. Department of Agriculture.

[a]HNIS was integrated into ARS in 1994.

U.S. adults show that the prevalence of elevated serum cholesterol levels[42] and of hypertension[43] decreased, whereas the prevalence of overweight increased.[44]

Food and nutrient consumption. Food and nutrient consumption measurements include estimates of individuals' intakes of foods and beverages (nonalcoholic and alcoholic) and nutritional supplements as well as intakes of nonessential nutrients such as dietary fiber. The USDA's Continuing Survey of Food Intakes by Individuals (CSFII) and HHS's NHANES, the two cornerstone NNMRRP surveys, provide national estimates of food and nutrient intakes in the general U.S. population and in subgroups. The CSFII emphasizes the food and nutrient intake of the general population and of subgroups of the population defined by various socioeconomic factors. In NHANES, dietary intake is related to health status in the same individuals. These surveys also provide the potential for assessing consumption of additives and pesticides in the diet.

USDA's Household Food Consumption Survey provides the only source of collective information on household food use, nutrient availability, and food expenditures. The survey, previously conducted in 1987–1988 as the Nationwide Food Consumption Survey, is proposed for the late 1990s.

Periodically, assessments are made of the food and nutrient consumption by specific subgroups of the population not adequately covered in national surveys. Such assessments have been conducted for military populations, American Indians, and schoolchildren. For example, the School Nutrition Dietary Assessment Study assessed the diets of American schoolchildren and the contribution of the National School Lunch Program to overall nutrient intake.[45]

Knowledge, attitudes, and behavior assessments. National surveys that measure knowledge, attitudes, and behavior about diet and nutrition and how these relate to health were added to the nutrition monitoring program in the past 10–15 years. In general, the Health and Diet Surveys focused on people's awareness of relationships between diet and risk for chronic disease and on health-related knowledge and attitudes.

The Diet and Health Knowledge Survey initiated by USDA in 1989 focused on the relationship of individuals' knowledge and attitudes about dietary guidelines and food safety to their food choices and nutrient intakes. The focus of the Behavioral Risk Factor Surveillance System, initiated by CDC in 1984, was on personal behavior and its relationship to nutritional and health status.

Surveys addressing specific topics such as the feeding practices of infants, weight-loss practices, and cholesterol awareness of health professionals have been periodically conducted to meet specific data needs. The National Cancer Institute conducted the 5 a Day for Better Health Baseline Survey in collaboration with the food industry to assess the public's knowledge, behavior, and attitudes about fruits and vegetables.

Food composition and nutrient databases. Since 1892, USDA has operated the National Nutrient Data Bank (NNDB) for the purpose of deriving representative nutrient values for foods consumed in the United States. Values from NNDB are released in Agriculture Handbook No. 8 and as part of the USDA Nutrient Data Base for Standard Reference. These values are used as the core of most nutrient databases developed in the United States for special purposes, such as those used in the commercially available dietary analysis programs. USDA produces the Survey Nutrient Data Base, which contains data for 28 food components and energy for each food item; the database is used for analyzing nationwide dietary intake surveys. A system is in place at USDA to periodically update this database with the most current information available from NNDB.

The Food and Drug Administration's (FDA's) Total Diet Study provides annual food composition analysis based on the foods consumed most frequently in the CSFII and NHANES. Representative foods are collected from retail markets, prepared for consumption, and analyzed individually for nutrients and other food components at the Total Diet Laboratory to estimate consumption of selected nutrients and organic and elemental contaminants.

Food supply determinations. Since the beginning of this century, U.S. food supply estimates have indicated levels of foods and nutrients available for consumption. These data, updated and published annually by USDA, are used to assess the potential of the U.S. food supply to meet the nutritional needs of the population and to monitor changes in the food supply over time. Proprietary data purchased from A.C. Nielsen Company are used to measure grocery store sales of all scannable packaged food products.

Progress and Challenges for Improving Nutrition Monitoring

A focused, comprehensive nutrition monitoring program involves more than just coordinating current activities in the five measurement component areas. It includes improving methodologies for the collection and interpretation of data, timely processing and release of data, expanding coverage of population subgroups, and addressing current nutrition issues. The 10-year plan encompasses a broad range of activities needed to achieve the primary goal and the objectives of a coordinated nutrition monitoring program.

Many surveys of NNMRRP are designed to collect data on various subgroups of the population, such as low-income people and minorities. The USDA food consumption surveys oversample low-income people to produce reliable estimates for the general and the low-income populations. USDA has increased efforts to improve survey response rates after the low response rates of 31–38% in the 1987–1988 NFCS.[30,36]

The most recent NHANES, in 1988–1994, included oversampling of children under age 6 years, people ages 60 years and older, African Americans, and Mexican Americans.[39] The National Health Interview Survey was redesigned in 1995 to produce improved estimates for minority groups in the population. However, NNMRRP data are currently limited or inadequate for some groups, including institutionalized people, American Indians, Alaska Natives, migrant farm workers, homeless people, and pregnant and lactating women. Focused studies are the most economical way to cover these and other minority groups, such as Asian and Pacific Islanders.[46]

In addition to expanded coverage of population subgroups, improved geographic coverage is needed to provide nutrition data at state and local levels. National surveys such as NHANES and CSFII provide data representative of the entire country and of its major geographic regions but cannot provide data representative of states, counties, and cities. The CDC surveillance systems provide data for participating states. Statistical methods have been applied to national surveys to produce model-based estimates for states and small areas. Further research is needed to improve the nutrition monitoring program's capability to produce reliable data for additional geographic areas, states, and small areas.

Continuous and coordinated data collection. Continuous collection of data in cross-sectional and longitudinal surveys and surveillance systems within NNMRRP is needed to evaluate and monitor the contribution that diet and nutritional status make to the health of the U.S. population, to plan national strategies for encouraging and assisting people to adopt healthy eating patterns, and to avoid duplication of efforts while meeting nutrition monitoring needs. Current efforts are aimed at conducting national surveys such as NHANES and CSFII more frequently or continuously to collect and produce timely, policy-relevant nutrition data.

A report completed under contract with the Research Triangle Institute in 1991 recommended options for increasing comparability of sampling designs and selected population descriptors in the two cornerstone surveys, NFCS and NHANES.[34] Recent survey coordination efforts have focused on planning the next round of NHANES and CSFII surveys, including design research to explore a joint sample design for future NHANES and CSFII surveys to improve population subgroup coverage[46] and the same dietary method being used in both surveys.[47,48] In 1994, a workshop was held to identify federal dietary data requirements, including the need for more descriptive specificity, such as brand name information. A continual goal is to expand and improve the food

composition database and achieve adequate representation of foods and nutrients for nutrition monitoring purposes.

Comparability and quality of nutrition monitoring data. Integral to the coordination of nutrition monitoring activities is the use of standardized or comparable methodologies for the collection, quality control, analysis, and reporting of data. Having basic criteria for sampling designs would allow data from different surveys—including data that assess dietary behavior, knowledge, attitudes about food and nutrient consumption, and nutrition-related health status—to be compared, linked, and combined.

Although many of the surveys in NNMRRP include nutrition and related health indicators, there is no standardized set of questions, assessments, and procedures that has been agreed on or used across surveys to measure nutrition and related health status. Without common definitions, the comparison of nutritional and related health findings among different surveys is limited.

An expert panel convened by the Life Sciences Research Office identified nutritional status core indicators for difficult-to-sample populations.[49] Their report developed a conceptual model but did not describe specific methods, questions, or indicators for nutritional status assessment. The IBNMRR Survey Comparability Working Group has begun to document similarities and differences for selected key nutrition and nutrition-related health variables across NNMRRP surveys and to identify the specific assessments that constitute a minimum set of indicators for measuring nutritional status. These efforts also include revising the National Center for Health Statistics (NCHS) growth charts,[50] which are used as the growth standard nationally and internationally; evaluating the methodologies for assessing nutritional status, such as folate status;[51] and developing standardized dietary indicators.[52]

Linkage of dietary survey data will be improved as the data collection methodologies for measuring dietary intake, coding, and analysis become more comparable. Since 1982, the same food codes and nutrient database have been used in HANES, NFCS, and CSFII for analysis and reporting of dietary intake data.[47,48] Survey differences related to how the data are collected, coded, and analyzed have been documented to aid interpretation of dietary estimates from different surveys. NCHS sponsored the Consensus Workshop on Dietary Assessment in 1992 to recommend guidelines for selection and use of dietary methods for nutrition monitoring and also for tracking of specific *Healthy People 2000* health objectives on intakes of fat, calcium, fruits and vegetables, and alcohol.[13,52] Implementation of these guidelines across the NNMRRP will improve the usefulness and interpretation of dietary data.

The interagency Working Group on Food Security, led by USDA's Food and Consumer Service and CDC's

NCHS, sponsored a 1994 conference to identify food security and hunger measurement and research issues.[53] Input from attendees representing federal agencies, academia, and public advocacy groups was critical to developing, testing, and fielding a standardized food security instrument sponsored by USDA in the April 1995 supplement to the Current Population Survey. Plans are being made to collect data using these core indicators of food security in the Survey of Income and Program Participation in late 1995–early 1996 and in other national surveys and state-based surveillance systems.[53,54]

Nutrition monitoring research. Research in the areas of survey design, questionnaire design, data collection methods, laboratory methods, data processing, and data analysis provides essential support for NNMRRP.[2,8,9,38] Research efforts should focus on identifying and developing methods and using computer technology that will enhance the monitoring of the nutritional status of the U.S. population and support the timely interpretation and release of information to users.

Reliable, valid, and cost-effective measures of nutritional status are needed along with appropriate interpretive criteria. Research is needed on methods (such as questionnaires, interviewing procedures, and physical measures) appropriate for subgroups at increased nutritional risk, practical and efficient measurement of dietary biochemical and clinical variables, and applied statistical methods for collecting and interpreting NNMRRP data. Research to develop and standardize questionnaires for valid and reliable estimation of knowledge, attitudes, and behavior will aid in the development of public health strategies at federal, state, and local levels to improve dietary status, promote health, and prevent nutrition-related disease.

Food composition values need to be continually evaluated and periodically updated as analytical methods are improved and as foods change over time. Even though NNDB contains thousands of individual food composition values, gaps and deficiencies still exist for some foods, food components, and specific nutrients. This situation will continue for the foreseeable future because of cost and the lack of reliable measurements of certain food components. A plan is needed for prioritizing the development of accurate and practical measurement systems for generating food composition data. A food composition database for nutritional supplements also needs to be developed so that total nutrient intakes can be estimated and the effect of nutritional supplements on nutritional status and health can be studied.

State and local activities. To create an effective and comprehensive NNMRRP, it is necessary to enhance state and local capacities to monitor nutritional status and dietary practices in a way that is coordinated with and complements national nutrition surveys. As national standardized indicators for population descriptors, food security, diet, nutritional and related health status, and knowledge, attitudes, and behavior assessments are developed, they should be incorporated into existing and planned surveillance systems. As states and localities strive to implement strategies and objectives comparable to the nutrition objectives in *Healthy People 2000*[13] and *Healthy Communities 2000: Model Standards*,[52,55,56] both baseline and continuing data will be necessary to monitor local progress. State laboratories must be able to support state and local monitoring efforts that are compatible with national efforts.

Planning for the development and implementation of a biennial school-based surveillance system, led by CDC and Food and Consumer Service, began in 1993. Progress has been made in developing monitoring tools, including behavioral and physical measures, support materials for nutrition education in classrooms, and data processing and analysis programs. Combined national and state-based survey designs would be used for survey modules. Progress to implement this system is dependent on the acquisition of additional resources.

The Survey of State Nutrition Surveillance Efforts carried out in 1988 by the Association of State and Territorial Public Health Nutrition Directors indicated that 80% of states rated participation in nutrition monitoring as very important or crucial. Major limitations to full participation in nutrition monitoring included insufficient professional staff, limited funding, and nonautomated data-collection systems.

For continuance of data quality at the state and local levels, periodic training in the collection, analysis, and use of nutrition monitoring data will be important. Success in using and disseminating state and local nutrition monitoring data will be key factors in assessing the usefulness of nutrition monitoring efforts. Periodic evaluation of state and local monitoring systems should be performed to ensure that state and local needs are met. State and local monitoring systems should also take advantage of new technology for electronic data transfer.

Information dissemination and timeliness of data. To increase awareness, cost-effective mechanisms that facilitate cooperation and collaboration, avoid duplication of efforts, and are easily accessible to practitioners, community workers, policy makers, journalists, and researchers are needed. Use of uniform statistical and reporting guidelines in interagency publications of survey findings, survey operations, and response rates has greatly facilitated the utility and linkage of nutrition information across NNMRRP.[33] Improvements have also been made in reporting national survey data in a more timely fashion, primarily through the use of automated data collection and processing, although further improvements are still needed. Coordinated, regular collection and analysis of survey data would facilitate more timely release of relevant data to meet public health and nutrition policy data needs.

Progress has been made in using electronic bulletin boards to announce or distribute survey data, survey reports, and nutrition monitoring publications and to distribute data in various electronic forms, such as tapes, diskettes, and CD-ROMs. In addition to preparing, promoting, and distributing survey reports and data tapes, increased efforts are being directed toward instructing users on how to access, process, and interpret data appropriately via the provision of training manuals, survey documentation on methods and quality-control procedures, and data user conferences at national and regional levels.[37]

Summary

The primary goal of the 10-year comprehensive plan is to establish a comprehensive nutrition monitoring and related research program by collecting quality data that are continuous, coordinated, timely, and reliable; using comparable methods for data collection and reporting of results; conducting relevant research; and efficiently and effectively disseminating and exchanging information with data users.[2] Given competing demands for limited national resources and resulting budget limitations, the goals for the NNMRRP will be evaluated against other competing national needs. Efforts and resources are critical to the efficient, continuing progress and research to expand and strengthen the nutrition monitoring program in the United States.

References

1. Mason JB, Habicht J-P, Tabatabai H, Valverde V (1984) Nutritional surveillance. World Health Organization, Geneva
2. US Department of Health and Human Services, US Department of Agriculture (1993) Ten-year comprehensive plan for the national nutrition monitoring and related research program. Fed Regist 58:32752–32806
3. Calloway CW (1984) National Nutrition Monitoring System. J Am Diet Assoc 84:1179–1180
4. Ostenso GL (1984) National Nutrition Monitoring System: a historical perspective. J Am Diet Assoc 84:1181–1185
5. Brown GE Jr. (1984) National Nutrition Monitoring System: a Congressional perspective. J Am Diet Assoc 84:1185–1188
6. Forbes AL, Stephenson MG (1984) National Nutrition Monitoring System: implications for public health policy at Food and Drug Administration. J Am Diet Assoc 84:1189–1193
7. Food and Agriculture Organization of the United Nations, World Health Organization Joint Secretariat for the International Conference on Nutrition (1992) The International Conference on Nutrition: world declaration and plan of action for nutrition, FAO, Rome, WHO, Geneva
8. Woteki CE (1993) Nutrition monitoring research. In The research agenda for dietetics. American Dietetic Association, Chicago, pp 39–48.
9. Sims LS (1993) Research aspects of public policy in nutrition generating research questions to determine the impact of nutritional, agricultural, and health care policy and regulations on the health and nutritional status of the public. In The research agenda for dietetics. American Dietetic Association, Chicago, pp 25–38
10. US Department of Agriculture, US Department of Health and Human Services (1995) Nutrition and your health: dietary guidelines for Americans, 4th ed. US Government Printing Office, Washington, DC
11. Human Nutrition Information Service (1983) The thrifty food plan. US Department of Agriculture, Hyattsville, MD
12. US Department of Health and Human Services (1986) The 1990 health objectives for the nation: a midcourse review. US Government Printing Office, Washington, DC
13. US Department of Health and Human Service (1991) Healthy People 2000: national health promotion and disease prevention objectives. DHHS Publication No. (PHS) 91-50212. US Government Printing Office, Washington, DC
14. National Research Council (1989) Recommended dietary allowances, 10th ed. National Academy Press, Washington, DC
15. Food and Nutrition Board (1993) Iron deficiency anemia: recommended guidelines for the prevention, detection, and management among US children and women of childbearing age. Earl R, Woteki CE (eds). National Academy Press, Washington, DC
16. National High Blood Pressure Education Program (1993) The fifth report of the Joint National Committee on Detection, Evaluation, and Treatment of High Blood Pressure. NIH Publication No. 93-1088. National Institutes of Health, Bethesda, MD
17. National Cholesterol Education Program (1993) Second report of the Expert Panel on Detection, Evaluation, and Treatment of High Blood Cholesterol in Adults (Adult Treatment Panel II). NIH Publication No. 93-3095. National Heart, Lung, and Blood Institute, Bethesda, MD
18. Pilch SM, Senti FR (eds) (1984) Assessment of iron nutritional status of the U.S. population based on data collected in the Second National Health and Nutrition Examination Survey (1976–1980). Life Sciences Research Office, Federation of American Societies for Experimental Biology, Bethesda, MD
19. Anderson SA (ed) (1988) Estimation of exposure to substances in the food supply. Life Sciences Research Office, Federation of American Societies for Experimental Biology, Bethesda, MD
20. Food Labeling (1990) Serving sizes, proposed rule, docket no. 90N-0165. Fed Regist 55(139):29517–29533
21. US Department of Health and Human Services (1988) The Surgeon General's report on nutrition and health. PHS Publication No. 88-50210. DHHS, Washington, DC
22. National Research Council (1989) Diet and health: implications for reducing chronic disease risk. National Academy Press, Washington, DC
23. Federation of American Societies for Experimental Biology, Life Sciences Research Office, prepared for the Interagency Board for Nutrition Monitoring and Related Research (1995) Third report on nutrition monitoring in the United States, vols 1 and 2. US Government Printing Office, Washington, DC, 365 and 354 pp
24. Committee on Military Nutrition Research, Food and Nutrition Board, Institute of Medicine (1991) Military nutrition initiatives. IOM Report-91-05. National Academy Press, Washington, DC
25. US Congress (1977) P. L. 95-113. The Food and Agriculture Act of 1997, Sec. 1428
26. Kuczmarski MF, Kuczmarski RJ (1994) Nutrition monitoring in the United States. In Shils ME, Olson JA, Shike M (eds), Modern nutrition in health and disease, 8th ed. Lea & Febiger, Philadelphia, pp 1506–1516

27. National Research Council (1984) National survey data on food consumption: uses and recommendations. National Academy Press, Washington, DC

28. US Department of Health and Human Services, US Department of Agriculture (1986) Nutrition monitoring in the United States: a progress report from the Joint Nutrition Monitoring Evaluation Committee. DHHS Publication No. (PHS) 86-1255. US Government Printing Office, Washington, DC

29. Interagency Committee on Nutrition Monitoring (1989) Nutrition monitoring in the United States: the directory of federal nutrition monitoring activities. DHHS Publication No. (PHS) 89-1255-1. US Government Printing Office, Washington, DC

30. Interagency Committee on Nutrition Monitoring (1992) Nutrition Monitoring in the United States: the directory of federal and state nutrition monitoring activities. DHHS Publication No. (PHS) 92-1255-1. US Government Printing Office, Washington, DC

31. Life Sciences Research Office, Federation of American Societies for Experimental Biology (1989) Nutrition monitoring in the United States: an update report on nutrition monitoring. DHHS Publication No. (PHS) 89-1255. US Government Printing Office, Washington, DC

32. U.S. Congress (1990) P.L. 101-445. National Nutrition Monitoring and Related Research Act

33. Interagency Board for Nutrition Monitoring and Related Research (1993) Nutrition monitoring in the United States. In Ervin B, Reed D (eds), Chartbook I: selected findings from the National Nutrition Monitoring and Related Research Program. DHHS Publication No. (PHS) 93-1255-2. Public Health Service, Hyattsville, MD

34. Research Triangle Institute (1991) Final report: sampling design and population descriptors of Nationwide Food Consumption Surveys and National Health and Nutrition Examination Surveys. Research Triangle Institute, Research Triangle Park, NC

35. US Department of Health and Human Services, US Department of Agriculture (1991) Proposed ten-year comprehensive plan for the National Nutrition Monitoring and Related Research Program. Fed Regist 91-25967:SS 716-55767

36. US General Accounting Office (1994) Nutrition monitoring: progress in developing a coordinated program. GAO/PEMD-94-23. General Accounting Office, Washington, DC

37. Kuczmarski MF, Moshfegh A, Briefel R (1994) Update on nutrition monitoring activities in the United States. J Am Diet Assoc 94:753–760

38. Woteki CE, Wong FL (1992) Interpretation and utilization of data from the National Nutrition Monitoring System. In Monsen ER (ed), Research: successful approaches. American Dietetic Association, Chicago, pp 204–219

39. US Department of Health and Human Services (1994) Plan and operation of the Third National Health and Nutrition Examination Survey 1988–1994. DHHS Publication No. (PHS) 94-1308. Vital Health Stat [32] 1:1–407

40. Centers for Disease Control and Prevention (1994) CDC's public health surveillance for women, infants and children. Wilcox LS, Marks JS (eds). US Public Health Service, Washington, DC

41. Lewis CJ, Crane NT, Moore BJ, Hubbard VS (1994) Healthy People 2000: report on the 1994 nutrition progress review. Nutr Today 29:6–14

42. Johnson CL, Rifkind BM, Sempos CT, et al (1993) Declining serum total cholesterol levels among US adults. JAMA 269(23):3002–3008

43. Burt VL, Whelton P, Roccella EJ, et al (1995) Prevalence of hypertension in the adult US population: results from the Third National Health and Nutrition Examination Survey, 1988–1991. Hypertension 25:305–313

44. Kuczmarski RJ, Flegal KM, Campbell SM, Johnson CL (1994) Increasing prevalence of overweight among US adults: NHANES 1960–91. JAMA 272(3):205–211

45. Burghardt JA, Devaney BL, Gordon AR (1995) The school nutrition dietary assessment study: summary and discussion. Am J Clin Nutr 61(suppl):252S–257S

46. Westat, Inc. (1994) Evaluation of design options in NHANES '97: a collection of first draft reports of selected topics. Westat, Inc, Rockville, MD

47. Briefel RR (1994) Assessment of the US diet in national nutrition surveys: national collaborative efforts and NHANES. Am J Clin Nutr 59(suppl):164S–167S.

48. Guenther PM (1994) Research needs for dietary assessment and monitoring in the United States. Am J Clin Nutr 59(suppl): 168S–170S

49. Life Sciences Research Office (1990) Core indicators of nutritional state for difficult-to-sample populations. J Nutr 120(suppl):1554–1600

50. National Center for Health Statistics (1994) Executive summary of the growth chart workshop, December 1992. National Center for Health Statistics, Hyattsville, MD

51. Raiten DJ, Fisher KD (eds) (1994) Assessment of folate methodology used in the third National Health and Nutrition Examination Survey (NHANES III, 1988–94). Life Sciences Research Office, Federation of American Societies for Experimental Biology, Bethesda, MD

52. Consensus Workshop on Dietary Assessment (1994) Nutrition monitoring and tracking the year 2000 objectives. Wright J, Ervin B, Briefel R (eds). National Center for Health Statistics, Hyattsville, MD

53. Food and Consumer Service, US Department of Agriculture; National Center for Health Statistics, Centers for Disease Control and Prevention, US Department of Health and Human Services (1995) Conference on Food Security Measurement and Research. Food and Consumer Service, Alexandria, VA

54. Briefel RR, Woteki CE (1992) Development of food sufficiency questions for the Third National Health and Nutrition Examination Survey. J Nutr Educ 24:24S–28S

55. American Public Health Association (1991) Healthy communities 2000 model standards: guidelines for community attainment of the year 2000 national health objectives. American Public Health Association, Washington, DC

56. Centers for Disease Control (1991) Report of the state and local input meeting: National Nutrition Monitoring and Related Research Plan. US Department of Health and Human Services, Atlanta, GA

Chapter 53

Enteral and Parenteral Nutrition

Stephanie Brooks and Patrick Kearns

This chapter focuses on the therapeutic modalities of enteral nutrition (EN) and parenteral nutrition (PN) whose use is typically limited to intervention in acute and chronic disease states. A historic background precedes a discussion of clinical applications. The model of nutritional intervention (Figure 1) is represented by a pyramid, which emphasizes the need to screen many people to identify those individuals who are at risk of complications from poor nutritional status. For them, our understanding of physiological, immunological, nutritional, and metabolic information can offer nutritional strategies designed to limit morbidity from malnutrition. Such information is integrated with existing practice and technologies currently applied to enteral and parenteral nutrition support. Placed atop this structure is the critical testing of each intervention to define its benefits, risks, and costs. The ideal is to use the randomized, controlled trial (RCT) as the ultimate arbiter of merit. With sufficient evidence from RCT, clinical nutrition moves toward the top of this structured approach in developing a comprehensive plan for improving nutritional status while limiting harm to the patient. This approach optimizes use of the limited resources available in health care. To emphasize material that is clinically relevant, references in this chapter are drawn from RCTs involving human subjects as well as authoritative reviews. The chapter highlights the change of emphasis from PN toward EN in clinical medicine on the basis of RCTs.

Historical Perspective

More than 2300 years ago, Egyptian physicians perceived that some patients were suffering from lack of nutrition.[1] These healers provided their patients with enemas and nutritional clysters. Greek physicians adopted these customs and administered rectal clysters consisting of wine, whey, milk, ptisan, and broth of spelt. Aquapendente[2] described forced feeding in 1617 and pictured a nasogastric tube. In 1879 Bliss[3] expounded the benefits of feeding per rectum via a tube-and-syringe

apparatus. Bliss was so satisfied with his apparatus that he conjectured it would be difficult to " . . . imagine that any further improvement in our present instruments will ever be made or needed." The aliments administered included beef extract, beef peptinoids, and whiskey. The materials were predigested by cooking and mixing with juice from pancreas of a freshly killed animal, yielding one of the first descriptions of a partially hydrolyzed enteral solution. Other references in the tradition of rectal alimentation include the 1878 work of Brown-Séquard,[4] who provided nutritional support to neurological patients via this route.

Alternative sites for delivery of nutrition include the stomach, small intestine, and veins. Each site enjoyed varying degrees of popularity over the last 200 years. During the 1770s John Hunter[5] favored the gastric route, as technology contributed leather tubing that allowed passage of nutrients directly into the stomach. Ewald[6] described a flexible gastric tube that used a stylet fashioned from whalebone to ease passage into the stomach.

Einhorn introduced delivery of nutrients into the duodenum in 1910. He described this as a remedy for patients unable to tolerate gastric or colonic feeding.[7] The concept of colonic alimentation revived when Rhoads[8] introduced a predigested peptone hydrolysate into isolated colonic loops and showed absorption of 25% of the nitrogen. This occurred in 1939, the same year that Elman and Weiner[9] described PN using a solution of casein hydrolysate delivered by venoclysis. Although neither route seemed adequate to satisfy nutritional requirements, the suggestion of combining methods anticipated developments occurring today.

In 1968 Wilmore et al.[10] and in 1970 Daily et al.[11] outlined procedures for delivery of nutrients into high-flow venous systems. This strategy avoided the thrombosis and sclerosis that hampered clinicians administering casein hydrolysate solutions by peripheral veins. As important as these procedural advancements were, they prompted only gradual changes in the practice of nutritional care. More rapid change followed the efforts by

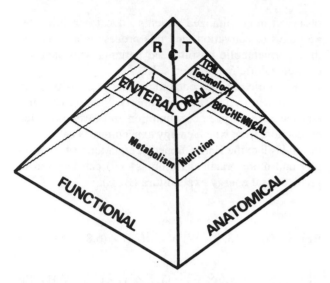

Figure 1. A model for the pyramidal structure of clinical nutrition.

Bistrian et al.,[12] who demonstrated the need for nutritional assessment of hospitalized patients. Their work stimulated an awareness of the beneficial influence of nutrition on patient recovery.

The combination of techniques for identifying patients in need with tools allowing successful intervention became the foundation for the design of a framework for clinical research in nutrition. The benefits of the parenteral route for nutritional support evolved to an appreciation of the physiological and nutritional advantages of enteral feeding. Hydrolyzed protein solutions administered intravenously were replaced by purified amino acid solutions almost exclusively. This happened at a time when complex or oligopeptide enteral solutions were favored over elemental enteral formulations.

The early acceptance of nutritional interventions may seem uncritical today, when advances in patient care require sophisticated scientific evidence from RCTs and meta-analysis before new therapies are implemented and established practices are discontinued. Guidelines for parenteral and enteral nutrition in adults and children rely on high levels of evidence, and 42% of recommendations are supported by randomized or controlled clinical trials.[13] Uncontrolled trials support 26% of guidelines, and the remaining practices have consensus or expert opinion as their basis.

Clinical Nutritional Assessment

Bistrian used simple assessment techniques to demonstrate the epidemic of malnutrition among hospitalized patients.[12,14,15] These techniques served to alert practitioners to the potential for preventable complications. The relevant issues in assessment are as follows. Does a nutritional deficit exist, and if so, to what degree? Will nutritional support help prevent or reverse progression of the malnourished condition? What route of delivery is best suited to accomplish this end?[16] It is difficult to answer the first question because of lack of agreement on the validity, accuracy, and reliability of the methods used to identify degrees of malnutrition and predict outcome.[17,18] The most widely used methods and those with the best testing characteristics will be discussed.

Anthropometrics. Body weight (BW) is the most important anthropometric measurement. Body weight is easily determined, inexpensive, and helpful in quantifying nutritional status. While the method is highly accurate, it is relatively insensitive to even moderate changes in nutritional status. A weight loss of >5% BW within 1 month or 10% over 6 months is likely to affect clinical outcome.[19] To compensate for genetic and geographic variability, weight measurements are standardized. Two such indices are percent ideal body weight (%IBW) and percent usual body weight (%UBW).

$$(\%IBW) = \frac{(Actual\ BW* 100\%)}{IBW}$$

$$(\%UBW) = \frac{(Actual\ BW* 100\%)}{UBW}$$

The %UBW method is more useful when assessing individual patients, but for patients without a weight history, the Hamwi equation[20] and height/weight tables can be used to estimate ideal body weight.

Men: 106 lb/5 ft + 6 lb/additional inch ± 10%
Women: 100 lb/5 ft + 5 lb/additional inch ± 10%

Body-weight measurements reflect contributions from many compartments. These compartments include adipose tissue, skeletal muscle, bone, and parenchymal organs. It may be difficult to identify changes in any one body compartment by composite measurement. Wang presents a lucid analysis and organizes the concepts in measuring body composition.[21] With this framework we can define the correlation between body-compartment change, nutritional status, and outcome. On the basis of this conceptual matrix, Royall et al.[22] demonstrated beneficial changes in nutritionally depleted patients with Crohn's disease who were fed an enteral diet for 3 weeks. The authors compared preintervention and postintervention measurements of body compartments in assessing nutritional products. Their study design is a model for the evaluation of nutritional therapy. With newer technologies, such as bioelectrical impedance analysis, systematic comparison of the effects of therapies on body composition is feasible.[23]

Biochemical indicators. Biochemical tools available for nutritional assessment rely on the body's ability to synthesize protein, which in turn depends on adequate nutrition. There are two classes of visceral proteins. Serum proteins such as albumin and transferrin are constitutive proteins and have a direct relationship with nutritional status and an inverse association with stress and inflammation. Proteins of the second class, globulins and ferritin, are acute-phase reactants and have a direct relationship with inflammation and stress.[24]

Among these proteins, serum albumin is a useful prognosticator of nutritional status and is relatively inexpensive to measure. Because of its 20-day half-life, however, albumin is too slow to reflect short-term nutritional changes and sluggish in showing response to adequate intervention. In addition, albumin levels fall rapidly in response to certain diseases, especially sepsis, and consequently low levels of serum albumin identify patients at increased risk of morbidity and mortality, but do not isolate malnutrition as the cause.[25] Serum albumin levels are helpful but must be used properly.[26] The probability that a particular albumin level is associated with malnutrition can be quantified experimentally, and is called the "likelihood ratio." Clinicians can apply this likelihood or weighting factor to their subjective estimation of the nutritional status to arrive at a stronger predictor of the degree of malnutrition and related morbidity, the posttest probability.

Visceral proteins other than albumin can be used in similar fashion, but albumin is the most widely used because of its low cost and ready availability. However, serum transferrin, with its shorter half-life of 8–10 days, does offer some advantages that make it a competitor as the standard tool for biochemical assessment. A recent prospective study affirmed that transferrin may be a better predictor of postoperative complications than albumin.[27] Regardless, since no perfect test is available, clinical wisdom uses anthropometrics and subjective clinical assessment, including the patient's functional status, to determine probability of malnutrition. This determination is made before biochemical tests, which are done subsequently to refine the clinical judgment.

Functional tests. Investigators have stressed the need for nutritional assessment techniques that reflect an individual's functional status.[28] Functional testing supplements other assessment techniques and offers great sensitivity in recognizing nutritional depletion. Typically functional tests are specific and highly sensitive.[29] Not only does functional testing offer earlier detection of nutritional depletion, it also identifies response to adequate intervention at an early stage. Christie et al.[30] used muscle function testing to show nutritional improvement before traditional methods reflected the improving clinical status.

Nutritional Needs

Energy requirements. Marasmus (protein-energy malnutrition) is the most common nutritional deficiency observed in hospitalized patients.[13] Death ensues after ≈60 days of starvation, and this process is accelerated in hypermetabolic hospitalized patients who have increased caloric requirements.[13,31]

The caloric intake needed to prevent malnutrition can be estimated by indirect calorimetry. Indirect calorimetry measures oxygen consumption and carbon dioxide production, from which energy expenditure is calculated. Formulas like the Harris-Benedict equation* (*A*) or simpler and more practical formulas* (*B*) can be used to predict basal energy expenditure (BEE).[32]

$$A$$
$$\text{Men}$$
$$\text{BEE} = [66 + (13.7 \times W) + (5 \times H) - (6.8 \times A)] \times SF$$

$$\text{Women}$$
$$\text{BEE} = [655 + (9.6 \times W) + (1.7 \times H) - (4.7 \times A)] \times SF$$

$$B$$
$$\text{General}$$
$$W \times 30 \text{ kcal} \cdot \text{kg}^{-1} \cdot \text{day}^{-1} \times SF$$

*where W = weight in kg; H = height in cm; A = age in years; SF = stress factor.

Proponents of measuring energy expenditure argue that assumptions made in formulating predictive equations frequently do not apply to individual patients, and accurate measurements are necessary. In response to this argument others question the need for this degree of accuracy in highly adaptable human metabolism. There are no studies comparing measured estimated energy expenditures in relation to clinical outcome. In practice, workers at institutions that have the equipment readily available tend to obtain indirect calorimetric measurements frequently. Until it is shown that outcome is improved by measuring energy expenditure, there is no basis for favoring measurements over the approximations given by the equations above and in Table 1.

Protein requirements. General recommendations for protein needs are based on consensus (Table 1). Protein requirements are met by administering protein or amino acid solutions. The demonstrable benefit of high-protein intake is improvement in nitrogen balance, rather than improved clinical outcome. Improvement in clinical outcome with high-protein intakes in stress conditions awaits substantiation.

Regarding protein requirements, controversy lingers over the benefits of administering albumin to partially meet the nitrogen needs of patients. Clinicians administer preformed albumin solutions as part of nutritional support in efforts to normalize serum albumin levels rapidly. There is no evidence that this strategy offers advantages in terms of fewer complications, lower mortality, or shorter hospital stays. Even tolerance of enteral feedings failed to improve after correction of oncotic pressure with serum albumin.[33] At present, evidence is

Table 1. Stress factors used in specific clinical conditions, as multipliers of the Harris-Benedict equation for prediction of caloric and protein needs

Clinical condition	Stress factor	Protein requirements (g·kg⁻¹·day⁻¹)
Spinal cord injury[79]	0.8–0.9	0.9
Alcoholism[44]	0.85–0.9	1.2
Liver transplant[80]	1.2	1.2
Head trauma[81]	1.35	1.5
Burn[82]	2.0–2.5	1.7–2.4

anecdotal and does not warrant routine administration of albumin in nutrition support.

Route of Nutritional Support

The routes chosen for delivery of protein and energy have changed over time. In antiquity Egyptians and Greeks chose to approach the alimentary tract via rectum. As early as 1598, feeding tubes were being passed via esophagus to deliver alimentation.[34] Randall's historical review of enteral feeding highlights the changing popularity of various approaches to the gastrointestinal (GI) tract.[35] Recently the emphasis has shifted, and clinicians now espouse the view that PN is a therapy used primarily when oral and tube feeding have failed.[36,37]

Enteral Nutrition

The advantages of feeding by the enteral route are financial as well as outcome based. Among studies showing advantages of EN is that of Gonzalez-Huix et al.[38] In this study of 42 patients being treated with steroids for ulcerative colitis, patients randomized to EN had a 75% reduction in adverse events—including postoperative infections—compared with patients receiving PN. The authors concluded that EN is safer than PN and equally effective in maintaining nutritional status.

Kudsk et al.[39] similarly found an advantage to enteral feeding over parenteral alimentation of trauma patients. Pneumonia, intraabdominal abscess, empyema, line sepsis, and fasciitis were reduced 73% with EN compared with PN. The authors noted that EN offered the greatest advantage to the more severely traumatized patients.[39]

Indications. "If the gut works and can be used safely, use it," is a rule routinely applied. This rule was introduced to offset the enthusiastic belief that PN offers an advantage for nutritional support. There is now increasing evidence, such as the above studies, supporting the superiority of EN.

The choice of enteral formula and the site of delivery are areas of active investigation. The choice of enteral formula will depend on the specific characteristics of the patient and the experience of the clinician. Information favoring one formula over another is not available. Each patient should be evaluated individu-

ally to determine disease state, nutritional needs, and available formulas.

Classification of enteral formulas. Formulas for enteral feeding are classified according to four features: caloric density, protein content, route of administration, and molecular complexity of nutrients.[40] This discussion uses the latter quality for primary differentiation, but other distinguishing features are equally important for clinical purposes and are summarized in Table 2.

Glucose polymers as carbohydrate source. Most critically ill patients can be fed enterally with lactose-free formulas containing oligosaccharides. Approximately 8360 kJ/day (2000 kcal/day) of a standard polymeric formula contains sufficient vitamins and minerals to meet 100% of the Recommended Daily Allowances. These glucose polymer products are isotonic and appropriate for undiluted delivery into stomach or jejunum. Some contain fiber, which delays gastric emptying and increases transit time through gut. These formulations tend to relieve or prevent diarrhea and to decrease fluctuations in serum glucose. Certain fibers serve as an added energy source by being fermented to absorbable short-chain fatty acids in colon.[41]

Partially hydrolyzed protein or elemental diets. These products bear a striking resemblance to those described by Bliss in the 1800s. Partially hydrolyzed formulas reduce the need for in vivo digestion. They are recommended for various conditions, including jejunostomy feedings; they tend to be more expensive. The carbohydrate substrate consists of disaccharides and monosaccharides while free amino acids and oligopeptides provide the nitrogen source. Medium-chain triacylglycerols (MCT) and polyunsaturated fatty acids supply the fat. Partially hydrolyzed formulas do not contain fiber, are relatively hypertonic, and require dilution prior to infusion. There is no clear advantage to the use of simple sugars and amino acids compared with oligosaccharides.[42,43]

Targeted formulations. Targeted formulations are enteral products designed to treat a particular disease state or organ failure. Examples of these formulas include products intended for use in liver failure, acquired immunodeficiency syndrome (AIDS), diabetes, respiratory failure, and critical illness such as burns and sepsis. Most of these formulas are expensive, and few have rigorous evidence to support their use.

Table 2. Classification of enteral products by characteristics of clinical application

	Osmolality (mOsmol/kg)	Energy (MJ/L) [kcal/mL])	Protein (g/MJ [g/1000 kcal])	Fat (g/MJ [g/1000 kcal])	Preferred route of delivery
Standard polymeric	300–500	4.2–5.0 [1–1.2]	7–11 [30–45]	6–11 [25–45]	Oral, gastric, or intestinal
High caloric density polymeric	>450	6.3–8.4 [1.5–2]	8–10 [35–42]	8–12 [33–52]	Oral, gastric, or intestinal
Partially hydrolyzed/ elemental	250–600	4.2–5.4 [1–1.3]	7–12 [30–50]	1–10 [3–40]	Intestinal
Targeted formulas	>450	4.2–8.4 [1–2]	2–14 [10–60]	1–14 [2–60]	Varied

The use of targeted formulations in liver disease is supported by RCTs. Patients who have liver failure experience improvement in symptoms of encephalopathy and an increase in functional hepatic mass when given a specialized enteral formula.[44] The formula's original design included a high branched-chain:aromatic-amino-acid ratio. The ratios found in simple soy protein-based formulas and vegetable diets are also effective when combined with lactulose.[45]

Recent formulations have targeted stressed patient populations. These solutions contain additives such as arginine (Arg), glutamine (Gln), ribonucleic acids (RNA), and n–3 fatty acids. Preliminary evidence suggests a reduction in length of hospital stay and frequency of infections in a subgroup of intensive-care patients;[46] this line of evidence is still developing. It seems likely that a group of patients benefiting from this supplementation exists and will be identified.

The enteral formulas discussed above are regulated as foods, and therefore must meet the standards of Good Manufacturing Practice required for all foods.[47] However, unlike drugs, manufacturers of enteral formulas are not required to submit evidence of the efficacy of products as long as marketing claims do not imply medical benefits. This area of regulation may change when nutritional products are accepted as offering primary and secondary therapeutic benefits.

Parenteral Nutrition

Parenteral nutrition involves the administration of nutrients intravenously. The terminology describing PN is not precise. Total parenteral nutrition (TPN) refers to provision of sufficient nutrients to maintain health and promote growth when appropriate. Partial parenteral nutrition (PPN) applies to solutions that deliver <85% of the major nutrients required to prevent deficiencies. The solutions for PN can be delivered via a central or peripheral vein, and give rise to the terms central and peripheral PN. The term hyperalimentation, of significant historical interest, pertains to an obsolete concept and is rarely used today.[48]

Relatively few RCTs demonstrate the benefits of PN. Studies conducted to date compare PN to EN or compare different PN solutions. However, some conditions have not required RCTs to establish the benefits of PN. These conditions, like short-bowel syndrome (SBS), were routinely fatal without the use of PN. With PN, even growth and development, let alone maintenance, are achieved. Now, with advances in transplant technology, PN will soon be challenged to prove its value in these conditions. Successful intestinal transplantation offers potential advantages over permanent PN, including improved quality of life and reduced costs.[49] As outcome improves with this modality, a trial comparing PN to intestinal transplantation may become necessary.

Indications. The primary use of PN is to prevent malnutrition. The primary indication for PN is the need for nutritional support in patients with limited intestinal absorption. A crucial RCT in establishing indications for use of PN looked at major postoperative complications in patients receiving 7–15 days of preoperative PN and in a control group receiving no nutritional intervention.[50] This study demonstrated a 2-fold greater risk of infectious complications with PN than in control patients (p<0.05), and a nonsignificant decrease (risk 0.75) in noninfectious complications with PN. Failure to demonstrate an overall benefit of PN in surgery and oncology patients has stimulated a reevaluation of the role of PN for nutritional support.[51]

One study demonstrating benefit from PN involved administration of glutamine-supplemented PN solutions to patients undergoing bone marrow transplantation.[52] Although the study demonstrated benefits to Gln supplementation, it did not demonstrate superiority of PN over EN or over no nutritional support. This type of control group is desirable because of inferior results seen in previous studies with PN.[53,54] Critical appraisal of PN continues and, while clarifying the role of PN, may further shift emphasis to EN.

Fat. Fat is necessary to prevent essential fatty acid deficiency and is also a rich energy source. To prevent essential fatty acid deficiency, 2–4% of the total energy requirement should come from linoleic acid. Commercially available lipid emulsions have concentrations of 10% and 20%, and provide 4.6 MJ/L (1.1 kcal/mL) and 8.4 MJ/L (2.0 kcal/mL), respectively.

Lipid emulsions consist of tiny droplets of long-chain triacylglycerols (LCT) and small amounts of cholesterol, emulsified by phospholipids and stabilized by glycerol. They are similar in size to chylomicrons, but are cleared from the circulation by the reticuloendothelial system (RES). Since the RES controls intravenous clearance of bacteria as well as lipid emulsions, this led to controversy regarding the safety of lipid emulsions in PN. Strong evidence suggests that inclusion of MCT improves outcome in patients undergoing hepatectomy.[55] The relative risk of morbidity was 0.66, and this reduction primarily reflected a lower infection rate. Increased complications from lipid-based PN are likely due to excessively rapid infusion rates.[56]

Minerals (electrolytes and trace elements). Mineral requirements in PN vary greatly depending on patient status. Electrolyte needs should be reviewed and adjusted on the basis of laboratory values and hydration status. In 1979 the AMA established guidelines for essential trace element solutions for PN use.[57] Trace elements should be provided in standard amounts except in diseases characterized by increased trace element losses, such as Crohn's disease. In these conditions plasma concentrations of zinc and selenium should be measured and, if necessary, these elements supplemented in PN or EN.

Nutrition in Specific Diseases

Cancer. There have been >70 RCTs evaluating the use of nutritional support of cancer patients. Klein and Koretz[51] reviewed those studies that defined clinically significant outcome measurements like duration of hospitalization, morbidity, and mortality. This review, although not a rigorous meta-analysis, concluded that studies do not support the routine use of nutritional therapy in cancer patients. As in any other disease, nutritional therapy in cancer must be tailored to the individual.

Inflammatory bowel disease. Inflammatory bowel disease offers great potential for nutritional intervention as a therapeutic modality. The benefits of nutritional support in Crohn's disease have been studied extensively. PN provides calories and protein necessary for growth and development in children and teens having frequent exacerbations. EN is also well tolerated and promotes remission even when steroid therapy fails. Lochs[58] and later Lindor[59] compared two primary treatments for Crohn's disease, an oligopeptide enteral formula and steroids plus sulfasalazine. The authors found the drug therapy to be more effective than EN, resulting in more rapid remission in larger numbers of patients. Nevertheless, 53% of patients treated with EN experienced remission during a 6-week observation period.

Gonzalez-Huix et al.[60] found remission rates of 88% and 80% in two groups of patients randomized to steroids or EN for acute Crohn's enteritis. The relapse rates favored the EN group, with a relative risk reduction of 36% compared with the steroid group. The authors concluded that, as suspected by Lochs, there appears to be a subgroup of patients with Crohn's disease who do as well with EN as with pharmacotherapy. How to identify this group has not been described.

Royall et al.[42] tried to determine which enteral formulas are most effective in inflammatory bowel disease. They examined the efficacy of elemental diets versus a peptide-based diet in the treatment of patients with Crohn's disease. Patients had equivalent outcomes regardless of the type of formula that was given, with remission rates of 84% in the elemental diet group and 75% in the peptide-based group. This high remission rate occurred despite a high fat intake in the peptide group.

Short-bowel syndrome. Short-bowel syndrome is characterized by maldigestion, malabsorption, dehydration, electrolyte abnormalities, and micronutrient deficiencies. To determine the type of nutritional support appropriate for patients with SBS, the practitioner needs to know the length, site, and mucosal integrity of remaining bowel. Patients who have had small intestinal resections of >75% usually require PN to avoid malnutrition and dehydration. Patients tolerate resection of up to 33% of the small bowel without changes in life-style. Resections up to 50% can be tolerated without PN, but require life-style changes to avoid deficiencies and dehydration.[13] With time, the remaining small bowel undergoes hyperplasia, resulting in increased absorptive capacity. As absorption increases, patients find that they need less PN. The wise selection of foods, attention to the quantity and frequency of feedings, and use of pharmacotherapy hasten the transition to oral or tube feedings.

In SBS, impaired absorption of vitamin B_{12} is common, and parenteral replacement is provided routinely. Oral calcium supplementation lowers oxalate absorption and helps prevent hyperoxaluria and renal stones. In addition, calcium supplementation improves calcium absorption, helping to avoid the disabling effects of osteoporosis. In patients with excessive fluid losses, replacement of potassium, zinc, selenium, and magnesium is essential to avoid cardiac arrhythmia, severe dermatitis, and infection.

Designer Nutrients

Immunonutrition. The use of nutrition to modulate the immune system arises from the observation that starving patients manifest reduced immunocompetence similar to that seen with human immunodeficiency virus (HIV) infection. When the immunologic dysfunction is due to malnutrition, nutritional intervention can improve humoral and cellular immunity. However, when immunosuppression is the result of infection, stress, or trauma, nutritional support has little effect.[61,62]

In well-nourished patients, the impact of nutrition on immunity is difficult to assess. Nonetheless, observations of immunologic effects of specific nutrients in stressed subjects have prompted controlled testing. Daly et al.[63] demonstrated a significant reduction in infections and wound complications in patients who were fed an enteral formula supplemented with Arg, RNA, and n–3 fatty acids. Bower and colleagues[46] found a decrease in length of hospital stay in septic patients who received an enteral formula with supplemental Arg, RNA, and n–3 fatty acids compared with patients who received an isonitrogenous, isocaloric standard formula. Although these finding are preliminary, they do suggest benefit from supplementation of EN with nutrients targeting particular immune functions.

Glutamine. Glutamine, the preferential fuel for the gut, is considered a conditionally essential amino acid in times of stress. Van der Hulst et al.[64] showed that in patients receiving PN, supplemental parenteral Gln had trophic effects on the gut. Decreased gut permeability and increased villus height was noted in the Gln-supplemented group. Glutamine-supplemented PN improved nitrogen balance in patients after bone marrow transplants or bowel surgery.[52,65,66]

Growth hormone. Growth hormone (GH) can improve nitrogen retention, maintain visceral protein levels, and promote lipid mobilization and protein synthesis in catabolic, critically ill patients.[67] Similar effects occur in patients with burns or GI dysfunction and after surgery.[68–70] There is a suggestion that the benefits of GH follow a dose-response curve with a threshold effect.[71] The use of GH in HIV wasting syndrome has also been explored, and it was found that when patients were treated with GH, weight gain was associated with increased lean body mass.[72,73] When GH therapy was terminated, patients lost weight. Hypertriglyceridemia and hyperglycemia were observed side effects of GH.[73,68,70] Short-term GH therapy improves nitrogen balance, but long-term outcome studies have not been done.

Structured lipids. Medium-chain triacylglycerols both enterally and parenterally help in the management of malabsorptive disorders. MCT are cleared and oxidized more rapidly than LCT.[74] Long-chain triacylglycerols contain linoleic acid, which is necessary to prevent essential fatty acid deficiency. Structured lipids are composed of a 50:50 mixture of long- and medium-chain fatty acids. Because structured lipids combine both LCT and MCT, they deliver the benefits of superior absorption and rapid clearance while providing essential fatty acids.[75,76]

Ethics

Given the ability to intervene with new technological advances, and accepting the conclusions of RCTs regarding nutritional support, the clinician must return to the base of the clinical pyramid to determine appropriate levels of intervention. The selection of optimal nutritional support is particularly important for patients suffering from a terminal illness or living in a permanent vegetative state, and imperative for patients refusing nutritional intervention. Providing food is symbolic of caring and comfort, especially to those who are dying. In the last two decades, U.S. courts have offered some direction to clinicians who are trying to resolve the moral and legal dilemma of feeding the dying or comatose patient. The Cruzan decision, rendered in 1990, held that the U.S. Supreme Court recognizes a competent person has "a constitutionally protected right to refuse life-saving hydration and nutrition." Although it affirms the accepted principle of respecting patient autonomy, in many cases the patient's wishes are not obvious. A consensus guideline outlines a reasonable approach for the clinician.[13] The guideline emphasizes the need to assess the wish of the patient through every source available, especially the patient's family. During the assessment, patients or surrogates should be apprised of the fact that PN and EN are medical treatments, and as such they impose burdens as well as benefits. The balance between these opposing forces should be presented in an attempt to obtain an informed decision. Recognizing a possible reluctance to initiate this deliberation, the Patient Self-Determination Act (1990) requires that patients be given written information on the law regarding advance directives and be told of their right to refuse treatment.[77] Finally, a prudent guideline comes from a court decision dating to 1891, which holds that "No right is held more sacred, or is more carefully guarded by the common law, than the right of every individual to the possession and control of his person, free from all restraint or interference of others, unless by clear and unquestionable authority of the law."[78]

Summary

This chapter attempts to provide the reader with an overview of parenteral and enteral nutrition. The historical review serves to illustrate that the past is a repository of useful ideas. As new technologies provide solutions to many aspects of nutritional therapy that were previously considered impediments, these ideas can be tapped and applied successfully. The clinical perspective presents an approach that attempts to support, through application of rules of evidence, a perceptible trend toward EN as a modality with therapeutic as well as nutritional benefits. The entire chapter assumes that successful use of PN and EN is based on recognition of the paramount importance of nutritional assessment focusing on the status and goals of the individual patient.

References

1. Cary H, transl (1855) Herodotus. Harper & Brothers, New York

2. Pareira MD, Conrad EJ, Hicks W, Elman R (1954) Therapeutic nutrition with tube feeding. JAMA 156:810–816

3. Bliss DW (1882) Feeding per rectum: as illustrated in the case of the late President Garfield and others. Med Rec 22:64–69

4. Brown-Séquard CE (1878) Feeding per rectum in nervous affections (letter). Lancet 1:144

5. Hunter J (1776) Proposals for the recovery of people apparently drowned. Philos Trans R Soc Lond 66(2):51–52

6. Ewald CA (1874) A ready method of washing out the stomach. Irish Hospital Gazette, August 15, pp 254–255

7. Einhorn M (1910) Duodenal alimentation. Med Rec 78:92–95

8. Rhoads JE, Stengel A, Riegal C, et al (1939) The absorption of protein split products from chronic isolated colon loops. Am J Physiol 125:707–712

9. Elman R, Weiner DO (1939) Intravenous alimentation. JAMA 112:796–802

10. Wilmore DW, Dudrick SJ (1968) Growth and development of an infant receiving all nutrients exclusively by vein. JAMA 203:860–864

11. Daily PO, Griepp RB, Shumway NE (1970) Percutaneous internal jugular vein cannulation. Arch Surg 101:534–536

12. Bistrian BR, Blackburn GL, Hallowell E, Heddle R (1974) Protein status of general surgical patients. JAMA 230:858–860

13. American Society of Parenteral and Enteral Nutrition (1993) Guidelines for the use of parenteral and enteral nutrition in adult and pediatric patients. JPEN 17:1SA–52SA

14. Bistrian BR, Blackburn GL, Bitale J, et al (1976) Prevalence of malnutrition in general medical patients. JAMA 235:1567–1570

15. Blackburn GL, Bistrian BR, Maini BS, et al (1977) Nutritional and metabolic assessment of the hospitalized patient. JPEN 1:11–22

16. Sitzmann JV, Pitt HA (1989) Statement on guidelines for total parenteral nutrition. Dig Dis Sci 34:489–496

17. Collins JP, McCarthy ID, Hill GL (1979) Assessment of protein nutrition in surgical patients—the value of anthropometrics. Am J Clin Nutr 32:1527–1530

18. Sullivan DH, Patch GA, Baden AL, Lipschitz DA (1989) An approach to assessing the reliability of anthropometrics in elderly patients. J Am Geriatr Soc 37:607–613

19. Roy L, Edwards P, Barr L (1985) The value of nutritional assessment in the surgical patient. JPEN 9:170–172

20. Hamwi, GJ (1964) Therapy: changing dietary concepts. In Danowski TS (ed), Diabetes mellitus: diagnosis and treatment. American Diabetes Association, Inc., New York, pp 73–78

21. Wang ZM, Heska A, Pierson RN Jr, Heymsfield SB (1995) Systematic organization of body composition methodology: an overview with emphasis on component-based methods. Am J Clin Nutr 61:457–465

22. Royall D, Greenberg FR, Allard JP, et al (1995) Total enteral nutrition support improves body composition of patients with active Crohn's disease. JPEN 19:95–99

23. Kushner RF (1992) Bioelectrical impedance analysis: a review of principles and applications. J Coll Nutr 11:199–209

24. Kudsk KA, Minard G, Wojtysiak SL, et al (1994) Visceral protein response to enteral versus parenteral nutrition and sepsis in patients with trauma. Surgery 116:516–523

25. Owen WF Jr, Lew NL, Liu Y, et al (1993) The urea reduction ratio and serum albumin concentration as predictors of mortality in patients undergoing hemodialysis. N Engl J Med 329:1001–1006

26. Jaeschke R, Guyatt GH, Sackett DL (1994) Users' guides to the medical literature: III. How to use an article about a diagnostic test. B. What are the results and will they help me in caring for my patients? JAMA 271:703–707

27. Dannhauser A, van Zyland JM, Nel JC (1995) Preoperative nutritional status and prognostic nutritional index in patients with benign disease undergoing abdominal operations. Part I. J Am Coll Nutr 14:80–90

28. Jeejeebhoy KN, Baker JP, Wolman SL, et al (1982) Critical evaluation of the role of clinical assessment and body composition studies in patients with malnutrition and after total parenteral nutrition. Am J Clin Nutr 35:1117–1127

29. Brough W, Horne G, Blount A, et al (1986) Effects of nutrient intake, surgery, sepsis, and long term administration of steroids on muscle function. Br Med J 293:983–988

30. Christie PM, Graham LH (1990) Effect of intravenous nutrition on nutrition and function in acute attacks of inflammatory bowel disease. Gastroenterology 99:730–736

31. Leiter LA, Marliss EB (1982) Survival during fasting may depend on fat as well as protein stores. JAMA 248:2306–2307

32. Harris JA, Benedict FG (1919) Standard basal metabolism constants for physiologists and clinicians: a biometric study of basal metabolism in man. Carnegie Institute of Washington, Washington, DC

33. D'Angio RG (1994) Is there a role for albumin administration in nutrition support? Ann Pharmacother 28:478–482

34. Capivacceus G (1598) Medicina practica. Sessae, Venice, pp 67–68

35. Randall HT (1984) Enteral nutrition: tube feeding in acute and chronic illness. JPEN 8:113–136

36. Howard L (1984) Parenteral nutrition. In Olson RE (ed), Present knowledge in nutrition, 5th ed. Nutrition Foundation, Washington, DC, pp 664–681

37. Ament ME (1990) Enteral and parenteral nutrition. In Brown ML (ed), Present knowledge in nutrition, 6th ed. International Life Sciences Institute, Washington, DC, pp 444–450

38. Gonzalez-Huix F, Fernandez-Banares F, Esteve-Comas M, et al (1993) Enteral versus parenteral nutrition as adjunct therapy in acute ulcerative colitis. Am J Gastroenterol 88:227–232

39. Kudsk KA, Croce MA, Fabian TC, et al (1992) Enteral versus parenteral feeding: effects on septic morbidity after blunt and penetrating trauma. Ann Surg 215:503–511

40. Heimburger DC, Young VR, Bistrian BR, et al (1986) The role of protein in nutrition, with particular reference to the composition and use of enteral feeding formulas: a consensus report. JPEN 10:425–430

41. Frankenfield DC, Beyer PL (1991) Dietary fiber and bowel function in tube-fed patients. J Am Diet Assoc 91:590–596

42. Royall D, Jeejeebhoy KN, Baker JP, et al (1994) Comparison of amino acid v peptide based enteral diets in active Crohn's disease: clinical and nutritional outcome. Gut 35:783–787

43. Rigaud D, Cosnes J, Le Quintree Y, et al (1991) Controlled trial comparing two types of enteral nutrition in treatment of active Crohn's disease: elemental v polymeric diet. Gut 32:1492–1497

44. Kearns PJ, Young HS, Garcia G, et al (1992) Accelerated improvement in the treatment of alcoholic liver disease with protein supplementation. Gastroenterology 102:200–205

45. Bianchi GP, Marchesini G, Fabbri A, et al (1993) Vegetable versus animal protein diet in cirrhotic patients with chronic encephalopathy: a randomized cross-over comparison. J Intern Med 233:385–392

46. Bower RH, Cerra FB, Bershadshy B, et al (1995) Early enteral administration of a formula (Impact) supplemented with arginine, nucleotides, and fish oil in intensive care unit patients: results of a multicenter, prospective, randomized, clinical trial. Crit Care Med 23:436–449

47. Life Sciences Research Office, Federation of American Societies for Experimental Biology (1991) Guidelines for the scientific review of enteral food products for special medical purposes. JPEN 15:99S–173S

48. Zaloga GP, Roberts P (1994) Permissive underfeeding. New Horiz 2:257–263

49. Asfar S, Zhong R, Grant D (1994) Small bowel transplantation. Surg Clin North Am 75:1197–1210

50. The VA total parenteral nutrition comparative study group (1991) Perioperative total parenteral nutrition in surgical patients. N Engl J Med 325:525–532

51. Klein S, Koretz RL (1994) Nutrition support in patients with cancer: what do the data really show? Nutr Clin Pract 9:91–100

52. Ziegler TR, Young LS, Benfell K, et al (1992) Clinical and metabolic efficacy of glutamine-supplemented parenteral nutrition after bone marrow transplantation. Ann Intern Med 116:821–828

53. American College of Physicians (1989) Parenteral nutrition in patients receiving cancer chemotherapy. Ann Intern Med 110:734–736

54. Klein S, Simes J, Blackburn GL (1986) Total parenteral nutrition and cancer clinical trials. Cancer 58:1378–1386

55. Fan ST, Lo CM, Lai EC, et al (1994) Perioperative nutritional support in patients undergoing hepatectomy for hepatocellular carcinoma. N Engl J Med 331:1547–1552

56. Miles JM (1991) Intravenous fat emulsions in nutritional support. Curr Opin Gastoenterol 7:306–311

57. Department of Foods and Nutrition, American Medical Association (1979) Guidelines for essential trace element preparations for parenteral use: a statement by an expert panel. JAMA 241:2051–2054

58. Lochs H, Steinhardt HJ, Klaus-Wentz B, et al (1991) Comparison of enteral nutrition and drug treatment in active Crohn's disease: results of the European Cooperative Crohn's Disease Study. IV. Gastroenterology 101:881–888

59. Lindor KD, Fleming CR, Burnes JU, et al (1992) A randomized, prospective trial comparing a defined formula diet, corticosteroids, and a defined formula diet plus corticosteroids in active Crohn's disease. Mayo Clin Proc 67:328–333

60. Gonzalez-Huix F, de Leon R, Fernandez-Banares F, et al (1993) Polymeric enteral diets as primary treatment of active Crohn's disease: a prospective steroid controlled trial. Gut 34:778–782

61. Daly JM, Lieberman MD, Goldfine J, et al (1992) Enteral nutrition with supplemental arginine, RNA, and omega-3 fatty acids in patients after operation: immunologic, metabolic, and clinical outcome. Surgery 112:56–67

62. Daly JM, Reynolds J, Thom A, et al (1988) Immune and metabolic effects of arginine in the surgical patient. Ann Surg 208:512–521

63. Daly JM, Weintraub FN, Shou J, et al (1995) Enteral nutrition during multimodality therapy in upper gastrointestinal cancer patients. Ann Surg 221:327–338

64. van der Hulst RR, van Kreel BK, von Meyenfeldt MF, et al (1993) Glutamine and the preservation of gut integrity. Lancet 341:1363–1365

65. MacBurney M, Young LS, Ziegler TR, Wilmore DW (1994) A cost-evaluation of glutamine-supplemented parenteral nutrition in adult bone marrow transplant patients. J Am Diet Assoc 94:1263–1266

66. Stehle P, Zander J, Mertes N, et al (1989) Effect of parenteral glutamine peptide supplements on muscle glutamine loss and nitrogen balance after major surgery. Lancet 1(8632):231–233

67. Jeevanandam M, Ali MR, Holaday NJ, Petersen SR (1995) Adjuvant recombinant human growth hormone normalizes plasma amino acids in parenterally fed trauma patients. JPEN 19:137–144

68. Ziegler TR, Rombeau JL, Young LS, et al (1992) Recombinant human growth hormone enhances the metabolic efficacy of parenteral nutrition: a double-blind, randomized controlled study. J Clin Endocrinol Metab 74:865–873

69. Wong WK, Soo KC, Nambiar R, et al (1995) The effect of recombinant growth hormone on nitrogen balance in malnourished patients after major abdominal surgery. Aust NZ J Surg 65:109–113

70. Hammarqvist F, Stromberg C, Decken A, et al (1992) Biosynthetic human growth hormone preserves both muscle protein synthesis and the decrease in muscle-free glutamine, and improves whole-body nitrogen economy after operation. Ann Surg 216:184–191

71. Tacke J, Bolder U, Lohlein D (1994) Improved cumulated nitrogen balance after administration of recombinant human growth hormone in patients undergoing gastrointestinal surgery. Infusionsther Transfusionsmed 21:24–29

72. Krentz AJ, Koster FT, Crist DM, et al (1993) Anthropometric, metabolic and immunologic effects of recombinant human growth hormone in AIDS and AIDS-related complex. J Acquir Immune Defic Syndr 6:245–251

73. Mulligan K, Grunfeld C, Hellerstein MK, et al (1993) Anabolic effects of recombinant human growth hormone in patients with wasting associated with human immunodeficiency virus infection. J Clin Endocrinol Metab 77:956–962

74. Jiang Z, Zhang S, Wang X, et al (1993) A comparison of medium-chain and long-chain triglycerides in surgical patients. Ann Surg 217:175–184

75. Bell SJ, Mascioli EA, Bistrian BR, et al (1991) Alternative lipid sources for enteral and parenteral nutrition: long- and medium-chain triglycerides, structured triglycerides, and fish oils. J Am Diet Assoc 91:74–78

76. Heyland DK, Cook DJ, Guyatt GH (1994) Does the formulation of enteral feeding products influence infectious morbidity and mortality rates in the critically ill patient? a critical review of the evidence. Crit Care Med 22: 1192–1202

77. LaPuma J, Orentilicher D, Moss RJ (1991) Advanced directives on admission: clinical implications and analysis of the Patient Self-determination Act of 1990. JAMA 266:402–405

78. White M, Fletcher J (1991) The Patient Self-Determination Act. JAMA 266:410–412

79. Kearns PJ, Thompson JD, Werner PC, et al (1992) Nutritional and metabolic response to acute spinal-cord injury. JPEN 16:11–15

80. Plevak DJ, DiCecco SR, Wiesner RH, et al (1994) Nutritional support for liver transplantation: identifying caloric and protein requirements. Mayo Clin Proc 69:225–230
81. Borzotta AP, Pennings J, Papasadero B, et al (1994) Enteral versus parenteral nutrition after severe closed head injury. J Trauma 37:459–468
82. Xie W-G, Li AN, Wang S-L (1993) Estimation of the caloric requirements of burned Chinese adults. Burns 19:146–149

Chapter 54

Nutrient-Drug Interactions

Howard R. Knapp

The distinction between chemicals ingested as micronutrients and as drugs is often not clearly drawn. Recent examples of toxic syndromes resulting from the overly enthusiastic use of vitamins[1] and amino acids[2] as health supplements remind us that the traditional emphasis on the importance of balance in nutrition continues to be valid. On the other hand, some drugs (e.g., niacin) are prescribed for ingestion in multigram daily dosages that can influence nutrient disposition on a mass basis. The purpose of this brief review is to outline the types of interactions that can take place between drugs and nutrients, with an emphasis on those of clinical relevance. Occasionally, comments will also be made about animal studies and theoretical considerations. Because of space limitations and because several books and symposia proceedings have been published on this subject,[3,4] reference will be made for the most part to other reviews of specific topics rather than to primary source articles. It is hoped that this approach will be most beneficial to students and clinicians alike.

Several important areas cannot be reviewed in an article of this size and have been dealt with elsewhere. These include the effects on nutritional status of antimetabolite drugs used for cancer chemotherapy and antibiotics that are relatively selective vitamin antagonists for microorganisms.[5] Limited reference will be made to interactions between drugs, nutrition, and alcohol, which have been reviewed elsewhere, and to electrolyte imbalances induced by diuretics and laxatives.[5–7] Finally, although the important appetite-stimulant and -suppressive effects of drugs is an area of great pharmacological interest in the management of eating disorders, this topic will not be covered here.[5,8]

Nutrients have been described as interacting with virtually every aspect of drug availability and action. Such effects can range from simple physical alteration of drug absorption to specific influences on the metabolic site of drug effect. Many of the nutrient-drug interactions that have been described in the past have proven to have little clinical relevance under normal conditions. However, careful observation and history-taking must be combined with a high index of suspicion if such interactions are to be detected outside the setting of a truly attention-getting clinical disaster. A working familiarity with the general details of drug availability, action, and disposal is necessary to appreciate the full range of possible nutrient interactions that can take place in an individual patient.[9]

That individuals may have dietary peculiarities is commonly acknowledged by every medical student who asks hypertensive patients whether they ingest large quantities of licorice; if licorice contains real plant extract, its mineralocorticoid activity can cause an increase in blood pressure.[10] This review will acquaint the reader with additional examples of how dietary components can alter the response to and need for drug therapy, as well as with the general pharmacological principles involved.

Physical Nutrient-Drug Interactions

Chemicals entering the gastrointestinal tract together may combine in a way that markedly alters their absorption (Table 1). Although the literature has emphasized the reduced bioavailability of the more important or the limited member of a pair of complexing molecules, there may be other effects. The failure of tetracyclines to be absorbed after complexing with di- and trivalent cations formed the basis of a number of publications, but this class of antibiotics is rarely administered orally for serious illnesses and is usually not given in high doses for long enough to have any clinical effect on iron or calcium balance.[11] The excessive use of antacids, however, has been found occasionally to cause clinically significant phosphate depletion by the formation of insoluble aluminum or magnesium phosphates.[12] A similar loss of dietary heavy metals occurs with the chronic ingestion of large quantities of plant-derived phytates, which are polyphosphate inositol derivatives that readily bind metals. Additional interactions of this type have been described.[13–15]

The interaction of neomycin with bile salts to form nonabsorbable precipitates is of use in hypercholesterolemia. Neomycin is enjoying renewed popularity in combination with the recently available cholesterol synthesis inhibitors.[16] By causing selective malabsorption of bile salts, neomycin enhances sterol excretion and

Table 1. Physical interactions between nutrients and drugs

Agents	Effects
Tetracyclines, phytates	Bind heavy metals into nonabsorbed complexes
Neomycin, cholestyramine	Bind bile acids and lower absorption of lipid-soluble vitamins
Mineral oil	Dissolves and removes lipophilic drugs, vitamins
Antacids (aluminum or magnesium)	Form insoluble phosphates

helps reduce the body's cholesterol pool. However, absorption of other lipophilic compounds, including vitamins and drugs, is also reduced.[17] Similar effects have been noted with cholestyramine and other bile acid–binding resins, which can have the additional effect of binding other acidic drugs.

It was shown in 1941 that ingestion of mineral oil, frequently used by the elderly to aid bowel function, will also impair absorption of lipid-soluble vitamins; this will obviously be true for drugs having this chemical property as well.[18] A further example of this type of interaction may evolve from the current emphasis on increasing the intake of bran and other vegetable polymers. Although several reported interactions between drugs and bran have been shown to be of little clinical relevance, there are suggestions that brans from different plant sources may have different properties.[19,20] Thus, the possibility of such an interaction should be considered when a patient appears to fail to absorb a drug. Nutrient-drug incompatibility may also be frequently overlooked in elderly, debilitated patients receiving tube-fed formula diets.[21]

Although it is frequently assumed that food reduces drug absorption, lipophilic drugs are in many cases more completely absorbed when ingested with a fatty meal.[22] This may be because of increased uptake in lipid micelles or better solubilization in the presence of increased concentrations of bile salts and lecithins (evoked by gall bladder emptying into duodenum in the presence of fat). Delayed gastric emptying by fatty food can lead to increased dispersion of granular drug preparations as well as to greater absorption of drugs from the stomach. In addition, drugs that are slowly removed from the duodenum by saturable transport processes may be more completely absorbed if their exit from the stomach is more gradual.[22] Finally, malabsorption syndromes are seen with drugs that directly injure a large proportion of the gastrointestinal epithelium. These include both antimetabolites used in cancer chemotherapy and colchicine used to treat gout.[23]

Metabolic Nutrient-Drug Interactions

The effects of both specific nutrients and general nutritional status on drug bioavailability (summarized in Table 2) begin in the gastrointestinal tract. Several cases have been described in which dietary protein has influenced the intestinal metabolism or absorption of drugs that are amino acid derivatives (e.g., methyl-dopa, L-dopa).[21] It is well known that intestinal bacteria metabolize L-dopa and sulfasalazine, and the ability of these bacteria to metabolize other drugs is now becoming more widely appreciated. Sulfasalazine is delivered to its site of action (colon) in prodrug form and is cleaved by colonic bacteria to an active drug (5-aminosalicylic acid) useful in inflammatory bowel disease.[24] However, the parent drug appears to impair folate absorption in the small intestine.[25]

The importance of drug metabolism by intestinal bacteria has not received a great deal of attention because it has been difficult to demonstrate significant, sustained changes in human intestinal flora via realistically achievable dietary manipulations. The most common clinical event demonstrating this process is the administration of an antibiotic to a patient who is on a stable dose of another drug; as a result, the other drug becomes toxic or ineffective.[26]

Despite the general resilience of our intestinal flora to dietary changes, it is possible that drastic or unusual dietary maneuvers, such as initiating a pure-formula diet regimen or consuming large doses of highly unsaturated fish oils for putative cardiovascular benefits, could alter the intestinal flora in a metabolically important way. The absorption and bacterial metabolism of some drugs has been found to depend upon intestinal transit time, which can be influenced by spicy or irritating foods, dietary fiber, and other food components.[21] Although one would not expect a marked change to take place over a prolonged period in fairly healthy patients, many patients with AIDS have markedly reduced transit times and generally poor bioavailability of orally administered drugs.[27]

Similar problems have been reported in patients who are chronic abusers of certain types of laxatives. Intermittent reductions in drug absorption for this reason may cause erratic plasma levels of rapidly metabolized drugs that need to be kept at a therapeutic level most of the time (e.g., drugs treating cardiac arrhythmias). Finally, the gastrointestinal tract itself has been shown to initiate the "first pass" metabolism of a number of drugs.[28] These processes may be influenced not only by dietary protein but also by the dietary fats that eventually

Table 2. Dietary factors affecting drug disposition and metabolism

- Dietary protein intake has effects on plasma albumin levels, drug-metabolizing enzymes in gut and liver, and intestinal microflora.
- Meal composition can alter intestinal activity and blood flow to accelerate or retard drug absorption or metabolism.
- Nutritional status also affects renal and biliary drug clearance rates, and can cause specific changes in drug action or toxicity.
- Excess body fat may increase volume of distribution of lipophilic drugs.
- Injection of drugs into subcutaneous adipose tissue may slow absorption of drugs into the circulation.

determine the types of fatty acids making up the membrane phospholipid environment of the drug-metabolizing enzymes.

Dietary protein has also been shown to influence splanchnic blood flow, which can be of importance for drugs that are largely metabolized by liver (first-pass effect). The rate of hepatic blood flow and the rapidity of drug absorption can determine what portion of the drug escapes first-pass metabolism via intrahepatic shunting or saturation of removal pathways.[29] Dietary protein also has important effects on the levels of drug-metabolizing enzymes in both intestine and liver.[30,31]

Interestingly, previous studies have shown that dietary carbohydrate or fat has little effect on the removal of drugs by these enzymes.[32] However, these studies did not include fish oils, which have recently received much attention because of their potential benefits in cardiovascular disease.[33,34] Because these highly unsaturated lipids induce peroxisome proliferation in rodents and alter the oxidation of fatty acids, in addition to prolonging bleeding time in humans, it will be surprising if they are not eventually found to have clinically important interactions with some drugs.[33] No such interactions have yet been reported, probably because detailed pharmacological studies with these lipids have been limited.

The activities of drug-metabolizing enzymes can be influenced by food components that are their substrates, which induce the formation of increased amounts of enzyme. This has been noted for indoles present in cabbage and brussels sprouts and for charcoal-broiled meats, but is probably also true for other smoked or preserved meats and vegetables that contain large amounts of chemicals metabolized by cytochrome P450 enzymes.[21]

Thus far, the effects of nutrients on drug-metabolizing enzymes have not been specific for particular drugs. However, different cytochrome P 450 enzymes (the major family of enzymes responsible for drug removal from the body) act on different types of drugs and have specific interactions with various nutrients.[31,35] As a result, particular drug-nutrient interactions have been noted in which a drug has stimulated or blocked the production of hormones or active forms of vitamins in the body. Examples include the reduction in availability of vitamins D and K by diphenylhydantoin and several other

drugs, with resultant lowering of calcium absorption or a bleeding diathesis.[5,21]

Interactions in Nutrient-Drug Disposition

The specific action of certain drugs to increase or decrease appetite has been mentioned. However, the nonspecific adverse effects of many drug therapies on patients' food ingestion is often unappreciated. In the hospital setting the dietary or nursing staff can follow this carefully, but doing so in an outpatient setting is difficult. Effects can vary from a bad taste in the mouth that makes all food unpalatable to nausea, a feeling of early satiety, or other gastrointestinal discomfort. In most patients the result is merely noncompliance with a drug regimen, but other patients (particularly those who are debilitated or elderly) may experience significant adverse effects on overall nutritional status.

Important differences in drug disposition can occur in patients who have significantly more or less than the average amount of body fat. The most obvious example of this phenomenon is in the administration of drugs by injection. In a cachectic patient, a subcutaneously administered drug such as heparin may be absorbed more rapidly and completely than normal. By contrast, absorption of drugs injected into fat rather than muscle will occur in a very delayed manner if at all. Most intravenously administered drugs are given on a per-unit-of-body-weight basis; to avoid overdosage it is important to use lean body weight to determine the dosage of drugs that do not distribute into adipose tissue. On the other hand, large amounts of very lipid soluble drugs or toxins may partition into the body fat of obese patients, requiring a prolonged period for removal.

The degree to which different drugs are protein-bound in plasma varies from low to nearly complete. This is important for metabolic removal because the unbound fraction is accessible to further metabolism.[9] Most such binding is to albumin, although some lipophilic drugs and vitamins are transported by lipoproteins or other special carrier proteins. A relative deficiency of protein intake results in a lowering of plasma albumin, which can be seen in the catabolic postoperative state as well as in cases of dietary inadequacy or severe malabsorption. This

NUTRIENT-DRUG INTERACTIONS/Knapp

Table 3. Specific nutrient-drug interactions

Action	Drugs	Food component
Inhibited nutrient metabolism	Monoamine oxidase inhibitors	Sympathomimetic amines
	Disulfiram	Ethanol
Increased drug loss	Lithium	Sodium, caffeine
Reversed drug effect	Diuretics	Sodium
Increased nutrient loss	n–3 fatty acids	Vitamin E
	Diphenylhydantoin	Vitamin D
	Isoniazid	Vitamin B-6
Drug-nutrient antagonism	Coumadin drugs	Vitamin K
Increased drug metabolism	L-dopa	Vitamin B-6

problem is being encountered with increasing frequency in patients with AIDS.[5,27]

Lower plasma albumin levels will influence the disposition of many drugs, but the degree and clinical importance of this effect will vary considerably. Penicillins, for example, are excreted more slowly in children with protein-calorie malnutrition because of reduced renal elimination; other drugs are metabolized more slowly by the liver in these patients.[36,37] There have been suggestions that postprandial increases in plasma free fatty acids can transiently displace drugs bound to albumin, but clinically important examples of this phenomenon have not been widely discussed.[30] On the other hand, the displacement of drugs or endogenous metabolites from albumin by other drugs is frequently an important interaction, which can result in more rapid elimination of particular vitamins or other nutrients from plasma.

Specific Nutrient-Drug Interactions

Several unexpected interactions between food items and drugs have been described clinically (Table 3). One of the best known involves the precipitation of hypertensive/hyperadrenergic crisis by the ingestion of foods containing tyramine (including matured cheeses and red wine) or other sympathomimetic amines during therapy with drugs that inhibit monoamine oxidase (MAO) enzymes.[38] Use of the drugs most involved in this interaction is now largely limited to psychiatry, and the dietary precautions necessary in this setting have been reviewed.[8,38] Occasionally, however, such reactions may be experienced with drugs that usually have weak MAO-inhibiting activity, such as isoniazid.[39]

The interaction of L-dopa and pyridoxine in patients with Parkinson's disease is another example of a nutrient altering drug metabolism.[9] Peripheral decarboxylation of L-dopa to dopamine causes severe side effects. Because the amino acid decarboxylase has pyridoxal phosphate as a cofactor, increased intake of pyridoxine caused greater enzyme activity and worse side effects from L-dopa therapy. This complication is less of a problem since the introduction of a decarboxylase inhibitor

(carbidopa) as concomitant therapy to lessen peripheral decarboxylation of L-dopa; this inhibitor is noncompetitive with pyridoxal phosphate. Although L-dopa therapy without carbidopa is now uncommon, this is a useful example of the kind of unexpected nutrient-drug interaction that may occur in sick patients receiving moderate amounts of vitamin supplements.

Lithium is now commonly used for the treatment of manic-depressive disorders. It has been appreciated for some time that sodium intake strongly influences lithium excretion. Sodium restriction in patients taking lithium has caused lithium accumulation and toxicity, whereas increased sodium intake leads to enhanced urinary lithium loss.[9] It has been reported that the renal effects of caffeine tend to increase lithium excretion and that cessation of coffee drinking in patients taking lithium has resulted in decreased lithium excretion and toxicity, with an apparently paradoxical increase in tremulousness.[40]

Although many interactions of alcohol, drugs, and nutrients are reviewed elsewhere, one that is pertinent to the present discussion is the flushing reaction that occurs in response to alcohol ingestion while taking disulfiram (Antabuse) or related aldehyde dehydrogenase-inhibiting drugs.[6–8,41] The accumulation of acetaldehyde in the body when ethanol is consumed causes flushing, nausea, and varying degrees of chest and abdominal discomfort. The syndrome is sufficiently unpleasant that disulfiram is used in aversion treatment of alcoholics. Similar symptoms have been reported with other drugs, particularly metronidazole and chlorpropamide.[9] The former is often prescribed for the sex partners of patients with trichomonal vaginitis or prostatitis; however, because the asymptomatic partner may not actually speak to the prescribing physician, he or she may be unaware of the frightening consequences of ingesting alcohol while taking the drug. Several widely used cephalosporin antibiotics can also cause Antabuse reactions in certain patients.

The intestinal flora of humans and other omnivores provides a much smaller proportion of calories (as short-chain fatty acids from carbohydrate polymer fermentation) than does that of ruminants. However, humans appear to receive a substantial supply of vitamins, especially vitamin K, from intestinal flora. It is not rare for patients with poor dietary intakes on prolonged antibiotic therapy to develop vitamin K deficiency and a bleeding diathesis.[42]

Changes in both dietary and intestinal-flora sources of vitamin K can precipitate either over- or under-treatment of patients on vitamin K–antagonist anticoagulants (e.g., warfarin).[43,44] Because the absorption, plasma binding, and metabolism of warfarin can be influenced by many other drugs to produce clinically serious effects, its drug-drug interactions are widely appreciated.[9] Patients are often on such anticoagulants for years, so it is important to avoid drastic changes in vitamin K availability. Occasionally patients may be unaware that they are taking vitamin K supplements, as in enteral formula feedings, which can antagonize the effects of the anticoagulant drug.[21]

Whereas vitamin K can cause problems in the clinical use of vitamin K antagonists, the use of vitamin A analogs can result in vitamin A toxicity when combined with excessive vitamin supplementation.[9] This is particularly true in children and in patients with liver disease.

Highly unsaturated marine oils containing n–3 fatty acids are the subject of a great deal of current medical research, especially in regard to their possible antiatherosclerotic and antithrombotic effects.[33] As mentioned above, the interaction of these nutrients (which are often studied in pharmacologic doses) with drugs is as yet unknown, but some concern has been expressed with regard to the oxidant stress exerted by such supplements in vivo. The classical method of inducing vitamin E deficiency in animals is to feed them high amounts of such polyunsaturated fats without antioxidants, including tocopherols.[45] Asymptomatic yellow-fat disease (caused by lipid peroxidation in vivo) has been noted in animals receiving a diet with a high fish content even though the animals were receiving vitamin E supplements.[46]

Vitamin E deficiency has not been noted in studies using unrefined fish oils in humans, but has recently been seen in studies involving the administration of highly purified n–3 polyunsaturated fatty acids.[47] Although this may be an adverse effect in some settings, some researchers are trying to take advantage of the vitamin E depletion caused by fish oil in circulating erythrocytes to cure malaria by oxidative destruction of parasites in blood. This effect was first noted in mice 30 years ago and was largely forgotten until recently.[48,49]

Specific chemical reactions of several drugs with pyridoxine have been found to result in depletion of this vitamin in humans, causing neuropathy.[9] The best-known examples are isoniazid and hydralazine; pyridoxine supplements are usually prescribed when the former is used as antituberculosis therapy. The problem is less common with hydralazine but illustrates another type of interaction that should be considered in the evaluation of possible medication side effects.

Final examples of nutrient-drug interactions involve sodium in the development of hypertension and congestive heart failure and potassium in regulating the electrical activity of cells. It is known from both population studies and clinical trials that excessive sodium ingestion leads to blood pressure elevation in susceptible individuals.[50] Diuretics are widely used to enhance sodium excretion in patients with hypertension, as well as in those with cardiac dysfunction associated with renal underperfusion and sodium retention (heart failure with resultant edema formation). Patients whose heart failure has been well compensated and others with histories of good blood pressure control are often seen in emergency rooms during the holiday season suffering from acute clinical deterioration caused by a high intake of heavily salted preserved meat products (e.g., in the southern United States, "country ham"). Likewise, the basis for taking digitalis preparations to improve cardiac contractility involves inhibition of the Na^+-K^+ pump.[9] Patients taking diuretics or having prolonged episodes of diarrhea without adequate dietary replacement can have sufficient potassium losses that digitalis toxicity results.[9] If dietary potassium via intake of fruits, vegetables, and juices is inadequate or not tolerated by the patient, potassium supplements are frequently prescribed.

Summary

Optimal pharmacologic therapy depends upon the predictable delivery and action of a prescribed drug. To assure this, one must take into account several aspects of the patient's general nutritional status and be aware of nutrient-drug interactions. These range from physical nutrient-drug complexation, causing altered drug and nutrient absorption, to effects on the disposition, metabolism, and site of action of drugs; effects of drugs on nutritional status, in altering nutrient requirements, and in antagonizing the actions of vitamins are also described. In addition to discussing general principles, examples of specific nutrient-drug interactions are given that can be of clinical relevance. These involve both nutrient-induced drug toxicity or ineffectiveness and drug-induced nutrient depletion.

Although the chapter does not present an exhaustive catalog, an attempt has been made to illustrate most of the possible types of nutrient-drug interactions so that readers will be more likely to appreciate the potential for such effects in their evaluation of clinical problems.

Nonpharmacological therapies for common diseases such as hypertension and cardiovascular disease have recently been emphasized. As this type of therapeutic intervention becomes more prevalent, clinically important nutrient-drug interactions will become more frequent.

It is hoped that this review, in illustrating a wide variety of possible interactions, will help to increase the reader's awareness of these processes when evaluating therapeutic options and results.

References

1. Schaumberg H, Kaplan J, Windebank A, et al (1983) Sensory neuropathy from pyridoxine abuse: a new megavitamin syndrome. N Engl J Med 309:445–448

2. Anonymous (1990) The clinical spectrum of the eosinophilia-myalgia-syndrome (EMS) in California. Morb Mortal Wkly Rep 39:89–91

3. Hathcock JN, Coon J, eds (1978) Nutrition and drug interrelations. Academic Press, New York

4. Hathcock JN, ed (1982) Nutritional toxicology. Academic Press, New York

5. Roe DA (1984) Nutrient and drug interactions. Nutr Rev 42:141–154

6. Seitz HK (1985) Alcohol effects on drug-nutrient interactions. Drug-Nutrient Interactions 4:143–163

7. Sexias FA (1975) Alcohol and its drug interactions. Ann Intern Med 83:86–92

8. Gray GE (1989) Nutritional aspects of psychiatric disorders. J Am Diet Assoc 89:1492–1498

9. Gilman AG, Rall TW, Nies AS, Taylor P, eds (1990) The pharmacological basis of therapeutics, 8th ed. Macmillan Publishing Co., New York

10. Epstein MT, Espiner EA, Donald RA, Hughes H (1977) Effects of eating licorice on the renin-angiotensin-aldosterone axis in normal subjects. Br Med J 1:488–490

11. Neuvonen PJ (1976) Interactions with the absorption of tetracyclines. Drugs 11:45–54

12. Baker LR, Ackrill P, Cattell WR, et al (1974) Iatrogenic osteomalacia and myopathy due to phosphate depletion. Br Med J 3:150–152

13. Ford JA, Colhoun EM, McIntosh WB, Dunnigan MG (1972) Rickets and osteomalacia in the Glasgow Pakistani community 1961–71. Br Med J 2:677–680

14. Berlyne GM, Ben Ari J, Nord E, Shainkin R (1973) Bedouin osteomalacia due to calcium deprivation caused by high phytic acid content of unleavened bread. Am J Clin Nutr 26:910–911

15. Welling PG (1977) Influence of food and diet on gastrointestinal drug absorption: a review. J Pharmacokinet Biopharm 5:291–334

16. Jones PH (1992) A clinical overview of dyslipidemias: treatment strategies. Am J Med 93:187–198

17. Jacobson ED, Chodos RV, Faloon WW (1960) An experimental malabsorption syndrome induced by neomycin. Am J Med 28:524–533

18. Morgan JW (1941) The harmful effects of mineral oil (liquid petrolatum) purgatives. J Am Med Assoc 117:1135–1136

19. Woods MN, Ingelfinger JA (1979) Lack of effect of bran on digoxin absorption. Clin Pharmacol Ther 26:21–23

20. Kasper H, Zilly W, Fassl H, Fehle F (1979) The effect of dietary fiber on postprandial serum digoxin concentrations in man. Am J Clin Nutr 32:2436–2438

21. Roe DA (1994) Medications and nutrition in the elderly. Nutr Old Age 21(1):135–147

22. Melander A (1978) Influence of food on the bioavailability of drugs. Clin Pharmacokinet 3:337–351

23. Race TF, Paes IC, Faloon WW (1970) Intestinal malabsorption induced by oral colchicine. Am J Med Sci 259:32–34

24. Peppercorn MA, Goldman P (1972) The role of intestinal bacteria in the metabolism of salicylazosulfapyridine (1972) J Pharmacol Exp Ther 181:555–562

25. Franklin JL, Rosenberg IH (1973) Impaired folic acid absorption in inflammatory bowel disease: effects of salicylazosulfapyridine (azulfidine). Gastroenterology 64:517–523

26. Hartiala K (1973) Metabolism of hormones, drugs and other substances by the gut. Physiol Rev 53:496–534

27. Gillin JD, Shike M, Alcock N, et al (1985) Malabsorption and mucosal abnormalities of the small intestine in the acquired immunodeficiency syndrome. Ann Intern Med 102:619–622

28. George CF (1981) Drug metabolism by the gastrointestinal mucosa. Clin Pharmacokin 6:259–274

29. Routledge PA, Shand DG (1979) Presystemic drug elimination. Annu Rev Pharmacol Toxicol 19:447–468

30. Hathcock JN (1985) Metabolic mechanisms of drug-nutrient interactions. Fed Proc 44:124–129

31. Guengerich FP (1984) Effects of nutritive factors on metabolic processes involving bioactivation and detoxication of chemicals. Annu Rev Nutr 4:207–231

32. Anderson KE, Conney AH, Kappas A (1979) Nutrition and oxidative metabolism in man: relative influence of dietary lipids, carbohydrate and protein. Clin Pharmacol Ther 26:493–501

33. von Schacky C (1987) Prophylaxis of arteriosclerosis with marine omega-3 fatty acids: a comprehensive strategy. Ann Intern Med 107:215–221

34. Knapp HR (1993) Dietary omega-3 fatty acids and blood pressure control. In Drevon CA, Baksaas I, Krokan HE (eds), Omega-3 fatty acids: metabolism and biological effects. Birkhäuser Verlag, Basel, pp 241–249

35. Campbell TC, Hayes JR (1974) Role of nutrition in the drug metabolizing enzyme system. Pharmacol Rev 26:171–197

36. Buchanan N, Robinson R, Koornhof HJ, Eyeberg C (1979) Penicillin pharmacokinetics in kwashiorkor. Am J Clin Nutr 32:2233–2236

37. Narang RK, Mehta S, Mathur VS (1977) Pharmacokinetic study of antipyrine in malnourished children. Am J Clin Nutr 30:1979–1982

38. McCabe BJ (1986) Dietary tyramine and other pressor amines in MAOI regimens: a review. J Am Diet Assoc 86:1059–1065

39. Smith CK, Durack DT (1978) Isoniazid and reaction to cheese. Ann Intern Med 88:520–521

40. Jefferson JW (1988) Lithium tremor and caffeine intake: two cases of drinking less and shaking more. J Clin Psychiatry 49:72–76

41. Hald J, Jacobsen E (1948) A drug sensitizing the organism to ethyl alcohol. Lancet 2:1001–1004

42. Ansell JE, Kuman R, Deykin D (1977) The spectrum of vitamin K deficiency. J Am Med Assoc 238:40–42

43. Kempin SJ (1983) Warfarin resistance caused by broccoli. N Engl J Med 308(20):1229–1230

44. Qureshi GD, Reinders TP, Swint JJ, Slate MB (1981) Acquired warfarin resistance and weight-reducing diet. Arch Intern Med 141:507–509

45. Dam H (1962) Interrelations between vitamin E and polyunsaturated fatty acids in animals. In Harris RS, Wool IG (eds), Vitamins and hormones, Vol 20. Academic Press, Orlando, FL, pp 527–540

46. Ruiter A, Jongbloed AW, van Gent CM, et al (1978) The influence of dietary mackerel oil on the condition of organs and on blood lipid composition in the growing young pig. Am J Clin Nutr 31:2159–2166

47. Sanders TA (1991) Effects of n-3 polyunsaturated fatty acids

on plasma lipids and lipoproteins. In Simopoulos AP, Kifer RR, Martin RE, Barlow SM (eds), Health effects of *n*-3 fatty acids in seafoods. Karger Verlag, Basel, pp 358–366

48. Godfrey DG (1957) Antiparasitic action of dietary cod liver oil upon plasmodium berghei and its reversal by vitamin E. Exp Parasitol 6:555–565

49. Levander OA, Ager AL, Morris VC, May OG (1989) Menhaden fish oil and a vitamin E deficient diet: protection against chloroquine-resistant malaria in mice. Am J Clin Nutr 50:1237–1239

50. Luft FC (1989) Salt and hypertension: recent advances and perspectives. J Lab Clin Med 114:215–221

Chapter 55

Alcohol: Medical and Nutritional Effects

Charles H. Halsted

Ethanol, a dietary substance with an energy value of 29.7 kJ/g (7.1 kcal/g), constitutes ≈5% of the daily energy intake of American adults when consumed in moderation.[1] When consumed in excess, ethanol is the most widely abused addictive drug worldwide, is unique in causing liver and other organ damage, and is responsible for ≈1 in 20 deaths in the United States.[2] Americans over the age of 14 years consume 9.5 L (2.5 gallons) of pure alcohol per capita per year, distributed among beer (one-half), spirits (one-third), and the rest as wine. About 30% of the American population abstains from alcohol, 60% are occasional to moderate drinkers, and the remaining 5–10% are heavy drinkers at risk for diseases of alcohol abuse.[3] In California, which represents 12% of the U.S. population, >13,000 persons died from alcohol-related causes in 1989, primarily motor vehicle accidents, alcoholic cirrhosis, homicides, suicides, and hemorrhagic strokes.[4] The economic loss contributed to these deaths was >$11 billion.[4] Given this wide spectrum of ethanol use and abuse, a discussion of alcohol and nutrition must address the health risks and benefits of ethanol as a dietary component when consumed in moderation and the interactions of excessive ethanol consumption with nutrient availability and metabolism in the pathogenesis of alcohol-related diseases.

Health Risks and Potential Benefits of Ethanol Consumption

The relation of ethanol consumption to mortality risk has been described as a J-shaped curve in numerous epidemiologic studies from different countries. In general, ethanol consumption was expressed in these studies as drinks per day, for which one drink provides ≈12 g ethanol as found in ≈270 mL (≈9 ounces) beer, 30 mL (1.0 ounce) of 80-proof spirits, or 100 mL (3.3 ounces) wine. After the results were standardized for smoking, age, and history of antecedent disease, a 13-year British survey of 12,321 male doctors aged 48–78 years showed lowest overall mortality in those consuming up to three drinks per day, but higher mortality in abstainers and those consuming greater amounts of ethanol.[5] A 12-year prospective study of 13,285 residents of Copenhagen aged 30–79 years and of both sexes found the lowest mortality in those consuming one to two drinks per day. Compared with this level, the relative risk of dying was significantly greater for abstainers and progressively greater for those consuming more than three drinks daily.[6] A follow-up study showed that the association of mortality with increased alcohol intake occurred mainly in consumers of spirits, whereas Danish wine drinkers had lower mortality at up to three to five drinks daily.[7] A 14-year follow-up of 8000 subjects in the original National Health and Nutrition Examination Survey (NHANES I) showed moderate protection at less than two drinks but increased mortality risk in men and women consuming more than two drinks daily.[8] An analysis of >120,000 adults in northern California found increased noncardiovascular mortality in men consuming more than six drinks daily, whereas women were at greater risk of dying at levels greater than three drinks per day.[9] Others found that males consuming more than three drinks per day were at specific increased risk for death from accidents, cirrhosis, and esophageal cancer.[10] A recent 12-year prospective study of >85,000 women showed that all mortality was decreased by "light" drinking (one to three drinks per week), but was increased at more than two drinks per day.[11] Thus, summarizing these data, mortality risk is somewhat greater in abstainers and appears to be decreased in those consuming up to two drinks per day; furthermore, the protective effect of alcohol is somewhat less in women, and overall mortality risk increases in both sexes above these levels. The health risk of ethanol consumption is disease-specific: increasing mortality from many diseases is offset by an apparent preventive effect on the risk of coronary heart disease. These data are summarized in Table 1.

Ethanol consumption and vascular disease. Abundant data indicate that the risk of severe coronary disease is diminished at all levels of ethanol intake, accounting for

Table 1. Benefits and risks of alcohol consumption

Disease	Potential benefit		Increased mortality risk (threshold)	
	Men	Women	Men	Women
Drinks/day[a]				
Overall[5-11]	2	1–2	3	2
Coronary heart disease[12-15]	3	2[b]	—	—
Ischemic strokes[13]	—	1–2	—	—
Hemorrhagic strokes[13]	—	—	—	All levels
Hypertension[16]	—	—	All	All
Cancer of oropharynx-esophagus[10,17]	—	—	2	2
Breast cancer[18]	—	—	—	2
Colorectal adenoma[19,20 c]	—	—	2	2
Liver cirrhosis[9,21]	—	—	6	3

[a]1 drink = 12 g ethanol as contained in 270 mL(9 oz) beer (4.5%), 100 mL wine (12%), or 30 mL(1 oz) 80-proof spirits (40%).

[b]Benefit only in postmenopausal women.[11]

[c]Protective effect of high-folate diet.[19,20]

recognized cardiac risk factors.[12] Examples of such data include the Nurse's Health Study, in which the risk of nonfatal myocardial infarction was 40% less in women consuming three or more drinks per day than in abstainers;[13] the Health Professionals Follow-up Study, in which the risk of nonfatal myocardial infarction in men was inversely related to progressively increasing ethanol intake independently of recognized cardiac risk factors;[14] and the Kaiser Permanente Study, in which protection against acute myocardial infarction was shown in men and women consuming up to three drinks daily.[15] However, the recent prospective follow-up of women in the Nurse's Health Study found that coronary protection by ethanol was limited to postmenopausal women who consumed no more than two drinks per day.[11] Furthermore, the overall mortality risk from all cardiac and vascular disease shows a J-shaped curve that increases at greater than three drinks daily because of the adverse effect of ethanol consumption on risk of cardiomyopathy and significant hypertension.[16] Other data showed a three- to fourfold increased risk of subarachnoid hemorrhage in women at all levels of ethanol consumption, which is in stark contrast to the protective effect of one to two drinks per day against more common ischemic strokes.[13]

Proposed mechanisms for the protective effect of moderate ethanol consumption on the development of atherosclerosis include effects on lipoprotein synthesis, altered eicosanoid metabolism with reduced thromboxane and platelet adhesiveness, and an antioxidant effect of nonalcoholic components of wine.[12] A recent study of patients with known coronary artery disease and of case-matched control subjects showed that both high-density lipoprotein fractions (HDL_2 and HDL_3) were elevated in relation to amounts of daily ethanol consump-

tion up to three drinks per day, and that each fraction correlated with reduced risk of adverse cardiac events.[22] Another study suggested a short-term benefit of moderate ethanol consumption on prevention of clot formation through stimulation of tissue plasminogen activator.[23]

Much interest was generated by a report from France on the paradoxical finding of reduced coronary disease in certain wine-consuming regions compared with other regions, despite similar regional consumption of dietary saturated fats and similar serum cholesterol levels.[24] These data led to a subsequent convincing demonstration that the oxidation of low-density lipoprotein, considered essential in atherosclerotic plaque formation, can be prevented by the in vitro addition of antioxidant phenolic compounds in diluted red wine.[25] However, reduction of cardiac risk cannot be exclusively ascribed to consumption of antioxidants in red wine because the regional increase in French red wine consumption was accompanied by increased dietary consumption of vegetables and fruit,[24] also known to be high in antioxidant potential. Furthermore, recent analysis of the Kaiser Health Questionnaire showed that the reduction of cardiac risk in wine-drinking northern California residents in relation to consumers of beer or spirits may relate to a lower incidence of other risk factors such as smoking, whereas the advantage of red wine was no different from that of white wine.[26] Overall, these data suggest that the life-style of wine drinkers is conducive to reduction of cardiac risk and that the protective antioxidant, phenolic compounds of red wine may be present in sufficient amounts in a variety of nondistilled fruits and other components of a healthy diet.

Ethanol consumption and cancer risk. A recent review of the world literature concluded that risk of cancers of the oropharynx and esophagus is definitively and progressively increased at all levels of ethanol consumption, that a probable association exists between ethanol consumption and colorectal cancer, and that cancers of the gastric cardia and pancreas may be increased as a result of chronic inflammation of these organs during or after excessive ethanol consumption.[27] The risk of oropharyngeal and esophageal cancers increases at consumption of more than two drinks per day[10,17] and is greatly accentuated by concurrent smoking,[17] but is possibly minimized by vegetable diets.[27] The mechanisms for the interaction of ethanol with potential carcinogens in the induction of oropharyngeal cancer and the protective effect of specific dietary compounds remain unclear. The risk of estrogen-sensitive breast cancer in women is increased nearly twofold by moderate drinking, and a prospective crossover study of premenopausal women showed a sensitive regulation of estrogen secretion in response to two drinks daily.[18]

Data from two large epidemiologic studies suggest that the increased risk of colorectal cancer during moderate ethanol consumption is linked to altered dietary folate intake or metabolism.[19,20] One case-control study showed a protective effect of high folate intake against rectal cancer, whereas high compared with low folate intake provided the greatest difference in cancer risk in men who consumed the greatest amount of daily ethanol.[19] Using data from the Nurses' Health Study and the Health Professionals Follow-up Study, others showed that the incidence of precancerous colorectal adenoma identified by flexible sigmoidoscopy was increased in those who consumed more than two drinks daily. Most striking, the incidence of adenoma at this level of ethanol intake was threefold greater in those with low folate intake than in those with high folate intake.[20] Because of the central role of folate as a cofactor for the synthesis of methionine from homocysteine and of thymidine from uracil, increased cancer risk in folate deficiency may be attributed to diminished DNA methylation and/or misincorporation of nucleotide bases in DNA synthesis. Ethanol is a known inhibitor of methionine synthase, and a recent study showed that reduced methionine synthase in Yucatan micropigs fed ethanol chronically correlated with elevated serum homocysteine levels, an abnormal ratio of hepatic uracil to thymidine, and precancerous abnormalities in programmed cell death and proliferation.[28]

Ethanol consumption and risk of alcoholic liver disease. Defining the risk of alcoholic liver disease as a function of ethanol consumption is complicated by the different stages of liver abnormality. For instance, whereas fatty liver, the earliest and reversible stage, occurs after only brief periods of sustained moderate drinking,[29] alcoholic hepatitis and its sequel cirrhosis usually occur after at least a decade of heavy alcohol consumption. Epidemiologic risk data are typically ex-

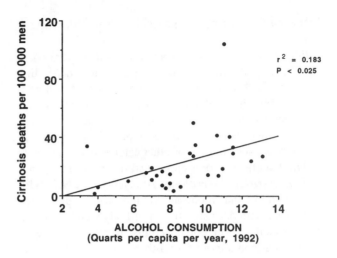

Figure 1. The relation of mortality from liver cirrhosis in men to per capita ethanol consumption worldwide, 1992. Each point represents one country. For example, in the United States, per capita absolute ethanol consumption per year was 7.0 L and cirrhosis mortality was 13.7 deaths per 100,000 men. Hungary had the highest mortality at 105 deaths per 100,000 men, with 10.5 L ethanol per capita. In France the per capita ethanol consumption was 11.0 L and alcoholic cirrhosis mortality was 24 deaths per 100,000 men. The country with the lowest recorded hepatitis was Norway with 5.6 deaths per 100,000 men and 3.8 L ethanol consumed per capita per year. Data from the World Health Organization.[30]

pressed for cirrhosis because this is the most unambiguous histological and clinical lesion of alcoholic liver disease. The incidence of cirrhosis according to hospital admission data was estimated at ≈20 persons per 100,000 in Denmark[30] and Ontario, Canada,[31] whereas the mortality rate from cirrhosis is ≈10 per 100,000 in the United States.[3] Abundant data indicate a direct relation of cirrhosis risk to the amount and duration of ethanol consumption. According to recent World Health Organization data, France and other wine-drinking countries have the highest mortality rates from alcoholic cirrhosis, and mortality correlates worldwide with national per capita ethanol consumption (Figure 1).[32] A study of German males in which elective liver biopsy was compared with careful retrospective drinking histories found liver cirrhosis in 50% of those consuming ≥160 g ethanol per day for 15 years.[33] A prospective study of Danish men followed for 10 years suggested a threshold of 75 g ethanol (6 drinks) per day as the minimal risk level for development of cirrhosis.[21] A similar and striking risk for cirrhosis death at more than six drinks per day was found in the Kaiser Permanente study, although risk was also statistically increased at lower levels of daily ethanol consumption.[9] Other factors known to contribute to cirrhosis risk include sex, with women having one-half the threshold risk of ethanol consumption of men;[34] genetics, with defined familial patterns; and potential modifying dietary factors,[35] as discussed below.

Ethanol Consumption and Energy Balance

Energy production and expenditure and body mass are significantly affected by chronic ethanol use, depending on the variables of sex and the amount of ethanol consumed. Experimental studies indicate that the net effect of ethanol consumption on energy balance and body weight is markedly influenced by patterns of consumption: ethanol substitution for other calories decreases body weight but ethanol addition may stimulate weight gain.[36]

Experimental observations. Analysis of the NHANES II data shows that moderate ethanol consumption was associated with only slightly lower body weights in men but markedly lower body weights in women.[37] A gender-comparison survey found that female drinkers who substituted ethanol for carbohydrate calories weighed less than did abstainers, whereas male drinkers weighed the same as abstainers despite adding ethanol calories to the diet.[38] Other studies have addressed the effect of moderate ethanol consumption on thermogenesis with conflicting results. The short-term isoenergetic substitution of moderate amounts of ethanol in the diet of women volunteers increased resting energy expenditure,[39] whereas in a long-term (1 month) crossover study of daily isoenergetic amounts of 750 mL wine (90 g ethanol or 7.5 drinks per day) or an equivalent amount of ethanol in juice, male volunteers lost weight and their urinary nitrogen losses increased.[40] Provision of isoenergetic diets that included 750 mL red wine or an equivalent amount of carbohydrate to healthy males for 2 weeks in a crossover design had no effect on resting energy expenditure or postprandial thermogenesis by indirect calorimetry but resulted in elevated serum HDL_2 levels.[41] By contrast, others showed in consecutive 24-hour studies of male volunteers living in metabolic chambers that either the addition or isoenergetic substitution of 90 g ethanol to the diet increased total energy expenditure by 7% and 4% while at the same time reducing the oxidation of dietary lipid.[42] Another metabolic chamber study confirmed the inhibitory effect of ethanol added to a single meal on postprandial fat oxidation, with somewhat lesser inhibition of carbohydrate oxidation.[43]

These studies must be placed in the context of an original observation that weight loss is induced by the substitution of dietary carbohydrate by excessive ethanol at 50% of energy whereas the addition of a similar amount of ethanol causes minimal weight gain compared with the equal addition of calories as carbohydrate.[44] Although originally interpreted as showing that ethanol provides "empty calories" that consume energy during metabolism,[44] later animal studies also showed an inhibitory effect of ethanol on weight gain in the presence of isoenergetic high-fat diets.[45,46] Others postulated that net energy dissipation during ethanol metabolism is caused by futile cycling of the initial metabolite acetaldehyde

back to ethanol.[47] In summary, it appears that ethanol consumption ≤90 g/day (7 or 8 drinks) may increase energy expenditure. Moderate ethanol consumption in women and excessive ethanol consumption in women and men promote weight loss due to the isoenergetic substitution of ethanol for carbohydrate. Conversely, the inhibitory effect of added ethanol on lipid oxidation may favor dietary lipid storage and weight gain, depending on the amount of fat in the diet, through the counteractive effect of inhibition of fatty acid oxidation. Added ethanol with excessive dietary energy from fat may accentuate obesity by favoring storage over oxidation of dietary lipids.

Ethanol metabolism summarized. Bomb calorimetry combustion of ethanol yields 29.7 kJ/g (7.1 kcal/g), but most alcoholic beverages are devoid of micronutrients. Furthermore, ethanol is metabolized completely and without storage, and as described above, its metabolism may waste energy while affecting the metabolism of other macronutrients. After the ingestion of an intoxicating dose of ethanol at 0.8 g/kg body weight by patient volunteers, gastric ethanol levels reached ≈1 mol/L (4–6 g/dL), whereas levels in the jejunum were 0.24–0.72 mol/L (1–3 g/dL), and levels in the remainder of the small intestine reflected those in the bloodstream as the result of back-diffusion after small intestinal absorption.[48]

Ethanol is initially metabolized in part by gastric alcohol dehydrogenase, a cytosolic enzyme with a relatively high K_m that accounts for "first pass" metabolism of ≈30% of ethanol in men but only 10% in women.[49] Gastric alcohol dehydrogenase is apparently inhibited by a variety of H_2 blocking agents and by chronic alcohol abuse, and decreases in activity with aging.[49] Within the liver, moderate amounts of ethanol are metabolized by hepatic alcohol dehydrogenase, a cytosolic enzyme with several genetically controlled isoforms and with a K_m up to 2 mmol/L (equivalent to ≈10 mg/dL blood ethanol). A second hepatic enzyme, purified as cytochromal (CYT) 2E1, is one of many inducible microsomal enzymes, and operates at a higher K_m of ≈10 mmol/L (equivalent to ≈50 mg/dL blood ethanol) and thus is operative during high-moderate to excessive ethanol consumption.[49] Although each hepatic enzyme produces acetaldehyde, which is then further metabolized by mitochondrial aldehyde dehydrogenase to acetate and acetyl-CoA, the two initial reactions have different effects on intermediary metabolism, each with different nutritional consequences. Cytosolic alcohol dehydrogenase reduces nicotine adenine dinucleotide (NAD) to NADH while oxidizing ethanol. Consequences of the increased ratio of NADH to NAD include suppression of the citric acid cycle with preferential production of lactate from pyruvate, reduced gluconeogenesis, reduced excretion of uric acid, and the potential clinical consequences of acidosis, hypoglycemia, and hyperuricemia. Increased NADH also favors

Table 2. Nutrient deficiencies associated with alcohol abuse

Micronutrients	Etiology	Consequences
Folate	Diet, malabsorption, oxidation	Anemia, diarrhea, cancer
Thiamine	Diet, malabsorption	Neurological (Wernicke), cardiomyopathy
Vitamin A	Diet, malabsorption, enhanced biliary excretion	Night blindness, immunity, cancer risk
Zinc	Diet, malabsorption, enhanced urine and fecal excretion	Anorexia, immunity, skin rash, poor wound healing
Protein	Diet, malabsorption, catabolism	Muscle wasting, immunity
Fat	Diet, malabsorption	Energy depletion

the synthesis of fatty acids, VLDL, and HDL_2 and HDL_3. Fatty acid and triacylglycerol synthesis is promoted by increased production of α-glycerophosphate. Reduced fatty acid oxidation favors obligatory ethanol oxidation, which results in net energy production of adenosine triphosphate (ATP).

The CYT 2E1 microsomal reaction predominates in the centrilobular portion of the liver lobule[50] and, rather than generating ATP, utilizes 2 mol reduced nicotine adenine dinucleotide phosphate (NADPH) for each 1 mol ethanol that is oxidized to acetaldehyde. Energy consumption by this predominating reaction may account for relative centrilobular hypoxia as one trigger of hepatic injury through enhancement of free radical generation. Furthermore, the increased production of acetaldehyde blocks mitochondrial respiration with further inhibition of fatty acid oxidation and promotion of fatty liver. Additional consequences of acetaldehyde production include enhanced catecholamine release, which favors peripheral lipolysis and ketoacidosis; binding and inactivation of the antioxidant glutathione; production of immunogenic acetaldehyde protein adducts; and stimulation of collagen synthesis. In addition, ethanol induction of other microsomal enzymes accelerates the metabolism and excretion of certain drugs such as warfarin, phenytoin, phenobarbital, and rifampin; the production of a toxic prooxidant metabolite of acetaminophen; the activation of certain procarcinogens and xenobiotics such as carbon tetrachloride and benzene; and the catabolism and accelerated biliary excretion of polar metabolites of vitamin A.[49]

Ethanol Consumption and Micronutrient Deficiencies

With few exceptions, very little is known about potential effects of moderate ethanol consumption on micronutrient status. On the other hand, abundant evidence from studies of binge-drinking alcoholics and animal models indicates that excessive ethanol consumption is probably the major cause of deficiencies of folate, thiamine, pyridoxine, vitamin A, and zinc in adult Americans (Table 2). These deficiencies are multiple in most instances and are more prevalent in the presence of alcoholic cirrhosis.[51]

Folate deficiency in alcoholism. As illustrated by reduced folate levels in red cells in about half of excessive drinkers with liver disease,[52] folate deficiency is a major cause of anemia in alcoholics.[53] Because of its role in cell replication in the small intestine, folate deficiency contributes to diarrhea in binge drinkers, a symptom that may be related to malabsorption of water-soluble nutrients that include folic acid and glucose.[54] Also, ethanol metabolism perturbs folate metabolism through inhibition of methionine synthase,[28] resulting in dysregulation of nucleotides and enhanced cancer risk.[19,20] The etiologies of folate deficiency in chronic alcoholism include poor diet,[52] intestinal malabsorption of the monoglutamyl form of the vitamin,[54] abnormal hepatobiliary metabolism,[55] and increased urinary loss due to reduced renal tubular reabsorption.[56] These multiple etiologies suggest that ethanol inhibits folate transporters known or presumed to exist in intestinal, hepatic, and renal tubular membranes.[52] Also, the acetaldehyde product of ethanol metabolism was shown in vitro to trigger oxidative catabolism of the folic acid molecule,[57] a possible explanation for a classic observation that the hematopoietic response of the bone marrow to therapeutic folic acid was inhibited by acute ethanol ingestion in alcoholic anemic patient volunteers.[58]

Thiamine deficiency in chronic alcoholism. The prevalence of thiamine deficiency in chronic alcoholism is not known, but the neuropathological lesion was found in 2.2% of consecutive autopsies.[59] The clinical features of thiamine deficiency in chronic alcoholism include the Wernicke-Korsakoff syndrome of ophthalmoplegia, ataxia, and altered memory, and alcoholic peripheral neuropathy.[60] Less obvious but functionally significant defects in judgment and concentration may result from thiamine deficiency.[61] The etiology of thiamine deficiency in chronic alcoholism includes poor diet together with intestinal malabsorption[62] due to inhibition of Na,K-ATPase at the basolateral membrane of the enterocyte.[63] Thiamine is required for transketolase reactions in carbohydrate metabolism, and others have postulated an additional genetic defect in transketolase synthesis or activity, or both, to explain selectivity in the clinical effects of thiamine deficiency.[64]

Pyridoxine deficiency in chronic alcoholism. Pyridoxine deficiency was responsible for sideroblastic changes in the bone marrow of about one-fourth of anemic alcoholics[53] and may contribute to findings of peripheral neuropathy. Because pyridoxine is essential for the activity of alanine transaminase (ALT), its deficiency may account for the well-known clinical finding of a lower serum level of this enzyme relative to aspartate transaminase (AST) in malnourished patients with alcoholic liver disease.[65] Pyridoxine deficiency in chronic alcoholism is caused in part by acetaldehyde displacement of the active form of the vitamin, pyridoxal-5-phosphate, from its protein binder with resultant accelerated urine losses.[66]

Vitamin A deficiency in chronic alcoholism. Although often unchanged in the serum of chronic alcoholics, liver vitamin A levels are progressively decreased according to the severity of alcoholic liver disease.[67] Deficiency of vitamin A probably results from its malabsorption as a fat-soluble vitamin in chronic alcoholic patients whose bile and pancreatic secretions are diminished[68] and also because of the effect of ethanol-induced microsomal oxidation on the turnover and biliary excretion of vitamin A metabolites.[69] Vitamin A deficiency may compromise immune function; may be procarcinogenic through effects on epithelial cell metaplasia in the oropharynx; impairs dark adaptation, thus increasing the risk of auto accidents; and causes lysosomal abnormalities in the hepatic ultrastructure.[70]

Zinc deficiency in chronic alcoholism. Low zinc levels in serum and liver tissue accompany the development of alcoholic liver disease in patients and in animal models.[71,72] The causes of zinc deficiency during chronic ethanol ingestion include inadequate dietary animal protein sources of zinc; decreased intestinal absorption, possibly due to increased trapping by intestinal metallothionein; and increased urine excretion related to low serum levels of zinc-binding albumin. Also, zinc pools are redistributed with greater tissue binding in response to various cytokine mediators of alcoholic liver injury.[73] The potential consequences of zinc deficiency in the setting of chronic alcoholism include acrodermatitis; altered taste and smell, which may contribute to anorexia; night blindness, because zinc is required for synthesis of retinol-binding protein and conversion of retinol to retinal; decreased testosterone production; altered cell-mediated immunity due to decreased thymulin production; and impaired wound healing.[74]

Nutrition in the Pathogenesis and Clinical Spectrum of Alcoholic Liver Disease

Alcoholic fatty liver results from ethanol metabolism with increased fatty acid and triacylclycerol synthesis and decreased fatty acid oxidation,[75] whereas alcoholic hepatitis and its sequel cirrhosis occur after many years of chronic ethanol abuse, typically in association with protein-energy malnutrition and multiple micronutrient deficiencies.[76] Although abundant epidemiologic data indicate that the risk of alcoholic liver disease relates to the amount and duration of ethanol consumption,[32] prospective studies in animal models of the baboon,[77] gavage-fed rat,[78] and micropig[79] showed that the pathogenesis of liver disease involves both ethanol metabolism and the modulating effects of several nutrients.

Nutrients in the pathogenesis of alcoholic liver disease. The pathogenesis of alcoholic liver disease is now understood to include complex relations among endotoxin-stimulated cytokines, oxidant injury to liver cell membranes, and increased collagen production from sinusoidal Ito cells surrounding the central vein of the liver lobule.[49] Typical histopathological features of alcoholic liver disease, including fat accumulation (steatosis), focal inflammation, and pericentral fibrosis, can be induced by feeding diets in which ethanol replaces carbohydrate at 35–50% of energy over 4 years in baboons,[77] over 6 months in gavage-fed rats,[78] and within 12 months in micropigs.[79] The severity of liver injury in animal models depends on the amount and composition of dietary fat. Thus, liver injury is accelerated when rats are fed diets high in polyunsaturated corn oil[80] because of stimulant effects of these diets on the activity of the centrilobular CYT 2E1 microsomal ethanol-oxidizing enzyme and on the promotion of collagen synthesis.[81] This observation is consistent with epidemiologic data correlating the incidence of alcoholic cirrhosis with the amount of dietary pork, known to be higher in polyunsaturated fat than is beef.[82]

These findings are relevant to oxidant liver injury because diets high in unsaturated lipids promote unsaturated liver membranes that are more susceptible to lipid peroxidation. Paradoxically, ethanol consumption by miniature pigs led to decreased fatty acid desaturation in liver cell mitochondrial and microsomal membranes, which appeared to be protective against lipid peroxidation.[83] Oxidant liver injury represents the balance between prooxidant effects of free radicals triggered by acetaldehyde and antioxidant protection. Nutrient regulation of antioxidant protection was shown by findings of decreased liver Zn-Cu–superoxide dismutase and selenium-dependent glutathione peroxidases in miniature pigs.[83] Chronic ethanol feeding reduces serum levels of the antioxidants vitamin E and liver mitochondrial glutathione in rats,[84,85] whereas glutathione levels were protected and liver injury was attenuated in baboons by provision of S-adenosylmethionine, a principal metabolic precursor of glutathione.[86]

Other data point to the essentiality of maintaining or enhancing membrane phosphatidylcholine for prevention of alcoholic liver injury. Thus, alcoholic liver injury was attenuated in ethanol-fed baboons by provision of polyunsaturated lecithin,[87] whereas provision of choline-deficient diets to human volunteers decreased phosphatidylcholine in red cell membranes and increased injury-specific serum aminotransferase levels in liver.[88] An imbalance of membrane phosphatidylcholine may occur during chronic ethanol exposure, which is known to inhibit the activities of three enzymes in phosphatidylcholine's synthetic pathway: methionine synthase,[28,89] S-adenosylmethionine synthetase, and phosphatidylethanolamine-N-methyl transferase.[90] Chronic ethanol exposure may also promote the salvage diversion of choline to methionine through increased activity of betaine homocysteine methyltransferase.[89] Overall, these data suggest a significant role of chronic ethanol exposure in disturbance of methylation pathways, with resultant abnormalities in production of phosphatidylcholine and glutathione that may be critical in membrane susceptibility to oxidation. Whereas collagen formation with eventual cirrhosis appears to be triggered by acetaldehyde,[91] ethanol-induced vitamin A deficiency produces lysosomal hepatocyte abnormalities.[70] Exogenous vitamin A is known to either inhibit collagen production in other settings[92] or to accelerate collagen production when provided together with ethanol.[93]

Effect of alcoholic liver disease on nutrition. Body composition, energy expenditure, and micronutrient status may be profoundly affected by alcoholic hepatitis and cirrhosis as the result of liver inflammation, loss of functional liver cells, and portal hypertension. By using a variety of parameters to assess visceral and skeletal protein status and balance, a multicenter Veterans Administration study of 284 patients hospitalized with alcoholic hepatitis identified one or more features of protein-energy malnutrition in virtually all patients.[76] Furthermore, the number of features of protein-energy malnutrition identified was correlated with the severity of liver disease. A follow-up study showed the significant predictive values of a composite of nutritional parameters on both 30-day and 12-month survival.[94] Etiologies of malnutrition in patients with alcoholic liver disease include poor diet, malabsorption, and energy and protein wastage. Thus, although these chronic alcoholics consumed >14.6 MJ/day (>3500 kcal/day), more than one-half of dietary energy was in the form of ethanol, and protein intake was only 8.1% of energy.[94]

As previously indicated, excessive ethanol consumption requires its metabolism by the energy-wasteful CYT 2E1 system.[44] Alcoholic beverages are essentially devoid of essential micronutrients, and chronic ethanol exposure limits the intestinal uptake and/or accelerates the turnover of folic acid, thiamine, pyridoxine, and folic acid. Furthermore, the digestion and intestinal absorption of dietary fat and fat-soluble vitamins is impaired

in more than one-half of patients with alcoholic cirrhosis as the result of diminished bile acid secretion[95] or pancreatic insufficiency.[96] Also, portal hypertension in cirrhotic patients results in significant losses of circulating protein from the intestine.[97] Body compositional studies of stable cirrhotic patients showed marked decrease in lean body mass. Whereas protein turnover was normal in these patients, protein degradation was increased when expressed according to functional lean body mass.[98] Using indirect calorimetry and labeled substrate turnover methods, others found that stable, nondrinking cirrhotics have normal fasting energy requirements but that more than two-thirds of energy is derived from endogenous fatty acids, analogous to the normal compensation for starvation.[99] Although these abundant data demonstrate a major role of protein-energy malnutrition in the clinical picture of decompensated alcoholic liver disease, the therapeutic role of aggressive nutritional support remains controversial owing to a multitude of studies with different designs and uncertain controls.[100]

References

1. Mitchell MC, Herlong HF (1986) Alcohol and nutrition: caloric value, bioenergetics, and relationship to liver damage. Annu Rev Nutr 6:457–474
2. McGinnis JM, Foege WH (1993) Actual causes of death in the United States. JAMA 270:2207–2212
3. National Institute on Alcohol Abuse and Alcoholism (1993) Eighth special report to the US Congress on alcohol and health. US Department of Health and Human Services, Rockville, MD
4. Sutocky JW, Shultz JM, Kizer KW (1993) Alcohol-related mortality in California, 1980–1989. Am J Public Health 83: 817–823
5. Doll R, Peto R, Hall E, et al (1994) Mortality in relation to consumption of alcohol: 13 years' observations on male British doctors. Br Med J 309:911–918
6. Grönback M, Deis A, Sorensen TIA, et al (1994) Influence of sex, age, body mass index, and smoking on alcohol intake and mortality. Br Med J 308:302–306
7. Grönback M, Deis A, Sorensen TIA, et al (1995) Mortality associated with moderate intakes of wine, beer, or spirits. Br Med J 310:1165–1169
8. Serdula M, Loong SL, Williamson DF, et al (1995) Alcohol intake and subsequent mortality: findings from the NHANES I follow-up study. J Stud Alcohol 56:233–239
9. Klatsky AL, Armstrong MA, Freidman GD (1992) Alcohol and mortality. Ann Intern Med 117:646–654
10. Boffeta P, Garfinkel L (1990) Alcohol drinking and mortality among men enrolled in an American Cancer Society prospective study. Epidemiology 1:342–348
11. Fuchs CS, Stampfer MJ, Colditz GA, et al (1995) Alcohol consumption and mortality in women. N Engl J Med 332: 1245–1250
12. Klatsky AL (1994) Epidemiology of coronary heart disease—influence of alcohol. Alcohol Clin Exp Res 18:88–96
13. Stampfer MJ, Colditz GA, Willett WC, et al (1988) Prospective study of moderate alcohol consumption and the risk of coronary disease and stroke in women. N Engl J Med 319:267–273

14. Rimm EB, Giovannucci EL, Willett WC, et al (1991) Prospective study of alcohol consumption and risk of coronary heart disease in men. Lancet 388:464–468

15. Klatsky AL, Armstrong MA, Friedman GD (1986) Relations of alcohol beverage use to subsequent coronary artery disease hospitalizations. Am J Cardiol 58:710–714

16. Klatsky AL, Friedman GD, Armstrong MA (1986) The relationships between alcoholic beverage use and other traits to blood pressure: a new Kaiser Permanente study. Circulation 73:628–636

17. Tuyns AJ, Pequinot G, Gignoux M, Valla A (1982) Cancers of the digestive tract, alcohol, and tobacco. Int J Cancer 30:9–11

18. Reichman ME, Judd JT, Longcope C, et al (1993) Effects of alcohol consumption on plasma and urinary hormone concentrations in premenopausal women. J Natl Cancer Inst 85:722–727

19. Freudenheim JL, Graham S, Marchall JR, et al (1991) Folate intake and carcinogenesis of the colon and rectum. Int J Epidemiol 20:368–374

20. Giovannucci E, Stampfer MJ, Colditz GA, et al (1993) Folate, methionine, and alcohol intake and risk of colorectal adenoma. J Natl Cancer Inst 85:875–884

21. Sorensen TIA, Orholm M, Bentsen KD, et al (1984) Prospective evaluation of alcohol abuse and alcoholic liver injury in men as predictors of development of cirrhosis. Lancet 2:241–244

22. Gaziano JM, Buring JE, Breslow JL (1993) Moderate alcohol intake, increased levels of high-density lipoprotein and its subfractions, and decreased risk of myocardial infarction. N Engl J Med 329:1829–1834

23. Ridker PM, Hennekens CH (1994) Association of moderate alcohol consumption and plasma concentration of endogenous tissue-type plasminogen activator. JAMA 272:929–933

24. Renaud S, de Lorgeril M (1992) Wine, alcohol, platelets, and the French paradox for coronary heart disease. Lancet 339:1523–1526

25. Frankel EN, Kanner J, German JB, et al (1993) Inhibition of oxidation of human low-density lipoprotein by phenolic substances in red wine. Lancet 341:454–457

26. Klatsky AL, Armstrong MA (1993) Alcoholic beverage choice and risk of coronary artery disease mortality: do red wine drinkers fare best? Am J Cardiol 71:467–469

27. Doll R, Forman D, La Vecchi C, Woutersen R (1993) Alcoholic beverages and cancers of the digestive tract and larynx. In Verschuren PM (ed), Health issues related to alcohol consumption. ILSI Press, Washington, DC, pp 125–166

28. Halsted CH, Villanueva J, Chandler CJ, et al (1996) Ethanol feeding of micropigs alters methionine metabolism and increases hepatocellular apoptosis and proliferation. Hepatology 23(3):497–505

29. Lane BP, Lieber CS (1966) Ultrastructural alterations in human hepatocytes following ingestion of ethanol with adequate diets. Am J Pathol 49:593–603

30. Almdahl TP, Sorensen TIA (1991) Incidence of parenchymal liver disease in Denmark, 1981 to 1985: analysis of hospitalization registry data. Hepatology 13:650–655

31. Hunter DJW, Halliday ML, Coates RA, Rankin JG (1989) Hospital morbidity from cirrhosis of the liver and per capita consumption of absolute alcohol in Ontario, 1978 to 1982: a descriptive analysis. Can J Public Health 79:243–248

32. Cronin A (1995) The tipplers and the temperate: drinking around the world. New York Times, News of the Week in Review, Jan 1, p 4

33. Lelbach WK (1975) Cirrhosis in the alcoholic and its relation to the volume of alcohol abuse. Ann NY Acad Sci 252:85–105

34. Ashler MJ, Olin JS, leRiche WH, et al (1977) Morbidity in alcoholics: evidence for accelerated physical disease in women. Arch Intern Med 137:883–887

35. Sorensen TIA (1989) Alcohol and liver injury: dose-related or permissive effect? Br J Addiction 84:581–589

36. Gruchow HW, Sobocinski KA, Barboriak JJ, Scheller JG (1985) Alcohol consumption, nutrient intake and relative body weight among US adults. Am J Clin Nutr 42:289–295

37. Williamson DF, Forman MR, Binkin NJ, et al (1987) Alcohol and body weight in United States adults. Am J Public Health 77:1324–1330

38. Colditz GA, Giovannucci E, Rimm EB, et al (1991) Alcohol intake in relation to diet and obesity in women and men. Am J Clin Nutr 54:49–55

39. Klesges RC, Mealer CZ, Klesges LM (1994) Effects of alcohol intake on resting energy expenditure in young women social drinkers. Am J Clin Nutr 59:805–809

40. MacDonald JT, Margen S (1976) Wine versus ethanol in human nutrition. I. Nitrogen and calorie balance. Am J Clin Nutr 29:1093–1103

41. Contaldo F, D'Arrigo E, Carandente V, et al (1989) Short-term effects of moderate alcohol consumption on lipid metabolism and energy balance in normal men. Metabolism 38:166–171

42. Suter PM, Schutz Y, Jequier E (1992) The effect of ethanol on fat storage in healthy subjects. N Engl J Med 326:983–987

43. Sonko BJ, Prentice AM, Murgatroyd PR, et al (1994) Effect of alcohol on postmeal storage. Am J Clin Nutr 59:619–625

44. Pirola RC, Lieber CS (1975) Energy cost of the metabolism of drugs, including ethanol. Pharmacology 7:185–196

45. Lieber CS, Lasker JM, DeCarli LM, et al (1988) Role of acetone, dietary fat and total energy intake in induction of hepatic microsomal ethanol oxidizing system. J Pharmacol Exp Ther 247:791–795

46. Lieber CS (1991) Perspectives: do alcohol calories count? Am J Clin Nutr 54:976–982

47. Lands WEM, Zakhari S (1991) The case of the missing calories. Am J Clin Nutr 54:47–48

48. Halsted CH, Robles EA, Mezey E (1973) The distribution of ethanol in the human gastrointestinal tract. Am J Clin Nutr 26:831–834

49. Lieber CS (1994) Alcohol and the liver: 1994 update. Gastroenterology 106:1085–1105

50. French SW, Wong K, Ju L, et al (1993) Effect of ethanol on cytochrome P450 2E1 (CYT2E1), lipid peroxidation, and serum protein adduct formation in relation to liver pathology pathogenesis. Exp Mol Pathol 58:61–75

51. Leevy CM, Baker H, TenHove W (1965) B-complex vitamins in liver disease of the alcoholic. Am J Clin Nutr 16:339–346

52. Halsted CH (1995) Alcohol and folate interactions: clinical implications. In Bailey LB (ed), Folate in health and disease. M Decker Inc, New York, pp 313–327

53. Savage D, Lindenbaum J (1986) Anemia in alcoholics. Medicine 65:322–328

54. Halsted CH, Robles EA, Mezey E (1973) Intestinal malabsorption in folate-deficient alcoholics. Gastroenterology 64:526–532

55. Tamura T, Romero JJ, Watson JE, et al (1981) Hepatic folate metabolism in the chronic alcoholic monkey. J Lab Clin Med 97:654–661

56. McMartin KE, Collins TD, Shiao CQ, et al (1986) Study of dose-dependence and urinary folate excretion produced by ethanol in humans and rats. Alcohol Exp Ther Res 10:419–424

57. Shaw S, Jayetilleke E, Herbert V, Colman N (1989) Cleavage of folates during ethanol metabolism: role of xanthine oxidase-generated superoxide dismutase. Biochem J 257:277–280

58. Sullivan LW, Herbert V (1964) Suppression of hematopoiesis by ethanol. J Clin Invest 43:2048–2062

59. Victor M, Laureno R (1978) The neurologic complications of alcohol abuse: epidemiologic aspects. Adv Neurol 19:603–617

60. Victor M (1992) The effects of alcohol on the nervous system. In Lieber CS (ed), Medical and nutritional complications of alcoholism. Plenum, New York, pp 413–457

61. Reuler JB, Girard DE, Cooney TG (1985) Wernicke's encephalopathy. N Engl J Med 312:1035–1039

62. Thomson AD, Baker H, Leevy CM (1970) Patterns of ^{35}S-thiamine hydrochloride absorption in the malnourished alcoholic patient. J Lab Clin Med 76:34–45

63. Hoyumpa AM, Nichols SC, Wilson FA, Schenker S (1977) Effect of ethanol on intestinal (Na, K) ATPase and intestinal thiamine transport in rats. J Lab Clin Med 101:1086–1095

64. Blass JP, Gibson GE (1977) Abnormality of a thiamine-requiring enzyme in patients with Wernicke-Korsakiff syndrome. N Engl J Med 297:1367–1370

65. Diehl AM, Potter JJ, Boitnott J, et al (1984) Relationship between pyridoxal 5'-phosphate deficiency and aminotransferase levels in alcoholic hepatitis. Gastroenterology 86:632–636

66. Veitch RL, Lumeng L, Li TK (1975) Vitamin B_6 metabolism in chronic alcohol abuse: the effect of ethanol oxidation on hepatic pyridoxal-5-phosphate metabolism. J Clin Invest 55:1026–1032

67. Leo MA, Lieber CS (1982) Hepatic vitamin A depletion in alcoholic liver injury in man. N Engl J Med 307:597–601

68. Mezey E, Kolman CJ, Diehl AM, et al (1988) Alcohol and dietary intake in the development of chronic pancreatitis and liver disease in alcoholism. Am J Clin Nutr 48:148–151

69. Leo MA, Lasker JM, Raucy JL, et al (1989) Metabolism of retinol and retinoic acid by human liver cytochrome P450IIC8. Arch Biochem Biophys 269:305–312

70. Leo MA, Sato M, Lieber CS (1983) Effect of hepatic vitamin A depletion on the liver in humans and rats. Gastroenterology 84:192–205

71. Bode JC, Hanisch P, Henning H, et al (1988) Hepatic zinc content in patients with various stages of alcoholic liver disease and in patients with chronic active and chronic persistent hepatitis. Hepatology 8:1605–1609

72. Zidenberg-Cherr S, Olin KL, Villanueva J, et al (1991) Ethanol-induced changes in hepatic free-radical defense mechanisms and fatty-acid composition in the miniature pig. Hepatology 13:1185–1192

73. McClain CJ, Cohen DA (1989) Increased tumor necrosis factor production by monocytes in alcoholic hepatitis. Hepatology 9:349–351

74. McClain CJ, Kasarskis EJ, Marsano L (1992) Zinc and alcohol. In Watson RR, Watzl B (eds), Nutrition and alcohol. CRC Press, Boca Raton, FL, pp 281–308

75. Lieber CS, Jones DP, DeCarli LM (1965) Effects of prolonged ethanol intake: production of fatty liver despite adequate diets. J Clin Invest 6:1009–1021

76. Mendenhall CL, Anderson S, Weesner RE, et al (1984) Protein-calorie malnutrition associated with alcoholic hepatitis. Am J Med 76:211–222

77. Lieber CS, DeCarli LM, Rubin E (1975) Sequential production of fatty liver, hepatitis, and cirrhosis in sub-human primates fed ethanol with adequate diets. Proc Natl Acad Sci USA 72:437–441

78. Tsukamoto H, Towner SJ, Cioffalo LM, French SW (1986) Ethanol induced liver fibrosis in rats fed high fat diet. Hepatology 6:814–822

79. Halsted CH, Villanueva J, Chandler CJ, et al (1993) Centrilobular distribution of acetaldehyde and collagen in the ethanol-fed micropig. Hepatology 18:954–960

80. Nanji AA, Mendenhall CL, French SW (1989) Beef fat prevents alcoholic liver disease in the rat. Alcohol Clin Exp Res 13:15–19

81. Takahashi H, Johansson I, French SW, Ingelman-Sundberg M (1992) Effects of dietary fat composition on activities of the microsomal ethanol oxidizing system and ethanol-inducible cytochrome P450 (CYT2E1) in the liver of rats chronically fed ethanol. Pharmacol Toxicol 70:347–351

82. Nanji AA, French SW (1985) Relationship between pork consumption and cirrhosis. Lancet 1:681–683

83. Zidenberg-Sherr S, Olin KL, Villanueva J, et al (1991) Ethanol-induced changes in hepatic free radical defense mechanisms and fatty-acid composition in the miniature pig. Hepatology 13:1185–1192

84. Kawase T, Kato S, Lieber CS (1989) Lipid peroxidation and antioxidant defense systems in rat liver after chronic ethanol feeding. Hepatology 10:815–821

85. Hirano T, Kaplowitz N, Tsukamoto H, et al (1992) Hepatic mitochondrial glutathione depletion and progression of experimental alcoholic liver disease in rats. Hepatology 16:1423–1427

86. Lieber CS, Casine A, DeCarli LM, et al (1990) S-Adenosyl-L-methionine attenuates alcohol-induced liver injury in the baboon. Hepatology 11:165–172

87. Lieber CS, DeCarli LM, Mak, KM, et al (1990) Attenuation of alcohol-induced hepatic fibrosis by polyunsaturated lecithin. Hepatology 12:1390–1398

88. Zeisel SH, DaCosta KA, Franklin PD, et al (1991) Choline, an essential nutrient for humans. FASEB J 5:2093–2098

89. Trimble KC, Molloy AM, Scott JM, Weir DG (1993) The effect of ethanol on one-carbon metabolism: increased methionine catabolism and lipotrope methyl-group wastage. Hepatology 18:984–989

90. Duce AM, Ortiz P, Cabrero C, Mato JM (1988) S-Adenosyl-L-methionine synthetase and phospholipid methyltransferase are inhibited in human cirrhosis. Hepatology 8:65–68.

91. Casini A, Cunningham M, Rojkind M, Lieber CS (1981) Acetaldehyde increases procollagen type I and fibronectin gene transcription in cultured rat fat-storing cells through a protein synthesis-dependent mechanism. Hepatology 13:758–765

92. Davis BH, Pratt BM, Madri JA (1987) Retinol and extracellular collagen matrices modulate hepatic Ito cell collagen phenotype and cellular retinol binding protein levels. J Biol Chem 262:10280–10286

93. Leo MA, Lieber CS (1983) Hepatic fibrosis after long-term administration of ethanol and moderate vitamin A supplementation in the rat. Hepatology 3:1–11

94. Mendenhall CL, Tosch T, Weesner RE, et al (1986) VA cooperative study on alcoholic hepatitis, II: prognostic significance of protein-calorie malnutrition. Am J Clin Nutr 43:213–218

95. Roggin GM, Iber FL, Kater RMH, Tabon F (1969) Malabsorption in the chronic alcoholic. Johns Hopkins Med J 125:321–330

96. Roggin GM, Iber FL, Linscheer W (1972) Intraluminal fat digestion in the chronic alcoholic. Gut 13:107–111

97. Bretagne JF, Lemee P, Esvant E, Gastard J (1982) Evaluation of protein-losing enteropathy in the cirrhotic patient by assessing the intestinal clearance of alpha 1 antitrypsin. Semin Hosp 58:575–577

98. McCullough AJ, Tavill AS (1991) Disordered energy and

protein metabolism in liver disease. Semin Liver Dis 11:265–277

99. Owens OE, Trapp VE, Reichard GA, et al (1983) Nature and quantity of fuels consumed in patients with alcoholic cirrhosis. J Clin Invest 72:1821–1832

100. Nompleggi DJ, Bonkowsky HL (1994) Nutritional supplementation in chronic liver disease: an analytical review. Hepatology 19:518–533

Chapter 56

Nutrition and Immunity: Disruption of Lymphopoiesis in Zinc-deficient Mice

Pamela Fraker

Extensive evidence from early as well as considerable recent literature indicates that zinc deficiency compromises host defense in both humans and animals, leading to increased morbidity and mortality.[1-4] Zinc-deficient mice may represent the best and most thoroughly characterized animal model of nutritional-immunological interaction. Because mice have for two decades proved to be reliable immunological models for humans, recent research using zinc-deficient mice will be the point of focus of this chapter.

Lymphopenia, Reduction of Host Defense Capacity, and Suboptimal Zinc Intake

Because the effects of zinc deficiency on the immune system are so rapid and profound, the underlying causes that created reduced defense capacity needed to be explored. As our own investigations in zinc-deficient adult mice proceeded, it became clear that the losses in antibody- and cell-mediated response capacity among zinc-deficient mice often correlated with reduction in absolute number of lymphocytes available to participate in immune responses.[2-6] For example, a degree of zinc deficiency that created a 25% loss in body weight in young adult mice caused a 50% loss in thymic weight while reducing by nearly half the number of lymphocytes populating the spleen and peripheral blood.[6] The antibody- and cell-mediated responses were also about half normal in these mice, correlating with the loss in absolute numbers of lymphocytes.[6] Interestingly, the phenotypic distribution or proportion of the major classes and subclasses of T and B cells in the spleen of zinc-deficient mice remained normal in spite of the 50% loss of splenocytes.[7] On a per cell basis, the residual splenocytes found in zinc-deficient mice gave normal responses to some antigens and mitogens as shown by our own and several other labs.[6,8] The amount of interleukin II produced per T cell as well as the amount of antibody pro-

duced per B cell was the same whether the cells came from mice fed zinc-deficient or zinc-adequate diets.[6,8] Thus, at the cellular level many functions remained intact in lymphocytes prepared from zinc-deficient mice. Because the total number of lymphocytes available to participate in an immune response were reduced, the intensity of the overall response to external challenges was also reduced in the zinc-deficient mice. This finding, along with the persistent observation by early investigators that thymic atrophy and lymphopenia accompany zinc deficiency as well as many other types of malnutrition in animals and humans, suggested that lymphopenia—reductions in the absolute number of lymphocytes in the peripheral immune system—plays a significant role in the observed reduction in host defense capacity.[2,4,6,9] New data that shed light on the underlying causes of lymphopenia are discussed below.

Production of B Cells by the Bone Marrow

The primary immune tissues, bone marrow and thymus, are responsible for the production of lymphocytes. The bone marrow is one of the largest tissues of the body and must produce billions of new lymphocytes each day in a process called lymphopoiesis.[10,11] Over 60% of the young lymphocytes die due to faulty rearrangements of the immunoglobulin chains or the T-cell receptor. These faulty cells are induced to undergo a form of cell suicide called apaptosis (programmed cell death) as a means of clearing them from the system.[12] The remaining lymphocytes survive only a few days before having to be replaced.[10,11] The large size of the marrow tissue and the high turnover and death rate of lymphoid cells suggest that this tissue requires substantial amounts of nutrients to maintain its functions. In the lymphopoietic processes precursor cells must not only mature, but proliferate as well.[10,11] Adequate zinc is, of course, essential to cell division, growth, and maturation.[13] It seemed probable

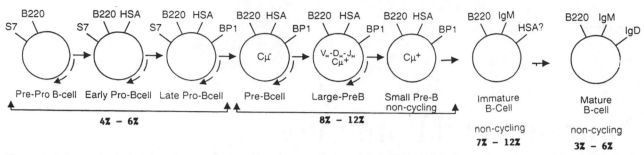

Figure 1. Scheme depicting the phenotypic or cell surface markers used to differentiate the various stages of B-cell development in murine bone marrow.

that as zinc deficiency advanced and zinc became limiting, the rate of lymphopoiesis would slow. Thus, we hypothesized that reductions in the rate of lymphopoiesis might be a central cause of lymphopenia.

Because of our heavy focus on lymphopoiesis the reader is provided with a short review. Figure 1 illustrates a scheme of the phenotypic or cell surface markers currently used to monitor development of murine marrow B cells from the earliest precursors that have unrearranged germ line immunoglobulin genes to mature cells that actively express IgM and IgD.[10,11,14] Because a sequential series of developmentally regulated surface markers are available for the study of developing B cells, we focused initially on B-lymphopoietic processes in zinc deficiency. All the major differentiation and maturation processes of B cells in adult mammals occur in the marrow.[10] By contrast, T cells begin development in the marrow but finish in the thymus, which complicates studies of T-cell lymphopoiesis, and gave us another reason for our initial focus on B-cell lymphopoiesis. It is thought that Thy1^{lo}Lin$^-$Sca$^+$Rh123^{lo} marrow cells are enriched with multipotent stem cells that are the precursors of all of the cells found in the blood including B cells.[15] These earliest of precursor cells are difficult to study because they constitute only 0.05% of the nucleated cells of the marrow.[15] One of the earliest markers to appear on a cell committed to the B-cell lineage is B220, which is a part of a large family of glycoproteins (CD45) that have tyrosine phosphatase activity.[10] B220 remains on the surface of B cells throughout their development and is also found on mature circu-

lating B cells. Collectively, the 220-bearing B cells constitute 25–30% of all nucleated cells in the murine bone marrow. Work from several laboratories indicates that some of the earliest B progenitors or pre-pro-B cells also bear the marker S7$^+$ or CD43 or leukosialin (B220$^+$S7$^+$) (Figure 1).[10,14] The heavy-chain immunoglobulin is basically in the germ line configuration in these very immature B cells. Gradually, the pro-B cells acquire HSA$^+$a third surface marker and become B220$^+$HSA$^+$S7$^+$.[14] HSA is the so-called heat-stable antigen. Hardy's lab recently demonstrated that a zinc-dependent metalloprotease, BP-1, is found on "late" pro-B cells as well as on all pre-B cells.[14] Of the late pro-B cells ≈80% have carried out the DJ$_H$ rearrangement, but do not yet have complete heavy chains (Table 1). Altogether the pro-B-cell population accounts for 4–6% of the nucleated cells of the marrow. Pre-B cells carry out extensive gene rearrangement and finally express cytoplasmic μ chain, or the heavy chain of IgM (μ) at the small or late-pre-B stage (B220$^+$HSA$^+$S7$^-$BP-1$^+$sμ$^-$cμ$^+$) (Figure 1 and Table 1). Eventually, these cells evolve into immature B cells which express IgM on their surface, and can respond to some antigenic challenges (B220$^+$IgM$^+$IgD$^-$). Finally, the mature B cells that express both IgM and IgD are generated (B220$^+$IgM$^+$IgD$^+$) and they eventually migrate out into the peripheral immune system. Mature cells constitute only 3–6% of the nucleated cells of the marrow. Clearly, these various surface markers can be used to monitor the effect of zinc deficiency on B-cell development in the marrow and to establish the relative sensitivity of each population to zinc deficiency.

Table 1. Phenotypic markers and state of rearrangement of the immunoglobulin heavy chain in pro- and pre-B cells

Early-pro-B cell	Late-pro-B cell	Pre-B cell	Late-pre-B cell
B220$^+$S7$^+$BP-1$^-$	B220$^+$S7$^+$BP-1$^+$	B220$^+$S7$^-$BP-1$^+$	B220$^+$S7$^-$BP-1$^+$
	D to J$_H$	V$_H$ to DJ$_H$	cμ
4–6% of cells of the bone marrow		8–14% of cells of the bone marrow	

Zinc Deficiency Disrupts Lymphopoiesis in the Marrow of Mice

To our knowledge the effect of malnutrition or zinc deficiency on lymphopoietic processes had not been examined using modern immunological tools. The general dietary protocol we used will be briefly described; more details are available in recent publications.[6,16] Young adult mice were placed on a synthetic egg white–based diet fortified with biotin. Zinc-adequate and zinc-restricted mice received 30 mg Zn/g diet. Zinc-deficient mice received <1 mg Zn/g diet. At day 30, zinc-deficient mice that exhibited moderate signs of parakeratosis on their tails and that were 70–75% the body weight of zinc-adequate mice were designated moderately zinc deficient.[6,16] Those mice that exhibited extensive parakeratosis of the tail, paws, ears, etc., and that weighed 65–68% of controls, were considered severely zinc deficient.[6,16] Though significant dermatological and immunological differences were noted, there were only modest differences in serum zinc levels between the moderately and severely zinc-deficient mice. This was not surprising, since serum and tissue zinc levels often provide only crude indications of zinc status.[3] Serum corticosterone (CS) levels were more elevated in severely zinc-deficient (1.88 µmol CS/L) mice than in moderately zinc-deficient (0.73 µmol CS/L) mice. The zinc-adequate controls had 0.35 µmol CS/L. The thymuses of moderately and severely zinc-deficient mice were, respectively, 50% and 20% the weight of zinc-adequate mice, showing that subdividing the mice by weight and degree of skin lesions provided immunological distinctions. Likewise, the spleens showed clear evidence of lymphopenia, having only half the normal number of lymphocytes in moderately zinc deficient and about one-third the normal number in severely zinc-deficient mice. Body, thymus weights, and serum zinc levels of zinc-restricted mice, which are a control for the inanition that accompanies zinc deficiency, were similar to zinc-adequate mice, with no statistical difference noted for most experiments.[6,16]

Both moderate and severe forms of zinc deficiency profoundly altered the marrow. In the marrow of young adult mice a moderate degree of zinc deficiency caused a 43% decline in the proportion of nucleated cells bearing B220 (all cells of the B lineage in the marrow), with a 91% decline noted among more severely zinc-deficient mice (Figure 2). Early B cells not yet expressing immunoglobulin (B220+Ig−) were reduced by almost 60% in moderately zinc-deficient mice and were barely detectable in severely zinc-deficient mice. Immature B cells (B220+IgM+IgD−) were similarly affected, declining 35–80% depending on the degree of the deficiency. Mature B cells (IgM+IgD+) were somewhat more resistant, exhibiting moderate losses among moderately zinc-deficient

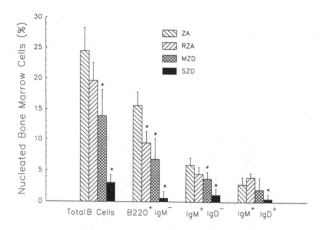

Figure 2. Phenotypic distribution of early (B220+Ig−), immature (B220+IgM+), and mature cells (IgM+IgD+) of the B lineage in the marrow of zinc-adequate, zinc-restricted, moderately zinc-deficient, and severely zinc-deficient young adult A/J mice at day 28 of a dietary study. Analyses were performed using flow cytometry. Six to eight mice per dietary group were individually assayed where the mean ± SD is given. *P=<0.05 when compared with the zinc-adequate group. Data are representative of two experiments.

mice but more significant losses in severely zinc-deficient mice (Figure 2). Flow cytometric scatter profiles also showed that zinc deficiency caused a sharp decline in the small nucleated marrow cells thought to contain a high proportion of developing lymphoid cells.[16] The lack of accumulation of any one subset of B cells tested suggested that zinc deficiency does not cause a specific block in development. This conclusion awaited three- and four-color analyses of pro- versus pre-B cells as well as kinetic studies where patterns of change in subsets of cells could be examined more thoroughly.

Effect of Zn Deficiency on Pro-B and Pre-B Cells

The next series of studies examined the effect of zinc deficiency on the development of pro- and pre-B cells. This is a very critical phase, since germ line genes begin to be rearranged in the late pro-B cells to form immunoglobulin heavy chains (µ), which are eventually expressed in the cytoplasm of late-phase pre-B cells (cµ) (Figure 1 and Table 1). The marker-molecular sequence shown in Table 1 made it possible to distinguish early pro-B cells (B220+S7+) that have just acquired S7 (or CD43) from late pro-B cells, which begin to express BP-1 (B220+S7+BP-1+). The majority of late pro-B cells (≈80%) have begun gene rearrangement (D to J_H) (Table 1).[14] The rearrangements proceed through the early pre-B-cell phase (B220+S7−BP-1+) (V_H to DJ_H), with these cells becoming the small noncycling pre-B cells that express cµ+ or cytoplasmic heavy chains of the IgM molecule.

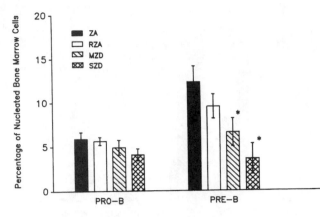

Figure 3. Effect of 30 days of suboptimal intake of zinc on pro-B cells. Dietary groups are as described for Figure 2. Most pro-B cells are in the germ line configuration or are just beginning rearrangements of the immunoglobulin heavy-chain genes. Extensive rearrangements are in progress among pre-B cells, which eventually express cμ. Means ± SD are shown where *denotes data significantly different from zinc-adequate mice at $P=<0.05$ and n=8–10 mice.

To determine effects of zinc deficiency on pro-B and pre-B cells, young adult A/J mice were again placed on zinc-adequate, zinc-restricted, or zinc-deficient diets using the typical dietary regimen, with zinc-deficient mice subdivided into moderately and severely zinc deficient.[6,16] Preliminary data from our first three-color protocol (anti-B220, S7, IgM) is shown in Figure 3. Moderate and severe zinc deficiency caused 50% and 70% depletion, respectively, of the pre-B-cell population that were actively undergoing gene rearrangements. As in the earlier studies, the greater the degree of deficiency, the greater the losses in the B-cell compartment of the marrow. Interestingly, neither moderate nor severe deficiency significantly affected the proportion of pro-B cells residing in the marrow. Pro-B cells appear more resistant to zinc deficiency than other cells of the B lineage. If early pro-B cells continue to show substantial resistance to zinc deficiency, this will represent an important finding. It may be that pro-B cells are less likely to enter an apoptotic state and have better "survival" mechanisms than pre and immature B-cells that are in the process of gene rearrangement of heavy chains and light chains.[14] Since pro-B cells have not yet made nonproductive or antiself rearrangements that need to be eliminated, they may not be as highly programmed to undergo cell death as the other B-cell stages. Pre-B cells that make numerous nonsense or nonproductive rearrangements may be programmed to undergo apoptosis more readily. This might also explain why pro-B cells are more resistant to zinc deficiency. The recent observation that pro-B cells contain higher levels than other B-cell progenitors of bcl-2, an oncogene-like protein that at high levels increases cell longevity and provides resistance to apoptosis, may

also apply to our problem.[17] If pro-B cells continue to show great resistance to zinc deficiency in subsequent experiments, we propose to see if this characteristic is more universal. In other words, are pro-B cells also more resistant than other B-cell precursors to glucocorticoid- or irradiation-induced cell death? A finding that pro-B cells are resistant to zinc deficiency would be one of several instances where nutritional studies make important contributions to our fundamental understanding of immunology.

In sum, the data clearly show that both moderate and severe zinc deficiency caused significant depletion of developing B cells in the bone marrow. The extent of loss was such that production of lymphocytes probably was also impaired by zinc deficiency. Studies of the effect of zinc deficiency on rate of lymphopoiesis and cell cycle status of proliferating pro- and pre-B cells are needed to demonstrate this point more clearly. Collectively, the data assembled to date lend further credence to our hypothesis that the lymphopenia observed in zinc deficiency is due, in part, to a reduction in the production of lymphocytes. These studies also clearly show that suboptimal nutriture can significantly alter B-cell lymphopoietic processes in the marrow, causing substantial depletion of early and immature precursor B cells.

Possible Role of Elevated Glucocorticoids Generated During Zinc Deficiency

We demonstrated several years ago that glucocorticoids, in particular corticosterone, were chronically elevated in zinc-deficient mice and that adrenalectomies, which removed the source of these steroids, prevented the thymus from atrophying during zinc deficiency.[18,19] Recently, a large body of literature indicated that corticosterone and other glucocorticoids readily induced cell death in immature thymocytes.[12,20] Indeed, glucocorticoid-induced apoptosis of thymocytes has become a classical system for the study of cell death.[12,20] Adrenalectomies were used to ascertain whether the chronically elevated glucocorticoids in zinc-deficient mice played any role in depletion of the marrow of developing B cells.[21] In two separate experiments, mice were adrenalectomized or sham operated and given 10–14 days to heal before being placed in the following dietary study: zinc-adequate sham-operated controls, zinc-adequate adrenalectomized, zinc-deficient sham-operated, or zinc-deficient adrenalectomized. The experiments were terminated when mice were only mildly zinc deficient (82% body weight of sham zinc-adequate mice) because we were concerned that adrenalectomized mice were more fragile and would not survive significant degrees of deficiency. At the time of sacrifice all adrenalectomized mice were checked to assure that there were no signs of residual adrenal glands, that the thymus was normal in size, and that the serum corticosterone levels were low. Zinc-deficient sham mice had a sixfold elevation of corticosterone levels and a thymus 65% the size of the adrenalectomized zinc-deficient mice. Moreover, the sham-operated zinc-deficient mice exhibited a reduction of 50% in the proportion of pre-B cells compared to adrenalectomized zinc-deficient mice.[21] Indeed, the adrenalectomized zinc-deficient mice had nearly normal levels of pre-B, immature, and mature B cells and were analogous to sham zinc-adequate mice for all these variables.[21] Removing corticosterone from the equation by adrenalectomy provided substantial protection for B-lineage cells developing in the marrow of mildly zinc-deficient mice and prevented atrophy of the thymus. These results suggest that chronically elevated corticosterone, generated as zinc deficiency advances, also plays a role in the observed lymphopenia and thymic atrophy of zinc deficiency.

To confirm these findings, we subsequently demonstrated that levels of corticosterone analogous to those produced during zinc deficiency but achieved by an implantation system also caused depletion of marrow B cells in a manner analogous to that seen in zinc-deficient mice.[22] Because of the rapid phagocytosis of apoptotic cells, it is difficult to measure the level of cell death in vivo. However, we suspect that the combination of suboptimal zinc and chronic elevation of corticosterone during zinc deficiency also heightens the level of apoptosis among precursor lymphocytes. This would also contribute to lymphopenia. Using recent advances in flow cytometry for measuring apoptosis, we hope to be able to assess the level of cell death among precursor cells in the marrow of zinc-deficient and zinc-adequate mice.[23]

Myelopoiesis

Bone marrow is the site of production of all blood cells including cells of the myeloid series.[24] The myeloid series includes phagocytic cells (e.g., monocytes, macrophages, neutrophils) as well as eosinophils and basophils. Data from the previous experiment indicated that as the B-cell compartment became depleted during zinc deficiency there was a concomitant accumulation or increase in cells bearing myeloid markers as well as an increase in the proportion of large, granular cells residing in the marrow of zinc-deficient mice as determined by flow cytometric scatter profiles.[16] In severe zinc deficiency there was as much as a 50–70% increase in the proportion of myeloid cells. This suggested that myelopoiesis was not as severely affected by zinc deficiency as was lymphopoiesis. Indeed, in an earlier study we found that neutrophils increased substantially in the blood of moderately and severely zinc-deficient mice (unpublished). In long-term marrow cultures the addition of glucocorticoids promotes development of

cells of the myeloid series.[25] The fact that myelopoiesis is fairly resistant to the suppressive apoptotic effects of glucocorticoids has already been shown. However, it is admittedly more difficult to understand why production of myeloid cells would be less affected by zinc unless they have greater stores of zinc and/or metallothionein. Nevertheless, since phagocytic cells are our first line of immune defense, it would be interesting if their production and longevity are greater during zinc deficiency. The system might represent a protective or fail-safe mechanism in place to provide minimal immune protection as zinc deficiency advances and the rest of the immune system is dismantled.

Future Consideration

From the data collected to date, we propose the following working hypothesis. As zinc becomes limiting, lymphopoiesis may need to be reduced in order to conserve the residual zinc for use by truly vital tissues like brain, heart, liver, kidney, etc. As zinc becomes limiting it induces the hypothalamus-pituitary-adrenocortical endocrine axis, which causes the production of chronically elevated levels of glucocorticoids.[18,19] We have shown that levels of glucocorticoids analogous to those found during zinc deficiency can cause substantial thymic atrophy and deplete the marrow of precursor B cells both in vitro and in vivo.[22] No doubt, suboptimal levels of zinc would also cause reduced proliferation and maturation of B and T cells because of the importance of zinc to cell division, growth, and proliferation.[3,13] It is also possible that modest declines in zinc might synergistically make precursor B and T cells more prone to glucocorticoid-initiated apoptosis. Though it is not currently possible to delineate precisely the effects on lymphopoiesis of suboptimal zinc versus glucocorticoids, we already have provided evidence that they both can and do play a role in the depletion of the marrow B cells. This might be a down-regulation mechanism in place so that during some forms of malnutrition lymphopoiesis is reduced, thereby saving large amounts of nutrients. Because myeloid cells are our first line of defense, it is also possible that they are more resistant to steroids and apoptosis. This could account for the fact that myeloid cells of the marrow seem less affected by zinc deficiency. The continued production and maintenance of myeloid cells might provide some form of basic or minimal level of immune protection.

Recognition that zinc deficiency alters lymphopoietic function will be important in the future when immunotherapy becomes more practical. It is already known that a number of specific cytokines contribute to B-cell and T-cell maturation and proliferation.[11] It may be that these cytokines could someday be used to boost the production of B and T cells in the marrow of malnourished subjects. Though it is difficult to quantitate the role that the chronically elevated glucocorticoids play in down-regulating lymphopoiesis in zinc-deficient mice, we feel that our recent steroid implantation studies and adrenal-ectomies show that glucocorticoids have a role to play in the depletion of B cells (as well as T cells), since they can readily induce apoptosis in precursor B cells.[22] It is also conceivable that some glucocorticoid antagonists, like RU40555 or other analogs, might be used to treat malnourished subjects in a way that could reduce the destruction of precursor lymphoid cells without undue alteration of essential metabolic functions.[20,22] Such treatments are already under consideration for AIDS patients where cortisol is also elevated.

Acknowledgment

The author would like to thank Farzaneh Osati for pro-B-cell data and Teresa Vollmer for preparation of the manuscript. This work was supported by a grant from the National Institutes of Health, HD10586-16.

References

1. Kuvibidila S, Yu L, Ode D, Warrier RP (1993) The immune response in protein-energy malnutrition and single nutrient deficiencies. In Klurfeld DM (ed), Human nutrition: a comprehensive treatise. Plenum Press, New York, pp 121–157
2. Fraker PJ, King L, Garvy B, Medina, C (1993) Immunopathology of zinc deficiency: a role for apoptosis. In Klurfeld DM (ed), Human nutrition: a comprehensive treatise. Plenum Press, New York, pp 267–283
3. Endre L, Beck F, Prasad A (1990) The role of zinc in human health. J Trace Elem Exp Med 3:337–375
4. Chandra R, Newberne P (1977) Nutrition, immunity and infection. Plenum Press, New York
5. Falutz J, Tsoukas C, Gold P (1988) Zinc as a cofactor in human immunodeficiency virus-induced immunosuppression. JAMA 260:1881–1883
6. Cook-Mills J, Fraker PJ (1993) Functional capacity of residual lymphocytes from zinc deficient adult mice. Br J Nutr 69:835–848
7. King LE, Fraker PJ (1991) Flow cytometric analysis of the phenotypic distribution of splenic lymphocytes in zinc deficient adult mouse. J Nutrition 121:1433–1438
8. Dowd PS, Kellher J, Guillou PJ (1986) T-lymphocyte subsets and interleukin-2 production in zinc-deficient rats. Br J Nutr 55:59–69
9. Wing EG, Magee DM, Barczynski LK (1988) Acute starvation in mice reduces number of T cells and suppresses the development of T-cell mediated immunity. Immunology 63: 677–682
10. Rolink A, Melchers F (1991) Molecular and cellular origins of B lymphocyte diversity. Cell 66:1081–1094
11. Kincade P, Lee G, Pietrangeli C, et al (1989) Cells and molecules that regulate B lymphopoiesis in bone marrow. Annu Rev Immunol 7:111–143
12. Cohen J, Duke R (1992) Apoptosis and programmed cell death in immunity. Annu Rev Immunol 10:267–293
13. Chesters J, Boyne R (1991) Nature of Zn^{2+} requirement for DNA synthesis by 3T3 cells. Exp Cell Res 192:631–636
14. Hardy RR, Carmack CE, Shinton SA, et al (1991) Resolution and characterization of pro-B and pre-pro-B cell stages in normal mouse bone marrow. J Exp Med 173:1213-1225
15. Uchida N, Weissman IL (1992) Searching for hematopoietic stem cells: evidence that Thy-1.1[lo] Lin- Sca-1+ cells are the only stem cells in C57BL/Ka-Thy-1.1 bone marrow. J Exp Med 175:175–184
16. King LE, Osati-Ashtiani F, Fraker P (1995) Depletion of cells of the B-lineage in the bone marrow of zinc deficient mouse. Immunology 85:69–73
17. Merino R, Ding L, Veis D, et al (1994) Development regulation of the Bcl-2 protein and susceptibility to cell death in B-lymphocytes. EMBO 13:683–691
18. DePasquale-Jardieu P, Fraker PJ (1979) The role of corticosterone in the loss in immune function in the zinc-deficient A/J mouse. J Nutr 109:1847–1855
19. DePasquale-Jardieu P, Fraker PJ (1980) Further characterization of the role of corticosterone in the loss of humoral immunity in zinc-deficient A/J mice as determined by adrenalectomy. J Immunol 124:2650–2655
20. Schwartzman R, Cidlowski J (1993) Apoptosis: the biochemistry and molecular biology of programmed cell death. Endocr Rev 14:133–151
21. Fraker P, Osati-Ashtiani F, Wagner M, King LL (1995) Possible roles for glucocorticoids and apoptosis in the suppression of lymphopoiesis during zinc deficiency. J Am Coll Nutr 14:11–17
22. Garvy B, King L, Telford W, et al (1993) Chronic levels of corticosterone reduce the number of cycling cells of the B-lineage in murine bone marrow and induce apoptosis. Immunology 80:587–592
23. Telford W, King L, Fraker PJ (1991) Evaluation of glucocorticoid induced DNA fragmentation in mouse thymocytes by flow cytometry. Cell Prolif 24:447–459
24. Leenen P, deBruijn M, Voerman J, et al (1994) Markers of mouse macrophage development detected by monoclonal antibodies. J Immunol Methods 174:5-19
25. Dexter T, Allen T, Lajtha L (1977) Conditions controlling the proliferation of hemopoietic stem cells in vitro. J Cell Physiol 91:335–341

Chapter 57

Toxic Substances in Foods

Michael W. Pariza

The term "food toxicology" does not refer to the toxicology of foods per se but rather to the study of toxic substances—particularly naturally occurring toxic substances—that may be associated with food.[1] Certain nonconventional foods, for example, puffer fish and bracken fern, contain levels of naturally occurring toxins that many would consider unacceptably high. Conventional foods (the kinds found typically in supermarkets) are on rare occasions contaminated with unacceptably high levels of naturally occurring toxins, but this is not the usual case. Hence, food toxicologists are not generally concerned with foods themselves but rather with toxic substances that may sometimes be found in foods. The two general types of naturally occurring toxicants—inherent toxicants, and contaminants—are described in Table 1.

It is important to distinguish between "toxic substance" and "toxic effect."[1,2] A toxic substance induces toxic effect, but will do so only if its concentration is sufficiently high. Hence, the terms toxic substance (toxicant) and toxic effect are not synonymous.

This distinction takes the form of a principle that underlies the science of toxicology. It was first presented as follows: "Everything is poison. There is nothing without poison. Only the dose makes a thing not a poison. For example, every food and every drink, if taken beyond its dose, is poison . . . ."[3,4] This observation is remarkable enough on its merits, but perhaps most surprising is that the author, the alchemist Paracelsus, penned it in 1564!

What we have learned of toxicology in the intervening 450 years has served only to reinforce Paracelsus' extraordinary insight. We recognize today that all chemicals are potentially toxic and that the dose alone determines whether or not a toxic effect occurs. Indeed, toxicant (or toxin) was recently defined as a "substance that has been shown to present some significant degree of possible risk when consumed in sufficient quantity by humans or animals."[5] We differ with Paracelsus only in reserving the term "poison" for the most potent substances (those which induce adverse effects at exposure levels of a few mg/kg body weight).

One expects drugs and household chemicals to exhibit at least some degree of toxicity, and these materials are ordinarily treated with the deference due them. However, even the most sophisticated might find it difficult to accept the notion that potentially toxic substances are commonly present in conventional foods. Some required nutrients, for example, vitamins A and D, induce toxic effects at intake levels not too much greater than those needed for optimal health. The safety margins for these and many other naturally occurring dietary substances are far smaller than the 100-fold safety factor customarily employed for food additives.[1]

The purpose of this chapter, then, is to provide an overview of toxicology as it relates to food. While all food chemicals (naturally occurring as well as synthetic) are potentially toxic, it is rare indeed to encounter a toxic effect induced as a result of consuming conventional foods.

Food Toxicology and the Law

The relationship between food safety and the science of toxicology is complex. Research in this area is done for two basic reasons: the pursuit of new knowledge and the evaluation of safety. The former is a true scientific goal, while the latter is a hybrid of science, politics, and law.[5]

By law, substances that are intentionally added to food must be shown to be safe under the intended conditions of their use. The methods and procedures for evaluating safety are matters of science, however, and additional considerations outside the purview of science also bear on the ultimate decision.

For example, substances may be classified as GRAS (generally recognized as safe). The decision as to whether something is GRAS is left to the scientific community, the people qualified as experts by training and experience. However, the Food and Drug Administration (FDA) reserves the right to challenge or affirm a GRAS determination.[5]

Reprinted and adapted, with permission, from *Food Chemistry*, Owen Fennema, ed., Marcel Dekker, Inc., New York, 1996.

Table 1. Types of food toxicants

Inherent toxicants
  — metabolites produced via biosynthesis by food
    organisms under normal growth conditions
  — metabolites produced via biosynthesis by food
    organisms that are stressed

Contaminants
  — toxicants that directly contaminate foods
  — toxicants that are absorbed from the environment
    by food-producing organisms
  — toxic metabolites produced by food organisms
    from substances that are absorbed from the
    environment
  — toxicants that are formed during food preparation

There are special considerations in the U.S. Food, Drug and Cosmetics Act (FD&C Act) for color additives, pesticide residues, prior-sanctioned ingredients (those in use prior to 1958, the year in which the FD&C Act was last amended), and substances for which FDA has issued formal food additive regulations. There is also the "constituents policy," which governs unavoidable contaminants.

Perhaps the best known provision of the FD&C Act is the Delaney clause, so-named for the congressman who chaired the congressional subcommittee that added the amendment to the FD&C Act. The Delaney clause, which bars the use of food additives shown to cause cancer in man or animals, actually appears in the FD&C Act three times, in sections 409 (Food Additives), 706 (Color Additives), and 612 (Animal Feeds and Drugs).

Pesticide residues on raw agricultural products are not subject to the Delaney clause, but concentrated residues that remain after a food is processed are subject to this legislation. In other words, it is legal to sell an apple that contains traces of a carcinogenic pesticide approved by the Environmental Protection Agency (EPA) but not to sell applesauce made from that apple. It is not even necessary to show that the applesauce actually contains the pesticide residue. Under the law, a processed food can be banned if a concentrated pesticide residue might theoretically be present.

By contrast, the Delaney clause does not apply to unavoidable contaminants that are present in a food or a food additive, even if the contaminants are carcinogens. Examples are traces of aflatoxin in peanuts and certain minor impurities that may occur in some chemically synthesized colors. For such contaminants, the courts have held that the FDA may use risk assessment methodologies coupled with the *de minimis* legal concept, a phrase meaning that the law does not deal with trifles.[5,6]

The result of all this is that an additive, for example, saccharin, that is very weakly carcinogenic in certain animal experiments and for which there is no evidence of human carcinogenicity, would be banned. (In fact, the only reason saccharin wasn't banned is because of a special congressional exemption). At the same time, theoretically "riskier" naturally occurring or synthetic carcinogens, which unavoidably contaminate food or color additives, are exempt from Delaney. For these, FDA sets limits on the amount of the contaminant that is to be tolerated.

Virtually all foods contain traces of carcinogenic substances, mostly from natural sources.[1,7,8] Examples are urethane in fermented beverages and certain naturally occurring components of spices such as safrole (the natural root beer flavor, banned as an intentional food additive in the 1960s) which is present in sassafras, sweet basil, and cinnamon.[9] A practical consequence of the federal law is that foods may be legally sold in the United States even if some of the constituents they contain cannot be intentionally added to a food.

Terms in Food Toxicology

Like all scientific disciplines, toxicology has a vocabulary of its own. Terms used by food toxicologists include acute toxicity, chronic toxicity, subchronic feeding test, maximum tolerated dose (MTD), no observable adverse effect level (NOAEL), and acceptable daily intake (ADI).

Acute toxicity refers to a toxic response, often immediate, induced by a single exposure. A lethal dose of hydrogen cyanide (50–60 mg) induces death within minutes. Cicutoxin, the toxic principal of water hemlock, kills so rapidly that cattle often die before the water hemlock they have eaten passes beyond the esophageal groove.[10] The acute toxicity of a substance is defined by its LD_{50}, the lethal dose of the substance that will kill 50% of a group of exposed animals.

Chronic toxicity refers to an effect that requires some time to develop, for example, cancer. Testing for chronic toxicity involves continuously feeding the test substance to rodents for 20–24 months. By analogy to LD_{50}, the amount of a carcinogen required to induce cancer in 50% of a group of exposed animals is referred to as the tumor dose (TD_{50}).[8]

Subchronic feeding test is a "ninety day toxicology study in an appropriate animal species."[5] It is often used to define the MTD and, for noncarcinogens, the NOAEL.

MTD is the acronym for "maximum tolerated dose." It is the highest level of a test substance that can be fed to an animal without inducing obvious signs of toxicity.[11] In chronic toxicity tests, the test substance is typically fed at its MTD and perhaps one or two lower doses. The MTD concept has been criticized because it is based solely on gross measures of toxicity such as weight loss. Subtle biochemical indicators of cellular toxicity, which may occur at lower doses, are ignored.[12]

NOAEL is the acronym for "no observable adverse effect level." For substances that induce a toxic response (other than cancer) in chronic feeding tests, the NOAEL is used to determine an acceptable daily intake (ADI).[6,12]

ADI is the acronym for "acceptable daily intake." By convention, for noncarcinogens, it is set at 1/100th of the NOAEL.

Potential food additives found to induce cancer are, of course, subject to the Delaney clause. The practical result is that such substances legally do not have a NOAEL. Hence, no amount can be added to food. (Whether this assumption is scientifically accurate is open to question.)

Evaluating Safety: The Traditional Approach

Rodent feeding tests are at the heart of traditional safety evaluations for new food ingredients. These tests were developed for the assessment of single chemicals, which could be fed at large multiples (100-fold or more) of proposed human consumption. High-dose feeding was needed, so the thinking went, to compensate for the relatively low number of test animals that practical considerations dictate can be used. (Low, that is, relative to the total number of potentially exposed humans. For example, the population of the United States is ≈250 million, yet one would be hard pressed to conduct a study with more than a few hundred rats. Hence each rat is a surrogate for a very large number of potentially exposed humans.)

The trade-off of feeding relatively small numbers of animal subjects relatively large amounts of test substances begged another question: how high should the exposure to test materials be? Thus was born the MTD, the greatest amount of a test substance that can be fed to a rat or mouse before overt signs of toxicity appear. Overt signs of toxicity were defined by a set of gross measurements, for example, failure of test animals to maintain at least 90% of the weight of controls.[11]

The traditional approach, then, is to determine the MTD for the test substance and feed the test substance at its MTD to rodents for 2 years. If the test group develops cancer in excess of the controls, then the substance may be judged a carcinogen and banned as a food additive under the Delaney clause.

If the substance is found not to induce cancer (or to induce it through secondary mechanisms that are not relevant to human experience), then its NOAEL is determined. The substance may then be permitted as a food additive at a concentration that is low enough so that humans will consume no more than 1/100th of the rodent NOAEL.

Evaluating Safety: New Approaches

The procedures discussed to this point were designed to evaluate the safety of substances, typically single chemicals but sometimes simple mixtures, that are intended to be used at relatively low levels in food. The qualification "relatively low levels" is critical in that the test substance is fed to experimental animals at large multiples of projected human exposure, usually 100-fold or more. Hence, by definition, the projected human exposure cannot be >1% of the diet, since at that point animals receiving a 100-fold multiple of human exposure would be consuming only the pure compound and nothing else. (In practice, the projected human dietary exposure must be considerably <1%, since feeding a substance to animals at more than a few percent of their diet risks creating a nutritional imbalance.) Obviously, a new approach is required for the evaluation of novel foods and "macro-ingredients" that are likely to represent >1% of the diets of at least some people (for example, genetically engineered tomatoes and novel edible oils).

In evaluating such materials, plausible substitutes for the standard high-dose animal feeding tests are required. One approach has its origins in the safety evaluation of enzymes used in food processing.[2]

Food-grade enzymes are in fact complex mixtures, not single entities. Typically there is little purification, so virtually everything the source organism produces may be present in a commercial enzyme preparation. Given this, one may reasonably ask how safety evaluation should be conducted. Should one focus on the active enzyme, or on all the components that constitute the product as it is marketed? Is it necessary to consider all possible adverse effects, or can the task be simplified by concentrating on those possible adverse effects that might reasonably occur as a result of the use of the specific source organism?

Fortunately, there is a sizable set of data for microbial toxins on which to base an evaluation system. It is possible, then, to evaluate a microbial enzyme preparation for its potential to produce adverse effects that might be anticipated given the production organism.[2]

A safety evaluation system based on these considerations begins with a thorough literature review to determine what (if any) adverse effects have been associated with the source organism and related organisms of same species or genus.[2] Particular attention is directed to finding reports of toxins active via the oral route (enterotoxins and certain neurotoxins). If such reports are found, it is then necessary to ensure that the enzyme preparation is free of the undesirable material.

The usual case is that the production organism will have been selected from those species with a prior history of safe use in food or food ingredient manufacture. In this case it is most probable that no adverse effects will have been reported for the organism. Limited animal testing may still be required to ensure that the proposed production organism does not produce unknown enterotoxins or other undesirable substances active via the oral route.

Table 2. Examples of toxicants inherent in plants

Toxins	Chemical nature	Main food sources	Major toxicity symptoms
Protease inhibitors	Proteins (mol. wt. 4000–24,000)	Beans (soy, mung, kidney, navy, lima); chick-pea; peas; potato (sweet, white); cereals	Impaired growth and food utilization; pancreatic hypertrophy
Hemagglutinins	Proteins (mol. wt. 10,000–124,000)	Beans (castor, soy, kidney, black, yellow, jack); lentils; peas	Impaired growth and food utilization; agglutination of erythrocytes in vitro; mitogenic activity to cell cultures in vitro
Saponins	Glycosides	Soybeans, sugarbeets, peanuts, spinach, asparagus	Hemolysis of erythrocytes in vitro
Glucosinolates	Thioglycosides	Cabbage and related species; turnips; rutabaga; radish; rapeseed; mustard	Hypothyroidism and thyroid enlargement
Cyanogens	Cyanogenic glucosides	Peas and beans; pulses; linseed; flax; fruit kernels; cassava	HCN poisoning
Gossypol pigments	Gossypol	Cottonseed	Liver damage; hemorrhage; edema
Lathyrogens	b-Aminopropionitrile and derivatives	Chick-pea; vetch	Neurolathyrism (CNS damage)
Allergens	Proteins?	Practically all foods (particularly grains, legumes, and nuts)	Allergic responses in sensitive individuals
Cycasin	Methylazoxymethanol	Nuts of *Cycas* genus	Cancer of liver and other organs
Favism	Vicine and convicine (pyrimidine-b-glucosides)	Fava beans	Acute hemolytic anemia
Phytoalexins	Simple furans (ipomeamarone)	Sweet potatoes	Pulmonary edema; liver and kidney damage
	Benzofurans (psoralins)	Celery; parsnips	Skin photosensitivity
	Acetylenic furans (wyerone)	Broad beans	
	Isoflavonoids (pisatin and phaseollin)	Peas, french beans	Cell lysis in vitro
Pyrrolizidine alkaloids	Dihydropyrroles	Families Compositae and Boraginaccae; herbal teas	Liver and lung damage; carcinogens
Safrole	Allyl-substituted benzene	Sassafras; black pepper	Carcinogens
a-Amanitin	Bicyclic octapeptides	*Amanita phalloides* mushrooms	Salivation; vomiting; convulsions; death
Atractyloside	Steroidal glycoside	Thistle (*Atractylis gummifera*)	Depletion of glycogen

From reference 14.

With slight modification this approach can accommodate enzymes produced by genetically engineered organisms.[5] Moreover, the proposition of focusing on potentially adverse substances that might be produced by the source organism (in contrast to a broader and largely unworkable approach of searching for any conceivable adverse effect via high-dose animal feeding tests) also forms the basis of safety evaluation systems for genetically engineered crops endorsed by government and industry.[5,13]

Comparative Toxicology and Inherent Toxicants

The traditional approach to safety evaluation is based on concepts developed in the middle of this century, some of which are now difficult to justify.[6,12] In particular, a basic assumption of the traditional approach, that dietary carcinogens are rare and therefore avoidable, is decidedly untenable.[7,8,12]

Table 3. Some naturally occurring carcinogens inherent in food

Rodent carcinogen	Plant food	Concentration (ppm)
5-/8-Methoxypsoralen	Parsley	14
	Parsnip, cooked	32
	Celery	0.8
	Celery, new cultivar	6.2
	Celery, stressed	25
p-Hydrazinobenzoate	Mushrooms	11
Glutamyl p-hydrazino-benzoate	Mushrooms	42
Sinigrin (allyl isothiocyanate)	Cabbage	35–590
	Collard greens	250–788
	Cauliflower	12–66
	Brussels sprouts	110–1560
	Mustard (brown)	16,000–72,000
	Horseradish	4500
Estragole	Basil	3800
	Fennel	3000
Safrole	Nutmeg	3000
	Mace	10,000
	Pepper, black	100
Ethyl acrylate	Pineapple	0.07
Sesamol	Sesame seeds (heated oil)	75
A-methylbenzyl alcohol	Cocoa	1.3
Benzyl acetate	Basil	82
	Jasmine tea	230
	Honey	16
	Coffee (roasted beans)	100
Caffeic acid	Apple, carrot, celery, cherry, eggplant, endive, grapes lettuce, pear, plum, and potato	50–100
	Absinthe, anise, basil, caraway, dill, marjoram, rosemary, sage, savory, tarragon, and thyme	>1000
	Coffee (roasted beans)	1800
	Apricot, cherry, peach, and plum	50–500
Chlorogenic acid (caffeic acid)	Coffee (roasted beans)	21,600
Neochlorogenicaicid (caffeic acid)	Apple, apricot, broccoli, brussels sprouts, cabbage, cherry, kale, peach, pear, and plum	50–500
	Coffee (roasted beans)	11,600

From Ames et al. (reference 7).

In contrast, the nontraditional approaches are more recent attempts to wed safety evaluation to the emerging realization that a quest for absolute safety is not only scientifically naive but also counter to the need to prioritize public health objectives in light of funding constraints.[7,8,12]

The focus of the new approaches proposed by the International Food Biotechnology Council and the FDA is comparative toxicology.[5,13] In this context, comparative toxicology refers to comparing the concentration of inherent toxins (e.g., those that are naturally and endogenously present) in the new food with the concentration of inherent toxins in the traditional counterpart of the new food. This is a fundamental conceptual shift from the traditional approach, which stresses the absence of toxicity over a wide safety margin (set arbitrarily at 100-fold). The new approach allows inherent toxicants in the new food if their levels do not exceed those contained in the traditional counterpart of the new food (the traditional counterpart is the food in current use that the new food will replace). Safety margins for the inherent toxicants would not ordinarily be of concern so long as the traditional counterpart is considered safe to eat.

Obviously, the credibility of these approaches depends on the existence of reliable, comprehensive databases of toxicants that occur naturally in commonly consumed foods.[5,13] Fortunately such databases exist, thanks to basic research that was conducted largely for the pursuit of knowledge without regard to the legal and regulatory aspects of food toxicology.[5] For example, we know that many kinds of inherent toxicants occur in plants (Table 2), and we also know that some of these substances are carcinogens in animal experiments (Table 3). However, we also know that only a few such inherent toxicants have actually caused harm to people consuming normal human diets (Table 4).

Inherent toxicants are a subset of the naturally occurring chemicals, a broad category that includes all substances except those that are not of biosynthetic origin

Table 4. Plant toxicants documented as causing harm in normal human diets

Substance (category/name/no. of substances)	Plant source	Methods of risk reduction
Honey toxicants (7)		
Acetylandromedel, andromedol, anhydroandromedol, and desacetylpireistoxin B	Rhododendron/Andromeda/Azalea family	Monitoring prohibition of beekeeping
Gelsamine	Yellow jasmine	
Tutin	Tutu tree	
Hyenanchin		
Forage and meat/milk toxicants (4)		
Cicutoxin	Water hemlock	Proper grazing and forage practices; avoidance
Coniine	Hemlock	
Methylconiine		
Conhydrine		
Toxicants from poor choice, handling, or processing of local diet (5+)		
Hypoglycin A	Ackee fruit (immature)	Avoidance
Linamarin and Lotaustralin	Lima beans and cassava root	Selection and breeding (and proper processing for cassava)
b-N-Oxalylamino-L-alanine	Chick-pea	Reduced use
(-)-Sparteine and related alkaloids	Lupine	Proper processing
Plant genetic factors/poor handling (1)		
Solanine	Potato	Selection and breeding, monitoring, proper handling
Human genetic factors (2)		
Vicine	Fava bean	Reduced use
Convivine		
Other (2)		
Cucurbitacin E	Squash, cucumber	Breeding isolation
Nitrates	Spinach and other green, leafy vegetables	Proper fertilizing practices and handling; monitoring
Total (21+)		

From International Food Biotechnology Council (reference 5) and Hall (reference 15).

and that are intentionally or accidentally introduced into food through human activity.[5] By this definition mycotoxins are naturally occurring even if they developed through mold growth due to careless handling of stored grain, but residues of synthetic pesticides used to kill insects harboring the mold spores are not naturally occurring. Arsenic is naturally occurring when in seafood (it is a natural component of sea water), but arsenic is not naturally occurring when present in produce from a field to which the element was intentionally applied as a pesticide (a custom no longer practiced in the United States).

Most chemicals in the environment (and of course this includes food) are naturally occurring in that they are not intentional products of synthetic chemistry. Very few substances are solely synthetic in that they are not known to exist in nature. Hence the number, variety, and concentration of naturally occurring chemicals in food far outweighs, by many orders of magnitude, synthetic substances.

A vast number of naturally occurring chemicals are present in food. No one knows precisely how many naturally occurring chemicals a typical consumer ingests each day, but an estimate of 1 million compounds is probably conservative. Cooking no doubt amplifies the total number, so that with more cooking, more chemicals are encountered.

Earlier we noted that all chemicals, whether synthetic or naturally occurring, exhibit toxicity at some level of exposure. Even pure water drunk to excess will kill through the induction of an electrolyte imbalance; there is, in fact, a condition of the elderly called "water toxicity" that is due in part to decreased renal capacity to excrete water.[16] The innumerable naturally occurring

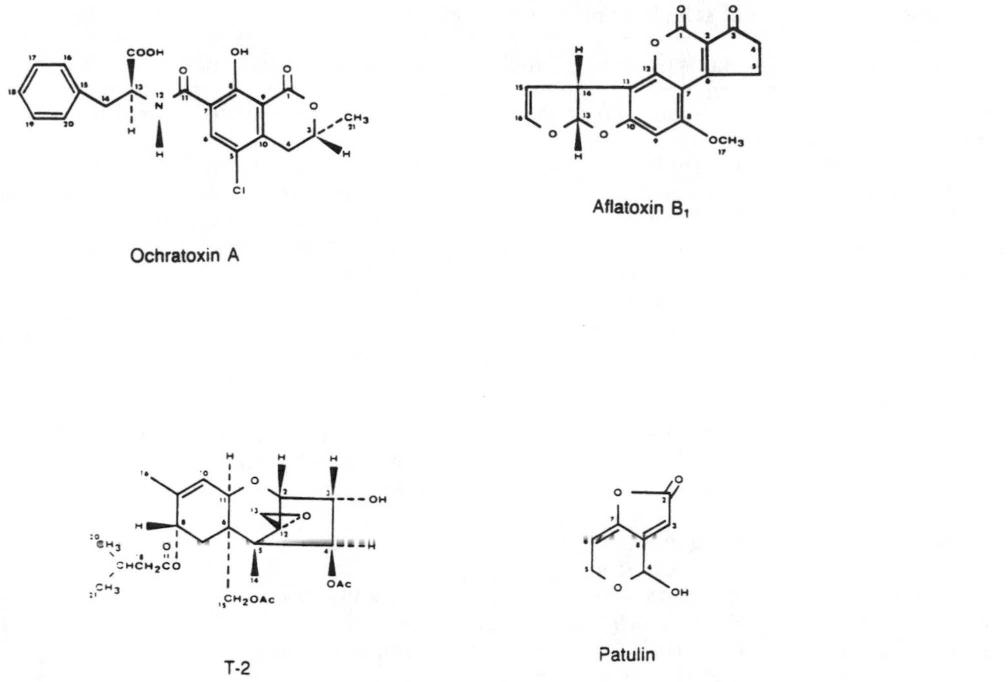

Figure 1. Chemical structures of four important mycotoxins. From Council on Agricultural Science and Technology.[17]

chemicals in food are all potentially capable of inducing toxic effects, but few are ordinarily present in sufficient concentration to do so.[1,5]

By one standard, a substance is of concern if it occurs in food within a narrow margin of safety; in other words, if a toxic effect results from ingesting no more than 25 times the amount typically found in food.[5] By this standard only a tiny fraction of food constituents (which is estimated to be less than one-tenth of 1%) are "toxicants."

Even so, the list of such toxicants is daunting. Table 2 is a listing of only 209 plant-derived food constituents classified as toxicants and/or carcinogens.[5] Many of these are inherent toxicants that form the basis for the comparative toxicology safety evaluation proposals.[5,13]

Hall[15] discusses 21 plant-derived toxicants that are documented to have harmed humans who were eating "ordinary" diets (as opposed to the consumption of toxic herbs or poisonous mushrooms, which are not ordinary dietary items). These are shown in Table 4. Of these 21 toxicants, only five are inherent toxicants of foods that are common in Western countries: solanine in potatoes (arguably the most important), cucurbitacin E in squash and cucumber, nitrates in spinach and other green leafy vegetables, and linamarin and lotaustralin in lima beans.

Contaminants

Inherent toxicants are not the only undesirable food constituents. One must also be concerned with contaminants, which may be synthetic or naturally occurring. The FDA makes few distinctions between these in terms of regulation, but there is general agreement among experts that naturally occurring contaminants are most important, particularly those produced by microorganisms.[12] This is not to minimize the potential consequences of contamination of food by synthetic toxicants, but rather to emphasize that contamination by pathogenic microorganisms or their toxins occurs far more frequently.

Two general kinds of microbial toxins are especially important: mycotoxins (mold toxins) and bacterial food poisoning toxins.

Mycotoxins are relatively small molecular weight organic molecules, i.e., almost all are smaller than 500 Da. In some cases the common name (e.g., patulin) signifies a single substance, while in other cases the common name (e.g., trichothecenes) signifies a class of chemically related substances. The chemical structures of four important mycotoxins are diagrammed in Figure 1.

Mycotoxins induce a wide range of acute and chronic toxic effects in humans and livestock, depending on the compound or compound class, the level of exposure, and the duration of exposure. Among the effects induced by different mycotoxins are tremors and hemorrhaging, immunological suppression, renal toxicity, fetal toxicity, or cancer.[17,18]

Toxigenic molds may enter the food and feed supply at numerous points, including production, processing, transport, and storage.[17] Substrate, moisture, pH, temperature, and crop stress are the major environmental

Table 5. Natural occurrence of selected common mycotoxins

Mycotoxins[a]	Major producing fungi	Typical substrate in nature	Biological effect
Alternaria (AM) mycotoxins	*Alternaria alternata*	Cereal grains, tomato, animal feeds	M, Hm
Aflatoxin (AF) B$_1$ and other aflatoxins	*Aspergillus flavus, A. parasiticus*	Peanuts, corn, cottonseed, cereals, figs, most tree nuts, milk, sorghum, walnuts	H, C, M, T
Citrinin (CT)	*Penicillium citrinum*	Barley, corn, rice, walnuts	Nh, C(?), M
Cyclopiazonic acid (CPA)	*A. flavus, P. cyclopium*	Peanuts, corn, cheese	Nr, Cv
Deoxynivalenol (DON)	*Fusarium graminearum*	Wheat, corn	Nr
Cyclochlorotine (CC)	*P. islandicum*	Rice	H, C
Fumonisins (FM)	*F. moniliforme*	Corn, sorghum	N, Nr, C(?), R
Luteoskyrin (LT)	*P. islandicum, P. rugulosum*	Rice, sorghum	H, C, M
Moniliformin (MN)	*F. moniliforme*	Corn	Nr, Cv
Ochratoxin A (OTA)	*A. ochraceus, P. verrucosum*	Barley, beans, cereals, coffee, feeds, maize, oats, rice, rye, wheat	Nh, T
Patulin (PT)	*P. patulum, P. urticae, A. clavatus*	Apple, apple juice, beans, wheat	Nr, C(?), D, T
Penicillic acid (PA)	*P. puberulum, A. ochraceus*	Barley, corn	Nr, C(?), M
Penitrem A (PNT)	*P. palitans*	Feedstuffs, corn	Nr
Roquefortine (RQF)	*P. roqueforti*	Cheese	Nr
Rubratoxin B (RB)	*P. rubrum, P. purpurogenum*	Corn, soybeans	H, T
Sterigmatocystin (ST)	*A. versicolor, A. nidulans*	Corn, grains, cheese	H, C, M
T-2 Toxin	*F. sporotrichioides*	Corn, feeds, hay	D, ATA, T
12-13,Epoxytrichothecenes (TCTC) other than T-2 and DON	*F. nivale*	Corn, feeds, hay, peanuts, rice	D, Nr
Zearalone (ZE)	*F. graminearum*	Cereals, corn feeds, rice	G, M

From Chu (reference 18).

ATA, alimentary toxic aleukia; C, carcinogenic; C(?), carcinogenic effect still questionable; Cv, cardiovascular lesion; D, dermatoxin; G, genitotoxin and estrogenic effects; H, hepatotoxic; Hr, hemorrhagic; M, mutagenic; Nh, nephrotoxin; Nr, neurotoxins; R, respiratory; T, teratogenic.

[a]The optimal temperatures for the production of mycotoxin are generally between 24 and 28 °C, except for T-2 toxin, which is generally produced maximally at 15 °C.

factors that affect mold growth and mycotoxin production.[17] Corn, peanuts, and cotton are the principal crops affected by mycotoxin contamination in the United States.[16]

Numerous mold species, belonging to more than 50 genera, are reported to produce toxic metabolites.[5] However, most of these toxic metabolites have not been associated with human or animal disease.[17] Species of mold belonging to three genera, *Aspergillus*, *Fusarium*, and *Penicillium*, produce the most important mycotoxins known to cause illness in humans and animals.[17]

Although a great number of mycotoxins have been identified they are not all equally important in terms of degree of toxicity and likelihood of human or animal exposure. Those that pose the greatest potential risk to human and animal health are listed in Table 5.[18]

In the United States and other countries with advanced food production systems, incidences of human illness induced by mycotoxins are extremely rare and virtually never traced to commercially processed foods.[17] The strict specifications set by food processors for amounts of

mycotoxins acceptable on grains and other ingredients used in food manufacture are based in part on tolerances established by regulatory agencies. Acceptable levels of mycotoxin contamination are determined using extremely conservative risk assessment analyses, so that public health is protected by wide safety margins.

By contrast, the chance contamination of animal feeds with harmful levels of mycotoxins is documented to occur in the United States and other developed countries.[17] Crop stress is an important contributing factor. For example, drought-induced stress enhances the probability of aflatoxin contamination of corn, whereas cold, wet weather that slows harvest may lead to contamination of grain with harmful levels of trichothecenes. Grain judged to be unacceptable for human consumption may end up being fed to livestock.

There is concern that mycotoxins in feeds might pass through to humans who consume animal products. For example, aflatoxin M is found in milk from cows that are fed aflatoxin-contaminated feed. The potential or actual extent of human harm from aflatoxin M or other mycotoxin metabolites in edible animal tissues is not known.

Bacterial food poisoning toxins are different from mycotoxins in three important ways. First, bacterial food-poisoning toxins with rare exception are proteins and not small organic molecules. Second, bacterial food-poisoning toxins are acute toxins. The onset of symptoms occurs a few hours to a few days after exposure. There is no counterpart among bacterial food-poisoning toxins to, for instance, the induction of liver cancer in rats by aflatoxin B$_1$. Finally, while bacterial food-poisoning toxins are important causes of human illness, such toxins are rarely associated with animal feeds. (Feeds can, however, harbor pathogenic bacteria that may infect livestock and be passed on to humans.) No doubt the absence of bacterial toxins in feeds has to do with low moisture content. Bacteria require higher moisture levels for growth and toxin synthesis than do molds.[19]

Bacterial toxins that cause food poisoning when ingested are listed in Table 6.

Staphylococcus aureus is the most common toxigenic foodborne bacterium. This organism is estimated to be responsible for >1 million cases of food poisoning in the United States each year.[20] *S. aureus* is also an important infectious agent of humans and other mammals, but staphylococcal food poisoning is caused by the ingestion of food containing preformed enterotoxin. (*Salmonella* species are estimated to produce almost 3 million cases of foodborne illness but they do so via infection, not toxin production.)

Staphylococcal enterotoxin is not a single entity but rather a group of more than seven single-chain proteins with molecular weights of 26,000–29,000.[21] The enterotoxins are antigenic and are detected using serological methods. Toxigenic strains of *S. aureus* may produce more than one enterotoxin. Symptoms of intoxication often include severe diarrhea and vomiting in addition to abdominal pain, headache, muscular cramping, and sweating.

The amount of a staphylococcal enterotoxin necessary to cause illness is not accurately known but is probably no more than a few hundred nanograms.[21] In general, it requires a million or more staphylococci to produce this amount of toxin. Foods most at risk for staphylococcal growth and enterotoxin production are those that are rich, moist, and subject to temperature abuse (custard or cream-filled bakery goods, cured meats such as ham, and salads containing egg, seafood, or meat).

The most feared toxigenic foodborne bacterium is *Clostridium botulinum*, the cause of botulism. Fortunately it is relatively uncommon, estimated at <300 cases per year in the United States.[20]

C. botulinum food poisoning is caused by a series of neurotoxins that cause symptoms including paralysis and death. Each of the seven different botulinal neurotoxins

Table 6. Bacterial toxins that cause foodborne illness

Toxin	Estimated cases of illness per year in U.S.
Staphylococcal enterotoxins	1,155,000
Bacillus cereus enterotoxins	84,000
Botulinal neurotoxins	270
Estimated total number of cases of foodborne illness in the U.S. per year from all causes	12,581,270

From Council on Agricultural Science and Technology (reference 20).

is a protein with molecular weight of ≈150,000 and with subunits linked by disulfide bonds. Botulinal neurotoxins are the most potent acute poisons known. Toxic potency ranges from 10^7 to 10^8 mouse LD_{50} units per mg of protein.[22]

C. botulinum is an anaerobic sporeformer, so it survives moderate heat treatments that kill vegetative cells. The neurotoxins, on the other hand, are readily destroyed by heating. Early in this century the canning industry developed procedures to ensure the complete destruction of *C. botulinum* spores in order to produce safe canned foods. In the United States today botulism is almost always associated with mishandling that occurs in food service establishments or the home.[20]

Bacillus cereus is a foodborne pathogen that produces two distinct enterotoxins. One causes diarrhea, the other induces vomiting. The mechanisms of action of these toxins are not known.[23]

As its name implies, *B. cereus* is a common soil microorganism that frequently contaminates cereal products. It is not a major cause of food poisoning in the United States but appears to be more common in Europe, particularly Great Britain.[20]

Less common forms of food poisoning are associated with bacterial metabolites that are not proteins. Examples include histamine poisoning, nitrite poisoning, and bongkrek food poisoning (caused by a toxic fatty acid produced by *Pseudomonas cocovenenans* and *Flavobacterium farinofermentans*).[24]

A number of foodborne bacterial pathogens produce toxins in association with gastrointestinal infections, including certain strains of *Escherichia coli* and *Clostridium perfringens*.[25,26] These illness are induced wholly or in part by toxin synthesized *in situ* following ingestion of the pathogenic microorganism.

Food Toxicology and Public Health: Setting Priorities

It is estimated that 12.5 million cases of food-associated illness occur each year in the United States, at a cost of ≈$8.5 billion.[20] The great majority of the illnesses are due to infectious agents: pathogenic bacteria like

Table 7. Prioritizing commonly encountered carcinogen exposures

Daily human exposure	HERP (%)
PCBs, daily dietary intake	0.0002
EDB[a], daily dietary intake	0.0004
Alar[b], one apple (230 g)	0.0002
Tap water, 1 liter (chloroform)	0.001
Cooked bacon, 100 g (nitrosamines)	0.003
Worst well water in Silicon Valley (trichloroethylene)	0.004
Peanut butter (one sandwich) (aflatoxin)	0.03
One glass of wine (ethanol)	4.7

Gold et al[8]

[a]EDB' refers to ethylene dibromide, a pesticide.

[b]Banned because of health concerns; HERP value based on exposure prior to ban.

Salmonella, viruses such as hepatitis A virus, and parasites such as *Toxoplasma gondii*. Foodborne toxins are estimated to account for <1.5 million of these cases of which >1 million are due to the staphylococcal enterotoxins.[20] The science of food toxicology indicates that while we should be vigilant in protecting foods against contamination by naturally occurring and synthetic toxins, by far the most common foodborne toxicologic risks in the United States and other developed countries come from certain bacterial toxins. Moreover, a great deal of scientific data are available to assist in controlling such contamination.

There still remains the dilemma of the public perception that toxicologic risk to our food supply is much greater than scientifically derived estimates indicate. Concern over perceived risks typically focuses on synthetic contaminants, pesticide residues, and food additives.[27]

There have been few attempts to address these concerns in a systematic, scientific manner. One such approach was developed by Ames and colleagues.[8] It involves ranking carcinogenic risks according to a ratio known by the acronym HERP (human exposure/rodent potency). A HERP can be calculated for any carcinogen so long as its human exposure level and potency in a rodent bioassay are known. To calculate a HERP, the human exposure level (mg/kg body weight) is divided by the TD_{50} (mg/kg body weight), and the result is then multiplied by 100.[8]

An example of some HERP values for common exposures to food substances is given in Table 7. As is evident, the concentration of synthetic pesticide residues and contaminants represents a far lower risk than many naturally occurring carcinogens. Ames and colleagues[7,8] estimate that 99.99% of the total mass of carcinogens typically ingested is of natural origin.

It is important that these conclusions be interpreted correctly. One should not infer that the level of exposure to naturally occurring dietary carcinogens is necessarily excessive, especially in developed countries.

Rather, the level of exposure to synthetic pesticide residues and contaminants is ordinarily so low as to be of no health significance whatever.

These considerations are of great importance in properly applying the results of food toxicology science to reducing public health risk.

References

1. Coon JM (1973) Toxicology of natural food chemicals: a perspective. In Committee on Food Protection, Food and Nutrition Board, National Research Council (eds), Toxicants occurring naturally in foods, 2nd ed. National Academy of Sciences, Washington, DC, pp 573–591
2. Pariza MW, Foster EM (1983) Determining the safety of enzymes used in food processing. J Food Prot 46:453–468
3. Deichmann WB, Henschler D, Holmstedt B, Keil G (1986) What is there that is not poison? a study of the Third Defense by Paracelsus. Arch Toxicol 58:207–213
4. Holmstedt B, Liljestrand G (1981) Readings in pharmacology. Raven Press, New York, p 29
5. International Food Biotechnology Council (1990) Biotechnologies and food: assuring the safety of foods produced by genetic modification. Regul Toxicol Pharmacol 12(3), part 2 of 2, pp S1–S196
6. Pariza MW (1992) Risk assessment. Crit Rev Food Sci Technol 31:205–209
7. Ames BN, Profet M, Gold LS (1990) Dietary pesticides (99.99% all natural). Proc Natl Acad Sci USA 87:7777–7781
8. Gold LS, Slone TH, Stern BR, et al (1992) Rodent carcinogens: setting priorities. Science 258:261–265
9. Miller EC, Swanson AB, Phillips DH, et al (1983) Structure-activity studies of the carcinogenicities in the mouse and rat of some naturally occurring and synthetic alkenylbenzene derivatives related to safrole and estragole. Cancer Res 43:1124–1134
10. Smith RA (1994) Poisonous plants. In Hui YH, Gorham JR, Murrell KD, Cliver DO (eds), Foodborne disease handbook. Marcel Dekker, New York, pp 187–226
11. Chhabra RS, Huff JE, Schwetz BS, Selkirk J (1990) An overview of prechronic and chronic toxicology/carcinogenicity experimental study designs and criteria used by the National Toxicology Program. Environ Health Perspec 86:313–321
12. Pariza MW (1992) A new approach to evaluating carcinogenic risk. Proc Natl Acad Sci USA 89:860–861
13. Kessler DA, Taylor MR, Maryanski JH, et al (1992) The safety of foods developed by biotechnology. Science 256: 1747–1749, 1832
14. Wogan GN, Marletta MA (1985) Undesirable or potentially undesirable constituents of foods. In Fennema OR (ed), Food chemistry. Marcel Dekker, New York, pp 694–695
15. Hall RL (1992) Toxicological burdens and the shifting burden of toxicology. Food Technol 46(3):109–112
16. Chernoff R (1994) Thirst and fluid requirements. Nutr Rev 52 (8, part 2):s3–s5
17. CAST (Council on Agricultural Science and Technology) (1989) Mycotoxins: economic and health risks. Task Force Report No. 116. Council on Agricultural Science and Technology, Ames, IA
18. Chu FS (1995) Mycotoxin analysis. In Jeon IJ, Ilkins WG (eds), Analyzing food for nutrition labeling and hazardous contaminants. Marcel Dekker, New York, pp 283–332
19. Cliver DO, ed (1990) Foodborne diseases. Academic Press, San Diego, CA, 395

20. CAST (Council on Agricultural Science and Technology) (1994) Foodborne pathogens: risks and consequences. Task Force Report No. 122. Council on Agricultural Science and Technology, Ames, IA

21. Bergdoll MS (1990) Staphylococcal food poisoning. In Cliver DO (ed), Foodborne diseases. Academic Press, San Diego, CA, pp 85–106

22. Sugiyama H (1990). Botulism. In Cliver DO (ed), Foodborne diseases. Academic Press, San Diego, CA, pp 85–106

23. Johnson EA (1990) *Bacillus cereus* food poisoning. In Cliver DO (ed), Foodborne diseases. Academic Press, San Diego, CA, pp 127–135

24. Taylor SL (1990) Other microbial intoxications. In Cliver DO (ed), Foodborne diseases. Academic Press, San Diego, CA, pp 159–170

25. Johnson EA (1990) *Clostridium perfringens* food poisoning. In Cliver DO (ed), Foodborne diseases. Academic Press, San Diego, CA, pp 1229–240

26. Doyle MP, Cliver DO (1990). *Escherichia coli*. In Cliver DO (ed), Foodborne diseases. Academic Press, San Diego, CA, pp 209–215

27. Foster EM (1990) Perennial issues in food safety. In Cliver DO (ed), Foodborne diseases. Academic Press, San Diego, CA, pp 127–135

Chapter 58

Nutrient-Gene Interactions
Carolyn D. Berdanier

From conception to death, living creatures are influenced by both internal and external factors. Among the internal factors of importance is the genetic material, DNA, which consists of a series of purine and pyrimidine bases linked together in a preset pattern, by phosphate and ribose groups. This preset pattern is divided into chromosomes, of which there are 46 in the human. These chromosomes are divided into specific units called genes, which dictate every feature and characteristic of life: the species, gender, life span, metabolic function, external characteristics, and the myriad responses to the external environment, which includes nutrition. Nutrient-gene interactions have the potential to influence conception, normal growth and development, and healthy life span, and, indeed, may determine the diseases that cause death. The purpose of this chapter is to discuss the current knowledge about these interactions in the context of nutrient needs and tolerances. Ultimately, as knowledge about individual genetic identity expands, nutritionists will be able to recommend nutrient intakes that enhance the expression of genes associated with good health and suppress the expression of genes associated with disease.

While nutrition (or specific nutrients) cannot negate one's ultimate genetic fate, it can modify the time frame during which the characteristics of this fate appear. This, then, is the theme of this chapter. The questions of how specific nutrients turn on or turn off the expression of specific genes will be addressed, as will the question of how specific genes affect the use of specific nutrients. Lastly, the question of how age and diet together influence these interactions will be approached as a means to explain why some disease-associated genetic signatures can be very subtle and take decades of human life to express themselves while others are devastatingly apparent at or before birth. Gene expression is a process that is still under investigation. Some genes have been completely sequenced and their location on specific chromosomes or on the mitochondrial genome has been mapped. Other genes are being discovered, sequenced, and mapped as the human genome project continues.

Nutrition, Genetic Heritage, Health, and Disease

While the DNA in all cells carries all of the genes for all of the body's characteristics, not all of these genes are expressed in all cells at all times. This implies that controls of gene expression exist that determine which codes are transcribed and translated into gene products. However, metabolic control mechanisms, which involve hormones, metabolites, ions, second messenger systems, and so forth, modify the phenotypic expression of these genes. Thus, a particular gene product having somewhat aberrant functional characteristics might have no discernible effect on health and well-being because of compensatory metabolic control mechanisms or dietary choices, or both, that have the same net effect. That is, the individual with this genetic "aberration" is totally normal. For example, more than 100 genetic aberrations have been identified as being associated with the many forms of diabetes mellitus.[1] Yet the number of new cases varies considerably from year to year in association with year-to-year variation in food supply, economics, or epidemics of certain communicable diseases.[2]

In the Great Depression, people in financial straits spent less money on food so that their limited resources could be used for other essential needs. The ongoing USDA Food Disappearance Survey shows that, during this period, people in the United States consumed less fat, protein, and energy per day than either before or after the depression.[3] Figure 1 shows the averages of the disappearance of the macronutrients as well as total energy for the period 1909 to 1990. After the depression, during World War II, economic constraints were relieved but there was a sharp reduction in food supply because of the need to send food to the European and Asian war theaters. Again, examination of the USDA Food Disappearance Data indicates a reduction in the total energy consumed by the American public.[3] However, in contrast to the food disappearance data from the depression period, all of the major macronutrient classes were affected, not just the fats and proteins. These constraints on food intake likely affected metabolism and

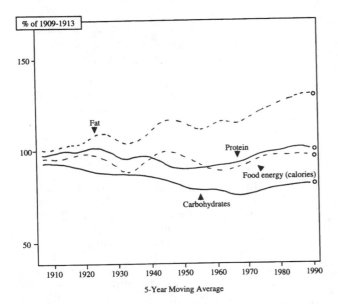

Figure 1. Food energy, protein, fat, and carbohydrate in the U.S. food supply.

the phenotypic expression of mutated genes that under abundant food intake conditions would result in non-insulin-dependent diabetes mellitus (NIDDM), obesity, or both conditions. During the depression and during World War II, obesity and the number of new cases of NIDDM probably declined. However, because of inadequate diagnostic criteria, the records for these time periods are not reliable.

More to the point are the reports of Cohen and co-workers.[4,5] They examined newly arrived Yemenite Jews and compared them with Yemenites who had lived in Israel for 20 years or more. Very few cases of NIDDM were found in the new arrivals, while the established immigrants had as many cases of the condition as Jews in other cultural groups. The Arabs living in the same region had an incidence of less than 5%.[6] The dietary habits of the established and newly arrived Yemenites, the native Israeli Jews, and the Arabs were similar with respect to their intake of macro- and micronutrients. What was different was that in Yemen the Yemenites had consumed very little refined carbohydrate. Upon arrival in Israel, their refined carbohydrate consumption rapidly increased to match that of the established Yemenite population. The new immigrants also increased their energy intake by about 10%. However, they had active lives and many were engaged in heavy work so that the increase in energy intake was matched by increase in energy expenditure. Obesity as we know it in the United States today was not a problem. Cohen and associates interpreted their observations as evidence of NIDDM arising as a result of an age-nutrient-gene interaction. They suggested that in the Yemenite population there was a genetic tendency for diabetes and that this tendency

was expressed when Yemenites consumed sugar-rich diets over extended periods of time.

The papers of Cohen and coworkers[4,5] were published well before the initiation of the human genome project. Their studies were an insightful observation of what happens in a given human population whose diet changes from a traditional low-sugar diet to one that contains a lot of sugar with a wide variety of raw and processed foods. Other populations might not have such a response.

The composition and quantity of the food consumed by Western societies have been linked to the development of hyperlipoproteinemia, atherosclerosis, and heart disease. Coronary vessel disease is a complex disorder characterized by incremental losses over time in vascular elasticity due to the development of atherosclerosis. While high-fat diets have been implicated in the atherosclerotic process, not all people (or animals) that consume such diets die of coronary vessel disease. There is a strong diet-genetic-age–dependent linkage among those who develop coronary vessel disease, and this linkage is lacking in those who do not develop this disease.[7] These observations of diet, age, and genetic factors suggest, therefore, that coronary vessel disease develops as a result of a nutrient-gene interaction. Ostensibly, this seems reasonable. Researchers seeking support for such a hypothesis have found a number of genes that are involved in the regulation of blood lipid levels. If any one of these mutate, there is a likelihood that blood lipid levels will be affected. These mutations and their consequences are listed in Table 1. However, genetically determined elevations in blood lipids do not always result in coronary vessel disease. Further, it is known that the influence of diet on blood lipids involves not only the amount of fat consumed but also the type of fat and the amount and type of carbohydrate. The nature of the diet effect on the expression of genes related to blood lipids ranges from influencing gene transcription to posttranslational effects on the gene products. Linking these effects to the atherogenic process and subsequent disease has been a challenge to researchers in this arena. While some progress has been made, we still do not know the details of this process.

The lipids of interest in coronary vessel disease are cholesterol and its esters and the triacylglycerides. Normal ranges of these lipids have been established as guidelines for interpreting blood assessments. Values in excess of "normal" ranges are considered risk factors for coronary vessel disease. That is, in people with higher than normal concentration of serum triacyglycerides or cholesterol, or both, the risk of dying from coronary vessel disease is increased. As research progressed, it was soon recognized that genetic factors dictate endogenous synthesis, transport, and storage of fat, and thus were important determinants of blood lipid levels in addition to dietary fat. For example, genetic defects in chylomi-

Table 1. Mutations in lipoprotein genes and their consequences

Gene	Function	Chromosome location	Mutation frequency	Consequences
apo B	Transport protein in chylomicrons	2 p 23–24	1:million	Abetalipoproteinemia or hypobetalipoproteinemia
LPL	Lipase that acts on chylomicrons	8p22	1:million	Defective chylomicron clearance
apo CII	Transport protein in chylomicrons	19	1:million	Defective chylomicron clearance
HTGL	Lipase that acts on IDL in liver Reduces size of HDL_2 to HDL_3	15 q 21	?	Defective LDL clearance
apo E	Required for chylomicron clearance	19	1:5000	Type III hyperlipoproteinemia
LDL receptor	Cell surface protein that binds LDL	19	1:500	Familial hypercholesterolemia
apo B-100	Lipid transport protein	2	1:500–1:1000	Familial defective apo B-100
LCAT	Reverse cholesterol transfer from periphery to liver	16q22.1	Rare	Familial lecithin:cholesterol transferase deficiency
apo A1	HDL and chylomicron transport	11	1:1,000,000 Rare	Defective HDL production Reduced HDL cholesterol and apo A-I levels (Milan variant)

Abbreviations: apo, apolipoprotein; LPL, lipoprotein lipase; IDL, intermediate-density lipoprotein; HDL, high-density lipoprotein; HTGL, hepatic triglyceride lipase; LDL, low-density lipoprotein; LCAT, lecithin cholesterol acyl transferase.

cron processing (Table 1) result in very high blood levels of both triacyglycerol and cholesterol, yet this disorder is rarely associated with atherogenesis. Chylomicron remnant clearance defects, of which there are several, likewise are characterized by elevated blood lipids. These defects are more frequent in the general population (~1 in 5000) than are defects in chylomicron processing (1 in 1 million), yet people with these defects also have very little increased risk for coronary vessel disease.

In contrast, genetic defects in the fat-carrying proteins—apo A-I, apo A-II, apo B, apo C-I, apo C-II, apo C-III, apo A-IV, apo D, apo (a), and apo E—and disorders in the cell surface receptors for these lipoproteins are associated with an increased risk for coronary vessel disease.[8] These defects are more prevalent in the general population than are the defects in chylomicron clearance and processing. The various defects and their associated mutations are listed in Table 1. Mutations in genes that encode the structural components of the heart and vascular tree also occur, and these also are probably involved in coronary vessel disease. Candidate genes for these structural components have yet to be proposed. Congenital defects of heart structure, such as septal defects and vascular malformations, may be due to an interaction of specific nutrients with specific genes or gene products.[9,10] Folacin, retinoic acid, and zinc are but a few of the nutrients that play important roles in morphogenesis and differentiation in the embryo. Should folacin be lacking in the diet of a newly pregnant woman, there is an increased risk of congenital neural tube malformation. Defective receptors for retinoic acid could also explain congenital heart defects. The details of these interactions have not been elucidated. For almost every disease process, be it as common as obesity or lipemia or as rare as congenital birth defects or errors in metabolism, resolution of the problem is approached by proposing candidate genes and, through the isolation and study of these genes, attempting to understand whether and how such genes can be manipulated by specific dietary ingredients. These studies require a thorough understanding of the entire process of gene transcription, translation, and posttranslational modification of the ultimate gene product. A brief review of gene expression follows.

Nutrient Control of Gene Expression

Research has shown that gene expression is regulated at each step in the pathway from DNA to RNA to protein. Figure 2 illustrates this pathway. The regulation of gene expression includes transcription control, RNA processing control, RNA transport control, translational control, messenger RNA (mRNA) stability control, and posttranslation control. Each of these control points are nutritionally responsive in some fashion. For most genes, the control of transcription is stronger than that of translation.[11–14] This control is exerted by that portion of the DNA called the promoter region. This region is responsible for binding the enzyme RNA polymerase II, plus a number of transcription factors. Promoters are located in the 5' flanking region upstream from the structural gene on the same strand of DNA. They are referred to as *cis*-acting elements and generally are located about −40 to −200 base pairs from the start site. Some promoters, e.g., the TATA, GC, and CCAAT boxes, are common to many

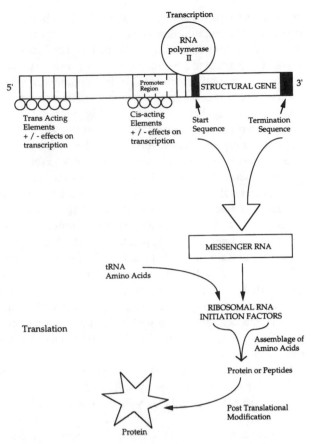

Figure 2. Schematic view of gene expression including transcription and translation.

genes transcribed by RNA polymerase II. These sequences interact with transcription factors that, in turn, form preinitiation complexes. The mechanisms of such transcriptional regulation have recently been reviewed by Semenza[15] and Johnson et al.[16] *Trans*-acting elements are those factors (usually proteins) produced by other genes that influence transcription. *Trans*-acting elements could be protein or peptide hormones, a steroid hormone–receptor protein complex, a vitamin-receptor protein, a mineral, or a mineral-protein complex. The mechanism of DNA binding by hormone receptors has been reviewed and described by Freedman and Luisi.[17]

The promoter contains the start site for RNA synthesis. When RNA polymerase II binds tightly to this specific DNA sequence, transcription begins. The RNA polymerase II opens up a local region of the DNA double helix so that the gene to be transcribed is exposed. One of the two DNA strands acts as the template for complementary base pairing with incoming ribonucleoside triphosphate monomers. The nucleotides are joined until the polymerase encounters a special sequence in the DNA called the termination sequence. At this point, transcription is complete and the mRNA is available for translation. This outline of transcription has omitted a number of important details with respect to transcription control.

For example, regulation of transcription is exerted by a group of proteins that determine which region of the DNA is to be transcribed. Cells contain a variety of sequence-specific DNA-binding proteins. Nutrients can bind to these proteins and have their effect in this way. These proteins are of low abundance, and they function by binding to specific regions on the DNA. These regions are variable in size but are usually between 8 and 15 nucleotides. Depending on the binding protein and the nutrient bound to it, transcription is either enhanced or inhibited and cell types may differ because of these proteins. Because all cells contain the same DNA, gene expression in discrete cell types is controlled at this point simply by the binding of these very specific DNA-binding proteins.[12] Thus, genes for the enzymes of gluconeogenesis, for example, could be turned on in the hepatocyte but not in the myocyte or adipocyte simply because the hepatocyte has the needed specific DNA-binding protein that the other cell types lack. At some point in differentiation, these cells failed to acquire sufficient amounts of these proteins so as to have the gluconeogenic capacity of the hepatocyte.

Actually, specific DNA-binding proteins as regulators of gene expression constitute only a part of this regulation. Most genes are regulated by a combination of regulatory elements.[11–17] In some, a group of DNA-binding proteins interact to control the activation and inhibition of transcription. Not all of these proteins are of equal power in all instances. There may be a master regulatory protein that serves to coordinate the binding of several lesser proteins.[11] This is important for the coordinate expression of genes in a single pathway. For example, in the lipogenic pathway, the genes that encode the enzymes of the fatty acid synthase complex are coordinately expressed.[18] That is, whether increased or decreased, all enzymes are synthesized to the same extent so that the pathway can function efficiently. The mammalian fatty acid synthase is an enzyme complex consisting of seven distinct enzymes. Shown in Figure 3 is the reaction sequence and the gene and its products. While each of the enzymes in the fatty acid synthetase complex has a specific catalytic function in the series of reactions that take methylmalonyl CoA to palmitate, in actuality this synthase comprises two polypeptide chains, each having discrete functional domains.[18] These domains are positioned head-to-tail such that two separate centers for fatty acid assembly are formed at the subunit interface. This spatial proximity of domains facilitates the transfer of intermediates from one enzyme to another.

Studies of the transcription and translation of all of the constituent components of this multifunctional complex have revealed that the fatty acid synthase is represented by a single gene that encodes seven gene products, the seven enzyme components of the fatty acid

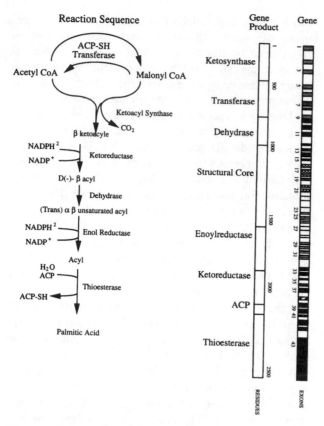

Figure 3. Fatty acid synthase: reaction sequence, gene products (enzymes in the fatty acid synthetase complex), and gene. Taken (with permission) from reference 18.

synthase complex. This enzyme complex is known to be regulated by nutrients at the levels of both transcription and translation. Arachidonic acid, a fatty acid with 20 carbons and four double bonds, suppresses gene transcription.[19] It is likely that the mechanism is one that involves a fatty acid binding protein that in turn binds to DNA as a *trans*-acting element. Where this binding takes place in the DNA is not known. However, S14, a protein that seems to be important in the regulation of mRNA transcription of not only fatty acid synthase but also a number of carbohydrate metabolic enzymes, also is suppressed by long-chain polyunsaturated fatty acids. The S14 gene has a carbohydrate-responsive element as well.[20] When diets rich in sugars are consumed, S14 mRNA increases, as do the mRNAs for glucokinase, glucose-6-phosphate dehydrogenase, 6-phosphogluconate dehydrogenase, and malic enzyme.[21] In each of these instances, nutrients (glucose, fatty acids) are actively involved as parts of transcription regulatory elements.

Mutations in genes that encode any one of these transcription factors could result in disease. Mutations in genes encoding transcription factors often have pleiotropic effects because these factors regulate a number of different genes. So too are the effects of nutrients that are required components of these transcription factors. Another example is the series of genes that encode the

enzymes needed for the conversion of a fibroblast to a myocyte. The mammalian skeletal muscle cell is very large and multinucleated. It is formed by the fusion of myoblasts (myocyte precursor cells) and contains characteristic structural proteins, as well as a number of other proteins that function in energy metabolism and nerve-muscle signaling. When muscle is being synthesized, all of these proteins must be synthesized at the same time. In proliferating myoblasts, very few of these proteins are present, yet as these myoblasts fuse, the mRNAs for these proteins increase, as does the synthesis of the proteins. This indicates that the expression of the genes for muscle protein synthesis is coordinated and controlled at the level of transcription and also that this process is responding to a single-gene regulatory DNA-binding protein. This protein (myo D1) has been isolated and identified and occurs only in muscle cells. Should this protein be inserted in some other cell type, a skin cell or an adipocyte, for example, the same expression will occur. That is, the skin or fat cell will look like a muscle cell; it will take on the characteristics of a myoblast and become a myocyte.

Of interest is the fact that although all of the genes needed for synthesis in the myocyte and its master controller are present, synthesis will not occur or will occur at a very limited rate if one or more of the essential amino acids needed for this synthesis is absent or deficient in the diet. Here is an example of a gene-nutrient interaction that has control properties with respect to muscle protein synthesis, and this interaction ultimately affects the overall process of growth. Turning this situation around, if the master regulator, myo D1, is aberrant or if one or more of the genes that encode the enzymes needed for protein synthesis in the myocyte have mutated such that the enzyme in question is nonfunctional or only partly functional, muscle development will cease or be retarded. In either instance, abnormal growth will result.

As mentioned, transcription is regulated by both the nearby upstream promoter region and the distant enhancer elements. The upstream enhancer element extends for about 100 base pairs. Enhancer fragments further upstream can bind multiple proteins that, in turn, can influence transcription. These proteins are labeled jun, AP2, ATF or CREB, SP1, OTF1, CTF or NF1, SRF, and others. One well-studied group of proteins are those that bind steroid hormones.[14] These are called the steroid receptors and bind to specific DNA sequences called steroid response elements. Steroids that enhance (or impair) transcription act by binding to one of these specific proteins that binds to DNA.[13–15] These elements thus enable cells to respond to a steroid hormone stimulus. The steroid response element has been well studied and consists of 100 amino acids and zinc. As mentioned, it recognizes a specific DNA sequence. For some members of this family of elements, the transcription-enhanc-

Table 2. Specific nutrient effects on specific genes

Nutrient	Gene	Effect
Glucose	Glucokinase	↑ Transcription
Retinoic acid	Retinoic acid receptor	↑ Transcription
Iron	Ferritin	↑ Translation
Vitamin B-6	Steroid hormone receptor	↓ Transcription
Zinc	Zinc-dependent enzymes	↑ Transcription
Ascorbic acid	Procollagen	↑ Translation ↑ Transcription
Vitamin K	Prothrombin	↑ Posttranslational carboxylation of glutamic acid residues
Cholesterol	HMG CoA reductase[a]	↓ Transcription

[a]Rate-limiting enzyme in the pathway for cholesterol synthesis.

ing domain is localized at the amino terminus of the polypeptide chain. At the carboxy terminus is the binding site for the steroid hormone.

Posttranscriptional regulation of gene expression is the next stage of control for many genes. The RNA transcription can be terminated prematurely, with the result of a smaller than expected gene product. The mRNA can also be split to produce different proteins from the same gene. These proteins may have comparable functions. Actually, most RNAs are far larger than the mature RNA generated from it by splicing and only 5% of this RNA ever leaves the nucleus. The remainder is degraded and the nucleosides reused or subject to further degradation. The RNA that leaves the nucleus does so through pores in the nuclear membrane. This is an active process, the details of which are not well known.

Not all of the mRNA that exits the nucleus is translated into protein. Translation can be blocked by specific proteins that bind at sites near the 5′ end of the molecule. This binding exerts negative translational control on gene expression. The mRNA has been made but the protein is not made. An example of this is seen in the regulation of the synthesis of ferritin.[22] Ferritin mRNA is not translated unless an iron response element binds to it. This allows for a rapid shift in ferritin synthesis when iron is present and an equally rapid shift away from ferritin synthesis when iron is in short supply. When iron is present, it binds to the iron response element, which then folds away from the start site for translation, making it available for use. When iron is absent, this start site is covered up by the iron response element that serves as a negative control element. Many mRNAs are subject to translational control by nutrients in this fashion.

The mRNAs have a very short half-life when compared with DNA and the other RNAs. If mRNA half-life is shortened or prolonged, gene expression is affected. Many of the very unstable mRNAs have half-lives in terms of minutes, including those that code for short-lived regulatory proteins such as the protooncogenes *fos* and *myc*. This instability is probably due to an A- and U-rich 3′ untranslated region. Stability of mRNA can be affected by steroid hormones, nutritional state, and drugs.

Once the mRNA has migrated from the nucleus to the cytoplasm and attaches to ribosomes, translation is ready to begin. All of the amino acids needed for the protein being synthesized must be present, attached to a transfer RNA. These transfer RNA amino acids dock on the mRNA again, using base pairing, and the amino acids are joined to one another via the peptide bond. The newly synthesized protein is released as it is made on the ribosome and changes to its conformation and structure occur. These changes depend on the constituent amino acids and their sequence. Posttranslational modification includes a wide variety of changes. For example, nuclear-encoded proteins needed for the respiratory chain are synthesized with a leader sequence that allows them to migrate into the mitochondria. This leader is then removed as the oxidative phosphorylation system is assembled. Another example is prothrombin, which is assembled with a large number of glutamic acid residues. In the presence of vitamin K these residues are carboxylated, and this posttranslational change results in a dramatic increase in the calcium-binding capacity of the resultant protein. Unless prothrombin can bind calcium, it cannot function in the clotting process. This is another example of how a nutrient can affect gene expression; in this instance, it is the expression of functional prothrombin. The site of the nutritional effect is that of posttranslational protein modification. Extending this further, one could argue that nutrients in surplus or excess also affect gene expression by altering the milieu in which gene products must function. For example, dietary fat intake can influence membrane composition that, in turn, can affect the activity and the conformational structure of the proteins embedded in these membranes that depend on membrane fluidity.[23]

Lastly, nutrition can affect the phenotypic expression of the genotype if certain nutrients are in short supply. This is the basis for the dietary management of a number of genetically determined disorders. For example, dietary phenylalanine is limited in the management of phenylketonuria to prevent the typical phenotypic expression of the defective genotype, mental retardation. A number of genetic diseases can be managed in this way:

lactose-lactase deficiency, galactose-galactosemia, carbohydrate-diabetes mellitus, and so forth.

Knowledge of single-gene defects in metabolism has contributed to and has been expanded by the scientific advances that are part of the human genome project. It is the purpose of this project to completely sequence and map the human genome. Even as this effort continues, progress is also being made in identifying the specifics of nutrient action vis à vis gene expression. Listed in Table 2 are examples of specific nutrient effects on specific genes. One of these nutrients, vitamin A (retinoic acid), has widespread effects on the synthesis of a variety of important proteins. These diverse effects are due largely to its combination with one or more nuclear receptors that serve as *trans*-acting factors that promote transcription. Several different receptors have been identified and each has a specific mode of action in growth and development.[24–26] For example, should a mutation occur in the α receptor, which would result in decreased retinoic acid binding, embryonic cell differentiation is affected, with the result of embryonic wastage or fetal malformation. Congenital heart malformation has been attributed to such a mechanism. Whether such actually occurs in man, however, has yet to be demonstrated. In avian embryos and in mouse embryos of transgenic mice, there are suggestions that this can occur.[9,10]

Summary

From the foregoing discussion it is apparent that nutrients not only serve as substrates for metabolic processes or as coenzymes or cofactors for these processes, but also serve to regulate the genes that encode the various proteins that are the enzymes, carriers, receptors, and structural elements of the living system. The considerable diversity in cell type and function depends on the appropriate intakes of nutrients. These nutrients sustain the metabolism and dictate the phenotypic expression of the individual's genotype. Manipulation of the nutrient intake (both specific nutrients and total nutrient supply) can manipulate this expression. While only a few examples could be discussed because of space constraints, these few illustrate how a specific nutrient could have effects on gene expression. Many more examples have been described in the rapidly expanding literature on nutrient-gene interactions.

References

1. Berdanier CD (1993) Diabetes mellitus: what have we learned from animals? Recent Progress Foods Nutr 17:261–285
2. Zimmet P (1983) Epidemiology of diabetes mellitus. In Ellenberg M, Rifkin H (eds), Diabetes mellitus: theory and practice, 3rd ed. Medical Examination Publishing Co, Hyde Park, NY, pp 451–469
3. USDA Food Disappearance Data, Human Nutrition Information Service, USDA, Hyattsville, MD
4. Cohen AM, Bavly S, Poznanski R (1961) Change of diet of Yemenite Jews in relation to diabetes and ischemic heart disease. Lancet 2:1399–1401
5. Cohen AM (1961) Prevalence of diabetes among different ethnic groups in Israel. Metabolism 10:50–58
6. Breguet D, Baczko A, Fabre J, et al (1981) Cardiovascular risk factors in headquarters staff of the World Health Organization. Schweiz Med Wochenschr 111:53–60
7. Barrett-Conner E, Khaw K-T (1984) Family history of heart attack as an independent predictor of death due to cardiovascular disease. Circulation 69:1065–1069
8. Breslow JL (1989) Genetic basis of lipoprotein disorders. J Clin Invest 84:373–380
9. Colbert MC, Robbins J (1996) Transgenic analysis of retinoic acid signaling in developing mouse heart. Cardiovasc Res, in press
10. Chien KR (1993) Molecular advances in cardiovascular biology. Science 260:916–917
11. Derman E (1981) Transcriptional control in the production of liver specific mRNA's. Cell 23:731–739
12. Maniatis T, Goodbourn S, Fischer JA (1987) Regulation of inducible and tissue specific gene expression. Science 236:1237–1245
13. Atchison ML (1988) Enhancers: mechanisms of action and cell specificity. Annu Rev Cell Biol 4:127–153
14. Yamamoto K (1985) Steroid receptor regulated transcription of specific genes and gene networks. Annu Rev Genet 19:209–252
15. Semenza GL (1994) Transcriptional regulation of gene expression: mechanisms and pathophysiology. Hum Mutat 3:180–199
16. Johnson PF, Sterneck E, Williams SC (1993) Activation domains of transcriptional regulatory proteins. J Nutr Biochem 4:386–398
17. Freedman LP, Luisi BF (1993) On the mechanism of DNA binding by nuclear hormone receptors: a structural and functional perspective. J Cell Biochem 51:140–150
18. Smith S (1994) The animal fatty acid synthase: One gene, one polypeptide, seven enzymes. FASEB J. 8:1248–1259.
19. Clark SD, Jump DB (1993) Regulation of hepatic gene expression by dietary fats: A unique role for polyunsaturated fatty acids. In Berdanier CD and Hargrove JL (eds), Nutrition and gene expression. CRC Press, Boca Raton, FL pp 227–246.
20. Shih H-M, Towle HC (1992) Definition of the carbohydrate response element of the rat S_{14} gene. Evidence for a common factor required for carbohydrate regulation of hepatic genes. J. Biol. Chem. 267:13222–13228.
21. Clarke SD, Abraham S (1992) Gene expression: nutrient control of pre and post transcriptional events. FASEB J 6:3146–3152
22. Munro HN, Kikinis Z, Eisenstein RS (1993) Iron dependent regulation of ferritin synthesis. In Berdanier CD, Hargrove JL (eds), Nutrition and gene expression. CRC Press, Boca Raton, FL, pp 525–545.
23. Berdanier CD (1992) Fatty acids and membrane function. In Chow CK (ed), Fatty acids in food and their health implications. Marcel Dekker, New York, p 531
24. Giguere V, Ong ES, Sigui P, Evans RM (1987) Identification of α receptor for the morphogen retinoic acid. Nature 330:624–630
25. Evans RM (1988) The steroid and thyroid hormone superfamily. Science 240:889–891
26. Jump DB, Lepar GJ, MacDonald OA (1993) Retinoic acid regulation of gene expression in adipocytes. In Berdanier CD, Hargrove JL (eds), Nutrition and gene expression. CRC Press, Boca Raton, FL, pp 431–454

Chapter 59

Macronutrient Substitutes

John W. Finley and Gilbert A. Leveille

Macronutrient substitutes comprise a wide variety of substances that are incorporated into foods to provide a potential health benefit, for example, reduction of calorie content. Another example is the reduction of dental caries when sugar alcohols replace sugar in confections. The Western diet is changing as technology provides new and unique reduced-calorie ingredients. This chapter will review macronutrient substitutes, with emphasis on their function, advantages, and nutritional effect.

Macronutrient substitutes are ingredients that are added to foods in lieu of normal macronutrients (e.g., carbohydrate and fat) to achieve specific effects, such as a reduction in fat or energy content. The most common macronutrient substitutes are carbohydrate and fat replacers. Carbohydrate replacements may replace starch or sugar. When sugar is replaced, the sweetening function is frequently provided by an intense sweetener, leaving the need for a bulking agent to replace the mass usually provided by sucrose or other sugars. Replacement of starch also requires the addition of bulking agents, but with different functionality than sucrose replacements.

Because fat is calorically dense, its replacement offers the greatest potential benefit for energy reduction. Three types of substitutes have been developed for fat: 1) mimetics, which are usually either protein or carbohydrates that provide some of the masticatory characteristics of fat when hydrated; 2) fat substitutes, which essentially replace the fat gram for gram but provide significantly fewer calories; and 3) low-calorie fats, which are true triacylglycerols that provide <38 kJ/g (9 kcal/g).

The replacement of sugars, complex carbohydrates, or fat with substitutes requires consideration of the benefits to the product and the consumer. Many of the substitutes allow the manufacturer to produce reduced-calorie products with organoleptic qualities similar to full-calorie products. The consumer benefits from the caloric reduction and increased fiber without having to compromise eating quality. As with any new ingredient, the risk versus the benefit of making the substitution must be considered.

New research suggests that foods can provide definite health benefits by preventing chronic disease or by enhancing the treatment of a variety of ailments. In the development of new foods or food components, appropriate testing is essential to demonstrate efficacy and ensure that the new foods or ingredients do not significantly increase consumer risk.

Carbohydrate Replacements

The main objective for the use of carbohydrate replacements is to obtain caloric reduction without loss of taste quality (sweetness). This can be achieved by replacing the usual sweetening carbohydrate (e.g., sucrose) with a carbohydrate of similar sweetness but lesser caloric density, or by replacing the carbohydrate by an intense sweetener plus a bulking agent. In liquid products such as soft drinks or sweeteners for coffee, sugar can be replaced by intense sweeteners. Because water is the bulk phase, the substitution is relatively simple. In solid foods such as cookies or cakes, sugar accounts for a considerable portion of the bulk phase. Thus, substitution with an intense sweetener would not fill the bulk missing from the food when sugars are deleted from the formula. Bulking agents are therefore required to make up this mass in product formulations.

Bulking agents can be any reduced-calorie or noncalorie carbohydrate from cellulose to sugar alcohols (polyols). Different bulking agents have different functions in foods. None acts precisely like sucrose or starch; thus numerous bulking agents have been explored.

Low-molecular-weight bulking agents. The simplest bulking agents are a group of sugar replacements referred to as polyols. Polyols are hydrogenated analogs of simple sugars. The polyols or sugar alcohols of simple carbohydrates are primarily produced by the hydrogenation of the corresponding reducing sugar. Examples of commercial polyols are summarized in Table 1. The primary use of polyols is in chewing gum, hard candies, and coatings for candies. In foods the sugar alcohols have

Table 1. Energy, taste, and function of polyols

Compound	Energy value (kj/g)	Taste of dry sugar	Sweetness relative to sucrose	Functional characteristics
Sorbitol	7.53–13.81	Cool	0.70	Sucrose free confections Less cariogenic than sucrose
Erythritol	0–1.67	Cool	0.65	
Mannitol	6.6976	Cool	0.50	
Maltitol	11.72–14.65	None	0.75	
Xylitol	~10.05	Very cool	0.90	
Reduced starch hydrolysates Less cariogenic than sucrose	11.72–13.39	None	0.75	Sucrose free confections
Lactitol	8.37 or less	Slightly cool	0.40	
Isomalt	8.37	None	0.60	
Fructooligo-saccahrides	8.37	~Sucrose	0.30	
Polydextrose	4.19	None	None	Bulking agent

similar functions and physical properties to those of sugars, particularly in liquid systems.

Sugar alcohols are present in fruits and vegetables, but for industrial purposes they are prepared by the catalytic hydrogenation of the parent sugars. This hydrogenation converts the aldehyde and ketone functions of the sugars to primary and secondary alcohols, respectively. The resultant sugar alcohols tend to be more hygroscopic and often are more difficult to crystallize than are the parent sugars.

Compared with that of sugars, the bioavailability of sugar alcohols in the upper gastrointestinal tract is dramatically reduced. As a consequence, significant quantities of ingested sugar alcohols reach the large intestine and the colon, where they are readily fermented by microflora (Figure 1). Fermentation in the colon generates less usable energy from the sugar alcohols than would be provided by the parent sugars. The microflora ferment the sugar alcohols to methane, hydrogen, and short-chain fatty acids by anaerobic fermentation. The production of short-chain fatty acids and of lactic acid (an intermediate in the pathway) lowers the pH of colonic material and thereby changes the species distribution of colonic microorganisms. The digestion, absorption, and metabolism of the various sugar alcohols are summarized in Table 2.

The absorption of monomeric sugar alcohols ranges from 50% for sorbitol to essentially 0 for erythritol. The fate of absorbed material varies greatly. For example, 100% of the absorbed xylitol is metabolized, whereas only a negligible proportion of absorbed mannitol is metabolized. The dimeric sugar alcohols exhibit ranges of digestibility and absorption on the basis of their monomeric components. All sugar alcohols are fermented in the colon. Thus, any nonabsorbed sugar alcohol is converted to short-chain fatty acids by the colonic bacteria when the sugar alcohol reaches the large intestine.

The caloric value (i.e., availability) of sugar alcohols has been estimated by a wide variety of approaches.[1-4] For the purpose of nutritional labeling, Dutch and French authorities have accepted a human test factorial system. The method consists of estimating the amount of test material that reaches the colon (by ileal intubation) and the amounts of sample recovered in the stool and urine. The fraction absorbed in the small intestine provides 17 kJ/g (4 kcal/g) and the portion fermented in the colon 8 kJ/g (2 kcal/g). The loss of recoverable energy with colonic fermentation is related to the formation of gas and short-chain fatty acids (acetic, propionic, and butyric) and the production of bacterial biomass and heat. The short-chain fatty acids are absorbed and either used by the intestinal mucosa or transported to the liver by the portal system for use in normal energy metabolism. Bornet[5] summarized data demonstrating that the sugar alcohols provide more calories when ingested with meals or in the postprandial period than during fasting.

For regulatory purposes the U.S. Food and Drug Administration allows the following energy values: 2.6 kcal/g for sorbitol, 3.0 kcal/g for starch hydrolysates, 2.4 kcal/g for xylitol, and 2 kcal/g for isomalt. The European

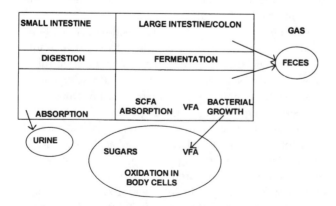

Figure 1. Fate of polyols in the gastrointestinal tract. SCFA = short-chain fatty acids; VFA = volatile fatty acids.

Table 2. Digestion and absorption of sugar alcohols

Sugar alcohol	Type	Digested	Absorbed	Metabolized	Fermented
Mannitol	Monomeric	No	~25%	Negligible	+
Sorbitol	Monomeric	No	~50%	Up to 85% of absorbed	+
Xylitol	Monomeric	No	25%	100% of absorbed	+
Erytritol	Monomeric	No	None	Negligible	+
Isomalt	Dimeric	20% to 75%	Up to 20%	+	+
Lactitol	Dimeric	Negligible	Negligible	Negligible	+
Maltitol	Dimeric	Partially	Up to 40%	+	+
Hydrogenated starch hydrolysates	Oligomeric	Partially	Incomplete	+	+

Community Nutritional Labeling Directive of 1990 assigned a value of 2.4 kcal/g to all polyols. Japan, on the other hand, has set individual values for the various polyols: isomalt,1.9 kcal/g; lactitol, 1.6 kcal/g; mannitol, sorbitol, and xylitol, 2.8 kcal/g; and maltitol, 1.8 kcal/g.

Sugar alcohols produce less dental caries than caloric sweeteners such as glucose and sucrose.[6] Xylitol and sorbose are more resistant to fermentation by oral microflora and produce less plaque than does glucose. Maltitol, platinate, platinose, sorbitol, and lycosin are fermented by Actinomyces, Lactobacillus, and Streptococcus. Although more acid is produced, these sugars seem to have no cariogenic effect with S. mutans in rodents. Fermentation-related changes in standard dental tests with sugar alcohols, glucose, and sucrose are summarized in Table 3.[7] These data show that glucose and sucrose have the greatest potential for producing adverse effects leading to dental caries, whereas lactitol and xylitol exhibited the lowest potential for adverse effects.

The caloric value of mannitol ranges from 6.3 to 16.7 kJ/g (1.5 to <4.0 kcal/g), with a calculated metabolizable energy of 8.33 kJ/g (1.99 kcal/g).[8,9] After ingestion, a portion of D-mannitol diffuses passively through the intestinal wall, where it is oxidized by mannitol dehydrogenase or L-iditol dehydrogenase to fructose, which is subsequently used in the normal fructose pathway.[10] Because the solubility of D-mannitol is low relative to other sugars and sugar alcohols, a substantial portion of the mannitol reaches the colon.[11] Bernier and Pascal[2] concluded that 25% of orally ingested mannitol is absorbed in the intestine, 75% is fermented in the colon,

and the energy value of mannitol is 6.3 kJ/g (1.5 kcal/g). In a weight-gain study with rats, Karimzadegan et al.[12] observed almost no weight gain when mannitol was fed as the sole source of dietary carbohydrate. In this study the growth-promoting effect of xylitol and sorbitol was 60% and 48% that of glucose, respectively. From the results of studies of ileostomy patients, an expert panel Life Science Research Office at the Federation of American Societies for Experimental Biology (LSRO)[8] concluded that the energy value of mannitol was ≈6.7 kJ/g (1.6 kcal/g). However, normal subjects may exhibit more than the 75% fermentation estimated for the ileostomy patients. If this is true, the caloric estimate may be slightly low.

Estimates of the caloric value of sorbitol range from 8.4 to 16.3 kJ/g (2.0 to 3.9 kcal/g). The metabolic fate of sorbitol has been studied extensively with reasonable agreement.[11,13–15] Sorbitol is absorbed by passive diffusion in the small intestine but at a slower rate than glucose.[16,17] Griem and Lang[18] found that rats consuming sorbitol exhibited enlarged ceca, which is characteristic of animals consuming slowly absorbed materials. Hyams[19] demonstrated that breath hydrogen increased significantly in subjects consuming 10 g of sorbitol in a single dose. The range of increase was from 0% to 98% of background, reflecting the variability in individual responses to sorbitol. Absorbed sorbitol is oxidized in the liver to fructose by L-iditol dehydrogenase. No increase in serum glucose or insulin concentration was observed in fasted subjects given 20 g sorbitol.[20] These observations indicate the direct oxidation of sorbitol to fructose. In both normal and diabetic subjects

Table 3. Order of fermentation-related changes in standard dental tests after 24 hours with various carbohydrates

Decrease in pH	Titratable acidity	Polysaccharide formation	Microbial growth	Calcium dissolving	Phosphorous dissolving
Glucose	Glucose	Glucose	Glucose	Sucrose	Sucrose
Sucrose	Sucrose	Sucrose	Sucrose	Glucose	Glucose
Mannitol	Mannitol	Mannitol	Sorbitol	Mannitol	Mannitol
Sorbitol	Sorbitol	Sorbitol	Mannitol	Sorbitol	Sorbitol
Xylitol	Lactitol	Lactitol	Lactitol	Lactitol	Lactitol
Lactitol	Xylitol	Xylitol	Xylitol	Xylitol	Xylitol

given sorbitol, ≈3% of the dose was found as sorbitol in the urine.[21] Of the orally administered sorbitol, 75% was metabolized to carbon dioxide and no sorbitol was detected in the feces. Thus, it appears that sorbitol is metabolized rather completely. Schnell-Dompert and Siebert[22] obtained similar results. Baugerie et al.[23] found that 79% of the ingested sorbitol was absorbed in the small intestine and that virtually all of the sorbitol that reached the colon was fermented. They estimated the caloric value of sorbitol at 14.98 kJ/g (3.58 kcal/g). Baugerie et al.[24] reported that subjects tolerated sorbitol well. Over an 8-hour period 66% of the sorbitol dose was unabsorbed, but the unabsorbed sorbitol was completely fermented in the colon. From these results they computed the metabolizable energy of sorbitol to be 11.3 kJ/g (2.7 kcal/g). An LSRO expert panel[8] concluded that the net energy available from sorbitol is highly dependent on the experimental conditions. The results of a number of studies show net energy values between 7.5 and 13.8 kJ/g (1.8 and 3.3 kcal/g).

When sorbitol is consumed in large quantities (25–50 g/day), a laxative effect has been observed. The effect is primarily due to the slow absorption of sorbitol from the gastrointestinal tract.[25,26] A dose-response study found that the no observable effect level (NOEL) for sorbitol was 0.15 g/kg body weight for males and 0.3 g/kg body weight for females.[27] The NOEL dose of maltitol was 0.3 g/kg body weight for both males and females. The 50% effective laxative dose for sorbitol was 0.4 g/kg body weight for males and 1.0 g/kg body weight for females. For maltitol the 50% effective laxative dose was 0.8 g/kg body weight for both males and females.

Xylitol is absorbed from the intestine by simple diffusion.[28–30] Its absorption ranges from 13% to 95% depending on experimental conditions.[20,31–35] Unabsorbed xylitol is completely fermented in the colon (A. Bar, unpublished observations, 1988, 1992).[31] The largest portion of absorbed xylitol is metabolized in the liver, with smaller amounts metabolized in the kidney and other tissues.[29,30,36] Xylitol is oxidized to xylulose by L-iditol dehydrogenase. D-Xylulokinase phosphorylates the xylulose for entry into the normal pentose pathway. From the study by Livesey[9] the LSRO panel[8] concluded that the energy value of xylitol is ≈12.1 kJ/g (2.9 kcal/g) and that the net energy is ≈10.0 kJ/g (2.4 kcal/g). Energy value is defined as the energy content of the macronutrient used by the body and net energy is the energy available from a nutrient to do physical or metabolic work.[8]

Erythritol is essentially completely absorbed in the small intestine and quantitatively excreted unchanged in the urine.[37,38] This results in a bulking agent with zero caloric value. Erythritol appears to have no detectable influence on the subject when it is absorbed and subsequently excreted. However, more testing should be conducted to ensure safety before extensive use of erythritol.

Isomalt is an equimolar mixture of α-D-glucopyranosyl-1-6-D-sorbitol (GPS) and α-D-glucopyranosyl-1,5-mannitol (GPM). Although both components are slowly hydrolyzed by various α-glucoamylases, including jejunal mucosal enzymes, most energy derived from GPS and GPM results from fermentation in the colon (A. Sentko, unpublished observation, 1992).[39,40] Kruger et al.[41] demonstrated that the caloric availability of isomalt was dose dependent, and they recommended that the caloric value be set at 13 kJ/g (3 kcal/g).

Lactitol is rapidly hydrolyzed to D-galactose and D-sorbitol by microbial enzymes. However, hydrolysis by β-galactosidase in the gastrointestinal tract is slow.[42] Most studies conclude that there is little or no absorption of lactitol in the upper intestinal tract. Lactitol appears to be transported to the colon, where it is readily fermented by the microflora.[8] In a crossover study with human volunteers, Van Es et al.[43] found that subjects consuming lactitol produced significant amounts of breath hydrogen and methane, confirming the colonic fermentation of lactitol. It was concluded that the net energy from lactitol was 6.7–7.1 kJ/g (1.6–1.7 kcal/g). The LSRO expert panel[8] concluded that the caloric value of lactitol was 8 kJ/g (2 kcal/g) or slightly less.

Maltitol is hydrolyzed in the stomach to glucose and sorbitol. However, a substantial portion reaches the colon, where it is fermented to short-chain fatty acids.[15,20,44,45] Hosoya (N. Hosoya, unpublished observation, 1972) found that only a small portion (0.1–0.2%) of labeled maltitol was expired as carbon dioxide within 24 hours. Initially, rats in the study exhibited considerable diarrhea, but they adapted after a few days. Lian-Loh et al.[46] concluded that the conversion of maltitol to short-chain fatty acids was key to the usable energy derived from this sugar alcohol. Estimates of the degree of maltitol utilization vary widely, but it is clear that some maltitol is utilized as such, as evidenced by the production of carbon dioxide, and some portion of the maltitol is fermented to short-chain fatty acids by the intestinal microflora and subsequently used as energy.[23,24,37,47–56] Most of these studies put the net energy value for maltitol between 11.7 and 13.4 kJ/g (2.8 and 3.2 kcal/g). However, Tsuji et al.[57] reported somewhat lower net energy values. LSRO[8] currently estimates the net energy of maltitol at 11.7–13.4 kJ/g, with the reservation that more work should be done to resolve the questions raised by Tsuji et al.

Reduced starch hydrolysates prepared by partial hydrolysis of starch followed by hydrogenation are mixtures of mono-, di-, and oligomeric polyols. Commercially available products contain various levels of sorbitol, maltitol, and oligosaccharides hydrogenated at the reducing end. Upon ingestion the reduced starch hydrolysates are hydrolyzed to glucose, sorbitol, and maltitol, with insignificant portions of the hydrolysis products reaching the colon.[20] Moskowitz[45] reviewed the human data and suggested that the available energy was ≈17 kJ/ g (4 kcal/g). Baugerie et al.[23] estimated energy values from 13.0 to 14.6 kJ/g (3.1 to 3.5 kcal/g), and Bernier and Pascal[2] proposed net energy values from 11.7 to 14.6 kJ/g (2.8 to 3.5 kcal/g). The LSRO[8] expert panel concluded that the net energy was probably below 13.4 kJ/ g (3.2 kcal/g).

The rate of absorption and metabolism of reduced starch hydrolysates is similar to that of maltitol but slower than that of sorbitol (Baugerie et al.[23]). This is presumably due to the slow hydrolysis of maltitol in the polymeric materials. When hydrogenated starch hydrolysates reach the colon, they are completely fermented to short-chain fatty acids which are ultimately absorbed and used for energy.

Fructo-oligosaccharides occur naturally in various plants, ranging from onion, asparagus, wheat, rye, and triticale to the Jerusalem artichoke.[58] Similar oligosaccharides can be prepared enzymatically from sucrose or inulin by fructosyl furanosidase. Functionally, fructo-oligosaccharides provide a sweet taste with intensity ≈30% that of sucrose but without the "cooling" effect experienced with crystalline sucrose. The water retention properties are slightly greater than those of sucrose but similar to those of sorbitol. The oligosaccharides are stable at low pH and heat-stable up to ≈140 °C.[59]

Fructo-oligosaccharides contain β(2→1) links and are not digested by the brush-border enzymes of the small intestine.[60] Therefore, these oligosaccharides do not elevate postprandial plasma glucose or fructose levels. The effects of dietary fructo-oligosaccharides were reviewed by Roberfoid.[61] Fructo-oligosaccharide polymers slow the digestion of other, digestible carbohydrates.[60,62–65] Hence, lower postprandial serum glucose levels are observed when substantial amounts of inulin or fructo-oligosaccarides are included in the diet. The colonic microflora easily and quantitatively hydrolyze and use inulin and fructo-oligosaccharides. The rapid use by the biofidogenic bacteria in the colon results in reduction in pH of the colon contents and increase of fecal mass proportional to the intake of fructo-oligosaccharides or inulin.[66–69] Hidaka et al.[69] demonstrated that patients who consumed fructo-oligosaccharides for 2 weeks exhibited higher *Bifidobacterium* populations. Concomitant with these changes there was a reduction in the production of putrefactive substances. The lowering of colonic pH is associated with increased production of lactic acid and short-chain fatty acids.[68–70] Fructo-oligosaccharides appear to have a caloric value of 4.2–6.3 kJ/g (1.0–1.5 kcal/g).[61]

As with other poorly absorbed ingredients that are fermented in the colon, flatulence and discomfort can occur after fructooligosaccharide consumption. Rusmessen et al.[63] reported minor gastrointestinal discomfort

in subjects consuming up to 50 g/day. Other workers have reported moderate symptoms at levels as low as 15 g/day.[70]

Polydextrose® is the product of the thermal polymerization of glucose, sorbitol, and citric acid. The water-soluble polymer is composed of randomly cross-linked glucose polymers with all types of glycosidic linkages, but 1→6 glycosidic linkages predominate. Commercially, polydextrose is available as a powder or as a liquid. Polydextrose solutions are Newtonian and slightly more viscous (viscosity is independent of shear rate) than the equivalent sucrose solution. Metabolic studies indicate that the caloric availability of polydextrose in humans is 4.1 kJ/g (1 kcal/g). Laxation can occur when polydextrose is consumed at high levels; thus, food products delivering >15 g per serving must be labeled accordingly.

Polydextrose is only partially metabolized by humans and, unlike sugar alcohols and fructo-oligosaccharides, it is not fermented by the microflora of the colon. Approximately 25% of polydextrose is metabolized, yielding ≈4.2 kJ/g (1 kcal/g) of net energy.[71] Allingham[72] reviewed the testing of polydextrose and reported that it is well tolerated at normal ingestion levels. There were no increases in blood glucose in diabetics consuming the product. The average threshold for laxative effects was 90 g/day compared with 70 g/day for sorbitol. Polydextrose was noncariogenic in standard tests.

Complex carbohydrate bulking agents (fiber). Complex carbohydrates, which are frequently classified as dietary fiber, can also be considered low-calorie bulking agents. Materials falling in this category include cellulose, hemicelluloses, pectins, gums, mucilages, and lignins. Unlike the lower-molecular-weight bulking agents, these materials are very complex mixtures of carbohydrate polymers. As a result of their complexity, they frequently are chemically somewhat ill-defined. Because they come from a variety of food sources, many are already common to our diets. The natural occurrence of these materials makes them attractive alternatives as bulking agents. It is the new and different applications of these materials that are of current interest. The chemical nature, source, and applications of some common polymeric carbohydrate bulking agents are summarized in Table 4.

Pectins are complex galacturonoglycans composed primarily of polymers of D-galacturonic acid. Pectins are linked in a linear chain of 1→4 linked α-D-galactopyranosyluronic acid. Frequently, the polymers include arabinans, arabinogalactans, and galactans.[73] Found primarily in cell walls of plants, the most abundant natural sources of pectins are apples, citrus fruits, sunflowers, and sugar beets. Pectins are slowly degraded by microflora in the colon. Pectin reportedly reduces total serum cholesterol without lowering high-density lipoprotein cholesterol.[71]

Table 4. Characteristics of complex carbohydrate bulking agents

Polysaccharide	Composition	Properties	Source	Applications
Agarose	β-D-galactose and 3,6-anhydro-β-L-galactose linked (1-3)	Gelling, emulsification, stabilization	Rhodophyceae	Baked products, confections, dairy products, desserts, meat analogs
Alginate	β-(1-4)-D-mannuronic acid and α-(1-4)-L-guluronic acid	Gelling, emulsions, thickening, water binding	Rhodophyceae	Baked products, beer foam stabilization, confections, dairy products, desserts, dietetic products, fabricated foods, salad dressing
Carrageenan	Sulfated polymers containing α-D-galactose and 3,6-anhydro-D-galactose	Gelling, complexing protein, thickening	Rhodophyceae	Bakery products, dairy products, desserts, meat products, jams and jellies
Cellulose	β-(1-4)-D-glucose polymers	Bulk	Most plants	Baked products
Galactomannans guar gum, locust bean gum	β-(1-4)-D-mannose backbone appended with α-(1-6)-D-Galactose	Stabilizing, thickening	*Cyanopsis tetragonolobus* (guar) *Ceratonia siliqua* (locust bean)	Ice cream, frozen foods, salad dresssing, sauces
D-glucans	β-(1-4)-D-glucose and β-(1-3)-D glucose			
Pectin	α-(1-4)-galacturonic acid partially esterified acid	Gelling, thickener	Fruits and vegetables	Dairy products, beverages, jams and jellies
Polydextrose	D-glucose, sorbitol and citric acid	Humectant, thickener, sugar replacement	Synthetic	Baked products, drinks
Xanthan gum	β-(1-4)-D-glucose appended with D-mannose, and D-glucuronic acid			

β-Glucans are glucose polymers containing both β(1→3) and β(1→4) linkages in various proportions depending on source.[74] Barley and oats are both excellent sources of β-glucans. Physiological effects associated with β-glucans are improved bowel activity and a lowering of serum cholesterol. These materials are not generally added to food directly but are a portion of cereal bran fractions.

Galactomannans are composed of β(1→4)-D-mannopyranosyl chains with β(1→6)-D galactopyranosyl units attached at carbon 6 of the mannose at various intervals, depending on the source.[75] Primary sources are guar gum and locust bean gum. Commercially, galactomannans are recovered from *Cyanopsis tetragonolobus* seeds and carob seeds.[73] Locust bean and guar gum are frequently used in low-calorie foods to emulate the texture of fat that has been removed. Galactomannans combined with carageenan simulate the spreadability of some fat products.

Cellulose refers to a group of complex carbohydrates whose primary structure is a β(1→4)-glucan. It also includes chemically modified celluloses, such as carboxymethyl cellulose, microcrystalline cellulose, and methyl cellulose. The cellulose derivatives can be used in foods as functional bulking agents, binders, stabilizers in frozen food systems, and thickeners. Cellulose acts as a noncaloric, insoluble bulking agent in a variety of food applications.

Resistant starch was discovered during the process of developing a procedure for measuring dietary fiber as nonstarch polysaccharide (NSP), that is, the non-α-glucan polysaccharides of plant material.[76] Unexpectedly, processed foods, such as white bread and potato, had a higher content of NSP than did their corresponding raw products. Further analysis determined that identical values for NSP content could be obtained for raw and processed foods when a glucan fraction, subsequently named resistant starch, was removed. Thus, heat processing of certain starchy foods caused a fraction of the starch to become resistant to digestive enzymes. On the basis of the probable rate of digestion in the small intestine, starches can be classified into three categories: rapidly digested starch, slowly digested starch, and resistant starch.[77]

Resistant starch was further classified into three types on the basis of intrinsic factors of the starch that render it indigestible. The undisrupted cell walls of partially milled grains and seeds present in some foods are physically inaccessible to digestive enzymes.[78,79] In plants, starch is closely packed into granules arranged in a partially crystalline form. Differences in the crystalline pattern of starch in the granule, as determined by x-ray diffraction, determine the susceptibility of starch to enzymic digestion. Fuwa et al.[80] reported starch fractions showing B- or C-type x-ray diffraction patterns to be the most resistant to pancreatic amylase, although the degree of resistance was dependent on the plant source. An example is the B-type starch found in raw banana and potato, which is poorly digested.[81] Cooking or processing disrupts the starch granule, leading to hydration and gelatinization. Thus, the resistant starch crystal of the potato is digestible when the food has been cooked. When cooled, however, the starch recrystallizes into a third, indigestible form. Formation of this type of resistant starch has been studied in potatoes, cereals, and legumes. Interestingly, the amylose fraction of starch retrogrades to a greater extent and is more firmly bound than the amylopectin fraction.[82–89] Resistant starch content is high in food products processed under relatively high moisture contents, such as boiling, baking, or autoclaving.[90–93]

Earlier it had been thought that starch, whose α-glucosidic linkages are susceptible to hydrolysis by pancreatic α-amylase, was completely digested in the small intestine. However, studies have clearly shown that significant amounts of dietary starch may escape digestion in the small intestine and pass into the colon, where the starch is fermented by anaerobic bacteria and the resulting volatile fatty acids are absorbed.[94–99] Resistant starch in the large intestine may share some of the characteristics and health benefits attributed to dietary fiber, such as amelioration of diabetes, cardiovascular disease, and colon cancer. Replacement of digestible starch with resistant starch in the diet of humans results in significant reductions in postprandial glycemia and insulinemia and in the subjective sensation of satiety.[100] Resistant starch lowers plasma insulin levels, lipogenesis, and postabsorptive cholesterol levels in rats.[101] In another study rats fed diets rich in resistant starch had lower serum triacylglycerol and cholesterol levels than did the control group.[102] However, the glycemic index, which is similar to the insulin response of carbohydrate-containing foods, did not correlate with percent resistant starch in most foods.[103] Results are inconclusive because some resistant-starch containing foods, such as bananas, contain large amounts of other simple carbohydrates that increase the glycemic index. A review article suggested that starch fermentation leads to the production of short-chain fatty acids, which decrease the concentration of carcinogenic agents in the intestinal mucosa, and that butyrate has a direct, protective effect on colonic cells against malignancy.[104] Van Munster et al.[105] reported that the decrease in colonic cell proliferation in humans may

result from a reduction in secondary bile acids and an increase in short-chain fatty acids resulting from dietary resistant starch.

The amount of starch reaching the large intestine is important in determining the extent of fermentation and effect on colonic function, which in turn may determine health benefits. The extent of starch malabsorption is estimated to be between 2% and 30%, as determined by breath hydrogen excretion and by intubation techniques.[94,106] The source of starch also appears to affect absorption. Anderson et al.[107] calculated that 10–20% of 100 g of wheat bread was not absorbed. Absorption values for starch from oat bread, corn bread, potato bread, and navy beans were 8%, 6%, 13%, and 18%, respectively. Other work showed that wheat or potato starch is also less absorbed than other starches.[108] However, in patients with ileostomies, Chapman et al.[109] found that unabsorbed wheat and potato starch ranged from only 1.3% to 5% of total ingested starch. Muir and O'Dea[110] reported that the amount of resistant starch in food decreased with increased chewing, indicating that the extent of chewing can affect the amount of starch escaping digestion. Unabsorbed starch was also found to be directly related to the quantity ingested and to the small intestine transit time.[94,109] Other work investigated the effect of food processing on glucose and insulin responses to starch.[111,112] Amylase inhibitors, the presence of NSP, and phytate also affect starch digestibility.[113–116]

The fate of polysaccharide bulking agents. "Nondigestible" polysaccharides are used in foods as bulking agents because they are more or less resistant to digestion in the small intestine. As with shorter-chain bulking agents, polysaccharides are partially fermented in the colon and bowel by intestinal microflora. The endogenous enzymes in the small intestine readily degrade amylose and amylopectin, polymers that make up starch, where they are found in various proportions. These enzymes hydrolyze the α-(1→4)-linkages of amylose and amylopectin. Other enzymes in the small intestine split the α-(1→6)-linkage of the amylopectin. Physical modification can render starch poorly digestible (resistant starch). Chemically modified starches, such as propoxylated starch, are resistant to digestion by normal intestinal enzymes. Table 5 summarizes the gastrointestinal effects of several complex carbohydrate bulking agents. Guar, pectin, and inulin are not digested in the small intestine but are readily fermented in the colon. The fermentable materials also demonstrate modest hypocholesterolemic activity. Nondigestible carbohydrates in wheat, bran, and cellulose cause predictable increase in stool weight and have little or no effect on serum cholesterol levels.

When carbohydrates enter the large intestine, they are fermented to various degrees by the intestinal microflora, yielding acetic, propionic, and butyric acids. Fleming and

Table 5. Gastrointestinal effects of complex carbohydrate bulking agents

Effects	Guar gum	Pectins	Cellulose	Wheat bran	Inulin and oligofructose
Fermentation	Large extent	Large extent	Limited or none	Partial	Large extent
Change in intra-luminal pH	⇓	⇓	No	=	⇓
Gastric emptying	Delay	Delay ?	Delay ?	0 ?	?
Weight of intestinal mucosa	⇑	⇑	?	?	?
Binding of bile acids	–	+/–	0	0 or weak	?
Stool weight	0	0	⇑	⇑	⇑
Cholesterolemia	⇓	⇓	0	0	⇓
Glucose absorption	Flattens tolerance	Delays	0	?	Flattens tolerance
Hepatic lipids & cholesterol	?	⇓	0	0	?

Rodriguez[117] reported that the average proportions of acetic, propionic, and butyric fatty acids produced from colonic fermentation was 54:29:17. Several other workers reported similar values.[118–120] The first step in the fermentation of complex carbohydrates to fatty acids is the hydrolysis of the complex polymers to monosaccharides. Saylers[121] showed that human feces contain lichenase, galacturonidase, xylanase, β-glucosidase, β-galactosidase, β-xylanase, and α-fucosidase activities. Bayliss and Houston[122] reported the presence of mannase, α-galactosidase, and β-glucosidase activities in human feces.

Generally, it can be stated that the more water soluble the polysaccharide, the greater the colonic digestibility. Cummings and MacFarlane[123] suggested that complete digestion of complex carbohydrates in the colon required considerable synergism between species of colonic microorganisms.

Livesey[124] concluded that ≈70% of the complex carbohydrates in the diet can be fermented in the colon. He also calculated that the energy conversion factor for simple sugars to fatty acids is ≈0.7. Thus, for each gram of simple sugar released from the complex carbohydrates in the colon, one would expect 11.7 kJ/g (0.7 × 16.7 kJ/g [2.8 kcal/g; 0.7 × 4 kcal/g]) of metabolizable energy to be available.

Monosaccharides entering or produced in the colon are taken up by the bacteria and metabolized anaerobically to fatty acids by the Embden-Meyerhof pathway to initially produce pyruvate, which is subsequently converted to short-chain fatty acids (formic, acetic, propionic, and butyric), succinate, lactate, ethanol, methane, carbon dioxide, and oxygen.[125] The short-chain fatty acids are not used by the microflora but are released for use by enterocytes.

Resistant starch is fermented to short-chain fatty acids in the colon.[126] The energy yield of resistant starch has been estimated at 9.2–9.6 kJ/g (2.2–2.3 kcal/g), depending on the route of fermentation.[126] The pattern of fermentation of resistant starch differs from that of other nondigestible polysaccharides and the sugar alcohols. Englyst and MacFarlane[99] reported a greater proportion of butyrate formation and an increase in microbial mass. The increased butyrate is potentially relevant because butyrate is an antiproliferative agent. One could therefore speculate that the increased bacterial cell mass that results in reduced transit time, combined with the antiproliferative effect of butyrate, may render resistant starch potentially protective against colonic cancer.[127,128]

Fat Replacements

There are three categories of fat replacers: fat mimetics, fat substitutes, and low-calorie fats. Generally, fat replacers are ingredients that are designed to replace all or part of the fat normally in a product with minimum effect on organoleptic quality of the food product. Examples include the addition of milk solids to reduced-fat or skim milk and frozen desserts, the addition of lean meat to low-fat and processed meat products, and the baking rather than frying of snack foods. In many low-fat baked products and other low-fat foods currently available, fat has been replaced by sugars and starches. To reduce the energy content of a food, the ideal fat replacers are water or air. However, fats and oils provide many important attributes to foods, including flavor, palatability, mouthfeel, creaminess, and lubricity. Frying oils are important as heat-transfer agents in the frying process, and in fried foods they impart crispness. Currently available fat replacers serve these functions to various degrees. The overall goal is to reduce the calories provided by fat. Regardless of the nature of fat replacers, they are intended to reduce the caloric contribution of fat in the diet.

Fat mimetics. Fat mimetics are materials that replace the bulk, body, and mouthfeel of fats but do not replace fat calories on a one-to-one basis. Typical fat mimetics are starch, cellulose, pectin, protein, hydrophilic colloids, dextrins, and polydextrose. These materials are frequently broken down to microparticles to emulate the particle size of fats. Many mimetic materials are fully digestible (e.g., starch, dextrins, and protein). Because they are highly hydrated, a caloric reduction in the food product ensues. Thus, fat mimetics provide a textural replacement of fat and a reduction in calorie content. Fat mimetics are generally limited to use in products with

Table 6. Fat mimetics

Mimetic	Producer	Protein	Carbohydrate
Amalean	American Maize		Corn starch
Avicel	FMC Corp.		Cellulose
Caprenin			
Carageenan			Seaweed
Cellulose gel			Cellulose
Dairylight	Pfizer	Whey	
Dairy-lo	Pfizer	Whey	
Enrich 301	Quest	Milk	
Fibercel	Alpha-Beta Technology		Yeast
Guar gum	Grinsted Products		Guar gum
Gum arabic			Gum arabic
Kelcogel	Kelco		Gellan gum
Leanmaker	Quaker Oats		Oat bran
Lita	Opta Food Ingredients	Zein	
Litese	Pfizer		Polydextrose
Locust bean gum			Locust bean
Maltrin	Grain Processing		Maltodextrin (corn starch)
Methocel	Dow Chemical		Cellulose
N-lite	National Starch		Starch
Guar gum			
N-oil	National Starch		Starch
Notsofat c			Maltodextrin
			Fiber
Nutralean	Webb Technologies		Oat bran
Oatrim	Quaker		Oat dextrin
Optagrade	Opta Food Ingredients		Starch
Paselli sa2	Avebe America Inc		Potato starch
Pectin			Pectin
Rhodilean sd	Rhone-Poulenc		Xanthan gum oatrim
Simplesse	Nutrasweet	Egg albumin	
		Milk protein	
Slenderlean			
Slendid	Hercules, Inc		Pectin
Solka-floc	James River		Cellulose
Sta-slim	A.E. Staley		Potato starch
Stellar	A.E. Staley		Corn starch
Trailblazer	Kraft Foods		Egg albumin
			Milk protein
Trim choice	Conagra		Oatrim
Ultracreme			
Ultra-freeze	A.E. Staley	Egg white	
		Milk protein	
Veri-lo	Pfizer		Emulsifiers
Wonderslim	Natural Food Technologies		Plums
Xanthan gum	Merck		Xanthan gum

a high degree of hydration, such as desserts and spreads, and are not applicable to fried products. Commercially available fat mimetics are listed in Table 6. The table includes the primary carbohydrate or protein source of the mimetic. Mimetics based on cellulose, seaweed, and gums are noncaloric, whereas those based on starch and protein provide 16.7 kJ/g (4 kcal/g). However, because most of these products are used in the hydrated form, their caloric contribution as fat replacers is reduced.

Low-calorie fats. Low-calorie fats are true triacylglycerols that are structured to provide <37.7 kJ/g (9 kcal/g). Commercial examples of low-calorie fats are Caprenin® (Procter & Gamble) and Salatrim® (Nabisco). Caprenin is specifically designed for use as a cocoa butter substitute in confections. Salatrim is useful in baked products, confections, dairy products, and spreads. Stepan Corporation has filed a generally recognized as safe (GRAS) petition for medium-chain triacylglycerols (MCTs). MCTs are triacylglycerols composed of 8–12 carbon fatty acids that provide 29.3–33.5 kJ/g (7–8 kcal/g). They are metabolized more like carbohydrate and are rapidly used as energy rather than stored as fat.

Caprenin is a reduced-calorie fat with properties similar to cocoa butter. Structurally, Caprenin differs from normal vegetable fats in that two fatty acids are medium-chain fatty acids (caprylic and capric) and the third is behenic acid. Caprylic and capric acids are primarily obtained by fractionation of palm kernel or coconut oil. Behenic acid, obtained by the complete hydrogenation of rapeseed oil, is poorly absorbed. As a result, the caloric value of Caprenin is ≈21 kJ/g (5 kcal/g).

Salatrim represents a family of low-calorie fats with various functional properties and food applications. Salatrim is a randomized triacylglycerol containing short- and long-chain fatty acids. The short-chain fatty acids can be acetic, propionic, and butyric acids, whereas the long- chain fatty acid is predominately stearic acid. These oils also contain small amounts of palmitic, arachidic, and behenic acids. The stearic acid and longer-chain fatty acids are poorly absorbed. On the basis of rat growth studies, Finley et al.[129] concluded that the caloric value of a range of Salatrim family members was 21 kJ/g (5 kcal/g). Hayes et al.[130] obtained similar results in a study using radiolabeled Salatrim, which also indicated that the short-chain fatty acids were rapidly hydrolyzed and converted to carbon dioxide. These investigators demonstrated that the stearic acid that was absorbed was largely converted to oleic acid. The caloric value estimates from rat studies were confirmed in a clinical study by Finley et al.[131]

Fat substitutes. Fat substitutes are physically similar to fats and oils and can theoretically replace fat on a one-to-one weight basis in foods. Generally, they are heat stable and provide 0–12.6 kJ/g (0–3 kcal/g).

Sucrose polyester (Olestra), developed at Procter & Gamble over the past 20 years, is a mixture of hexa-, hepta-, and octa-fatty acid esters of sucrose. The fatty acid distribution can range from 8- to 22-carbon fatty acids, either saturated or unsaturated. The wide range of available fatty acids allows the development of various sucrose polyesters with a wide range of functionality. This functionality includes fats that are liquid, plastic, or hard. Taste, viscosity, heat stability, functionality, and appearance are claimed to be indistinguishable from normal vegetable fats. Sucrose polyesters with at least six esterified fatty acids are virtually indigestible. Because of this indigestibility, they act as organic solvents in the digestive track. Clinical tests have shown that when fat-soluble vitamins are mixed with Olestra, a reduction in their absorption occurs. Thus, supplementation of Olestra with vitamin E may be necessary.[132] The same property that inhibits the absorption of fat-soluble vitamins is an advantage in that it sequesters and removes cholesterol from the gastrointestinal tract. The digestion and absorption of Olestra are reviewed in detail by Swanson et al.[133] When liquid forms of Olestra reach the anal sphincter, they are not well retained and some anal leakage has been reported. This issue has been addressed by developing Olestra variations that melt above 37 °C, thus remain-ing solid throughout their passage through the gastrointestinal tract. In January 1996 the Food and Drug Administration (FDA) approved Olestra for use in snacks and crackers. Products containing Olestra will carry a warning about potential gastrointestinal discomfort.

Pfizer is investigating a noncaloric fat called Sorbestrin®, the hexa-fatty acid ester of sorbitol. Like Olestra it is indigestible, with the fatty acid composition determining functionality.

Esterified propoxylated glycerol esters (EPG), a family of noncaloric fats, have been developed by Arco Chemical Corporation. EPGs are made from naturally occurring fats with 1–4 propylene oxide units inserted between the glycerol and the fatty acids. The EPGs can be made from any common fat or oil, including soy, cottonseed, corn oil, tallow, lard, or canola. The physical properties range from oils through plastic to solid fats. Like Olestra the EPGs are not significantly digested or fermented in the gastrointestinal tract. The potential benefits and negatives are similar to those of Olestra.

CPC International has developed a fat substitute based on polycarboxylate esters, with trialkoxytricarballylate (TACTA) as the primary representative. Proposed uses include addition to mayonnaise and margarine. TACTA basically reverses the esters of the glycerol and appends the backbone with long-chain fatty alcohols. The resultant molecule is not digested and, similarly to other noncaloric fat substitutes, is likely to act as an organic solvent in the gastrointestinal tract. Liquid forms potentially cause anal leakage.

An outgrowth of the CPC technology is the carboxy-carboxylate ester technology patented by Klemann and Finley.[134] These materials are low-calorie rather than noncaloric fat substitutes. The backbone of the molecules are either malonic or tartaric acids that have fatty acids esterified to the hydroxyl groups and fatty alcohols esterified to the acid groups. The result is a family of fat substitutes whose functionality ranges from oil-like to hard fat. The materials are heat stable and partially digestible. Caloric values range from 4.2 to 12.6 kJ/g (1 to 3 kcal/g), depending on the fatty alcohols and fatty acids appended to the backbone.

Safety Testing of Macronutrient Substitutes

Depending on the nature of the proposed macronutrient, two approaches toward approval by FDA can be considered. One is a full food additive petition (FAP) where essentially all Redbook requirements are addressed. Alternatively, when macronutrient substitutes represent less radical changes from normal foods, such as Salatrim, a petition can be filed declaring the ingredient to be GRAS.

The primary guide for safety testing of new ingredients or food additives is the Redbook or the newly re-

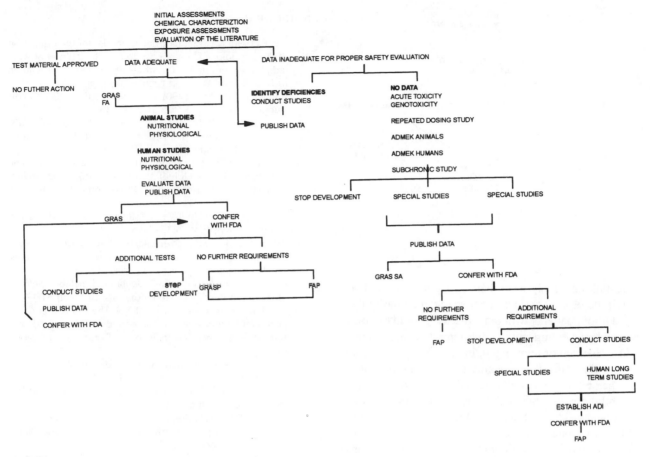

Figure 2. Procedure for evaluating the safety of macronutrient substitutes. FAP, food additive petition; GRAS P, GRAS petition; GRAS SA, GRAS scientific assessment.

vised Redbook II.[135] This FDA publication describes the traditional toxicological studies, including genetic, toxicological, and animal studies, to establish either a no observed effect level or a no observed adverse effect level. These levels can then be used to derive an acceptable daily intake based on the integration of safety data and exposure estimates. Although testing is generally conducted with exposures that are orders of magnitude greater than anticipated exposures, for macronutrient substitutes testing can usually be done at intake levels that only moderately exceed usual intake levels.

A general flow sheet for assessing macronutrient substitutes is shown in Figure 2. Borzelleca[136] proposed a more detailed process for assessing macronutrients. The general approach not only assists with the nature of the testing to be done, but also provides a decision tree that helps decide whether to approach the testing as GRAS material or as a food additive petition. Nabisco Inc. took a slightly modified approach in safety testing for the low-calorie fat Salatrim. It was determined that, because Salatrim was a triacylglycerol with no unusual characteristics other than the presence of short-chain fatty acids, a GRAS petition was appropriate. The Nabisco testing program is outlined in Figure 3. The Borzelleca[136] approach

in Figure 2 is a comprehensive program covering the safety testing of either a GRAS or a food additive type of macronutrient substitute. The Nabisco approach provides an example of a carefully conducted safety program in line with Borzelleca's recommendations.

Assuming that the basic animal and initial clinical safety testing is successfully completed, there are several other considerations required before approaching the FDA with either a GRAS or food additive petition. One must conduct extensive exposure estimates. These estimates need to include not only average use but also 90th percentile use. The potential exposure by various age groups should also be considered. For example, is there a risk that the product could be fed to infants or small children where exposure per unit of body mass can be larger than may have been tested in animals? Although it is often difficult to anticipate, the potential for abuse of the ingredient must also be considered. What if a new noncaloric macronutrient were so readily available that it became a major dietary item? Some individuals could overuse the material and produce dietary imbalances or deficiencies of essential nutrients. Sensitive subpopulations also present concerns. One must consider how to deal with subjects with malabsorption syndromes or

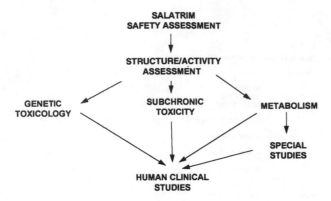

Figure 3. Salatrim® safety assessment.

potential food allergies. Either subpopulation could be at risk if the new macroingredient were dangerous to them. In addition, patients with renal disease should be considered when dealing with ingredients that are excreted, either changed or unchanged, in the urine. Either testing or warnings must be considered with these subjects.

When adding macronutrient substitutes to the diet, the potential for causing malabsorption of other nutrients must be considered. For example, the early formulations of Olestra appeared to reduce the absorption of fat-soluble vitamins, particularly vitamin E. These problems can be overcome by fortification or modification of the formula.

The influence of new macronutrients on intestinal function in children, adults, and patients with modified gastrointestinal function must be considered. This is a case where there is potential for either a positive or a negative effect from a macronutrient. For example, fiber and other bulking agents such as sugar alcohols have a positive effect on gut function. They provide the substrate for fermentation by colonic bacteria. This fermentation supplies short-chain fatty acids to the intestinal mucosa. The fermentation also results in greater bulk of the feces, thus decreasing transit time. In healthy patients these are all desirable effects. However, in particularly sensitive subjects, especially on initial exposure, laxation or gastrointestinal upset may occur.

Conclusions

A number of macronutrient substitutes are currently available and many more are on the horizon. They offer immense potential for the production of reduced-calorie foods. With a population where >30% are obese, there is a need for low-caloric-density foods that provide satisfaction and are consumed long enough to provide public health benefits. These foods must taste good and must have familiar textures. Macronutrient substitution helps the food processor achieve these objectives.

References

1. Bar A (1990) Factorial calculation model for the estimation of the physiological caloric value of polyols. In Hosoya N (ed), Caloric evaluation of carbohydrates. Japan Association of Dietetic and Enriched Foods, Tokyo, pp 209–257
2. Bernier J, Pascal G (1990) Valeur energetique des polyols (sucres alcools). Med Nutr 26:221–238
3. Voedingsraad (1987) The energy value of sugar alcohols: recommendations of the Committee on Polyalcohols. Netherland Nutrition Council, The Hague
4. Bornet FRJ (1993) Low calorie bulk sweeteners: nutrition and metabolism. In Khan R (ed), Low calorie foods and food ingredients. Blackie Academic & Professional, New York, pp 36–52
5. Bornet FRJ (1994) Undigestible sugars in food products. Am J Clin Nutr 59(suppl):763S–769S
6. Birkhed D, Kalfas S, Svensater G, Edwardsson S (1985) Microbiological aspects of some caloric sugar substitutes. Int Dent J 35:9–17
7. Grenby TH, Phillips A (1989) Dental and metabolic effects of lactitol in the diet of laboratory rats. Br J Nutr 51:17–24
8. Life Sciences Research Office (1994) The evaluation of the energy of certain sugar alcohols used as food ingredients. Federation of American Societies for Experimental Biology, Bethesda, MD
9. Livesey G (1992) The energy values of dietary fiber and sugar alcohols for man. Nutr Res Rev 5:61–84
10. Senti FR (1986) Health aspects of sugar alcohols and lactose. NTIS, Springfield, VA
11. Dwivedi BK (1991) Sorbitol and mannitol. In Nabors LO, Gelardi RC (eds), Alternative sweeteners, 2nd ed. Marcel Dekker, New York, pp 333–348
12. Karimzadegan E, Clifford AJ, Hill FW (1979) A rat bioassay for measuring the comparative availability of carbohydrates and its application to legume foods, pure carbohydrates and polyols. J Nutr 109:2247–2259
13. Allison RG (1979) Dietary sugars in health and disease. III. Sorbitol. PB-295 775. NTIS, Springfield, VA
14. Dwivedi BK (1977) Absorption, metabolism, and application of polyols. In Hood LF, Wardrip EK, Bollenback GN (eds), Carbohydrates and health. AVI, Westport, CT, pp 27–38
15. Sicard PJ (1982) Hydrogenated glucose syrups, sorbitol, mannitol, and xylitol. In Birch GG, Parker KJ (eds), Nutritive sweeteners. Applied Sciences Publishers, London, pp 145–170
16. Herman RH (1974) Hydrolysis and absorption of carbohydrates and adaptive responses of the jejunum. In Sipple HL, McNutt KW (eds), Sugars in nutrition. Academic Press, New York, pp 145–172
17. Wick AM, Almen MC, Joseph L (1951) The metabolism of sorbitol. J Am Pharm Assoc 40:542–544
18. Griem W, Lang K (1960) Versuche zur parenteralen Ernahrung mit Aminosauren-Sorbit- Losungen. Klin Wochenschr 38: 336–337
19. Hyams JS (1983) Sorbitol intolerance: an unappreciated cause of functional gastrointestinal complaints. Gastroenterology 84:30–33
20. Nguyen NU, Dumoulin G, Henriet MT, et al (1993) Carbohydrate metabolism and urinary excretion of calcium and oxalate after ingestion of polyol sweeteners. J Clin Endocrinol Metab 77:388–392
21. Adcock LH, Gray CH (1957) The metabolism of sorbitol in the human subject. Biochem J 65:554–560
22. Schnell-Dompert E, Siebert,G. (1980) Metabolism of sorbitol in the intact organism. Hoppe Seylers Z Physiol Chem 361:1069–1075

23. Baugerie L, Flourie B, Marteau P, et al (1990) Digestion and absorption in the human intestine of three sugar alcohols. Gastroenterology 99:717–723

24. Baugerie L, Flourie B, Marteau P, et al (1991) Clinical tolerance, intestinal absorption, and energy value of four polyols ingested after fasting. Gastroenterol Clin Biol 15:929–32

25. Ellis FW, Krantz JC (1941) Sugar alcohols. XXII. Metabolism and toxicity studies with mannitol and sorbitol in man and animals. J Biol Chem 141:147–154

26. Peters R, Lock RH (1958) Laxative effects of sorbitol. Br Med J 5097:677–678

27. Koizumi N, Fuji M., Ninomiya R, et al (1983) Studies on transitory laxitive effects of sorbitol and maltitol. I. Estimation of 50% effective dose and maximum non-effective dose. Chemosphere 12:45–53

28. Bassler KH (1969) Adaptive processes concerned with absorption and metabolism of xylitol. In Horecker BL, Lang K, Takagi Y (eds), International symposium on metabolism physiology, and clinical use of pentoses and pentitols. Springer-Verlag, Berlin, pp 190–196

29. Bassler KH, Stein G, Belzer W (1966) Xylitstoffwechsel und Xylitresorption: Stoffwechseladaptation als Ursache fur Resorptionsbeschleunigung. Biochem Z 346:171–185

30. Muller F, Strack E, Kuhfahl E, Dettmer D (1967) Der Stoffwechsel von Xylit bei normalen und alloxandiabetischen Kaninchen Z Gesamte Exp Med 142:338–350

31. Schmidt B, Fingerhut M, Lang K (1964) Uber den Stoffwechsel von radioaktiv markiertem Xylit bei der Ratte. Klin Wochenschr 42:1073–1077

32. Dehmel KH, Forster H, Mehnert H (1969) Absorption of xylitol. In Horecker BL, Lang K, Takagi Y (eds), Pentoses and pentitols. Springer-Verlag, Berlin, pp 177–181

33. Asano T, Levitt MD (1973) Xylitol absorption in healthy man. Diabetes 22:279–281

34. Muller-Hess R, Geser CA, Bonjour JP, et al (1975) Effects of oral xylitol administration on carbohydrate and lipid metabolism in normal subjects. Infusionstherapie 2:247–252

35. Mehnert H (1976) Zuckeraustauschstoffe in der Diabetesdiaet. Int J Vitam Nutr Res (suppl 15):295–324

36. Wang MC, Meng HC (1971) Xylitol metabolism in extrahepatic tissues. Z Ernahrungswiss Suppl 11:8–16

37. Hiele M, Ghoos Y, Rutgeerts P, Vantrappen G (1993) Metabolism of erythritol in humans: comparison with glucose and lactitol. Br J Nutr 69:169–176

38. Bornet F, Dauchy F, Chevalier A, Slama G (1992) Etude du devenier metabolique, aprPs ingestion chez l'homme sain, d'un nouvel edulcorant de charge basse calorie: l'erythritol [abstract]. Gastroenterol Clin Biol 16:69

39. Grupp U, Siebert G (1978) Metabolism of hydrogenated palatinose, an equimolar mixture of alpha-D-glucopyranosido-1, 6-sorbitol and alpha-D-glucopyranosido-1,5-mannitol. Res Exp Med (Berl) 173:261–278

40. Strater PJ, Irwin WE (1991) Isomalt. In Nabors LO, Gelardi RC (eds), Alternative sweeteners, 2nd ed. Marcel Dekker, New York, pp 309–332

41. Kruger D, Grossklaus R, Klingebiel L, et al (1991) Caloric availability of Palatinit (isomalt) in the small intestine of rats: implications of dose dependency on the energy value. Nutr Res 11:669–678

42. Linko P (1982) Lactose and lactitol. In Birch GG, Parker KJ (eds), Nutritive sweeteners. Applied Publishers, London, pp 109–131

43. Van Es AJH, de Groot L, Vogt JE (1986) Energy balances of eight volunteers fed on diets supplemented with either lactitol or saccharose. Br J Nutr 56:545–554

44. Oku T, Kim SH, Hosoya N (1981) Effect of maltose and diet containing starch on maltitol hydrolysis in rat. J Japan Soc Food Nutr 34:145–151

45. Moskowitz AH (1991) Maltitol and hydrogenated starch hydrosylate. In Nabors LO, Gelardi RC (eds), Alternative sweeteners, 2nd ed. Marcel Dekker, New York, pp 259–282

46. Lian-Loh R, Birch GG, Coates ME (1982) The metabolism of maltitol in the rat. Br J. Nutr 48:477–481

47. Rennhard HH, Bianchine JR (1976) Metabolism and caloric utilization of orally administered maltitol-14C in rat, dog and man. J Agric Food Chem 24:287–291

48. Maranesi M, Gentili P, Carenini G (1984) Nutritional studies on maltitol. Part I. Acceptability, energy yield, effects on growth and blood biochemical parameters. Acta Vitaminol Enzymol 6:3–9

49. Felber JP, Tappy L, Vouillamoz D, et al (1987) Comparative study of maltitol and sucrose by means of continuous indirect calorimetery. JPEN J Parenter Enteral Nutr 11:250–254

50. Wursch P, Schweizer TF (1987) Sugar substitutes and their energy value for the human body. Dtsch Zahnarztl Z 42: S151–S153

51. Wursch P, Koellreutter B, Schweizer TY (1989) Hydrogen excretion after ingestion of five different sugar alcohols and lactulose. Eur J Clin Nutr 43:819–825

52. Baugerie L, Flourie, B, Franchisseur C, et al (1989) Absorption intestinale et tolerance clinique au sorbitol, maltitol, lactitol et isomalt [abstract]. Gastroenterol Clin Biol 13:102

53. Akiba M, Nakamura S, Hosoya N, et al (1990) Metabolism of 14C-U-maltitol in man. In Hosoya N (ed), Caloric evaluation of carbohydrates. Tokyo, Japan Association of Dietetic and Enriched Foods, pp 91–108

54. Oku T (1990) Evaluation of bioavailable energy of maltitol. In Hoysoya N (ed), Caloric evaluation of carbohydrates. Tokyo, Japan Association of Dietetic and Enriched Foods, pp 109–124

55. Oku T (1991) Caloric evaluation of reduced-energy bulking sweeteners. In Romsos DR, Himms-Hagen J, Suzuki M (eds), Obesity: dietary factors and control. S Karger, Basel, pp 169–180

56. Tamura Y, Furuse M, Matsuda S, et al (1991) Energy utilization of sorbose in comparison with maltitol in growing rats. J Agric Food Chem 39:732–735

57. Tsuji K, Osada Y, Shimada N, et al (1990) Energy evaluation of sorbitol and maltitol in healthy men and rats. In Hosoya N (ed), Caloric evaluation of carbohydrates. Tokyo, Japan Association of Dietetic and Enriched Foods, pp 77–90

58. Clevenger MA, Turnbull D, Inoue H, et al (1988) Toxicological evaluation of neosugar: genotoxicity and chronic toxicity. J Am Coll Toxicol 5:643–662

59. Drevon T, Bornet F (1992) Les fructo-oligosaccharides: ACTILIGHT. In Multon JL (ed), Le sucre, les sucres, les édulcorants et les glucides de charges dans les IAA. TEC & DOC Lavoisier, pp 313–338

60. Oku T, Tokunaga R, Hoysoya N (1984) Non-digestibility of a new sweetener "Neosugar" in the rat. J Nutr 114:1574–1581

61. Roberfoid M (1993) Dietary fiber, inulin, and oligofructose: a review comparing their physiological effects. Crit Rev Food Sci Nutr 33:103–148

62. Stone-Dorshow T, Levitt MD (1987) Gaseous response to ingestion of poorly absorbed fructo-oligosaccharide sweetener. Am J Clin Nutr 46:61–65

63. Rusmessen JJ, Bode S, Hamberg O, Gudmand-Hoyer E (1990) Fructans from Jerusalem artichokes: intestinal transport, absorption, fermentation and influence on blood glucose, insulin and C-peptide response in healthy subjects. Am J Clin Nutr 52:675–681

64. Oku T, Tokunaga R (1986) Improvement of metabolism by

"Neosugar": effect of fructo-oligosaccharides in rat intestine. In Proc. 2nd Neosugar Research Conf. Neosugar Res. Soc. Meiji-Seika Publ. 1986; 53

65. Tokunaga T, Oku T, Hoysoya N (1989) Utilization and excretion of a new sweetener, fructooligosaccharide (Neosugar), in Rats. J. Nutr. 119:553–559

66. Tsuji Y, Yamada K, Hoysoya N, Moriuchi S (1986) Digestion and absorption of sugars and sugar substitutes in rat small intestine. J Nutr Sci Vitaminol (Tokyo) 32:92–100

67. Tokunaga R, Oku T (1989) Utilization and excretion of a new sweetener, fructooligosaccharide (Neosugar), in rats. J Nutr 119:553–559

68. Hidaka H (1983) Fructosyloligosaccharides. A new material for dietary food. Attention to the improvement balance and the effect of lowering cholesterol in the blood. Kagaku to Seibustu 21:291–293

69. Hidaka H, Eida T, Takizawa T, et al (1986) Effects of fructooligosaccahrides on intestinal flora and human health. Bifido-bacteria Microflora 5:37–47

70. Hidaka H, Eida T (1988) Roles of fructo-oligosaccharides for the improvement of intestinal flora and suppression of production of putrid substances. Shokuhin-Kogyo (Food Engineering) 31:52–55

71. Annison G, Bertocchi C, Khan R (1993) Low-calorie bulking ingredients: nutrition and metabolism in low calorie foods and food ingredients. In Khan R (ed), Low calorie food and food ingredients. Blackie Academic & Professional, New York, pp 51–76

72. Allingham RP (1982) Polydextrose—a new food ingredient: technical aspects. In Charalambous G, Inglett G (eds), Chemistry of foods and beverages: recent developments. Academic Press, New York, pp 293–303

73. Khan R, Wold JK, Paulsen BS (1983) In Ansell MF (ed), Rodds chemistry of carbon compounds, Vol. I FG. Elsevier, pp 231–343

74. Aspinall GO, Carpenter KJ (1984) Structural investigations on the non-starchy polysaccharides of oat bran. Carbohydr Polym 4:271–278

75. Gidley MJ, McArthur AJ, Underwood DR (1991) ^{13}C-NMR characterization of molecular structure in powder, hydrates and gels of galactomannans and glucomannans. Food Hydrocolloids 5:129–140

76. Englyst HN, Trowell HW, Southgate DAT, Cummings JH (1987) Dietary fiber and resistant starch. Am J Clin Nutr 46:873–874

77. Englyst HN, Kingman SM, Cummings JH (1992) Classification and measurement of nutritionally important starch fractions. Eur J Clin Nutr 46(suppl 2):S33–S50

78. Snow P, O'Dea, K (1981) Factors affecting the rate of hydrolysis of starch in food. Am J Clin Nutr 34:2721–2727

79. Wursch P, Vedovo SD, Koellreutter B (1986) Cell structure and starch nature as key determinants of the digestion rate of starch in legume. Am J Clin Nutr 43:25–29

80. Fuwa H, Takaya T, Sugimoto Y (1980) Degradation of various starch granules by amylases. In Marshall JJ (ed), Mechanisms of saccharide polymerization and depolymerization. Academic Press, New York, pp 73–100

81. Englyst HN, Cummings JH (1990) Non-starch polysaccharides (dietary fiber) and resistant starch. In Furda I, Brine CJ (eds), New developments in dietary fiber. Plenum Press, New York, pp 205–225

82. Berry CS (1986) Resistant starch: formation and measurement of starch that survives exhaustive digestion with amylolytic enzymes during the determination of dietary fiber. J Cereal Sci 4:301–314

83. Berry CS, Iíanson I, Miles MJ, et al (1988) Physical chemical characterization of resistant starch from wheat. J Cereal Sci 8:203–206

84. Ring SC, Gee JM, Whittam M, et al (1988) Resistant starch: its chemical form in foodstuffs and effect on digestibility in vitro. Food Chem 28:97–99

85. Siljestrom M, Eliasson AC, Bjorck I (1989) Characterization of resistant starch from autoclaved wheat starch. Starch/Staerke 41:147–151

86. Sievert D, PomeranzY (1990) Enzyme-resistant starch. II. Differential scanning calorimetry studies on heat-treated starches and enzyme-resistant residues. Cereal Chem 68: 86–91

87. Czuchajowska Z, Sievert D, Pomeranz Y (1991) Enzyme-resistant starch. IV. Effects of complexing lipids. Cereal Chem 68:537–542

88. Eerlingen RC, Crombez M, Delcour JA (1993) Enzyme-resistant starch. I. Quantitative and qualitative influence of incubation time and temperature of autoclaved starch on resistant starch formation. Cereal Chem 70:339–344

89. Sterling C (1978) Textural qualities and molecular structure of starch products. J Texture Stud 9:225–255

90. Kingman SM, Englyst HN (1994) The influence of food preparation methods on the in vitro digestibility of starch in potatoes. Food Chem 49:181–186

91. Eerlingen RC, Van Haesendonck IP, De Paepe G, Delcour JA (1994) Enzyme-resistant starch. III. The quality of straight-dough bread containing varying levels of enzyme-resistant starch. Cereal Chem 71:165–170

92. Lin P-Y, Czuchajowska Z, Pomeranz Y (1994) Enzyme-resistant starch in yellow layer cakes. Cereal Chem 71:69–75

93. Ranhotra GS, Gelroth JA, Eisenbraun GJ (1991) High-fiber white flour and its use in cookie products. Cereal Chem 68:432–434

94. Stephen AM, Haddad AC, Phillips SF (1983) Passage of carbohydrate into the colon: direct measurements in humans. Gastroenterology 85:589–595

95. Englyst HN, Cummings JH (1985) Digestion of polysaccharides of some cereal foods in the human small intestine. Am J Clin Nutr 42:778–787

96. Englyst HN, Cummings JH (1986) Digestion of the carbohydrates of banana (Musa paradisiaca sapientum) in the small intestine. Am J Clin Nutr 44:42–50

97. Englyst HN, Cummings JH (1987) Digestion of polysaccharides of potato in the small intestine of man. Am J Clin Nutr 44:423–431

98. Englyst HN, Cummings HN (1987) Fermentation in the human large intestine and the available substrates. Am J Clin Nutr 45:1243–1255

99. Englyst HN, MacFarlane GT (1986) Breakdown of resistant starch and readily digestible starch by the human gut. J Sci Food Agric 37:699–706

100. Raben A, Tagliabue A, Christensen NJ, et al (1994) Resistant starch: the effect on postprandial glycemia, hormonal response, and satiety. Am J Clin Nutr 60:544–551

101. Morand C, Levrat MA, Besson C, et al (1994) Effects of a diet rich in resistant starch on hepatic lipid metabolism in the rat. J Nutr Biochem 5:138–144

102. deDecker EAM, Kloots WJ, Van Amelsvoort JMM (1993) Resistant starch decreases serum cholesterol and triacylglycerol concentrations in rats. J Nutr 123:2142–2151

103. Truswell AS (1992) Glycemic index of foods. Eur J Clin Nutr 46(suppl 2):S91–S102

104. Scheppach W (1994) Effects of short-chain fatty acids on gut morphology and function. Gut 35(1, suppl):S35–S38

105. Van Munster IP, Tangerman A, Nagengast FM (1994) Effect of resistant starch on colonic fermentation, bile acid metabolism, and mucosal proliferation. Dig Dis Sci 39:834–842

106 Levitt MD (1983) Malabsorption of starch: a normal phenomenon. Gastroenterology 85:769–770

107. Anderson IH, Levine AS, Levitt, MD (1981) Incomplete absorption of the carbohydrate in all purpose wheat flour. N Engl J Med 304:891–892

108. Levine AS, Levitt MD (1981) Malabsorption of starch moiety of oats, corn and potatoes. Gastroenterology 80:1209–1213

109. Chapman RW, Sillery JK, Graham MM, Saunders DR (1985) Absorption of starch by healthy ileostomates: effect of transit time and carbohydrate load. Am J Clin Nutr 41:1244–1248

110. Muir JG, O'Dea K (1992) Measurement of resistant starch: factors affecting the amount of starch escaping digestion in vitro. Am J Clin Nutr 56:123–127

111. Collings P, Williams C, Macdonald I (1981) Effects of cooking on serum glucose and insulin responses to starch. Br Med J 282:1093–1101

112. Jenkins DJA, Thorne MJ, Camelon K (1982) Effect of processing on digestibility and blood glucose response: a study of lentils. Am J Clin Nutr 36:1093–1101

113. Layer P, Carlson GL, DiMagno EP (1985) Partially purified white bean amylase inhibitor reduces starch digestion in vitro and inactivates intraduodenal amylase in humans. Gastroenterology 88:1895–1902

114. Levitt MD, Ellis CJ, Fetzer CA, et al (1984) Causes of malabsorption of flour. Gastroenterology 86:1162–1167

115. Wolever TMS, Jenkins DJA (1986) Effect of dietary fiber and foods on carbohydrate metabolism. In Spiller GA (ed), CRC handbook of dietary fiber in human nutrition. CRC Press, Boca Raton, FL, pp 87–119

116. Yoon JH, Thompson LU, Jenkins DJA (1983) The effect of phytic acid on in vitro rate of starch digestibility and blood glucose response. Am J Clin Nutr 38:835–842

117. Fleming SE, Rodriguez MA (1983) Influence of dietary fiber on fecal excretion of volatile fatty acids by human adults. J Nutr 113:1613–1625

118. Rubinstein R, Howard AV, Wrong AM (1969) In vivo dialysis of faeces as a method of stool analysis. IV. The organic anion component. Clin Sci 37:549–553

119. Cummings JH, Southgate DA, Branch WJ, et al (1979) The digestion of pectin in the human gut and its effect on the absorption of calcium and large bowel function. Br J Nutr 41:477–482

120. Spiller GA, Chernoff MC, Hill RA, et al (1980) Effect of purified cellulose, pectin, and a low residue diet on fecal volatile fatty acids, transit time, and fecal weight in humans. Am J Clin Nutr 33:754–759

121. Saylers AA (1979) Energy sources of intestinal anaerobes. Am J Clin Nutr 32:158–169

122. Bayliss CE, Houston AP (1985) The effect of guar gum on microbial activity in the human colon. Food Microbiol 2:53–62

123. Cummings JH, MacFarlane GT (1991) The control and consequences of bacterial fermentation in the human colon. J Appl Bacteriol 70:443–459

124. Livesey G (1991) Determinants of energy density with conventional foods and artificial feeds. Proc Nutr Soc 50:371–382

125. Miller TL, Wolin MJ (1979) Fermentations by saccharolytic intestinal bacteria. Am J Clin Nutr 32:164–172

126. Mathers JC (1992) Energy value of resistant starch. Euro J Clin Nutr 46(suppl 2):S129–S130

127. Krih J (1982) Effects of sodium butyrate, a new pharmacolgical agent, on cells in culture. Mol Cell Biochem 42:65–82

128. Smith PJ (1986) n-Butyrate alters chromatin accessibility to DNA repair enzymes. Carcinogenesis 7:423–529

129. Finley JW, Leveille GA, Klemann LP (1994) Growth method for estimating the caloric availability of fats and oils. J Agric Food Chem 42:489–494

130. Hayes JH, Finley JW, Leveille GA (1994) In vivo metabolism of Salatrim in the rat. J Agric Food Chem 42:500–514

131. Finley JW, Leveille GA, Dixon RM, et al (1994) Clinical assesment of Salatrim, a reduced calorie triacylglycerol. J Agric Food Chem 42:581–596

132. LaBarge RG (1988) The search for a low-calorie oil. Food Technol 42:84–86

133. Swanson BG, Boutte TT, Akoh CC (1994) Digestion and absorption of carbohydrate polyesters. In Akoh CC, Swanson BG (eds), Carbohydrate polyesters as fat substitutes. Marcel Dekker, New York, pp 183–196

134. Klemann LP, Finley JW (1989) Low calorie fat mimetics comprising carboxy/carboxylate esters. US Patent 4,830,787

135. Bureau of Foods (1982) Toxicological principles for the safety assessment of direct food additives used in food. US Food and Drug Administration, Washington, DC

136. Borzelleca JF (1992) Macronutrient substitutes: safety evaluation. Regul Toxicol Pharmacol 16:253–264

Chapter **60**

Antioxidants

Barry Halliwell

Free radicals and antioxidants are widely discussed in the clinical and nutritional literature and even in the lay press. The assumption is that free radicals are bad and antioxidants good. By contrast, a recent clinical trial suggested that giving the "antioxidant" β-carotene to smokers accelerated the development of lung cancer.[1] The purpose of this article is to provide some scientific background to help nutritionists evaluate such claims and counterclaims.

Why Do We Need Antioxidants?

When living organisms first appeared on the earth, they did so under an atmosphere containing very little O_2, which means that they must have been essentially anaerobes. Anaerobic microorganisms still survive to this day, but their growth is inhibited and they can often be killed by exposure to 21% O_2, the current atmospheric level. As the O_2 content of the atmosphere rose (as a result of the evolution of photosynthetic organisms that used light energy to split water), many primitive organisms may have died out. Present-day anaerobes are presumably the descendants of those primitive organisms that followed the evolutionary path of adapting to rising atmospheric O_2 levels by restricting themselves to environments that the O_2 did not penetrate. However, other organisms began the evolutionary process of evolving antioxidant defense systems to protect against O_2 toxicity. In retrospect, this was a fruitful path to follow, because organisms that tolerated the presence of O_2 could also evolve to use it for metabolic transformations (e.g., by cytochrome P450) and for efficient energy production by using electron transport chains with O_2 as the terminal electron acceptor, such as those present in mitochondria. Mitochondria make >80% of the ATP we need, and the lethal effects of inhibiting this production, for example, by cyanide, show how important the mitochondria are.[2]

We have developed antioxidant defenses to protect against 21% O_2, but no greater than that. This limitation is evidenced by all aerobes suffering demonstrable injurious effects if exposed to O_2 at concentrations >21%.[2] For example, the incidence of eye damage, to an extent sometimes causing complete blindness, increased abruptly in the early 1940s among infants born prematurely. Not until 1954 was it realized that this retinopathy of prematurity is associated with the use of high O_2 concentrations in incubators for premature babies. More careful control of O_2 concentrations (continuous transcutaneous O_2 monitoring, with supplementary O_2 given only where necessary) and administration of the lipid-soluble antioxidant α-tocopherol to babies have decreased its incidence. However, the problem has not disappeared, because many premature infants need high levels of O_2 in order to survive.[3]

The earliest suggestion made to explain O_2 toxicity was that O_2 is a direct inhibitor of enzymes, thereby interfering with metabolism.[2] However, few targets of direct damage by O_2 have been identified in aerobes. In 1954, Gerschman et al.[4] proposed that the damaging effects of O_2 could be attributed to the formation of oxygen radicals. This hypothesis was popularized and converted into the superoxide theory of O_2 toxicity after the discovery of superoxide dismutase (SOD) enzymes that specifically remove the superoxide free radical.[5] In its simplest form, this theory states that O_2 toxicity is due to excess formation of superoxide radical ($O_2^{\cdot-}$) and that the SOD enzymes are important antioxidant defenses.

What Is a Radical?

We need antioxidants to scavenge and prevent the formation of free radicals such as superoxide, but what exactly is a radical?

In the structure of atoms and molecules, electrons usually associate in pairs, with each pair moving within a defined region of space around the nucleus. This space is referred to as an atomic or molecular orbital. One electron in each pair has a spin quantum number of $+\frac{1}{2}$, the other $-\frac{1}{2}$. A free radical is any species capable of independent existence (hence the term "free") that contains one or more unpaired electrons, that is, one that is alone in an orbital.[6] The simplest free radical is an atom of the element hydrogen, with one proton and a single electron. Table 1 gives examples of other free radicals (a superscript dot is used to denote free radical species).

Table 1. Examples of free radicals

Name	Formula	Comments
Hydrogen atom	H$^\bullet$	The simplest free radical.
Trichloromethyl	CCl$_3$$^\bullet$	A carbon-centered radical (i.e., the unpaired electron resides on carbon). CCl$_3$$^\bullet$ is formed during metabolism of the solvent carbon tetrachloride in liver and contributes to the toxic effects of this solvent. Carbon-centered radicals usually react quickly with O$_2$ to make peroxyl radicals, e.g., CCl$_3$$^\bullet$ + O$_2$ → CCl$_3$O$_2$.
Superoxide	O$_2$–	An oxygen-centered radical. Has limited reactivity.
Hydroxyl	OH$^\bullet$	A highly reactive oxygen-centered radical. Very reactive indeed: attacks all molecules in the human body.
Peroxyl, alkoxyl	RO$_2$$^\bullet$, RO$^\bullet$	Oxygen-centered radicals formed (among other routes) during the breakdown of organic peroxides.
Oxides of nitrogen	NO$^\bullet$, NO$_2$$^\bullet$	Nitric oxide (NO$^\bullet$) is formed in vivo from the amino acid L-arginine. Nitrogen dioxide (NO$_2$$^\bullet$) is made when NO$^\bullet$ reacts with O$_2$ and is found in polluted air and smoke from burning organic materials (e.g., cigarette smoke).

What Radicals Are Made in the Human Body?

Humans are exposed to electromagnetic radiation from the environment, both natural (e.g., radioactive radon gas and cosmic radiation) and man made. Low-wavelength electromagnetic radiation (e.g., gamma rays) can split water in the body to generate hydroxyl radical OH$^\bullet$. This viciously reactive radical, once generated, attacks whatever it is next to.[6,7]

The human body also makes the superoxide radical O$_2$$^{\bullet-}$.[5] Some superoxide is made by accidents of chemistry, in that many molecules in the body react directly with O$_2$ to make O$_2$$^{\bullet-}$. Examples are the catecholamines (e.g., adrenalin, dopamine), tetrahydrofolates, and some compounds found in mitochondrial and endoplasmic reticular electron transport chains.[5] Such O$_2$$^{\bullet-}$ generation is an unavoidable consequence of having these molecules in a body that needs oxygen.[5,8] However, in addition, some O$_2$$^{\bullet-}$ is made deliberately. For example, the phagocytic cells (neutrophils, monocytes, macrophages, and eosinophils) that defend the body against bacteria, viruses, and fungi generate large amounts of O$_2$$^{\bullet-}$ as part of the mechanism by which foreign organisms are killed.[9] This is an essential defense mechanism against infection. However, it can go wrong: there are several diseases (examples being rheumatoid arthritis and inflammatory bowel disease) in which there is excessive phagocyte activation. This inappropriate phagocyte activation causes tissue damage, to which oxygen radicals contribute.[6]

It has been estimated that 1–3% of the oxygen breathed in is used to make O$_2$$^{\bullet-}$ in the human body.[5] Because humans consume a lot of O$_2$, a simple calculation shows that we make >2 kg of O$_2$$^{\bullet-}$ in the human body every year;[8] people with chronic infections may make much more.

Another physiological free radical is nitric oxide, NO$^\bullet$. It performs many useful physiological functions, such as regulation of blood pressure and intercellular signaling,[10] but too much NO$^\bullet$ (like too much O$_2$$^{\bullet-}$) can be toxic: excess NO$^\bullet$ production is thought to be an important tissue injury mechanism in several diseases, including chronic inflammation, stroke, and septic shock.[10]

Hydrogen Peroxide, a Nonradical

Most of the O$_2$$^{\bullet-}$ generated in vivo probably undergoes a nonenzymatic or SOD-catalyzed reaction to generate H$_2$O$_2$, as represented by the overall equation below:

$$2O_2^{\bullet-} + 2H^+ \rightarrow H_2O_2 + O_2.$$

Hydrogen peroxide has no unpaired electrons and so is a nonradical. H$_2$O$_2$ resembles water in its molecular structure and is very diffusible within and between cells.[6] As well as arising from O$_2$$^{\bullet-}$, H$_2O_2$ is produced by the action of several oxidase enzymes in vivo, including amino acid oxidases and the enzyme xanthine oxidase.[11] Xanthine oxidase catalyzes the oxidation of hypoxanthine to xanthine and of xanthine to uric acid, whereas oxygen is simultaneously reduced both to O$_2$$^{\bullet-}$ and to H$_2$O$_2$. Only low levels of xanthine oxidase are normally present in mammalian tissues, but these levels often increase when tissues are subjected to insult, such as trauma or deprivation of oxygen.[12]

Some metabolic roles for H$_2$O$_2$ are known and others have been proposed. For example, H$_2$O$_2$ generated in the thyroid gland is used by a peroxidase enzyme to iodinate the thyroid hormones.[13] H$_2$O$_2$ may up-regulate the expression of certain genes: one mechanism is by directly or indirectly leading to the displacement of an inhibitory subunit from the cytoplasmic gene transcription factor NF-κB.[14] Displacement of the inhibitory subunit causes the active factor to migrate to the nucleus and activate many different genes. Thus H$_2$O$_2$ and other peroxides (such as lipid peroxides) can induce expression of genes controlled by NF-κB.[15] This is of particular interest because in cell culture systems, H$_2$O$_2$

can activate NF-κB and induce expression of the provirus of human immunodeficiency virus-1. This virus is the most common cause of acquired immunodeficiency syndrome, and its expression in cell culture can sometimes be prevented by antioxidants.[14]

How Do Radicals React?

Reactivity depends on the radical and what the radical is presented with. If two free radicals meet, they can join their unpaired electrons to form a covalent bond. Thus atomic hydrogen forms diatomic hydrogen. A more biologically relevant example is the very fast reaction of $NO^{\cdot}$ and $O_2^{\cdot-}$ to form a nonradical product, peroxynitrite:[16,17]

$$NO^{\cdot} + O_2^{\cdot-} \rightarrow ONOO^- \text{ (peroxynitrite).}$$

However, when a free radical reacts with a nonradical, a new radical results, and a chain reaction is set up. Because most biological molecules are nonradicals, the generation of reactive radicals such as $OH^{\cdot}$ in vivo usually starts chain reactions. For example, attack of reactive radicals on fatty acid side chains in membranes and lipoproteins can abstract hydrogen, leaving a carbon-centered radical and initiating the process of lipid peroxidation.[6,8] There is growing evidence that lipid peroxidation occurs in human blood vessel walls and contributes to the development of atherosclerosis, often leading to stroke and myocardial infarction.[18]

When $OH^{\cdot}$ is generated adjacent to DNA, it attacks both the deoxyribose sugar and the purine and pyrimidine bases, forming a wide range of products. This multiplicity of products is characteristic of attack by $OH^{\cdot}$ and may be used to show that such attack has occurred in vivo.[19] These products are present at low levels in human tissue DNA,[19] and their amounts are greater in DNA from cancerous tumors.[20,21] This could be due to increased $OH^{\cdot}$ formation in cancers. In healthy cells, repair enzymes remove damaged bases from DNA constantly;[22] an alternative possibility is that this process is less efficient in cancer cells.

Toxicity of Superoxide, Hydrogen Peroxide, and Nitric Oxide

Experimental results show that removal of $O_2^{\cdot-}$ and H_2O_2 by antioxidant defense systems (see below) is essential for life. Why is this? In organic media, $O_2^{\cdot-}$ can be very reactive, but in aqueous media it is not, mainly acting as a moderate reducing agent.[6] However, $O_2^{\cdot-}$ does react rapidly with a few targets. These include some bacterial iron-sulfur proteins, including enzymes essential to metabolism, such as aconitase.[23] Whether similar $O_2^{\cdot-}$-sensitive targets exist in human cells remains to be established. However, in isolated submitochondrial particles, $O_2^{\cdot-}$ has been claimed to inactivate the NADH dehydrogenase complex of the mitochondrial electron transport chain.[24]

One important molecule in humans that reacts with $O_2^{\cdot-}$ is $NO^{\cdot}$. $NO^{\cdot}$ is useful in human metabolism, but an excess can be cytotoxic; this mechanism of tissue injury has been implicated in several human diseases.[10] Excess $NO^{\cdot}$ can be directly toxic, e.g., by damaging iron-sulfur proteins[10] and inhibiting the enzyme ribonucleoside diphosphate reductase.[25] However, evidence is increasing to show that $NO^{\cdot}$-$O_2^{\cdot-}$ interactions are also involved.[10,17,26] Because $NO^{\cdot}$ acts upon smooth muscle cells in blood vessel walls to produce relaxation and lower blood pressure, then $O_2^{\cdot-}$, by removing $NO^{\cdot}$, can act as a vasoconstrictor, which might have deleterious effects in some clinical situations. For example, excess vascular $O_2^{\cdot-}$ production could lead to hypertension,[27,28] and peroxynitrite produced when $O_2^{\cdot-}$ and $NO^{\cdot}$ react could promote atherosclerosis.[29] Peroxynitrite can oxidize essential -SH groups on proteins and lead to nitration of aromatic amino acids (such as phenylalanine and tyrosine), perhaps interfering with cell signal transduction.[17,26,29,30]

Like $O_2^{\cdot-}$, H_2O_2 at micromolar levels also appears poorly reactive, but higher (>50 μmol/L) levels can attack certain cellular targets.[31] For example, H_2O_2 oxidizes an essential -SH group on the glycolytic enzyme glyceraldehyde-3-phosphate dehydrogenase, blocking glycolysis. H_2O_2 also interferes with other aspects of cell energy metabolism.[31]

It is widely thought that much of the toxicity of $O_2^{\cdot-}$ and H_2O_2 involves their conversion into $OH^{\cdot}$.[32] Three mechanisms have been proposed to explain this. One is the interaction of $O_2^{\cdot-}$ and $NO^{\cdot}$ to form $ONOO^-$, which can decompose to generate some $OH^{\cdot}$.[30] An earlier proposal was the superoxide-driven Fenton reaction:

$$O_2^{\cdot-} + Fe(III) \rightarrow Fe(II) + O_2$$
$$Fe(II) + H_2O_2 \rightarrow OH^{\cdot} + OH^- + Fe(III).$$

Copper ions also catalyze formation of $OH^{\cdot}$ from $O_2^{\cdot-}$ and H_2O_2.[32] A third mechanism for making $OH^{\cdot}$ is the reaction of $O_2^{\cdot-}$ with hypochlorous acid, an antibacterial product generated by activated neutrophils:[33]

$$O_2^{\cdot-} + HOCl \rightarrow OH^{\cdot} + OH^- + O_2.$$

Do Metal Ion Catalysts of Free Radical Reactions Exist In Vivo?

Iron and copper ions in chemical forms that can decompose H_2O_2 to $OH^{\cdot}$ are in very short supply in vivo. The human body is very careful to ensure that as much iron and copper as possible are kept safely bound to transport or storage proteins. Indeed, this sequestration of metal ions is an important antioxidant defense mechanism.[32,34]

Hence, an important determinant of the nature of the damage done by excess generation of $O_2^{\cdot-}$ and H_2O_2 in vivo is the availability and location of metal ion catalysts of $OH^{\cdot}$ radical formation. If, for example, catalytic iron ions are bound to DNA in one cell type and to membrane lipids in another, then excessive formation of H_2O_2 and $O_2^{\cdot-}$ will, in the first case, damage the DNA and in the second case could initiate lipid peroxidation. Evidence for $OH^{\cdot}$ formation in the nucleus of cells treated with H_2O_2 has been obtained by showing that all four DNA bases are modified in the way expected from $OH^{\cdot}$ attack.[35] If this $OH^{\cdot}$ is formed by metal ion-dependent reactions, then the catalytic metal ions must be bound to the DNA itself, since $OH^{\cdot}$ is so reactive that it cannot migrate within the cell: it reacts at its site of formation.

Escherichia coli mutants lacking SOD activity are hypersensitive to damage by H_2O_2[36] and, if able to enter cells, SOD can protect against damage by H_2O_2.[37] These and much other data are consistent with a role of $O_2^{\cdot-}$ in facilitating damage by H_2O_2, and the superoxide-driven Fenton reaction provides a possible explanation. Superoxide also plays an important role in the provision of the iron required for $OH^{\cdot}$ generation. Thus $O_2^{\cdot-}$ can release iron ions from the iron-storage protein ferritin.[38] Because the amount of $O_2^{\cdot-}$-releasable iron is very small, ferritin-bound iron is much safer than an equivalent amount of free iron.[39] Superoxide may also release iron if it attacks iron-sulfur proteins,[23] and H_2O_2 can release iron ions by degrading the heme rings of proteins such as myoglobin, cytochrome c, and hemoglobin.[40,41]

Antioxidant Defenses

All organisms suffer some exposure to $OH^{\cdot}$, because it is generated during the splitting of O-H bonds in water, driven by ionizing radiation from the environment.[7] Hydroxyl radical is so reactive with all biological molecules that it is impossible to evolve a scavenger specific for it. Once $OH^{\cdot}$ has been formed, damage is probably unavoidable and is dealt with by repair systems, including DNA repair enzymes.[22] Many of our antioxidant defenses minimize the production of $OH^{\cdot}$.

Enzymes. SODs remove $O_2^{\cdot-}$ by accelerating the rate of its conversion to H_2O_2 by $\approx$40-fold at pH 7.4. Mammalian cells have a SOD enzyme containing manganese (MnSOD) at its active site in the mitochondria. A SOD with copper and zinc (CuZnSOD) at the active site is also present but largely in the cytosol.[5] It has recently been shown that the familial dominant form of amyotrophic lateral sclerosis, a fatal degenerative disorder of motor neurons in the brain and spinal cord, is somehow related to mutations affecting the CuZn enzyme protein.[42] These mutations decrease activity somewhat but may also somehow cause this normally protective protein to become toxic.[42,43] One possibility is that the mutant enzymes easily release copper, a powerful prooxidant.[44]

Because SOD enzymes generate H_2O_2, they work in collaboration with H_2O_2-removing enzymes. Catalases convert H_2O_2 to water and O_2 and are located in the peroxisomes of mammalian cells, probably serving to destroy H_2O_2 generated by oxidase enzymes located within these subcellular organelles.[11] However, it is likely that the most important H_2O_2-removing enzymes in mammalian cells are the glutathione peroxidase (GSHPX) enzymes, which contain the element selenium at their active sites.[11]

Sequestration of transition metals. As already stated, an additional important antioxidant defense system is the presence of metal ion storage and transport proteins. For example, iron bound to the plasma protein transferrin will not catalyze damaging free radical reactions.[45] The same is true of iron bound to the protein lactoferrin, found in secretory fluids, including milk.[45] However, in a high percentage of preterm babies and a lower percentage of apparently normal full-term babies, transferrin is iron-saturated and plasma contains iron that can catalyze damaging free radical reactions, such as $OH^{\cdot}$ formation.[46-48] Such babies are presumably at high risk of free radical damage.

The human body also contains molecules that remove free radicals by reacting directly with them in a noncatalytic manner, such as reduced glutathione (GSH), α-tocopherol, and ascorbate.

Vitamin E and vitamin C. Alpha-tocopherol, the major constituent of the fat-soluble vitamin E, is the most important (but by no means the only) free radical scavenger within membranes and lipoproteins.[49-51] Alpha-tocopherol inhibits lipid peroxidation by scavenging peroxyl radical (Table 1) intermediates in the chain reaction

$$\alpha TH + LOO^{\cdot} \rightarrow \alpha T^{\cdot} + LOOH.$$

The resulting α-tocopherol radical ($\alpha T^{\cdot}$), although not completely unreactive, is much less efficient at attacking unmolested fatty acid side chains than are peroxyl ($LOO^{\cdot}$) radicals, so the overall effect of α-tocopherol is to slow the chain reaction of lipid peroxidation.[52] Several mechanisms may exist for recycling $\alpha T^{\cdot}$ back to α-tocopherol (none yet rigorously proved to operate in the human body). Likely mechanisms include the reaction of $\alpha T^{\cdot}$ with ascorbic acid (vitamin C) at the surface of membranes and lipoproteins.[49,51] Ascorbic acid may also have multiple other antioxidant properties, especially in the respiratory tract, where it may help to detoxify inhaled oxidizing air pollutants, such as ozone and nitrogen dioxide.[53,54] By contrast, in the presence of transition metal ions, such as iron and copper, ascorbate can become prooxidant, acting as a reducing agent and generating $O_2^{\cdot-}$, H_2O_2, and $OH^{\cdot}$. Normally, because such metal ions are available in very limited amounts in vivo,

Table 2. Dietary antioxidants: where are we now?

A diet rich in fruits, nuts, grains, and vegetables seems to be protective against several human diseases. This may be due to the antioxidants they contain, to the many other compounds present, or both.

1. Known to be important as antioxidants

Vitamin E (fat soluble)	General name for a group of compounds, of which α-tocopherol is the most important. Found in membranes and lipoproteins. Block the chain reaction of lipid peroxidation by scavenging intermediate peroxyl radicals.

$$O_2^{\bullet} \qquad\quad O_2H$$
$$\mid \qquad\qquad\quad \mid$$
$$-\,C\!-\, +\, TH \,\rightarrow\, -\,C\!-\, +\, T^{\bullet}$$

The tocopherol radical ($T^{\bullet}$) is much less reactive in attacking adjacent fatty acid side chains and can be converted back to TH by vitamin C. Important in protection against atherosclerosis and, in babies, retinopathy of prematurity and, perhaps, intracranial hemorrhage.[60] Severe vitamin E deficiency in adults causes neurodegeneration.

2. Widely thought to be important as an antioxidant

Vitamin C (ascorbic acid)	Plays several metabolic roles, e.g., in collagen synthesis and hormone production. Inhibits the carcinogenicity of dietary nitrosamines. Probably assists α-tocopherol in inhibiting lipid peroxidation by recycling the tocopherol radical $T^{\bullet}$ + ascorbate → TH + ascorbate$^{\bullet}$. Good scavenger of many free radicals and may help to detoxify certain air pollutants (ozone, oxides of nitrogen, cigarette smoke) in the respiratory tract. Some potential prooxidant effects (see text).

3. Probably important in human health, but not necessarily by acting as antioxidants

β-carotene, other carotenoids, related plant pigments	Increasing epidemiologic evidence that high body levels are associated with diminished risk of cancer and cardiovascular disease, particularly in smokers.[61] Often simplistically grouped with vitamins E and C as antioxidants. Although many carotenoids exert antioxidant events in vitro under certain conditions,[61] it remains to be proved that this is their mechanism of action in vivo.

4. Possibly important as antioxidants

Flavonoids, other plant phenolics	Plants contain many phenolic compounds that inhibit lipid peroxidation and lipoxygenases in vitro (e.g., flavonoids), although (like ascorbate) they can sometimes be prooxidant if mixed with copper or iron ions in vitro.[62-64] It has been speculated that flavonoids in red wine could partly explain the "French paradox."[63] We do not know how many plant phenolic compounds are absorbed from the gut and become available in vivo to act as antioxidants. Many of them are being considered as antioxidant food additives.

the antioxidant properties of ascorbate predominate.[53,55] However, ascorbate can be toxic if given to patients with iron overload diseases unless iron ion chelators are administered simultaneously.[56] There is considerable argument about the net effect of ascorbate in premature babies: is it antioxidant or prooxidant?[57-59]

Other dietary antioxidants. Alpha-tocopherol and ascorbate are normally obtained from the diet. Many other dietary constituents have been speculated to be important free radical scavengers, but the evidence is not always good. Table 2 summarizes the author's views.

Despite all these antioxidants, some free radicals still escape to do damage in the human body. Thus DNA undergoes constant oxidative damage and has to be repaired.[22] Free radicals attack proteins, and the damaged products have to be degraded. End products of lipid peroxidation are measurable in human body fluids, in atherosclerotic lesions, and in the "age pigments" that accumulate in old tissues.[6,8]

Oxidative Stress

Because production of reactive oxygen species and antioxidant defenses are approximately balanced, it is easy to tip this balance in favor of the reactive oxygen species and create the situation of oxidative stress.[65]

Oxidative stress can result from 1) depletions of dietary antioxidants caused by malnutrition (e.g., through inadequate dietary intakes of α-tocopherol, ascorbic acid, sulfur-containing amino acids [needed for GSH manufacture], or riboflavin [needed to make the FAD cofactor of glutathione reductase]) and 2) excess production of O_2^{-} and H_2O_2 (e.g., by exposure to elevated O_2 concentrations, the presence of toxins that are metabolized to produce free radicals, or excessive activation of natural radical-producing systems [e.g., inappropriate activation of phagocytic cells in chronic inflammatory diseases, such as rheumatoid arthritis and ulcerative colitis]).[6] One particular area of interest is the possibility that the side effects of several drugs involve increased oxidative damage, often because the drugs are metabolized to free radical species.[66]

Cells can tolerate mild oxidative stress, which often results in up-regulation of the synthesis of antioxidant defense systems in an attempt to restore the balance.[67] However, severe oxidative stress can produce major derangements of cell metabolism, including DNA damage, rises in intracellular "free" Ca^{2+} and "free" iron ions, damage to membrane ion transporters and other proteins, and lipid peroxidation. Cell injury and death may result.[6,65,68]

Oxidative Stress and Human Disease: Prevention By Diet?

Damaged tissues undergo more free radical reactions than do healthy tissues.[69] As a result, in most human diseases, oxidative stress is a secondary phenomenon, not the primary cause of the disease.[69] This does not mean that oxidative stress is not important. Its importance varies in different disease states. For example, oxidative damage to lipids in blood vessel walls is a significant contributor to the development of atherosclerosis.[18] Oxidative DNA damage probably contributes to the age-related development of cancer.[70,71] Excess production of radicals probably contributes significantly to tissue damage in rheumatoid arthritis, inflammatory bowel diseases (such as Crohn's disease and ulcerative colitis), and neurodegenerative diseases.[72]

There is growing evidence that the major killers, cardiovascular disease and cancer, can be prevented or delayed to some extent by dietary changes, such as reduction in fat intake and increased consumption of fruits, grains, and vegetables. We obtain several compounds from a healthful diet that act (or may act) to diminish oxidative damage in vivo. Table 2 summarizes the author's view of our current state of knowledge. Because our endogenous antioxidant defenses are not 100% efficient, it seems reasonable to propose that dietary antioxidants are particularly important in diminishing the cumulative effects of oxidative damage over the long human life span and that they account for some of the beneficial effects of fruits, grains, and vegetables. For example, if continuous free radical damage to DNA, perhaps not always efficiently repaired, is involved in the development of spontaneous cancers, then more dietary antioxidants might help.[70,71] There is growing evidence that an increased dietary intake of vitamin E will decrease death from myocardial infarction.[73] Dietary vitamin E requirement is probably raised if the percentage of polyunsaturated fatty acids in the diet is increased.

What Do We Know?

Perusal of Table 2 shows that many unanswered questions remain. Vitamin E seems protective against cardiovascular disease, retinopathy of prematurity, and possibly intracranial hemorrhage, but what is the optimal dietary intake? Does it relate to the polyunsaturated fatty acid content of the diet? Carotenoids may be important anticancer agents, but is this action really related to an antioxidant effect? A good daily intake of vitamin C probably helps protect against cardiovascular disease and some forms of cancer (e.g., stomach cancer), but could much higher intakes do good or harm? Are prooxidant effects biologically relevant? Is ascorbate good for adults but bad for some babies? Is there too much iron supplementation?

Fortunately, experimental tools to answer these questions are now becoming available. Thus methods exist for measuring both ongoing and steady-state (i.e., the balance between damage and repair) oxidative damage to DNA, proteins, and lipids in the human body. These methods may help us to gain information about optimal nutritional intakes. If the major killers, cancer and vascular disease, could be delayed by even a few years by dietary changes, the social and economic benefits would be enormous.

References

1. α-Tocopherol, β-Carotene Prevention Study Group (1994) The effect of vitamin E and beta carotene on the incidence of lung cancer and other cancers in male smokers. N Engl J Med 330:1029–1035
2. Balentine J (1982) Pathology of oxygen toxicity. Academic Press, New York
3. Ehrenkranz RA (1989) Vitamin E and retinopathy of prematurity: still controversial. J Pediatr 114:801–803
4. Gerschman K, Gilbert DL, Nye SW, et al (1954) Oxygen poisoning and x-irradiation: a mechanism in common. Science 119:623–626
5. Fridovich I (1986) Superoxide dismutases. Methods Enzymol 58:61–97.
6. Halliwell B, Gutteridge JMC (1989) Free radicals in biology and medicine, 2nd ed. Clarendon Press, Oxford
7. von Sonntag C (1987) The chemical basis of radiation biology. Taylor and Francis, London
8. Halliwell B (1994) Free radicals and antioxidants: a personal view. Nutr Rev 52:253–265

9. Babior BM, Woodman RC (1990) Chronic granulomatous disease. Semin Hematol 27:247–259

10. Moncada S, Higgs A (1993) The L-arginine-nitric oxide pathway. N Engl J Med 329:2002–2011

11. Chance B, Sies H, Boveris A (1979) Hydroperoxide metabolism in mammalian organs. Physiol Rev 59:527–605

12. Granger DN (1988) Role of xanthine oxidase and granulocytes in ischemia-reperfusion injury. Am J Physiol 255:H1269–H1275

13. Dupuy C, Virion A, Ohayon R, et al (1991) Mechanism of hydrogen peroxide formation catalyzed by NADPH oxidase in thyroid plasma membrane. J Biol Chem 266:3739–3743

14. Schreck R, Albermann KAJ, Baeuerle PA (1992) Nuclear factor κB: an oxidative stress-responsive transcription factor of eukaryotic cells (a review). Free Radic Res Commun 17:221–237

15. Collins T (1993) Endothelial nuclear factor-κB and the initiation of the atherosclerotic lesion. Lab Invest 68:499–508

16. Huie RE, Padmaja S (1993) The reaction of NO with superoxide. Free Radic Res Commun 18:195–199

17. Beckman JS, Chen J, Ischiropoulos H, Crow JP (1994) Oxidative chemistry of peroxynitrite. Methods Enzymol 233: 229–240

18. Steinberg D, Parthasarathy S, Carew TE, et al (1989) Beyond cholesterol: modifications of low-density lipoprotein that increase its atherogenicity. N Engl J Med 320:915–924

19. Halliwell B, Aruoma OI (eds) (1993) DNA and free radicals. Ellis-Horwood, Chichester, United Kingdom

20. Malins DC (1993) Identification of hydroxyl radical-induced lesions in DNA base structure: biomarkers with a putative link to cancer development. J Toxicol Environ Health 40:247–261

21. Olinski R, Zastawny T, Budzbon, et al (1992) DNA modification in chromatin of human cancerous tissues. FEBS Lett 309:193–198

22. Demple B, Harrison L (1994) Repair of oxidative damage to DNA: enzymology and biology. Annu Rev Biochem 63:915–948

23. Flint DH, Tuminello JF, Emptage MH (1993) The inactivation of Fe-S cluster containing hydrolyases by superoxide. J Biol Chem 268:22369–22376

24. Zhang Y, Marcillat O, Giulivi C, et al (1990) The oxidative inactivation of mitochondrial electron transport chain components and ATPase. J Biol Chem 265:16330–16336

25. Lepoivre M, Flaman JM, Bobé P, et al (1994) Quenching of the tyrosyl free radical of ribonucleotide reductase by nitric oxide. J Biol Chem 269:21891–21897

26. Darley-Usmar V, Wiseman H, Halliwell B (1995) Nitric oxide and oxygen radicals: a question of balance. FEBS Lett 369:131–135

27. Laurindo FRM, Da Luz PL, Uint L, et al (1991) Evidence for superoxide radical-dependent coronary vasospasm after angioplasty in intact dogs. Circulation 83:1705–1715

28. Nakazono K, Watanabe N, Matsuno K, et al (1991) Does superoxide underlie the pathogenesis of hypertension? Proc Natl Acad Sci USA 88:10045–10048

29. Beckman JS, Ye YZ, Anderson PG, et al (1994) Extensive nitration of protein tyrosines in human atherosclerosis detected by immunohistochemistry. Biol Chem Hoppe Seyler 375:81–88

30. Van der Vliet A, O'Neill CA, Halliwell B, et al (1994) Aromatic hydroxylation and nitration of phenylalanine and tyrosine by peroxynitrite: evidence for hydroxyl radical production from peroxynitrite. FEBS Lett 339:89–92

31. Cochrane CG (1991) Mechanisms of oxidant injury of cells. Mol Aspects Med 12:137–147

32. Halliwell B, Gutteridge JMC (1990) Role of free radicals and catalytic metal ions in human disease. Methods Enzymol 186:1–85.

33. Candeias LP, Patel KB, Stratford MRL, Wardman P (1993) Free hydroxyl radicals are formed on reaction between the neutrophil-derived species superoxide anion and hypochlorous acid. FEBS Lett 333:151–153

34. Halliwell B, Gutteridge JMC (1991) The antioxidants of human extracellular fluids. Arch Biochem Biophys 200:1–8

35. Dizdaroglu M, Nackerdien Z, Chao BC, et al (1991) Chemical nature of in vivo DNA base damage in hydrogen peroxide-treated mammalian cells. Arch Biochem Biophys 285:388–390

36. Touati D (1989) The molecular genetics of superoxide dismutase in E. coli: an approach to understanding the biological role and regulation of SODs in relation to other elements of the defense system against oxygen toxicity. Free Radic Res Commun 8:1–9

37. Kyle ME, Nakae D, Sakaida I, et al (1988) Endocytosis of superoxide dismutase is required in order for the enzyme to protect hepatocytes from the cytoxicity of hydrogen peroxide. J Biol Chem 263:3784–3789

38. Biemond P, Van Eijk HG, Swaak AJG, Koster JF (1984) Iron mobilization from ferritin by superoxide derived from stimulated polymorphonuclear leukocytes: possible mechanism in inflammation diseases. J Clin Invest 73:1576–1579

39. Bolann BJ, Ulvik RJ (1990) On the limited ability of superoxide to release iron from ferritin. Eur J Biochem 193:899–904

40. Gutteridge JMC (1986) Iron promoters of the Fenton reaction and lipid peroxidation can be released from haemoglobin by peroxides. FEBS Lett 201:291–295

41. Harel S, Salan MA, Kanner J (1988) Iron release from metmyoglobin, methaemoglobin and cytochrome c by a system generating hydrogen peroxide. Free Radic Res Commun 5:11–19

42. Robberecht W, Sapp P, Viaene MK, et al (1994) Cu/Zn superoxide dismutase activity in familial and sporadic amyotrophic lateral sclerosis. J Neurochem 62:384–387

43. Gurney ME, Pu H, Chiu AY, et al (1994) Motor neuron degeneration in mice that express a human Cu, Zn superoxide dismutase mutation. Science 264:1772–1775

44. Spencer JPE, Jenner A, Aruoma OI, et al (1994) Intense oxidative DNA damage promoted by L-DOPA and its metabolites: implications for neurodegenerative disease. FEBS Lett 353:246–250

45. Aruoma OI, Halliwell B (1987) Superoxide-dependent and ascorbate-dependent formation of hydroxyl radicals from hydrogen peroxide in the presence of iron: are lactoferrin and transferrin promoters of hydroxyl-radical generation? Biochem J 241:273–278

46. Moison RMW, Palinckx JJS, Roest M, et al (1993) Induction of lipid peroxidation of pulmonary surfactant by plasma of preterm babies. Lancet 341:79–82

47. Evans PJ, Evans RW, Kovar IZ, et al (1992) Bleomycin-detectable iron in the plasma of premature and full-term neonates. FEBS Lett 303:210–212

48. Kaur H, Halliwell B (1994) Aromatic hydroxylation of phenylalanine as an assay for hydroxyl radicals: measurement of hydroxyl radical formation from ozone and in blood from premature babies using improved HPLC methodology. Anal Biochem 220:11–15

49. Burton GW, Traber MG (1990) Vitamin E: antioxidant activity biokinetics and bioavailability. Annu Rev Nutr 120: 357–382

50. Kagan VE, Serbinova EA, Packer L (1990) Antioxidant effects of ubiquinones in microsomes and mitochondria are

mediated by tocopherol recycling. Biochem Biophys Res Commun 169:851–857

51. Esterbauer H, Striegl G, Puhl H, Rotheneder M (1989) Continuous monitoring of in vitro oxidation of human low density lipoprotein. Free Radic Res Commun 6:67–75

52. Mukai K, Morimoto H, Okauchi Y, Nagaoka S (1993) Kinetic study of reactions between tocopheroxyl radicals and fatty acids. Lipids 28:753–756

53. Bendich A, Machlin LJ, Scandurra O, et al (1986) The antioxidant role of vitamin C. Adv Free Radic Biol Med 2:419–444

54. Cross CE, Van der Vliet A, O'Neill CA, et al (1994) Oxidants, antioxidants and respiratory tract lining fluids. Env Health Perspec 102(suppl 10):185–191

55. Halliwell B (1990) How to characterize a biological antioxidant. Free Radic Res Commun 9:1–32

56. Burt MJ, Halliday JW, Powell LW (1993) Iron and coronary heart disease. Br Med J 307:575–576

57. Gopinathan V, Miller NJ, Milner AD, Rice-Evans CA (1994) Bilirubin and ascorbate antioxidant activity in neonatal plasma. FEBS Lett 349:197–200

58. Powers HJ, Loban A, Silvers K, Gibson AT (1995) Vitamin C at concentrations observed in premature babies inhibits the ferroxidase activity of caeruloplasmin. Free Radic Res 22:57–65

59. Berger HM, Mumby S, Gutteridge JMC (1995) Ferrous ions detected in iron-overloaded cord blood plasma from preterm and term babies: implications for oxidative stress. Free Radic Res 22:555–559

60. Fish WH, Cohen M, Franzek D, et al (1990) Effect of intramuscular vitamin E on mortality and intracranial hemorrhage in neonates of 1000 grams or less. Pediatrics 85:578–584

61. Krinksy NI (1993) Action of carotenoids in biological systems. Annu Rev Nutr 13:561–587

62. Hertog MGL, Feskens EJM, Hollman PCH, et al (1993) Dietary antioxidant flavonoids and risk of coronary heart disease: the Zutphen elderly study. Lancet 342:1007–1011

63. Kanner J, Frankel E, Granit R, et al (1994) Natural antioxidants in grapes and wines. J Agric Food Chem 42:64–69

64. Laughton MJ, Evans PJ, Moroney MA, et al (1991) Inhibition of mammalian 5-lipoxygenase and cyclo-oxygenase by flavonoids and phenolic dietary additives: relationship to antioxidant activity and to iron ion-reducing ability. Biochem Pharmacol 42:1673–1681

65. Sies H (ed) (1991) Oxidative stress, oxidants and antioxidants. Academic Press, London

66. Halliwell B, Evans PJ, Kaur H, Chirico S (1993) Drug derived radicals: mediators of the side effects of anti-inflammatory drugs? Ann Rheum Dis 51:1261–1263

67. Iqbal J, Clerch LB, Hass MA, et al (1989) Endotoxin increases lung Cu, Zn superoxide dismutase mRNA: O_2 raises enzyme synthesis. Am J Physiol 257:L61–L64

68. Orrenius S, McConkey DJ, Bellomo G, Nicotera P (1989) Role of Ca^{2+} in toxic cell killing. Trends Pharmacol Sci 10:281–285

69. Halliwell B, Gutteridge JMC, Cross CE (1992) Free radicals, antioxidants, and human disease: where are we now? J Lab Clin Med 119:598–620

70. Totter JR (1980) Spontaneous cancer and its possible relationship to oxygen metabolism. Proc Natl Acad Sci USA 77:1763–1767

71. Ames BN, Shigenaga MK, Hagen TM (1993) Oxidants, antioxidants and the degenerative diseases of aging. Proc Natl Acad Sci USA 90:7915–7922

72. Jenner P (1994) Oxidative damage in neurodegenerative disease. Lancet 344:796–798

73. Byers T (1993) Vitamin E supplements and coronary heart disease. Nutr Rev 51:333–345

Chapter 61

Adverse Reactions to Foods

John M. James

Adverse symptoms following the ingestion of a food have been discussed for centuries. Scientific advances in the understanding of these reactions were almost non-existent until the early 1900s, when a serologic substance responsible for allergic reactions to ingested fish was discovered.[1] This substance could be transferred to a fish-tolerant individual, resulting in fish sensitivity. Fortunately, the past 15 years have witnessed significant advances in our understanding of adverse reactions to foods and food additives. Recent scientific milestones, including the use of well-controlled, blinded food challenges, have enhanced our understanding of these adverse reactions.[2]

Sorting out whether these symptoms are caused by immunologically mediated reactions or are secondary to normal physiologic processes can be a challenge. Therefore, the foundation for implicating foods and food additives as the cause of these adverse reactions should rest on controlled scientific observations, not on anecdotal experiences. This chapter provides a practical, scientific approach to adverse reactions to foods and food additives. Epidemiologic information regarding the incidence and prevalence of these reactions will be reviewed; this information will be followed by a basic overview of the immune response to food allergens. Next, the most common clinical manifestations of food allergy and the diagnosis of these disorders will be presented in detail. Currently accepted treatment and prophylactic measures for these reactions will be discussed, and present thinking on the natural history of food allergy will be critically examined.

Epidemiology

The labeling of every symptomatic reaction to ingested foods as an allergic reaction has been a frustrating, recurring problem. To address this, uniform definitions for adverse food reactions were published.[3,4] An adverse food reaction encompasses any abnormal clinical response following the ingestion of a food or food additive. Adverse food reactions are divided into two categories: food allergy (hypersensitivity), which is an immunologically mediated food reaction (e.g., peanut anaphylaxis) unre-

lated to any physiologic effect of the food or additive, and food intolerance, which is an abnormal physiological response to food that is not immunologically mediated. Food intolerance reactions include metabolic reactions (e.g., lactose intolerance), food toxicity (e.g., bacterial food poisoning), pharmacological reactions (e.g., caffeine), and idiosyncratic reactions. This nomenclature has helped standardize the clinical approach to adverse food reactions and has strengthened the design and interpretation of research studies in this clinical area.

There are no universally accepted prevalence figures for food allergy and other adverse reactions to foods, but generalizations can be made from the few well-designed epidemiologic studies. One survey reported that ≈30% of households had at least one member who believed they were allergic to some food ingredient.[5] Although >10% of Dutch adults reported adverse reactions to foods, the prevalence of these reactions was ≈2% when clinical histories were confirmed with blinded food challenges.[6] Adverse food reactions have been documented by blinded challenge in 8% of children <6 years of age.[7] Two separate reports demonstrated that in about one-third of children with histories suggestive of food allergy, blinded food challenges confirmed the clinical impression.[7,8] Overall, the actual prevalence of adverse reactions to foods and food additives in the general population is estimated to be <2%.[9]

The actual incidence of food allergy has also been investigated. Four prospective studies have examined the incidence of cow milk allergy in the first 3 years of life.[7,10–12] Clinical reactivity to this protein source was determined by oral challenge. The incidence, 2.3–2.8%, was very similar in all of the study populations. Most of the infants developed allergy to cow milk in the first year of life, and over three-fourths of the patients became tolerant to cow milk by their third birthday.

Immunopathogenesis

Mucosal immunity. Food allergens usually gain access to the body at all levels of the gastrointestinal tract, enter the circulation, and travel to distal target organs.[13] Antibodies of all immunoglobulin classes can be produced after oral administration of antigen, but immunoglobulin A (IgA) production predominates.[14] Secretory IgA forms complexes with foreign food antigens preventing their absorption.[15] Although low concentrations of serum IgG, IgG subclasses, IgM, and IgA antibodies and antigen-antibody complexes are formed to specific food allergens and are detectable in normal and atopic individuals,[16–20] their significance is unknown.[21,22] Likewise, the significance of proliferative responses of peripheral blood mononuclear cells to food allergens remains to be determined.[23]

Of all the adverse food reactions, food hypersensitivity or IgE-mediated reactions are understood in the greatest detail. A susceptible host produces food-specific IgE antibodies that bind high-affinity IgE receptors on mast cells and basophils, as well as low-affinity receptors on macrophages, monocytes, lymphocytes, eosinophils, and platelets. On subsequent allergen exposure, allergen binds to IgE antibodies on mast cells or basophils, stimulating the release of mediators such as histamine, prostaglandins, and leukotrienes. This results in vasodilation, smooth muscle contraction, and mucus secretion.[24] Significant increases in plasma histamine have been reported during positive blinded food challenges in patients with atopic dermatitis.[25] With repeated ingestion of food allergen, mononuclear cells are stimulated to secrete an IgE-dependent cytokine that stimulates basophils through surface-bound IgE, increasing basophil releasability.[26] These results have implicated mast cells and basophils in the pathogenesis of food hypersensitivity in atopic dermatitis.

Food allergens. Food allergens comprise glycoproteins that are largely resistant to degradation by proteases, acid, and heat.[27] They are water-soluble proteins with molecular weights <70,000. These features facilitate their absorption across mucosal surfaces. Foods implicated most often in IgE-mediated food hypersensitivity reactions include egg, peanut, milk, soy, wheat, fish, tree nuts, and shellfish.[7,9,28,29] Multiple food hypersensitivities are rare. Chicken egg, a common food allergen in children, contains several major allergens, including ovalbumin, ovomucoid, and ovotransferrin.[30] Cow milk, another common food allergen in infants,[31] contains >20 protein fractions subdivided into the casein (70–80%) and whey fractions, mainly β-lactoglobulin, α-lactalbumin, and bovine serum albumin,[32] that may trigger antibody production in humans.[33] Multiple allergenic fractions have been identified in peanuts, but two major allergens, *Ara h* I and *Ara h* II, predominate.[34,35]

Soybeans cause food allergic reactions mainly in children. Although extensive immunological cross-reactivity to more than one legume has been demonstrated, symptomatic reactivity to more than one is rare.[36] Tree nuts are also major food allergens, but nut-allergic patients do not necessarily need to avoid peanut, a legume.

Fish are another common cause of food allergy in adults and children. The immunodominant allergen in codfish, *Gad c* I, is a calcium-binding glycoprotein found in fish muscle tissue.[37] Shellfish consist of a wide variety of mollusks (clams, oysters, and scallops) and crustacea (crabs, lobster, and shrimp) and have been associated with allergic reactions. A major shrimp allergen, *Pen a* I, has been isolated that appears to be a tropomyosin.[38] Wheat and other cereal grains compose the last major group of food allergens in children.[39]

Food additives. Several different classes of food additives have been implicated in adverse reactions.[40] Food preservatives include such agents as benzoates and parabens. Bisulfites and metabisulfites are antioxidants commonly added to foods. In addition, several colorants, including many azo and nonazo dyes, are added to foods and medications to enhance appearance and processing. Monosodium glutamate and aspartame are popular food additives for flavoring and sweetening, respectively. Finally, emulsifiers and fillers are added to many food products.

Common food allergen structures. Allergen structures have been identified that are common to related and unrelated foods as well as to certain food and inhalant allergens. The major allergen in codfish, *Gad c* I, and its homologues in other fish species are probably responsible for multiple fish sensitivity.[41,42] As mentioned above, extensive immunological cross-reactivity among legumes exists, but symptomatic clinical reactivity to more than one is rare.[36] Clinically insignificant cross-reactivity also exists for the major cereal grains.[43] Studies of the oral allergy syndrome have identified shared allergen sensitivities for ragweed and melons and for birch and raw fruits and vegetables.[44–46] Finally, immunochemical cross-reactivity was reported for latex, an inhalant allergen, and several foods; some of the implicated foods are banana, chestnut, and avocado.[47]

Tolerance. Processing of food antigens by the gastrointestinal system is an essential factor for the development of oral tolerance. Food proteins capable of triggering an immune response enter the circulation but do not normally cause clinical symptoms because tolerance has developed. Suppression of systemic IgM, IgG, and IgE antibody responses and cell-mediated immune responses may be important in this process.[48] In mice, ovalbumin can be recovered in the serum after ingestion. This processed protein, similar in molecular weight to native ovalbumin, induces suppression of cell-mediated responses to native ovalbumin in recipient mice.[49] A failure in this process, including immaturity of the immune system of the gut, may increase the chances of food allergies developing in infancy. For example, the combination of low concentrations of secretory IgA and large loads of ingested proteins lead to an enormous antigenic load presented to the immune system.[50] These factors may stimulate overproduction of IgE antibodies, especially in those infants with a genetic predisposition of atopy.

Clinical Manifestations

Clinical symptoms of adverse food reactions typically involve the skin, gastrointestinal tract, and respiratory system. These symptoms may occur alone or in combination, and in some cases there can be generalized anaphylaxis.

IgE-mediated adverse food reactions: food allergy. Cutaneous reactions are the most common clinical finding of food hypersensitivity and can range from an erythematous, pruritic rash to exacerbations of atopic dermatitis. Urticaria and angioedema are among the most common acute skin symptoms,[9] but food allergy is rarely responsible for chronic urticaria.[51] Finally, food allergy has been identified as a significant pathogenic factor in ≈30% of children with atopic dermatitis presenting in an outpatient clinic setting.[29]

Gastrointestinal reactions are the second most common clinical symptoms of food allergy. These findings include nausea, vomiting, abdominal pain, and cramping; diarrhea is found less frequently.[52] Symptoms typically occur within 1 hour of the food ingestion but may appear within minutes after food ingestion. The presence of blood in stools is another clinical sign indicating the possibility of a food allergy. Growth delay and failure to thrive are clinical findings that can accompany food allergy.

The oral allergy syndrome, a form of contact urticaria from ingested allergens, is mainly limited to the oropharynx.[44-46] Pruritus and angioedema of the lips, tongue, palate, and throat transiently appear and resolve rapidly. Fresh fruits and raw vegetables are often implicated in patients with specific sensitizations to other inhalant allergens. A suggestive history and positive skin tests using fresh fruits or vegetables as test material are needed for this diagnosis.[46]

Allergic eosinophilic gastroenteropathy is a disorder characterized by infiltration of the gastric wall, the intestinal wall, or both with eosinophils and peripheral blood eosinophilia without the occurrence of vasculitis. Patients with this disease commonly present with postprandial nausea and vomiting, abdominal pain, diarrhea, weight loss, or, in infants, failure to thrive. The food-induced, IgE-mediated form of this disease is characterized by a history of atopy, elevated serum IgE concentrations, and positive prick skin tests to a variety of foods and inhalants.[53]

Food hypersensitivity as a trigger mechanism for infantile colic has been recently entertained and supported by double-blind crossover trials.[54-56] Through use of a sensitive radioimmunoassay, the presence of bovine IgG

was detected in human breast milk and infant formula.[57] More bovine IgG was found in the breast milk of mothers with colicky babies than breast milk of mothers with babies who were not colicky, suggesting a role of this protein in infantile colic. Only 10–15% of colic, however, is likely to be secondary to IgE-mediated food allergy.[58]

Both upper and lower respiratory tract reactions were reported during blinded food challenges, but isolated respiratory symptoms as the sole clinical finding of food hypersensitivity are uncommon.[28,59] Nasal congestion, sneezing, and rhinorrhea were observed. In a study of 140 asthmatic children, eight (5.7%) had a positive food challenge including bronchospasm.[60] In another report, 300 asthmatic patients were screened for possible food allergy by the use of history, skin tests, and radioallergosorbent tests (RASTs).[61] Twenty-five patients had either a history, skin test, or RAST suggestive of food allergy, and six of these patients had positive blinded food challenges with documented wheezing. Food hypersensitivity increasing nonspecific bronchial hyperresponsiveness was studied but no consensus was reached.[62,63]

Severe anaphylactic reactions including fatalities can occur following the ingestion of foods and food additives.[64-66] Peanut, milk, egg, and tree nuts have been implicated in most of the IgE-mediated reactions reported to date. Common features in these reactions include presence of asthma, previous episodes of anaphylaxis with the incriminated foods, failure to recognize early symptoms of anaphylaxis, and delay or lack of immediate use of emergency medications such as subcutaneous epinephrine to treat the reaction.

A food-dependent form of exercise-induced anaphylaxis was reported.[67,68] This severe reaction initially requires the ingestion of a specific food or meal. In some patients the reaction is associated with a specific food allergen against which the patient has IgE antibodies, and in other patients the reaction follows a certain meal. In both groups, exercise after ingestion of the food is the triggering event for the systemic reaction. Either factor alone does not provoke anaphylaxis.

Various food additives have been implicated in adverse reactions.[40,69] Tartrazine, an azo dye (FD & C yellow #5), was incriminated as an aggravating agent for asthma as well as urticarial reactions.[40,69,70] Double-blind testing in large groups of patients has not completely substantiated these associations. Antioxidants such as sulfites provoke exacerbations in asthmatic patients undergoing blinded challenges.[40,69,71] In addition, flavoring agents have been investigated, but further controlled studies are needed to evaluate the effect of monosodium glutamate and delayed asthmatic responses. Aspartame, a common sweetener, does not appear to be responsible for any significant adverse reactions.[72] There may be a small subset of patients in whom food additives will have an effect on behavior, but the problem appears to be much smaller than originally proposed.[73]

Non IgE-mediated adverse food reactions. Several adverse food reactions have been described that do not appear to be IgE-mediated. Food-induced enterocolitis syndrome commonly presents in infants younger than 3 months of age and is most often triggered by cow milk and soy protein. This syndrome presents with protracted vomiting and diarrhea with secondary dehydration.[74] The reaction usually occurs a few hours after the protein is ingested. Prick skin tests and RASTs of the suspected food allergen are usually negative. A food-induced allergic colitis has also been reported secondary to cow milk or soy protein.[75] Infants with this disorder generally do not appear ill and are usually identified because of occult or gross blood in their stool. Patients usually become tolerant to the offending protein in childhood. Celiac disease is a malabsorption syndrome resulting from a sensitivity to gluten found in wheat, rye, oat, and barley. The specific mechanism of this intestinal hypersensitivity reaction has not been resolved. Life-long elimination of gluten-containing foods is imperative for both symptomatic relief and decreasing the malignancy risk.

Other symptoms associated with food ingestion have been reported.[73] Anemia and occult gastrointestinal blood loss have been associated with consumption of large volumes of cow milk, but the mechanism is unknown. Recurrent diarrhea precipitated by the ingestion of fruit and fruit juices during infancy has also been reported. The mechanism is thought to be related to malabsorption of natural carbohydrates contained in these foods. Finally, some cases of fatigue and hyperactivity have been attributed to adverse food reactions, but these symptoms have not been substantiated in well-controlled clinical studies.

Diagnosis

A thorough medical history is helpful in the differentiation of food allergy and food intolerance. A detailed description of each symptom provoked by the food ingestion (especially skin, gastrointestinal, respiratory, and generalized symptoms) should be obtained. The timing of the reaction in relation to food ingestion, the minimum quantity of food required to trigger symptoms, the reproducibility of the symptoms, and the length of time since the previous reaction occurred are very important historical points. Documentation of the location of the reaction, the type of treatment received, and the response observed are also very useful. Unfortunately, a patient's history is not always reliable in chronic disorders such as atopic dermatitis and chronic urticaria.

Diet diaries are prospective chronological records of all ingested foods and any associated symptoms experienced. These are occasionally helpful in identifying the

Table 1. Differential diagnosis of adverse reactions to foods

---

Gastrointestinal disorders
    Structural abnormalities
        Hiatal hernia
        Pyloric stenosis
        Hirshsprung's disease
        Tracheoesophageal fistula
    Metabolic and enzyme deficiencies
        Lactose intolerance
        Phenylketonuria
        Pancreatic insufficiency
    Peptic ulcer disease
Contaminants and additives
    Flavoring and preservatives
    Dyes
    Toxins and infectious organisms
    Accidental contaminants
Pharmacological agents
    Caffeine
    Histamine
    Serotonin
Psychologic reactions

---

food most likely responsible for an adverse reaction. Occasionally, an unrecognized adverse food reaction is discovered. An atopic family history can be useful in identifying patients at increased risk of food allergy. For example, if one parent has a history of atopy, a child's risk is ≈20–40%; if both parents have such a history, the risk rises to 50–80%.[76]

A physical examination is useful in the assessment of overall nutritional status and signs of any allergic disorder, such as asthma, allergic rhinitis, and atopic dermatitis. Moreover, this examination helps to rule out other conditions that may mimic food allergy. Four major categories of disorders should be included in the differential diagnosis of adverse food reactions: gastrointestinal disorders, contaminants and additives, pharmacological agents, and psychological reactions to ingested foods (Table 1).[77]

Prick skin tests are frequently used to screen patients for IgE-mediated food allergies, and when used in conjunction with standard criteria of interpretation, give useful clinical information quickly. Food allergen extracts are applied by the prick or puncture technique along with positive (histamine) and negative (saline) controls. Wheals of ≥3 mm larger than the negative control are interpreted as positive.[78] Pricking with some fresh fruits and vegetables (apples, melons, carrots, and celery) becomes necessary because of the lability of extracts prepared from these foods.[46] If high-quality extracts are used, the prick skin test is excellent for excluding IgE-mediated food allergies because of the >95% negative predictive accuracy. However, the overall positive predictive accuracy is generally <50%, limiting the clinical interpretation of positive skin tests.[79-81] Intradermal skin testing has an increased risk of inducing a systemic reaction compared with the prick method and is even less specific than prick skin testing when compared with blinded food challenges.[79] Elimination diets, usually for 7–14 days, can also be used in the diagnosis of food allergy. Their success depends on identifying the correct allergen and completely eliminating all forms of the allergen from the diet. Elimination diets used alone, however, are rarely diagnostic of food allergy.

Laboratory assessment of food allergy includes measuring food-specific IgE in the serum, which provides information similar to prick skin tests but is less specific.[82] Basophil histamine release assays have not been shown conclusively to be a reproducible diagnostic test for food allergy.[9] The clinical utility of these assays remains controversial, and they have been limited mainly to research settings. Objective measures have been noted during intragastric provocation with food allergens under endoscopy,[83] but confirmatory studies are needed.

The double-blind placebo-controlled food challenge is considered the "gold standard" for diagnosing food allergies and adverse reactions to food additives.[28,29,80,81,84,85] Such challenges should be conducted in a clinic or hospital setting, especially if an IgE-mediated reaction is suspected; trained personnel and equipment for treating systemic anaphylaxis must be present.[86] A published guide reviewed the combined experience of six centers doing blinded challenges and highlighted useful information such as preparing challenges, scoring reactions, and blinding methods.[87] In brief, suspected foods are eliminated and antihistamines are discontinued for 1–2 weeks before the challenge. A system for scoring clinical symptoms and appropriate emergency medical equipment to treat anaphylaxis are necessary. The food challenge substance, blinded in either liquid or a safe food, is administered to the fasting subject, and the dose (500 mg) is doubled every 15–60 minutes. Once 10 g of the challenge substance has been tolerated, clinical reactivity is ruled out. All negative, blinded food challenges must be confirmed by an open feeding of the food prepared as usual. Foods unlikely to provoke allergic reactions (negative history and negative skin test) may be screened with open, nonblinded challenges.

The diagnostic value of food-specific IgG or IgG4 antibody concentrations and food antigen-antibody complexes is not supported by objective evidence. A carefully controlled trial of subcutaneous provocation and neutralization clearly demonstrated a lack of efficacy for this method.[88]

In summary, a thorough medical history supplemented by skin test or RAST data, an appropriate exclusion diet, and blinded food challenges all contribute to the diagnostic evaluation of food allergy. A presumptive diagnosis of food allergy based on history and skin test or RAST alone is not acceptable. If no foods are implicated

in the history and if prick skin tests are negative, further work-up for IgE-mediated allergy is generally not indicated. With positive skin tests or symptoms associated with food, an elimination diet may be tried for 7–14 days. If symptoms persist, food is not likely to be the problem, except possibly in atopic dermatitis or chronic asthma. Symptoms recurring after a regular diet is resumed should be evaluated with a double-blind placebo-controlled food challenge after a short list of most likely foods is identified.

Treatment

Strict elimination of the responsible food allergen or food additive is the only proven therapy for food hypersensitivity.[4,28,39,84] Restriction diets should exclude only foods proven to provoke food allergy.[28,36,39] A properly managed elimination diet can lead to resolution of food reaction problems and avoid malnutrition and other undesirable outcomes.[89,90] Educating parents about the words commonly used on food labels for the allergen of concern (e.g., for milk: casein and whey) is crucial and will help in avoiding ingestion of hidden ingredients.[91,92] Diet counseling will ensure a balanced elimination diet, provide appropriate substitutes for avoided allergens, and help to prevent anticipated deficiencies, such as calcium deficiency in a milk-elimination diet. Diet sheets or pocket-sized cards are also useful references for food-allergic patients.[91] Finally, the Food Allergy Network (Fairfax, VA) is a lay organization that serves as a resource to patients with food allergies and their families, caretakers, physicians, and other health care providers.

Milk protein hydrolysates are available for use by infants with cow milk hypersensitivity. These formulas have provided safe substitutes for patients allergic to cow milk and soy. Several casein hydrolysates have been tested in milk-allergic patients and are labeled hypoallergenic on the basis of clinical data as well as the final size of protein after hydrolysis.[93] There have been only a few reports of isolated reactions to casein hydrolysate formulas.[94,95] Use of an amino acid–based nutritionally complete formula has provided another alternative for these clinical situations.[96] Finally, oral cromolyn sodium has been extensively studied as a potential therapy for adverse food reactions, but the results are conflicting.[97,98]

The influence of dietary manipulation on the incidence of food allergy has been studied extensively. In one study of prophylaxis, the introduction of solids to atopy-prone infants in the first 6 months of life increased the prevalence of atopic dermatitis and food hypersensitivity at 2 years of age.[99] In a large prospective study of infants at high risk for developing atopic disease, maternal and infant avoidance of major allergenic foods (cow milk, egg, and peanut) resulted in a decreased prevalence of atopic dermatitis and cow milk allergy compared with infants who did not avoid the same major food allergens.[100] The ultimate development of rhinitis or asthma does not seem to be affected by these dietary changes.[100,101]

Natural History

Several themes have emerged regarding the natural history of adverse reactions to foods and food additives. Prolonged elimination of food is usually unnecessary because children often "outgrow" food allergy, even severe reactions. One study of adverse reactions to foods reported that 80% of confirmed symptoms occurred in the first year of life[7] and that almost all of the patients returned to a normal diet by age 3 years. Another group reported that 80-90% of cow milk allergy appearing in infancy was lost before age 3 years.[11] Those with early IgE sensitization were more prone to have persistent milk sensitivity and to develop allergies to other foods and inhalants. Key factors involved in the development of tolerance include the food antigen involved[28,102,103] and the ability to completely restrict the allergen in the diet.[103,104] Overall, approximately one-third of children and adults lose their clinical reactivity after 1–2 years of allergen avoidance.[84] Unfortunately, allergies to peanut, tree nuts, fish, and shellfish rarely appear to be "outgrown."[102,105]

Conclusions

Specific terminology and controlled studies have helped distinguish food hypersensitivity from food intolerance and have provided a better overall understanding of adverse food reactions. The main clinical manifestations have been confirmed by several investigators, and new insights into reactions precipitated by foods and food additives have been reported. Blinded food challenges remain the diagnostic tool of choice for food hypersensitivity, and strict elimination of the responsible food remains the only proven therapy. Future investigations should provide a better understanding of these reactions.

Acknowledgments

I wish to thank Hugh A. Sampson, M.D., for his insightful direction during my fellowship training at Johns Hopkins Hospital and A. Wesley Burks, M.D., for his support and encouragement during my academic experience at the Arkansas Children's Hospital.

References

1. Prausnitz C, Küstner H (1921) Studies on supersensitivity. Centralbl Bakteriol 86:160–161

2. Anderson JA (1994) Milestones marking the knowledge of adverse reactions to food in the decade of the 1980s. Ann Allergy 72:143–154

3. American Academy of Allergy and Immunology, National Institute of Allergy and Infectious Diseases; Anderson JA, Sogn DD (eds)(1984) Adverse reactions to foods. NIH Publication 84-2442. National Institutes of Health, Bethesda, MD, pp 1–6

4. Sampson HA (1989) Food allergy. J Allergy Clin Immunol 84:1062–1067

5. Sloan AE, Powers ME (1986) A perspective on popular perceptions of adverse reactions to foods. J Allergy Clin Immunol 78:127–133

6. Niestijl Jansen JJ, Kardinaal AFM, Huijbers G, et al (1994) Prevalence of food allergy and intolerance in the adult Dutch population. J Allergy Clin Immunol 93:446–456

7. Bock SA (1987) Prospective appraisal of complaints of adverse reactions to foods in children during the first 3 years of life. Pediatrics 79:683–688

8. Kajosaari M (1982) Food allergy in Finnish children aged 1 to 6 years. Acta Pediatr Scand 71:815–819

9. James JM, Sampson HA (1992) An overview of food hypersensitivity. Pediatr Allergy Immunol 3:67–78

10. Hide DW, Guyer BM (1983) Cow's milk intolerance in Isle of Wright. Br J Clin Prac 37:285–287

11. Host A, Halken S (1990) A prospective study of cow milk allergy in Danish infants during the first 3 years of life. Allergy 45:587–596

12. Schrander JJP, van den Bogart JPH, Forget PP, et al (1993) Cow's milk protein intolerance in infants under 1 year of age: a prospective epidemiology. Eur J Pediatr 152:640–644

13. Walzer M (1941) Allergy of the abdominal organs. J Lab Clin Med 26:1867–1877

14. Gearhart PJ, Cebra JJ (1979) Differentiated B-lymphocytes: potential to express particular antibody variable and constant regions depends on site of lymphoid tissue and antigen load. J Exp Med 149:216–227

15. Kleinman RE, Walker A (1979) The enteromammary immune system: an important new concept in breast milk host defense. Dig Dis Sci 24:876–882

16. Johansson SGO, Dannaeus A, Lilha G (1984) The relevance of anti-food antibodies for the diagnosis of food allergy. Ann Allergy 53:665–672

17. Morgan JE, Daul CB, Lehrer SB (1990) The relationships among shrimp-specific IgG subclass antibodies and immediate adverse reactions to shrimp challenge. J Allergy Clin Immunol 86:387–392

18. James JM, Sampson HA (1992) Immunologic changes associated with the development of tolerance in children with cow's milk allergy. J Pediatr 121:371–377

19. Paganelli R, Levinsky RJ, Brostoff J, et al (1979) Immune complexes containing food proteins in normal and atopic subjects after oral challenge and effect of sodium cromoglycate on antigen absorption. Lancet 1:1270–1272

20. Paganelli R, Quiti I, D'Offizi GP, et al (1987) Immune-complexes in food allergy: a critical reappraisal. Ann Allergy 59:157–161

21. Falth-Magnusson K, Kjellman NIM, Magnusson KE (1988) Antibodies IgG, IgA, and IgM to food antigens during the first 18 months of life in relation to feeding and development of atopic disease. J Allergy Clin Immunol 81: 743–749

22. Kemeny DM, Urbanek R, Amlot PL, et al (1986) Sub-class of IgG in allergic disease. I. IgG sub-class antibodies in immediate and non-immediate food allergy. Clin Allergy 16:571–581

23. Kondo N, Fukutomi O, Agata H, et al (1993) The role of T

lymphocytes in patients with food-sensitive atopic dermatitis. J Allergy Clin Immunol 86:253–260

24. Lemanske RF, Kaliner MA. (1988) Late-phase allergic reactions. In Middleton RE, Reed CE, Ellis EF, et al (eds), Allergy: principles and practice. CV Mosby, St. Louis, pp 12–30

25. Sampson HA, Jolie PL (1984) Increased plasma histamine concentrations after food challenges in children with atopic dermatitis. N Engl J Med 311:372–376

26. Sampson HA, Broadbent KR, Bernhisel–Broadbent J (1989) Spontaneous release of histamine from basophils and histamine-releasing factor in patients with atopic dermatitis and food hypersensitivity. N Engl J Med 321:228–232

27. Lemanske RF, Taylor SL (1987) Standardized extracts, foods. Clin Rev Allergy 5:23–36

28. Bock SA, Atkins FM (1990) Patterns of food hypersensitivity during sixteen years of double-blind placebo-controlled oral food challenges. J Pediatr 117:561–567

29. Burks AW, Mallory SB, Williams LW, Shirrell MA (1988) Atopic dermatitis: clinical relevance of food hypersensitivity reactions. J Pediatr 113:447–451

30. Holen E, Elsayed S (1990) Characterization of four major allergens of hen egg white by IEF/SDS-PAGE combined with electrophoretic transfer and IgE-immunoautoradiography. Int Arch Allergy Appl Immunol 91:136–141

31. Savilahti E (1981) Cow's milk allergy. Allergy 36:73–88

32. Swaisgood HE (1982) Chemistry of milk protein. In Fox PF (ed), Developments in dairy chemistry—1. Applied Science, London, pp 1–59

33. Bleumink E, Young E (1968) Identification of the atopic allergen in cow's milk. Int Arch Allergy 34:521–543

34. Burks AW, Williams LW, Helm RM, et al (1991) Identification of a major peanut allergen, Ara h I, in patients with atopic dermatitis and positive peanut challenges. J Allergy Clin Immunol 88:172–179

35. Burks AW, Williams LW, Connaughton C, et al (1992) Identification and characterization of a second major peanut allergen, Ara h II, with use of sera of patients with atopic dermatitis and positive peanut challenges. J Allergy Clin Immunol 90:962–969

36. Bernhisel-Broadbent J, Sampson HA (1989) Cross-allergenicity in the legume botanical family in children with food hypersensitivity. J Allergy Clin Immunol 83:435–440

37. O'Neil C, Helbling AA, Lehrer SB (1993) Allergic reactions to fish. Clin Rev Allergy 11:183–200

38. Daul CB, Slattery M, Lehrer SB (1993) Shared antigenic/allergenic epitopes between shrimp Pen a I and fruit fly extract [abstract]. J Allergy Clin Immunol 91:341

39. Sampson HA, McCaskill CM (1985) Food hypersensitivity and atopic dermatitis: evaluation of 113 patients. J Pediatr 107:669–675

40. Weber RW (1993) Food additives and allergy. Ann Allergy 70:183–192

41. Bernhisel-Broadbent J, Sampson HA. (1992) Fish hypersensitivity. I. In vitro and oral challenge results in fish allergic patients. J Allergy Clin Immunol 89:730–737

42. Bernhisel-Broadbent J, Sampson HA (1992) Fish hypersensitivity. II. Clinical relevance of altered fish allergenicity caused by various preparation methods. J Allergy Clin Immunol 90:622–629

43. Jones SM, Cooke SK, Sampson HA (1993) Immunologic cross-reactivity among cereal grains and grasses in children with food hypersensitivity [abstract]. J Allergy Clin Immunol 91:343

44. Enberg RN, Leickly FE, McCullough J, et al (1987) Watermelon and ragweed share allergens. J Allergy Clin Immunol 79:867–875

45. Calkhoven PG, Aalbers M, Koshte VL, et al (1987) Cross-reactivity among birch pollen, vegetables and fruits as detected by IgE antibodies is due to at least three distinct cross-reactive structures. Allergy 42:382–390

46. Ortaloni C, Ispano M, Pastorello EA, et al (1989) Comparison of results of skin prick tests (with fresh foods and commercial food extracts) and RAST in 100 patients with oral allergy syndrome. J Allergy Clin Immunol 83:683–690

47. Slater JE (1994) Latex allergy. J Allergy Clin Immunol 94:139–150

48. Mowat AM (1987) The regulation of immune responses to dietary protein antigens. Immunol Today 8:93–98

49. Bruce MG, Ferguson A (1986) Oral tolerance to ovalbumin in mice: studies of chemically modified and "biologically filtered" antigen. Immunology 57:627–630

50. Burgio GR, Lanzavecchia A, Plebani A, et al (1980) Ontogeny of secretory immunity: levels of secretory IgA and natural antibodies in saliva. Pediatr Res 14:1111–1114

51. Champion RH, Roberts SO, Carpenter RG, Roger JH (1969) Urticaria and angioedema: a review of 554 patients. Br J Dermatol 81:588–597

52. Bock SA (1991) Food hypersensitivity. In Fireman P, Slavin RG (eds), Atlas of allergies. Lippincott, Philadelphia, pp 13.2–13.12

53. Kettlehut BV, Metcalfe DD (1988) Adverse reactions to foods. In Middleton E, Reed CE, Ellis EF, et al (eds), Allergy: principles and practice. CV Mosby, St Louis, pp 1481–1502

54. Jakobsson I, Lindberg T (1983) Cow's milk proteins cause infantile colic in breast-fed infants: a double-blind crossover study. Pediatrics 71:268–271

55. Lothe L, Lindberg T (1989) Cow's milk whey protein elicits symptoms of infantile colic in colicky formula-fed infants: a double-blind crossover study. Pediatrics 83:262–266

56. Forsyth BWC (1989) Colic and the effect of changing formulas: a double-blind multiple-crossover study. J Pediatr 115:521–526

57. Clyne PS, Kulczycki A (1991) Human breast milk contains bovine IgG: relationship to infant colic. Pediatrics 87:439–444

58. Sampson HA (1989) Infantile colic and food allergy: fact or fiction. J Pediatr 115:583–584

59. James JM, Bernhisel-Broadbent J, Sampson HA (1994) Respiratory reactions provoked by double-blind food challenges in children. Am J Respir Crit Care Med 149:59–64

60. Novembre E, de Martino M, Vierucci A (1988) Foods and respiratory allergy. J Allergy Clin Immunol 81:1059–1065.

61. Silverman M, Wilson N. Clinical physiology of food intolerance in asthma. In Reed CE (ed), Proceedings of the XIIth International Congress of Allergology and Clinical Immmunology. CV Mosby, St Louis, pp 457–462

62. Zwetchkenbaum JF, Skufca R, Nelson HS (1991) An examination of food hypersensitivity as a cause of increased bronchial responsiveness to inhaled methacholine. J Allergy Clin Immunol 88:360–364

63. Sampson HA, James JM (1992) Respiratory reactions induced by food challenges in children with eczema. Pediatr Allergy Immunol 3:195–200

64. Yunginger JW, Sweeney KG, Sturner WQ, et al (1988) Fatal food-induced anaphylaxis. J Am Med Assoc 260:1450–1452

65. Sampson HA, Mendelson L, Rosen JP (1992) Fatal and near-fatal food anaphylaxis reactions in children. N Engl J Med 327:380–384

66. James JM, Burks AW (1995) Food-induced anaphylaxis. Immunol Clin North Am 15:477–488

67. Dohi M, Suko M, Sugiyama H, et al (1991) Food-dependent, exercise-induced anaphylaxis: a study on 11 Japanese cases. J Allergy Clin Immunol 87:34–40

68. Novey HS (1993) Exercise-induced asthma and anaphylaxis. West J Med 158:613

69. Taylor SL, Bush RK, Nordlee JA (1991) In Metcalfe DD, Sampson HA, Simon RA (eds), Food allergy: adverse reactions to foods and food additives. Blackwell Scientific, Boston, pp 332–354

70. Bosso JV, Simon RA (1991) Urticaria, angioedema, and anaphylaxis provoked by food additives. In Metcalfe DD, Sampson HA, Simon RA (eds), Food allergy: adverse reactions to foods and food additives. Blackwell Scientific, Boston, pp 288–300

71. Taylor SL, Bush RK, Selner JC, et al (1988) Sensitivity to sulfited foods among sulfite-sensitive subjects with asthma. J Allergy Clin Immunol 81:1159–1167

72. Garriga MM, Berkebile C, Metcalfe DD (1991) A combined single-blind, double-blind, placebo-controlled study to determine the reproducibility of hypersensitivity reactions to aspartame. J Allergy Clin Immunol 87:821–827

73. Bock SA, Sampson HA (1994) Food allergy in infancy. Pediatr Clin North Am 41:1047–1067

74. Powell GK (1978) Milk and soy induced enterocolitis of infancy: clinical features and standardization of challenge. J Pediatr 93:553–560

75. Jenkins HR, Pincott JR, Soothill JG, et al (1984) Food allergy: the major cause of infantile colitis. Arch Dis Child 59:326–329

76. Fireman P (1991) Immunology of allergic disorders. In Fireman P, Slavin RG (eds), Atlas of allergies. Lippincott, Philadelphia, pp 1.2–1.24

77. Sampson HA. (1986) Differential diagnosis in adverse reactions to foods. J Allergy Clin Immunol 78:212–219

78. Bock SA, Lee W-Y, Remigio LK, et al (1978) Studies of hypersensitivity reactions to foods in infants and children. J Allergy Clin Immunol 62:327–334

79. Bock SA, Buckley J, Holst A, May CD (1978) Proper use of skin tests with food extracts in diagnosis of food hypersensitivity. Clin Allergy 8:559–564

80. Sampson HA (1983) Role of immediate food hypersensitivity in the pathogenesis of atopic dermatitis. J Allergy Clin Immunol 71:473–480

81. Atkins FM, Steinberg SS, Metcalfe DD (1985) Evaluation of immediate adverse reactions to foods in adult patients. I. Correlation on demographic, laboratory, and prick skin test data with response to controlled oral food challenge. J Allergy Clin Immunol 75:348–355

82. Wraith DG, Merret J, Roth A, et al (1979) Recognition of food-allergic patients and their allergens by the RAST technique and clinical investigation. Clin Allergy 9:25–36

83. Reimann HJ, Ring J, Ultsch B, Wendt P. (1985) Intragastric provocation under endoscopic control (IPEC) in food allergy: mast cell and histamine changes in gastric mucosa. Clin Allergy 15:195–202

84. Pastorello EA, Stocchi L, Pravetonni V, et al (1989) Role of the elimination diet in adults with food allergy. J Allergy Clin Immunol 84:475–483

85. Sampson HA. (1988) Immunologically mediated food allergy: the importance of food challenge procedures. Ann Allergy 60:262–269

86. Executive Committee of the Academy of Allergy and Immunology (1986) Personnel and equipment to treat systemic reactions caused by immunotherapy with allergic extracts. J Allergy Clin Immunol 77:271–273

87. Bock SA, Sampson HA, Atkins FM, et al (1988) Double-blind placebo-controlled food challenge as an office procedure: a manual. J Allergy Clin Immunol 82:986–997

88. Jewett DL, Gein G, Greenberg MH (1990) A double-blind study of symptom provocation to determine food sensitivity. N Engl J Med 323:429–433

89. Lloyd-Still JD (1979) Chronic diarrhea of childhood and the misuse of elimination diets. J Pediatr 95:10–13

90. David TJ, Waddington E, Stanton RHJ (1984) Nutritional hazards of elimination diets in children with atopic dermatitis. Arch Dis Child 59:323–325

91. Barnes-Koerner C, Sampson HA (1991) Diets and nutrition in food allergy. In Metcalfe DD, Sampson HA, Simon RA (eds), Food allergy: adverse reactions to foods and food additives. Blackwell Scientific Publications, Boston, pp 332–354

92. Gern J, Sampson HA (1991) Allergic reactions to milk-contaminated "nondairy" products. N Engl J Med 324:976–979

93. Drebord S, Bjorksten B, Sampson HA (1993) Use of hydrolyzed cow's milk formulae for prevention of early sensitization and signs of atopy must be further documented [editorial]. Pediatr Allergy Immunol 4:99–100

94. Bock SA (1990) Probable allergic reaction to casein hydrolysate formula. J Allergy Clin Immunol 84:272

95. Saylor JD, Bahna SL (1991) Anaphylaxis to casein hydrolysate formula. J Pediatr 118:71–74

96. Sampson HA, James JM, Bernhisel-Broadbent J (1992) Safety of an amino acid-derived infant formula in children allergic to cow milk. Pediatrics 40:463–465

97. Sogn DD (1986) Medications and their use in the treatment of adverse reactions to foods. J Allergy Clin Immunol 78:238–243

98. Burks AW, Sampson HA (1988) Double-blind placebo-controlled trial of oral cromolyn in children with atopic dermatitis and documented food hypersensitivity. J Allergy Clin Immunol 81: 417–423

99. Kajosaari M, Saarinen UM (1983) Prophylaxis of atopic disease by six months' total solid food elimination. Arch Paediatr Scand 72:411–414

100. Zeiger RS, Heller S, Mellon MH, et al (1989) Effect of combined maternal and infant food-allergen avoidance on development of atopy in early infancy: a randomized study. J Allergy Clin Immunol 84:72–89

101. Hill DJ, Hosking CS (1993) Preventing childhood allergy. Med J Aust 158:367–369

102. Bock SA, Atkins FM (1989) The natural history of peanut allergy. J Allergy Clin Immunol 83:900–904

103. Sampson HA, Scanlon SM (1989) Natural history of food hypersensitivity in children with atopic dermatitis. J Pediatr 115:23–27

104. Businco L, Benincori N, Cantani A, et al (1985) Chronic diarrhea due to cow's milk allergy: a 4- to 10- year follow-up study. Ann Allergy 55:844–847

105. Daul CB, Morgan JE, Lehrer SB (1990) The natural history of shrimp hypersensitivity. J Allergy Clin Immunol 86:88–93

Chapter 62

Nutrient Status and Central Nervous System Function

John Beard

The main emphasis of this chapter is on the effects of selected nutrient deficiency states on central nervous system (CNS) function and development. Of necessity, coverage of the topic is often superficial, but the approach will focus on building the associations of nutrient status, nutrient function in brain development and maintenance, and sequelae when the proper amount of nutrient is unavailable. The specific nutrients addressed are those that have the highest prevalence of deficiency states in the world. The model of organization includes function, location, and consequences as we understand them at this time.

Iron

Function. The topic of iron deficiency and cognitive functioning has been the focus of a number of reviews in the recent past.[1-4] The rate at which individual tissues and cellular organelles within those tissues develop a true deficit in iron depends on the rate of turnover of these iron-containing proteins, the intracellular mechanisms for recycling iron, and the rate of delivery of iron to tissue from the plasma pool.[5] Manifestations of depletion of body iron are readily apparent. Besides anemia, there are significant decreases in mitochondrial iron-sulfur content, in mitochondrial cytochrome content, and in total mitochondrial oxidative capacity.[5-8] Iron is not only an essential element and important nutrient, but also a potent toxin. Thus, an elegant system has evolved that regulates the delivery of iron to brain cells and has as its best-known components transferrin and its receptor. Iron is an essential component of a number of general cellular functions as well as functions more specific to neurological activity, such as the synthesis of dopamine, serotonin, catecholamines, and possibly γ-aminobutyric acid (GABA) and myelin formation.[9-12] When iron is stored, it is incorporated into ferritin with a heterogeneous distribution in the brain by both region and cell type.[1]

There is sparse documentation of iron-dependent electron transport alterations in the brain due to iron defi-

ciency; it appears that the brain is partially protected from the effects of nutritional iron deprivation, although it has been found that there is still a profound decrease in brain iron content of young rats deprived of iron.[13] There is little information regarding the developmental aspects of brain iron deprivation on neurological dysfunction; however, investigators have noted that the reduction in brain iron is irreversible with later refeeding of iron in adulthood.[13-16]

Iron is a cofactor for tyrosine hydroxylase, tryptophan hydroxylase, xanthine oxidase, and ribonucleoside reductase.[17] Thus, the expectation would be that nutritional iron deficiency would lead to decreased activities of these enzymes. This is not the consistent observation, however. When brain iron levels were reduced by as much as 40% by dietary restriction in postweanling rats, there was no change in the activity of tyrosine hydroxylase, tryptophan hydroxylase, monoamine oxidase, succinate hydroxylase, or cytochrome c oxidase.[18,19] Other studies showed that whole-brain concentrations of norepinephrine and dopamine were unaltered by iron deficiency while concentrations of serotonin and 5-hydroxyindoleacetic acid were decreased.[19-21] More recently, in vivo microdialysis has been used by our laboratory to demonstrate that caudate putamen interstitial dopamine and norepinephrine are significantly elevated in awake, freely moving, iron-deficient rats.[22]

Location. The highest levels of iron in the brain are found in the basal ganglia, but iron is found throughout the brain, including the white matter.[23] Indeed, both biochemical and histochemical studies reveal white matter throughout the brain as a major site of iron concentration.[24-28] Iron uptake into the brain is maximal during the period of rapid brain growth, which coincides with the peak of myelinogenesis.[29-32] However, iron uptake into the brain continues throughout life.[33,34] This iron uptake is reportedly homogeneous, followed by a redistribution to the basal ganglia.[35] The mechanism of transport of iron within the CNS is not understood; both transferrin-mediated and axoplasmic flow have been suggested. There is at least one observation in the literature that suggests that cerebrospinal fluid iron concentration exceeds that of the iron-binding capacity of the transferrin present in this fluid.[36] Thus, other proteins may play a role in iron transport in the brain, as they do in the placenta, but the exact nature of these nontransferrin iron transport proteins is unknown. Transferrin immunostaining is generally absent in neurons following colchicine treatment.[37] An intracellular transport mechanism for iron may not involve transferrin. Questions concerning iron transport and accumulation in basal ganglia are important clinical considerations because iron accumulation in this brain region is reportedly associated with a number of disease states such as Alzheimer's disease, multiple sclerosis, and Parkinson's disease.[38]

Dallman and coworkers[39,40] demonstrated two decades ago that young rats deprived of iron in early postnatal life have significantly lower (27%) whole-brain iron contents than controls 28 days postnatally; they were quite resistant to restoration of their normal complement of brain iron (still 20% lower) despite aggressive dietary repletion for 45 days.[39,40] This finding is in contrast to the prompt normalization of hepatic iron content and hemoglobin concentration. The regional distribution of iron and responsiveness of various brain regions to iron nutritional states in these conditions have not been documented and remain underexplored. Magnetic resonance imaging has recently been used to map the distribution of iron in brains of children and adolescents.[41] The highest concentrations are found in the globus pallidus, caudate nucleus, putamen, and substantia nigra; substantially lower concentrations are found in the cortex and cerebellum.

The involvement of iron in neurological disease, particularly as it relates to oxidative damage, is receiving increasing attention. Recently, data were presented on the brain iron content of postmortem brains of individuals who had Parkinson's disease.[38] Total iron was increased 176% and ferric iron increased 255% in the substantia nigra, but there were no changes in the cortex, hippocampus, putamen, or globus pallidus. The timing of this acquisition of iron by the brain is unknown.

Consequences. Iron deficiency is the most common single-nutrient deficiency disease in the world and is a major concern for approximately 15% of the world's population.[42–44] The World Health Organization estimates that 1.3 billion people are anemic, with iron deficiency as the causal agent in many cases. Perhaps as many as 40–45% of children are iron-deficient and anemic. Recent reviews have covered the growing research area relating iron nutrition to cognition and behavior.[1–4,45,46] The studies reviewed demonstrate a consistency in the observation that iron-deficient children have alterations in attention span, lower intelligence scores, and some

degree of perceptual disturbance. Although there is some reason to believe that the relationship of iron to cognition is developmentally linked, some studies have shown alterations in brain functions in adults with variations in iron status. The biochemical alterations that occur in the brains of children with chronic iron deficiency may also occur in adults in similar fashion as in children, but this also remains unexplored. Oski et al.[47] first observed increases in urinary norepinephrine in iron-deficient infants 9–26 months of age. These children also had significantly lower psychomotor Bayley scores than controls. Both the Bayley scores and urine catecholamine excretions were normalized after a short period of iron treatment.

Studies in older children have shown decreased attentiveness, narrow attention spans, and perceptual restriction.[48–50] Lozoff and colleagues[48–50] observed a significant impact of anemia on affective behavior. Low affect in iron-deficient children was significantly related to poor performance on the Bayley Mental Index (BMI) in the model proposed by these investigators. Infants were considered abnormal in affect if their infant behavior records showed at least two of the following patterns: withdrawal from or hesitance with the examiner, unhappiness all or part of the session, easy fatigability or restlessness, and increased body tension. With moderate anemia, many of the children were considered to have abnormal affective behavior. In severe anemia (<9 g/dL), all of the children were classified as abnormal. Lozoff et al.[50] argued that the significantly greater amount of close contact between anemic child and mother is a manifestation of affect, energy, and activity. Their Costa Rican studies and those of Walter and coworkers[51,52] in Chile noted a failure to improve performance in many of the anemic children with active iron therapy despite prompt hematologic response and normalization. In addition, children with storage iron depletion, but no anemia, showed no measurable behavioral abnormalities.

In a treatment trial with older children or adolescents, investigators demonstrated a decreased efficiency in visual discrimination tests that was significantly improved with oral iron therapy.[53–55] An important point, however, is that the cognitive domains tested by these achievement-oriented tests are far different from the developmental constructions applied to infants.[46] More recently, Idjradinata and Pollitt[54] demonstrated that the cognitive deficits in iron deficiency can be reversed with iron supplementation in infants. This finding, which needs to be verified in other populations, provides evidence that in some settings cognitive deficits are not always permanent.

Iron excess. The involvement of iron in neurological disease, particularly as it relates to oxidative damage, is receiving increasing attention. This is partly because of the aging of the U.S. population. One aspect of the concern about a possible increase in iron status is its possible relationship to oxidative pathologies, such as cardiovascular disease, aging, and brain abnormalities.[1,3,57]

Brain dysfunction in patients with Alzheimer's disease may relate to iron content since iron is a significant component of senile plaques, and iron encrustation of brain blood vessels in Alzheimer's disease is a common observation.[3,58] Iron levels are elevated in brains of patients with Alzheimer's disease in the hippocampus, amygdala, nucleus basalis of Meynert, and the cerebral cortex.[59,60] By virtue of its reactive ability with hydrogen peroxide and oxygen, high amounts of iron can initiate lipid peroxidation, leading to membrane damage and ultimately cell death.[60,61] A decrease in cell membrane fluidity within the CNS is considered part of the pathogenesis of aging, and an increase in free radical production has been demonstrated in Alzheimer's disease brain tissue.[3,58]

Iodine

Function. On a worldwide basis, iodine deficiency is as prevalent as iron deficiency. Iodine deficiency leads to a dramatic impairment in brain development when it occurs in utero.[62,63] More than 70% of the body's iodine content is concentrated in the thyroid gland and is associated with the various iodoproteins that comprise the storage or precursor forms and the secreted forms of thyroid hormone, thyroxine and triiodothyronine. The thyroid hormones are essential for proper brain development and functioning. Lack of sufficient thyroid hormone for the brain during fetal and early postnatal development leads to permanent neurological damage.[63–64] Fetal hypothyroidism is associated with alterations in neurotransmitter metabolism as evidenced by a decrease in protein kinase C, ornithine decarboxylase, choline acetyltransferase, and dihydroxyphenylaline decarboxylase.[64]

Location. The defects are located largely in the cerebral cortical association areas, basal ganglia, and motor control pathways.[65,66] There is a decrease in the number of neurons, an irregular arrangement of cells, larger ventricles, and decreases in numbers of dendrites from pyramidal cells in the cortical motor area.[66,67] Thyroid hormones are essential for normal neuroblastogenesis; especially affected are the interhemispheric connections of the anterior commissure, corpus callosum, and callosal connections.[68,69] A decrease in thyroid hormone during development leads to a decrease in the maturation of the commissural axons, with only partial reversibility. When severely iodine-deficient pregnant ewes were given a single injection of iodized oil, there was a rapid restoration of the number of axons and the amount of myelination in both cerebellum and cerebral hemispheres.[70] There was, however, persistence of a lower density of synapses in the cortex. Thus, a critical period of nutritional insult is present and not all alterations in function are reversible when iodine restoration occurs after a certain point in time. A role for iodide apart from its functioning in thyroid hormone is uncertain. Thus, it is the deficiency in thyroid hormones secondary to iodine deficiency that leads to alterations in CNS function.[64]

In iodine deficiency there is an upregulation of the Type II 5'-deiodinase enzyme in brain and in other tissues in an attempt to maintain local concentrations of the active hormone triiodothyronine.[71] This mechanism of local triiodothyronine production from thyroxine appears to reach a maximum at 15–18 weeks of gestational age in cerebral cortex and corresponds to the timing of peak neuroblastogenesis. Iodine deficiency in rats leads to an increase in deiodinase activity in pituitary, cerebellum, brain stem, and cortex of adult rats but not in hypothalmus.[72] The increase in cortex Type II deiodinase activity is in response to hypothyroidism.[73,74] The production of this triiodothyronine appears to be neuronal but is not strictly developmentally dependent.

DeLong and others[64] make a convincing argument that, given the timing of the neurodevelopmental alterations (10–18 weeks gestational age), the onset of fetal thyroid function (12–20 weeks gestational age), and the appearance of thyroid receptors in the brain at 10 weeks, an especially critical period for iodine deficiency is during the second and third trimesters of human gestation. Thus, maternal thyroid and iodine status are significant determinants of fetal brain development.[75] There is a negative correlation between severity of maternal iodine deficiency and outcome of pregnancy with regard to either stillbirth or cretinism.[76–78] In iodine deficiency, there is evidence that the fetal thyroid is not able to compensate for this lack of maternal thyroxine despite the attempt of the fetal brain to increase local triiodothyronine production through the cortical Type II deiodinase.

Consequences. Neurological cretinism is characterized by mental deficiency, deafness, mutism, and motor disorders accompanied by basal ganglia calcification in some patients with severe hypothyroidism.[79–81] In extreme cases, there are reports of autism and muscle wasting.[63,64] There is a characteristic cochlear lesion, and while exhaustive pathological studies are not available, there are suggestions of alterations in medial temporal structures, the hippocampus, and the amygdala. The duration and timing of the hypothyroidism during development may be critical in determining the extent of the severity of symptoms. Recently, the timing of the nutritional insult was examined in an intervention trial in China with staging of iodine administration at each trimester and at each year for 3 years of postnatal life.[82] Treatment later than the second trimester improved brain growth and developmental achievement, but did not improve neurological status. While the clinical sequalae of iodine deficiency in later stages of development are classically defined as goiter with complications (hypothyroidism), there are reports of impaired mental function in these adults and adolescents.[83] The clear causal relationship is lacking, as specific tests that focus on visual or auditory acuity, primary or secondary memory, processing, and attention were not reported. Thus, while we characterize patients with hypothyroidism as having a certain degree of "apathy" and lassitude, the biological explanation is lacking.

Intervention projects of many forms have been attempted throughout the world, and the elimination of iodine deficiency remains a high priority for the international nutrition community.[84]

Protein-Energy Malnutrition

Function. The developing nervous system of the young child is vulnerable to a shortage of protein and calories when these nutrients become limiting either in utero or postnatally.[85] As noted in the cited review, in the real world it is unlikely that protein-energy malnutrition (PEM) occurs without concurrent micronutrient deficiency states; thus, the assignment of specific alterations in brain or CNS function to PEM is very difficult. Nonetheless, some generalizations can be ventured. Protein-energy malnutrition is associated with a decrease in total brain lipid, cholesterol, phospholipid, and ganglioside.[86–88] Sastry[88] also reported that increased lipid peroxidation contributed to a 27% decrease in myelin. As would be expected, there is decreased DNA and RNA content throughout the brain as cell growth and differentiation are slowed in PEM.[89] Neurotransmitter alterations in the GABAergic, monoaminergic, and serotoninergic systems have all been reported.[88,90–92] While the specifics of these alterations are often unclear, they are likely related to alterations in membrane characteristics, receptor expression, and energy-dependent processes of ion transport.[93] Of recent interest is the possibility of alterations in the excitatory amino acids such as glutamate.[85] While not explicitly examined in the current literature, it is likely that the excitatory amino acids are dramatically altered by PEM. Structural, organizational, and ongoing functions are all likely to be affected by PEM; the timing of the insult, its duration, and the vigor of refeeding will determine the reversibility of these alterations.[85]

Location. The impact of PEM is felt in most of the CNS during early development, although the most recognizable alterations are in cortical regions. Neuromuscular dysfunction is a common sign in both kwashiorkor and marasmus, suggesting both motor neuron effects and sensory nerve defects. There is a 40–50% decrease in nerve conduction velocity, a marked demyelination in peripheral nerves, myelin sheath folding, and axonal shrinkage in PEM.[94,95] In one study, the diameter of myelinated fibers was smaller and less dense in malnourished animals than controls.[96] Much of the damage is in the neocortex and cerebellum, with hippocampus also implicated.[97] The number of myelinating fibers usually increases about fourfold between birth and 5 years of age in healthy growing children. This process is limited in PEM. Glial multiplication and neuronal growth and differentiation are sensitive to limiting effects of PEM between 13 weeks of gestational age and year 1 or 2 of postnatal life. A failure to provide sufficient protein or calories or both during these periods leads to gross morphological changes.[85]

Consequences. The important events of cell growth, migration, dendritic arborization, myelination, and synaptogenesis can all be negatively affected by PEM, with resulting alterations in motor control, learning capacity, and mental functioning.[85,97] Apathy, irritability, attention deficit, and poor tertiary memory are a part of the functional consequences associated with early-life PEM.[98–101] Galler and colleagues[101,102] have repeatedly argued that motor coordination and soft neurological signs are characteristic of early PEM, and that with refeeding there is some lessening of the impact although fine motor skills are still diminished. Poor achievement test scores can be attributed to the attention deficits of the children as well as a strong influence of environmental factors in the home and community that lead to a less stimulating environment for the developing child.[103–106] Biological alterations are not limited to decreased synaptic function, pyramidal cell loss in the neocortex, electroencephalographic abnormalities, and previously mentioned alterations in cerebellar and cerebral cortex.[97,107–109] Specific examinations of aspects of arousal and components of cognition, such as attention and processing, would provide additional insights, although it is already clear that profound PEM in early life usually results in some degree of irreversible change in CNS functioning.

Selenium

Function and consequences. Selenium function in the brain is a relatively new topic of investigation and generally revolves around the functions of the selenium-dependent glutathione peroxidase (Se-GPX) and the selenocysteine-containing enzyme Type I thyroxine deiodinase.[110–112] The biosynthesis and functioning of various selenoproteins has been recently described elsewhere.[113] While many of the effects of selenium deficiency can be attributed to a loss of Se-GPX activity, not all consequences are clearly linked to this important part of the oxidative damage-protection system.[114–120] Cellular Se-GPX isozymes are thought to play a role in the regulation of peroxide concentration and potentially play a role in the biology of aging. There is a decline in brain Se-GPX with aging, although Nistico and colleagues[121] showed that the content of Se-GPX in brain regions of aging (24-month-old) rats could be prevented with the administration of nerve growth factor. Thus, regulatory control of brain Se-GPX is not strictly a function of selenium status. The Se-GPX activity is highest in myelin fractions of the brain, followed by the synaptosomes. This is also the subcellular fraction that has the highest concentration of selenite.[122] A large amount of polyunsaturated fatty acids in the synaptic membrane compartment are thus protected from peroxidation by this Se-GPX activity. In contrast, injected ^{75}Se methionine is distributed fairly evenly across subcellular fractions. Other reports note that neurotoxicity of N-methyl-1,2,3,6 tetrahydropyridine and methyl-mercury are related to brain Se-GPX activity and selenium status.[123–125] Oxidative damage is implicated in the toxic effects of both of these compounds—the former is a model of neuropathology of Parkinsonian syndrome and the latter is a potent environmental toxin.

The role of selenium in brain development and functioning has been reexamined recently because of the observations that peripheral conversion of thyroxine to the active hormone triiodothyronine depends on the selenocysteine-containing enzyme type I 5′-deiodinase.[110,126,127] In selenium deficiency, the activity of this enzyme, located primarily in liver and kidney, decreases and leads to an increased concentration of the prohormone thyroxine and a lowering of the active hormone triiodothyronine. In brain cerebral cortex and anterior pituitary, a second form of the protein, type II deiodinase, is not selenium-containing and primarily produces triiodothyronine for local consumption.[110] This is true both in neonatal brain and in adult brain of rats.[128] Thus, despite a functional state of hypothyroidism elsewhere in the body, the brain may be protected in selenium deficiency.[126]

In combination with iodine deficiency, selenium status may play a role in the pathogenesis of myxedematous cretinism. As noted previously in the section on iodine metabolism, hypothyroidism in the developing brain leads to disorders of neural process growth.[129] There is reduced axonal size and dendritic complexity that may also include changes in the neuronal cytoskeleton.[130] Indeed, interventions in populations with both deficiencies with the provision of selenium may dramatically increase clinical expression of cretinism.[131] Selenium deficiency in rats is associated with a decrease in brain type II deiodinase activity, although this is secondary to the elevated thyroxine and not a direct effect of selenium.[71,132] In a study to determine the early developmental dependency on selenium, fetuses were not affected by maternal selenium deficiency.[71] Within 14 days of postnatal life, however, there was a significant decline in brain type II deiodinase activity while plasma triiodothyronine concentration remained near normal. This suggests that brain type II deiodinase could be a major vehicle for protecting the neonatal brain from low thyroid status and the resulting irreversible poor neural development. In a mouse model, neonatal selenium deficiency resulted in a 95% reduction in liver selenium and only a 40% reduction in brain selenium.[133] There was no regional or cellular distribution of selenium reported, so it is unclear if all regions of the brain were equally affected.

When selenium becomes limiting in the diet, there is a hierarchy established such that 5′-deiodinase activity is maintained at the expense of Se-GPX activity.[127] Neonatal selenium deficiency is associated with decreased motor function in a mouse model in one study, although specific effects on the development or functioning of motor tracts were not investigated.[133]

Poor selenium status may also alter neurotransmitter metabolism in an undetermined fashion, as suggested by a recent paper by Castano et al.[134] The turnover of dopamine, noradrenaline, and serotonin was increased in caudate putamen or substantia nigra in selenium-deficient adult rats. At the same time, Se-GPX activities in these brain regions were significantly decreased. The authors postulate that oxidative damage was responsible for the increase in neurotransmitter turnover, although direct proof that synthesis release and reuptake are directly altered is lacking. This study suggests some behavioral alterations could be expected in subjects with low selenium status, as all three of the neurotransmitters mentioned are critical to processes of attention, arousal, and memory, in addition to their roles in motor activities. In another study, two children were shown to have low selenium status and intractable seizures.[135] The older child was given selenium (3–5 μg/kg body weight) to reduce the frequency of epileptic seizures, which suggests that selenium status may play a role in the neurobiology of epileptic patients.

Location. There is little recent work on the distribution of selenium and selenoproteins in the brain apart from what has already been mentioned.[121] Highest concentrations are in cerebellum, followed by a fairly uniform distribution in white and gray matter, and in spinal cord.[136] Radiolabeled selenoproteins appear to turn over more slowly than brain selenium when the tracer is introduced as selenite. It is not certain that there was equilibration of label with slowly turning over brain pools; thus, the dynamics of selenium movement in the brain are still largely unknown. The uptake of selenium into the brain is greater than into other tissues, with a selective sequestration into seven subcellular selenoprotein bands. Brain distributions of selenoproteins are not well defined with regard to cell types (oligodendrocytes, glial cells, astrocytes, neurons), distributions in the brain, and their dependence on selenium status or age.[123] Selenoprotein W is distributed in brain, muscle, spleen, and testes; this concentration has been found to decline when rats are fed a selenium-deficient diet.[137] The distribution within brain is unreported. In addition, binding of plasma selenoprotein P is greatest to brain cell membranes compared with other organs.[138,139] An increase in dietary selenium led to an increased binding. The role of selenoprotein P in brain function is not known, nor are the mechanisms of distribution elucidated.

Zinc

Function. In contrast to the relatively few functional roles just described for selenium with regard to CNS function, zinc is one of the most ubiquitous nutrients; it is a constituent of more than 200 enzymes and is widely distributed in various forms.[140–143] Such important enzymes as carbonic anhydrase, alkaline phosphatase, copper-zinc superoxide dismutase, and ribonucleotide polymerase are zinc-containing enzymes. Zinc deficiency leads to both primary and secondary alterations in brain development and brain growth. In some cases, this is related to reduced thymidine incorporation into DNA, reduced polyribosomes, and alterations in zinc-finger–regulated gene transcription.[144–146] Low availability of zinc to the developing fetus has tremendous impact on the developing brain as well as other tissues; one of the most striking alterations is a primary neural tube defect.[147] As reviewed and described by Keen and colleagues,[144] "The teratogenic effects of zinc deficiency may be attributed to reductions in protein or nucleic acid synthesis, reduction in the rate of tubulin polymerization, oxidative damage, gene expression, and altered cell cycles, and morphoregulatory molecules."

Location. Zinc is heterogeneously distributed in the brain and is concentrated within groups of neurons; it is more abundant in gray matter than in white matter, and is in three distinct pools of free zinc, vesicular zinc, and protein-bound zinc.[142] Zinc-containing pathways are located in the cerebral hemisphere, and the best characterized are the mossy fiber projections running from hippocampus granule cells to the CA3 pyramidal neurons.[148] Other nerve fibers also contain zinc in abundance with projections to cerebrocortical paths. There is also staining in hypothalmus, pons, and cerebellum.[142] The zinc in these neurons is usually contained in synaptic vesicles and may be present in as high a concentration as 300 μM. Studies of the mossy fiber system of the hippocampus clearly show that zinc is released from these neurons and synaptic vesicles.[149] There is active transport of zinc into these neurons.[150] One study of the normal distribution of zinc showed that it may be altered by magnesium deficiency, although careful brain cytology was not performed.[151] Since the concentration of zinc in the hippocampus, amygdala, and perirhinal regions of the brain are important focal points for opera-

tion of the limbic system, it is presumed that appropriate amounts of zinc are necessary for proper plasticity and experiential learning.[143] Metallothionein-rich regions of the brain generally correspond to zinc-rich regions of the brain. Hao et al.[152] developed cDNA probes for two brain forms of metallothionein, I and III, and used these probes to examine brain distribution of this important zinc protein. Northern blot analysis of brain mRNA showed that metallothionen I mRNA content was particularly responsive to increased dietary zinc, with the greatest responses in cerebellum and hippocampus. Metallothionein III is more abundant in cerebral cortex, hippocampus, amygdala, and deep cerebellar nuclei, and the cellular location corresponds to those neurons that have synaptic vesicles of zinc.[153] Primary cell cultures show that metallothionen III is present in both neurons and astrocytes, and responds to induction by traditional inducers such as zinc, copper, and glucocorticoids.[154]

Takeda and colleagues[155] used radiolabeled zinc and manganese injected in the third ventricle compared with systemic injections to demonstrate that zinc and manganese travel freely through the cerebrospinal fluid compartments. It is only after 7 days that the characteristic specific localization in the hippocampus appears on autoradiographs. Vera-Gil and Perez-Castejon[156] have recently reviewed the literature on the use of ^{65}Zn as a tool to investigate the distribution and dynamics of zinc movement in the brain.

Consequences. Zinc is in the highest concentrations in the hippocampus, but effects of zinc deprivation are most strongly seen in poor growth of the cerebellum and Purkinje cells.[142,157,158] Indirect effects of zinc deficiency may also be observed in the lipid content of the developing fetal brain, which may suggest alterations in functioning due to changes in membrane characteristics.[159] A role for zinc in neurotransmission is strongly inferred from the neuronal location of the metal, its active uptake by neurons, storage in synaptic vesicles, and release with depolarization due to Ca^{2+} stimulation.[141,143] These neurons are now thought to be a subclass of glutamate-secreting neurons and respond to Ca^{2+} stimulation for neurotransmission. A recent paper by Browning and O'Dell[145] has shown that zinc deficiency impairs calcium uptake in brain synaptosomes of guinea pigs. The co-release of zinc with glutamate provides a mechanism of modulation of postsynaptic membrane excitability. The excitatory amino acid receptors, especially the N-methyl-$_D$-aspartate (NMDA) receptor, have zinc as a particularly potent antagonist.[160,161] Zinc provides a window of control of membrane excitability by depressing postsynaptic action when firing rates become very high.[141,143] Some authors propose that zinc may enter into neurons by binding to NMDA receptors.[162] Alcoholic brain dysfunction is possibly related to low cerebral cortical zinc and, hence, enhanced NMDA excitotoxicity; zinc treatment in chronic alcoholics may thus provide some benefit in withdrawal seizures.[163]

The recent literature also describes the role of zinc in modulation of GABA receptors and in the synchronization of release of GABA from neurons.[141,143] The addition of zinc to the media-bathing cultured neurons led to a pulsatile release of GABA. While many causal relationships are not well established, changes in brain zinc concentration have been observed in a number of diseases including Alzheimer's disease, Down's syndrome, epilepsy, multiple sclerosis, retinal dystrophy, and schizophrenia.[164,165] A study of transgenic mice with an altered copper-zinc superoxide dismutase showed rapid neurodegeneration of motor neurons within the spinal cord, brain stem, and neocortex.[166] Constantinidis[167] suggests that amyloid production in Alzheimer's disease is related to a disturbance in zinc metabolism. The fundamentals of this theory are that amyloid protein formed in the capillaries of the brain alters the permeability of the blood-brain barrier, which then increases its permeability to aluminum, iron, and mercury. These metals can displace zinc from enzymes, leading to abnormal DNA synthesis and the production of abnormal proteins like paired helical filaments and neurofibrillary tangles. In addition, there may be alterations in the zinc modulation of glutamate excitation of postsynaptic membranes and possible changes in superoxide dismutase and carbonic anhydrase activity.[167]

Summary

This brief review is by no means comprehensive for any of the five nutrients considered, nor is it comprehensive with regard to nutrients that affect the functioning of the CNS. Other very important nutrients with a highly visible impact on brain development and perhaps functioning include folic acid and specific fats. In actuality, all essential nutrients impact on the functioning of the brain and play critical roles in proper neonatal and postnatal development, daily functioning, and perhaps for some nutrients in the prevention of neuropathologies. The reader is urged to consult the many excellent review and original articles published each year regarding individual nutrients and brain function. While I have tried to focus on the nutrients that have the higher prevalence rates for deficiency states, this does not diminish the importance of other nutrients; it only reflects my limited time, space, and grasp of some of the intricacies of the brain.

Acknowledgments

I am indebted to my colleague James R. Connor for his willingness to spend many hours talking with me about iron and neuroanatomy over the recent 4–5 years and also to my students who have spent many hours working on some of the information in the section pertaining to iron in this chapter.

References

1. Sheard NF (1994) Iron deficiency and infant development. Nutr Rev 52:137–140
2. Beard JL, Connor JR, Jones BC (1993) Iron in the brain. Nutr Rev 51:157–170
3. Connor JR (1992) Proteins of iron regulation in the brain in Alzheimer's disease. In Lauffer RB (ed), Iron and human disease. CRC Press, Ann Arbor, MI, pp 365–393
4. Pollitt E (1993) Iron deficiency and cognitive function. Annu Rev Nutr 13:521–537
5. Dallman PR (1982) Manifestations of iron deficiency. Semin Hematol 19:19–30
6. Maguire JJ, Davies KJA, Dallman PR, Packer L (1982) Effects of dietary iron deficiency on iron-sulfur proteins and bioenergetic functions of skeletal muscle mitochondria. Biochim Biophys Acta 679:210–220
7. McKay RH, Higuchi DA, Winder WW, Fell RD, Brown EB (1983) Tissue effects of iron deficiency in the rat. Biochim Biophys Acta 757:352–358
8. McLane JA, Fell RD, McKay RH, et al (1981) Physiological and biochemical effects of iron deficiency on rat skeletal muscle. Am J Physiol 241:C47–C54
9. Wigglesworth JM, Baum H (1988) Iron dependent enzymes in the brain. In Youdim MBH (ed), Brain iron: neurochemical and behavioral aspects. Taylor & Francis, New York, pp 25–66
10. Youdim MBH (1990) Neuropharmacological and neurobiochemical aspects of iron deficiency. In Dobbing J (ed), Brain, behaviour, and iron in the infant diet. Springer-Verlag, London, pp 83–106
11. Hill JM (1985) Iron concentration reduced in ventral pallidum, globus pallidus, and substantia nigra by GABA-transaminase inhibitor, gamma-vinyl GABA. Brain Res 342:18–25
12. Larkin EC, Rao GA (1990) Importance of fetal and neonatal iron: adequacy for normal development of central nervous system. In Dobbing J (ed), Brain, behaviour and iron in the infant diet. Springer-Verlag, London, pp 43–63
13. Dallman PR (1986) Biochemical basis for the manifestations of iron deficiency. Annu Rev Nutr 6:13–40
14. Beard JL, Finch CA (1984) Iron deficiency. In Clydesdale F, Weimer KL (eds), Iron fortification of foods. Academic Press, New York, pp 3–16
15. Baynes RD, Bothwell TH (1990) Iron deficiency. Annu Rev Nutr 10:133–148
16. Scrimshaw NS (1984) Functional consequences of iron deficiency in human populations. J Nutr Sci Vitaminol (Tokyo) 30:47–63
17. Sourkes TL (1973) Influence of specific nutrients on catecholamine synthesis and metabolism. Pharmacol Rev 24:359–379
18. Youdim MBH, Ben-Schachar D, Yehuda S (1989) Putative biological mechanisms on the effects of iron deficiency on brain biochemistry. Am J Clin Nutr 50:607–617
19. Youdim MBH, Green AR (1978) Iron deficiency and neurotransmitter synthesis and function. Proc Nutr Soc 37:173–179
20. Ben-Shachar D, Ashkenazi R, Youdim MBH (1986) Long term consequences of early iron-deficiency on dopaminergic neurotransmission. Int J Dev Neurosci 4:81–88

21. Ashkenazi R, Ben-Shachar D, Youdim MBH (1982) Nutritional iron deficiency and dopamine binding sites in the rat brain. Pharmacol Biochem Behav 17:43–47

22. Beard JL, Chen Q, Connor JR, Jones BC (1993) Altered monoamine metabolism in caudate putamen of iron deficient rats. Pharmacol Biochem Behav 48:621–624

23. Hallgren B, Sourander P (1958) The effect of age on the nonhaem iron in the human brain. J Neurochem 3:41–51

24. Rajan KS, Colburn RW, Davis JM (1976) Distribution of metal ions in the subcellular fractions of several rat brain areas. Life Sci 18:423–432

25. Levine SM, Macklin WB (1990) Iron-enriched oligodendrocytes: a reexamination of the spatial distribution. J Neurosci Res 29:413–419

26. Connor JR, Menzies SM, Martin SM, Mufson EL (1990) Cellular distribution of transferrin, ferritin and iron in normal and aged human brains. J Neurosci Res 27:595–611

27. Francois C, Mguyen-Legros J, Percheron G (1981) Topographical and cytological localization of iron in rat and monkey brains. Brain Res 215:317–322

28. Dwork AJ, Schon EA, Herbert J (1988) Non-identical distribution of transferrin and ferric iron in human brain. Neuroscience 27:333–345

29. Taylor EM, Morgan THE (1990) Developmental changes in transferrin and iron uptake by the brain in the rat. Dev Brain Res 55:35–42

30. Jacobson S (1963) Sequence of myelinization in the brain of the albino rat. A. Cerebral cortex, thalamus and related structures. J Comp Neurol 121:5–29

31. Morris CM, Candy JM, Bloxham CA, Edwardson JA (1992) Distribution of transferrin receptors in relation to cytochrome oxidase activity in the human spinal cord, lower brainstem and cerebellum. J Neurol Sci 111:158–172

32. Morris CM, Candy JM, Oakley AE, Bloxham CA, Edwardson JA (1992) Histochemical distribution of non-haem iron in the human brain. Acta Anat (Basel) 144:235–257

33. Fishman JB, Rubin JB, Handrahan JV, Connor JR, Fine RE (1987) Receptor mediated uptake of transferrin across the blood brain barrier. J Neurosci Res 18:299–304

34. Partridge WM, Eisenberg J, Yang J (1987) Human blood brain barrier transferrin receptor. Metabolism 36:892–895

35. Dwork AJ, Lawler G, Zybert PA, Schon EA (1990) An autoradiographic study of the uptake and distribution of iron by the brain of the young rat. Brain Res 518:31–39

36. Bleijenberg BG, von Eijk HG, Leijnse B (1971) The determination of non-heme iron and transferrin in cerebrospinal fluid. Clin Chim Acta 31:277–281

37. Connor JR, Fine RE (1986) The distribution of transferrin immunoreactivity in the rat central nervous system. Brain Res 368:319–328

38. Sofic E, Riederer P, Heinsen H, et al (1988) Increased iron (III) and total iron content in postmortem substantia nigra of Parkinsonian brain. J Neural Transm 74:199–208

39. Dallman PR, Siimes MN, Manies EC (1975) Brain iron: persistent deficiency following short term iron deprivation in the young rat. Br J Haematol 31:209–215

40. Dallman PR, Spirito RA (1977) Brain iron in the rat: extremely slow turnover in normal rat may explain the long-lasting effects of early iron-deficiency. J Nutr 107:1075–1081

41. Aoki S, Okada Y, Nishimura K, et al (1989) Normal deposition of brain iron in childhood and adolescence: MR imaging at 1.5 T. Radiology 172:381–385

42. DeMaeyer E, Adiels-Tegman M (1985) The prevalence of anemia in the world. World Health Stat Q 38:302–316

43. Expert Scientific Working Group (1985) Summary of a report on assessment of the iron nutritional status of the United States population. Am J Clin Nutr 42:1318–1330

44. Seoane NA, Roberge AG, Page M, Allard C, Bouchard C (1985) Selected indices of iron status in adolescents. J Can Diet Assoc 46:298–303

45. Dobbing J (1990) Vulnerable periods in the developing brain. In Dobbing J (ed), Brain, behaviour and iron in the infant diet. Springer-Verlag, London, pp 1–17

46. Pollitt E, Metallinos-Katsaras E (1990) Iron deficiency and behavior: constructs, methods, and validity of the findings. In Wurtman RJ, Wurtman JJ (eds), Nutrition and the brain, vol 8. Raven Press, New York, pp 101–146

47. Oski FA, Honig AS, Helu B, Howanitz P (1983) Effect of iron therapy on behavioral performance in nonamenic, iron deficient infants. Pediatrics 71:877–880

48. Lozoff B, Brittenham GM (1986) Behavioural aspects of iron deficiency. Prog Hematol 14:23–53

49. Lozoff B, Brittenham GM, Viteri FE, Wolf AW, Urrutia JJ (1982) Developmental deficits in iron deficient infants: effects of age and severity of iron lack. J Pediatr 100:351–357

50. Lozoff B, Brittenham GM, Wolf AW, et al (1987) Iron deficiency anemia and iron therapy: effects on infant developmental test performance. Pediatrics 79:981–995

51. Walter T, Kowalskys J, Stekel A (1983) Effect of mild iron deficiency on infant mental development scores. J Pediatr 102:519–522

52. Walter T (1990) Iron deficiency and behaviour in infancy: a critical review. In Dobbing J (ed), Brain, behaviour and iron in the infant diet. Springer-Verlag, London, pp 133–150

53. Soemantri AG, Pollitt E, Kim I (1985) Iron deficiency anemia and educational achievement. Am J Clin Nutr 42:1221–1228

54. Pollitt E, Soemantri AG, Yunis F, Scrimshaw NS (1985) Cognitive effects of iron deficiency anemia. Lancet 1:158–162

55. Groner JA, Holtzman NA, Charney E, Mellits ED (1986) A randomized trial of oral iron on tests of short-term memory and attention span in young pregnant women. J Adolesc Health Care 7:44–48

56. Idjradinata P, Pollitt E (1993) Reversal of developmental delays in iron deficient anemic infants treated with iron. Lancet 341:1–4

57. Benkovic S, Connor JR (1993) Ferritin, transferrin and iron in normal and aged rat brains. J Comp Neurol 337:97–113

58. Olanow CW, Marsden D, Perl D, Cohen G, eds (1992) Iron and oxidative stress in Parkinson's disease. Ann Neurol 32(suppl 3):S17–S20

59. Thompson CM, Marksberry WR, Ehmann WD, Mao Y-Y, Vance DE (1988) Regional brain trace-element studies in Alzheimer's disease. Neurotoxicology 9:1–7

60. Zaleska MM, Floyd R (1985) Regional lipid peroxidation in rat brain in vitro: possible role of endogenous iron. Neurochem Res 10:397–410

61. Halliwell B (1991) Reactive oxygen species in living systems: source, biochemistry, and role of human disease. Am J Med 91(suppl 3c):14S–22S

62. Hetzel B (1989) The story of iodine deficiency: an international challenge in nutrition. Oxford University Press, Oxford, pp 84–101

63. Delange F (1984) The disorders induced by iodine deficiency. Nutr Rev 4:107–128

64. DeLong GR (1993) Effects of nutrition on brain development in humans. Am J Clin Nutr 57(suppl):286S–290S

65. Ekins RP, Sinha AK, Pickard MR, Evans IM, al Yatama F (1994) Transport of thyroid hormones to target tissues. Acta Med Austriaca 21:26–34

66. Yan Y, Guan C, Leng L, Li J (1989) Quantitative histology study on brain nerve cells of neurological cretins. In Delong

GR, Robins J, Condliffe PG (eds), Iodine and the brain. Plenum Press, New York, pp 359–377

67. Chaouki ML, Maoui R, Benmiloud M (1988) Comparative study of neurological and myxoedematous cretinism associated with severe iodine deficiency. Clin Endocrinol 28:399–408

68. Berbel P, Guadano-Ferraz A, Angulo A, Ramon Cerezo J (1994) Role of thyroid hormones in the maturation of interhemispheric connections in rats. Behav Brain Res 64:9–14

69. Berbel P, Guadano-Ferraz A, Martinez M, Quiles JA (1993) Organization of auditory callosal connections in hypothyroid adult rats. J Neurochem 5:1465–1478

70. Potter BJ, Mano MT, Bellin GB, et al (1984) Restoration of brain growth in fetal sheep after iodized oil administration to pregnant iodine-deficient ewes. J Neurosci 66:15–26

71. Chanoine JP, Safran M, Farwell AP, Tranter P (1992) Selenium deficiency and type II 5′-deiodinase regulation in the euthyroid and hypothyroid rat: evidence of a direct effect of thyroxine. Endocrinology 131:479–484

72. Serrano-Lozano A, Montiel M, Morell M, Morata P (1993) 5′ Deiodinase activity in brain regions of adult rats modifications in different situations of experimental hypothyroidism. Brain Res Bull 30:611–616

73. Chanoine JP, Alex S, Stone S, et al (1993) Placental 5-deiodinase activity and fetal thyroid hormone economy are unaffected by selenium deficiency in the rat. Pediatr Res 34:288–292

74. Beckett GJ, Arthur JR (1994) Hormone-nuclear receptor interactions in health and disease: the iodothyronine deiodinases and 5′-deiodination. Baillieres Clin Endocrinol Metab 8:285–304

75. Escobar GM, Obregon MJ, Calvo R, Escobar de Rev F (1993) Effects of iodine deficiency on thyroid hormone metabolism and the brain in fetal rats: the role of the maternal transfer of thyroxin. Am J Clin Nutr 57(suppl):280S–285S

76. Pharoah POD, Connolly KJ (1989) Maternal thyroid hormones and fetal brain development. In DeLong GR, Robins J, Condliffe PG (eds), Iodine and the brain. Plenum Press, New York, pp 333–354

77. Pharoah POD, Ellis SM, Ekins RP, Harding AG (1976) Maternal thyroid function, iodine deficiency and fetal development. Clin Endocrinol 5:159–166

78. Pharoah POD, Connolly KJ, Ekins RP, Harding AG (1984) Maternal thyroid hormones in pregnancy and the consequent cognitive and motor performance of the children. Clin Endocrinol 21:265–270

79. DeLong GR, Stanbury JB, Fierro-Benitez R (1985) Neurological signs in congenital iodine-deficiency disorder (endemic cretinism). Dev Med Child Neurol 27:317–324

80. Halphern JP, Boyages SC, Maberly GF, et al (1991) The neurology of endemic cretinism: a study of two endemias. Brain 114(Pt 2):825–841

81. Eastman CJ, Phillips DI (1988) Endemic goitre and iodine deficiency disorders—aetiology, epidemiology and treatment. Baillieres Clin Endocrinol Metab 2:719–735

82. Cao XY, Jiang XM, Dou ZH, et al (1994) Timing of vulnerability of the brain to iodine deficiency in endemic cretinism. J Med 331:1739–1744

83. Dodd NS, Samuel AM (1993) Iodine deficiency in adolescents from Bombay slums. Natl Med J India 6:110–113

84. Dunn JT (1993) Iodine supplementation and the prevention of cretinism. Ann NY Acad Sci 678:158–168

85. Chopra JS, Arun Sharma (1992) Protein energy malnutrition and the nervous system. J Neurosci 110:8–20

86. Wiggins RC (1982) Myelin development and nutritional insufficiency. Brain Res Rev 4:151–175

87. Yusuf HKM, Mozaffar Z (1979) Raised level of cholesterol ester in the brain of protein undernourished mice. J Neurochem 32:273–275

88. Sastry PS (1985) Lipids of nervous tissue: composition and metabolism. In Holman RT (ed), Progress in lipid research. Pergamon Press, Oxford, pp 69–176

89. Azzolin IR, Bernard EA, Trindade VMT, Ganmallo JLG, Penny MLS (1991) Effect of protein malnutrition on glycoprotein, protein and lipid synthesis in the rat cerebellum during the period of brain growth spurt. Ann Nutr Metab 35:82–88

90. Telang SD, Fuller G, Wiggins R, Enna SJ (1984) Early undernutrition and H-GABA binding in rat brain. J Neurol 43:640–645

91. Seidler FJ, Bell JM, Slotkin TA (1990) Undernutrition and overnutrition in the neonatal rat: long-term effects on noradrenergic pathways in brain regions. Pediatr Res 27:191–197

92. Detering N, Collins RM, Hawkins RL, Ozand PT, Karahasan A (1980) Comparative effects of ethanol and malnutrition on the development of catecholamine neurons. J Neurochem 34:1587–1593

93. Olorunsogo OO (1989) Changes in brain mitochondrial bioenergetics in protein-deficient rats. Br J Exp Pathol 70:607–619

94. Chopra JS (1991) Neurological consequences of protein and protein-calorie undernutrition. Crit Rev Neurobiol 6(2):99–118.

95. Chopra JS, Dhand UK, Mehta S, et al (1986) Electrophysiological, histopathological and morphometric studies in peripheral nerves of protein calorie malnourished (PCM) rhesus monkeys. Brain 109:307–323

96. Hedley-Whyte ET (1973) Myelination of rat sciatic nerve: comparison of undernutrition and cholesterol biosynthesis inhibition. J Neuropath Exp Neurol 32:284–302

97. Dobbing J, Smart JL (1974) Vulnerability of developing brain and behaviour. Br Med Bull 30:164–168

98. Lozoff B (1989) Nutrition and behaviour. Am Psychol 44:231–236

99. Galler JR, Ramsey F, Salt P, Archer E (1987) The long term effects of early kwashiorkor compared with marasmus. I. Physical growth. J Pediatr Gastroenterol Nutr 6:841–846

100. Galler JR, Ramsey F, Salt P, Forde V (1987) The long term effects of early kwashiorkor compared with marasmus: intellectual performance. J Pediatr Gastroenterol Nutr 6:847–854

101. Vega-Franco L (1990) Behavioural development and nerve conduction velocity during recovery from malnutrition. Bol Med Hosp Infant Mex 47:85–90

102. Galler JR, Ramsey F, Salt P, Archer E (1987) The long term effects of early kwashiorkor compared with marasmus: fine motor skills. J Pediatr Gastroenterol Nutr 6:835–859

103. Galler JR, Ramsey F, Morley SD, Archer E, Salt P (1990) The long term effects of early kwashiorkor compared with marasmus. IV. Performance on the National High School Entrance Examination. Pediatr Res 28:235–239

104. Sigman M (1989) Cognitive abilities of Kenyan children in relation to nutrition, family characteristics and education. Child Dev 60:1463–1474

105. Waber DP, Christiansen L, Nelson O, Clement JR (1981) Nutritional supplementation maternal education and cognitive development of infants at risk of malnutrition. Am J Clin Nutr 34:797–803

106. Grantham-Mcgregor SG, Stewart ME, Schofield WN (1980) Effect of long term psychological stimulation on mental development in severely malnourished children. Lancet 11:785–789

107. Austin K, Bronzino JD, Morgane PJ (1986) Prenatal protein malnutrition affects synaptic potentiation in the dentate gyrus of rats in adulthood. Dev Brain Res 29:267–273

108. Medvedev DI (1989) Possibilities of restoring glial population of the neocortex after protein-energy insufficiency. Arkh Anat Gistol Embriol 97:25–30

109. Bronzino JD, Austin K, LaFrance RJ, Morgane PJ, Galler JR (1983) Spectral analysis of neocortical and hippocampal EEG in the protein malnourished rat. Electroencephalogr Clin Neurophysiol 55:699–709

110. Arthur, JR, Nicol F, Beckett GJ (1993) Selenium deficiency, thyroid hormone metabolism, and thyroid hormone deiodinases. Am J Clin Nutr 57(suppl):236S–239S

111. Burk RF, Hill KE (1993) Regulation of selenoproteins. Annu Rev Nutr 13:65–81

112. Behne D, Kyriakopoulos (1993) Effects of dietary selenium on the tissue concentrations of type I iodothyronine 5'-deiodinase and other selenoproteins. Am J Clin Nutr 57(suppl):310S–312S

113. Stadtman TC (1991) Biosynthesis and function of selenocysteine-containing enzymes. J Biol Chem 266:16257–16260

114. Burk RF (1983) Biological activity of selenium. Annu Rev Nutr 3:53–70

115. Burk RF (1989) Recent developments in trace element metabolism and function: newer roles of selenium in nutrition. J Nutr 119:1051–1054

116. Sunde RA (1990) Molecular biology of selenoproteins. Annu Rev Nutr 10:451–474

117. Arthur JR (1991) The role of selenium and thyroid hormone metabolism. Can J Physiol Pharmacol 69:1648–1652

118. Reiter R, Wendel A (1984) Selenium and drug metabolism. II. Independence of glutathione peroxidase and reversibility of hepatic enzyme modulations in deficient mice. Biochem Pharmacol 33:1923–1928

119. Reiter R, Wendel A (1985) Selenium and drug metabolism. II. Relation of glutathione peroxidase and other hepatic enzyme modulations to dietary supplements. Biochem Pharmacol 34:2287–2290

120. Arthur JR, Nicol F, Boyne R, et al (1987) Old and new roles for selenium. In Hemphill DD (ed), Trace substances in environmental health XXI. University of Missouri, Columbia, MO, pp 487–498

121. Nistico G, Ciriolo MR, Fiskin K, et al (1992) NGF restores decrease in catalase activity and increases superoxide dismutase and glutathione peroxidase activity in the brain of aged rats. Free Radic Biol Med 12:177–181

122. Clausen J (1991) Uptake and distribution in rat brain of organic and inorganic selenium. Biol Trace Elem Res 28:39–45

123. Buckman TD, Sutphin MS, Eckhert CD (1993) A comparison of the effects of dietary selenium on selenoprotein expression in rat brain and liver. Biochim Biophys Acta 1163:176–184

124. Glynn AW, Ilback NG, Brabencova D, et al (1993) Influence of sodium selenite on 203Hg absorption, distribution and elimination in male mice exposed to methyl-mercury. Biol Trace Elem Res 39:91–107

125. Moller-Madsen B, Danscher G (1991) Localization of mercury in CNS of the rat. IV. The effect of selenium on orally administered organic and inorganic mercury. Toxicol Appl Pharmacol 108:457–473

126. Corvilain B, Contempre B, Longombe AO, et al (1993) Selenium and the thyroid: how the relationship was established [review]. Am J Clin Nutr 57:244S–248S

127. Kohrle J (1992) The trace components—selenium and flavonoids—affect iodothyronine deiodinases, throid hormone transport and TSH regulation [review]. Acta Med Austriaca 19(suppl 1):13–17

128. Santini F, Chopra IJ, Hurd RE, Solomon DH, Teco GN (1992) A study of the characteristics of the rat placental iodothyronine 5-monodeiodinase: evidence that it is distinct from the rat hepatic iodothyronine 5'-monodeiodinase. Endocrinology 130:2325–2332

129. Garza R, Paymirat J, Dussault JH (1990) Influence of soluble environmental factors on development of fetal brain acetylcholinesterase-positive neurons cultured in a chemically defined medium: comparison with effects of L-T3. Brain Res 56:160–168

130. Stein SA, Kirkpatrick LL, Shanklin DR, Adams PM, Brady ST (1991) Hypothyroidism reduces the rate of slow component A (Sca). J Neurosci Res 28:121–133

131. Vanderpas JB, Contempre B, Duale NL, et al (1993) Selenium deficiency mitigates hypothroxinemia in iodine-deficient subjects. Am J Clin Nutr 57(suppl):271S–275S

132. Meinhold H, Campos-Barros A, Behne D (1992) Effects of selenium and iodine deficiency on iodothyronine deiodinases in brain, thyroid and peripheral tissue. Acta Med Austriaca 19(suppl)1:8–12

133. Watanabe C, Satoh H (1994) Brain selenium status and behavioral development in selenium-deficient preweanling mice. Physiol Behav 56:927–932

134. Castano A, Cano J, Machado A (1993) Low selenium diet affects monoamine turnover differentially in substantia nigra and striatum. J Neurochem 61:1302–1307

135. Ramaekers VT, Calomme M, Vanden Berghe D, Makropoulos W (1994) Selenium deficiency triggering intractable seizures. Neuropediatrics 25:217–223

136. Gronbaek H, Thorlacius-Ussing O (1992) Selenium in the central nervous system of rats exposed to 75Se L-selenomethionine and sodium selenite. Biol Trace Elem Res 35:119–127

137. Yeh JY, Beilstein MA, Andrews JS, Whanger PD (1995) Tissue distribution and influence of selenium status on levels of selenoprotein W. FASEB J 9:392–396

138. Wilson DS, Tappel AL (1993) Binding of plasma selenoprotein P to cell membranes. J Inorg Biochem 51:707–714

139. Burk RF, Hill KE, Read R, Bellew T (1991) Response of rat selenoprotein P to selenium administration and fate of its selenium. Am J Physiol 261:E26–E30

140. Ebadi M, Elsayed MA, Aly MH (1994) The importance of zinc and metallothionein in brain. Biol Signals 3:123–126

141. Smart TG, Xie X, Krishek BJ (1994) Modulation of inhibitory and excitatory amino acid receptor ion channels by zinc. Neurobiology 42:393–441

142. Frederickson C (1989) Neurobiology of zinc and zinc-containing neurons. In Smythies J, Bradley R (eds), International review of neurobiology. Academic Press, New York, pp 145–238

143. Cousins RJ (1994) Metal elements and gene expression. Annu Rev Nutr 14:449–469

144. Keen CL, Taubeneck MW, Daston GP, Rogers JM, Gershwin ME (1993) Primary and secondary zinc deficiency as factors underlying abnormal CNS development. Ann NY Acad Sci 378:37–47

145. Browning JD, O'Dell BL (1993) Low zinc status in guinea pigs impairs calcium uptake by brain synaptosome. J Nutr 124:436–443

146. Dreosti IE (1983) Zinc and the central nervous system. In Dreosti IE, Smith RM (eds), Neurobiology of the trace elements: trace element neurobiology and deficiencies. Humana Press, Totowa, NJ, pp 135–162

147. Hurley LS, Gordon P, Keen CL, Merkhofer L (1982) Circa-

dian variation in rat plasma zinc and rapid effect of dietary zinc deficiency. Proc Soc Exp Biol Med 170:48–52

148. Slomianka L (1992) Neurons of origin of zinc-containing pathways and the distribution of zinc-containing boutons in the hippocampal region of the rat. Neuroscience 48:325–352

149. Charlton G, Rovira C, Ben-Ari Y, Leviel V (1985) Spontaneous and evoked release of endogenous Zn²⁺ in the hippocampal mossy fibre zone of the rat in situ. Exp Brain Res 58:202–205

150. Howell GA, Welch MG, Frederickson CJ (1984) Stimulation-induced uptake and release of zinc in hippocampal slices. Nature 308:736–738

151. Planells E, Aranda P, Lerma A, Llopis J (1994) Changes in bioavailability and tissue distribution of zinc caused by magnesium deficiency in rats. Br J Nutr 72:315–323

152. Hao R, Cerutis DR, Blaxall HS, Rodriguez-Sierra JF, Pfeiffer RF, Ebadi M (1994) Distribution of metallothionein mRNA in rat brain using in situ hybridization. Neurochem Res 19:761–767

153. Masters BA, Quaife CJ, Erickson JC, et al (1994) Metallothionein III is expressed in neurons that sequester zinc in synaptic vesicles. J Neurosci 14:5844–5857

154. Hidalgo J, Gasull T, Giralt M, Armario A (1994) Brain metallothionein in stress. Biol Signals 3:198–210

155. Takeda A, Sawashita J, Okada S (1994) Localization in rat brain of the trace metals, zinc and manganese, after intracerebroventricular injection. Brain Res 658:252–254

156. Vera-Gil A, Perez-Castejon MC (1994) ⁶⁵Zn in studies of the neurobiology of zinc [review]. Histol Histopathol 9:413–420

157. Buell SJ, Fosmire GJ, Ollerich DA, Sanstead HH (1977) Effects of postnatal zinc deficiency on cerebellar and hippocampal development in the rat. Exp Neurol 55:199–210

158. Dvergsten CL, Fosmire GJ, Ollerich DA, Sandstead HH (1983) Alterations in the postnatal development of the cerebellar cortex due to zinc deficiency: impaired acquisition of granule cells. Brain Res 271:217–226

159. Yang J, Cunnane SC (1994) Quantitative measurements of dietary and [1-14C] linoleate metabolism in pregnant rats: specific influence of moderate zinc depletion independent of food intake. J Physiol Pharmacol 72:1180–1185

160. Reynolds IJ (1992) Interactions between zinc and spermidine on the N-methyl-D-aspartate receptors: similarities to the action of zinc. Br J Pharmacol 95:95–102

161. Hollmann M, Boulter J, Maron C, et al (1993) Zinc potentiates against-induces currents at certain splice variants of the NMDA receptor. Neuron 10:943–954

162. Koh JY, Choi DW (1994) Zinc toxicity on cultured cortical neurons: involvement of N-methyl-D-aspartate receptors. Neuroscience 60:1049–1057

163. Menzano E, Carlen PL (1994) Zinc deficiency and corticosteroids in the pathogenesis of alcoholic brain dysfunction—a review. Alcohol Clin Exp Res 18:895–901

164. Ebadi M, Murrin LC, Pfeiffer RF (1990) Hippocampal zinc thioim and pyridoxal phosphate modulate synaptic functions. Ann NY Acad Sci 585:189–201

165. Ebadi M, Hama Y (1986) Zinc-binding proteins in the brain. Adv Exp Biol 203:557–570

166. Ripps ME, Huntley GW, Hof PR, et al (1995) Transgenic mice expressing an altered murine superoxide dismutase gene provide an animal model of amyotrophic lateral sclerosis. Proc Natl Acad Sci USA 92:689–693

167. Constantinidis J (1991) Hypothesis regarding amyloid and zinc in the pathogenesis of Alzheimer disease: potential for preventive intervention [review]. Alzheimer Dis Assoc Disord 5:31–35

Chapter 63

Inborn Errors of Metabolism
William J. Rhead

Inborn errors of metabolism are human genetic disorders resulting from enzymatic deficiencies involving substrate conversion. The first of these disorders to be discovered, alkaptonuria, was identified by Garrod[1] around the turn of the century. Since that time, several hundred metabolic disorders have been described;[2,3] entire new families of disorders, i.e., those involving intramitochondrial fatty acid β-oxidation, peroxisomal function, and cholesterol biosynthesis, have been described only in the past 2–15 years.[4-8] For the most part, only those disorders involving the enzymes and pathways of general and intermediary metabolism are accessible to dietary treatment. Inborn errors of metabolism affecting enzymes that catabolize complex glucolipids or glycolipoproteins, especially disorders involving enzymes in the central nervous system, such as the mucopolysaccharidoses, gangliosidoses, and sphingolipidoses, have proven refractory to dietary treatment. For a comprehensive review of all these disorders, their biochemistry, pathogenesis, molecular genetics, and treatment, the reader is referred to the exhaustive reference work edited by C.R. Scriver, A.L. Beaudet, W.S. Sly, and D. Valle: *The Metabolic and Molecular Bases of Inherited Disease,* 7th edition.

Inborn errors of metabolism can affect anabolic pathways that are involved in the synthesis of compounds important for cell metabolism and health or in the interconversion of substrates, as well as catabolic pathways that are involved in the metabolic conversion and disposal of essential and nonessential nutrients. However, most inborn errors of metabolism involve catabolic pathways, in which the accumulation of toxic intermediates negatively interferes with or destroys essential functions of specific tissues and organs. Principles of treatment include complete avoidance of nonessential nutrients that generate toxic metabolites, for example in the treatment of hereditary fructose intolerance[9] and galactosemia[10] (Table 1). In other disorders, essential nutrients become toxic in and of themselves at high intracellular concentrations or they generate toxic metabolites; thus, their intakes must be restricted to the minimum adequate for normal growth and development. Examples of such disorders include the hyperphenyl-

alaninemias (phenylketonuria) and the hyperammonemias of the urea cycle disorders.[11,12] In other diseases, essential or nonessential nutrients become necessary and therapeutic when ingested in far greater than normal amounts: examples are carbohydrate therapy in glycogen storage disease type I and nicotinamide therapy in Hartnup disease.[13,14]

In certain disorders, nutrients, cofactors, or vitamins become therapeutic either in doses that are pharmacological rather than physiological or when administered parenterally rather than enterally. Examples include the entire family of vitamin- and cofactor-responsive inborn errors of metabolism, such as vitamin B-12–responsive methylmalonic acidemia;[15,16] vitamin B-6–responsive homocystinuria;[17] the disorders of biotin metabolism and usage,[18] including biotinidase and holocarboxylase synthetase deficiencies; and certain disorders of folate metabolism.[19] In many diseases, effective dietary treatment requires that natural foods be replaced with artificial nutrient mixtures in diets that lower intakes of potentially toxic nutrients while meeting essential nutritional requirements. Examples of such diseases include phenylketonuria, the urea cycle disorders, branched-chain ketoacidemia, methylmalonic acidemia, and propionic acidemia.[11,12,15,16,20] In certain disorders, the enzymatic deficiency blocks anabolic pathways, thus rendering nutrients essential that are not usually so or raising the dietary requirements necessary to avoid nutritional deficiency and clinical disease. Nutrient deficiencies considered here include cholesterol in Smith-Lemli-Optiz syndrome,[8] arginine in the urea cycle disorders,[12] nicotinamide in Hartnup disease,[14] and biotin in biotinidase deficiency.[18]

In many disorders the provision of pharmacological amounts of specific nutrients activates alternate metabolic pathways, thus disposing of the accumulated toxic intermediates in the blocked primary metabolic pathway. Examples include glycine therapy in isovaleric acidemia[21] and carnitine therapy in disorders of fatty acid β-oxidation.[4,5] Some new classes of nutritional therapies involve altering normal pathways of metabolism to avoid endogenous synthesis and accumulation of toxic compounds, such as using erucic and oleic acids

Table 1. Dietary therapy of inborn errors of metabolism

Principle	Disorder	Nutrient
Complete avoidance of nonessential nutrients rendered toxic by the enzymatic deficiency	Galactosemia; hereditary fructose intolerance; urea cycle disorders	Galactose; fructose; nonessential amino acids
Reduction of essential nutrient intake to a minimum to avoid toxicity	Hyperphenylalaninemias; urea cycle disorders; branched-chain ketoacidemia	Phenylalanine; protein, essential amino acids; leucine, isoleucine, valine
Increased requirement for essential or nonessential nutrients	Hartnup disease; urea cycle disorders; biotindase, Smith-Lemli-Opitz; prolidase deficiency; hereditary orotic acidemia	Nicotinamide; essential amino acids, arginine; biotin; cholesterol, essential fatty acids; glycine, proline, hydroxylproline; uridine
Vitamin- and cofactor-responsive disorders	Methylmalonic acidemia; homocystinuria; holocarboxylase synthetase; fatty acid oxidation disorders; hyperphenylalaninemias (rare)	Cobalamin (vitamin B-12); pyridoxine (vitamin B-6); biotin; riboflavin; biopterin, and tetrahydrobiopterin
Provision of specific nutrients to activate alternative pathways for toxic metabolite disposal	Isovaleric acidemia; fatty acid oxidation disorders	Glycine, carnitine
Nutrients that inhibit normal metabolic pathways to prevent accumulation of toxic metabolites	Urea cycle disorders; adrenoleukodystrophy; hereditary orotic aciduria	Arginine, citrulline; erucic and oleic acids; uridine
Provision of modified biochemicals that have become essential nutrients due to an enzymatic deficiency	Functional methionine synthetase deficiency; glutathione synthetase deficiency	Hydroxycobalamin; glutathione alcohol esters

in adrenoleukodystrophy patients to prevent synthesis of toxic very-long-chain fatty acids from shorter-chain precursors.[7]

Disorders of Amino Acid Metabolism

The inborn errors of amino acid metabolism present classic examples of the successful treatment and avoidance of medical complications through the use of nutritional therapies. The prototype of these successes is phenylketonuria, which is due to either a deficiency of phenylalanine hydroxylase or, more rarely, a deficiency of the enzymes synthesizing or recycling the reduced tetrahydrobiopterin cofactor essential for function of this enzyme.[11] Since the 1950s, phenylketonuria has been successfully treated with diets containing all essential macro- and micronutrients but that are low in or free of phenylalanine. Phenylalanine levels are regulated by adding normal protein foods to the diet in amounts that permit normal growth and development but prevent phenylalanine accumulation in cells and tissues. Dietary restriction of phenylalanine has been highly successful in preventing the severe progressive mental retardation

found in individuals with phenylketonuria. Untreated persons with phenylketonuria have intellectual quotients in the range of 10–30, whereas treated individuals have intellectual quotients only a few points below those of their normal, unaffected siblings. In those rare hyperphenylalaninemia variants involving synthesis or recycling of the tetrahydrobiopterin cofactor, therapy involves providing pharamacological amounts of either biopterin or tetrahydrobiopterin coupled with pharmacological supplementation of neurotransmitters or their precursors. The latter therapies are designed to correct the functional central nervous system consequences resulting from the deficient tetrahydrobiopterin-mediated hydroxylation reactions of neurotransmitter synthesis.[22]

A similar approach has been used in maple syrup urine disease, more correctly termed branched-chain ketoacidemia, which results from deficiency of the branched-chain ketoacid dehydrogenase involved in the catabolism of all three branched-chain amino acids.[20] However, because metabolic imbalance and accumulation of branched ketoacid intermediates produce generalized metabolic acidosis and life-threatening episodic crises, in contrast with phenylketonuria, in which toxicity is largely confined to the central nervous system, therapeutic approaches in branched-chain ketoacidemia have been less successful in preventing long-term medical and neurological sequelae than in phenylketonuria. Providing adequate energy intake as carbohydrate and fat helps to prevent tissue protein catabolism, which occurs during fasting and illness, and thereby ameliorates chronic acidosis and reverses metabolic crises in those disorders involving amino acid catabolic pathways. Similarly, propionic and methylmalonic acidemias,[15] when not responsive to vitamins or cofactors,[16] are treated with diets low in valine, isoleucine, threonine, and methionine—precursors to both methylmalonyl- and propionyl-CoA. Leucine restriction in isovaleric acidemia due to isovaleryl-CoA dehydrogenase deficiency decreases the frequency and severity of metabolic decompensations and clinical crises.[21]

In the hyperammonemias due to urea cycle disorders, dietary protein restriction is a mainstay of therapy.[12] Severe enzymatic blocks in the urea cycle also interfere with arginine synthesis, converting this amino acid from a nonessential to an essential one in these patients. Arginine supplementation also has the benefit of decreasing tissue protein catabolism and, as a result, the flux of nitrogen moieties through the urea cycle, which synthesizes urea from excess dietary nitrogen for urinary excretion. In carbamyl phosphate synthetase and ornithine transcarbamylase deficiencies, citrulline supplementation permits arginine synthesis, promotes excretion of 1 mol tissue waste nitrogen per mol urea excreted, and inhibits tissue protein catabolism. Essential amino acid supplementation and synthetic low-protein diets help lower total nitrogen intake and forestall hyperammonemic crises.

In many disorders, supplementing essential or nonessential nutrients at either physiological or pharmacological levels may correct acquired nutrient deficiencies or divert, conjugate, or inhibit the production of otherwise toxic metabolic intermediates. In Hartnup disease, decreased gastrointestinal absorption and increased urinary excretion of α-monoamino-monocarboxylic amino acids lead to systemic deficiency of several essential amino acids, notably tryptophan, a precursor for nicotinamide synthesis.[14] In this disorder, therefore, intakes of essential amino acids must be raised to permit positive nitrogen balance, and nicotinamide supplements must be provided. In isovaleric acidemia, glycine supplementation promotes conjugation of accumulated isovaleryl-CoA by N-glycine acylase to yield isovalerylglycine, which is effectively excreted in the urine, improving the clearance of isovaleryl moities.[21]

Similarly, in prolidase deficiency, which results from the absence of the dipeptidase-cleaving imidodipeptides, the total body balance of glycine, proline, hydroxyproline, and other essential and nonessential amino acids may be altered by the increased urinary losses of these compounds as glycylproline and other imidodipeptides.[23] The increased collagen turnover noted in patients with prolidase deficiency may reflect systemic attempts to maintain normal intracellular pools of these precursor amino acids. However, the increased collagen turnover could theoretically be related to the potentially severe dermatological manifestations of this disease. To date, supplementation with essential and nonessential amino acids has not been shown to be effective in this rare, autosomal-recessive disorder, although such therapies may merit further investigation.

Disorders of Carbohydrate Metabolism

Treating disorders of carbohydrate metabolism involves several different nutritional approaches. In galactosemia, which results from deficiency of galactose-1-phosphate uridyl transferase, ingestion of galactose or any galactose-containing disaccharide leads to the production of galactitol and other toxic metabolites.[10] Toxic manifestations include rapidly progressive hepatic dysfunction that leads to hepatic necrosis if galactose ingestion is not stopped, as well as the development of cataracts and renal tubular dysfunction. The mainstay of treatment is lifetime avoidance of galactose ingestion, which prevents the development of the potentially fatal hepatic complications. However, galactosemic individuals detected by neonatal screening programs and treated with galactose restriction starting in the first week of life still exhibit largely unexplained late sequelae. These include specific expressive speech delays, subtle intellectual dysfunction, and premature ovarian failure in females. It has been widely debated whether intracellular uridine deficiency plays a role in the pathogenesis of these late complications; to date, this hypothesis has not been confirmed and no consensus has been reached regarding treatment of galactosemic individuals with uridine. In hereditary fructose intolerance due to deficiency of fructose aldolase B, the clinical presentation is generally more chronic than that in galactosemia and consists of failure to grow, mild hepatotoxicity, and proximal renal tubular dysfunction.[9] As in galactosemia, in hereditary fructose intolerance, lifetime avoidance of fructose largely prevents the development of symptoms.

The first described of the glycogen storage diseases, type I or von Gierke disease, which results from a deficiency of glucose-6-phosphatase, is the carbohydrate disorder with the most protean effects on hepatic and total body glycogen and glucose metabolism.[13] Glucose-6-phosphatase is a key regulatory enzyme of glucose homeostasis. Almost all hepatic glucose production and output into the circulation by either glycogenolysis, gluconeogenesis, or hexose interconversion is mediated by this microsomal enzyme. The primary biochemical consequence of this enzymatic deficiency is severe, chronic, and unremitting hypoglycemia, which results in activation of pathways of lipolysis, and, futilely, gluconeogenesis and glycogenolysis, either directly by biochemical or indirectly by endocrinological mechanisms. The functional result is an influx of carbon moieties to the liver, leading to the overproduction of acetyl-CoA and other compounds, such as lactic acid, cholesterol, triacylglycerol, and uric acid.

Formerly, children affected with von Gierke disease either died of lactic acidosis in early infancy or developed severe failure to grow associated with the metabolic and physiologic abnormalities mentioned above, as well as late-onset renal dysfunction. Initially, therapy consisted of frequent carbohydrate feedings during the waking hours. However, a major therapeutic advance was the provision of continuous nocturnal glucose administration via nasogastric tubes to normalize blood glucose levels uniformly during the hours of sleep. Normalization of blood glucose levels decreases lactic acid production, inhibits futile gluconeogenesis and glycogenolysis, and lowers circulating levels of catabolic hormones, such as glucocorticoids, epinephrine, and glucagon. More recently, intermittent enteral dosing with carbohydrate in the form of cornstarch at doses approximating normal hepatic glucose production has largely replaced nocturnal nasogastric therapy.[24] Blood glucose levels can be normalized both day and night with this technique, with the result that lactic acid, uric acid, triacylglycerol, and cholesterol levels fall, hepatomegaly resolves, and growth improves. In this disorder, normalization of blood glucose levels by nutritional therapy, which is easily postulated but often difficult to achieve, should permit effective treatment of most affected individuals.

In glycogen storage disease type III, which is due to a deficiency of the amylo-1,6-glucosidase debrancher enzyme, hepatic glucose production from glycogen is largely interrupted, although gluconeogenesis from other carbon sources remains intact. In early infancy the clinical presentation of these individuals—failure to thrive, hepatomegaly, and hypoglycemia—is similar to but often less severe than that of individuals with glycogen storage disease type I. In later childhood and adolescence, these symptoms generally spontaneously resolve and clinical status improves. However, later in adult life, affected individuals may develop a debilitating myopathy, presumably due, at least in part, to increased muscle protein turnover during fasting and sleep, with the resultant amino acid flux utilized to maintain blood glucose levels via gluconeogenesis. In these individuals, avoidance of fasting and the provision of cornstarch therapy and protein and amino acid supplements could theoretically prevent the progression of or even reverse the myopathic process, although this therapy remains unproved.

Vitamin- and Cofactor-responsive Disorders

There are many well-documented cofactor-dependent metabolic disorders. In general, these disorders are characterized by unequivocal biochemical and/or clinical responses to orally administered supraphysiological doses of a vitamin or cofactor, or to parenterally administered native or modified cofactors. Examples include the pyridoxine (vitamin B-6)-responsive homocystinurias,[17] cobalamin (vitamin B-12)-responsive methylmalonic acidemias,[15,16] biotin-responsive propionic acidemia,[15,18] thiamine-responsive branched-chain ketoacidemia,[20] riboflavin-responsive disorders of β-oxidation,[4,5] and other, very rare defects, such as those involving plasma transport proteins, for example, transcobalamin II deficiency.[25] Another related disorder is biotinidase deficiency, a metabolic disorder characterized by functional tissue biotin deficiency resulting from the defective release of covalently protein-bound biotin. Biotinidase deficiency can be treated effectively with high doses of biotin.[18]

In all these disorders, either supranormal amounts of normal vitamins and cofactors are needed, as in the pyridoxine-responsive homocystinurias,[17] or physiologic but modified forms of the vitamins must be provided, as in the methylmalonic acidemias resulting from defective conversion of hydroxycobalamin to adenosyl- and methyl-cobalamins[16] or in the folate cycle disorders.[19] Marked genetic and biochemical heterogeneity underlie many of these disorders. In many cases, the clinical and biochemical differentiation of vitamin-responsive from vitamin-unresponsive variants is very difficult. In the methylmalonic acidemias, molecular genetic techniques have helped define specific mutations associated with vitamin-responsive and nonresponsive phenotypes.[26]

The treatment of other disorders, such as a defect of the electron transport chain due to deficiencies of the individual enzyme complexes of the mitochondrial respiratory chain, is much more problematic.[27,28] In many of these disorders, even when specific deficiencies of individual respiratory chain complexes are defined, which are most commonly those of complex I (NADH:coenzyme Q oxidoreductase) or complex IV (cytochrome c oxidase), only nonspecific and unproven therapies are available that make use of combinations of the vitamins and cofactors involved primarily or secondarily in mitochondrial electron transport or that may shunt electron transfer around the defective complex. These cofactor combinations include thiamine, lipoic acid, biotin, riboflavin, nicotinamide, coenzyme Q_{10}, menadione (vitamin K_3), ascorbic acid, and vitamin E. In certain defects of the electron transport chain, attempts can be made to circumvent the metabolic block by providing nutrients that can be metabolized despite the block. For example, in complex I deficiency, succinic acid supplementation has been attempted, as has menadione and ascorbic acid therapy in complex III deficiency (coenzyme Q_{10}:cytochrome c oxidoreductase).[29]

Similar approaches are used to treat lactic acidemias due to pyruvate dehydrogenase deficiency.[30] These disorders involve the major entry point for carbon moieties from the glycolytic pathway into the tricarboxylic acid cycle. Similar approaches are used in the related gluconeogenic disorders pyruvate carboxylase deficiency and phosphoenolpyruvate carboxykinase deficiency. Riboflavin, thiamin, and lipoic acid supplementation are used with limited success in pyruvate dehydrogenase deficiency, as is biotin supplementation in pyruvate carboxylase deficiency. These disorders are also treated, with varying effectiveness, by dietary manipulations delivering a diet relatively low in carbohydrate energy and high in fat and protein. However, given the critical biochemical roles played by both the enzymes of pyruvate metabolism and of the mitochondrial electron transport chain in intermediary and energy metabolism, therapies based on cofactors and on diet are only marginally successful in a minority of cases.

Inborn Errors of Fatty Acid β-Oxidation

The enzymatic deficiencies producing defective mitochondrial β-oxidation have become more prominent since 1982, when medium-chain acyl-CoA dehydrogenase deficiency was first identified.[31] β-Oxidation disorders have a broad clinical spectrum, with marked heterogeneity even within a single enzymatic deficiency.[4,5] For example, short-chain acyl-CoA dehydrogenase deficiency has been associated with either clinical normalcy or death in the neonatal period or with early onset of significant neuromuscular retardation. Similarly, palmityl carnitine transferase I deficiency produces a complete inability of the mitochondria to transport and β-oxidize long-chain (C16) fatty acids, and leads to markedly impaired ketogenesis and hypoglycemia with prolonged fasting. However, individuals with this deficiency are clinically normal if they have not suffered sequelae due to severe hypoglycemia during an episode of fasting. In contrast, very-long-chain acyl-CoA dehydrogenase deficiency can result in significant neuromuscular and cardiac complications.[32]

The clinical hallmark of most, but not all, of these disorders is hypoglycemia and reduced ketogenesis during fasting. Dietary therapy includes providing diets that are low in fat, avoiding hypoglycemia by frequent feedings and, more rarely, supplementation with carbohydrate or cornstarch. In those disorders that affect only the β-oxidation of long-chain fats, such as very-long-chain acyl-CoA dehydrogenase deficiency, medium-chain triacylglycerols can be oxidized normally and are given therapeutically. In many of these disorders, riboflavin is given orally in the hopes of increasing levels of intramitochondrial flavin adenine dinucleotide, and thus raising the activity of β-oxidation flavoproteins, such as the acyl-CoA dehydrogenases. However, clinically and biochemically confirmed cases of riboflavin-responsive β-oxidation disorders are few in number.[4,5,33] Dietary supplementation with carnitine and glycine may promote disposal of accumulated intramitochondrial acyl-CoA as either acyl-carnitines or acyl-glycines.[34] Carnitine supplementation also appears to be effective in the treatment of other disorders characterized by intramitochondrial acyl-CoA accumulation, such as methylmalonic and propionic acidemias[15] and, possibly, branched-chain ketoacidemia.[20] The acyl-carnitines and acyl-glycines excreted in the urine generally reflect the chain length of the accumulated intramitochondrial acyl-CoAs. The oxidation of these acyl-CoAs is blocked by the enzymatic deficiency, although, most commonly, the acids excreted in the urine are metabolically modified derivatives of the parent compound.[21]

Smith-Lemli-Opitz syndrome is a genetic disorder characterized by microcephaly, characteristic facial features, severe psychomotor retardation, genital anomalies in males, and cutaneous syndactyly.[35] This disorder was long thought to result from disturbed embryogenesis, although its inheritance in an autosomal recessive manner would imply that an important catalytic polypeptide, i.e., an enzyme, is absent. This possibility was recently confirmed by the finding that the syndrome results from defective cholesterol synthesis due to a deficiency of the enzyme 7-dehydrocholesterol reductase.[8] This enzymatic block leads to the accumulation of 7-dehydrocholesterol and systemic cholesterol deficiency. Therapeutic trials are now underway to treat this disorder with cholesterol supplementation, as well as with bile acids, essential fatty acids, and the fat-soluble vitamins A, D, E, and K.[36] Smith-Lemli-Opitz syndrome is therefore an enzymatic deficiency that blocks an important anabolic, rather than a catabolic, pathway, although the toxic effects of the accumulated 7-dehydrocholesterol are difficult to delineate at present.

Adrenoleukodystrophy is a peroxisomal disorder inherited in an X-linked recessive fashion.[7] The enzymatic deficiency involves activation and transport of very-long-chain fatty acids across the peroxisomal membrane, after which the fatty acid chain would normally be shortened by the peroxisomal β-oxidation system. Systemic accumulation of very-long-chain fatty acids affects both central nervous system function and adrenal function to varying degrees in different affected males, even in brothers in the same family. The early-onset (before the age of 10), rapidly progressive, and fatal disease is termed adrenoleukodystrophy, whereas the later-onset (adult), slowly progressive form is called adrenomyeloneuropathy. The reason for the clinical and phenotypical heterogeneity in related males with presumably identical biochemical defects remains unknown. However, the provision of diets high in triacylglycerols containing erucic and oleic acids and low in long-chain fat prevents chain elongation of dietary long-chain (C16) fatty acids to very-long-chain (C22–C32) fatty acids. Thus, glycerol-trioleate and -trierucate therapy hold some promise for the treatment of this devastating disease; therapeutic trials of these compounds are currently under way. This therapy incorporates the interesting feature of using a normal nutrient in unusually high amounts to inhibit an anabolic synthetic pathway, the end products of which, if accumulated, are deleterious.

In other disorders, such as glutathione synthetase deficiency, also termed 5-oxoprolinuria, provision of normal intracellular metabolites that are not usually micro- or macronutrients may be necessary.[37] In glutathione synthetase deficiency, progressive mental retardation, retinal damage and dysfunction, spasticity, chronic metabolic acidosis, and hemolytic anemia all result from an intracellular deficiency of the essential tripeptide antioxidant glutathione. Raising intracellular glutathione levels may mitigate many, and possibly all, of these clinical manifestations. However, glutathione itself cannot be absorbed at either the intestinal, cellular, or tissue level. The pioneering work of Meister[38] and coworkers on the effective cellular uptake of simple glutathione alcohol esters suggested a potential means of treatment, and we are currently conducting a clinical trial of glutathione monoethyl ester therapy in patients with this disorder. This treatment illustrates another therapeutic approach involving use of simple derivatives of essential biochemical compounds as nutrients in and of themselves. Although there is no dietary requirement for glutathione as such, an adult theoretically would require between 50 and 200 g glutathione/day absorbed into the intracellular compartment to replace endogenous glutathione synthesis. Similarly, in hereditary orotic aciduria due to uridine monophosphate synthetase deficiency, which is characterized by macrocytic megaloblastic anemia and orotic acid crystalluria, correction of the uridine deficiency with supplements of this pyrimidine has generally yielded clinical improvement.[39]

Summary

Certain disorders of carbohydrate, amino acid, and fatty acid metabolism can be treated with nutritional approaches, as can various other disorders that involve vitamin and cofactor metabolism. The general principles include the use of conventional nutrients in either unusually high or low amounts or in chemically modified forms. Many potential treatments may involve the provision of metabolic intermediates not usually thought of as micro- or macronutrients in pharmacological quantities to correct deficiency states, to prevent synthesis of potentially toxic intermediates, or to bypass metabolic blocks produced by enzymatic deficiencies. As our understanding of metabolic pathways and alternative routes of metabolism increases, other possibilities for effective therapy of inherited metabolic disorders should become apparent. These developments underscore the need for close cooperation and collaboration among nutritionists, biochemists, geneticists, and molecular biologists in elucidating the etiology of these disorders and in developing effective nutritional therapies for them.

References

1. Garrod AE (1908) The Croonian lecturers on inborn errors of metabolism. Lecture II. Alkaptonuria. Lancet 2:73
2. Beaudet AL, Scriver CR, Sly WS, Davlle D (1995) Genetics, biochemistry, and molecular basis of variant human phenotypes. In Scriver CR, Beaudet AL, Sly WS, Valle D (eds), The metabolic and molecular bases of inherited disease, 7th ed. McGraw-Hill, New York, pp 53–228
3. Childs B (1995) A logic of disease. In Scriver CR, Beaudet AL, Sly WS, Valle D (eds), The metabolic and molecular bases of inherited disease, 7th ed. McGraw-Hill, New York, pp 229–258
4. Rhead WJ (1991) Inborn errors of fatty acid oxidation in man. Clin Biochem 24:319–329
5. Roe CR (1995) Mitochondrial fatty acid oxidation disorders. In Scriver CR, Beaudet AL, Sly WS, Valle D (eds), The metabolic and molecular bases of inherited disease, 7th ed. McGraw-Hill, New York, pp 1501–1534
6. Lazarow PB, Moser HW (1995) Disorders of peroxisome biogenesis. In Scriver CR, Beaudet AL, Sly WS, Valle D (eds), The metabolic and molecular bases of inherited disease, 7th ed. McGraw-Hill, New York, pp 2287–2324
7. Moser HW, Smith KD, Moser AB (1995) X-linked adrenoleukodystrophy. In Scriver CR, Beaudet AL, Sly WS, Valle D (eds), The metabolic and molecular bases of inherited disease, 7th ed. McGraw-Hill, New York, pp 2325–2350
8. Irons M, Elias E, Tint GS, et al (1994) Abnormal cholesterol metabolism in the Smith-Lemli-Opitz syndrome: report of clinical and biochemical findings in four patients and treatment in one other. Am J Med Genet 50:347–352
9. Gitzelmann R, Steinmann B, Van den Berghe G (1995) Disorders of fructose metabolism. In Scriver CR, Beaudet AL, Sly WS, Valle D (eds), The metabolic and molecular bases of inherited disease, 7th ed. McGraw-Hill, New York, pp 905–934
10. Segal S, Berry GT (1995) Disorders of galactose metabolism. In Scriver CR, Beaudet AL, Sly WS, Valle D (eds), The metabolic and molecular bases of inherited disease, 7th ed. McGraw-Hill, New York, pp 967–1000
11. Scriver CR, Kaufman S, Eisensmsith RC, Woo SLC (1995) The hyperphenylalaninemias. In Scriver CR, Beaudet AL, Sly WS, Valle D (eds), The metabolic and molecular bases of inherited disease, 7th ed. McGraw-Hill, New York, pp 1015–1076
12. Brusilow SW, Horwich AL (1995) Urea cycle enzymes. In Scriver CR, Beaudet AL, Sly WS, Valle D (eds), The metabolic and molecular bases of inherited disease, 7th ed. McGraw-Hill, New York, pp 1187–1232
13. Chen Y-T, Burchell A (1995) Glycogen storage diseases. In Scriver CR, Beaudet AL, Sly WS, Valle D (eds), The meta-

bolic and molecular bases of inherited disease, 7th ed. McGraw-Hill, New York, pp 935–968

14. Levy HL (1995) Hartnup disorder. In Scriver CR, Beaudet AL, Sly WS, Valle D (eds), The metabolic and molecular bases of inherited disease, 7th ed. McGraw-Hill, New York, pp 3629–3642

15. Fenton WA, Rosenberg LE (1995) Disorders of propionate and methylmalonate metabolism. In Scriver CR, Beaudet AL, Sly WS, Valle D (eds), The metabolic and molecular bases of inherited disease, 7th ed. McGraw-Hill, New York, pp 1423–1450

16. Fenton WA, Rosenberg LE (1995) Inherited disorders of cobalamin transport and metabolism. In Scriver CR, Beaudet AL, Sly WS, Valle D (eds), The metabolic and molecular bases of inherited disease, 7th ed. McGraw-Hill, New York, pp 3129–3150

17. Mudd SH, Levy HL, Skovy F (1995) Disorders of transsulfuration. In Scriver CR, Beaudet AL, Sly WS, Valle D (eds), The metabolic and molecular bases of inherited disease, 7th ed. McGraw-Hill, New York, pp 1279–1328

18. Wolf B (1995) Disorders of biotin metabolism. In Scriver CR, Beaudet AL, Sly WS, Valle D (eds), The metabolic and molecular bases of inherited disease, 7th ed. McGraw-Hill, New York, pp 3151–3180

19. Rosenblatt DS (1995) Inherited disorders of folate transport and metabolism. In Scriver CR, Beaudet AL, Sly WS, Valle D (eds), The metabolic and molecular bases of inherited disease, 7th ed. McGraw-Hill, New York, pp 3111–3128

20. Chuang DT, Shih VE (1995) Disorders of branched chain amino acid and keto acid metabolism. In Scriver CR, Beaudet AL, Sly WS, Valle D (eds), The metabolic and molecular bases of inherited disease, 7th ed. McGraw-Hill, New York, pp 1239–1278

21. Sweetman L, Williams JC (1995) Branched chain organic acidurias. In Scriver CR, Beaudet AL, Sly WS, Valle D (eds), The metabolic and molecular bases of inherited disease, 7th ed. McGraw-Hill, New York, pp 1387–1422

22. McInnes RR, Kaufman S, Warsh JJ, et al (1984) Biopterin synthesis defect: treatment with L-dopa and 5-hydroxytryptophan compared with therapy with a tetrahydropterin. J Clin Invest 73:458–469

23. Phang JM, Yeh GC, Scriver CR (1995) Disorders of proline and hydroxyproline metabolism. In Scriver CR, Beaudet AL, Sly WS, Valle D (eds), The metabolic and molecular bases of inherited disease, 7th ed. McGraw-Hill, New York, pp 1125–1146

24. Chen Y-T, Cornblath M, Sidbury JB (1984) Cornstarch therapy in type I glycogen storage disease. N Engl J Med 31:171–175

25. Seligman PA, Steiner D, Allen RH (1980) Studies of a patient with megaloblastic anemia and an abnormal transcobalamin II. N Engl J Med 303:1209–1212

26. Wilkemeyer MF, Crane AM, Ledley FD (1991) Differential diagnosis of *mut* and *cbl* methylmalonic aciduria by DNA-mediated gene transfer in primary fibroblasts. J Clin Invest 87:915–918

27. Shoffner JM, Wallace DC (1995) Oxidative phosphorylation diseases. In Scriver CR, Beaudet AL, Sly WS, Valle D (eds), The metabolic and molecular bases of inherited disease, 7th ed. McGraw-Hill, New York, pp 1535–1610

28. Frerman FE, Goodman SI (1995) Nuclear-encoded defects of the mitochondrial respiratory chain, including glutaric acidemia type II. In Scriver CR, Beaudet AL, Sly WS, Valle D (eds), The metabolic and molecular bases of inherited disease, 7th ed. McGraw-Hill, New York, pp 1611–1630

29. Argov Z, Bank WJ, Maris J, et al (1986) Treatment of mitochondrial myopathy due to Complex III deficiency with vitamins K_3 and C: a 31P-NMR follow-up study. Ann Neurol 19:598–602

30. Robinson BH (1995) Lactic acidemia (disorders of pyruvate carboxylase, pyruvate dehydrogenase). In Scriver CR, Beaudet AL, Sly WS, Valle D (eds), The metabolic and molecular bases of inherited disease, 7th ed. McGraw-Hill, New York, pp 1479–1500

31. Divry P, David M, Gregersen N, et al (1983) Dicarboxylic aciduria: evidence due to medium-chain acyl-CoA dehydrogenase defect: a cause of hypoglycemia in childhood. Acta Paediatr Scand 72:943–946

32. Aoyama T, Uchida Y, Kelley RI, et al (1995) A novel disease with deficiency of mitochondrial very-long-chain acyl-CoA dehydrogenase. Biochem Biophys Res Commun 191: 1369–1372

33. Rhead W, Roettger V, Marshall T, Amendt B (1993) Multiple acyl-coenzyme A dehydrogenation disorder responsive to riboflavin: substrate oxidation, flavin metabolism, and flavoenzyme activities in fibroblasts. Pediatr Res 33:129–135

34. Rinaldo P, Welch RD, Previs SF, et al (1991) Ethylmalonic/adipic aciduria: effects of oral medium-chain triglycerides, carnitine, and glycine on urinary excretion of organic acids, acylcarnitines, and acylglycines. Pediatr Res 30:216–221

35. Smith DW, Lemli L, Opitz JM (1964) A newly recognized syndrome of multiple congenital anomalies. J Pediatr 64:210–217

36. Acosta PB (1995) Theoretical and practical aspects of dietary treatment of Smith-Lemli-Opitz syndrome. Int Pediatr 10:37–40

37. Meister A, Larrson A (1995) Glutathione synthetase deficiency and other disorders of the γ-glutamyl cycle. In Scriver CR, Beaudet AL, Sly WS, Valle D (eds), The metabolic and molecular bases of inherited disease, 7th ed. McGraw-Hill, New York, pp 1461–1478

38. Meister A (1991) Glutathione deficiency produced by inhibition of its synthesis, and its reversal: applications in research and therapy. Pharmacol Ther 51:155–194

39. Webster DR, Becroft DMO, Suttle DP (1995) Hereditary orotic aciduria and other disorders of pyrimidine metabolism. In Scriver CR, Beaudet AL, Sly WS, Valle D (eds), The metabolic and molecular bases of inherited disease, 7th ed. McGraw-Hill, New York, pp 1799–2160

Chapter 64

Nutrient Standards, Dietary Guidelines, and Food Guides

Susan Welsh

Nutrient standards, dietary guidelines, and food guides each define aspects of a healthful diet, but in different ways (Figure 1). Since the chapter that covered these topics in the 1990 edition of *Present Knowledge in Nutrition* was written, there have been significant changes in each of these areas.[5] A major revision of the approach to determining nutrient standards is being formulated, dietary guidelines for the general population were revised and released in 1995, and a new food guide has become well established.[1,2,6,7] However, probably the most significant change over the past 5 years is that the development processes and uses of nutrient standards, dietary guidelines, and food guides have begun to come together.

Nutrient standards for diets are defined as the average daily amounts of essential nutrients estimated on the basis of available scientific knowledge to be sufficiently high to meet the physiological needs of nearly all healthy persons. The discoveries of essential nutrients and their functions, which occurred rapidly during the first half of the century, led to the establishment of nutrient standards. Their research base usually involves experimental studies in which quantities of nutrients needed to support growth, maintain weight, and prevent nutrient deficiencies are determined. Nutrient standards are intended for use by the professional nutrition community as reference points, most often for planning diets and also as a base for evaluating the dietary status of groups. In the United States, nutrient standards are essentially synonymous with the recommended dietary allowances (RDAs) developed by the Food and Nutrition Board of the National Academy of Sciences since 1941.[8]

Dietary guidelines have been distinguished from nutrient standards in several ways: they give advice on consumption of types of foods or food components for which there is a related public health concern; they frequently are established for food components for which RDAs have not been available; they include recommendations for nonessential food components; they are often expressed in relation to the total diet and in qualitative terms, e.g., to eat more; and they are intended for the public directly or indirectly through educators, health professionals, and policy makers. The research base for dietary guidelines relies more on clinical and epidemiologic research relating the composition of the diet, either in terms of nutrients, food components, or types of foods, to the risk of diet-related diseases of public health significance. Although there are some notable exceptions, most dietary guidelines have been released over the past 15 years. The U.S. Department of Agriculture (USDA) and the Department of Health and Human Services (DHHS) released four editions of *Dietary Guidelines for Americans* in 1980, 1985, 1990, and 1995.[2] These guidelines are important for two reasons. First, they are a statement of federal nutrition policy and, as such, form the basis of all federal nutrition programs directed to the general healthy population. Second, they are widely accepted by the scientific community as a consensus of research findings relating diet and health; therefore, they are widely used by both the public and private sectors.

Food guides are a translation of both nutrient standards and dietary guidelines into recommendations on daily food intake. A food guide is a conceptual framework for selecting the kinds and amounts of foods of various types that together provide a nutritionally satisfactory diet. Science-based food guides depend on several types of research, including research that establishes nutrient standards and dietary guidelines as well as research on the composition of food, food intake patterns, and the factors that influence food choice in the population for which the food guide is being developed. A different body of research is needed to effectively communicate food guides in ways that actually change the eating behavior of the target audience. In the United States, science-based food guides were first published in 1916, but probably the most widely known have been the Basic Four and, currently, the Food Guide Pyramid.[1,9,10]

Over the past century, the differences between nutrient standards, dietary guidelines, and food guides sometimes have been more apparent than the connection between them. At the beginning of the century, basic and applied nutrition research were integrated. Single reports covered research on quantities of essential nutrients to include in daily diets, qualitative guidance on avoiding nutritional excesses, data on food composition and consumption, and practical advice on appealing, cost-efficient menus.[11,12] As the research base grew, these topics

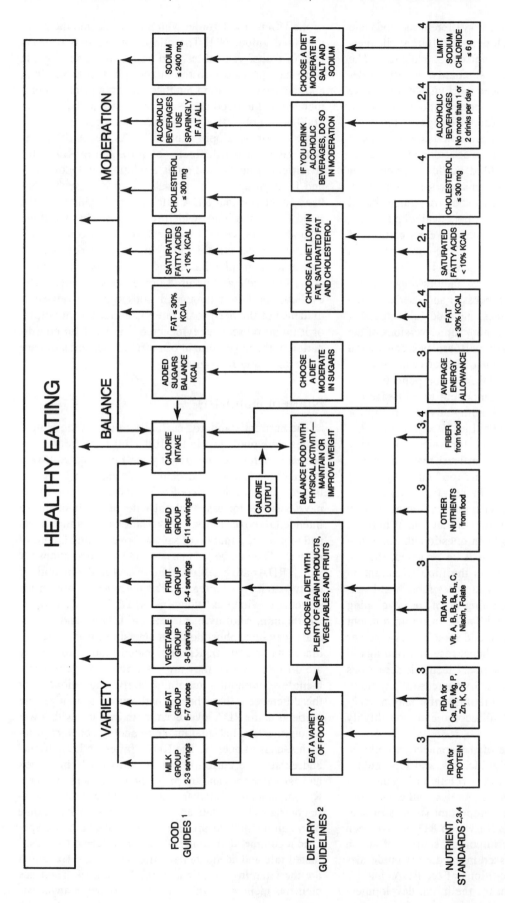

Figure 1. The relationship of specified nutrient standards, dietary guidelines, and food guidelines to healthy eating.

became compartmentalized, with different methods and expertise required for development, different channels of communication, and different target audiences. The connections between nutrient standards, dietary guidelines, and food guides have been most visible when there has been a need to balance concerns about nutritional adequacy and excesses. The food shortages of the Great Depression and World War II prompted concerns about nutritional adequacy, bringing the development processes for nutrient standards and food guides together. For example, Hazel Stiebeling and an associate[13,14] published nutrient standards and family food buying guides based on these standards to help consumers deal with the economic stress of the depression; and the early editions of the RDAs included food guides to help consumers deal with the food shortages of World War II.[8]

Over the past 5 years, several factors appear to be bringing the development processes and uses of nutrient standards, dietary guidelines, and food guides together again. In deliberations concerning future versions of the RDAs, the Food and Nutrition Board has considered expanding the RDAs to include quantitative dietary recommendations for nonessential food components when adequate data relating the component to a disease exist.[6] Also considered was including advice directly for the public, perhaps as a food guide. The 1990 and 1995 editions of the dietary guidelines for Americans already include quantitative limits for at least two nutrients—fat and saturated fatty acids—and food guide–type recommendations for three food groups—fruits, vegetables, and grain products. The process of developing dietary guidelines on the basis of research that relates nutrient intake to function has also been questioned. Some nutrition authorities suggest that it be reversed, that is, "natural experiments" in which the food consumption patterns of groups of people with a desirable health status would be used as the starting point for developing dietary guidelines.[15] Another factor bringing nutrient standards, dietary guidelines, and food guides together is consumer demand for the latest research findings to be translated into practical advice. Electronic access has and will continue to dramatically increase the rapidity and breadth of communication of all information, making conflicting or impractical recommendations highly visible.

The growing importance of the connection between nutrient standards, dietary guidelines, and food guides is perhaps best illustrated by the evolution of recommendations for intakes of fruits, vegetables, and grain products. These food groups are important sources of specific vitamins and minerals for which RDAs have been established. They are also important sources of starch and fiber, which are addressed in the dietary guidelines for Americans. The 1980 editions of the RDAs and dietary guidelines were input for the initial development of the USDA food guide, which later became the pyramid food guide.[1,2,16,17] The minimum numbers of servings of fruits, vegetables, and grains in the food guide were incorporated into the dietary guidelines in 1990, and the same minimum numbers of servings are recommended by the Food and Nutrition Board and are a year 2000 health objective.[4,18] In discussions concerning the methods for developing future RDAs, recognition has been given to the difficulty of formulating RDAs for specific nutrients based on data relating intake of foods and food groups to the prevalence of disease.[19] It has been suggested that RDA calculations begin "from the Food Guide Pyramid, which represents what we think a good diet delivers."[20] In effect, the Food Guide Pyramid, which was considered by its developers to be one way of implementing RDAs and dietary guidelines, could come full circle and be used in their development. The evolution of these recommendations might be viewed as evidence of the need to differentiate input from output, or it might be seen as evidence of the need for coordination in the development of nutrient standards, dietary guidelines, and food guides.

Nutrient Standards

The nutrient standards currently in use in the United States were published in the 10th edition of the *Recommended Dietary Allowances* by the Food and Nutrition Board of the National Academy of Sciences in 1989 (see Figure 1).[3] Since they were first published in 1941, RDAs have been set for essential nutrients at levels of intake intended to cover individual variations in requirements and to provide a margin of safety above minimal requirements.[6,8] The number of nutrients and subpopulations for which RDAs are established increased as the breadth of the research base increased. Currently RDAs are set for protein, 11 vitamins (vitamins A, D, E, K, C, B-6, B-12, thiamin, riboflavin, niacin, and folate), and 7 minerals (calcium, phosphorus, magnesium, iron, zinc, iodine, and selenium). Recommended intakes of energy are different in that they are set at the average requirement level without a margin of safety. The rationale for this difference is that while no harm comes from ingesting nutrients at the RDA level even for individuals with lower requirements, a habitual intake of energy above requirements leads to obesity. The RDAs for essential nutrients and energy are currently set for individuals in 15 sex and age categories and for pregnant and lactating women. Recommendations also are established for certain essential nutrients when data are sufficient to estimate a range of requirements but are insufficient to establish a specific recommended intake. These are referred to as estimated safe and adequate daily dietary intakes. Examples are the vitamins biotin and pantothenic acid. The trace elements included in this category—copper, manganese, fluoride, chromium, and molybdenum—bear the additional caution that the upper level set for them should not be habitually exceeded because of concerns about potential toxicity. Minimum requirements have been established for three electrolytes: sodium, potassium, and chloride. Neither recommended intakes nor recommended upper limits of intake have been set for these electrolytes, but the 10th edition of the publication listing the RDAs indicates that there is no evidence of health benefits from higher intakes of sodium or chloride.

Ideally, the methods for establishing RDAs follow a process of first estimating the average physiological requirement for an absorbed nutrient by healthy individuals representative of a sex and age group. The requirement for a nutrient is defined as the minimum intake that will maintain normal function and health. An amount is then added, sometimes referred to as a safety factor, which is intended to compensate for the variance in nutrient requirements among individuals and for the variance in the bioavailability of nutrients in commonly consumed foods. The criteria used to set RDAs differ according to the function of the nutrient, the ability of the body to store the nutrient, the age, sex, and physiological status of the subpopulation for which RDAs are being defined, and the scientific judgment of the researchers involved.

Various kinds of evidence are used to establish RDAs: 1) nutrient depletion and repletion studies in which subjects are maintained on diets containing low or deficient levels of a nutrient, followed by correction of the deficit with measured amounts of the nutrient; 2) nutrient balance studies that measure nutrient status in relation to intake; 3) biochemical measurements of tissue saturation or adequacy of molecular function in relation to nutrient intake; 4) nutrient intakes of fully breastfed infants; 5) epidemiologic observations of the nutritional status of populations in relation to nutrient intake; and 6) in some cases, extrapolation of data from animal experiments. In practice, for most nutrients only some of these types of data are available on which estimates of nutrient requirements can be based.

Most revisions of the RDAs have been based on new scientific data rather than on changes in definition or development criteria. For example, between the ninth and 10th editions listing the RDAs, relatively large changes were made in the RDAs for folate and vitamin B-12, and RDAs were established for the first time for vitamin K and selenium. Another major change in the 10th edition of the RDAs was that heights and weights of reference adults in each age and sex class are actual medians for the U.S. population as reported in the second National Health and Nutrition Examination Survey. In the earlier editions listing the RDAs, reference heights and weights were set at an abritrary ideal. This change in methods had the potential to affect RDAs that correlate with body weight or caloric intake, or both, but in practice, the effect was very small.

From their original application in the early 1940s as a guide for advising on the adequacy of the food supply in connection with national defense, the RDAs have become the most well-known and used standard for nutrient intake. Probably their most frequent use is in planning diets. Another important use is as a base for evaluating diets. Specific uses include procuring food supplies for population subgroups such as the military, interpreting food consumption records of individuals and populations, establishing standards for food assistance programs, evaluating the adequacy of food supplies in meeting national nutritional needs, designing nutrition education programs, developing new products by the food industry, and establishing guidelines for nutrition labeling of foods.

As the name implies, RDAs are the amounts of nutrients intended to be consumed as part of a diet. The rationale is that a diet composed of a variety of foods from diverse food groups, as opposed to diet in which RDAs are met by supplements or a few highly fortified foods, is likely to be adequate in nutrients and other food components for which RDAs have not been established. When RDAs are met through the usual American diet, the ingestion of toxic levels of nutrients would be highly unlikely. Pharmacological actions of nutrients or undesirable toxic effects are generally possible only by high use of supplements or highly fortified foods. In addition, the development process for RDAs ideally involves an upward adjustment from the requirement level to compensate for variations in the bioavailability of nutrients among food sources. The level of adjustment needed for a nutrient depends on the degree to which digestion and absorption are affected by the form in which the nutrient occurs in food or by other components of the diet. In the United States, it is assumed that the usual mix of foods in the American diet is consumed. Significant departures from this pattern can affect the bioavailability of nutrients and the adequacy of the diet.

Although RDAs are not set for several important components of the diet, such as carbohydrate and fat, it is recommended that diets be planned on the combined basis of the RDAs and the dietary guidelines of the Food and Nutrition Board's report *Diet and Health*.[4] Even though RDAs are expressed on a per day basis, they are intended to represent an average intake over time. The length of time over which averaging should be done depends on the nutrient, the size of the body pool, and the rate of turnover of the nutrient. Therefore, it is not necessary for each day's diet to contain full RDAs for all nutrients, nor is it necessary for each meal to contain a fixed percentage of RDAs. Intakes for most nutrients can be averaged over 3 days, whereas intakes for some nutrients—such as vitamins A and B-12—could be averaged over several months. The practical recommendation given in the 10th edition of the RDAs is to plan menus that meet RDAs over 5 to 10 days.

Using the RDAs to evaluate diets poses special problems.[21] Diets that meet RDAs are generally assumed to be adequate in those nutrients. The risk of nutritional deficiency increases the further dietary intakes fall below the RDAs. However, quantifying the risk is complicated by the fact that RDAs are set above average requirements to ensure that the needs of practically all healthy people are met. How far above the requirement level the RDAs are set differs by nutrient because both the bioavailability of nutrients and the variance in requirements differ by nutrient. Therefore, a fixed cutoff point below the RDA is not indicative of the same degree of deficiency risk across nutrients. In addition to data on the variance in nutrient requirements, data on the distribution of usual nutrient intakes are needed to estimate the risk of deficiency. For a population group, a few days of dietary intake data can provide reasonable estimates of usual intakes. On the other hand, to estimate usual intake of a nutrient by an individual requires long periods of data collection, especially for nutrients that are more concentrated in a few less-frequently consumed foods. One study found that 30–50 days of dietary records could give an accurate measure (defined as being within 10% of the 365-day average 95% of time) for an individual's intake of energy, protein, carbohydrate, phosphorous, and potassium.[22] However, more than 200 days were needed to estimate vitamin C to the same level of precision and 400 or more days were needed for vitamin A. Since individuals with low intakes can also have low requirements, only statements about the probability of deficiency can be made. Physiological or biochemical data would be needed for a diagnosis of deficiency.

Even for food consumption surveys for which the response rate is high enough to alleviate concerns about nonresponse bias and for which the sample size and number of days of intake data are large enough to estimate usual intakes, the potential for a systematic bias in reporting food intake presents further problems for evaluation. It is commonly believed that adults underreport food and especially alcoholic beverage consumption.[3,4,21] National surveys indicating energy intakes only slightly higher than basal energy requirements in conjunction with data showing high prevalences of obesity have raised concerns.[23] Even under highly controlled conditions, the magnitude of the underreporting for total energy intake has been estimated to average almost 20%.[24] A uniform correction of nutrient intake data is not advisable because the magnitude and direction of bias may differ by the type of food reported and by the sex, age, and physiological status of the subject. The practical implication is that a failure to address the random variance in nutrient requirements and food intake, and the potential for systematic bias in reporting food intake, may exaggerate problems of underconsumption and minimize problems of overconsumption.[21]

Future editions of RDAs. A serious debate concerning the fundamental purpose and scientific criteria used to develop RDAs began before release of the 10th edition of *Recommended Dietary Allowances* and has continued in the scientific community. The Food and Nutrition Board has taken this as an opportunity to seek input from the nutrition community regarding uses of and methods for determining RDAs. The decision that is likely to have the greatest impact will be whether or not the traditional focus on preventing nutritional deficiencies will be expanded to include recommendations that take into account reducing the risk of nutrition-related chronic diseases. If the board decides to so expand the RDA concept, it will need to address issues related to setting recommended upper limits on the intake of food components such as fat, saturated fatty acids, or sodium, which in the past have been addressed by other National Academy of Sciences committees and by federal agencies. Decisions also will be needed concerning whether the role of essential nutrients in reducing the risk of chronic diseases as well as in preventing deficiency diseases will be considered. The most important technical decision for all RDAs will be what functional endpoints or indicators should be used in relation to nutritional adequacy and chronic disease. For example, what criteria would be used to establish recommended intakes of the antioxidant nutrients, fiber, or other food components such as bioflavonoids and carotenoids? In addition, assessments of the feasibility of simultaneously meeting all the RDAs with the current U.S. food supply may need to be considered.

The tentative decision of the Food and Nutrition Board, as reported in 1994, is to broaden the RDA concept to include the reduction in risk of chronic disease.[6] The development of multiple reference points is being considered; for example, deficient, average requirement, RDA, and upper safe levels. A similar approach was adopted in the United Kingdom.[25] Present thinking is that panels of experts should be formed to address groups of related nutrients rather than trying to cover all nutrients simultaneously. One of the first projects planned focuses on four related nutrients: calcium, vitamin D, magnesium, and phosphorus. Publications would be released as the data warrant. A separate publication that addresses appropriate uses of the recommendations by policy makers and practitoneers in diet planning and evaluation is under discussion. Also under discussion is the possible development of a report in which the standards for nutrients and food components would be translated into food-based dietary guidelines and food guides for the general population and population subgroups.

No doubt the changes under consideration for the RDAs increase the need for and complexity of nutrition research. In 1993 a cabinet-level advisory body, the National Science and Technology Council, was formed and was followed by a presidential statement that emphasized the need for a long-term public investment in fundamental scientific research and education and the need for enhanced cooperation in solving broad interdisciplinary problems.[26] Based on work done to identify national research priorities, three primary themes for nutrition research have been identified: basic studies of nutritional modulation of gene expression and metabolic processes, energy balance and its implications in obesity and related conditions, and research on how to improve behavior related to nutrition and fitness.[27] There are two other reports that may have implications for future nutrition research: one is from the Food and Nutrition Board and emphasizes new opportunities in nutrition research and the need for well-trained scientists, and one is from the National Association of State Universities and Land-Grant Colleges in which food production and consumption are viewed as part of an integrated system with a single goal of enhancing health.[28,29] This latter report is intended to serve as a reference for future food and agriculture legislation, in particular future farm bills. These activities and reports emphasize the importance of science in general or of nutrition research in particular and the effect it can have on improving the nation's health and well-being while reducing health care costs.

Dietary Guidelines

Beginning in the early 1960s, a series of publications from the American Heart Association began to link diet and heart disease.[30] During the next two decades, an intense interest in the role of diet as a controllable risk factor in the etiology of several chronic diseases developed. Interpreting the research and coming to conclusions regarding appropriate dietary guidance was strongly debated in the scientific literature. The debate was covered by the media, and both public interest and confusion were high. In 1977, Congress took action, resulting in the release of the landmark *Dietary Goals for the United States.*[31] The quantitative standards set for total fat, saturated and polyunsaturated fatty acids, total carbohydrate, added sugars, cholesterol, sodium, and protein were controversial. In 1980, USDA and DHHS released the first edition of *Nutrition and Your Health: Dietary Guidelines for Americans,* and a second, very similar, edition was released in 1985.[2] These guidelines addressed issues for which there was considerable consensus and which were thought to have the greatest potential effect on public health. The guidelines were written for the public and gave guidance in qualitative

terms, such as "avoid excess . . . ." However, the controversy continued and numerous organizations developed new sets of dietary guidelines. Without understanding the sometimes subtle differences in purpose, new guidelines were often viewed as a repudiation of past guidelines. While the scientific debate continued, diet books and products proliferated.

In the late 1980s, two major reviews of dietary guidance for the public and of the evidence relating diet to health and disease were conducted, one by the U.S. Surgeon General and one by a committee established by the Food and Nutrition Board of the National Academy of Sciences.[4,32] These reports came to very similar conclusions regarding dietary guidance for the public. They were the primary resources in developing the 1990 edition of the *Dietary Guidelines for Americans,* thereby increasing the acceptance of these guidelines by the scientific community.[2] Another factor that had a major impact on support for the 1990 edition of the guidelines was the passage of the National Nutrition Monitoring and Related Research Act of 1990 (PL 101-445). This law requires that the Secretaries of DHHS and USDA jointly issue the dietary guidelines at least every 5 years and that all federal dietary guidance for the general public be consistent with these guidelines. In addition, the development of dietary guidelines was one of the commitments made in the World Declaration on Nutrition formulated at the International Conference on Nutrition sponsored by the Food and Agriculture Organization of the United Nations and the World Health Organization.[33]

As now required by law, the 1990 edition of the *Dietary Guidelines for Americans* was revised and reissued by USDA and DHHS in 1995.[7] To this purpose, an 11-member advisory committee of nutrition experts had been established in 1994 to advise both the USDA and DHHS on revisions needed in the guidelines.[7] The committee's meetings were open to the public and written comment was sought. Although the major thrust of earlier guidelines remained unchanged, several changes were recommended. The committee was concerned that in the new edition of the guidelines more emphasis should be given to the total diet as opposed to specific foods and that the positive as opposed to the negative effects of diet be emphasized. The committee recommended that the new guidelines include information on using the Food Guide Pyramid and the nutrition facts label as tools in implementing the guidelines and that such information be included in supplemental educational materials as well. Considerably more emphasis is given to the benefits of physical activity in the new guidelines. Weight maintenance for all ages is stressed; weight gain with age is discouraged. Considerably more prominence is given to the guideline on grain products, vegetables, and fruits. A statement is included for the first time that vegetarian diets can be compatible with the dietary guidelines.

The quantitative guidelines on fat (no more than 30% of energy) and saturated fatty acids (less than 10% of energy) were retained. In effect, the guidelines on cholesterol and sodium were quantified for the first time by referencing the nutrition facts label on which they are quantified. The limit set for cholesterol is 300 mg/day and for sodium, 2400 mg/day.

In the 5 years between the 1990 and 1995 editions of the dietary guidelines, only a few major reports that include new dietary guidance were released in the United States. Reports from the National Cholesterol Education Program provided population strategies for controlling blood cholesterol in adults and children, and the National High Blood Pressure Education Program issued primary prevention strategies for high blood pressure.[34–36] A report on optimal calcium intakes included recommendations for calcium intakes that are higher than current RDAs and considerably higher than the usual American diet.[37] In addition to providing dietary recommendations related to specific diseases and food components, these reports showed the consistency of their recommendations with the more general dietary guidelines for Americans. Dietary guidelines established by other countries are generally consistent with the U.S. Dietary Guidelines (Table 1).

The focus of the nutrition and health community between 1990 and 1995 appears to have been more on the implementation of dietary guidance rather than on the development of new or different guidelines. The concepts expressed in the dietary guidelines are incorporated in the 21 nutrition-related objectives that are part of the comprehensive year 2000 health objectives.[18] Targets are set for achieving specific guidelines or the guidelines in general. For example, one objective is to increase to at least 90% the proportion of school lunch services with menus consistent with the dietary guidelines. In 1991, a Food and Nutrition Board committee recommended strategies that policy makers, health professionals, the food industry, educators, and others could use to implement dietary guidance.[67] In 1995, another Food and Nutrition Board committee reported on the prevention and treatment of obesity.[68] The National Cancer Institute has focused its nutrition education research and promotion efforts on the "Five a Day" program, which is designed to increase fruit and vegetable consumption. The USDA, in June 1995, issued a final rule requiring school meal programs to conform to the dietary guidelines by 1996–1997.[69]

Future dietary guidlines. The advisory committee established to make recommendations on the content of the 1995 edition of the dietary guidelines also made recommendations for the future development of the guidelines, their use, and their implementation. The committee identified the major scientific reports on diet and health done by the surgeon general and the National

Academy of Sciences as essential to the development of dietary guidelines, and they recommended that such reports be updated as necessary.[4,32] They specifically cited the need for research on the long-term health effects of fat intake during childhood, body weight loss versus body weight maintenance, and alcoholic beverage consumption especially in relation to cardiovascular disease. Other research needs cited included the relationship between electrolyte balance and hypertension, the function and bioavailability of compounds in plant foods important to health, and the best ways to educate the public and implement dietary change. The committee strongly recommended that dietary guidelines be developed for children including those under 2 years of age. Another strong recommendation was for research on consumer understanding of guideline messages.

The advisory committee also commented on the development process for dietary guidelines and recommended that two reports be developed by two different committees in the future. The first report would focus on the scientific rationale for dietary guidance and would be written for policy makers and health professionals; the second one would focus on effectively communicating the dietary guidance message to consumers. Presumably these reports would be released in 2000. Other major reports scheduled for release in 1996 are the *Surgeon General's Report on Dietary Fat and Health* and a review and revision of guidance from the American Heart Association. It is anticipated that both of these reports will provide the scientific basis for dietary recommendations related to intake of total fat, specific fatty acids including *trans* fatty acids, and cholesterol. Although the direction that this guidance is likely to take seems clear, the specific goals and to whom they apply are still being debated. For example, the Canadian Paediatric Society recommends that the goal of 30% or less of calories from fat should not apply until late adolescence.[70]

In the foreseeable future, it is anticipated that the general consistency of dietary guidance will allow policy makers and practitioners to focus on implementation issues. Examples include the types of changes that will need to occur in school food services to implement the Healthy Meals for Healthy Americans Act (PL 103-448) of 1994, which requires that meals served in schools meet the dietary guidelines for Americans, including the limits set for total fat and saturated fatty acids. It is anticipated that the Food Guide Pyramid will continue to be widely used in public and private sector nutrition education and promotion programs as an implementation strategy for the dietary guidelines. Under the leadership of the U.S. Agency for International Development, DHHS, and USDA, a national implementation plan to improve nutrition is being developed and it, along with implementation plans from other countries, will be submitted to the Food and Agricultural Organization of the United

Table 1. General dietary recommendations in other countries

	Adequacy		Balance		Moderation					Other recommendations
	Variety of foods	Foods high in complex CHO and fiber	Calories/ activity/ body weight	Fat, total	Saturated fatty acid	Cholesterol	Sugars, added	Salt/ sodium	Alcohol	
Australia[38]	+	+	+	+	+	−	+	+	+	a
Canada[39,40]	+	+	+	+	+	−	−	+	+	b
China[41]	−	+	+	+	+	+	+	+	+	c
Czechoslovakia[42]	+	+	+	+	−	−	+	+	+	
France[43]	+	+	+	+	+	−	+	+	+	d
Germany, Federal Republic[44]	+	+	+	+	−	−	+	+	+	e
Greece[45]	−	+	+	+	−	−	+	+	−	f
Hungary[46]	+	+	+	+	−	−	+	+	+	g
Ireland[47]	−	+	+	+	+	+	−	+	+	
Italy[48]	+	+	+	+	+	+	+	+	+	h
Japan[49,50]	+	+	+	−	+	−	+	+	+	
Korea[51]	+	−	+	+	−	+	+	+	+	i
Mexico[52]	+	+	+	+	+	−	+	+	+	
The Netherlands[53,54]	+	+	+	+	+	+	+	+	+	j
New Zealand[55]	+	−	+	+	+	+	+	+	+	k
The Nordic Countries[56] (Finland, Denmark, Iceland, Norway, Sweden)	+	+	+	+	+	+	+	+	+	l
Panama[57]	+	+	+	+	+	+	+	+	+	
The Phillipines[58]	+	−	−	−	−	+	−	+	−	n
Portugal[59]	−	+	+	+	+	+	+	+	+	o
Singapore[60]	−	+	+	+	+	+	+	+	+	p
Slovenia[61]	−	+	+	+	−	−	+	+	+	
South Africa[62]	+	+	+	+	+	−	+	+	+	q
Switzerland[63]	+	+	+	+	+	+	+	+	+	r
United Kingdom[64]	+	+	+	+	+	−	+	+	−	s
USSR[65]	+	−	−	+	+	−	−	−	−	t
Venezuela[66]	+	+	+	−	+	−	+	+	+	u

a Promote breastfeeding. Eat foods containing Ca and Fe.
b Limit caffeine. Fluoridate water.
c Distribute calorie intake among 3 meals.
d Know your risk factors, cholesterol. Do not smoke.
e Less animal protein. More frequent smaller meals, cook well, conserve nutrients.
f More milk. Eat 4–5 times/day. Do not smoke.
g Sufficient Ca. Pleasant family meals. Do not smoke.
h More legumes, fish, milk. Pleasant family meals.
i Promote breastfeeding. Moderate additives. Do not smoke.
j Replace part of the saturated fat with various unsaturated fats in the cis configuration.
k Plenty of water.
m Sufficient essential fatty acids. Protein 10–15% of calories. Distribute energy between 3 meals and snacks.
n Promote breastfeeding. Food safety. Healthy lifestyle.
o Promote breastfeeding. Fluoridate water. More milk, fish.
p Promote breastfeeding. Reduce intake of salt-cured, preserved, smoked food. Modify fat intake to equal parts saturated, monounsaturated, and polyunsaturated.
q Drink at least one litre of fluid. Restrict caffeine.
r More milk. More fluids. Cook well.
s Enjoy food. Look after vitamins and minerals in food.
t Eat at least 3 meals/day.
u Promote breastfeeding. Food economy. Moderate animal fats. Eat family meals. Drink water.

Nations and the World Health Organization as a follow-up to the World Declaration and Plan of Action for Nutrition.[33]

Food Guides

A science-based approach to the development of food guides began about 100 years ago with the work of Atwater,[11,12] in which the essential connection among health, diet, and food composition was made. As the research base developed, food guides changed.[64,65] Table 2 shows some features of the more prominent food guides used in the United States. The first food guide consisting of familiar food groups was issued by Caroline Hunt in 1916.[9] Similar food guides issued over the following decade and those food guides issued during the 1930s were actually food-buying guides providing advice on the amounts of foods to purchase and use over a specified period of time. The Basic Seven food guide issued in the 1940s and the familiar Basic Four issued in the 1950s suggest amounts of foods to eat.[10,74–76] Both the Basic Four and the Basic Seven, like other food guides of the time, were guides for foundation diets; that is, they were designed to meet only a portion, although the major portion, of calorie and nutrient needs. The Basic Four was designed to provide about 80% of the RDAs for nine nutrients (protein, vitamins A, C, and D, thiamin, riboflavin, niacin, calcium, and iron) for which there were RDAs in 1953.[79] It was assumed that people would eat more food than the guide recommended to satisfy their full needs. The focus was on avoiding nutritional deficiencies.

By the 1970s, the focus of dietary recommendations had begun to shift to concerns about dietary excesses. The turning point for food guides came in 1977 with the release of the dietary goals by the U.S. Senate Select Committee on Nutrition and Human Needs, popularly known as the "McGovern Committee."[31] In response, the USDA released the *Hassle-Free Daily Food Guide* in which a small but important revision to the Basic Four food guide was made.[77] Foods that provide primarily energy from fat and added sugars with few other nutrients were separated into a fifth food group called fats, sweets, and alcohol. The intent was to highlight the need for moderation; however, more specific advice on how to balance adequacy and moderation was not given. With the joint release by USDA and DHHS of the *Dietary Guidelines for Americans* in 1980, the USDA began work on a new food guide. There was a strong conviction that if a new food guide was to be accepted by consumers, it had to be evaluated and accepted by the professional community first. Therefore, it was considered essential that the development process be fully documented and open for peer review, and that the documentation include the purpose or under-lying goals of the food guide, the specific nutritional objectives, the food composition and food consumption databases used, and data to show that the goals and objectives specified could be achieved.[17,72,78,80,81]

The underlying goals of USDA's new food guide were based on a study of the evolution of food guides and on a needs assessment of the professional community conducted in 1983.[82,83] Approximately three fourths of the nutritionists surveyed wanted the Basic Four replaced. The criticisms of the Basic Four related to failure to assure nutrient adequacy for the full array of nutrients for which RDAs had been established by 1980, failure to address nutritional concerns about excess intake of food components, and failure to communicate effectively. Two thirds of the nutritionist surveyed indicated that they would prefer a food guide for a total diet rather than a foundation diet. Other studies indicated that the very familiarity of the Basic Four negatively influenced its ability to communicate.[84] Consumers regarded the Basic Four as old fashioned, something they already knew. As a result of this review process, the underlying goals established for development of a new food guide were to

- focus on overall health, rather than on single diseases;
- be based on up-to-date scientific research;
- address the total diet, including concerns about both adequacy and moderation;
- be realistic by meeting nutritional objectives with ordinary foods;
- be flexible by allowing for maximum consumer choice;
- be useful by reflecting the way consumers think about and use food;
- be practical by accommodating to feeding families or other groups; and
- be evolutionary and anticipate the direction of future dietary recommendations.

Nutritional objectives for the food guide were established and updated in accordance with current RDAs, dietary guidelines, and recommendations of other authoritative groups (see Figure 1).[78,81] Concerns about both adequacy and moderation were addressed. Related to adequacy concerns, the objectives for energy, protein, vitamins, and minerals were 100% of the RDAs for healthy people aged 2 and older. The objectives for carbohydrate and fiber were to provide amounts greater than usual intake through increased use of vegetables, fruits, and grains, especially whole-grain products. Related to moderation concerns, the limit for total fat was set at 30% or less of energy, and for saturated fatty acids the limit was set at <10% of energy. The limit for cholesterol was 300 mg, and for sodium it was 2400 mg. The intent was for added sugars to provide the balance of energy needed without exceeding usual intakes. The objective for total energy was to cover the range

Table 2. Major U.S. food guides: food groups and numbers of servings (daily unless noted otherwise)

FOOD GUIDE	NUMBER OF FOOD GROUPS	PROTEIN-RICH FOOD — MILK	PROTEIN-RICH FOOD — MEAT	BREADS	VEGETABLES	FRUIT	OTHER — FATS	OTHER — SUGARS
1916 Caroline Hunt [9,75] buying guides	5	MEATS AND OTHER PROTEIN-RICH FOOD (10% cal. milk, 10% cal. other) 1 C milk + 2-3 svgs other, (based on 3 oz svg)		CEREALS AND OTHER STARCHY FOODS (20% cal) 9 (based on 1 oz or 3/4 C dry cereal svg)	VEGETABLES AND FRUIT (30% cal) 5 (based on average 8oz svg)		FATTY FOODS (20% cal.) 9 (based on 1 Tbsp svg)	SUGARS (10% cal) 10 (based on 1 Tbsp svg)
1933 Stiebeling [13,14] buying guides	12	MILK 2 C	LEAN MEAT, POULTRY, FISH, 9-10/wk — DRY MATURE BEANS, PEAS, AND NUTS 1/wk — EGGS 1	FLOURS, CEREALS — As desired	LEAFY GREEN YELLOW 11-12/wk — POTATOES SWEET POTATOES 1	OTHER VEGETABLES & FRUIT 3 — TOMATOES & CITRUS 1	BUTTER ∶ — OTHER FATS ∶	SUGARS ∶
1943 Basic Seven [74,75] foundation diet	7	MILK AND MILK PRODUCTS 2 C or more	MEAT, POULTRY, FISH, EGGS, DRIED BEANS, PEAS, NUTS 1-2	BREAD, FLOUR, AND CEREALS every day	LEAFY GREEN YELLOW 1 or more — POTATOES & OTHER FRUIT & VEGETABLES 2 or more	CITRUS, TOMATO, CABBAGE SALAD GREENS 1 or more	BUTTER-FORTIFIED MARGARINE some daily	
1956 Basic Four [10,76] foundation diet	4	MILK GROUP 2 C or more	MEAT GROUP 2 or more (2-3 oz svg)	BREAD, CEREAL 4 or more (1 oz dry, 1 slice; 1/2-3/4 C cooked)	VEGETABLE-FRUIT GROUP 4 or more incl. dark green/yellow vegetables frequently and citrus daily (1/2 C or average size piece)			
1979 Hassle-Free [77] foundation diet	5	MILK-CHEESE GROUP 2 (1 C, 1-1/2 oz cheese)	MEAT, POULTRY, FISH AND BEANS GROUP 2 (2-3 oz svg)	BREAD-CEREAL GROUP 4 (1 oz dry, 1 slice; 1/2-3/4 C cooked)	VEGETABLE-FRUIT GROUP 4 or more (incl. dark green/yellow vegetables frequently and citrus daily; 1/2 C or typical portion)		FATS, SWEETS, ALCOHOL GROUP use dependent on calorie needs	
1985 Food Guide Pyramid [17,78] total diet	6	MILK, YOGURT, CHEESE 2-3 (1 C, 1-1/2 oz cheese)	MEAT, POULTRY, FISH, EGGS, DRY BEANS, NUTS 2-3 (5-7 oz total/day)	BREADS, CEREALS, RICE, PASTA 6-11 whole grain enriched (1 slice, 1/2 C cooked)	VEGETABLE 3-5 dark green/deep yellow starchy/legumes other (1 C raw, 1/2 C cooked)	FRUIT 2-4 citrus other (1/2 C or average)	FATS, OILS, SWEETS total fat not to exceed 30% cal., sweets vary according to caloric need	

recommended for moderately active individuals older than 2 years of age.

Food groups were formed primarily on the basis of nutrient content, but the way foods are generally used in meals and the way foods were grouped in past food guides also were considered. Within some of the major food groups, subgroups of foods were identified to give emphasis to nutrients of concern. For example, vegetables were separated into five subgroups to focus on their specific contributions of vitamins, minerals, and fiber; grain products were separated into enriched and whole-grain products to emphasize fiber. As in the *Hassle-Free Food Guide,* foods relatively high in fat or added sugars and relatively low in vitamins and minerals were classified into a separate group; the group was called fats, oils, and sweets. Although alcoholic beverages are included in this group, they were not highlighted in the name of the group, so that the food guide could be more easily used with audiences for whom discussion of alcoholic beverages is not appropriate.

Serving sizes were assigned to foods taking four factors into consideration: typical portion sizes reported in food consumption surveys; ease of use, for example, household units that could easily be multiplied or divided; similar nutrient content, for example, one-half cup of pasta, one-half cup of rice, and one slice of bread provide about the same amounts of nutrients; and tradition—serving sizes used in other food guides. Sometimes the factors considered in assigning serving sizes pointed in different directions. For example, a typical serving for grain products reported in national surveys more nearly equates to two slices of bread or one cup of pasta. However, serving sizes used in education materials and past food guides traditionally have been one slice of bread and one-half cup of cereal or pasta. If the larger serving sizes were used in the new food guide, the minimum number of servings from the grain group would have been three rather than six. This might have given the erroneous impression that, compared to the Basic Four, with its specified four servings from the grain group, the new food guide called for a reduction in consumption. In this case, the decision was made to retain one slice of bread as a serving size. No serving sizes were specified for the fats, oils, and sweets group because the message was to use these foods sparingly.

Determining the numbers of servings of food groups and the allowances for fat and added sugars in the total diet was a two-phase process. First, nutrient profiles were established that defined the quantities of nutrients that one could expect to obtain on average from a serving of a food group or subgroup. Therefore, the nutrient profile for each group primarily reflects the foods that are most frequently consumed within it. For example, large proportions of the grain products consumed by Americans are breads and rolls; nutrient profiles of both enriched and whole-grain subgroups reflect this. In keeping with the original goal of developing a highly flexible food guide, only lean or low-fat forms of foods without added fats or sugars were used to develop the nutrient profiles. For example, the nutrient profile for the milk group includes only skim milk; the meat group includes lean cuts of meat trimmed of all fat and poultry without skin; fruits and vegetables are without added fats or sugars. This approach allowed determination of the numbers of servings of food groups needed to meet the objectives for nutritional adequacy while keeping low the levels of food components for which overconsumption is a concern. Ranges in numbers of servings of food groups were established to cover the range of RDAs appropriate for different sex and age groups. The energy provided by these food groups composed of low-fat, lean choices without added fats or sugars ranged from 1220 to 1990 kcal (5.104 to 8.326 MJ).

In the second phase of the process, the differences between the energy calculated as coming from the nutrient-dense food groups in phase one and the energy intakes recommended by the Food and Nutrition Board (≈1300 to ≈3000 kcal [5.439 to 12.552 MJ]) were used to determine the amounts of fat and sugars that could be added to the diet.[3] The amount of discretionary fat that could be added was constrained to keep the total, which includes "nondiscretionary fat" from lean meats, poultry, and fish, and even the small amounts from grains, vegetables, and skim milk, to below 30% of energy. A nutrient profile was developed for discretionary fat to reflect the expectation that consumers would get some discretionary fat from foods in the fats, oils, and sweets group and some by selecting foods relatively high in fat from other food groups, such as spareribs, cheese, and muffins. Therefore, the fat composite was comprised of one-third animal fats including meat fat, poultry fat, butter, and lard; one-third margarine and other vegetable shortening; and one-third vegetable oils. The allowance for added sugars was the residual balance in energy. The nutrient profile for added sugars reflected the carbohydrate and calorie content of sucrose. The fats, oils, and sweets group was not considered a significant source of protein, vitamins, or minerals, with the exception of vitamin E.

Estimates of the nutrient levels provided by the food guide indicate that the goal of 100% of the RDA for protein, vitamins, and minerals will be met if it is assumed that the usual variety of foods within food groups is consumed and that people eat at least the number of servings that provide calorie levels appropriate for their age and sex group (Table 3). For example, the recommended calorie intake for 4- to 6-year-old children is 1800 kcal (7.531 MJ), close to the amount provided by the minimum number of servings in the food guide; 2200 kcal (9.205 MJ) for adult females, about the amount provided by the middle number of servings; and 2900

Table 3. Levels of nutrients and other food components provided by the Food Guide Pyramid

Food component	Numbers of servings[1]	
	Minimum	Maximum
Energy (kcal)	1600	2800
Macronutrients (% of calories)		
Protein	20	16
Fat	30	30
Saturated fat	9	9
Monounsaturated fat	10	10
Polyunsaturated fat	8	8
Carbohydrate	52	55
Minerals (mg)		
Calcium[2]	880	1095
Iron	11.5	19.2
Magnesium	273	399
Phosphorus	1244	1654
Zinc	11.4	16.1
Potassium	2780	4130
Sodium	1350	2210
Copper	1.1	1.9
Vitamins		
Vitamins A (RE)	1973	3059
Vitamins E (mg)	7.6	13.7
Thiamin (mg)	1.3	2.2
Riboflavin (mg)	1.8	2.5
Preformed niacin (mg)	15.8	25.8
Vitamin B-6 (mg)	1.5	2.4
Vitamin B-12 (ug)	7.2	9.4
Ascorbic acid (mg)	104	191
Folate (ug)	256	423
Other components		
Cholesterol (mg)	256	348
Fiber (g)	17	27.5

[1]For minimum and maximum numbers of servings, see Food Guide Pyramid graphic.

[2]Based on 2 servings of milk; 3 servings would provide the additional nutrients in 8 oz skim milk e.g. 302 mg Ca.

kcal (12.134 MJ) for adult males, close to the amount provided by the highest number of servings. The exception was the RDA for iron of 30 mg/day for pregnant women, which was not met even at the upper end of the range of servings recommended in the food guide; however, iron supplements are usually recommended for pregnant women.[3] The fiber estimates assume that half of the minimum number of servings from the grain group are whole grains. The cholesterol estimates depend on limiting egg yolks to three or four per week. The sodium estimates assume that no salt is added in home preparation or at the table, but these estimates do include some sodium added in processing, such as salt added to breads, margarine, and lean cured meats. Keeping cholesterol and sodium within the limits set is more difficult at higher calorie levels because of the greater amounts of foods eaten.

In 1988, cooperative work began with a market research company (Porter Novelli) to develop and test a consumer bulletin devoted entirely to the new food guide and including an illustration of its key principles. Several graphics were developed and tested with the target audience of average American adults. A circle graphic was perceived as unimaginative, old-fashioned, or providing information already known. Participants thought two graphics that used blocks to depict the minimum numbers of servings for the food groups did not convey enough information, since neither the ranges in the numbers of servings for food groups nor the fats, oils, and sweets group was shown. An inverted pyramid design showing grains in the top, wide band, and fats, oils, and sweets at the bottom tip, was disliked by many as it was perceived as precarious or off-balance. On the other hand, the pyramid design was well received; it was seen as new, interesting, and easy to remember (Figure 2). It was selected for further development because it was thought to best convey the three key guidance principles of variety, balance, and moderation. Variety among food groups was shown by the names of the food groups and by the separate sections of the pyramid. Variety within food groups was shown by the pictures of several foods within each group. Balance between food groups or proportionality was conveyed by the size of the food group sections and the text indicating numbers of servings. Moderation of foods high in fat and added sugars was shown by the small size of the tip of the pyramid and the "use sparingly" text. Moderation related to food choices within food groups was shown by the density of the fat and added sugars symbols in the food groups.

Further testing of the pyramid graphic and other alternatives was done in 1991 with more than 3000 respondents including blacks, whites, Hispanics, low-income adults, adults with less than a high school education, participants in food assistance programs, and children from the second grade through high school. Teachers, consumer advocacy groups, food industries, and trade associations were also represented in the survey. Final testing was done on two designs, a bowl and a pyramid. The differences between the designs in communicating the concepts of balance and moderation were large and highly significant. The relatively simple variety concept was tested by only one question, which involved reading the names of the food groups. This question did not show differences between the bowl and the pyramid designs. Earlier concerns that consumers would incorrectly see foods at the top of the pyramid as being superior to those as the bottom were not supported. In fact, the bowl design was found to convey more misinformation. The conclusion that the pyramid was the more effective graphic was consistent for all the subpopulations tested.

Release of the Food Guide Pyramid graphic was jointly announced by USDA and DHHS in 1992, followed by a consumer bulletin and research reports.[1,72,74] In 1993, the development process was awarded the President's Circle Award for nutrition education by the American Dietetic Association. To date, the extensive use of the Food Guide Pyramid by nutrition and health professionals, educators, media, and the food industry has made it an effective educational tool. The pyramid has been widely used on food labels and incorporated into a host of promotional and educational materials. A database to help professionals access research studies and educational materials that use the pyramid is maintained at USDA's National Agricultural Library and is accessible via the Internet.

Future food guides. One of the goals in developing the Food Guide Pyramid was for it to be evolutionary, that is, for it to accommodate potential changes in RDAs and dietary guidelines. Because the food guide was developed to meet multiple nutritional objectives simultaneously and because foods provide patterns of nutrients, some potential changes in RDAs or dietary guidelines could be more easily accommodated than others. However, it is important to bear in mind that determining the types of changes that could be accommodated by the food guide does not indicate desirability or easy implementation by consumers.

For some nutrients, considerable change could be made in the RDAs before a change in the food guide would be needed. For example, the food guide provides enough protein, ascorbic acid, folate, vitamin A, thiamin, riboflavin, niacin, vitamin B-12, and phosphorus to accommodate an increase in RDAs of at least 50%. Decreasing the RDAs for any one of these nutrients also is not likely to impact on the food guide because multiple factors affect the number of servings of food groups. For example, decreasing the RDA for ascorbic acid is not likely to decrease the recommended number of servings for fruit because fruit is also low in energy and fat and high in vitamin A, folate, and fiber. However, the establishment of upper limits of intake for some of these nutrients might be problematic. For example, an upper limit on protein intake might be easily exceeded in food guide patterns for young females. In this case, the numbers of servings of the meat, milk, and grain groups, which are primary sources of protein, are driven by factors other than protein, such as the RDAs for zinc, iron, calcium, and vitamin B-6. Switching from meat to legumes as a source of minerals would not be a solution in that both meat and legumes are high in protein. Changes in recommendations related to dietary fiber would be relatively easy to accommodate in the food guide by providing greater specificity in guidance on selecting high-fiber foods within food groups. In estimating fiber levels provided by the food guide (see Table 3), it was assumed that high-fiber foods like legumes would be consumed several times per week and that at

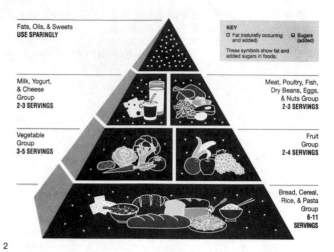

Figure 2. Food Guide Pyramid.

least half of the minimum number of servings from the bread group would be whole grains. Higher intakes of these foods would have a significant effect on fiber intake. If all six to 11 servings of grains, for example, were whole grains, the estimated total fiber level of food guide diets would rise to 21–35 g.

Changes in RDAs necessitating changes in the Food Guide Pyramid might be anticipated for nutrients that are provided by the current food guide at close to the RDA level for some sex and age groups. This is especially true for nutrients that are more concentrated in certain food groups rather than being relatively evenly distributed throughout the food supply. Examples of changes in RDAs that would be more difficult to accommodate with the current food guide are increases in the RDAs for iron, zinc, vitamin E, and vitamin B-6 for some sex and age groups, and increases in the RDA for calcium above 1400 mg. Even among these nutrients, some increases in RDAs could be accommodated relatively easily by emphasizing subgroups within several major food groups that are especially good sources. For example, additional guidance could be given to increase consumption of subgroups within the grain, vegetable, and meat groups that are especially good sources of iron and vitamin B-6. On the other hand, large increases in RDAs for calcium, which is most concentrated in the milk group, or for vitamin E, which is most concentrated in higher-fat foods, might require major changes in the way foods are grouped or in the numbers of servings recommended.

The potential for change in dietary guidance related to moderation was a major consideration in the development of the food guide. Within certain parameters, changes in dietary guidance can be accommodated without major changes in the current food guide. The minimum calorie levels that could be achieved while following the food guide can be estimated by assuming that all low-fat, lean foods without added sugars are selected. With this assumption, the minimum number of servings in the pyramid would provide ≈1200 kcal (5.021 MJ) and the maximum number of servings would provide about ≈2000 kcal (8.368 MJ). These diets contain about 16% of energy from fat. The minimum percentage of energy from fat that could be achieved while following the food guide can be estimated by assuming that all low-fat, lean foods are selected from the major food groups and that the balance in energy comes from nonfat sources such as sugars. With this assumption, diets providing 1600–2800 kcal (6.694–11.715 MJ) would contain about 12% of energy from fat. At the other end of the spectrum, if the balance in energy in these diets came only from fat, they would contain about 37% of energy from fat. Going below 12% of energy from fat would require changes in the mix of foods within the food groups. For example, replacing all the beef in the meat, poultry, fish group with poultry and fish could further lower the estimated percentage of energy from fat from 12% to 9%, but some of the nutrients provided by beef, such as zinc, would be below RDAs. Replacing all the meat, poultry, and fish with legumes could further lower the estimated fat level to 6% of energy, but fiber levels could increase to 44–65 g.

Some changes in dietary guidance concerning the distribution of fatty acids in the diet could be accommodated by changing the source of discretionary fat. In the current food guide, it is assumed that about one-half of the total fat is essentially nondiscretionary from low-fat, lean foods in the major food groups and about one-half is discretionary fat, which is assumed to be a mixture of animal fats, vegetable shortening, and oil. These assumptions result in an estimated percentage of energy from saturated, monounsaturated, and polyunsaturated fatty acids of 9%, 10%, and 8%, respectively. If the objective were to further lower saturated fatty acids, changing the discretionary fat to include only vegetable fats, such as corn oil and margarine, would decrease the estimated percentage of energy from saturated fatty acids to 6–7% with a reciprocal rise in polyunsaturates. If the objective were to increase monounsaturated fatty acids, as one might assume is an objective of the Mediterranean diet, all discretionary fat might be changed to olive oil.[15,85] With this assumption, the estimated percentage of energy from saturated, monounsaturated, and polyunsaturated fatty acids would be 7%, 18%, and 4%, respectively. If the objective were get fat as low as possible while still using the Food Guide Pyramid, all discretionary fat could be replaced by sugar. The result would be to change the estimated distribution of the fatty acids to 4%, 4%, and 2% of energy, respectively.

Changes in dietary guidance related to cholesterol could be accommodated by the current food guide by changing recommendations on the primary sources of cholesterol. In the current food guide, it is assumed that no more than three to four egg yolks are consumed per week. If egg yolks were eliminated completely, the estimated cholesterol level of food guide patterns would be decreased by ≈90 mg/day. Changing the discretionary fat assumed in the food guide from a mix of animal and vegetable to only vegetable fats would eliminate another 20–35 mg of cholesterol. Together these changes would lower the estimated cholesterol levels in Food Guide Pyramid patterns to ≈150–230 mg/day. Lower quantitative limits on cholesterol intake could require major changes in the current food guide, since estimates already assume that skim milk is the selection from the milk group and that low-fat, lean meats and poultry without skin are selected from the meat group. Changes in dietary guidelines that would further limit sodium intake would be especially difficult to accommodate with the current food guide. Even though the estimates of sodium levels in food guide patterns do not include discretionary salt, condiments, or most processed foods, they range from 1350 to 2210 mg/day.

Commentary

Recent research on the relationship between diet, genes, and disease suggests that a time may come when recommendations for a healthful diet can be tailored to the individual, but this probably will not be in the near future. Over the next decade, the resolution of the policy debates on the definition and criteria for RDAs and on how nutrient standards, dietary guidelines, and food guides are integrated are likely to have significant effects on population-based recommendations for healthful eating. Future recommendations may call for higher intakes of certain vitamins and minerals and lower intakes of total fat and saturated fatty acids than currently recommended. Regardless of the numbers, however, the primary difficulty in implementation will remain the balancing of the competing goals of achieving nutritional adequacy while avoiding nutritional excesses in a diet that is palatable, convenient, safe, and affordable. Dietary intake data and even casual observations indicate that progress in implementing recommendations has been slow. Research needs for the future development of nutrient standards, dietary guidelines, and food guides seem relatively clear. The greater challenge for the future will be in finding ways of putting into practice what is already known about healthful eating.

References

1. US Department of Agriculture, Human Nutrition Information Service (1992) The Food Guide Pyramid. Home and Garden Bulletin No. 252. US Government Printing Office, Washington, DC

2. US Department of Agriculture/Department of Health and Human Services (1990) Nutrition and your health: dietary guidelines for Americans, 4th ed. Home and Garden Bulletin No. 232. US Government Printing Office, Washington, DC

3. Food and Nutrition Board (1989) Recommended dietary allowances, 10th ed. National Academy Press, Washington, DC

4. Food and Nutrition Board (1989) Diet and health: implications for reducing chronic disease risk. National Academy Press, Washington, DC

5. Harper AE (1990) Dietary standards and dietary guidelines. In Brown ML (ed), Present knowledge in nutrition. International Life Sciences Institute, Washington, DC, pp 491–501

6. Food and Nutrition Board (1994) How should the recommended dietary allowances be revised? National Academy Press, Washington, DC

7. US Department of Agriculture, US Department of Health and Human Services (1995) Dietary guidelines for Americans, 4th ed. US Government Printing Office, Washington, DC

8. Food and Nutrition Board (1941) Recommended dietary allowances. National Research Council, Washington, DC

9. Hunt CL (1916) Food for young children. US Department of Agriculture Farmers' Bulletin No. 717. US Government Printing Office, Washington, DC

10. Page L, Phipard EF (1956) Essentials of an adequate diet...facts for nutrition programs. US Department of Agriculture, Agricultural Research Service Bulletin No. 62-4. US Government Printing Office, Washington, DC

11. Atwater WO (1894) Foods: nutritive value and cost. US Department of Agriculture, Farmers' Bulletin No. 23. US Government Printing Office, Washington, DC

12. Atwater WO (1902) Principles of nutrition and nutritive value of food. US Department of Agriculture Farmers' Bulletin No. 142. US Government Printing Office, Washington, DC

13. Stiebeling HK (1933) Food budgets for nutrition and production programs. US Department of Agriculture Misc. Publication No. 183. US Government Printing Office, Washington, DC

14. Stiebeling HK, Ward M (1933) Diets at four levels of nutrition content and cost. US Department of Agriculture Circular No. 296. US Government Printing Office, Washington, DC

15. World Health Organization, Regional Office for Europe, Nutrition Unit (1994) Background to the WHO regional office for Europe's involvement in the development of the traditional healthy Mediterranean diet pyramid [statement distributed at Oldways symposium, June 20–25]. Changing American Appetites, San Francisco

16. Food and Nutrition Board (1980) Recommended dietary allowances, 9th ed. National Academy Press, Washington, DC

17. US Department of Agriculture, Human Nutrition Information Service (1985) Developing the food guidance system for better eating for better health, a nutrition course for adults. USDA, Human Nutrition Information Service Administrative Report No. 377. US Government Printing Office, Washington, DC

18. Department of Health and Human Services (1990) Healthy people 2000: national health promotion and disease prevention objectives. Public Health Service No. 91-50 212. US Government Printing Office, Washington, DC

19. Block G (1993) Impact of new research on optimal health on the RDAs. In Proceedings of a workshop on future recommended dietary allowances. Rutgers, New Brunswick, NJ, pp 45–55

20. Willett W (1993) Commentary. In Proceedings of a workshop on future recommended dietary allowances. Rutgers, New Brunswick, NJ, p 100

21. Food and Nutrition Board (1986) Nutrient adequacy: assessment using food consumption surveys. National Academy Press, Washington, DC

22. Basiotis PP, Welsh SO, Cronin FJ, et al (1987) Number of days of food intake records required to estimate individual and group nutrient intakes with defined confidence. J Nutr 117:1638–1641

23. Van Itallie TB, Woteki CE (1985) Health implications of overweight and obesity. In Health implications of obesity [National Institutes of Health consensus development conference, program and abstracts]. Department of Health and Human Services, Washington, DC

24. Mertz W, Tsui JC, Judd JT, et al (1991) What are people really eating? the relation between energy intake derived from estimated diet records and intake determined to maintain body weight. Am J Clin Nutr 54:291–295

25. Committee on Medical Aspects of Food Policy, United Kingdom (1991) Dietary reference values for food energy and nutrients for the United Kingdom. Department of Health Report on Health and Social Subjects No. 41, HMSO, London

26. National Science and Technology Council (1994) Science in the national interest. Office of Science and Technology Policy, Executive Office of the President, National Science and Technology Council, Washington, DC

27. Committee on Health, Safety and Food, National Science and Technology Council (1994) Meeting the challenge: health, safety and food for America [forum]. Office of Science and Technology Policy, Executive Office of the President, National Science and Technology Council, Washington, DC

28. Food and Nutrition Board (1994) Opportunities in nutrition and food sciences, research challenges and the next generation of investigators. National Academy Press, Washington, DC

29. National Association of State Universities and Land-Grant Colleges (1994) Food systems for consumer health workshop. Washington, DC.

30. American Heart Association (1961) Dietary fat and its relation to heart attacks and strokes. Circulation 23:133–135

31. US Senate Select Committee on Nutrition and Human Needs (1977) Dietary goals for the United States, 2nd ed. US Government Printing Office, Washington, DC

32. Department of Health and Human Services (1988) The Surgeon General's report on nutrition and health. Public Health Service No. 88-50210. US Government Printing Office, Washington, DC

33. Food and Agricultural Organization of the United Nations and World Health Organization (1992) International conference on nutrition: world declaration and plan of action for nutrition. FAO/WHO, Rome

34. National Cholesterol Education Program (1990) Report of the expert panel on population strategies for blood cholesterol reduction. Department of Health and Human Services, National Institutes of Health Publication No. 90-3046. NIH, Bethesda, Md

35. National Cholesterol Education Program (1991) Report of the expert panel on blood cholesterol levels in children and adolescents. Department of Health and Human Services, National Institutes of Health Publication No. 91-2732. NIH, Bethesda, MD

36. National High Blood Pressure Education Program (1993) Working group report on primary prevention of hypertension.

Department of Health and Human Services, National Institutes of Health Publication No. 93-2669. NIH, Bethesda, MD

37. National Institutes of Health Consensus Statement (1994) Optimal calcium intake. Department of Health and Human Services, NIH Consensus Statement 12:4. NIH, Bethesda, MD

38. National Health and Medical Research Council, Commonwealth of Australia (1992) Dietary guidelines for Australians. Commonwealth Department of Human Sciences and Health. Australia Government Publishing Service, Canberra, Australia

39. Health and Welfare Canada (1990) Nutrition recommendations: the report of the scientific review committee. Minister of Supply and Services, Ottawa, Canada

40. Health and Welfare Canada (1990) Action towards healthy eating...Canada's guidelines for healthy eating and recommended strategies for implementation. Report of the Communications/Implementation Committee. Minister of Supply and Services, Ottawa, Canada

41. Chinese Nutrition Society (1990) Recommended dietary allowances for nutrients and dietary guidelines of China. Acta Nutrimenta Sinica 12:10–17

42. Berger S (1989) Dietary guidelines in East European countries. In Dietary guidelines: proceedings of an international conference. Cornell International Nutrition Monograph Series No. 21. Cornell University, Ithaca, NY, pp 112–157

43. Conseil National de l'Alimentation (1990) Eat well for better health—ten guidelines. Conseil National de l'Alimentation, Paris, France

44. German Society of Nutrition (1991) Recommendations on nutrient intake, 5th ed. German Society of Nutrition, Federal Republic of Germany, Franfurt, Germany

45. Greek Society of Nutrition (1989) Dietary guidelines for Greece. Greek Society of Nutrition, Athens, Greece

46. Hungarian Society of Nutrition (1987) Dietary guidelines for Hungarians. National Institute of Food, Hygiene and Nutrition, Budapest, Hungary

47. Food Advisory Committee (1984) Guidelines for preparing information and advice to the general public on healthy eating. Department of Health, Dublin, Ireland

48. Italian Society for Human Nutrition (1986) Livelli di assunzione giornalieri raccomandati di engeria e nutrienti per la popolazione Italiana Revisione 1986–87. Nutrition Foundation of Italy, Milan

49. Japanese Ministry of Health and Welfare (1985) Dietary guidelines for health promotion. Health Promotion and Nutrition Division, Health Services Bureau, Tokyo, Japan

50. Japanese Ministry of Health and Welfare (1990) Dietary guidelines for preventing chronic disease. Health Services Bureau, Tokyo, Japan

51. Korean Nutrition Institute (1988) Korean dietary guidelines. Seoul, Korea

52. Chavez M, Chavez A, Madrigal H, Rios E (1993) Guias de Alimentacion Mexico. Instituto Nacional de la Nutricion, Mexico

53. Food and Nutrition Council, Netherlands (1986) Guidelines for a healthy diet. Ministry of Health, Welfare and Culture, Ministry of Agriculture, and the Ministry of Economics, The Hague, Netherlands

54. Netherlands Nutrition Council (1991) Reassessment of the advice on fat consumption contained in guidelines of a healthy diet 1986. Minister of Welfare, Health and Cultural Affairs, Minister of Agriculture, and Nature Management and Fisheries, The Hague, Netherlands

55. New Zealand Food and Nutrition Policy Taskforce (1991) Food for health. Department of Health, Te Tari Ora, Wellington, New Zealand

56. Nordisk Ministerrad (1989) Nodic nutrition recommenda-

tions, 2nd ed. Standing Nordic Committee on Food (PNUN); Updated: Expert Group for Diet and Health 1992, Stockholm

57. Asociacion Nurticionistas de Panama (1994) Guias de Alimentacion Panama (version preliminar). Asociacion Nutricionistas de Panama, Panama

58. Interagency Committee on Nutrition (1990) Nutritional guidelines for Filipinos. Interagency Committee on Nutrition, The Phillipines

59. Nutrition Research Centre of National Institute of Health, Portugal (1982) Revista do Centro de Estudos de Nutricao. Ministry of Health, Portugal. Eur J Clin Nutr (1990) 44(suppl 2):95–96

60. National Advisory Committee on Food and Nutrition, Training and Health Education Department, Ministry of Health, Singapore (1989) Guidelines for a healthy diet. Ministry of Health,Singapore

61. Ministrstvo za Zdravstvo (1993) Zdravstvenega Varstva Republike Slovenije do leta 2000. Ministrstvo za Zdravstvo, Ljubljana, Zaloska

62. Nutrition Services Subcommittee, Health Matters Advisory Committee, Department of Health, South Africa (1992) Sensible diet-guidelines for South Africa. Department of Health, South Africa

63. Swiss Federal Office of Public Health (1990) Dietary recommendations for the general population of Switzerland. Swiss Federal Office of Public Health, Berne, Switzerland

64. Health of the Nation—Nutrition Panel (1992) Eight guidelines for a healthy diet. Health Education Authority, London

65. Institute of Nutrition, USSR Academy of Medical Sciences, Ministry of Health (1990) Dietary guidelines. Eur J Clin Nutr 44(suppl 2):99–100

66. Instituto Nacional de Nutricion, Fundacion Cavendes (1991) Guias de Alimentacion para Venezuela. Fundacion Cavendes, Caracas, Venezuela

67. Food and Nutrition Board (1991) Improving America's diet and health, from recommendations to action. National Academy Press, Washington, DC

68. Food and Nutrition Board (1995) Weighing the options: criteria for evaluating weight-management programs. National Academy Press, Washington, DC

69. US Department of Agriculture, Food and Nutrition Service (1995) Nutrition guidance for child nutrition programs. USDA: school meals initiative for healthy children (final rule). Fed Register 60:31188–31222

70. Health and Welfare Canada (1993) Nutrition recommendations update...dietary fat and children. Report of the Joint Working Group of the Canadian Paediatric Society and Health Canada. Minister of Supply and Services, Ottawa, Canada

71. Welsh S, Davis C, Shaw A (1992) A brief history of food guides in the United States. Nutrition Today, Nov/Dec, pp 6–11

72. Welsh S (1994) Atwater to the present: evolution of nutrition education. J Nutr 124(9S):1799S–1807S

73. Hunt CL (1921) A week's food for an average family. US Department of Agriculture Farmers' Bulletin No. 1228. US Government Printing Office, Washington, DC

74. US Department of Agriculture, War Food Administration (1943) National Wartime Nutrition Guide. USDA Leaflet. US Government Printing Office, Washington, DC

75. US Department of Agriculture, Agricultural Research Service (1946) National food guide. USDA Leaflet No. 288. US Government Printing Office, Washington, DC

76. US Department of Agriculture (1958) Food for fitness—a daily

food guide. USDA Leaflet No. 424. US Government Printing Office, Washington, DC

77. US Department of Agriculture, Science and Education Administration (1979) Food, Home and Garden Bulletin No. 228. US Government Printing Office, Washington, DC

78. Welsh S, Davis C, Shaw A (1992) Development of the Food Guide Pyramid. Nutrition Today 27:12–23

79. Food and Nutrition Board (1953) Recommended dietary allowances, revised 1953. Publication No. 302. National Research Council, Washington, DC

80. Cronin FJ, Shaw A, Krebs-Smith SM, et al (1987) Developing a food guidance system to implement the dietary guidelines. J Nutr Educ 19:281–302

81. US Department of Agriculture, Human Nutrition Information Service (1993) USDA's food guide, background and development. Human Nutrition Information Service Misc. Publication No. 1514. US Government Printing Office, Washington, DC

82. Light L, Cronin F (1981) Food guidance revisited. J Nutr Educ 13:57–62

83. Gillespie AH (1987) A survey of nutritionists' opinions on objectives of a dietary guidance system. J Nutr Educ 19: 220–224

84. Shepherd SK, Sims LS, Cronin FJ, et al (1989) Use of focus groups to explore consumers' preferences for content and graphic design of nutrition publications. J Am Diet Assoc 89:1612–1614

85. American Dietetic Association (1994) ADA supports USDA Food Guide Pyramid, not Mediterranean diet pyramid [press release]. June 20. American Dietetic Association, Chicago

Index

Note: An "f" or a "t" following a page number designates a figure or a table, respectively.